PLURAL+PLUS

COMPANION WEBSITE

Purchase of *Cochlear Implants: Audiologic Management and Considerations for Implantable Hearing Devices* comes with access to supplementary student and instructor materials on a PluralPlus companion website.

The companion website is located at:
http://www.pluralpublishing.com/publication/cimp

STUDENTS:

To access the **student** materials, you must register on the companion website and log in using the access code below.*

Access Code: **CIMP-WA3CDR**

INSTRUCTORS:

To access the **instructor** materials, you must contact Plural Publishing, Inc. to be verified as an instructor and receive your access code.

   Email: information@pluralpublishing.com
   Tel: 866-758-7251 (toll free) or 858-492-1555

Note for students: If you have purchased this textbook used or have rented it, your access code will not work if it was already redeemed by the original buyer of the book. Plural Publishing does not offer replacement access codes for used or rented textbooks.

COCHLEAR IMPLANTS

*Audiologic Management and Considerations
for Implantable Hearing Devices*

COCHLEAR IMPLANTS

*Audiologic Management and Considerations
for Implantable Hearing Devices*

Jace Wolfe, PhD

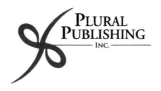
PLURAL
PUBLISHING
INC.

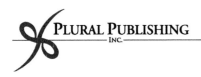

5521 Ruffin Road
San Diego, CA 92123

e-mail: information@pluralpublishing.com
Website: http://www.pluralpublishing.com

Copyright 2020 © by Plural Publishing, Inc.

Typeset in 10/12 Garamond by Flanagan's Publishing Services, Inc.
Printed in the United States of America by Integrated Books International
21 20 19   2 3 4 5

All rights, including that of translation, reserved. No part of this publication may be reproduced, stored in a retrieval system, or transmitted in any form or by any means, electronic, mechanical, recording, or otherwise, including photocopying, recording, taping, Web distribution, or information storage and retrieval systems without the prior written consent of the publisher.

For permission to use material from this text, contact us by
Telephone: (866) 758-7251
Fax: (888) 758-7255
e-mail: permissions@pluralpublishing.com

Every attempt has been made to contact the copyright holders for material originally printed in another source. If any have been inadvertently overlooked, the publishers will gladly make the necessary arrangements at the first opportunity.

Library of Congress Cataloging-in-Publication Data

Names: Wolfe, Jace, author.
Title: Cochlear implants : audiologic management and considerations for
    implantable hearing devices / Jace Wolfe.
Description: San Diego, CA : Plural Publishing, [2020] | Includes
    bibliographical references and index.
Identifiers: LCCN 2018028888| ISBN 9781597568920 (alk. paper) | ISBN
    1597568929 (alk. paper)
Subjects: | MESH: Cochlear Implants | Cochlear Implantation—methods |
    Hearing Loss—surgery | Correction of Hearing Impairment—instrumentation
Classification: LCC RF305 | NLM WV 274 | DDC 617.8/8220592—dc23
LC record available at https://lccn.loc.gov/2018028888

Contents

Preface

All in One Place, for Audiologists

Almost 30 years ago, the multiple-channel cochlear implant was approved by the United States Food and Drug Administration (FDA) for clinical use with adults. Other implantable hearing devices, such as implantable bone conduction devices, middle ear implants, and auditory brainstem implants have been in clinical use for over 20 years. Over the past 20-plus years, these implantable hearing technologies have been covered in several excellent textbooks. However, no textbook has comprehensively addressed the audiologic considerations pertaining to each of the implantable hearing technologies available for children and adults with hearing loss. The objective of this textbook is to fill that void. Specifically, this textbook aspires to provide comprehensive coverage pertaining to the audiologic management of cochlear implants, implantable bone conduction devices, hybrid cochlear implants, middle ear implants, and auditory brainstem implants. This book is intended to serve as a text for AuD and PhD courses covering implantable hearing technologies and also as a resource to guide audiologists who are providing patient care in clinical settings. Although this book is primarily written for and by audiologists, it also will hopefully be helpful for other clinicians and researchers who are interested in implantable hearing technologies.

This book is intended to be a practical, "how-to" book. For each of the implantable hearing technologies discussed in this text, the author has sought to provide a summary of the assessment battery used to determine candidacy for the implantable hearing device, the audiologic procedures used to program the device to optimally meet the recipient's unique needs, and the assessment battery used to evaluate the outcomes achieved with each type of implantable hearing device. Audiologic management of hearing technologies is discussed in general terms, but for implantable hearing technologies that are approved for commercial distribution by the United States FDA, detailed, manufacturer-specific information is also provided.

This textbook is also unique because it is primarily written by a single author who has substantial experience in both the clinical and research arenas associated with implantable hearing technologies. The potential advantage of a singular voice is to avoid redundancy across chapters while also avoiding the omission of information that is vitally important in regard to the audiologic management of implantable hearing technologies. Of note, however, the expertise of a handful of gifted clinicians was accessed to cover four topics that did not directly fall within the scope of the primary author's personal experience including the medical aspects pertaining to cochlear implantation (which was authored by an experienced cochlear implant surgeon), considerations for radiologic imaging of implantable hearing device recipients (which was authored by a physician who is trained both as a medical radiologist and an otologist), considerations pertaining to the relationship of vestibular function and cochlear implantation (which was authored by an audiologist who specializes in the clinical and research aspects related to vestibular assessment and management), and the medical aspects pertaining to implantable bone conduction devices (which was authored by an otologic surgeon who has considerable experience with bone conduction implants).

The first chapter of this textbook summarizes the fascinating history of cochlear implant technology. The second and third chapters provide basic information pertaining to the physics and physiology associated with implantable hearing technology. Chapters 4 through 6 address matters associated with cochlear implant candidacy assessment. Chapters 7, 8, 14, 20, and 23 discuss basic principles pertaining to the management of cochlear implant recipients. Chapters 7, 8, 9, 15, 16, and 17 provide manufacturer-specific information regarding the hardware, signal processing, and programming of modern cochlear implant systems. Chapters 12 and 13 provide information pertaining to medical considerations associated with cochlear implantation. Chapter 18 provides a thorough overview of objective measures that may be used to evaluate the function of cochlear implant technology and the recipient's auditory responsiveness to electrical stimulation from the cochlear implant, whereas Chapter 19 provides an excellent overview of the important points to consider regarding vestibular function and cochlear implantation. Chapter 24 provides a summary of electric-acoustic stimulation and hybrid cochlear implant technology. Chapter 25 provides a brief overview of the basics pertaining to auditory brainstem implants. Chapters 26 and 27 provide information pertaining to the assessment and management of recipients with implantable bine conduction devices. Chapter 28 provides a basic overview of middle ear implantable devices.

A relatively larger portion of this text is devoted to cochlear implant technology because the typical audiologist is more likely to encounter cochlear implant recipients than auditory brainstem implants or middle ear implant recipients. Although bone conduction implants are fairly commonplace, an argument can be reasonably made that the management of cochlear implant recipients is more complex than the management of bone conduction implant recipients. As a result, the author has made an attempt to

provide the reader with a thorough knowledge base that will facilitate the clinical management of recipients of each of the implantable hearing technologies discussed in this textbook.

Although no book can provide an exhaustive, detailed coverage of all of the information pertaining to implantable hearing technologies, it does provide comprehensive basic information that is supported by extensive references. The book certainly provides a robust foundation that will allow an audiologist to build a skillset that will capably serve recipients of implantable hearing technologies. However, the clinician should strive to stay current with advances that will inevitably occur with implantable hearing technologies. Medical knowledge is always evolving and advancing. The astute clinician never ceases to be an eager student. Finally, this book includes a tangible demonstration of clinical practices associated with implantable hearing technologies in a supplemental video that is available on a PluralPlus companion website.

Acknowledgments

Several of my former professors and mentors influenced the development of this book, either in the knowledge that they imparted over the past 20 years or in the support and encouragement they provided as I wrote the manuscript. I will always be grateful for my "audiology heroes," a group of professors, researchers, and master clinicians who have shared their expertise with me. These generous and ingenious individuals include Stephen Painton, Richard Talbott, Michael Grim, J. Michael Dennis, James W. Hall III, Francis Kuk, Christine Jones, Stefan Launer, Rene Gifford, and Richard Seewald. I am grateful from Teresa Caraway, Stan Baker, and Mark Wood who coaxed me into working with children with cochlear implants and who continue to serve as valuable colleagues and friends today. I am also grateful to the countless pioneers and visionaries who have contributed to the development and refinement of the cochlear implant and other implantable technologies. Many of these surgeons, clinicians, and scientists are mentioned throughout this book.

I am also very indebted to a large group of people who have directly contributed to the development of this book. I am grateful for a host of talented healthcare professionals who have generously sacrificed their time and energy to share their expertise as chapter authors. Stan Baker, Mark Wood, and Anthony Alleman are gifted physicians who wrote excellent chapters summarizing the medical aspects associated with implantable hearing technologies. Jamie Bogle is one of the brightest young minds in vestibular assessment, and she was gracious enough to write a terrific chapter on the factors pertaining the vestibular function and cochlear implantation. Elizabeth Musgrave is a talented audiologist and electrophysiologist who co-authored an informative chapter on regulatory considerations pertaining to cochlear implantation. Also, my long-time colleague and friend, Professor Erin Schafer contributed to several chapters in this book. Dr. Schafer is one of the most intelligent audiologists I have ever known. I am fortunate to be able to work with her. Laura Schadt, Sarah McCullough, and Skyler Thompson are all students who study under Dr. Schafer. They were kind enough to assist in the formatting of the references that were cited in this text. Without their help, this book may still be "in process."

Several representatives from implantable hearing technology companies also helped to contribute information and images specific to each of their technologies. These helpful colleagues include Smita Agrawal, Erin Nelson, Sarah Downing, Leo Litvak, Darla Franz, Scott Hansson, Nathalie Davis, Amy Donaldson, Amy Popp, Pete Arkis, Aaron Parkinson, Leigh Ann Monthey, Christy Miller-Gardner, Jessica Ballard, Darren Knowles, George Cire, Phil Guyer, Kimberlee Griffey, and Chrissy Parlacoski. I also am thankful for Kalie Koscielak, Valerie Johns, and numerous other team members at Plural Publishing, Inc. for their tireless and capable efforts to bring this book to print.

I am continually thankful for the team of colleagues with whom I get to work at Hearts for Hearing. I know that I am biased, but I truly believe that I work with the best implantable hearing technology team in the world! Not a week goes by that I do not personally benefit from the talents and generosity of my excellent colleagues at Hearts for Hearing. I am also grateful for thousands of patients I have been privileged to serve. Without a doubt, much of the information in this book has been influenced by the lessons I have learned as I have strived to optimize the outcomes of recipients of implantable hearing technologies. Additionally, I am forever indebted to Joanna Smith, the Chief Executive Officer of Hearts for Hearing and my boss, friend, mentor, counselor, and colleague. Joanna has constantly encouraged me to shoot for the stars when working with recipients of implantable hearing technologies. She also continually inspires me to honor Him by maximizing the opportunities of individuals with hearing loss to listen and talk for a lifetime.

I owe a heartfelt thanks to my wonderful family. I am so proud of my three children, Hayden, Harper, and Henley. I love them with all of my heart, and I often felt like I should scrap the whole idea of this book because it interfered with time I could be spending with them. I appreciate their patience. I hope this book makes them proud of me and instills in them the importance of making sacrifices and working hard to hopefully make life better for others. Finally, I am most grateful for and indebted to my soulmate, life partner, and wife, Lynnette, whose love, support, sacrifice, and constant encouragement are the driving force that inspires me to convince her that she made the right choice in blessing me with the incredible opportunity to do life with her.

Contributors

Anthony M. Alleman, MD, MPH
Bob G. Eaton Chair in Radiological Sciences
Associate Professor
Department of Radiological Sciences
The University of Oklahoma Health Sciences Center
Oklahoma City, Oklahoma
Chapter 13

R. Stanley Baker, MD
Otologic Medical Clinic
Oklahoma City, Oklahoma
Chapter 12

Jamie M. Bogle, AuD, PhD
Assistant Professor
Mayo Clinic
College of Medicine and Science
Scottsdale, Arizona
Chapter 19

James W. Heller, MSEE, BSEE, PE
Director of Clinical Technical Services (retired)
Cochlear Corp.
Englewood, Colorado
Chapter 2

Elizabeth Musgrave, AuD, CCC-A
Clinical Audiologist
Hearts for Hearing Foundation
Oklahoma City, Oklahoma
Chapter 4

Sara Neumann, AuD
Clinical Audiologist
Audiology Research Manager
Deaf Education Consultant
Hearts for Hearing Foundation
Oklahoma City, Oklahoma
Chapter 17

Erin C. Schafer, PhD
Professor
University of North Texas
Department of Speech and Hearing Sciences
Denton, Texas
Chapters 7, 8, 9, 10, 15, and 16

Mark Wood, MD
Oklahoma Otolaryngology Associates, LLC
Oklahoma City, Oklahoma
Chapter 27

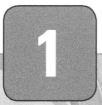

1

Basic Operation and History of Cochlear Implant Technology

Jace Wolfe

Introduction

The multiple-channel cochlear implant is the most successful sensory prosthetic device in the history of medicine. Many persons who develop severe to profound hearing loss in adulthood are able to achieve excellent open-set speech recognition (Gifford, Shallop, & Peterson, 2008; Helms et al., 2004), and many are also able to communicate over the telephone (Anderson et al., 2006; Wolfe et al., 2016a, 2016b). Additionally, children who are born with severe to profound hearing loss and receive a cochlear implant during the first year of life frequently develop age-appropriate spoken language abilities (Ching et al., 2013a; Dettman et al., 2016; Geers, 2004; Geers, Brenner, & Davidson, 2003; Geers, Moog, Biedenstein, Brenner, & Hayes, 2009). For instance, Dettman and colleagues (2016) evaluated spoken language outcomes in 403 children who used cochlear implants and were entering kindergarten and reported that almost 81% of those implanted before 12 months of age had normal vocabulary development.

Cochlear implants bypass the sensory function of the cochlea and stimulate the cochlear nerve directly. The primary function of the cochlea is to convert acousto-mechanical energy into neural impulses that may be delivered from the cochlear nerve to the auditory nuclei in the brainstem. Specifically, cochlear sensory cells, known as hair cells, serve as transduc-

ers that convert the hydrodynamic energy of cochlear fluid displacement (in response to acoustic stimulation) into neuro-electric impulses. In most cases of sensorineural hearing loss, the primary site of lesion is localized to the cochlear hair cells (i.e., auditory sensory cells) or to the structures that support the electrochemical environment within the cochlea that is necessary to allow for effective stimulation of the hair cells (e.g., genetic mutations that interfere with the development of the stria vascularis, which is instrumental in the production of K+ ions that maintain the highly positive endocochlear resting potential necessary for normal hair cell function).

The term "nerve deafness" is often used to describe sensorineural hearing loss, but this term usually does not accurately describe the primary underlying etiology of the hearing loss. The cochlear nerve is typically intact for the most part and functional, but in the case of severe to profound hearing loss and the concomitant loss of cochlear hair cells, the cochlear nerve does not receive adequate stimulation from the cochlear sensory cells. As a result, the cochlear nerve delivers a severely impoverished signal to the auditory nervous system. Cochlear implants are of substantial benefit to many persons with severe to profound hearing loss, because electrical stimulation is directly delivered to the functional cochlear nerve, resulting in the provision of a more robust auditory signal that includes components spanning the entire speech frequency range (Figure 1–1).

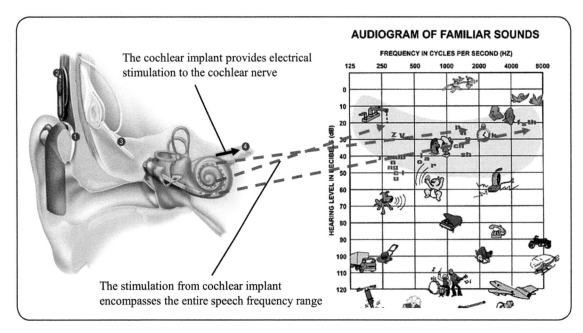

FIGURE 1–1. An illustration of a behind-the-ear cochlear implant sound processor and cochlear implant providing stimulation to the cochlear nerve so that audibility is restored throughout the speech frequency range. The image of the auditory system with cochlear implant is provided courtesy of Cochlear Americas, ©2018. The image of the familiar sounds audiogram is provided courtesy of Advanced Bionics, LLC.

It should also be noted that cochlear implants may also be beneficial for some persons who have cochlear nerve pathology. For instance, many researchers have shown that cochlear implants may provide significant improvements in speech recognition of persons with auditory neuropathy, many of whom likely have cochlear nerve abnormalities (e.g., demyelination of the cochlear nerve) (Ching et al., 2013b; Rance & Barker, 2008). In cases of demyelination of the cochlear nerve, it is possible that the high level of neural synchronization provided by electrical stimulation of the cochlear nerve results in a more robust signal than may be elicited by acoustical stimulation.

Furthermore, post-mortem studies have shown rather sparse populations of surviving spiral ganglion cells in some persons who achieved good benefit from and high levels of open-set speech recognition with a cochlear implant (Khan et al., 2005; Linthicum & Fayad, 2009). Additionally, research has shown that some (but certainly not all) children with deficient cochlear nerves, as indicated by magnetic resonance imaging (MRI), achieve open-set speech recognition and develop spoken language abilities after cochlear implantation, albeit with outcomes that are diminished compared with a child with a normally

developed cochlear nerve (Peng et al., 2017). Taken collectively, the studies mentioned in this paragraph suggest that it is possible to achieve a relatively modest amount of benefit from cochlear implantation in the presence of a fairly small population of functional cochlear nerve elements.

Basic Hardware of Cochlear Implants

There are certainly numerous differences in the hardware of cochlear implant systems produced by the various implant manufacturers, but all cochlear implant systems possess some basic components that are common across manufacturers. Every cochlear implant system comprises two general components: an external sound processor and the cochlear implant, which is sometimes referred to as the internal device. An example of external sound processors are shown in Figure 1–2, and an example of a cochlear implant is shown in Figure 1–3. Of note, the unique technologies and differences across cochlear implant manufacturers will be discussed in Chapters 9, 10, and 11.

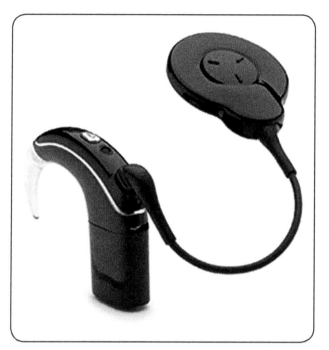

FIGURE 1–2. A Nucleus CP1000 behind-the-ear sound processor. Image provided courtesy of Cochlear Americas, ©2018.

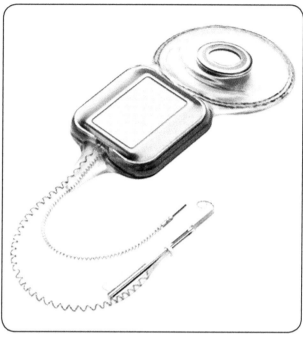

FIGURE 1–3. A Nucleus Profile cochlear implant. Image provided courtesy of Cochlear Americas, ©2018.

Cochlear Implant External Sound Processor

The external sound processor typically consists of five basic components: a microphone (or microphones), a digital signal processor, a power source (i.e., a battery), an external transmitting/receiving coil (i.e., external antenna), and an external magnet. The sound processor depicted in Figure 1–2 is behind the ear and, as shown, possesses a cable that exchanges information between the sound processor and the external coil. Sound processors are now available in a wide variety of configurations. Figure 1–4 provides examples of behind-the-ear, body-worn, and off-the-ear/single unit sound processors. As shown, the off-the-ear/single-unit sound processors do not contain a transmitting cable, because the microphone, digital signal processor, power source, and transmitting/receiving coil are housed in the same unit. Most sound processors are operated by lithium-ion rechargeable batteries. Lithium-ion technology has several advantages over other types of rechargeable batteries, including a flat voltage discharge curve, a long shelf life, a relatively robust voltage capacity, as well as the fact that it has little to no memory effect (i.e., it does not lose its ability to accept a full charge

if it is not charged from a mostly depleted state during each charging cycle). Of note, many modern sound processors may also be powered by zinc-air #675 hearing aid batteries or alkaline disposable batteries.

Cochlear Implant

The cochlear implant consists of six basic components, (1) the internal receiving/transmitting coil (i.e., internal antenna), (2) an internal magnet, (3) a digital signal processor, (4) a stimulator for electric pulse generation, (5) electrode leads, and (6) an electrode array. Together, the internal coil, digital signal processor, and stimulator are sometimes referred to as the receiver/stimulator. The digital signal processor and stimulator are housed in a biocompatible titanium case. Recently, there has been a general trend toward reducing the size (primarily the thickness) of the case in order to reduce the need for the surgeon to create a deep recession in the skull to accommodate the case as well as to reduce the tension/stretching placed on the skin that resides above the implant.

The electrode leads deliver the electric current from the stimulator to the electrode array that is

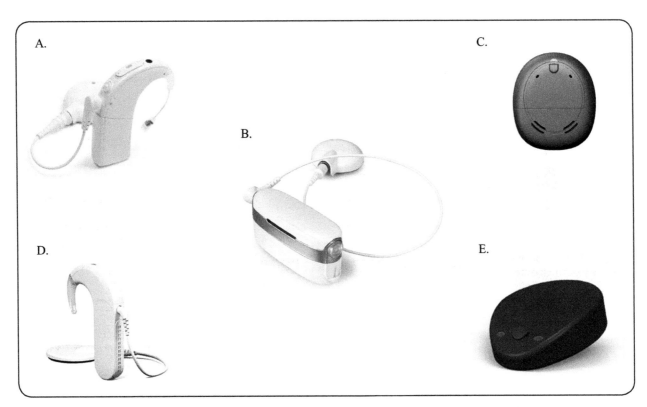

FIGURE 1–4. An illustration of several different types of cochlear implant sound processors including ear-level, body-worn, and on-the-head sound processors. **A.** Advanced Bionics Naida CI Q series sound processor, image provided courtesy of Advanced Bionics, LLC. **B.** Advanced Bionics Neptune sound processor, image provided courtesy of Advanced Bionics, LLC. **C.** Cochlear Nucleus Kanso sound processor, image provided courtesy of Cochlear Americas, ©2018. **D.** MED-EL SONNET sound processor, image provided courtesy of MED-EL Corporation. **E.** MED-EL RONDO sound processor, image provided courtesy of MED-EL Corporation.

housed within the cochlea. The electrode array consists of multiple (e.g., 12 to 22) electrode contacts. Collectively, the electrode leads and electrode array are sometimes referred to as the electrode.

There are numerous differences in the design and philosophy underlying the design of electrode arrays developed by the different cochlear implant manufacturers. Some electrode arrays are designed to be inserted close to the neural elements innervating the cochlea, whereas other electrode arrays are designed to be positioned remotely from the neural elements in an attempt to avoid trauma to the delicate sensory cells and supporting structures of the organ of Corti. Additionally, some electrode arrays are designed to be inserted to a relatively shallow depth in the cochlea (e.g., just beyond the first turn), while other electrode arrays are much longer and designed to be inserted toward the most apical end of the cochlea.

Basic Operation of Cochlear Implants

As with cochlear implant hardware, several differences exist in the way in which cochlear implant systems process and code incoming audio signals and provide stimulation to the cochlear nerve, but there are also some fundamental similarities in the manner in which cochlear implant systems operate. Figure 1–5 provides an illustration of the basic function of a cochlear implant system. The reader should note that the signal coding strategy described in Figure 1–5 and in the following paragraphs is a simplified explanation of the *Continuous Interleaved Sampling* (CIS) signal coding strategy, which essentially serves as a foundation for modern cochlear implant signal coding strategies. However, there are numerous differences between the original CIS signal coding strategies and signal coding strategies that are

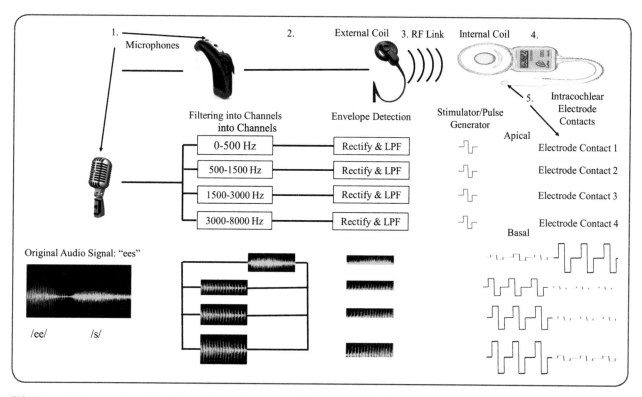

FIGURE 1–5. A block schematic of the Continuous Interleaved Stimulation (CIS) signal coding strategy.

used in most contemporary cochlear implant systems. The reader can find greater detail on cochlear implant signal coding strategies in Chapter 8.

As shown in Figure 1–5, the microphone(s) of the external sound processor captures the incoming audio signal and converts it into an electrical signal. The electrical signal is delivered to a preamplifier that increases the amplitude of the signal in order to improve the signal-to-noise ratio prior to further processing. The preamplifier typically provides a greater increase to the high-frequency components of the audio signal, because high-frequency speech sounds, such as /s/, are usually less intense and are more susceptible to masking from the relatively high-level, low-frequency speech and environmental sounds.

Next, the signal is analyzed by the sound processor's digital signal processor to determine the composition of the audio input in the frequency, temporal, and intensity domains. At this stage of operation, the signal is divided into different analysis bands (e.g., frequency bands or channels) to allow for frequency-specific processing and eventual stimulus delivery. The process of parsing the broadband input signal into spectral analysis bands is typically accomplished

with digital filtering (e.g., fast Fourier transformation, Hilbert transformation). During this stage of signal analysis, the sound processor may attempt to classify the signal as speech, noise, or some other type of acoustic signal, and signal processing may take place with the goal of optimizing signal delivery to the recipient (e.g., reduction in signal intensity in analysis bands mainly comprising noise along with an enhancement of the signal intensity within the analysis bands determined to primarily comprise speech). However, it is prudent to clarify that audio signal classification is not a component of the original CIS signal coding strategy.

It is important to note that prior to the recipient's use of the cochlear implant system, an audiologist typically programs the sound processor with the goal of determining the magnitude of electrical current required at each electrode contact (as noted later, an electrode contact usually corresponds to a particular analysis band associated with the contact in the spectral domain) to facilitate audibility as well as to produce a sensation that is loud but not uncomfortable, a process that is sometimes referred to as MAPping (i.e., determining the implant recipient's electrical dynamic range so that the desired range of acoustic inputs may be MAPped into the recipient's electrical range of hearing with the end goal of restoring audibility and normalizing loudness).

After the audio signal has been spectrally analyzed and assigned to different analysis bands, the output from the different bands is subjected to rectification and low-pass filtering in order to capture the amplitude envelope (i.e., boundary across each of the spectral bands) of the input signal (note that Figure 1–5 depicts the process of rectification (i.e., only the components above baseline are preserved, but low-pass filtering has not yet been completed because the fine temporal structure of the original signal remains). Then, based on the information that was obtained during the MAPping process, the sound processor determines the magnitude of stimulation that should be delivered to elicit audibility and a loudness percept that is appropriate for the input level of the audio signal).

Next, the digital signal processor converts the processed signal to a coded electrical signal that is delivered to the external coil, which delivers the signal across the recipient's skin to the internal coil of the cochlear implant via digital electromagnetic induction/radiofrequency (RF) transmission with a carrier frequency ranging from approximately 2.5 to 50 MHz. The signal delivered from the processor to the cochlear implant determines how the implant should deliver electrical stimulation to the cochlear nerve. Furthermore, the cochlear implant does not contain its own power source, so the RF signal delivered from the sound processor is also used to operate the cochlear implant.

Once the cochlear implant receives the digitized RF signal, it is analyzed by the digital signal processor of the implant. The cochlear implant possesses a stimulator that continuously produces biphasic electrical pulses at a fixed, moderate to fast rate (e.g., typically in the range of 800 to 1600 pulses per second) (the term "continuous" in CIS refers to the fact that electrical pulses are continuously delivered at a fixed rate). The amplitude of these electrical pulses is modulated (i.e., varied) by the magnitude of the amplitude envelope of the signal in each analysis band (see Figure 1–5). In other words, the amplitude of the electrical pulses is directly proportional to the magnitude of the amplitude envelope of the original signal (the term "sampling" indicates that the amplitude envelope of the original audio signal is captured or sampled and used to determine the magnitude of the stimulation delivered to the cochlear nerve).

Then, the amplitude-modulated electrical pulses are delivered to electrode contacts that correspond to a given analysis band. More specifically, multiple channel cochlear implants take advantage of the natural tonotopic organization that exists in the cochlea by delivering high-frequency signals to electrodes located toward the basal end of the cochlea and low-frequency signals toward more apical locations. As shown in the Figure 1–5, the electrical pulses delivered across each of the electrodes are slightly staggered in time so that an electrical pulse is never simultaneously delivered to two different electrode contacts, hence the term "interleaved."

The History of Cochlear Implants

Antecedents to the Development of the Cochlear Implant

Advances in understanding electricity and basic electronics in the late 1700s and early 1800s led to rudimentary experiments in which physicists explored the potential to stimulate the auditory system with electrical current. In 1752, a physicist, Benjamin Wilson, described a rather crude attempt at electrical stimulation to elicit auditory sensation in a woman who was deaf:

> *The covered vial being electrised by two turns of the wheel only, I applied the end of a thick wire, which was fastened to the covering of the vial, to the left temple, just above the ear; then, I brought the end of that wire, which was in the vial, towards the opposite side of her head, and there ensued a small explosion. She was much surprised and perceived a small warmth in her head, but chiefly across it from ear to ear. I repeated the experiment four times and made the electrical shock stronger on each trial.*

Quite obviously, Wilson's method of electrically stimulating the auditory system of a person with hearing loss is no longer in use in research laboratories or clinical settings today.

In the same vein, the noted Italian physicist Alessandro Volta (pictured in Figure 1–6), who is credited with the invention of the battery and for whom the SI unit of electrical force (i.e., volt) is named, also described a primitive attempt to electrically stimulate his own auditory system. Around the year 1800, Volta

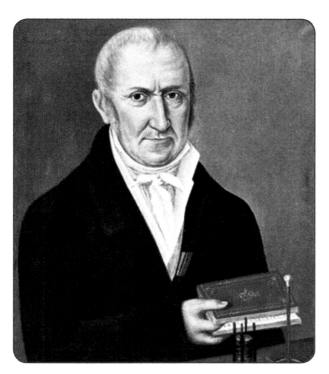

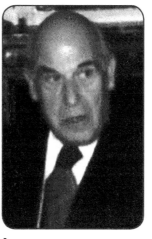 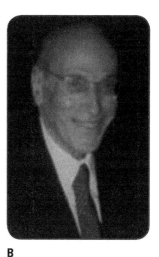

A   **B**

FIGURE 1–7. A. Charles Eyriès. **B.** André Djourno. Images provided courtesy of Claude-Henri Chouard, M.D.

FIGURE 1–6. Alessandro Volta. Image provided courtesy of Encyclopedia Britannica, Inc.

inserted leads from each end of a 50-volt battery into each ear, completing a circuit for electric current to travel through his auditory system. He described the resulting experience as follows:

> *At the moment when the circuit was complete, I received a shock in the head, and some moments after, I began to hear a sound, or rather a noise in the ears, which I cannot well define: it was kind of crackling with shocks, as if some paste or tenacious matter had been boiling. . . . This disagreeable sensation, which I believe might be dangerous because of the shock in the brain, prevented me from repeating the experiment.*

Volta's description of his experience with electrical stimulation of the auditory system seems far from pleasant, and indeed, there was a paucity of reports describing electrical stimulation of the ear for a considerable period of time.

The Nascent Stage of Cochlear Implantation

André Djourno and Charles Eyriès (pictured in Figure 1–7) are generally recognized as the first per-

sons to develop an implantable prosthesis designed to electrically stimulate the cochlear nerve. Djourno was an electrophysiologist who developed an interest in the use of electrical stimulation for medical purposes. For instance, he explored the possibility of providing artificial respiration through electrical stimulation of the phrenic nerve. Additionally, his research focused on the use of implantable induction coils, which would allow for stimulation to be delivered electromagnetically across the skin (i.e., transcutaneously) to an implanted coil which would then deliver electrical current to peripheral nerves or muscles. An example of one of Djourno's induction coils is shown in Figure 1–8.

Eyriès was an otolaryngologist who developed an expertise in facial nerve reconstruction. In 1957, while Eyriès and Djourno were both working at the L'Institut Prophylactique in Paris, Eyriès sought to provide a facial nerve graft for a patient who had bilateral cholesteatomas requiring temporal bone resection and bilateral severance of the facial and cochlea-vestibular nerves. Eyriès visited the medical center's cadaver laboratory in search of tissue that could be used to support a facial nerve graft. While seeking suitable grafting tissue, Eyriès discussed the case with Djourno, who suggested implantation of an induction stimulator in order to provide electrical stimulation of the cochlear nerve. Considering the fact that the patient, who was deaf, had nothing to lose from this novel procedure conducted in conjunction with the facial nerve repair, Eyriès agreed to implant Djourno's device.

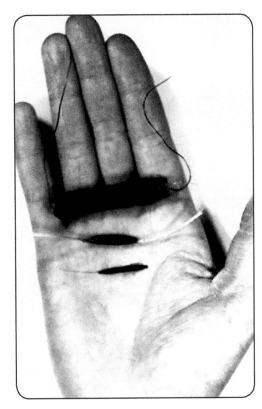

FIGURE 1–8. An example of induction coils used by Charles Eyriès and André Djourno. Image provided courtesy of Claude-Henri Chouard, M.D.

Upon examination of the cochlear nerve during surgery, Eyriès noted that most of the cochlear nerve had been resected, leaving a small stump near the brainstem. He placed the stimulating lead from Djourno's induction coil in the base of the remaining cochlear nerve and the ground electrode in the temporalis muscle. Following surgery, Djourno was able to deliver stimulation to the implanted device via electromagnetic induction. The patient was able to astutely distinguish changes in the intensity of stimulation but could only differentiate broad differences in the frequency of stimulation. Although the patient was enthused by the ability to be able to hear again, he was unable to understand speech presented in open-set without visual cues. Unfortunately, the device malfunctioned after a short period of use. Eyriès implanted a second device, which also quickly malfunctioned. Eyriès and Djourno parted company at that point.

To be completely accurate, Eyriès and Djourno's device was not a cochlear implant. First, the stimulating lead was not placed in the cochlea. Second,

because the cochlear nerve was essentially destroyed by the previous temporal bone resection, electrical stimulation was possibly provided directly to the cochlear nuclei in the brainstem rather than to an intact and functional cochlear nerve. However, their collaborative work represented the first successful endeavor in which an implantable device was used to electrically stimulate the auditory nerve. Furthermore, their work served as motivating impetus for William F. House and Claude Henri-Chouard, two persons who eventually became pioneers of cochlear implantation.

Development of the Cochlear Implant System

William F. House: The First Cochlear Implant Surgeon

William F. House earned degrees in dentistry and medicine. He was a successful otologist who was a pioneer in temporal bone surgery, including middle fossa approaches to access the internal auditory meatus. In 1958, a patient brought Dr. House a newspaper article that described how Eyriès and Djourno had created an implantable device that allowed persons with profound hearing loss to hear (House, 1974, 2011). Dr. House was very intrigued by Eyriès and Djourno's work and decided to explore the development of implantable hearing technology. In his memoirs, Dr. House noted,

I had seen deaf children with some residual hearing who could hear a degraded signal with a hearing aid and could learn lip-reading. It seemed possible that if an implant could give totally deaf children some hearing, they could learn lip-reading, be successful in an oral school, understand English language, and learn to read. (House, 2011, p. 67)

In January 1961, in collaboration with John Doyle, a Los Angeles neurosurgeon, Dr. House implanted a single wire into an opening anterior to the round window of a man who was profoundly deaf. The recipient was able to hear crude sounds when the wire, which protruded from the skin just behind the ear, was electrically stimulated, but the wire was removed after a few weeks because of concerns regarding infection. Another patient was implanted with a single wire in the cochlea and, once again, the recipient reported hearing sound upon stimulation, but the wire was removed after a short period of time for fear of infection. Of note, Dr. Doyle's brother, Jim Doyle, was an electrical engineer who assisted Drs.

House and Doyle in the development of instrumentation necessary to provide electrical stimulation to the cochlea (Mudry & Mills, 2013).

In February 1961, Drs. House and Doyle implanted a five-wire implant into the scala tympani of the first patient they had originally implanted a month earlier (House, 1976; House & Urban, 1973). The induction coils of the five-electrode system were seated in the skull just behind the auricle. The patient was able to detect different frequencies with stimulation to the different electrodes, which were placed at varying depths in the cochlea. The device was removed without complication in March 1961.

The positive initial experiences of House and the Doyles generated excitement among persons with hearing loss after the Doyles reported details of their cochlear implants to the media. Dr. House was upset with what he perceived to be the Doyle brothers' premature release of information about their preliminary experiences with electrical stimulation to the public. According to Dr. House (2011):

We began to be deluged by calls from people who had heard about the implant and its possibilities. The engineer who had constructed the implant exercised bad judgment and encouraged newspaper articles about the research we were doing.

Dr. House and the Doyles also disagreed on how the team should proceed toward commercialization of their cochlear implant work and who owned the intellectual property associated with their cochlear implant technology (Mudry & Mills, 2013). Dr. House also had concerns about the threat of infection and adverse reaction to the materials that were used in their early cochlear implants (Eshraghi et al., 2012; House, 2011; Hyman, 1990). As a result of these factors, Dr. House and the Doyle brothers ceased their collaborative endeavor. The Doyle brothers continued to implant patients until 1968, when a lack of finances prevented them from proceeding (Eshraghi et al., 2012). Dr. House did not resume his work to develop a cochlear implant until 1967. At that point in time, he was convinced that the success of other biomedical devices, such as pacemakers, which included hermetic sealing technology developed for the NASA space program and prevented body fluids from damaging electronic components, indicated that a cochlear implant could be created of materials and with methods that would allow for long-term durability of the device and safety of the recipient (House, 2011).

Dr. House began a collaboration with Jack Urban, an electrical engineer, in the late 1960s (Eshraghi et al., 2012; House, 1976; House & Urban, 1973; Mudry & Mills, 2013). They began implanting patients with a single-channel cochlear implant in 1969. At that time, their single-channel cochlear implant possessed a percutaneous plug that was implanted in the skull and protruded through the recipient's skin. Over the next several years, Dr. House implanted several patients with similar devices. In 1973, House and Urban reported on their early experiences with cochlear implantation in one patient in the journal *Annals of Otology, Rhinology, and Laryngology*. At this point in time, great interest in cochlear implantation was emerging in the otology and audiology communities, although many prominent clinicians, scientists, and researchers were skeptical that cochlear implantation could ever allow recipients to achieve open-set speech recognition. For example, noted otology surgeon Harold Schuknecht, M.D., Chief of Otolaryngology at the Massachusetts Eye and Ear Infirmary, attended the First International Conference on Electrical Stimulation of the Acoustic Nerve (held at the University of California San Francisco [UCSF]), where he saw videos of cochlear implant recipients responding to sound and heard case reports describing outcomes from early recipients. Dr. Schuknecht exclaimed (Henkel, 2013):

I interpreted the movies and the case presentations to confirm my suspicion that the prostheses as they are now designed are of very little use.

Schuknecht also stated (Wilson & Dorman, 2008):

I have the utmost admiration for the courage of those surgeons who have implanted humans, and I will admit that we need a new operation in otology, but I am afraid this is not it.

Merle Lawrence, a prominent hearing scientist, may have been even more skeptical than Dr. Schuknecht. Lawrence noted (Wilson & Dorman, 2008):

Direct stimulation of the auditory nerve fibers with resultant perception of speech is not feasible (Lawrence, 1964).

In spite of the skepticism surrounding his work and that of other pioneers conducting similar work in the 1960s and 1970s, Dr. House forged ahead. With the assistance of Jack Urban, in 1972, one of Dr. House's patients became the first cochlear implant recipient to be provided with a wearable sound processor that could be used outside of the clinic (Figure 1–9). As a result of the fact that Dr. House was the first surgeon to implant an electrode into the cochlea as well as the first to assist in the development of a wearable cochlear implant system, he is often called the "father of cochlear implantation" (Eshraghi et al., 2012). Dr. House went on to lead several multicenter trials exploring the safety and efficacy of cochlear implantation in adults and children. Additionally, Dr. House and Urban partnered with the 3M Company to commercially develop the House/3M single-channel cochlear implant system (Figure 1–10). In 1982, the House/3M cochlear implant was the first cochlear implant to be evaluated in a multicenter U.S. Food and Drug Administration (FDA) clinical trial (Eisenberg, 2015). In 1984, the House/3M device became the first cochlear implant to be approved by the FDA for commercial distribution in the United States (Eisenberg, 2015).

Furthermore, Dr. House implanted his single-channel cochlear implant in a 3-year-old child in 1981, who at the time was the youngest child to receive a cochlear implant (Eisenberg & House, 1982). Buoyed by his desire to assist children with profound hearing loss to listen to and develop spoken language, Dr. House led the first FDA trial exploring cochlear implantation in children. By 1985, the House/3M cochlear implant was provided to 164 children (Eisenberg, 2015). The average age of implantation of the children in the study was 8 years, and as a result, the benefits were modest. However, the study did demonstrate the safety and reliability of cochlear implantation for children with severe to profound hearing loss. By 1987, two hundred sixty-five children had been implanted with the House/3M cochlear implant (Berliner et al., 1990). The trial allowed investigators to learn that several factors influenced the benefit children obtained from cochlear implantation, including age of implantation, family involvement, mode of communication/intervention type, and child-specific factors (e.g., neuro-cognitive factors, additional disabilities, cochlear anatomy). In 1987, an FDA panel reviewed data from the large, multicenter pediatric cochlear implant trial led by Dr. House and recommended commercial approval of his device. The House/3M device was sold to another company in 1987, and final FDA commercial approval was never obtained (Eisenberg, 2015). Altogether, just over 1000 persons received a House/3M single-channel cochlear implant.

Contributions from Blair Simmons and the Stanford Cochlear Implant Team

In the 1960s, otolaryngologist Blair Simmons, M.D., explored the potential of treating deafness with electrical stimulation of the cochlear nerve in both animals and humans (Figure 1–11). In 1962, Dr. Simmons performed a posterior craniotomy and placed a single wire with an electrode on the tip on the cochlear nerve. The patient, who received a local anesthetic during the procedure, reported hearing sound with electrical stimulation of the cochlear nerve (Simmons et al., 1964). In 1964, Simmons implanted a six-wire/electrode device into the modiolus of a deafened adult. Simmons and colleagues performed extensive psychoacoustic testing with this recipient and determined that the recipient could detect different pitches with stimulation of different electrodes, which were placed at varying depths in the cochlea (Simmons, 1966). Also, Simmons showed that pitch changed with stimulation rate from about 30 to 300 electrical pulses per second. Additionally, the recipient reported that the device elicited a speech-like sound when broad-

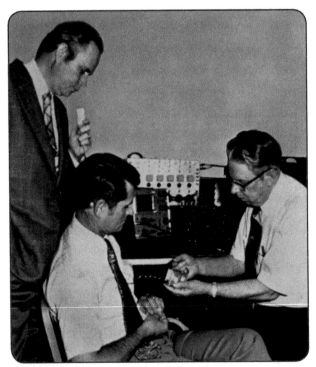

FIGURE 1–9. William F. House, M.D., cochlear implant surgeon, and colleagues at the House Ear Institute. Image provided courtesy of Laurie Eisenberg and the House Ear Institute archives.

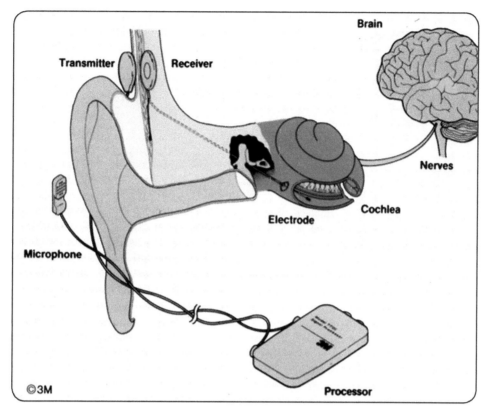

FIGURE 1–10. The House/3M single channel cochlear implant system. Image provided courtesy of Laurie Eisenberg and the House Ear Institute archives.

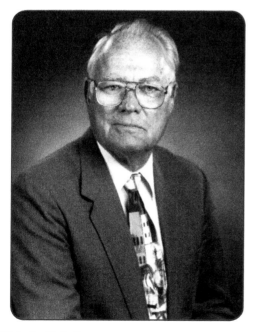

FIGURE 1–11. Blair Simmons, M.D., cochlear implant surgeon. Image provided courtesy of Stanford University's Department of Otolaryngology-Head & Neck Surgery.

band electrical stimulation was provided. However, the recipient was unable to understand speech presented in an open set, a fact that discouraged Simmons, who ceased evaluation of electrical stimulation in humans in the late 1960s. Of note, Simmons did present and publish throughout the mid to late 1960s on his findings with electrical stimulation of the auditory system, and he is believed to be the first person to use the term "cochlear implant" (Simmons, 1969).

Contributions from the University of California San Francisco Cochlear Implant Group

Robin Michelson, M.D., an otolaryngologist at UCSF, implanted several patients with a single-channel wire ensheathed in a silicone molding that was inserted into the basal end of the scala tympani in the late 1960s and early 1970s (Merzenich, 2015). Michael Merzenich, a physiologist, was recruited to UCSF in 1971 to collaborate with Dr. Michelson on the development of a multichannel device (Figure 1–12). Merzenich was initially skeptical that a cochlear implant could provide open-set speech recognition. However,

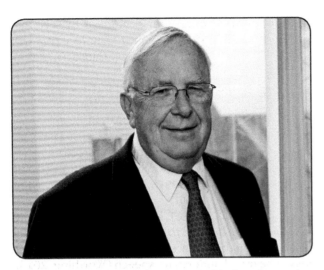

FIGURE 1–12. Michael Merzenich, Ph.D., physiologist and researcher. Image provided courtesy of Michael Merzenich.

he conducted psychophysical studies with some of Simmons' early recipients and was surprised to find that they could detect changes in frequency/pitch with changes in electrical stimulation rate through several hundred hertz. Merzenich felt that the low-frequency cues provided via changes in electrical stimulation rate could be paired with high-frequency place cues obtained from stimulation to several electrode contacts positioned throughout the cochlea (Merzenich, 2015).

Although Michelson's early recipients could not understand speech in open set, Merzenich was encouraged by the restoration of basic auditory abilities offered by the crude single-channel device. Merzenich conducted several studies to evaluate electrical stimulation of the cochlear nerve in cats in an effort to better understand the complexities involved in supporting speech recognition with cochlear implantation in humans. Merzenich's studies with animals and Michelson's early implant recipients convinced the San Francisco team to pursue development of a multi-channel cochlear implant system (Merzenich et al., 1973, 1974).

Otolaryngologist Robert Schindler, M.D., spearheaded the San Francisco group's efforts to develop a cochlear implant with biocompatible materials that would allow for a device that was safe to implant in the human body and that could function over the long term in an environment (i.e., the head) that was hostile to electronics (e.g., moist, mobile, susceptible to impact damage). Schindler was joined by scientist Birgitta Bjorkroth and anatomist Patricia Leake,

who also sought to identify safe methods to provide long-term electrical stimulation of the cochlear nerve (Merzenich, 2015). The group of researchers demonstrated that electrodes encased in silicone were safe to implant in the temporal bone. They also demonstrated that long-term charge-balanced electrical stimulation of the cochlear nerve in animals not only was safe (Leake-Jones, 1981) but actually promoted survival of cochlear neural elements (Wong-Riley, 1981).

Merzenich and colleagues collaborated with Blake Wilson and Charles Finley's team at the Research Triangle Institute (RTI) in North Carolina. Based on their collective findings in numerous research studies, they developed an eight-channel cochlear implant with independent/isolated channels (Merzenich, 2015). A CIS-type signal coding strategy was employed in the UCSF device. Much of the work conducted at UCSF and at the RTI was financially supported by the Neural Prosthesis Program (NPP) of the United States National Institutes of Health (NIH) (Wilson & Dorman, 2008). The results obtained with recipients who used the UCSF device and/or the RTI signal coding strategies were very encouraging, and as a result, the Storz Medical Instruments Company partnered with UCSF with the goal of developing a cochlear implant system for commercial/clinical use (Eshraghi et al., 2012). Storz produced a prototype of the UCSF cochlear implant system, but the device was plagued by issues with reliability. In 1986, UCSF entered into an agreement with another company, Minimed, which was owned by entrepreneur Alfred Mann, who provided substantial financial backing to the development of a commercial cochlear implant system (Eshraghi et al., 2012; Merzenich, 2015). Mann formed the Advanced Bionics Company, which eventually developed the Clarion cochlear implant system. The Clarion cochlear implant system was approved by the FDA for commercial distribution in the United States in 1996 for adults and in 1997 for children. Advanced Bionics was eventually acquired by the Boston Scientific medical manufacturer in 2004. Mann and colleague Jeffrey Greiner reacquired Advanced Bionics from Boston Scientific after the latter expressed concern about the profitability and quality control of the company. Mann and Greiner later sold Advanced Bionics to Sonova Holding AG in 2009.

Graeme Clark: The Father of the Modern Multiple-Channel Cochlear Implant

Graeme Clark, M.D., became an otolaryngologist after watching his father struggle with significant hearing loss (Figure 1–13). Dr. Clark's father was a pharmacist, and as a teenager, the junior Clark often assisted his father in his pharmacy clinic. Dr. Clark has often reminisced about the awkwardness that existed when his father's clients would have to speak loudly about their private health needs so that his father could hear and understand his customers' needs (Worthing, 2015).

Inspired to improve the lives of persons with hearing loss, Dr. Clark earned a medical degree and became a successful otolaryngology surgeon in Melbourne, Australia. His clinical practice was quite successful and provided considerable financial means for his wife and young daughters. By 1966, he had become the head of the clinic and the Royal Victorian Eye and Ear Hospital (Worthing, 2015, p. 68). In his clinical practice, he saw many patients who had severe to profound hearing loss. He lamented the fact that he was unable to provide them with substantial improvement in their communication abilities. Dr. Clark has acknowledged that the futility that he experienced when serving persons with severe to profound hearing loss served as an inspiration to develop the cochlear implant. An example of this

inability to provide help for persons with severe to profound hearing can be seen in a note written by one of Dr. Clark's colleagues, Les Caust, M.D. (see the box below).

Toward the later part of 1966, Dr. Clark read of Dr. Blair Simmons' work with cochlear implants, which was published in the *Archives of Otolaryngology*. After reading Simmons' promising report, Dr. Clark conferred with his wife and trusted mentors about the possibility of moving to Sydney, Australia in order to pursue a Ph.D. and research electrical stimulation of the auditory system with the goal of treating deafness. In 1967, Dr. Clark commenced with his studies and his goal to develop a cochlear implant to allow persons with severe to profound hearing loss to hear and understand speech (Worthing, 2015).

Dr. Clark's early research focused on answering basic questions such as could electrical stimulation reproduce the auditory system's typical coding of frequency and intensity. In animal studies, he was able to demonstrate increases in the magnitude of the auditory system's response with increases in electrical stimulation of the cochlear nerve. However, increases in the frequency of electrical stimulation

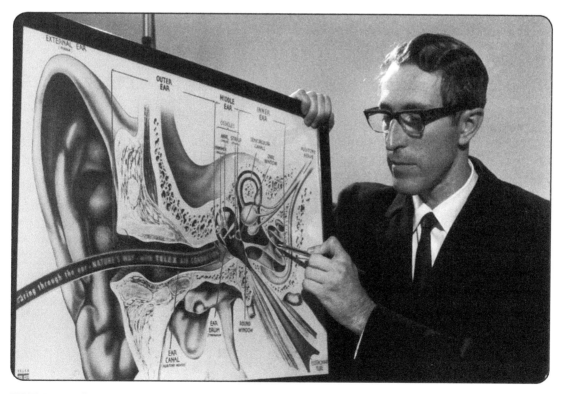

FIGURE 1–13. Graeme Clark, M.D., cochlear implant surgeon and co-developer of the multiple-channel cochlear implant. Image provided courtesy of Graeme Clark.

An example of a chart note written by Les Caust, M.D., one of Dr. Clark's medical colleagues. Dr. Clark noted that chart notes like these served as a motivator to create the cochlear implant. Provided courtesy of Graeme Clark.

4th April, 1967

Dear Mr. Kearton,

Thank you very much for going along to the Acoustic Laboratory and having their somewhat more sophisticated tests....

It does appear that you have a complete bilateral sensori-neural hearing loss and that no surgical or any other attack would be of any avail to you. I would agree entirely with this that you rejoin the Australian Association for Better Hearing and I have enclosed a form for you to fill out to this end. It was disappointing that nothing surgical can help, but I'm sure with your perseverance and continued attack on it with the ability that you have got then you will make the most of a pretty bad lot.

as Chair of the Otolaryngology Department at the University of Melbourne. Dr. Clark formed a multi-disciplinary team of professionals (e.g., engineers, physiologists, audiologists) who worked to develop a multiple-channel cochlear implant that would be available for clinical use. Dr. David Dewhurst and Jim Patrick, both electrical engineers, provided the expertise necessary to develop signal coding strategies designed to electrically convey the necessary acoustic properties of speech and to develop the hardware of a multiple-channel cochlear implant system. Dr. Clark's team also included hearing science and audiology luminaries Field Rickards, Richard Dowell, and Yit Chow (Joe) Tong (Worthing, 2015).

Because Dr. Clark devoted the majority of his time to the development of administrative responsibilities within the academic department and to his cochlear implant research, funding for his research endeavors was in short supply. Dr. Clark led a grassroots effort to raise money to fund his research with legend suggesting that he resorted to begging on the streets (Figure 1–14). He delivered numerous presentations describing his research and objectives to local organizations that may have been able to offer finan-

(i.e., electrical pulses per second) could not be faithfully coded by the response properties of the cochlear nerve beyond about 400 Hz (Clark, 1969). Due to the limitations of temporal coding of frequency, Dr. Clark concluded that a multiple-channel cochlear implant would be required to support open-set speech recognition (Clark et al., 1977, 1978).

Dr. Clark's research and clinical experience made him aware of several obstacles that had to be surpassed in order for cochlear implantation to allow for a successful outcome. First, Clark's research indicated that the dynamic range of electrical hearing (i.e., range between threshold of electrical hearing and upper limit of tolerance to electrical stimulation) was much less (e.g., 5–10 dB) than the dynamic range of speech (Clark et al., 1978). Also, Dr. Clark postulated that in order to thoroughly represent the spectral range of speech across the cochlea, an electrode lead would have to be inserted at least 20 to 25 mm into the cochlea (Clark, 2015). Dr. Clark also acknowledged that there was no consensus regarding the proper coding strategy necessary to represent the spectral and temporal properties of speech to allow for open-set speech recognition.

After graduating with a Ph.D. from the University of Sydney in 1969, Dr. Clark accepted a position

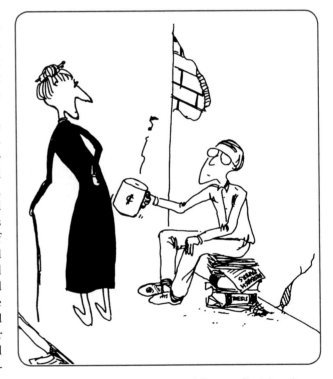

FIGURE 1–14. A cartoon depiction of Graeme Clark begging on the streets to raise money for his research to develop a cochlear implant. Image provided courtesy of Graeme Clark.

cial support. The Apex Club, a local service organization, donated $2000 to support Clark's research, and the Australian Broadcasting Commission featured a story on the donation on the evening news. Sir Reginald Ansett, the founder of Ansett Airways and the owner of an Australian television station, saw the story on the news and offered to host a telethon on his station to raise money for cochlear implant research. Ultimately, Ansett hosted multiple telethons throughout the mid-1970s which not only raised considerable money to fund Dr. Clark's research but also enhanced public awareness of cochlear implantation as a means to improve hearing in persons who are deaf (Worthing, 2015).

Clark studied speech perception on a sabbatical in England from 1975 to 1976. Dewhurst, Patrick, and Ian Forster completed a bench version of a multiple-channel cochlear implant in 1976. Indeed, the work of developing the electronics necessary to support multiple-channel stimulation and signal coding to support speech recognition was tedious and required arduous study, but progress was steadily achieved. However, Clark noted that the team continued to struggle with the task of inserting an array of wires and electrode contacts 20 to 25 mm into the scala tympani of the cochlea. Specifically, Dr. Clark noted that his team explored the development of a suitable electrode array without success from 1975 throughout 1976. In 1977, Dr. Clark was on vacation with his family at a beach in Melbourne. While his children were playing on the beach, Dr. Clark picked up a nearby snail shell and marveled at its structural similarities to the human cochlea. He then picked up a blade of grass and inserted it into the shell. He quickly noted that blades of grass that became progressively thinner from the base to the tip and progressively stiffer from the tip to the base easily slid into the shell (Figure 1–15). Unable to contain his excitement with his newfound discovery, he packed up his family and left their vacation two days earlier than planned. He then conveyed his observations to his team of engineers, who were able to develop an electrode array that could be inserted to the desired depth of approximately 25 mm into the cochlea (Worthing, 2015).

In August 1978, Rod Saunders was the first person to receive one of Dr. Clark's multiple-channel cochlear implants (Figure 1–16). Because the activation of Mr. Saunders' cochlear implant was the culmination of over 10 years of research, development, and fundraising, it was a big event that was covered by the Australian media, including the television station that hosted telethons to support the development of the cochlear implant. To everyone's dismay and disappointment, Saunders was unable to hear anything when Clark's team attempted to activate his cochlear implant. Saunders returned to the clinic a short time later, but once again, he was unable to hear when his cochlear implant was activated. Eventually, Clark's team discovered a faulty lead from the

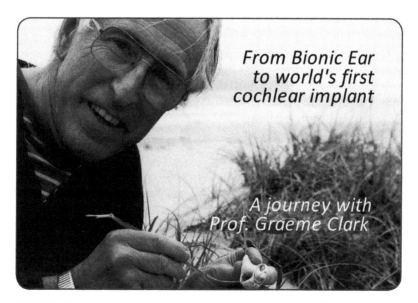

FIGURE 1–15. Graeme Clark inserting a reed of grass into a sea shell. Image provided courtesy of Graeme Clark.

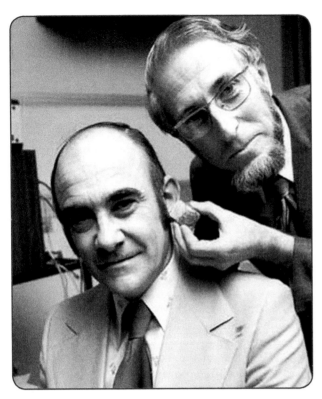

FIGURE 1–16. Graeme Clark with Rod Saunders, the first recipient of Clark's multiple-channel cochlear implant. Image provided courtesy of Graeme Clark.

activating computer to the external transmitting coil of the cochlear implant. Ironically enough, one of the main culprits of faults in modern cochlear implants are faulty cables that deliver the signal from the recipient's sound processor to the external transmitting coil. The faulty lead on Clark's equipment was replaced, and Saunders returned for a third time for activation of his cochlear implant. As the old saying goes, the third time was the charm. Saunders' cochlear implant was activated, and the Australian national anthem was played over a loudspeaker. Saunders, who was a veteran of the Australian armed forces, slowly but dramatically rose from his chair, stood at attention, and saluted to the sound of the anthem that he had not heard in years. Needless to say, Clark and his team were elated. It soon became apparent that Saunders was also able to understand speech presented in open set with the use of his cochlear implant. Dr. Clark describes his emotional reaction to the point in time at which he realized that all of his efforts and sacrifices to develop a cochlear implant had come to fruition and his new development that would allow persons with severe to profound hearing

loss, like his father, to hear sound and understand speech (Worthing, 2015):

> *It was the moment I had been waiting for. I went into the adjoining room and cried for joy.*

Additional patients were implanted with Dr. Clark's multiple-channel cochlear implant, and Clark became convinced that his device would allow for better hearing for persons with severe to profound hearing loss. He entered into a partnership with medical device manufacturer Telectronics, with the goal of manufacturing the multiple-channel cochlear implant for commercial distribution. Engineers at Telectronics initially expressed doubts that Clark's cochlear implant could be commercially produced so that it possessed long-term reliability. Specifically, the pacemakers that Telectronics specialized in manufacturing had only one lead that had to pass through a hermetically sealed port from the pacemaker's processor/stimulator. In contrast, Clark's cochlear implant required 20 leads to pass from a ceramic-to-metal seal. Telectronic engineers worried that such a small device with so many leads could not be developed without the almost certain threat of body fluid entering into the cochlear implant and causing electronic failure (Worthing, 2015).

In his biography on the life and contributions of Graeme Clark, Mark Worthing (2015) described the dilemma and Clark's response as follows:

> *So the company* [Telectronics] *hired a specialist engineer, Januz Kuzma, to work specifically on this problem. He worked for several months with no solution.*
>
> *Graeme was becoming frustrated with the delays and the claims that it couldn't be done, so he did what he always had done in such circumstances. He decided he would attempt to solve the problem himself. He asked his own engineer, Jim Patrick, to help him. Graeme got some clays and metals and fired up his pottery kiln at the back of his house in Eltham. About this time, Kuzma at Telectronics, who had heard that Professor Clark was attempting to do it himself in his backyard pottery kiln, began making some genuine progress and Graeme and Jim Patrick put their work on hold. Graeme likes to think that the risk of having amateurs working with a backyard kiln come up with a solution provided an added incentive to creativity. In any event, a ceramic solution to the problem was found.*

In September 1982, Telectronics manufactured a commercial prototype of Clark's cochlear implant. Graham Carrick was the first recipient of a commercial version of Clark's device. Because the research and development of Clark's cochlear implant was now being funded by the Australian government, the activation of Carrick's implant was once again a significant event which was covered by the Australian media. Similar to the experience with Rod Saunders, Carrick was unable to hear with his new cochlear implant throughout the first 15 minutes of the activation session. Eventually, Carrick heard a sound through his implant. Carrick noted (Worthing, 2015):

It hit me, I heard a "ding dong" and I said to myself "bloody hell!" To get this sound was fascinating and mind boggling. Tears ran down my face.

By 1983, Clark's cochlear implant was being trialed by surgeons in Australia, the United States, and Europe. Clark's team developed methodical research studies to develop the data necessary to seek FDA approval for commercial distribution. Telectronics became known as Nucleus, which later developed a subsidiary company called Cochlear Limited. In short, Graeme Clark's multiple-channel cochlear implant became the Cochlear Nucleus 22 cochlear implant system. Cochlear Ltd. is now the world's largest manufacturer of cochlear implant technology. The FDA granted approval for commercial distribution of the Nucleus 22 cochlear implant for adults in 1985 and for children in 1990.

Contributions from Claude Chouard and Other French Cochlear Implant Researchers

In 1972, Claude-Henri Chouard, an otolaryngology surgeon in France, was informed of the advances that William House and Robin Michelson had made with their cochlear implant research (Figure 1–17). Inspired by the notion of developing a treatment for deafness, Dr. Chouard, who had previously served as a student in Charles Eyriès' laboratory during the time that Eyriès and Djourno explored electrical stimulation of the cochlear nerve, partnered with Patrick MacLeod to develop an interdisciplinary team to conduct research on and develop a multiple-channel cochlear implant (Chouard, 2015). Chouard and MacLeod made several significant contributions to the development of the cochlear implant. In their early efforts, they established a frequency map of almost the entire length of the human cochlea, which

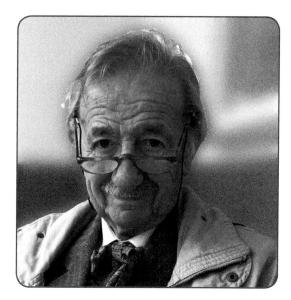

FIGURE 1–17. Claude-Henri Chouard, M.D., cochlear implant surgeon. Image provided courtesy of Claude-Henri Chouard.

allowed researchers to determine where electrode contacts would need to be located to elicit a desired frequency/pitch percept.

Chouard and MacLeod also explored the biocompatibility of various materials that could be used to create a cochlear implant. In the 1970s, Chouard showed that Teflon-coated platinum-iridium electrode contacts and silicone Silastic™ insulation were safe to implant in the human cochlea and possessed physical characteristics that promoted long-term durability (Chouard, 2015). Chouard and MacLeod also explored signal coding strategies and were one of the first groups to suggest that sequential digital, pulsatile electrical stimulation may be preferable to analog stimulation because of the former's ability to lessen channel interaction (Chouard & MacLeod, 1976).

In September 1976, Drs. Chouard and Bernard Meyer implanted a patient with an eight-electrode cochlear implant (Meyer, 1974). Chouard noted that the performance of their early multiple-channel cochlear implant recipients was very favorable relative to results reported at the time for single-channel implant recipients (Chouard, 2015). Chouard and colleagues also reported on the need to determine signal parameters (e.g., stimulation levels) based on the electrophysiologic characteristics of each electrode contact, and they described rehabilitative strategies that facilitated a successful response to cochlear implantation (Chouard et al., 1983a). Furthermore, Chouard et al. (1983b) demonstrated the importance of early implantation for congenitally deafened recipients by showing greater neural atrophy in the brainstems of guinea pigs implanted later in life relative to those implanted earlier.

Led by Chouard, the French cochlear implant group developed a 12-channel cochlear implant that was originally known as the Chlorimac-12. The early Chlorimac-12 implants were manufactured by Bertin®, which later sold the patent for the Chlorimac-12 implant to the French company MXM Neurelec® (Chouard, 2015). In 2013, the MXM Neurelec cochlear implant was eventually acquired by the William Demant Group, the holding company of Oticon Medical and of the Oticon hearing aid company. At the time of this writing, the Oticon Medical cochlear implant had not been approved by the FDA for commercial distribution in the United States.

Contributions of the Vienna Cochlear Implant Group

Spurred by reports on electrical stimulation of the auditory system emerging from France and the United States, a team of researchers led by Ervin Hochmair at the Technical University of Vienna in Austria began work toward the development of a cochlear implant in the 1970s (Eshraghi et al., 2012). Ingeborg (Desoyer) Hochmair was also a promi-

nent member of the Vienna cochlear implant team (Figure 1–18). In 1975, The Hochmairs received a research grant to develop a multiple-channel cochlear implant, and within 18 months they had developed an eight-channel system complete with Teflon-insulated platinum electrodes encased in a silicone carrier. In 1977, a patient was implanted with the Vienna multiple-channel device. Initially, the Vienna team experimented with single-channel analog stimulation, but most recipients experienced difficulty understanding speech. Eventually, the Hochmairs collaborated with Blake Wilson at the RTI in North Carolina and incorporated CIS into their multiple-channel cochlear implant. Of note, the Hochmairs were convinced that a long electrode array (e.g., ~31 mm) would optimize speech recognition performance and sound quality by accessing the most apical regions of the cochlea, where low-frequency sounds are naturally coded. In 1990, the Hochmair team created the private company MED-EL to facilitate the commercial development of their multiple-channel cochlear implant. Ingeborg Hochmair left the University of Vienna to operate the MED-EL company, which is located in Innsbruck, Austria. In 2001, the MED-EL COMBI 40+ cochlear implant system was approved by the FDA for commercial distribution in the United States for adults and children.

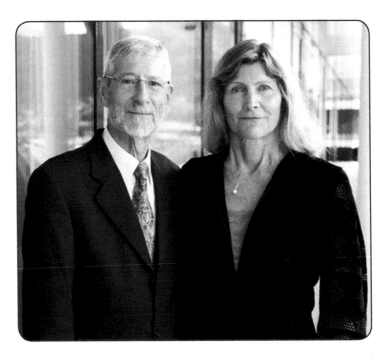

FIGURE 1–18. Ervin and Ingeborg Hochmair, researchers and developers of the MED-EL cochlear implant. Image provided courtesy of Ingeborg Hochmair.

Several researchers at the University of Utah contributed substantially to the development of modern cochlear implant technology. Michael Dorman and James Parkin (2015) have provided an excellent summary of the various contributions of the Utah Artificial ear project to the development of cochlear implant technology. The Dorman and Parkin (2015) review serves as the source of most of the information that is presented here in regard to the Utah Artificial Ear Project.

The University of Utah was home to the prolific Division of Artificial Organs, which was led by William J. "Pimm" Kolff, who developed the first artificial kidney. Kolff's team was exploring the possible development of visual and auditory prostheses with initial interest directed toward stimulation of the auditory cortex. They eventually turned their interest toward intracochlear stimulation, because cochlear surgery was "less drastic" compared with implanting electrodes in the cerebrum, and they could potentially take advantage of the tonotopic organization that naturally exists within the cochlea.

The Utah group partnered with the Ear Research Institute in Los Angeles to pursue the development of a cochlear implant. The joint program included the Ear Research Institute surgeon Derald Brackmann and Utah's James Parkin (surgeon), Michael Mladejovsky, (engineer), William Dobelle (physiologist), Geary McCandless (audiologist), and Don Eddington (who was a graduate student in engineering at the beginning of the project). Work on the Utah Artificial Ear Project began in the early 1970s.

One of the early decisions made by the Utah group that was largely responsible for the impact it made on cochlear implant technology was the commitment to percutaneous signal delivery via an implanted pedestal. Most researchers at the time had chosen to develop cochlear implant systems that used electromagnetic induction to deliver signals across the skin (i.e., transcutaneous delivery) to the cochlear implant. Although transcutaneous systems have the benefit of housing all of the implantable components entirely underneath the recipient's skin, there are constraints to the amount of information that may be delivered via electromagnetic induction/RF delivery.

In contrast, a percutaneous pedestal basically serves as an outlet to which an external processor may be connected to deliver stimulation directly to electrodes that are wired to the pedestal. As a result of this direct connection, there are essentially no lim-

its to the amount of information that may be delivered from an external processor to the implanted electrode contacts. Additionally, the electrode leads and contacts may be continuously monitored for faults, and there are no implanted electronics that could critically fail. Because of the inherent flexibility of the percutaneous design, the Utah Ear group was able to conduct a series of psychophysical studies designed to explore how recipients respond to electrical stimulation of the cochlear nerve. Of note, the Utah percutaneous implant was originally marketed by Symbion, Inc. under the name Ineraid. The Ineraid cochlear implant system is shown in Figure 1–19.

Utah's Ineraid cochlear implant possessed six electrode leads that were coupled to the pedestal at the lateral end and to six electrode contacts at the medial end. The electrode leads were intended to be inserted into the cochlea at different depths in order to code six different frequencies/pitch percepts. Dr. Brackmann implanted two patients with the Ineraid device in 1975. Of note, one of these patients was

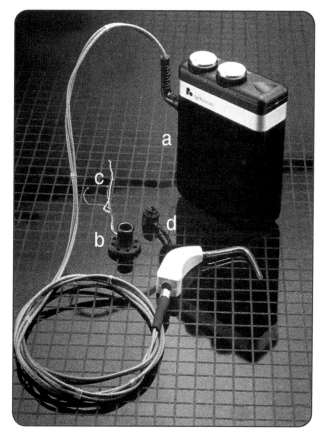

FIGURE 1–19. The Ineraid percutaneous cochlear implant system. Image provided courtesy of Michael Dorman.

bilaterally deafened and the other was unilaterally deafened. Two additional patients were implanted in 1977. The initial cohort of Ineraid implant recipients included persons who were prelingually deafened and others who lost their hearing as adults. The varied backgrounds of the Utah subjects allowed the researchers to gain keen insights into variables that influence outcomes obtained with a cochlear implant.

Eddington and Mladejovsky conducted exhaustive psychophysical studies with the initial Ineraid recipients. They were able to gain a preliminary understanding of many fundamental concepts pertaining to electrical stimulation of the cochlear nerve, including the relationship of place of stimulation (i.e., location/depth of the electrode in the cochlea) and pitch percept, the relationship of stimulus current amplitude, duration (pulse width), and rate to loudness percept, the pros and cons of bipolar versus monopolar electrode coupling, electrode impedance changes over time, etc. Their experiments greatly advanced the understanding of electrical stimulation of the human cochlea and the association to recipient experience.

Additionally, the Utah group capitalized on the unique opportunity afforded by the inclusion of a recipient with normal hearing in the non-implanted ear. Specifically, Eddington noted that they completed studies to match the pitch elicited by electrical stimulation at various depths in the implanted ear to the pitch elicited by pure tones presented to the opposite ear. Their measures confirmed that the implant place-to-pitch relationship corresponded to frequency-by-distance maps of the cochlea. The tonotopic information gleaned from the Utah group's research assisted other researchers in the development of multiple-channel cochlear implant systems and the application of pitch to electrode contact location.

In 1978, Eddington began to explore speech recognition obtained with single- and multiple-channel stimulation. At the time, there was still disagreement among researchers as to whether multiple-channel implants would allow for better performance than single-channel devices. In particular, some researchers contended that an electric current analogous to the acoustic input signal could be delivered to a single electrode contact in order to comprehensively provide the signal captured by the microphone. Eddington compared speech recognition obtained with a single channel to a four-channel stimulation (electric analog stimulation delivered in each condition). He reported that performance was unequivocally better with multiple-channel stimulation. However, the subjects were generally unable to understand speech presented in open set, a finding that may have been attributed to the fact that a wearable processor was unavailable, so recipients were only able to hear with their cochlear implants when they came to the laboratory for research. As a result, they were unable to acclimate to electrical stimulation.

Between 1977 and 1984, no new patients were implanted with the Ineraid device. During that period, Eddington developed a wearable sound processor. Symbion, Inc. used Eddington's design to produce the first portable Ineraid sound processor, which was fitted to a recipient in 1983. Notably, the first recipient to use the Ineraid sound processor was implanted in 1977 and had gone six years with only being able to hear while visiting the laboratory for research sessions.

In 1984, the FDA granted permission to Symbion, Inc. to conduct a clinical trial of the Ineraid, and Dr. Parkin began to implant the Ineraid device at the University of Utah. Implantation of the Ineraid device eventually was performed at 19 different centers in the United States. Many recipients obtained substantial benefit and open-set speech recognition with the Ineraid implant. For instance, Scott Shepard was the first recipient of an Ineraid cochlear implant as part of the FDA clinical trial. Mr. Shepard achieved a score of 73% correct on the CNC monosyllabic word recognition test just a few months after the activation of his cochlear implant. Of note, these recipients were using a signal coding strategy that divided the input signal into four analysis bands centered at 500, 1000, 2000, and 4000 Hz, and an electric analog of the audio signal within each of the four bands was delivered to four electrode contacts located 4 mm apart within the cochlea.

In 1983, Blake Wilson and a team of his researchers located in North Carolina received funding from the NIH to develop signal coding strategies for cochlear implants. Wilson and colleagues were unable to effectively test many of their experimental strategies with recipients using implants with transcutaneous transmission, because at that time the electromagnetic link would not allow for delivery of the coded information. Consequently, Wilson began to study his new signal coding strategies with Ineraid recipients in 1989. The percutaneous connection of the Ineraid proved to be highly beneficial to Wilson's research, because Wilson and colleagues were able to deliver complex coded information to the Ineraid electrode contacts via the pedestal.

Wilson's work with the Ineraid recipients resulted in the development of the CIS signal coding strategy mentioned earlier in this chapter. As previously noted, the CIS strategy served as the foundation on which all modern signal coding strategies were developed. Additionally, during their signal coding research with Ineraid recipients, Wilson and colleagues explored the potential benefit of other signal processing schemes that would eventually become mainstays in modern cochlear implant systems. Their work included assessment of *n-of-m* strategies, fine structure processing (FSP), current steering, and high-rate CIS stimulation.

Furthermore, researchers working with Ineraid recipients were able to make direct recordings of the compound action potential generated by the cochlear nerve in response to electrical stimulation. This research eventually led to the development of "onboard" systems in commercial implants to allow for measurement of the electrically evoked compound action potential (e.g., neural response telemetry [NRT]) (see Chapter 18). Also, because the Ineraid did not have the magnet necessary in transcutaneous implants, researchers were able to conduct functional MRI with Ineraid recipients and evaluate activity in the auditory cortex elicited by electrical stimulation from the implant.

Despite the numerous merits and contributions of the Ineraid system, the FDA never approved it for commercial distribution. In 1989, the FDA raised concerns regarding safety associated with a percutaneous pedestal. Specifically, the FDA was concerned that the percutaneous outlet would allow for infection in adjacent skin or in the brain. The FDA also expressed concern regarding "administrative issues" in the Symbion, Inc. company. Later, in the early 1990s, reports began to emerge of recipients experiencing a sensation of electric shock while using the Ineraid implant. Engineers determined that the check was likely arising from static electricity discharge collected at the long cable of the sound processor. In other words, the cable was essentially acting as an antenna to collect static electrical discharge. Design changes were made to the cable, and the problem was resolved. Also, a review of adverse effects associated with the Ineraid device indicated that there was no serious threat to complication, such as infection, with use of the percutaneous pedestal. Nevertheless, Symbion, Inc. grew weary of the process of seeking commercial approval from the FDA, and the Ineraid technology was sold to Cochlear Ltd. The pursuit of commercial approval was extinguished, but the remarkably positive legacy of the Ineraid implant (along with its designers, such as Don Eddington) and the positive

influence on modern cochlear implant technology are undeniable.

Prominent Milestones in the Development of Cochlear Implant Technology

The Neural Prosthesis Program (NPP) of the NIH was developed in 1970 and was under the leadership of Dr. F. Terry Hambrecht and later Dr. William J. Heetderks (Wilson & Dorman, 2008). Dr. Hambrecht hosted an annual workshop comprising scientists conducting research with neural prostheses. In 1973, Michelson, House, Merzenich, and Simmons shared their preliminary results from and experiences with their trials with electrical stimulation of the cochlear nerve in their patients with profound hearing loss. The outcomes were impressive enough to convince the NIH to provide federal funding of the research that was being conducted at the various sites in the United States.

In 1975, the NIH funded a study to evaluate the outcomes of 13 single-channel cochlear implant recipients. Eleven of these recipients were implanted by Dr. William House and two were implanted by Dr. Robin Michelson. The study was led by Robert Bilger, an audiologist and physiologist at the University of Pittsburgh. The 13 single-channel implant recipients were flown to the University of Pittsburgh for extensive assessment by Bilger and his colleagues. The findings of the study were published in a paper that is often referred to as the Bilger Report (Bilger & Black, 1977). In the summary, Dr. Bilger noted,

Although the subjects could not understand speech through their prosthesis, they did score significantly higher on tests of lipreading and recognition of environmental sounds with their prostheses activated than without them (Wilson & Dorman, 2008).

and

To the extent that the effectiveness of single-channel auditory prostheses has been demonstrated here, the next step lies in the exploration of a multichannel prosthesis (Mudry & Mills, 2013).

The Bilger Report was a watershed moment in the development of the cochlear implant, because it served to legitimize cochlear implantation in the scientific community, and it resulted in the provision of substantial NIH funding to researchers in the

United States, such as Michelson, Simmons, House, Blake Wilson, and so forth as well as Graeme Clark's program in Australia. The support of NIH for cochlear implantation was critical in advancing the state of the technology. At the time, there were still numerous opponents of the notion that electrical stimulation could prove to be beneficial for persons with severe to profound hearing loss. For example, in 1978, prominent auditory physiologist Professor Rainer Klinke said (Wilson, 2017),

> *From a physiological point of view, cochlear implants will not work.*

The support NIH offered to fund cochlear implant research around the world fueled impressive advances that defied the expectations of skeptics. The NIH hosted a consensus conference in cochlear implants in 1988 and suggested that multiple-channel cochlear implants were likely to provide better performance than single-channel cochlear implants and that 1 in 20 recipients could understand speech in open set without speechreading. At a second consensus conference in 1995, the group concluded (NIH, 1995):

> *A majority of those individuals with the latest speech processors for their implants will score above 80% correct on high-context sentences, even without visual cues.*

In the late 1980s, Richard Tyler, hearing scientist, traveled throughout the world to evaluate outcomes of recipients with a variety of different types of single- and multiple-channel cochlear implants. Tyler reported a wide range of outcomes across recipients but did show that good to excellent open-set speech recognition without visual cues was possible for some recipients (Tyler, Moore, & Kuk, 1989).

We would be remiss to discuss cochlear outcomes without inclusion of Margaret Skinner, an audiologist and hearing scientist at Washington University in Saint Louis, Missouri (Figure 1–20). Dr. Skinner was instrumental in the evaluation of cochlear implant outcomes in children and adults. She conducted research to show the benefits and limitations of cochlear implant technology in quiet and in noise for both children and adults. Her research was essential in identifying the variety of factors that influence outcomes experienced by cochlear implant recipients. She also developed the SPEAK signal coding strategy, and she explored the use of high-resolution CT scan assessment to evaluate the scalar position of cochlear implant electrode array. She was one of the first examiners to show the importance of electrode array placement in scala tympani (rather than dislocation in the scala vestibuli and/or scala media), and she demonstrated the benefit of close proximity of the electrode conducts to the cochlear neural elements in the modiolus (Holden et al., 2013).

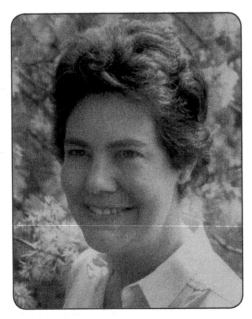 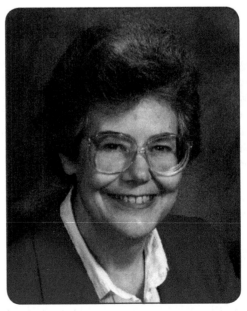

FIGURE 1–20. Margaret Skinner, cochlear implant researcher. Images provided courtesy of Laura Holden.

Any discussion of the history of cochlear implants would be incomplete without mention of the extraordinary contributions of Blake Wilson and colleagues at the Research Triangle Institute in North Carolina (see Better Hearing with Cochlear Implants: Studies at the Research Triangle Institute by Wilson and Dorman [2012] for a comprehensive review). In 1983, the RTI team received the first of numerous NIH funding awards to support the development of cochlear implant signal coding strategies. Of note, the RTI cochlear implant team had consecutive funding from the NIH for over 20 years. Throughout the next 25 years, Blake Wilson collaborated closely with several luminaries in the cochlear implant research arena, including Charles Finley, Don Eddington, Michael Dorman, Dewey Lawson, and more (Figure 1–21).

One of the most important contributions of the RTI cochlear implant group was the development of the CIS signal coding strategy in 1989. CIS, which serves as the foundation for most signal coding strategies found in modern cochlear implant systems, provided a sizable leap forward in the open-set speech recognition obtained by cochlear implant users in the early 1990s. Wilson and colleagues also developed the so-called *n-of-m* signal coding strategy, which is the basis for what eventually became the *Advanced Combination Encoder* (ACE) signal coding strategy, which continues to be the primary signal coding strategy used in Cochlear Nucleus cochlear implants (see Chapter 8 for more information on signal coding). Furthermore, Wilson and colleagues developed the concept of electrical current steering to create "virtual channels/sites" of stimulation, a concept which figures prominently in modern Advanced Bionics and MED-EL signal coding strategies. Wilson et al. also explored the use of a roving stimulation rate across low-frequency channels in an effort to provide fine temporal structure cues, a concept that is prevalent in contemporary MED-EL signal coding strategies. Additionally, Wilson, Dorman, and colleagues have exhaustively explored the benefits and limitations of electric-acoustic stimulation for recipients who have preservation of low-frequency acoustic hearing following cochlear implant surgery (Dorman et al., 2008, 2015).

Expanding Cochlear Implantation to the Chinese
Market and Other Developing Countries

At the time of this writing, several hundred thousand people with severe to profound hearing loss have received cochlear implants. Unfortunately, most of

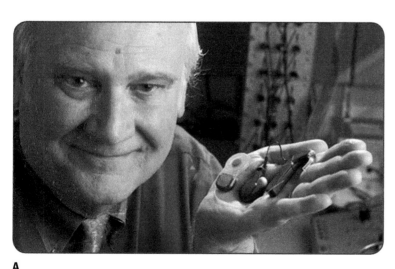

A

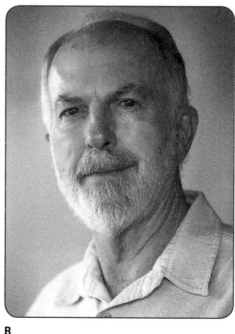

B

FIGURE 1–21. A. Blake Wilson. **B.** Michael Dorman. Cochlear implant researchers and developers. Images provided courtesy of Blake Wilson and Michael Dorman.

these recipients have resided in the United States, western Europe, and Australia, whereas many persons with hearing loss in developing parts of the world have had limited access to cochlear implants. China was an example of a market that went quite some time without access to cochlear implant technology. Prominent cochlear implant researcher Fan-Geng Zeng, M.D., Ph.D., partnered with researchers and medical technologists in China and in the United States to develop the Nurotron cochlear implant system (Zeng et al., 2015). The Nurotron is a 26-electrode cochlear implant system which was developed with two objectives, to allow similar outcomes obtained with cochlear implants that are currently approved by the FDA for commercial distribution but to provide the system at a lower cost than existing cochlear implants. In 2011, the Nurotron cochlear implant received approval for commercial distribution in China by the Chinese equivalent of the Food and Drug Administration, and in 2012, Nurotron received the European Conformitè Marketing designation. At the time of this writing, the Nurotron was not approved for commercial distribution in the United States by the FDA.

Key Concepts

- The multiple-channel cochlear implant is the most successful sensory prosthetic device developed in the field of medicine. A multiple-channel cochlear implant allows many adults with severe to profound hearing loss to develop open-set speech recognition abilities and to understand speech in occupational and social situations and when presented over the telephone and television. Cochlear implants also allow children who are born with severe to profound hearing loss to develop age-appropriate spoken language abilities.
- Published reports describing attempts to stimulate the auditory system date back to the 1700s and 1800s.
- Several researchers and surgeons worked around the globe in the 1960s and 1970s to develop the multiple-channel cochlear implant.

References

Berliner, K. I., Luxford, W. M., House, W. F., & Tonokawa, L. L. (1990). Cochlear implants in children. In E. Myers, C. Blue-
stone, D. Brackmann, & C. Krause (Eds.), *Advances in otolaryngology–head and neck surgery* (Vol. 4, pp. 61–79). St. Louis, MO: Mosby Year Book.

Bilger R. C., & Black, F. O. (1977). Auditory prostheses in perspective. *Annals of Otology, Rhinology, and Laryngology, 86*(Suppl. 38), 3–10.

Ching, T. Y., Day, J., Dillon, H., Gardner-Berry, K., Hou, S., Seeto, M., . . . Zhang, V. (2013). Impact of the presence of auditory neuropathy spectrum disorder (ANSD) on outcomes of children at three years of age. *International Journal of Audiology, 52*(Suppl. 2), S55–S64.

Ching, T. Y., Dillon, H., Marnane, V., Hou, S., Day, J., Seeto, M., . . . Yeh, A. (2013a). Outcomes of early- and late-identified children at 3 years of age. *Ear and Hearing, 34*(5), 535–552.

Chouard, C. H. (2015). The early days of the multi-channel cochlear implant: efforts and achievement in France. *Hearing Research, 322*, 47–51.

Chouard, C. H., & MacLeod, P. (1976). Implantation of multiple intracochlear electrodes for rehabilitation of total deafness: Preliminary report. *Laryngoscope, 86*(11), 1743–1751.

Chouard, C. H., Fugain, C., Meyer, B., & Lacombe, H. (1983b). Long–term results of the multichannel cochlear implant. *Annals of the New York Academy of Sciences, 405*, 387–411.

Chouard, C. H., Meyer, B., Josset, P., & Buche, J. F. (1983a). The effect of the acoustic nerve chronic electric stimulation upon the guinea pig cochlear nucleus development. *Acta Otolaryngologica, 95*(5–6), 639–645.

Clark, G. M. (1969). Responses of cells in the superior olivary complex of the cat to electrical stimulation of the auditory nerve. *Experimental Neurology, 24*(1), 124–136.

Clark, G. M. (2015). The multi-channel cochlear implant: Multidisciplinary development of electrical stimulation of the cochlea and the resulting clinical benefit. *Hearing Research, 322*, 4–13.

Clark, G. M., Black, R., Dewhurst, D. J., Forster, I. C., Patrick, J. F., & Tong, Y. C. (1977). A multiple-electrode hearing prosthesis for cochlea implantation in deaf patients. *Medical Progress through Technology, 5*(3), 127–140.

Clark, G. M., Black, R., Forster, I. C., Patrick, J. F., & Tong, Y. C. (1978). Design criteria of a multiple-electrode cochlear implant hearing prosthesis [43.66.Ts, 43.66.Sr]. *Journal of the Acoustical Society of America, 63*(2), 631–633.

Dettman, S. J., Dowell, R. C., Choo, D., Arnott, W., Abrahams, Y., Davis, A., . . . Briggs, R. J. (2016). Long-term communication outcomes for children receiving cochlear implants younger than 12 months: A multicenter study. *Otology and Neurotology, 37*(2), e82–e95.

Djourno, A., Eyries, C., & Vallancien, B. (1957). De l'excitation électrique du nerf cochléaire chez l'homme, par induction à distance, à l'aide d'un micro–bobinage inclus à demeure [Electrical excitation of the cochlear nerve in humans, by remote induction, using a micro-coil included at home]. *C R Socity of Biology, 151*, 423–425.

Eisenberg, L. S. (2015). The contributions of William F. House to the field of implantable auditory devices. *Hearing Research, 322*, 52–56.

Eisenberg, L. S., & House, W. F. (1982). Initial experience with the cochlear implant in children. *Annals of Otology, Rhinology and Laryngology Supplement, 91*(2 Pt. 3), 67–73.

Eshraghi, A. A., Gupta, C., Ozdamar, O., Balkany, T. J., Truy, E., & Nazarian, R. (2012). Biomedical engineering principles of modern cochlear implants and recent surgical innovations. *Anatomical Record (Hoboken), 295*(11), 1957–1966.

Geers, A. E. (2004). Speech, language, and reading skills after early cochlear implantation. *Archives of Otolaryngology–Head and Neck Surgery, 130*(5), 634–638.

Geers, A., Brenner, C., & Davidson, L. (2003). Factors associated with development of speech perception skills in children implanted by age five. *Ear and Hearing, 24*(1 Suppl.), 24S–35S.

Geers, A. E., Moog, J. S., Biedenstein, J., Brenner, C., & Hayes, H. (2009). Spoken language scores of children using cochlear implants compared to hearing age-mates at school entry. *Journal of Deaf Studies and Deaf Education, 14*(3), 371–385.

Helms J., Weichbold V., Baumann U., von Specht H., Schön F., Müller J., . . . D'Haese P. (2004). Analysis of ceiling effects occurring with speech recognition tests in adult cochlear-implanted patients. *ORL Journal Otorhinolaryngology Related Specialties, 66*(3), 130–135.

Henkel, G. (2013). *History of the cochlear implant.* ENT today, April, 2013. Retrieved from http://www.enttoday.org/article/history-of-the-cochlear-implant/

House, W. F. (1974). Goals of the cochlear implant. *Laryngoscope, 84*(11), 1883–1887.

House, W. F. (1976). Cochlear implants. *Annals of Otology, Rhinology and Laryngology, 85*(Suppl. 27, 3Pt. 2), 1–93.

House W. (2011). *The struggles of a medical innovator: Cochlear implants and other ear surgeries.* Lexington, KY: CreateSpace.

House, W. F., & Urban, J. (1973). Long term results of electrode implantation and electronic stimulation of the cochlea in man. *Annals of Otology, Rhinology and Laryngology, 82*(4), 504–517.

Holden, L. K., Finley, C. C., Firszt, J. B., Holden, T. A., Brenner, C., Potts, L. G., . . . Skinner, M. W. (2013). Factors affecting open-set word recognition in adults with cochlear implants. *Ear and Hearing, 34*(3), 342–360.

Hyman. S. (1990). For the *world to hear: A biography of Howard P. House.* Pasadena, CA: Hope.

Khan, A. M., Handzel, O., Burgess, B. J., Damian, D., Eddington, D. K., & Nadol, J. B., Jr. (2005). Is word recognition correlated with the number of surviving spiral ganglion cells and electrode insertion depth in human subjects with cochlear implants? *Laryngoscope, 115*(4), 672–677.

Lawrence, M. (1964). Direct stimulation of auditory nerve fibers. *Archives of Otolaryngology, 80,* 367–368.

Leake-Jones, P. A., Walsh, S. M., & Merzenich, M. M. (1981). Cochlear pathology following chronic intracochlear electrical stimulation. *Annals of Otology, Rhinology and Laryngology Supplement, 90*(2 Pt 3), 6–8.

Linthicum, F. H., Jr., & Fayad, J. N. (2009). Spiral ganglion cell loss is unrelated to segmental cochlear sensory system degeneration in humans. *Otology and Neurotology, 30*(3), 418–422.

Merzenich, M. M. (2015). Early UCSF contributions to the development of multiple-channel cochlear implants. *Hearing Research, 322,* 39–46.

Merzenich, M. M., Michelson, R. P., Pettit, C. R., Schindler, R. A., & Reid, M. (1973). Neural encoding of sound sensation evoked by electrical stimulation of the acoustic nerve. *Annals of Otology, Rhinology and Laryngology, 82*(4), 486–503.

Merzenich, M. M., Schindler, D. N., & White, M. W. (1974). Feasibility of multichannel scala tympani stimulation. *Laryngoscope, 84*(11), 1887–1893.

Meyer, B., 1974. *Contribution _ala rehabilitation chirurgicale des surdit_es totales par implantation intracochleaire d'electrodes multiples. These Medecine.* Univ. Paris–VII, Paris.

Mudry, A., & Mills, M. (2013). The early history of the cochlear implant: A retrospective. *JAMA Otolaryngology–Head and Neck Surgery, 139*(5), 446–453.

National Institutes of Health (1995). Cochlear implants in adults and children. *NIH Consensus Statement, 13*(2), 1–30.

Peng, K. A., Kuan, E. C., Hagan, S., Wilkinson, E. P., & Miller, M. E. (2017). Cochlear nerve aplasia and hypoplasia: Predictors of cochlear implant success. *Otolaryngology–Head and Neck Surgery, 157*(3), 392–400.

Rance, G., & Barker, E. J. (2008). Speech perception in children with auditory neuropathy/dyssynchrony managed with either hearing AIDS or cochlear implants. *Otology and Neurotology, 29*(2), 179–182.

Simmons, F. B. (1966). Electrical stimulation of the auditory nerve in man. *Archives in Otolaryngology, 84*(1), 2–54.

Simmons, F. B. (1969). Cochlear implants. *Archives in Otolaryngology, 89*(1), 61–69.

Simmons, F. B., Mongeon, C. J., Lewis, W. R., & Huntington, D.A. (1964). Electrical stimulation of the acoustic nerve and inferior colliculus. *Archives in Otolaryngology, 79,* 559–568.

Tyler, R. S., Moore, B. C., & Kuk, F. K. (1989). Performance of some of the better cochlear implant patients. *Journal of Speech and Hearing Research, 32*(4), 887–911.

Volta, A. (1800). On the electricity excited by mere contact of conducting substances of different kinds. *Philosophical Transactions of the Royal Society, 90,* 403–431

Wilson B. A. (1752). *Treatise on electricity* (2nd ed., pp. 202–208). London, UK: Davis.

Wilson, B. S. (2017). The modern cochlear implant: a triumph of biomedical engineering and the first substantial restoration of human sense using a medical intervention. *IEEE Pulse, 8*(2), 29–32.

Wilson, B. S., & Dorman, M. F. (2008). Cochlear implants: a remarkable past and a brilliant future. *Hearing Research, 242*(1–2), 3–21.

Wilson, B., & Dorman, M. (2012). *Better hearing with cochlear implants: Studies at the Research Triangle Institute.* San Diego, CA: Plural.

Wolfe, J., Morais, M., & Schafer, E. (2016a). Speech recognition of bimodal cochlear implant recipients using a wireless audio streaming accessory for the telephone. *Otology and Neurotology, 37*(2), 20–25.

Wolfe, J., Morais Duke, M., Schafer, E., Cire, G., Menapace, C., & O'Neill, L. (2016b). Evaluation of a wireless audio streaming accessory to improve mobile telephone performance of cochlear implant users. *International Journal of Audiology, 55*(2), 75–82.

Wong-Riley, M. T., Walsh, S. M., Leake-Jones, P. A., & Merzenich, M. M. (1981). Maintenance of neuronal activity by electrical stimulation of unilaterally deafened cats demonstrable with cytochrome oxidase technique. *Annals of Otology, Rhinology and Laryngology Supplement, 90*(2 Pt. 3), 30–32.

Worthing, M. (2015). *Graeme Clark: The man who invented the bionic ear.* Allen & Unwin, Crows Nest NSW, Australia.

Zeng, F., Rebscher, S. J., Fu, Q., Chen, H., Sun, X., Yin, L, . . . Chi, F. (2015). Development and evaluation of the Nurotron 26-electrode cochlear implant system. *Hearing Research, 322,* 188–199.

Physics and Electronics of Cochlear Implantation

Jace Wolfe and James W. Heller

Introduction

In order to fully understand the principles and practices associated with implantable hearing technology and to maximize the outcomes of the recipients of these technologies, the audiologist must have an understanding of several basic sciences associated with auditory implantable devices. Specifically, the audiologist must have a basic knowledge pertaining to the fundamentals of electricity, modern electronics, auditory physiology and pathophysiology, and neuronal physiology. A detailed discussion of these topics is beyond the scope of this chapter. However, an overview will be provided on these topics so that the reader will have a solid foundation on which to build an understanding of how to best manage the care of recipients of implantable auditory devices. Chapter 2 will provide a brief review of the physics and electronics associated with cochlear implant technology, and Chapter 3 will discuss auditory anatomy and physiology associated with cochlear implantation.

Fundamentals of Electricity

Cochlear implants bypass the impaired cochlea and stimulate the cochlear nerve with electrical current. Fundamentally, electricity is the flow of charged particles. More specifically, in electronics, electricity is the flow of electrons. All forms of matter comprise elements, which are defined as substances that cannot be broken down into a simpler component and that are made up entirely from one type of atom. At the time of this writing, there are 118 known unique elements, each of which is defined by the number of protons within its atoms (also known as its atomic number). For instance, hydrogen atoms contain one proton, whereas copper atoms contain 29 protons.

Atoms possess a nucleus made up of protons and neutrons and an electron or electrons that orbit the nucleus. Protons possess a positive electrical charge, electrons possess a negative electrical charge, and neutrons possess a neutral charge. Like charges repel one another, while opposite charges attract one another (i.e., Newton's third law). As a result, an electron is electrically attracted to the positive charge of the atom's nucleus (which is the mechanism that causes electrons to orbit around the nucleus) and tends to repel other electrons.

When an atom is in its neutral state, the number of protons and electrons are equal to one another. The electrons orbit around the nucleus in three-dimensional shells with a certain number of electrons within each shell. The innermost shell contains no more than 2 electrons, whereas the second, third, fourth, and fifth shells contain as many as 8, 18, 32, and 50 electrons, respectively. The outermost orbital or shell is called the valence shell.

Figure 2–1 provides an elementary example of the atomic structure of three different elements,

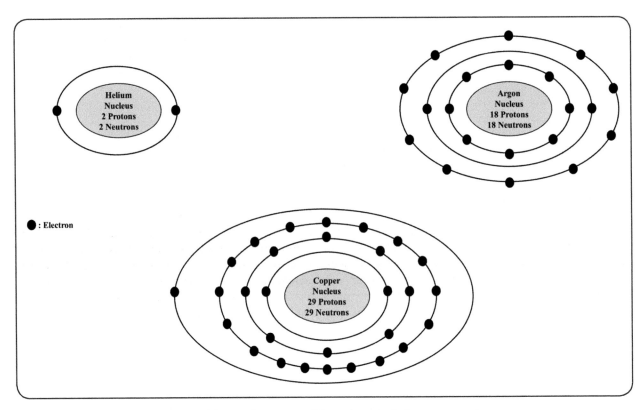

FIGURE 2–1. An elementary illustration of the atomic structure of three elements: helium, argon, and copper.

helium, argon, and copper. Please note that electrons actually revolve around an atom's nucleus in complex three-dimensional orbits, but two-dimensional orbits are displayed for the sake of simplicity. As shown in Figure 2–1, helium and argon, both of which are referred to as inert gases, contain the maximum possible number of electrons in their valence shells. In contrast, copper, which is makes up a solid metal, only contains one electron in its valence shell. Most metals, such as copper, are good conductors of electricity, because the valence electron is alone in its own orbital shell and far removed from the nucleus. Platinum and titanium are two metals used in cochlear implants for their properties of electrical conductivity as well as biocompatibility. Because good conductors like platinum and gold have one electron in the outermost shell of each atom, the valence electron can be easily dislodged from the atom and distributed to a neighboring atom. In contrast, insulators are materials such as ceramics and plastics that contain elements that have electrons that are tightly bound together. As a result, the electrons are not easily displaced from the atom.

Electrical charge is attributed to the number of electrons present relative to the atom's resting state. If an atom has lost an electron or electrons to another atom, then it possesses a positive charge. If an atom has gained an electron or electrons, then it possesses a negative charge. The magnitude of charge present at a particular location is determined by the number of electrons an atom has gained or lost as well as the quantity of these charged atoms at the given location. The unit of measurement of electrical charge is the coulomb (C); one coulomb is equal to the amount of electrical charge present on $6.24 * 10^{18}$ electrons (6,240,000,000,000,000,000 electrons!). Electrical charge is an important parameter for electrical auditory stimulation. Within the typical stimulation parameters, perceived loudness is proportionate to the delivered charge.

A physical property of matter is its tendency to seek a state of balance or equilibrium in which its different components are distributed uniformly across space. For instance, air molecules seek to "spread out" as much as possible within a given space and move randomly throughout that space (e.g., brownian motion). Similarly, atoms that possess a surplus of electrons will seek to distribute their excess electrons to surrounding electrons, whereas atoms with an electron deficit will seek to attract electrons from neighboring electrons. You are already familiar with the law of physics that states that opposite charges attract, whereas like charges repel. When one location possesses an excess or abundance of electrons, there is a tendency for the excess of electrons to seek out a location in which there is a scarcity of electrons. The greater the charge difference between two existing points in space (i.e., the larger the difference between the excessive concentration of electrons at one location, the relative scarcity of electrons at another location), the higher the potential for the excess electrons to seek out the space with a smaller concentration of electrons. The tendency for molecules, ions, substances, and electrons to move from an area of great concentration to an area of deficient concentration is referred to as "moving down their concentration gradient."

In their natural state, electrons in a conductor, such as a copper wire, will move freely and randomly from one atom to another, much like air molecules move randomly in a state of brownian motion. However, the electrons will all move in one direction when acted upon by an external force. **Electromotive force** is the technical name for the force that acts upon electrons and causes them to move or flow in a certain way. Electromotive force, which is abbreviated as EMF or more commonly as "E," is more commonly known as **voltage**. This parameter is commonly used to specify electrical power sources such as batteries, solar panels, and generators.

Voltage

Voltage is simply a difference in charge between two locations (e.g., between a location of interest and a reference location) and can possess a positive or negative value. Figure 2–2A provides a visual representation of the concept of voltage. As shown in Figure 2–2A, location "X" possesses a greater concentration of electrons than location "Y," which possesses a greater concentration of electrons that location "Z." Relative to location "Y" as a reference point, "X" has a voltage of –20 volts. Relative to location "Z," "X" has a voltage of –40 volts. In contrast, location "Z" has a voltage of +40 and +20 volts relative to points "X" and "Y," respectively. Additionally, it is important to note

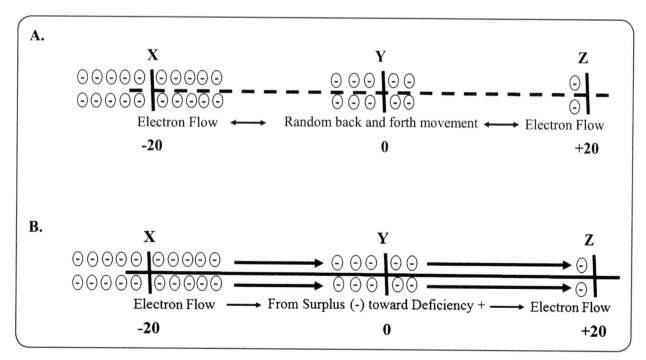

FIGURE 2–2. A. An elementary example of the concept of voltage (see text for an explanation). **B.** An elementary example of current flow with electrons moving from an area of high concentration to an area of low concentration.

that location "Y" has a voltage of +20 volts relative to "X" and a voltage of −20 volts relative to "Z." Again, voltage is a relative measure and is dependent on the difference charge (i.e., concentration of electrons) between two locations.

The concept of voltage represents potential energy. The excess of electrons located at "X" will be attracted to the deficiency of electrons located at "Y" and "Z." In Figure 2–2A, there is not a path for the excess electrons to travel to the locations at which there is a deficiency, because the two points are not physically connected (as represented by the dashed line in Figure 2–2A). As a result, the difference in charge between the two locations creates the condition for electrons to **potentially** (hence, the reference to potential energy) move down their concentration gradient. Voltages used in electrical auditory stimulation power sources range from approximately 3 to 12 V.

Electrical Current

When two points in Figure 2–2A are physically connected, a path is created for electrons to flow from the location with an electron surplus to the location at which a deficiency exists. The flow of electrons is technically referred to as **electrical current** and is measured in amperes. One ampere is equal to the movement of 1 coulomb per 1 second. In most biomedical and hearing technology applications, electrical current is delivered in fractions of an ampere, and as a result, current is often measured in milliamperes (10^{-3} A) or microamperes (10^{-6} A).

Figure 2–2B represents the flow of electrons from point "X" to "Z" as they move down their concentration gradient toward a location with a more positive charge (i.e., a surplus of electrons). Figures 2–2A and 2–2B represent an electrical circuit, which is a path in which electrical current moves. In Figure 2–2A, the electrical circuit is **open**, because there is no path for electrons to flow from the place at which there is a surplus ("X") to the place at which there is a deficiency ("Z"). With an open circuit condition, no work is done by the electricity. An example of an open circuit in cochlear implants is a broken electrode lead wire. In Figure 2–2B, the circuit is **closed**, because there is an intact path which allows electron flow. In Figure 2–2B, the intact path is present in the form of a continuous copper wire (i.e., a conducting lead) that physically connects "X" to "Z." Electrical switches are typically used to change a circuit from the open

(OFF) to closed (ON) condition. Electrical circuits will be discussed at greater length below.

The copper wire depicted in Figure 2–2B serves as an excellent conductor of electric current, because the copper atoms naturally have one valence electron that may easily be displaced from one atom to the next. However, a physical conducting lead, such as the copper wire shown in Figure 2–2B, is not required for electrical current to travel from one location to another. In fact, electrical current will travel across a medium that is a relatively poor conductor if the difference in charge is great enough between two different locations across the medium. For instance, lightning will strike from a thunderstorm cloud toward the ground when a large imbalance in charge is created between the surplus of electrons at the base of the cloud and the relative deficiency of electrons on the ground. Additionally, electric current will readily pass through human tissue and body fluids. For example, the positively charged particles in perilymph and extracellular fluid (e.g., Na+) makes body fluid a good conductor of electrical current. A comparison of the electrical conductivity of common biological and engineered materials relevant to cochlear implants is shown in Table 2–1.

TABLE 2–1. Comparison of the Electrical Conductivity of Selected Biological and Engineered Materials Relevant to Cochlear Implants

Material	Resistivity (ohm-m)
Copper	1.7×10^{-8}
Gold	2.4×10^{-8}
Platinum	1.1×10^{-7}
Titanium	4.4×10^{-7}
Stainless steel	6.9×10^{-7}
Saline	7.0×10^{-1}
Blood	4.0
Muscle	1.0×10^{1}
Fat	3.0×10^{1}
Bone	1.0×10^{2}
Glass	1.0×10^{13}
Air	1.3×10^{16}
Teflon	1.0×10^{23}

Source: Reference for Biological Materials: Webster, J., *Encyclopedia of Biomedical Engineering*, Wiley & Sons, 2006.

Many students find it difficult to distinguish between voltage and current, because the electrical charge and current flow are typically invisible and somewhat of an abstract phenomenon. It is often helpful to establish an analogy between voltage and current and water flow through a hose. The flow of water through the hose is analogous to the flow of electrons in a conducting lead/wire, and the water pressure is analogous to the voltage. The faucet is analogous to the electrical switch.

It is important to note that the valence electron of one copper atom moves toward the positive charge and displaces a valence electron of a neighboring atom, which moves toward the positive charge and displaces a neighboring valence electron and so on. Essentially, electronic current represents a propagation of electrons through a conducting lead/wire, and as a result, current travels almost instantaneously through a circuit once two points of disparate charge are connected to one another. Additionally, if the electron movement shown in Figure 2–2B simply occurred across a conducting lead between points "X" and "Z," the electrons would eventually stop moving in one direction, would distribute evenly across the space between "X" and "Z," and settle into random motion throughout that space.

Ohm's Law

In order to maintain a voltage difference between two endpoints in a circuit, the circuit must contain a component that impedes current flow. As a result, electrical current is dependent not only on the voltage driving electron flow but also on the amount of opposition present in the circuit. This opposition to current flow is typically referred to as **resistance**. German physicist Georg Ohm is credited with describing the relationship between voltage, resistance, and current. Specifically, Ohm's law states:

Equation 2–1: Voltage (Volts) =
Current (Amperes) * Resistance (Ohms)

Stated differently, electrical current is directly proportional to voltage (i.e., current increases as voltage increases) and inversely proportional to resistance (i.e., current decreases as resistance increases.

Application of Ohm's Law to Cochlear Implants

Ohm's law has important implications in the electrical stimulation delivered by a cochlear implant. The maximum voltage provided by a cochlear implant system is determined by the battery of the sound processor and the radiofrequency link between the processor and the implant. Remember, there is no power source present in contemporary cochlear implants, so the power required to operate the cochlear implant is supplied by electromagnetic induction from the external sound processor, which is powered by a battery. The voltage of the sound processor battery is fixed at a known value (e.g., 4 volts).

Because the voltage of the power source is known, Ohm's law may be used to measure the impedance present at each electrode contact. Electrode impedance simply refers to the opposition of current flow through an electrode contact. Impedance is different from resistance. Resistance refers to direct current (DC) or current that flows in one direction, such as the current from a battery. Impedance refers to alternating current (AC) or current that flows alternately in both directions, such as the current from electrical utilities or as used in cochlear implant stimulation. Electrode impedance measurements are completed by delivering a relatively small controlled electrical current between each electrode contact and the return electrode and measuring the voltage drop across the electrodes. Because voltage and current are known entities during the electrode impedance measurement, Ohm's law may be used to calculate electrode contact impedance.

Electrode impedance is affected not only by the integrity of the electrode lead and electrode contact and the return electrode (i.e., the physical electrical circuit) but also by the cochlear fluids and tissues between the active and return electrodes. As previously mentioned, electrical current can travel through fluids (e.g., cochlear perilymphatic fluid) and human tissue (e.g., scar tissue, supporting cells, basilar membrane). As a result, the electrical current passing through the electrode contact is also distributed to surrounding cochlear fluids and tissues and to the cochlear nerve. The conductivity of fluids and tissues adjacent to the active and indifferent electrode contacts affect electrode impedance. For example, if an electrode contact is immersed in cochlear fluid, the electrode impedance is typically lower than what would be measured if the electrode contact is surrounded by air or by fibrous scar tissue (Clark et al., 1995). Of note, an **open circuit** was previously described as an electrical pathway that is not physically intact, and consequently, electrical current cannot travel through the circuit. The term *open* is typically used to describe the situation in which electrode impedance is infinitely high as what would occur when an electrode lead is broken.

Additionally, the maximum current available for stimulation at each electrode contact may also be calculated via Ohm's law. Specifically, the maximum current available at an electrode contact is determined by dividing the available voltage by the impedance (i.e., impedance of the active electrode, tissue, and indifferent electrode). These three impedance components are connected in series. A series circuit is one in which the electrical current must pass through different elements sequentially in order to complete the circuit. In series circuits, the total impedance is equal to the sum of the individual impedances. Thus, changes in the electrode surfaces or the tissue can change the measured electrode impedance.

Equation 2–2: Current = Voltage/Resistance

It is important for the audiologist to be aware of the maximum current available for stimulation at an electrode contact in order to be certain that satisfactory loudness can be provided. Loudness is related to the electrical charge delivered to the nerve. Charge

(typically in units of nano-coulombs for cochlear implant stimulation) is defined as the product of the electrical current (in microamperes) and the duration (in milliseconds). The arrows in Figure 2–3 provide an example of the maximum current available at each electrode contact. The arrows in Figure 2–3 point to dashes that indicate the maximum current the programming audiologist may provide at each electrode contact. The current level cannot be increased beyond the value signified by each dash, because the limits available from the voltage source (typically 5–10 volts direct current [VDC] for a cochlear implant) have been reached. Attempting to provide a higher level of stimulation will not result in an actual increase in the current provided. This condition is referred to as "reaching the compliance limit" of the cochlear implant. As will be discussed further in Chapter 7, the audiologist must instead increase the pulse width (i.e., duration of the electrical pulse) to increase the electrical charge and loudness. The dashes noted by the arrows in Figure 2–3 represent a cochlear implant programming term referred to as **voltage compliance levels**, which indicate the maximum amount of

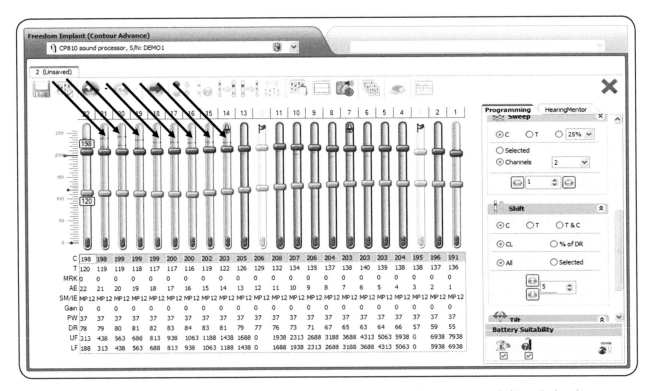

FIGURE 2–3. An example of voltage compliance levels for a cochlear implant recipient. The arrows are pointing to dashes that represent the maximum amount of electrical current that can be provided on each channel. The channels that are highlighted (i.e., channels 2–13) provide examples in which the current levels for a particular channel exceed to maximum current that may be provided by the voltage limits of the system. Image provided courtesy of Cochlear Americas, ©2018.

electrical current that may be provided by the voltage limits of the cochlear implant system.

In Figure 2–3, channels 2 through 13 are highlighted because the voltage compliance levels have been exceeded. In this case, the audiologist should increase the pulse width of the stimulus. As one would anticipate from Ohm's law, recipients with relatively high electrode impedance and/or high "C" levels are more likely to require increased pulse width due to reaching the compliance limit. Consequently, when working with a recipient with higher electrode impedance values, the audiologist must be aware that lesser amounts of current will be available and the pulse width of the stimulus may need to be increased. Alternately, the audiologist may program in a wider pulse width from the onset or recommend use of a battery with a higher voltage capacity, if available.

The Concept of Electrical Circuits and Cochlear Implants

Electricity does no work unless it passes through a circuit. A circuit is an uninterrupted path between the two poles of the electrical power source. In a cochlear implant, the stimulation circuit consists of the active electrode wire, active electrode, tissues between the

active and indifferent electrodes, indifferent electrode, and indifferent electrode wire (Figure 2–4). The energy is provided by a current generator circuit within the cochlear implant. A break anywhere in the circuit will stop current flow. A change in impedance in any of the elements will change the overall impedance to the current generator.

Figure 2–5 provides an example of a direct current electrical circuit in which electrical current travels from one terminal of a battery, through electrical components, and back to the opposite terminal of the battery. In household appliances, electrical current travels from the outlet contacts through the power cord and through the appliance and then back through the power cord and outlet contacts.

In cochlear implant systems, electrical current cannot travel back to the battery of the sound processor. Instead, the indifferent electrode provides a return path and destination point for electrical current after the current travels through the stimulating electrode contact in the cochlea. Figure 2–6 provides an example of the path that electrical current takes when traveling through a cochlear implant. As shown, electrical current travels from the current generator down a lead wire toward the active electrode contact. Once it reaches the electrode contact, the current travels through the surrounding cochlear fluid and/

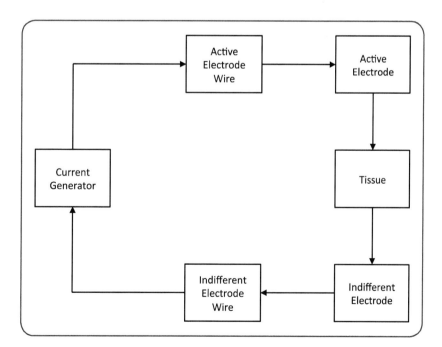

FIGURE 2–4. An elementary block schematic representing the components that exist in the "circuit" through which electrical current travels in a cochlear implant.

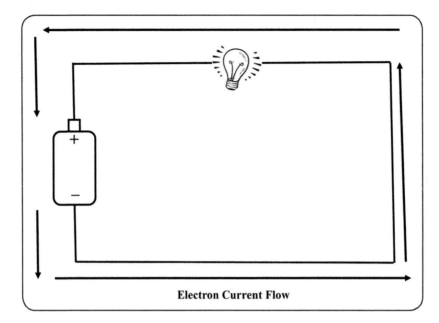

Electron Current Flow

FIGURE 2–5. An elementary example of how direct current travels through a circuit.

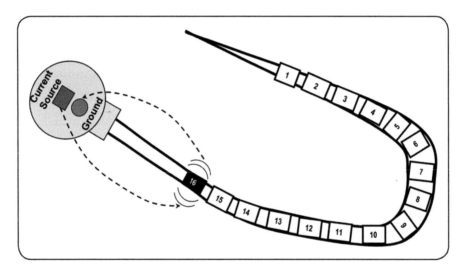

FIGURE 2–6. A visual illustration of how electrical current travels from the current source of a cochlear implant to an intracochlear electrode contact and then back to an extracochlear ground electrode.

or tissue and eventually to the cochlear nerve. The indifferent ground electrode and its lead wire provide a return path to the current generator.

Direct Current Versus Alternating Current

The electrical circuit shown in Figure 2–5 is known as a **direct current** circuit, because current travels in only one direction through the circuit. The power provided from an electrical wall outlet is an **alternating current** source. In other words, the direction of the current flow continuously alternates back and forth at a rhythmic rate. In the United States of America, alternating current electricity fluctuates at a rate of 60 Hz, whereas in many other countries, alternating current electricity fluctuates at 50 Hz. There are many practical points to note in our discussion of alternating current electricity. First, although the electrons move back and forth at 60 Hz, current moves through a circuit. As previously discussed, this occurs because electrons are lined up throughout the conducting leads of a circuit and will immediately move (like box cars in a train) when acted upon by a voltage. Second, many electronic devices require direct current but are powered by a cable and plug inserted into an alternating current electrical outlet. In these cases, the power cord is connected to a circuit that converts alternating current to direct current, a process which is discussed later in this chapter. Third, alternating current can be transmitted through the air by the process of electromagnetic induction, which will also be discussed later in this chapter.

Electricity in the Form of Ionic Flow

As previously noted, electricity is the flow of charged particles. In electronic devices, electricity is the flow of electrons through a circuit. However, electricity is also present in many organs in the human body in the form of the flow of charged particles. In particular, electric responses from a physiologic perspective occur in the form of the movement of ions. An ion is an atom or molecule that possesses an electrical charge because it has lost or gained an electron. Ions that have gained an electron or electrons have a negative charge (e.g., Cl–, which is a chloride ion that has lost three electrons; HCO3–, which is a bicarbonate ion, whose oxygen molecule has lost three electrons), whereas ions that have lost electrons have a positive charge (e.g., Na^+, K^+, Ca^{2+}).

Newton's third law governing actions and reactions (i.e., opposites attract and like charges repel) also applies to ionic distribution. Ions tend to try to distribute evenly throughout a space. When ions with a particular type of charge (e.g., Na+) is gathered together in a large group, they tend to spread apart, because the ions are repelled by their like charge. In particular, ions with a positive charge will seek out areas where a negative charge exists and vice versa, a phenomenon referred to as moving down their charge gradient. Additionally, substances are composed of the same element (e.g., K^+) will try to spread out the areas in which there is not as high a concentration of that particular element, a phenomenon referred to as moving down their concentration gradient.

In the human body, extra- and intracellular fluids are often comprised of molecules/ions that possess a charge. For instance, the fluid inside the neuron is often composed of K+, whereas the fluid outside the neuron comprises Na+. In the normal resting state, there are typically more Na+ ions outside the neuron than there are K+ inside the neuron. Because there are a greater number of positively charged ions outside the neuron, the extracellular fluid has a positive charge relative to the intracellular fluid, creating a difference in charge between the inside and the outside of the neuron (also, it should be noted that the intracellular fluid has a negative charge relative to the extracellular fluid). As previously discussed, a difference in charge between two locations creates the potential to move electrons and is represented by voltage. For example, the internal environment of a neuron at rest is typically about –70 millivolts. Because of the difference in charge and chemical composition that exists between the internal and external environments of the neuron, the Na+ ions outside of the cell are attracted to the internal environment of the neuron (i.e., the Na+ ions seek to move down their electrical and concentration gradient). When a neuron responds (i.e., fires in response to a stimulus), gates open that allow the Na+ ions to rush into the neuron, causing it to suddenly possess a positive voltage. This movement of charged ions is another form of electrical activity that has important implications for implantable hearing technologies, because it influences cochlear hair cell transduction and neuronal function. A more detailed discussion of this topic will follow in the section of this book discussing physiology of the auditory system (see Chapter 3).

Modern Electronics

Modern medical and consumer electronics are composed of several electrical components that work together to allow electronic devices to achieve their desired function. Of course, a full description of electronics is beyond the scope of this textbook, but some of the more basic components and principles of modern electronics germane to cochlear implants will be discussed here.

Resistance

Electrical resistance occurs when electrons encounter other atoms, resulting in a reduction in energy or electrical current flow. The unit of resistance is the ohm (named after Georg Ohm). A resistor is an electric component that provides opposition to electrical current flow. Resistors are comprised of materials that contain atoms that are bonded together so that the electrons are tightly packed together and fully occupied in the valence shell. As a result, electrical current does not flow easily through a resistor.

Examples of tissues around a cochlear implant that offer higher resistance to electrical current are cartilage and bone. For example, ossification of the cochlea can cause a significant increase in impedance through which a cochlear implant must deliver current. This physiologic change can result in an out-of-compliance condition.

Resistance also depends on the cross-sectional area and length of the conducting apparatus (i.e., the conducting lead). Specifically, the resistance increases as the cross-sectional diameter decreases and/or the length increases. In a light bulb, current is passed through a very thin tungsten wire called a filament. The small cross-sectional area of the wire filament and the properties of tungsten provide resistance to electrical current flow, and the current flow produces heat, which causes the filament to glow and produce light. In electric circuits, resistors are used to control the level of current flowing through a circuit.

Constant Voltage and Constant Current Sources

Batteries are an example of a constant voltage source. The battery provides a fixed voltage and the current flow is dependent on the resistance of the circuit connected to the battery. Cochlear implants utilize constant current sources for the stimuli. This is because loudness is a function of electrical charge (the product of electrical current and time). So, by accurately controlling the current and the duration of the stimulus, the charge is also controlled. In a constant current source, the current remains constant and the voltage is dependent on the impedance of the load. All constant current sources have a limited voltage. This voltage determines the maximum current that can be delivered for any given impedance.

Capacitance

Capacitance refers to the ability of an electrical circuit to hold a charge. A capacitor is an electronic component that is comprised of two conducting plates which are separated by an insulator called a dielectric (Figure 2–7). Electrons travel from the power source of a circuit down a lead that is connected to one of the plates and collect on that plate, resulting in a buildup of electrical charge. The dielectric, which may be air or an insulating substance such as glass, between the two plates prevents the electrical charge from traveling from one plate to the other. In Figure 2–4, the plate that is connected to the negative terminal of the battery collects electrons supplied by the battery because the electrons move down their

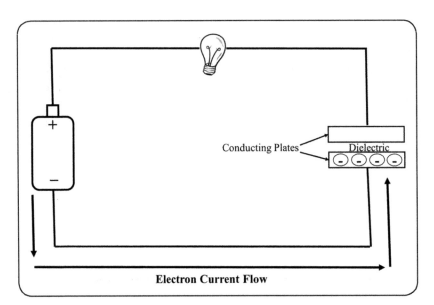

Electron Current Flow

FIGURE 2–7. An elementary example of a capacitor. The direct current travels from one pole of the battery toward the other but "builds up" at one plate of the dielectric (i.e., capacitor).

electrical concentration gradient. Also, electrons from the other plate are attracted to the positive terminal of the battery. Eventually, a surplus of electrons will compile at the plate connected to the negative terminal, resulting in a capacitor that is charged (i.e., there is a difference in electrical charge between the two plates). If the battery in Figure 2–7 is replaced with a conducting lead, the charge that has built up on the plate closest to the negative terminal of the battery will suddenly rush through the circuit toward the opposite plate (Figure 2–8).

A common example of the use of a capacitor may be found in a flash camera. A capacitor stores a relatively large charge, and when a photo is taken in a dimly lit room, a switch is closed allowing that large charge to be released in a fraction of a second, resulting in the bright illumination of the flash bulb. Capacitors may also be used to prevent direct current in a circuit. When current travels in one direction, as it would in a battery-powered, direct current circuit, all of the electrons build up on the plate nearest to the negative terminal of the battery but are prevented from traveling to the opposite plate and traveling through the circuit. With an alternating current power supply, current flow moves back and forth in a circuit and can alternately travel between the two plates of the capacitor. As a result, capacitors prevent or reduce electrical transmission in direct current circuits but allow for transmission in alternating current circuits. In other words, the impedance offered by a capacitor

is inversely proportional to the frequency of the electric current. This application is of great importance in cochlear implant systems, because even a very small imbalance of charge (i.e., negative or positive residual charge) in the cochlea can result in electrotoxicity and subsequent damage to the delicate cochlear structures and cochlear nerve tissue. Of note, the unit of measurement of capacitance is the farad (named after the English physicist Michael Faraday), and capacitance in a cochlear implant system is typically measured in microfarads. Capacitors are used in cochlear implants to store charge. This allows the implant to remain powered during brief pauses in the signal from the processor. They are also used in the indifferent electrode lead to block direct current flow to the cochlea.

Induction

Electromagnetic induction is of great significance in implantable hearing technologies. Electromagnetic induction occurs in two basic forms. In the transmission form of electromagnetic induction, the delivery of an electrical current through a conducting lead (e.g., copper or gold wire) generates magnetic lines of flux which surround the lead (Figure 2–9). In many electrical circuits, this form of electromagnetic induction is created by arranging the conducting lead into the shape of a coil, which results in an enhancement

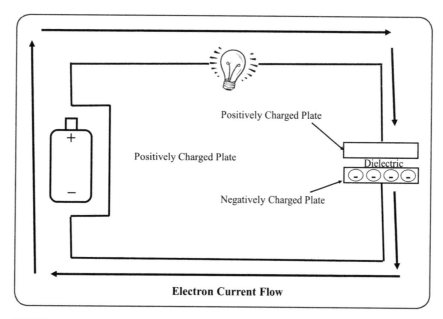

FIGURE 2–8. An elementary example illustrating how current flows from one side of the dielectric to the other with the provision of a conductive path.

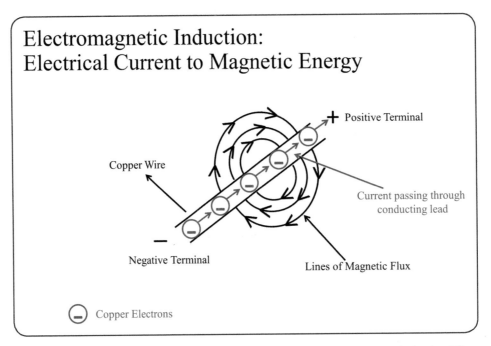

FIGURE 2–9. An elementary example depicting the concept of electromagnetic induction. When electrical current passes through the conducting lead, magnetic lines of flux emanate around the conducting lead.

of the strength of the magnetic lines of flux as current passes through the coil. Additionally, placing a ferrous (i.e., magnetic) rod in the middle of the coil further enhances the inductance of the coil. This is used in radio transmitters and motors. In the receiving form of electromagnetic induction, when a conducting lead passes through magnetic lines of flux (or when the magnetic lines of flux pass across a conducting lead), an electrical current is induced through the conducting lead (Figure 2–10). This is used for radio receivers and electrical generators. Both electrical power and control signals are sent from the processor to the implant using electromagnetic transmission and reception.

Electromagnetic Induction for Cochlear Implant Telemetry

Electromagnetic induction is used to deliver the signals between the sound processor and the cochlear implant as well as to deliver power from the sound processor to the cochlear implant. As shown in Figure 2–11, the digital code from the sound processor is converted to an electrical signal. This electrical signal is delivered to the external transmitting coil of the sound processor. Of note, the external transmitting coil comprises wire arranged in a coil around the entire perimeter of the coil. The electrical current traveling through the wire in the transmitting coil induces magnetic lines of flux which emanate from the coil and across the recipient's skin. These magnetic lines of flux then cross the coiled wire in the internal coil of the cochlear implant and induce an electrical signal within the implant coil. This electrical signal is carried to the digital signal processor within the cochlear implant. In a similar fashion, reverse transmission occurs when the digital signal processor of the cochlear implant converts digital code into an electrical signal that may also be delivered to the coil of the cochlear implant, resulting in magnetic lines of flux that induce an electrical current in the external sound processor coil. As such, electromagnetic induction may be used to deliver information both to and from the external sound processor and cochlear implant.

The magnetic lines of flux emanating from the sound processor transmitting coil are also used to power the cochlear implant by inducing electrical current within the implant. In fact, the majority of the power of the battery of the external sound processor is used to power the cochlear implant. Thus, the skin flap thickness and the efficiency of the electromagnetic link are critical factors to enable the use of a small battery in the sound processor. The process of

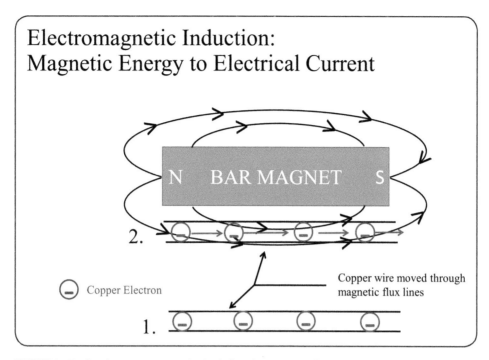

FIGURE 2–10. An elementary example depicting the concept of electromagnetic induction. When a conducting lead (e.g., copper wire) passes through magnetic lines of flux, an electrical current is induced through the conducting lead.

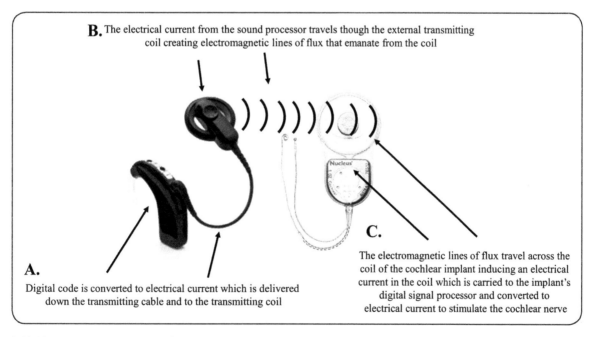

FIGURE 2–11. A visual example of how electromagnetic induction is used to deliver a signal from the coil of the cochlear implant sound processor to the coil of the cochlear implant. Image provided courtesy of Cochlear Americas, ©2018.

delivering information and power via electromagnetic induction is often referred to as **telemetry**. When information is exchanged in two different directions, this process is typically referred to as bidirectional telemetry. The telemetry used in cochlear implant systems is a form of near-field magnetic induction (NFMI). NFMI is a form of short-range radio transmission. Due to the relatively short distance of transmission relative to conventional radio transmission, NFMI is not subject to interference between two devices that are both using NFMI unless the two devices are in very close proximity to one another. Another advantage of NFMI is that it allows for the provision of a wide spectrum of information between the transmitter and receiver. Information transmissions from the processor contain a check sum after each packet of data. The implant tests the validity of the check sum against the received data. If it does not check, the implant takes no action. This is used to prevent other ambient electromagnetic signals from causing unintended stimulation.

Use of Electromagnetic Induction to Create Radio Signals

Electromagnetic induction is also used to deliver radio signals. Figure 2–12 provides an example of the elec-

tromagnetic spectrum. The electromagnetic spectrum, including radio, television, satellite communication, cell phones, WiFi, infrared, metal detectors, and Bluetooth, is made up of electromagnetic signals encompassing a wide range of different frequencies. For example, AM (amplitude-modulated) radio signals possess an electromagnetic carrier frequency that oscillates at a frequency between about 500,000 Hz (500 kHz) to 1.6 million Hz (1.6 MHz), whereas the FM (frequency-modulated) bandwidth spans from about 88 to 108 MHz for broadcast radio applications and between 216 and 217 MHz for FM radio devices used specifically for persons with hearing loss. Infrared light transmission is also a signal on the electromagnetic spectrum that is used to deliver information. Infrared light oscillates at about 13 trillion Hz and is just below the visible light spectrum.

When the electrical signal is delivered to an antenna, the antenna acts as a radiating apparatus for electromagnetic waves. If the electrical signal traveling through the antenna oscillates between 500,000 to 1.6 million Hz, 88 to 108 million Hz, or at 0.9, 2.4, or 5 billion Hz, the electromagnetic waves emanating from the antenna are AM, FM, or digital radio waves, respectively. Figure 2–13 provides an elementary example of how an audio signal can be transmitted

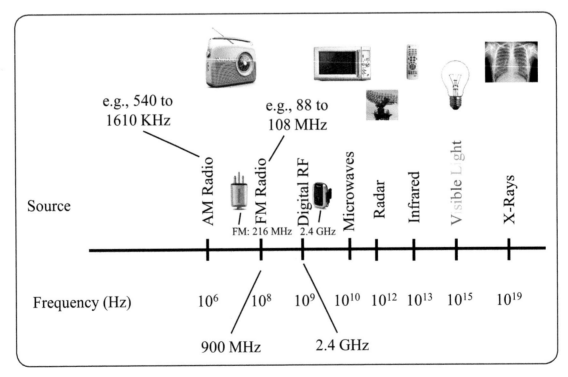

FIGURE 2–12. A representation of the electromagnetic spectrum.

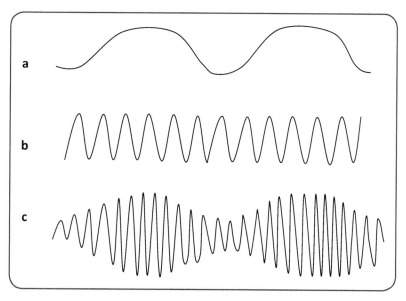

FIGURE 2–13. A. The waveform of an audio signal of interest. **B.** The carrier wave of an electromagnetic radio signal. **C.** The radio wave is amplitude modulated based on the physical properties of the audio signals.

via AM radio. Figure 2–13A depicts an audio signal (e.g., speech transduced from a microphone). Figure 2–13B shows an example of a carrier frequency, which for AM radio would be within the 500,000 to 1.6 million Hz bandwidth. Figure 2–13C shows an example of the carrier frequency being amplitude-modulated by the audio signal. As shown, the peaks of the amplitude-modulated carrier frequency coincide with the peaks of the original audio signal, and the fluctuation in the amplitude modulations occur at the same rate (i.e., frequency) as the fluctuations of the audio signal. Thus, the intensity, frequency, and temporal characteristics of the audio signal are captured in the amplitude-modulation pattern superimposed on the carrier frequency. The amplitude-modulated electrical signal is delivered to the antenna at a high voltage, resulting in emanation of an electromagnetic radio wave that is analogous to the carrier signal. This electromagnetic radio signal is transmitted throughout the environment. When the electromagnetic signal crosses over a receiving antenna, which is essentially a conducting lead, an electric current is induced in the receiving antenna. The electric signal that is induced in the receiving antenna can be converted to an audio signal that is analogous to the original audio signal.

An example of FM radio is provided in Figure 2–14. The audio signal is displayed in Figure 2–14A, and the carrier frequency, which falls in the 216 million

Hz band for hearing assistance technology, is shown in Figure 2–14B. As can be seen in Figure 2–14C, the carrier frequency is modulated in the frequency domain based on the characteristics of the audio signal. The peaks in the original audio signal coincide with increases in the frequency of the carrier signal, while the lower-amplitude components of the audio signal coincide with decreases in the frequency of the carrier signal.

Digital Radio Frequency Transmissions

Modern radio applications typically use digital radio transmission. In digital radio systems, the audio signal is first converted to a digital code (Figure 2–15). Then, the digital code is transmitted on a carrier frequency, which is most commonly within the 2.4 billion Hz band. Of note, the 2.4 GHz band is one of several bands that are reserved globally for the use of radio transmission for industrial, science, and medical (ISM) applications other than telecommunications. Figure 2–16 provides an example of a digital radiofrequency transmission technology referred to as amplitude-shift keying (ASK). For digital radio applications using ASK, the carrier frequency is pulsed off and on to convey the digital code of "0s" and "1s," respectively. The radio receiver received the electromagnetic representation of the digital code and delivers it to a digital-to-analog converter that translates the

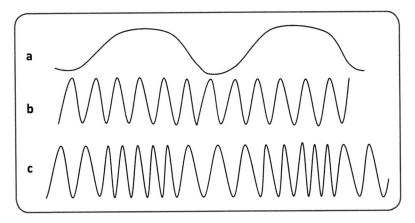

FIGURE 2–14. **A.** The waveform of an audio signal of interest. **B.** The carrier wave of an electromagnetic radio signal. **C.** The radio wave is frequency modulated based on the physical properties of the audio signals.

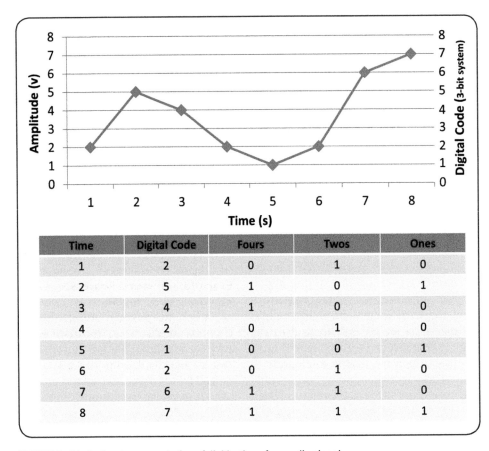

Time	Digital Code	Fours	Twos	Ones
1	2	0	1	0
2	5	1	0	1
3	4	1	0	0
4	2	0	1	0
5	1	0	0	1
6	2	0	1	0
7	6	1	1	0
8	7	1	1	1

FIGURE 2–15. A visual representation of digitization of an audio signal.

digitized signal to an electrical signal which may be transduced to the original audio signal. Figure 2–17 provides an example of another type of digital radio transmission known as frequency-shift keying (FSK), which alters cycles in the carrier frequency to represent "0s" and "1s."

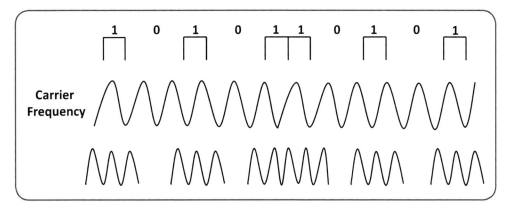

FIGURE 2–16. An example of digital radiofrequency transmission using amplitude-shift keying. The digital code (i.e., "1s" and "0s") is represented by the presence ("1") or absence ("0") of the carrier frequency.

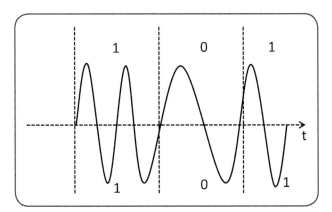

FIGURE 2–17. An example of digital radiofrequency transmission using frequency-shift keying. The digital code (i.e., "1s" and "0s") is represented by leaving the cycle of the carrier frequency intact ("1") or by altering a cycle ("0").

Modern digital radio systems utilize a principle called *frequency hopping*, which alternately varies the carrier frequency across the transmission band (e.g., 2.4 GHz, 2.425 GHz, 2.45 GHz, 2.425 GHz, 2.475 GHz). The digital radio transmitter and receiver are paired together in order to establish the devices that are intended to be used for transfer of information. This pairing process basically creates a password between the transmitter and the receiver. The digitally transmitted code contains not only the relevant audio information but also this password to ensure the devices should communicate. The digitally transmitted code also contains a protocol to determine the sequence of the frequency-hopping behavior. One (of several) advantages of digital radio over analog radio (AM or FM) is the ability to implement frequency-hopping technology, because the instantaneous changes in carrier frequency avoid interference between devices that historically plagued AM and FM systems.

Applications of Digital Radio Transmission in Cochlear Implants

Digital radiofrequency technology is very pertinent to cochlear implants for multiple reasons. For instance, as previously discussed, NFMI is used to deliver power and information to and from the sound processor transmitting/receiving coil to the receiving/transmitting coil of the cochlear implant. However, the information delivered via NFMI is typically transmitted in the form of a digitized code on a carrier frequency ranging from 5 to almost 50 million Hz. Use of a digital code allows for several useful features. For example, the sound processor and cochlear implant may be paired together so that the sound processor will only provide stimulation to the designated cochlear implant (e.g., the right ear sound processor will not stimulate the left ear cochlear implant; John Doe's sound processor will not stimulate Jane Doe's cochlear implant). Secondly, digital transmission allows the sound processor and cochlear implant to exchange information regarding the status of implant function (e.g., how much power is required to operate the implant) and of the recipient's physiologic function (e.g., the cochlear nerve's response in the form of the electrically evoked compound action potential).

Additionally, digital radio transmission is also used to deliver information from hearing assistive technology (HAT) to the cochlear implant sound processor. The most contemporary sound processors of the major cochlear implant manufacturers possess a digital radio antenna that may be used to receive digital signals (typically on the 2.4 GHz band). As a result, digital radio may be used to deliver an audio signal from a remote microphone to the sound processor or to deliver audio information from consumer electronics (e.g., mobile telephone, television, tablets, computers) to the sound processor. The use of these integrated wireless HATs are often of great benefit to cochlear implant recipients in challenging listening situations. Chapter 20 provides additional information on HAT for cochlear implant recipients. Of note, digital radio transmission is also used to deliver information between the cochlear implant sound processors and remote controls, allowing recipients to adjust the settings of their cochlear implants and to access information about the status of their hardware (e.g., battery life). Sound processors will also be able to communicate with other devices using WiFi or Bluetooth protocols.

Induction Coils and Loops

Electromagnetic induction may play another important role for cochlear implant recipients. Most modern cochlear implant sound processors contain a telecoil that may be used to capture signals from telephones, induction neckloops, and induction room loops. Telephones possess a receiver (i.e., a miniature loudspeaker) that operates on the principle of electromagnetic induction. The audio signal from the telephone is delivered in the form of an analogous electric current to a coiled wire. Electromagnetic lines of flux emanate from the coil as the current travels through the coil. The fluctuating magnetic field attracts and repels an adjacent magnet that is physically coupled to the diaphragm of the receiver. The magnet-driven movement of the diaphragm creates an audio signal.

When a telephone is held close to a sound processor, the electromagnetic lines of flux emanating from the receiver cross the telecoil, which is typically a coil of copper wire, in the processor. When this occurs, an electrical current is elicited in the coil and can be delivered to an analog-to-digital converter for further processing. With an induction loop system, an audio signal is converted to an analogous electrical current, amplified, and delivered through a coiled, conducting wire (i.e., loop) that surrounds a room or that is worn around the user's neck. Magnetic lines of flux are created as the electrical current travels

through the loop, and these magnetic lines of flux emanate around the loop. Once again, these magnetic lines of flux are proportionally analogous (in frequency, intensity, temporal characteristics) to the original audio signal. The magnetic line of flux will then induce an electrical current through the telecoil, and the current will be delivered to the analog-to-digital converter of the processor and processed according to the signal processing within the instrument and the individual programming completed by the user's audiologist.

Inductors

Electromagnetic induction is also used in an electronic component called an inductor. An inductor is comprised of a wire formed into a spiral shape. When electrical current travels through the coil, a magnetic field builds up and eventually reaches a maximum value. The magnetic field around the coil impedes the flow of current. Once the magnetic field reaches its maximum value, current may travel through the circuit as it would if the inductor were not present. When the current is removed, the magnetic field around the inductor collapses, and as the magnetic field temporarily persists, current continues to travel through the coil. Current will cease traveling through the coil when the magnetic field is eliminated. The primary function of an inductor is to resist changes in current in a circuit. As a result, inductors may be used to attenuate fluctuations in electrical signals. More specifically, inductors may be used to preferentially allow low-frequency signals and not high frequencies.

Transistors and Integrated Circuits

The transistor is the essential electronic component in all modern electronics. Transistors consist of silicon, an element known as a semi-conductor. The valence shell of atoms known as semi-conductors typically are half-full of electrons. As a result, semi-conductors are able to receive and give electrons to neighboring atoms. Figure 2–18 provides an elementary example of the atomic structure of silicon.

Silicon can be "doped" (i.e., treated) with other elements such as arsenic or phosphorous and boron or aluminum. When silicon is doped with arsenic or phosphorous, it receives additional electrons in its valence shell and consequently possesses additional "free electrons" that it can share with nearby atoms. When silicon is doped with a substance that pro-

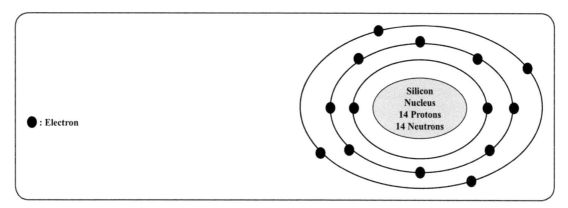

FIGURE 2–18. An elementary example of the atomic structure of silicon.

vides additional free electrons, it is referred to as an n-type. The additional free electrons of n-type silicon readily allow electric current to travel out of the silicon, because the excess free electrons are easily displaced and are moved down or away from their concentration and electrical gradient. When silicon is doped with boron or aluminum, it gives up some of its valence electrons to the doping agent, resulting in fewer free electrons for current to travel. Silicon doped with boron or aluminum is referred to as a p-type silicon, and because of its reduced number of free electrons, electric current is attracted into it.

Transistors are created by creating alternating layers of n-type and p-type silicon (Figure 2–19). In general, transistors are created by aligning silicon layers in a p-n-p (i.e., n-type silicon is surrounded by two layers of p-type silicon) or n-p-n configuration (i.e., p-type silicon is surrounded by two layers of n-type silicon) (see Figure 2–19). Each end of the transistor is connected to a conducting lead, and a third lead is also connected to the middle layer as well. The middle layer is known as the base and one far side of the transistor is known as the emitter and the other far side as the collector. When a small electric current is applied to the base, electrons will flow out of the n-type silicon and into the p-type silicon. This small current applied to the base results in a larger current elicited through the layers of the transistor, and as a result, transistors can serve as an electrical component that amplifies an electrical current (i.e., transistors as amplifiers). Furthermore, when the small current to the base results in the transistor passing electrical current (i.e., the transistor "turns on"), the transistor is essentially functioning as an electronic switch. The ability to function as an

on/off switch allows transistors to convey the binary digital code, with a "0" represented by the switch in the off position and a "1" being represented by the on position.

Digital signal processing has become pervasive in almost all medical and consumer electronics. In these applications, thousands, millions, or possibly billions of transistors are combined to allow for complex signal processing. In modern electronics, these transistors are all housed on one chip that contains other electronics components as well and is referred to as an integrated circuit. Moore's law, named after the engineer Gordon Moore, states that due to advances in technology, the number of transistors that developers can fit on an integrated circuit approximately doubles every two years. Increasing the number of transistors in the circuit allows for the development of hearing technology that is more efficient and effective.

Of note, early digital systems contained multiple functional blocks with an integrated circuit or circuits which processes signals in a sequential fashion (i.e., one block completed a dedicated task, and then a second block completed its designated task, and so on). For instance, in a cochlear implant signal processor, one component of a digital circuit may function to control the directional properties of a dual-microphone directional system. After directional processing is completed, then another block may determine the amount of compression that should be applied to the signal. Once compression is determined, yet another block within the digital circuit may seek to determine whether the signal is speech or noise and provide attenuation if the signal is noise. This type of sequential processing is less than ideal, because

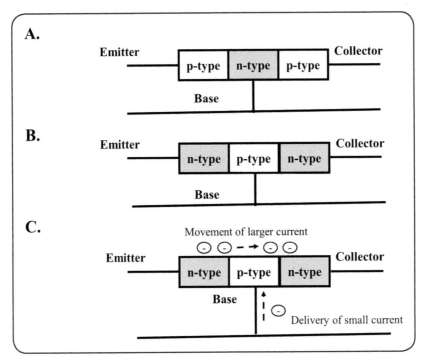

FIGURE 2–19. A. An elementary example of a pnp transistor. **B.** An elementary example of an npn transistor. **C.** An elementary example depicting how the delivery of a small electrical current to the base of a transistor can result in the creation of a much larger electrical current being passed through the transistor.

it is inefficient, and various processing decisions are made without respect to the function of other types of processing.

Modern circuits are more likely to incorporate integrated digital signal processing. Integrated signal processing allows for multiple blocks of processing to occur simultaneously. Additionally, the function of each processing block is analyzed by an integrator so that the processing decisions at each block are made to optimize the final signal the user will receive.

Key Concepts

- The audiologist should possess a working knowledge of the fundamentals of electricity in order to comprehend the operation of implantable hearing devices.
- Cochlear implants deliver electrical current to the cochlear nerve to elicit an auditory percept.

The leads (i.e., wires) and electrode contacts of the cochlear implant along with the tissues in the cochlea make up an electrical circuit through which current passes.

- Electromagnetic induction is prevalent throughout all implantable hearing technologies. Electromagnetic induction is used to deliver signals via radiofrequency transmission as well as to transduce (i.e., change) a signal from one state (e.g., magnetic) to another (e.g., electrical current).

References

Clark, G. M., Shute, S. A., Sheperd, R. K., & Carter, T. D. (1995). Cochlear implantation: Osteoneogenesis, electrode-tissue impedance, and residual hearing. *Annals of Otology, Rhinology and Laryngology Supplement, 166,* 40–42.

Webster, J. (Ed.) (2006). *Encyclopedia of biomedical devices and instrumentation.* Hoboken, NJ: Wiley-Interscience.

3

Anatomy and Physiology Associated with Cochlear Implantation

Jace Wolfe

Auditory Physiology and Pathophysiology

Introduction

A full description of the anatomy and physiology of the auditory system is beyond the scope of this book and is not a prerequisite for the reader to gain an understanding of the concepts presented in this book. This chapter will focus on the aspects of auditory anatomy and physiology that are most relevant to implantable hearing technologies. For the purpose of presentation in this book, the auditory system will be categorized into four sections which include the: (1) external ear, (2) middle ear, (3) cochlea and cochlear nerve, and (4) auditory nervous system (Figure 3–1).

External Ear

Influence of the Auricle and External Auditory Meatus on Acoustics

Although the external ear is the most familiar part of the auditory system, it does possess the least significant role in hearing function. With that said, the contribution of the external ear to auditory function is not entirely trivial. The external ear is comprised of two general structures: the auricle and the external auditory meatus (Figure 3–2). The auricle contributes to auditory function in two different ways. First, the auricle serves to funnel high-frequency sounds arriv-

ing from in front of a listener toward the ear canal, and enhances the amplitude of incoming sound at certain frequencies. Specifically, the concha resonance provides about a 5 dB increase at approximately 5000 Hz to the incoming acoustic signal (Shaw, 1966). The concha resonance is primarily due to the size of its ridges and folds relative to the size of the wavelength of the incoming sound. Second, the auricle contributes to localization in both the horizontal and vertical planes. As will be discussed later in this chapter, localization in the horizontal plane is primarily supported by interaural time and intensity differences, which are both minimal for sounds arriving from 0 and 180 degrees azimuth because there are no interaural differences (given the fact that the sound arrives from a location that is equidistant between the right and left ears).

The external auditory meatus also influences the sound arriving at the tympanic membrane. The external auditory meatus essentially functions as a tube that is closed at one end. A tube closed at one end will resonate to a sound that has a wavelength that is four times the length of the tube (note that **resonant frequency/resonance** refers to a system's natural or best frequency of oscillation/vibration, i.e., the frequency at which a system naturally oscillates at a maximum amplitude). The adult external auditory meatus is approximately 2.5 cm in length, and as a result, it will produce a resonance at a frequency with a 10 cm wavelength. Given a sound propagation velocity of 340 m/sec, the resonant frequency of the

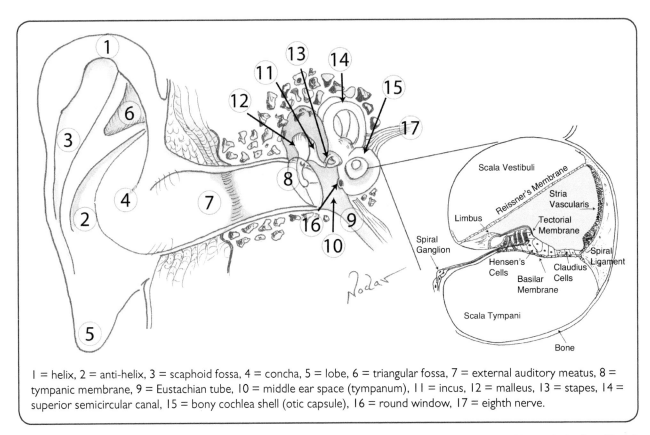

1 = helix, 2 = anti-helix, 3 = scaphoid fossa, 4 = concha, 5 = lobe, 6 = triangular fossa, 7 = external auditory meatus, 8 = tympanic membrane, 9 = Eustachian tube, 10 = middle ear space (tympanum), 11 = incus, 12 = malleus, 13 = stapes, 14 = superior semicircular canal, 15 = bony cochlea shell (otic capsule), 16 = round window, 17 = eighth nerve.

FIGURE 3–1. An illustration of the peripheral auditory system and a cross section of the cochlea. Reprinted with permission from Musiek and Baran, *The Auditory System: Anatomy, Physiology, and Clinical Correlates* (2016). Copyright © Plural Publishing, Inc.

average adult external auditory meatus is expected to occur at approximately 3400 Hz (Equation 3–1).

Equation 3–1: Frequency =
propagation velocity of sound/wavelength of sound

Frequency = 340 m/sec/0.1 m

Frequency = 3400 Hz

In reality, the resonant frequency of the average adult ear canal is approximately 2700 Hz because the tympanic membrane is compliant to sound, which prevents the external auditory meatus from behaving exactly like a tube that is closed at one end. It is also important to note that the listener's head also influences the spectrum of sound. The combined effect of the head, auricle, and external auditory meatus on the spectrum of sound arriving at the tympanic membrane is referred to as the *head related transfer function* (HRTF). The HRTF is determined by measuring the difference in sound pressure level (SPL) for a microphone suspended alone in a sound field versus the sound pressure level measured at the tym-

panic membrane when the listener's head is located at the same place at which the initial measure was completed. Figure 3–3 provides an example of the combined resonance of the head, auricle, and ear canal (Shaw, 1974).

The effect of the head, auricle, and external auditory meatus is pertinent to implantable hearing technologies because many implantable hearing technologies incorporate the use of a sound processor with a microphone that is located at the top of the auricle or on the side of the head. Consequently, the HRTF is considerably altered, a fact that may or may not impact the listener's experience dependent on the type of technology the listener is using. Furthermore, placing a microphone on the top of the auricle or at the side of the head will alter the localization cues typically provided by the auricle. The impact of these localization cues and of the HRTF associated with the use of various implantable hearing technologies will be addressed when each implantable hearing technology is discussed in isolation in upcoming chapters.

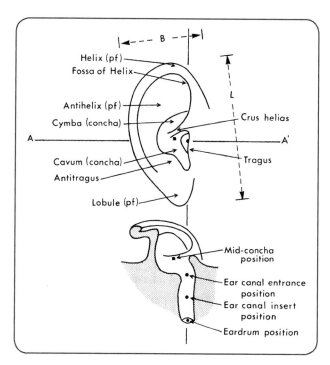

FIGURE 3–2. An illustration of the external ear. Reprinted with permission from Møller, *Hearing: Anatomy, Physiology, and Disorders of the Auditory System, Third Edition* (2013). Copyright © Plural Publishing, Inc.

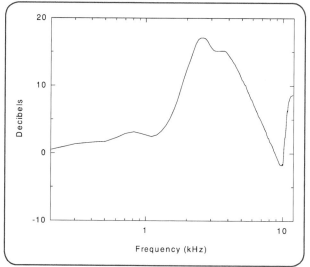

FIGURE 3–3. A visual representation of the acoustic resonance of the auricle, external auditory meatus, and the head. Reprinted with permission from Møller, *Hearing: Anatomy, Physiology, and Disorders of the Auditory System, Third Edition* (2013). Copyright © Plural Publishing, Inc.

The External Auditory Canal and the Occlusion Effect

The outer half of the external auditory meatus is composed of cartilage, whereas the inner half is made up of bone (continuous with the tympanic portion of the temporal bone). During vocalization, the oscillations from the vocal tract radiate throughout the head with considerable vibration of the cartilaginous portion of the external auditory meatus. The movement of the cartilaginous portion of the external auditory meatus results in areas of compression and rarefaction of the air in the external auditory meatus (i.e., sound oscillations). These oscillations are normally not bothersome because they escape the open ear canal. However, when the ear canal is blocked with a hearing aid, an acoustic component of a hybrid cochlear implant sound processor, or the processor of a middle ear implantable hearing device, these sound oscillations are trapped in the external auditory meatus. Because the closed external auditory meatus is a relatively small cavity and the level of the voice radiating through the head is fairly high (e.g., 100 dB SPL), these trapped sound oscillations can become quite intense. The increase in sound pressure level that occurs when the opening of the

external auditory meatus is closed is referred to as the occlusion effect. Figure 3–4 provides an objective example of the occlusion effect. The measure was made while the subject vocalized the vowel /i/ ("ee") at a sustained level (65 dBA at one meter away). The trace which has a lower sound pressure level in the low-frequency range was obtained from a measure in which the external auditory meatus is open, whereas the trace with the higher sound pressure level in the low-frequency range was obtained from a measurement completed with the external auditory meatus occluded. The increase in low-frequency sound pressure level at the tympanic membrane is a representation of the occlusion effect and occurs not only during vocalization but also during eating (e.g., chewing on crunchy food) and for various body movements (e.g., stepping on a hard floor while wearing shoes, swallowing). Of note, the reduction in sound pressure level that occurs around 3000 Hz in the ear occluded condition occurred because the resonance of the external auditory meatus was reduced when the ear canal was occluded.

The occlusion effect can be quite annoying to the listener. In fact, the occlusion effect has historically been a factor for why persons with hearing loss reject hearing aids (Flynn, 2004; Kochkin, 2000) and for the rise in popularity of receiver-in-the-canal hearing aid technology that leaves the external auditory

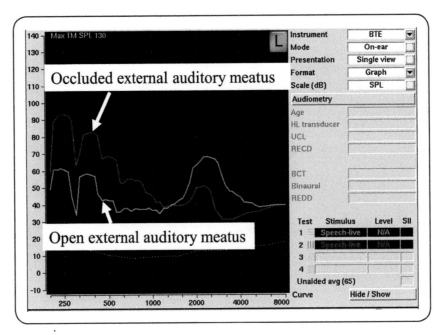

FIGURE 3–4. A visual representation of the occlusion effect.

meatus relatively open (Flynn, 2004). Avoidance of the occlusion effect can be difficult when attempting to provide amplification for persons with relatively good low-frequency hearing and significant high-frequency hearing loss. Specifically, it is challenging to keep the external auditory meatus open while delivering substantial high-frequency gain. The provision of satisfactory high-frequency gain while leaving the external auditory meatus open is one attractive feature of many middle ear implantable hearing devices. Of note, the audiologist will want to consider the occlusion effect when fitting the acoustic component for a recipient who has normal to near normal low-frequency hearing after cochlear implantation and who uses electric-acoustic stimulation. In particular, the audiologist will likely need to keep the external auditory meatus relatively open with an open dome or a shell with sizable venting in order to avoid the occlusion effect.

Middle Ear

The audiologist must have a thorough understanding of middle ear anatomy and physiology in order to optimize outcomes with many implantable hearing technologies. A simplified illustration of the most important structures of the middle ear is shown in Figure 3–5. Sound is collected at the tympanic mem-

brane, which resides in the annulus, a bony ring that exists in the tympanic portion of the temporal bone. The tympanic membrane is composed of three layers, an outer layer that is consistent with the epithelial lining of the external auditory meatus, a middle layer made up of tough fibers, and an inner layer comprised of mucous tissue that is continuous with the lining of the middle ear space (Zemlin, 1998). The middle fibrous section is actually made up of two layers, one with fibers that radiate from the middle of the tympanic membrane to the edges, much like the spokes of a bicycle wheel, and a second with fibers arranged in circles. A small section in the upper middle portion of the tympanic membrane possesses a small number of fibers and is more flaccid than the rest of the tympanic membrane. This section is known as the pars flaccida. The fibrous portion of the tympanic membrane is known as the pars tensa and is the portion of the tympanic membrane that primarily oscillates in response to sound. The stiffness of the tympanic membrane is determined by the arrangement of the fibers in the tympanic membrane, the connection of the tympanic membrane to the annulus and to the ossicular chain. The overall stiffness of the tympanic membrane plays an important role in auditory transmission. If the tension of the tympanic membrane is too little or too great, then the efficiency of sound transmission will diminish.

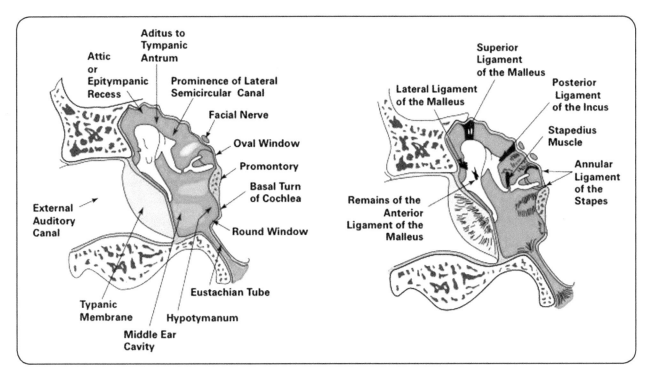

FIGURE 3–5. An illustration of the middle ear. Image provided courtesy of James W. Hall, III.

Ossicular Chain

The tympanic membrane is coupled to the malleus, which is the most lateral of the three middle ear ossicles (i.e., a small chain of bones residing within the middle ear space). The manubrium of the malleus is intimately coupled to the middle of the tympanic membrane, whereas the lateral process of the manubrium attaches to the tympanic membrane superiorly. The malleus is then coupled to the incus by an articular facet joint, and the incus is coupled to the head of the stapes by an articular facet joint. The stapes is coupled to the oval window of the cochlea by an annular ligament, which is larger in the anterior region, a fact that causes the footplate to be held more firmly in place in the posterior region. The difference in the rigidity of the connection between the anterior and posterior ends causes the footplate to rock back and forth in the oval window rather than push in and out like a piston (Zemlin, 1998). The crura (i.e., legs) of the stapes are hollow, which reduces its mass. However, the crura of the stapes are arranged in the shape of a gothic arch, which architects recognize as a structurally sound and durable configuration.

Of note, the ossicular chain is suspended in the middle ear cavity by several ligaments (Figure 3–6) (Moller, 2013). It is also connected to the tendons of

two different middle ear muscles, the tensor tympani muscle, which connects by way of a tendon to the malleus where the manubrium meets the neck, and the stapedius muscle, which connects by way of a tendon to the head of the stapes. The network of ligaments and tendons places the ossicular chain under a certain amount of tension which assists in determining the overall stiffness of the middle ear system. As with the tympanic membrane, sound transmission will suffer if the stiffness of the ossicular chain is too little or too great.

The Role of the Middle Ear in Auditory Function

The primary job of the middle ear is to convert acoustic signals to mechanical energy and transmit the mechanical analog of the acoustic signal to the cochlea. A large impedance mismatch exists between air (the primary medium for sound transmission) and the fluids within the cochlea. You have likely experienced the consequence of this mismatch when someone speaks while you are submerged in a swimming pool. Because the water has a higher impedance than air, much of the sound from the speaker's voice reflects off the surface of the water, and it is difficult to understand what is said. A similar experience

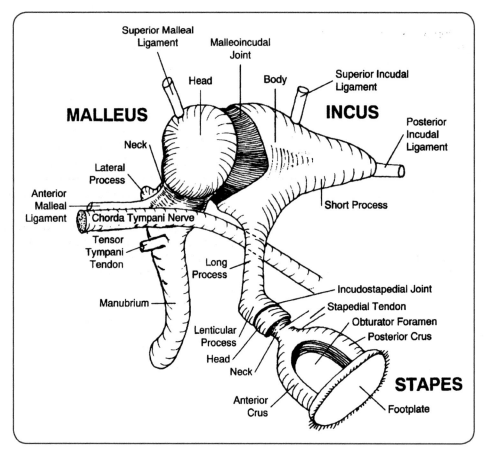

FIGURE 3–6. An illustration of the middle ear ossicles. Reprinted with permission from Møller, *Hearing: Anatomy, Physiology, and Disorders of the Auditory System, Third Edition* (2013). Copyright © Plural Publishing, Inc.

would occur if sound had to travel from the outside world directly to the fluids within the cochlea. In fact, the impedance mismatch between air and cochlear fluids results in about a 35 dB reduction in sound transmission (Lipscomb, 1996). As a result, the middle ear is often referred to as a transformer because it functions to overcome the loss of energy as sound is transformed from acoustic oscillations (i.e., air movement) to fluid displacement (i.e., hydrodynamic oscillations).

Three properties of the middle ear partially overcome this impedance mismatch. First, the surface area of the tympanic membrane is much larger than the surface area of the footplate of the stapes. von Békésy estimated almost a 17:1 ratio between the effective vibrational surface of the tympanic membrane and the surface of the stapes footplate (von Békésy, 1941). This areal relationship between the tympanic membrane results in a relatively large amount of energy

collected at the tympanic membrane being focused on the small destination of the oval window. This configuration is similar to what occurs when a sledge hammer drives a spike into the ground. The areal relationship between the tympanic membrane and stapes footplate overcomes about 23 dB of the loss that occurs because of the impedance mismatch between air and the cochlear fluids (Lipscomb, 1996).

Two additional properties of the middle ear help overcome the impedance mismatch between air and the cochlear fluids. Because of the difference in length of the manubrium of the malleus and the long process of the incus, the ossicular chain possesses a lever action when oscillating. This lever action of the ossicular chain assists in overcoming almost 2.5 dB of the transmission loss that would occur as sound travels from air to the cochlear fluids (Lipscomb, 1996; Moller, 2013). Finally, the tympanic membrane is more firmly attached to the annulus at its superior edge compared with the inferior border. As a result, it buckles or swings laterally rather than pushing in and out of the middle ear space with a piston-like motion. This buckling action of the tympanic membrane results in an almost two-fold increase in force, which provides almost a 6 dB enhancement in middle ear transmission. Collectively, the areal relationship of the tympanic membrane to the stapes footplate, the lever action of the ossicles, and the buckling effect of the tympanic membrane serve to overcome about 31 of the 35 dB lost to the impedance mismatch between air and cochlear fluids.

Middle Ear Impedance and Hearing Function

"Impedance" is a term that is often used to describe the efficiency and effectiveness of sound conduction through the middle ear. In the context of sound transmission through the middle ear, impedance refers to the opposition of acoustic energy flow through the system. Impedance is composed of three components: mass reactance, stiffness reactance, and resistance. Mass reactance influences the transmission of high-frequency energy through a system. An increase in mass results in a decrease in the transmission of high-frequency energy. Stiffness reactance results influence the transmission of low-frequency energy through a system. An increase in stiffness results in a decrease in the transmission of low-frequency energy. Resistance is frequency independent (i.e., an increase in resistance reduces sound transmission similarly across a broad frequency range).

From a perspective of sound transmission, it is important to recognize that the middle ear is a mechano-acoustic system. In other words, the middle ear is a combination of a mechanical and acoustic system. The tympanic membrane and ossicular chain are physical components that make up a mechanical system. The air in the middle ear space and mastoid air cell system behave as an acoustic system. As depicted in Figure 3–7, mechanical and acoustic systems each possess resistance, mass reactance, and stiffness reactance. As a result, the response of the middle ear to sound conduction is complex because it is influenced by the physical properties of the mechanical and acoustical components. Increases in the mass of the tympanic membrane or ossicles will result in a high-frequency conductive hearing loss. Increases in the stiffness of the tympanic membrane or ossicles will result in a low-frequency conductive hearing loss. A reduction in the volume of the air-filled middle ear space that occurs in the presence of a partial middle

ear effusion results in an increase in acoustic stiffness reactance and a reduction in low-frequency sound transmission. Of note, a thick effusion also influences high-frequency sound transmission because of the mass effect.

As previously noted, the tympanic membrane and the ossicular chain are under a given amount of tension or stiffness, which is determined by the physical coupling of these structures at their attachment points as well as the network of ligaments and tendons that suspend the ossicular chain within the middle ear space. Furthermore, the mass of the tympanic membrane is determined by its three layers, and the mass of the ossicles is determined by their physical composition (e.g., the crura of the stapes are hollow). These physical properties and characteristics of the middle ear system determine its mass reactance, stiffness reactance, and resistance. The collective impedance present in the middle ear mechano-acoustic system determines the resonant response of the middle ear. The mature middle ear most efficiently transmits sound across a broad frequency range with a resonant frequency that typically falls between 800 and 1200 Hz (Zemlin, 1998). Additionally, the resonant frequency of the ossicular chain in isolation is around 2000 Hz.

Eustachian Tube Dysfunction

Any discussion of middle ear function would be remiss without mention of the eustachian tube. The role of the eustachian tube is to equalize the air pressure in the middle ear space with the atmospheric air pressure. The mucous lining of the middle ear space is vascularized and requires oxygen to support its function. As the oxygen is consumed, negative air pressure builds up in the middle ear space relative to atmospheric air pressure. Likewise, changes in elevation and/or changes in atmospheric air pressure related to weather changes can result in a difference in air pressure in the middle ear space relative to the ambient environment. When negative middle ear pressure exists within the middle ear space, the tympanic membrane is retracted into the middle ear. When positive pressure exists within the middle ear space, the tympanic membrane is pushed toward the external auditory meatus. In either case, an imbalance between ambient and middle ear pressure causes the tympanic membrane to be displaced from its neutral position, resulting in an increase in stiffness of the tympanic membrane. This increase in stiffness results in a reduction of low-frequency sound transmission.

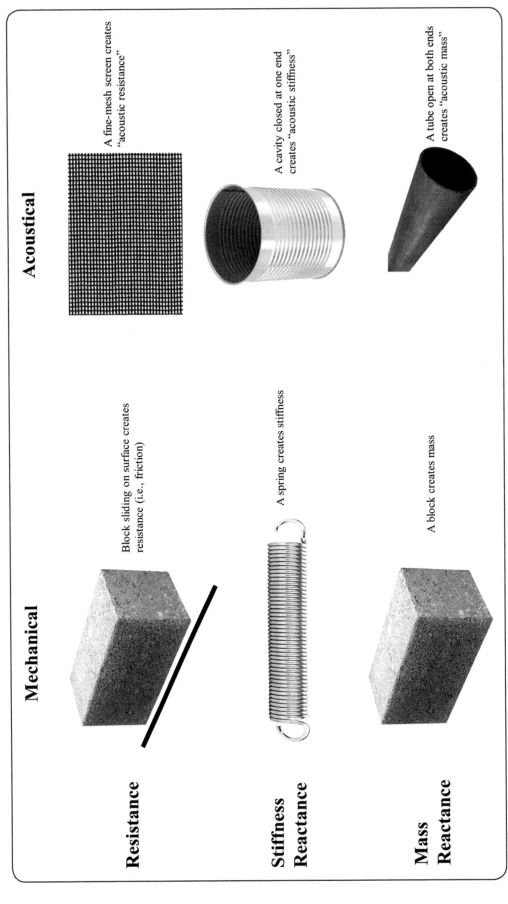

Mechanical

Acoustical

Block sliding on surface creates resistance (i.e., friction)

A fine-mesh screen creates "acoustic resistance"

Resistance

A spring creates stiffness

A cavity closed at one end creates "acoustic stiffness"

Stiffness Reactance

A block creates mass

A tube open at both ends creates "acoustic mass"

Mass Reactance

FIGURE 3–7. A visual representation of resistance, stiffness reactance, and mass reactance of a mechanical and an acoustical system.

If negative pressure persists in the middle ear space, the mucous lining of the middle ear space will become inflamed (i.e., otitis media) and begin to secrete fluid, which is commonly referred to as a middle ear effusion. If the middle ear effusion persists, bacteria invading the middle ear space may result in a thick, purulent (i.e., infected) effusion. The presence of a middle ear effusion can increase the stiffness and mass present in the middle ear.

The eustachian tube opens to equalize pressure in the middle ear space. When functioning correctly, negative middle ear pressure cannot persist in the middle ear space, and a middle ear effusion will not occur. Additionally, the eustachian tube may serve to allow for middle ear secretions to drain into the nasopharynx.

Chorda Tympani Nerve

The chorda tympani is a small branch of the facial nerve that passes just behind the tympanic membrane near the lateral neck of the malleus and leaves the middle ear space through an opening called the iter chordae anterius. The chorda tympani innervates the tongue and is involved with taste sensation. Its typical course places it toward the top of the middle ear space. In rare circumstances, the chorda tympani nerve may be injured during surgical procedures involving the middle ear space (e.g., cochlear implant, middle ear implantable hearing devices). In such cases, the recipient may complain of an altered sensation of taste following surgery. In most cases, normal taste sensation returns within several weeks to months (Lloyd et al., 2007).

The Influence of the Middle Ear on Outcomes with Implantable Auditory Technology

The implications of mechano-acoustic properties for implantable hearing technology are widespread. For implantable middle ear devices, adding transducers to the ossicular chain contributes mass, which may decrease high-frequency transmission. Likewise, the surgeon must balance the contradicting needs of intimately coupling a transducer to the ossicular chain to facilitate long-term retention while avoiding excessive coupling that unnecessarily increases stiffness, resulting in a reduction of low-frequency transmission.

Additionally, surgeons are typically reluctant to proceed with cochlear implantation in the presence of an active middle ear effusion for fear that bacteria will spread to the cochlea and onto the meninges (result-ing in bacterial meningitis). Many cochlear implant surgeons proactively treat middle ear dysfunction in cochlear implant candidates prior to the implant surgery. Otologic intervention may include the provision of antibiotics and/or the placement of pressure equalization (PE) tubes in the tympanic membrane. Of note, conventional wisdom would suggest that otitis media would not affect the auditory function of cochlear implant recipients, because the cochlear implant bypasses the middle ear and stimulates the cochlear nerve directly. However, anecdotal experience suggests that many cochlear implant recipients complain of decreased hearing during episodes of Eustachian tube dysfunction (i.e., negative middle ear pressure) and otitis media. It is possible that negative middle ear pressure acts upon the round window of the cochlea and results in a change in pressure in the cochlear scalae. A subtle change in the pressure within the cochlear scalae may affect the position of the cochlear implant electrode array relative to the cochlear nerve, which may subsequently result in a change in hearing function. A middle ear effusion may also exert pressure on the round window, which may alter cochlear mechanics and electrode array positioning.

Additionally, a middle ear effusion is often present for several weeks following cochlear implant surgery, a fact that may result in a temporary conductive hearing loss that influences any residual hearing capacity preserved after the operation. This temporary conductive hearing loss may hinder immediate benefit for persons who have preservation of low-frequency cochlear function and wish to use low-frequency acoustic stimulation from an electric-acoustic processor. The audiologist may need to wait for middle ear effusion to resolve before the recipient is able to benefit from low-frequency acoustic access. Furthermore, for electric-acoustic cochlear implant users, the surgeon should avoid placing the lead of the cochlear implant on the ossicular chain to avoid altering the transmission of low-frequency acoustic stimulation.

Implantable bone conduction hearing devices are often used as a technological intervention for persons with permanent middle ear dysfunction. Implantable bone conduction devices convert the sounds captured at the processor microphone to mechanical oscillations/vibrations that are transmitted to the skull and on to the cochlea via bone conduction. Bone conduction signal delivery bypasses the dysfunctional middle ear, effectively overcoming conductive hearing loss.

Cochlea

The inner ear consists of the cochlea, the vestibule, and the semicircular canals (Figure 3–8). The vestibule and semicircular canals house the sensory organs of the vestibular system, which assists in the maintenance of balance and spatial orientation. Because the focus of this book is implantable hearing technologies, this chapter will focus on the cochlea, with minimal discussion of the vestibule and semicircular canals. The cochlea obviously plays an important role in most implantable hearing devices. The cochlea resides deep within the petrous portion of the temporal bone. In order to conceptualize the position of the cochlea, the reader can imagine drawing two imaginary lines, one extending from one external auditory meatus to the other and another line coursing from just below the eyeball directly toward the back of the skull. The cochlea resides at the approximate intersection of those two lines (Figure 3–9). Of note, the cochlea is continuous with the vestibule of the peripheral vestibular system. The oval window, which houses the stapes footplate, resides in the vestibule.

The cochlea is generally 2⅝ turns and resembles a snail shell with approximately 2⅝ turns and is coiled into a tight spiral that wraps around a bony core called the modiolus (Figure 3–10). The cochlea is typically about 35 mm in length, but it should be noted that substantial variability is observed in cochlear duct length. For instance, Stakhovska et al. (2007) reported a range spanning from 30.5 to 36.87 mm in nine adult cadavers. The cochlea is composed of three chambers called scalae. The three scalae are best observed when the cochlea is "unwound" so that it resembles an elongated tube. For the purpose of explanation, let's pretend that the cochlea has been unwound to resemble a tube of cookie dough. Then, let's pretend that you took a knife and cut through the width of the tube of cookie dough (i.e., a cross-sectional cut) (Figure 3–11A). If you picked up one of the halves of the newly sectioned tube and looked into it much like you would a picture box (i.e., you looked down the tube in a lengthwise direction, Figure 3–11B), you would see an image similar to what is shown in Figure 3–11C. As seen in Figure 3–11C, the cochlea contains three chambers: the scala tympani, scala media, and scala vestibuli.

Each of these chambers is filled with a cochlear fluid. A fluid called perilymph exists in the scala tympani and scala vestibuli, whereas a fluid called endolymph exists in the scala media. Perilymph possesses a chemical composition similar to extracellular fluid and is relatively high in Na+ ions and low in K+ ions. In contrast, endolymph is composed of relatively high levels of K+ ions and low levels of Na+ ions. Of note, the concentration of K+ ions is higher than the concentration of positively charged ions in neighboring fluids and tissues. As a result, the endolymph is attracted to the relatively negative charge of neighboring areas.

The scala vestibuli and scala media are separated by the flexible Reissner's membrane, which is made up of one layer of ectodermal epithelium and one layer of mesothelial tissue (Zemlin, 1998). The boundary between the scala media and scala vestibuli consists of three structures, a thin bony shelf called the spiral lamina, the basilar membrane, and the spiral ligament, which attaches to the lateral bony wall of the cochlea. The organ of Corti is the primary sensory organ of the cochlea and houses the cochlear sensory cells (i.e., cochlear hair cells). Figure 3–12 provides a close-up representation of the organ of Corti from a cross-section cut of the cochlea (i.e., similar to the orientation described in Figure 3–11).

The inferior boundary of the organ of Corti consists of the spiral lamina medially and the basilar membrane laterally. The segment that is primarily made up of the bony spiral lamina is rigid and known as the pars tecta, while the segment made up of the basilar membrane is flexible and known as the pars pectinata.

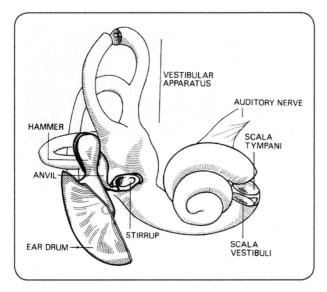

FIGURE 3–8. An illustration of the inner ear. Reprinted with permission from Møller, *Hearing: Anatomy, Physiology, and Disorders of the Auditory System, Third Edition* (2013). Copyright © Plural Publishing, Inc.

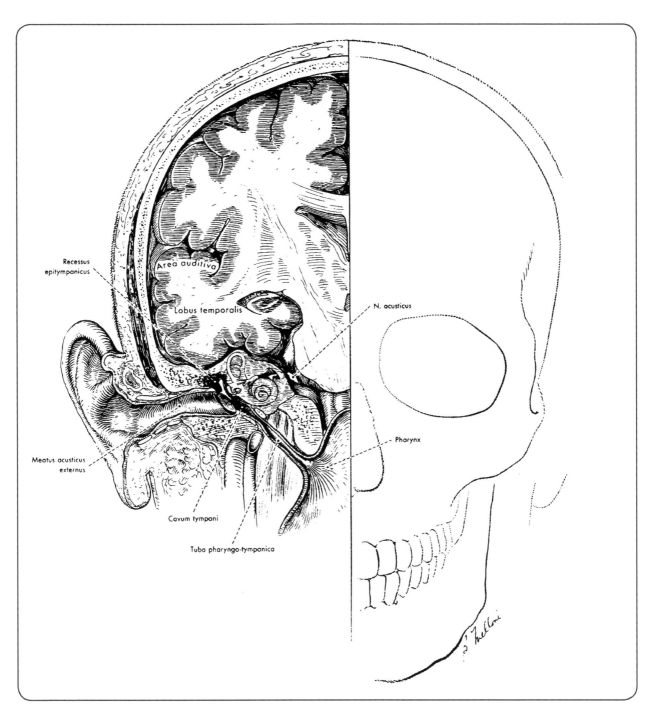

FIGURE 3–9. An illustration of the location of the inner ear within the temporal bone. Reprinted with permission from Møller, *Hearing: Anatomy, Physiology, and Disorders of the Auditory System, Third Edition* (2013). Copyright © Plural Publishing, Inc.

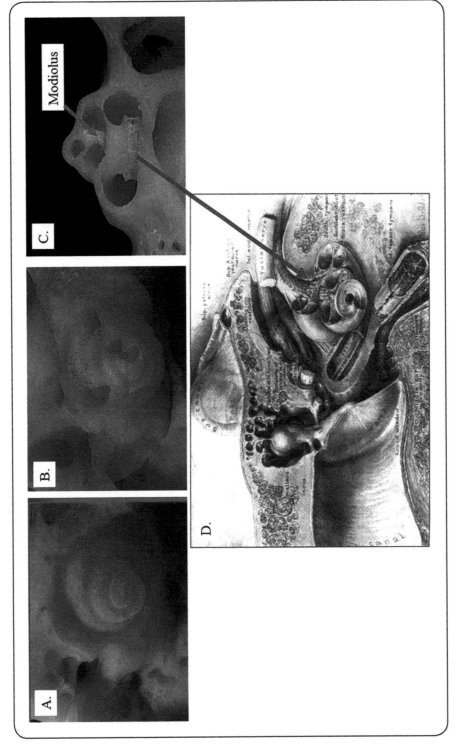

FIGURE 3–10. A. A visual representation of the bony cochlea. **B.** The bony cochlea with the superior half removed to expose the scalae and multiple turns. **C.** The image shown in Figure 3–10B is inverted. **D.** The peripheral auditory system with the superior half of the bony cochlea removed to expose the scalae and multiple turns. *A–C,* Reprinted with permission from Acland's Video Atlas of Human Anatomy (aclandanatomy.com), Volume 4:4.11.11. Copyright © Wolters Kluwer Health, Inc. *D,* Reprinted with permission from Møller, Hearing: Anatomy, Physiology, and Disorders of the Auditory System, Third Edition (2013). Copyright © Plural Publishing, Inc.

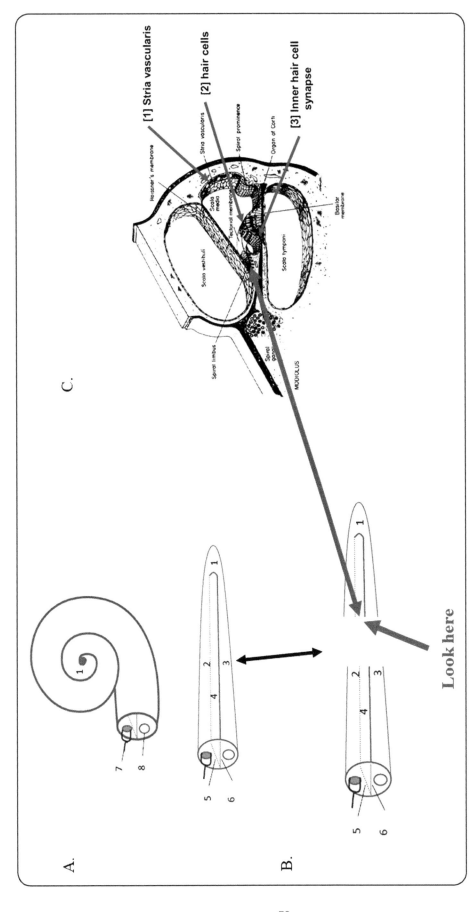

FIGURE 3–11. A visual representation of a cross-section of cochlea showing the three scalae. **A.** A schematic of the cochlea unfolded into a long tube. Key: 1 = helicotrema, 2 = scala vestibuli, 3 = scala tympani, 4 = scala media, 5 = Reissner's membrane, 6 = basilar membrane, 7 = stapes and oval window, 8 = round window. **B.** A representation of a cross-sectional cut made through the middle of unfolded cochlea. **C.** A representation of all three scalae if an observer was able to look into the cochlea at the point at which the cross-sectional cut was made. *A* and *B,* Adapted with permission from Musiek and Baran. *The Auditory System: Anatomy, Physiology, and Clinical Correlates, Third Edition* (2020). Copyright © Plural Publishing, Inc. *C,* Adapted with permission from Tremblay and Burkard, *Translational Perspectives in Auditory Neuroscience: Normal Aspects of Hearing* (2012). Copyright © Plural Publishing, Inc.

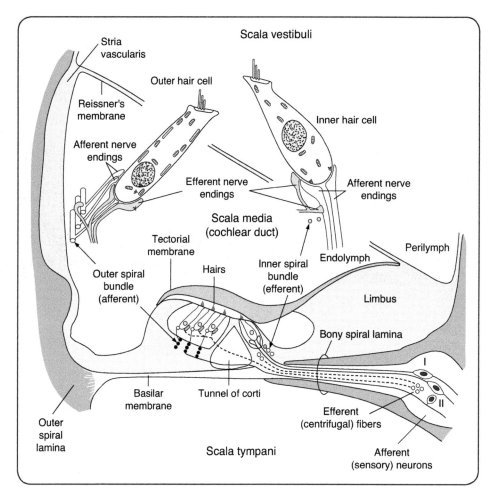

FIGURE 3–12. A cross-section of the cochlea with each scala and the organ of Corti. Reprinted with permission from Møller, *Hearing: Anatomy, Physiology, and Disorders of the Auditory System, Third Edition* (2013). Copyright © Plural Publishing, Inc.

The basilar membrane is relatively flexible because it is composed of fibrous tissue. The organ of Corti consists of two types of sensory hair cells (inner and outer hair cells), multiple supporting cells (outer pillar cells, inner phalangeal cells, Deiters' cells, cells of Hensen, border cells, etc.), the reticular lamina, and the tectorial membrane (Figure 3–13).

When the ossicular chain oscillates in response to sound stimulation, the footplate of the stapes rocks back and forth into the oval window, resulting in a displacement of the perilymph in the underlying vestibule. The vestibule is continuous with the scala vestibuli, so the perilymphatic displacement that occurs in response to the movement of the stapes footplate is transmitted through the scala vestibuli and toward the scala media. Because the scala media is composed of endolymphatic fluid and is bound superiorly and

inferiorly by flexible membranes (i.e., Reissner's and basilar membrane, respectively), the fluid displacement in the scala vestibuli produces oscillations in the scala media. The oscillations of the scala media are also transferred to the scala tympani. The membrane of the round window, which resides at the base of the scala tympani, serves as a pressure relief valve by moving inward and outward in response to the displacements transmitted through the cochlea.

Physical Properties of the Organ of Corti

The physical characteristics of the basilar membrane, the supporting cells, the stereocilia, and the tectorial membrane change in a continual gradient from the base to the apex of the cochlea. Specifically, all of these structures are relatively stiff and narrow

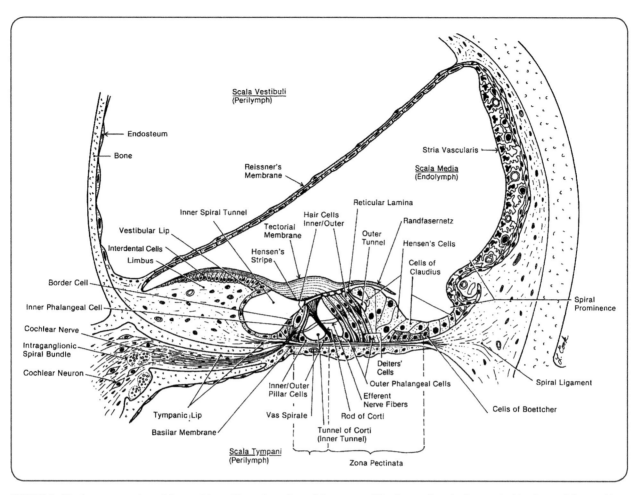

FIGURE 3–13. A cross-section of the cochlea with each scala and the organ of Corti as well as the bony spiral lamina and the cochlear nerve. Reproduced from H. Davis, "Advances in the neurophysiology and neuroanatomy of the cochlea," *Journal of the Acoustical Society of America* (1962), 34(9B), 1377–1385, with permission of the Acoustical Society of America.

at the basal end (i.e., the base of the cochlea) and become more flaccid and possess more mass toward the apical end. The gradient change in physical characteristics of the organ of Corti from base to apex influences how the cochlea responds to sound as a function of frequency. As previously noted, the part of a mechanical system that is stiffness dominated will provide opposition to the transmission of low-frequency oscillations and will respond more freely to high-frequency oscillations. In contrast, the part of the systems that is mass dominated will impede the transmission of high-frequency oscillations while being more receptive to the transmission of low-frequency oscillations.

Additionally, for any mechanical system with a stiffness gradient, the stiffest part of the system will initially respond to displacement (i.e., oscillation),

whereas a time lag in responsiveness will occur for the part of the system that is mass dominant. As a result, high-frequency sounds produce maximum displacement at the basal end of the cochlea, and low-frequency sounds produce maximum displacement toward the apical end of the cochlea. Furthermore, oscillations in the cochlear fluids cause a stimulation wave to gradually build in amplitude beginning at the base and moving toward the apex. This roving wave of displacement occurring across the flexible basilar membrane as well as other cochlear structures (e.g., supporting cells, stereocilia, tectorial membrane) will reach a maximum amplitude at a point at which the effects of stiffness and mass are equal. At this point, stiffness and mass will effectively offset one another, and the system will oscillate with minimal opposition. Once again, the resonant frequency describes the frequency of oscillation at which a system vibrates with greatest amplitude. In essence, the resonant frequency of the cochlea changes from base to apex.

Georg von Békésy and the Traveling Wave

Georg von Békésy, a Hungarian physicist who won a Nobel Prize for his research exploring auditory physiology, was the first to describe the vibratory response of the cochlea in response to stimulation. Von Békésy described the frequency-specific displacement of the basilar membrane as a traveling wave, and noted that the traveling wave provides the basis for spectral (i.e., frequency) analysis in the auditory system (von Békésy, 1960). Tonotopic organization refers to the fact that sounds are coded at different locations on the basis of frequency (e.g., high-frequency sounds are coded at the base of the cochlea, whereas low-frequency sounds are coded at apical locations). The tonotopic organization that begins in the cochlea is present in the cochlear nerve and throughout the auditory nervous system. Von Békésy noted that the traveling wave begins at the basal end of the cochlea, gradually builds in amplitude as it overcomes the effects of stiffness, reaches a maximum amplitude when the stimulating sound encounters a point where the effects of stiffness and mass are equal (i.e., resonance), and then rapidly dissipates as it encounters mass effects beyond the point of maximum displacement (Figure 3–14). Von Békésy's traveling wave is associated with the place principle, which indicates that frequency/pitch are coded on the basis of location of the auditory neurons that respond to the sound. Donald Greenwood (1961) studied data from psychophysical masking studies (e.g., critical band research) and calculated the physical location of cochlear hair cells associated with a given frequency of acoustic stimulation. The Greenwood function has played an important role in determining the appropriate location to place a cochlear implant electrode to provide stimulation for a desired acoustic frequency. The place principle

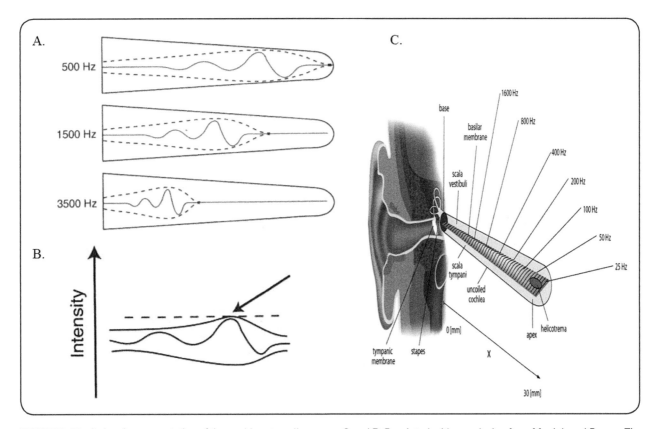

FIGURE 3–14. A visual representation of the cochlear traveling wave. **A** and **B.** Reprinted with permission from Musiek and Baran, *The Auditory System: Anatomy, Physiology, and Clinical Correlates* (2016). Copyright © Plural Publishing, Inc. **C.** Reprinted with permission from Moller, *Hearing: Anatomy, Physiology, and Disorders of the Auditory System, Third Edition* (2013). Copyright © Plural Publishing, Inc.

of stimulation certainly plays a role in spectral processing and has important implications in the design of implantable hearing technologies. It is, however, unlikely to be the auditory system's sole mechanism of spectral/pitch processing. An additional mechanism of spectral processing will be proposed later in this chapter during the discussion of phase-locked responses of the cochlear nerve.

Cochlear Sensory Cells

At each cross-sectional cut in the cochlea, there are one row of inner hair cells and three to five rows of outer hair cells. The inner hair cells are shaped like a flask, while the outer hair cells have a cylindrical "test tube" shape (Figure 3–15). Furthermore, the inner hair cells are completely surrounded along the entire axis of their body by supporting cells, whereas the outer hair cells are only supported at their base and apex by Deiters' cells. More specifically, the entire lateral wall of each outer hair cell is free from physical contact from supporting cells and is in contact with

a cochlear fluid called cortilymph. Protein filaments called stereocilia sit atop both the inner and outer hair cells. On average, inner hair cells possess about 40 to 80 stereocilia arranged in a flattened U-shaped configuration, whereas outer hair cells have about 65 to 150 stereocilia arranged in a W or V shape (Figure 3–16). The stereocilia of outer and inner hair cells are arranged in a stairstep configuration, with the tallest members positioned toward the lateral wall of the cochlea and the shortest members located medially.

Additionally, about 95% of the afferent cochlear nerve fibers (i.e., the cochlear nerve fibers that carry auditory information from the cochlea to the brainstem) innervate the inner hair cells, whereas only the remaining 5% of afferent nerve fibers innervate the outer hair cells (Musiek & Baran, 2007). Furthermore, the afferent nerve fibers innervating the inner hair cells are relatively large and myelinated, but the afferent fibers innervating outer hair cells are thinner and unmyelinated. In contrast, myelinated efferent cochlear nerve fibers directly innervate the base of outer hair cells, whereas thinner unmyelinated effer-

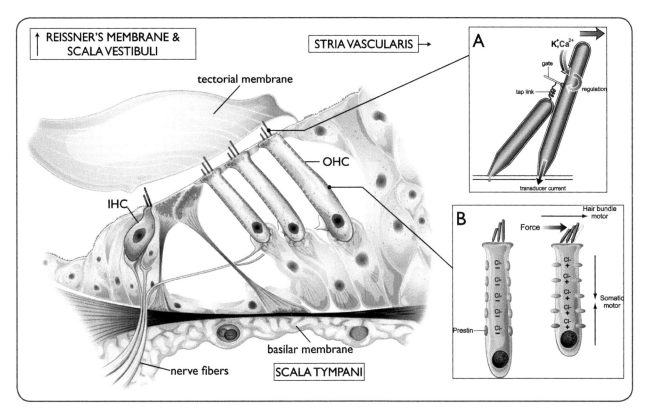

FIGURE 3–15. A close-up cross-sectional view of the organ of Corti with three rows of outer hair cells and one row of inner hair cells. Reprinted with permission from Dhar and Hall, *Otoacoustic Emissions: Principles, Procedures, and Protocols* (2012). Copyright © Plural Publishing, Inc.

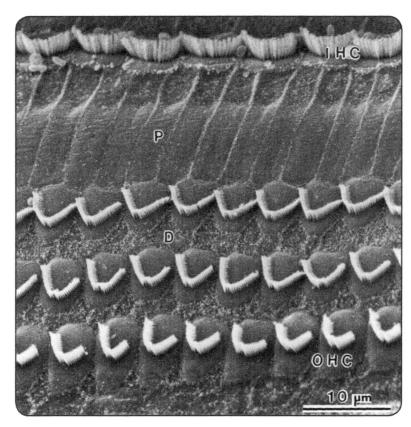

FIGURE 3–16. A visual depiction of the stereocilia of outer hair cells arranged in rows of three and inner hair cells arranged in a single row. Reprinted with permission from Møller, *Hearing: Anatomy, Physiology, and Disorders of the Auditory System, Third Edition* (2013). Copyright © Plural Publishing, Inc.

ent fibers do not directly innervate the inner hair cells but instead innervate the afferent nerve fibers that innervate the inner hair cells.

The reticular lamina is a rigid structure composed of several supporting cells, including the inner phalangeal cells, the rods of Corti, and the apex of the Deiters' cells, and makes up the superior boundary of the organ of Corti. The stereocilia of the hair cells extend just beyond the reticular lamina. The tectorial membrane is a fibrogelatinous structure that is firmly attached to the spiral limbus medially and rather loosely connected to the cochlear supporting cells (i.e., cells of Hensen) laterally. The tectorial membrane possesses a similar density to endolymph, and as a result, it essentially floats above to the organ of Corti. Of note, the stereocilia of the outer hair cells are intimately connected to the underside of the tectorial membrane at a region known as Hardesty's membrane; however, the stereocilia of the inner hair cells are not connected with the tectorial membrane.

Von Békésy and Thomas Gold

Although von Békésy's traveling wave provided a basis for how sounds are spectrally processed in the cochlea, the observations von Békésy made of basilar membrane movement in cadavers did not fully explain auditory function. Von Békésy conducted his measures in the 1940s and 1950s, a time at which limitations in microscope technology would only allow for observation of basilar membrane movement in response to very high-level stimulation (e.g., 120 dB SPL and greater). When the amplitude of basilar membrane displacement observed at high levels was linearly extrapolated downward to predict basilar membrane vibration at lower stimulation levels, no movement of the basilar membrane was estimated in response to stimulation levels consistent with normal hearing sensitivity. Additionally, the broad displacement patterns von Békésy observed at high stimulation levels was inconsistent with the auditory system's ability to discriminate small changes in frequency at low to moderate stimulation levels as measured in psychoacoustical studies (von Békésy, 1960). Collectively, the disparities between von Békésy's observations of cadaver basilar membrane displacement at high levels and auditory function measured in behavioral studies suggested the presence of a biologically active, non-linear mechanism that enhanced cochlear sensitivity and spectral resolution.

In the late 1940s, Austrian physicist Thomas Gold proposed the idea of an active mechanism within the cochlea that would contribute energy to the traveling wave at low stimulation levels (Hall, 2000). He discussed his theory with von Békésy, but von Békésy dismissed it and suggested that a neural mechanism was responsible for enhancing and tuning the response of the cochlea to account for its fine sensitivity and selectivity. Because of von Békésy's prominent stature amongst auditory physiologists, Gold's theory was largely dismissed by the auditory science community. A dejected Gold turned his interest toward the field of astronomy.

The Active Cochlea

Research advances in the 1970s and 1980s further accelerated the understanding of cochlear physiology. David Kemp, an English physiologist, was the first to report on otoacoustic emissions (OAEs), which are low-level sounds recorded in the ear canal after stimulation of the ear with moderate-level sound (e.g., 45–65 dB SPL) (Kemp, 1978). Kemp noted that OAEs were only present in persons with normal to near normal hearing sensitivity, and he theorized that OAEs were produced by outer hair cells. Also, Kemp postulated that OAEs may be a by-product of an active feedback system within the cochlea that contributes energy to enhance responsiveness to low- to moderate-level sounds.

In the 1980s, another physiologist, William Brownell, was the first to demonstrate that outer hair cells moved up and down in response to electrical stimulation, a function he referred to as electromotility (Brownell, 1984). Specifically, Brownell noted that outer hair cells lengthened along their vertical axis when stimulated and shortened (i.e., contracted) when stimulation was withdrawn (i.e., upon hyperpolarization). In fact, outer hair cells are capable of changing length at a rate that spans the entire frequency range of the normal auditory system (e.g., up to at least 20,000 Hz). For instance, outer hair cells are able to change length 500 times per second in response to a 500 Hz stimulus, but outer hair cells are also able to change shape 20,000 times per second in response to a 20,000 Hz audio signal. Brownell's observation provided an explanation for both the production of OAEs as well as the auditory system's responsiveness to low-level sounds.

Cochlear Transduction

As previously stated, the endolymphatic fluid surrounding the organ of Corti is highly comprised of K+ ions. As a result, the endolymph has a highly positive charge relative to surrounding cochlear tissues and structures. Specifically, the endolymphatic resting potential is approximately +80 mV (Musiek & Baran, 2007). The highly positive resting charge of endolymph is attributed to the stria vascularis, a structure that is located on the lateral wall of the scala media and that actively pumps K+ into the scala media. The outer and inner hair cells possess a resting potential of −70 and −45 mV, respectively (Musiek & Baran, 2007) (Figure 3–17). The 150 mV difference in electrical potential between the endolymph and outer hair cells is greater than any other biologic electrical gradient in the rest of the body. Once again, opposites attract, so the endolymphatic fluid is drawn to the internal environment of both the outer and inner hair cells (i.e., the K+ ions of endolymph seek to move down their electrical and concentration gradients).

Auditory physiologists have identified the stereocilia of the hair cells as the transduction gates through which endolymph may move into the hair cells (Hudspeth, 1989). When the basilar membrane is deflected upward (i.e., toward the scala vestibuli), the stereocilia are all displaced toward the tallest member (i.e., laterally). When the basilar membrane is deflected downward (i.e., toward the scala tympani), all of the stereocilia are displaced to the shortest members of the group (i.e., medially). The stereocilia move in unison upon displacement because they are coupled to one another at their sidewalls by protein filaments called side-links. They are also coupled by tip-links, which connect from the apex of an individual stereocilium to the upper sidewall of its next tallest neighbor (Figure 3–18). When the stereocilia move toward their tallest members (upward deflection), tension on the tip-links pulls open a gate located at the top of the stereocilia, and endolymph rushes into the hair cell. When the stereocilia swing back toward their shortest members, the tension on the tip-links relaxes and the transduction gates close. As a result, the hair cells are depolarized (i.e., stimulated) and produce a response

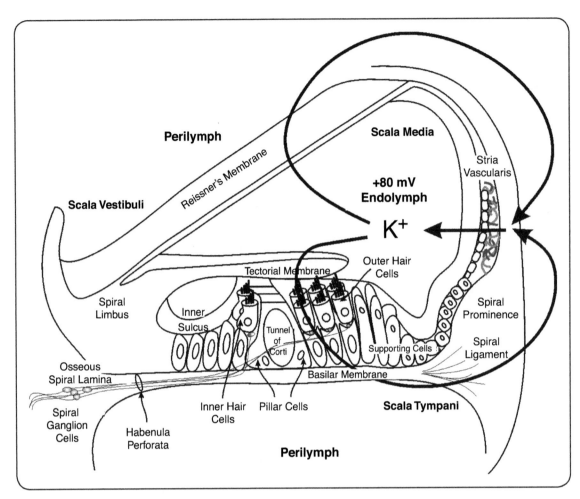

FIGURE 3–17. A visual representation of the resting electrical potentials of the cochlea and the passage of positively charged potassium ions from the stria vascularis to the endolymph. Reprinted with permission from Musiek and Baran, *The Auditory System: Anatomy, Physiology, and Clinical Correlates* (2016). Copyright © Plural Publishing, Inc.

each time the basilar membrane oscillates upward. Stated differently, the hair cells can be depolarized at the same rate as the stimulating sound. If a 12,000 Hz sound causes the basilar membrane to oscillate up and down at a rate of 12,000 cycles per second, then stereocilia will swing back and forth 12,000 times per second, and the hair cell will be stimulated 12,000 times per second. After the transduction gates open and the hair cell is depolarized (i.e., becomes positively charged), the gates quickly close and the hair cell is restored to its negative resting potential. The restoration to the negative resting potential is likely facilitated by the outflow of K+ ions. Specifically, when the hair cell becomes positively charged, voltage-sensitive (i.e., gates that open in response to the voltage becoming positive) Ca^{2+} gates open, allowing CA^{2+} to rush into the cell. These CA^{2+} ions bind to the receptors of K+-selective channels, which allows K+ to depart the cell as it gravitates away from the positive charge in the cell and toward a neutral charge of the cortilymph surrounding the cell and or the perilymph at the base of the cell.

For several reasons, the outer hair cells are more likely to be stimulated in response to low-level stimulation. First, the physical connection of the tectorial membrane to the sterocilia of the outer hair cells results in a shearing of the former over the latter during stimulation. This shearing facilitates movement of the back-and-forth movement of the outer hair cell stereocilia. Second, the outer hair cells are located over the relatively flexible basilar membrane, while the inner hair cells are located above the fairly rigid spiral lamina. Consequently, the outer hair cells are better positioned to oscillate up and down in

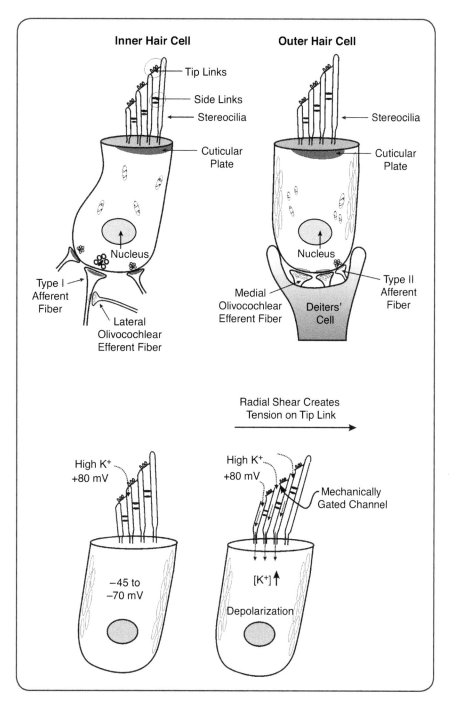

FIGURE 3–18. A visual representation of the cochlear transduction process occurring at the stereocilia. Reprinted with permission from Musiek and Baran, *The Auditory System: Anatomy, Physiology, and Clinical Correlates* (2016). Copyright © Plural Publishing, Inc.

response to cochlear stimulation. Third, a larger electrical potential difference exists between endolymph and outer hair cells (around 150 mV) compared with endolymph and inner hair cells (around 125 mV).

Inner Hair Cell Function

When endolymph rushes into an inner hair cell, the hair cell becomes positively charged (i.e., depolarized), which triggers the opening of voltage-sensitive calcium gates. Ca^{2+} moves down its concentration gradient and into the base of the hair cell. The influx of Ca^{2+} facilitates the fusing of synaptic vesicles located at the base of the inner hair cell to the cell membrane by the process of exocytosis. The synaptic vesicles then release the neurotransmitter, glutamate, into the synaptic cleft between the hair cell and the cochlear nerve (Moller, 2013). Glutamate is an excitatory neurotransmitter, and as a result, it can elicit a response in the cochlear nerve. It should be emphasized that the inner hair cells are the only sensory cell within the cochlea that provides afferent stimulation of the cochlear nerve. When inner hair cells are absent or devoid of function, auditory information from that area of the cochlea will not be transmitted to the auditory nervous system. Of note, the Ca^{2+} also binds to the receptors of K+ gates inside the inner hair cell, allowing these gates to open and K+ to leave the cell. The efflux of K+ aids in the restoration of the cell's resting potential.

Outer Hair Cell Function

The outer hair cell does not directly stimulate the afferent cochlear nerve fibers to provide auditory information to the nervous system. Instead, the outer hair cell serves to modulate the cochlear response across a wide range of input sound levels. When the basilar membrane is displaced upward, the transduction gates at the stereocilia open and endolymph rushes into and depolarizes the outer hair cell. Upon depolarization, the outer hair cell contracts along its longitudinal axis. When the basilar membrane deflects downward, the transduction gates close, the resting electrical potential of the hair cell is restored, and the outer hair cell elongates along its longitudinal axis. This movement of the outer hair cell can occur at the same frequency of the stimulating sound. Once again, if a 12,000 Hz sound causes the basilar membrane to move up and down 12,000 times per second, the outer hair cells will also move up and down 12,000 times per second. "Electromotility" is a term used to describe the outer hair cell's ability to change shape in response to a change in its electrical charge.

The movement of the outer hair cell contributes energy into the cochlea and enhances the cochlea's response to low-level sounds. In particular, the movement of the outer hair cells enhances the likelihood that the inner hair cells, which reside above the more rigid spiral lamina and whose stereocilia are not embedded in the tectorial membrane, will respond to low-level sounds. Several possibilities exist for how the electromotile function of the outer

hair cells might facilitate a response from the inner hair cell. First, the oscillating movement of the outer hair cells may contribute mechanical energy to the oscillations of the organ of Corti. However, this possibility likely plays a minimal role in facilitating a response from the inner hair cell, because again, the inner hair cell is relatively incapable of mechanical oscillation due to its position over the relatively rigid pars tecta portion of the cochlea. A second way in which the electromotile function of the outer hair cells may facilitate the response of the inner hair cells is by pulling the tectorial membrane onto the stereocilia of the inner hair cells during the contraction that occurs when the outer hair cell is depolarized. However, this explanation is also unlikely, as the distance between the inner hair cell stereocilia and the tectorial membrane is unlikely to be closed by contraction of the outer hair cells (Hall, 2000). A third and the most plausible explanation for how the outer hair cell electromotility facilitates inner hair cell responses is that the movement of the outer hair cells introduces oscillations into the endolymphatic fluid immediately adjacent to the outer hair cell. The increase in the velocity of fluid displacement subsequent to outer hair cell movement likely facilitates a back-and-forth movement of the inner hair cell stereocilia. Because the energy enhancing the fluid displacement occurs at the same frequency as the stimulating sound, the inner hair cell stereocilia also oscillate at the same frequency, causing the inner hair cell to respond at the stimulating frequency as well.

Without the addition of energy from the electromotile response of the outer hair cells, the inner hair cells would not be stimulated by low-level to moderately low-level sounds (e.g., below 60 dB SPL). In other words, the electromotile function of the outer hair cells serves to enhance audibility for low-level sounds by facilitating stimulation of the inner hair cells. Additionally, because the energy from outer hair cell electromotility is introduced only in the immediate area of the oscillating outer hair cells, the facilitation of inner hair cell stimulation occurs in a relatively localized area of the cochlea corresponding to the frequency of the stimulating sound. Because the energy introduced by the outer hair cell is frequency specific, the electromotile function of the outer hair cell also serves to enhance the frequency selectivity of the cochlea at low to moderate stimulation levels.

At moderate to high levels of stimulation, the displacement of the organ of Corti is rather large and results in endolymphatic displacement with a high enough velocity to sufficiently stimulate the inner hair cells without assistance from the outer hair cells.

At these moderate to high levels, the electromotile response of the outer hair cells reduces or ceases to exist in response to the opening and closing of the transduction channels. The term "saturation" is used to describe the lack of an electromotile response at high levels. Outer hair cell saturation likely occurs because of inhibitory signals received from the efferent auditory system. Specifically, at moderate to high stimulation levels, the efferent auditory fibers from the lower brainstem innervate the outer hair cells with the delivery of the neurotransmitters acetylcholine (ACh) and gamma-aminobutyric acid (GABA) (Musiek & Baran, 2007). ACh likely binds to a receptor that allows Ca^{2+} to enter the outer hair cell and subsequently bind to receptors that open K+ channels, allowing K+ to exit the cell. GABA likely binds to receptors that allow negatively charged Cl– to enter the cell, which also serves to restore the negative resting potential of the cell. The restoration of the negative electrical potential of the outer hair cell causes it to remain in an elongated position, which ceases the electromotile response. The stabilization of the outer hair cell in the elongated position may serve to stabilize the basilar membrane, which may assist in tuning the cochlear response in moderate- to high-level stimulation.

Brief Summary of Cochlear Transduction Process

The primary function of the cochlea is to convert the middle ear's mechanical energy from auditory stimulation into a neuroelectric potential that stimulates the cochlear nerve. The footplate of the stapes rocks back and forth in the oval window of the vestibule when the middle ear ossicles move in response to sound. The stapes movement displaces the perilymphatic fluid in the vestibule, resulting in hydrodynamic oscillations that are transmitted to the organ of Corti via the scala vestibuli. The organ of Corti is bound by the flexible Reissner's membrane superiorly and the basilar membrane inferiorly. The physical characteristics of the organ of Corti change from the base to the apex of the cochlea. The basilar membrane, supporting cells, tectorial membrane, and stereocilia are narrow and stiff at the basal end and wide with greater mass at the apical end. These changes in physical characteristics from base to apex cause high-frequency sounds to be delivered to the base of the cochlea and low-frequency sounds to be delivered to the apex of the cochlea. Von Békésy described a "traveling wave" of displacement that occurs along the basilar membrane, with displacement gradually building from the basal end, reaching a maximum amplitude, and then quickly dissipating. As the organ of Corti oscillates up and down, the stereocilia of the outer hair cells are moved back and forth from the shearing of the tectorial membrane. When the basilar membrane is deflected upward, the stereocilia move medially (i.e., toward the tallest members of their group), and the tension on the stereocilia tiplinks opens transduction gates at the apex of the stereocilia. When the transduction gates open, endolymphatic fluid rushes into the hair cell causing it to be depolarized. When outer hair cells are depolarized, they change in length (i.e., electromotility) and are able to do so at the same frequency as the stimulating sound. The electromotile response of the outer hair cells introduces energy into the adjacent endolymph, which produces oscillations in the endolymphatic fluid. Oscillations of endolymphatic fluid displace the stereocilia of the inner hair cells. When the stereocilia of the inner hair cells are displaced medially, transduction gates open, and endolymph rushes into the cell. The inner hair cell is depolarized and glutamate is released into the synaptic cleft, resulting in stimulation of the cochlear nerve. Low to moderately low level sounds do not produce sufficient oscillation of the endolymphatic fluid to facilitate inner hair cell stimulation. However, the electromotile response of the outer hair cells introduces energy into the adjacent endolymphatic fluid, and the increased velocity in fluid displacement enhances the displacement of the inner hair cell stereocilia. Consequently, the inner hair cell is able to respond in a very frequency-specific manner to low-level sounds (e.g., below 60 dB SPL). As the sound level increases to moderate to high levels (e.g., greater than 60 dB SPL), outer hair cell electromotility saturates, and the endolymphatic displacement is intense enough to sufficiently stimulate the inner hair cells without assistance from the outer hair cells. At moderate to high stimulation levels, outer hair cell saturation likely contributes to stabilization of the organ of Corti.

Cochlear Nerve

The adult cochlear nerve is approximately 2.5 cm in length when measured from the internal auditory meatus to the point where it enters the brainstem at the dorsolateral junction of the pons at its juncture with the medulla oblongata (Moller, 2013). After leaving the brainstem, the cochlear nerve (along with the vestibular and facial nerves) courses anterolaterally through the internal auditory meatus, which is located in the petrous portion of the temporal bone (Figure 3–19).

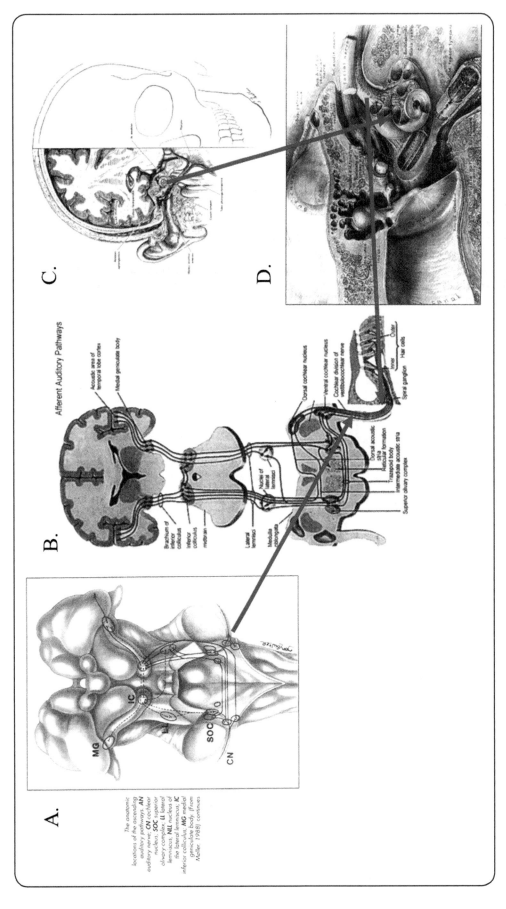

FIGURE 3–19. A visual representation of the location of the modiolus and the entry of the cochlear nerve into the modiolus. **A.** The cochlear-vestibular nerve leaving the brainstem at the dorsolateral junction of the medulla oblongata and pons. Reprinted with permission from Moller, *Hearing: Anatomy, Physiology, and Disorders of the Auditory System, Third Edition* (2013). Copyright © Plural Publishing, Inc. **B.** The cochlear nerve projecting from the auditory nervous system to the cochlea. Reprinted with permission from Tharpe and Seewald, *Comprehensive Handbook of Pediatric Audiology, Second Edition* (2016). Copyright © Plural Publishing, Inc. **C.** The bony cochlea shown in the skull. Reprinted with permission from Moller, *Hearing: Anatomy, Physiology, and Disorders of the Auditory System, Third Edition* (2013). Copyright © Plural Publishing, Inc. **D.** Cross-section of the cochlea with cochlear nerve projecting into the modiolus. Reprinted with permission from Moller, *Hearing: Anatomy, Physiology, and Disorders of the Auditory System, Third Edition* (2013). Copyright © Plural Publishing, Inc.

The internal auditory meatus transitions into the modiolus, the bony core on which the cochlea is wrapped (see Figure 3–19). It can sometimes be difficult to conceptualize anatomy that is not viewed on a daily basis (such as the cochlea and modiolus). Figure 3–19 attempts to provide the reader with a clear perspective of cochlear anatomy in order to allow for a better understanding of how the cochlear nerve travels from the internal auditory meatus to the modiolus to the spiral lamina of the cochlea.

The human cochlear nerve is composed of approximately 30,000 afferent nerve fibers (Moller, 2013). Type I fibers make up 95% of the afferent cochlear nerve fibers. Type I fibers are large, myelinated bipolar nerve fibers, which innervate the inner hair cells

(Moller, 2013). Figure 3–20 provides an illustration of a bipolar cochlear nerve fiber, including the spiral ganglion cell body, the dendritic fiber that innervates the inner hair cell, and the axon that travels through the internal auditory meatus on its way to the cochlear nucleus in the pons of the brainstem.

The remaining 5% of the cochlear nerve fibers are called Type II fibers and are thin, unmyelinated nerve fibers which innervate the outer hair cells. Auditory information from the cochlear nerve is transmitted to the brainstem via Type I nerve fibers. The function of Type II nerve fibers is unclear. Recent research has suggested that the Type II fibers may transmit pain signals when auditory stimulation occurs at levels high enough to cause cochlear damage (Liu et al., 2015).

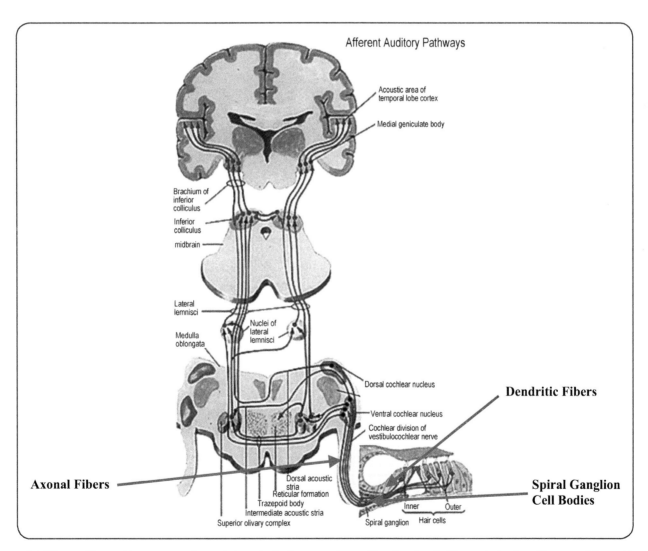

FIGURE 3–20. The cochlear nerve as it travels from the brainstem to the cochlea. Reprinted with permission from Tharpe and Seewald, *Comprehensive Handbook of Pediatric Audiology, Second Edition* (2016). Copyright © Plural Publishing, Inc.

As the cochlear nerve axon fibers leave the modiolus, they are often referred to as radial fibers, because they radiate outward in the direction of the organ of Corti. This radial displacement is similar to the spokes of a bicycle wheel radiating from the center of the wheel to the periphery. The axonal fibers travel from the modiolus into Rosenthal's canal, which is a slightly enlarged opening that branches off from the modiolus and extends from the cochlea (see Figure 3–20). The cochlear spiral ganglion cell bodies reside in Rosenthal's canal (see Figure 3–20). The dendritic fibers extend from the spiral ganglion cell bodies in Rosenthal's canal toward the spiral lamina of the cochlea. At the point at which the spiral lamina enters into the organ of Corti, there are small holes known as habenulae perforata. The Type I afferent cochlear nerve fibers course through habenulae perforata and make a one-to-one connection with an individual inner hair cell. In other words, each individual Type I afferent cochlear nerve fiber innervates only one inner hair cell. However, each inner hair cell is innervated by approximately 20 cochlear nerve fibers (Moller, 2013). Of note, the dendrites of the Type I cochlear nerve fibers are unmyelinated as they course from the habenulae perforata to the hair cell. The Type I fibers are myelinated with Schwann cells from the habenulae perforata to the brainstem, where the myelin sheath is made up of oligodendrocytes.

The Type II cochlear nerve fibers also extend radially from the modiolus through the spiral lamina and into the organ of Corti. Type II fibers pass through the rod of Corti and then abruptly turn and head in a longitudinal direction toward the apex (i.e., perpendicular to the direction of the Type I fibers) (Figure 3–21). The Type II fibers eventually innervate outer hair cells. Because there are substantially more outer hair cells than Type II fibers, the Type II fibers branch out, and each fiber innervates several outer hair cells.

Neuronal Anatomy and Physiology

In order to fully understand the physiology of the cochlear nerve, it is necessary for the reader to possess a basic understanding of neuronal physiology. A knowledge of neuronal physiology will assist the reader in understanding how the auditory system responds to implantable hearing technologies. A basic understanding of neuronal physiology is also necessary for the reader to fully comprehend the application of electrophysiologic measures (e.g., auditory brainstem response [ABR], electrically evoked compound action potential, electrically evoked ABR).

Neuronal Anatomy

The neurons of the cochlear nerve and auditory nervous system are bipolar cells. Bipolar neurons possess a cell body (i.e., soma), dendritic fibers that receive stimulation from hair cells or neighboring neurons, and an axon that delivers stimulation from the neuron's cell body to neighboring neurons (Figure 3–22). The dendritic fibers branch out extensively in several directions in order to expand the area that is able to receive stimulation from nearby sensory cells or neurons. Because the dendritic fibers represent the branches or roots of a tree, the term "arborization" (derived from the Latin word *arbor*, which refers to a tree) is often used to refer to development of the extensive branching of the dendrites that occurs during the first few years of life.

The cell body possesses the neuron's organelles (e.g., nucleus, mitochondria) and cytoplasm. The cytoplasm possesses a high composition of K+ ions and a low composition of Na+ ions. The fluid outside of the neuron (i.e., extracellular fluid) possesses a high composition of Na+ and a low composition of K+. The neuron's plasma membrane possesses ATP-driven protein pumps that actively pump Na+ out of the cell and K+ into the cell. About three Na+ ions are pumped out of the neuron for every two K+ ions that are pumped into the neuron (Figure 3–23). The difference in ionic composition between the internal and external environment of the neuron results in a difference in charge between the two locations. Specifically, at rest, the high composition of Na+ ions outside of the neuron create a positive voltage in the extracellular fluid immediately outside the cell and a negative electrical potential of about −70 mV inside the neuron (see Figure 3–23).

The cell body gives rise to the neuron's axon. The base of the axon is known as the axon hillock. The axon extends away from the cell body, eventually terminating in small branches known as telodendria, and synaptic knobs exist at the tips of the telodendria (see Figure 3–22). Synaptic vesicles, which possess neurotransmitter substance, reside within the synaptic knobs. The synaptic knobs typically reside adjacent to the dendrites of neighboring neurons. A small gap, called a synaptic cleft, exists between the axon of one neuron and the dendrite or cell body of a neighboring neuron.

The axon is insulated by a fatty substance known as myelin. Supporting cells called Schwann cells make up the myelin of neurons in the peripheral nervous system, and supporting cells called oligodendrocytes make up the myelin present in the central nervous system. The myelin sheath completely wraps around the

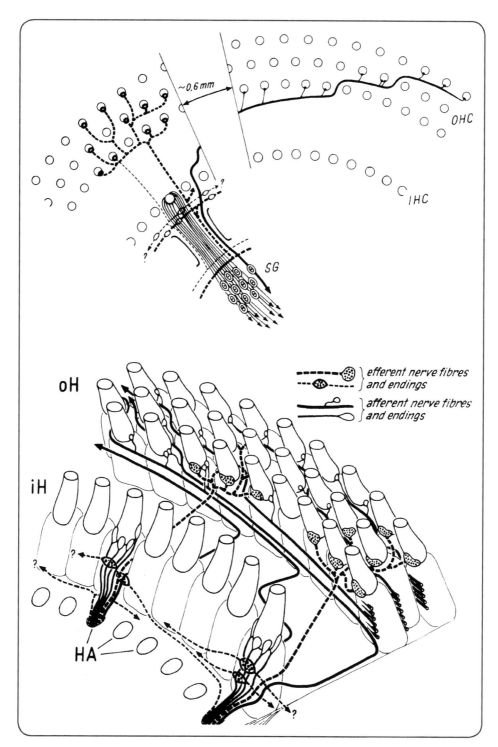

FIGURE 3–21. A visual illustration of how the cochlear nerve fibers innervate the cochlear hair cells. Reprinted with permission from Møller, *Hearing: Anatomy, Physiology, and Disorders of the Auditory System, Third Edition* (2013). Copyright © Plural Publishing, Inc.

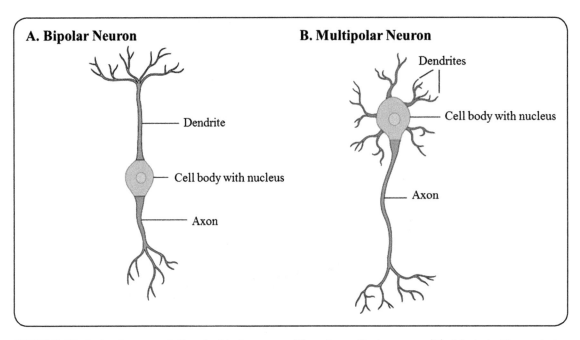

FIGURE 3–22. A visual representation of a bipolar neuron (**A**), and a multipolar neuron (**B**). Adapted with permission from Andreatta, *Neuroscience Fundamentals for Communication Sciences and Disorders* (in press). Copyright © Plural Publishing, Inc.

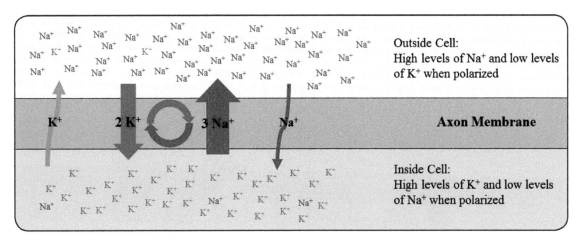

FIGURE 3–23. A visual representation of the sodium-potassium pump.

axon like the breading of a corn dog or a jelly roll. However, there are small gaps or voids in the myelin sheath throughout the length of the axon. These gaps in the myelin insulation are called nodes of Ranvier and along with the myelin sheath give the axon the appearance of sausages that are strung together (see Figure 3–22).

Neuronal Physiology

When a neuron is at rest, Na+ ions are attracted to the internal environment of the cell because they seek to move down their electrical and concentration gradients. In other words, opposites attract, and the abundance of Na+ ions are attracted to the negative electrical environment and low composition of Na+ inside the neuron. However, the cell membrane is relatively impermeable to these Na+ ions and the sodium-potassium pumps within the neuron's plasma membrane work to keep Na+ outside of the cell. Several types of stimuli can alter the permeability of the cell membrane to Na+. These stimuli include chemical, electrical, thermal, physical, light, and so forth. When Na+

ions enter into the neuron, the neuron's electrical potential becomes more positive. A graded potential occurs when a stimulus acts upon a cell to temporarily alter its membrane permeability, allow Na+ to enter, and make the electrical potential more positive.

If the stimulus is strong enough, the neuron's electrical potential will reach a voltage threshold (approximately 50 mV) that will trigger the open-

ing of numerous voltage-sensitive gates that allow the entry of positively charged Na+ ions, which rush down their electrical and concentration gradients (Figure 3–24). The sudden opening of these gates and the subsequent entry of Na+ ions cause the electrical potential inside the neuron to quickly and temporarily assume a positive value (e.g., 35 mV). The opening of the voltage-sensitive gates, the sudden influx of

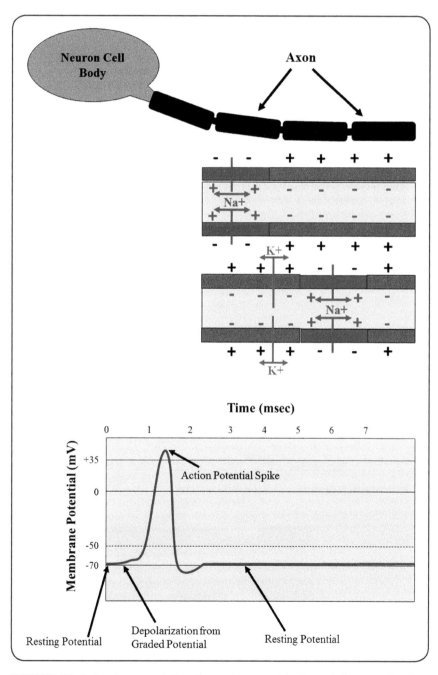

FIGURE 3–24. A visual representation of an action potential spike and of propagation of an action potential along an axon.

Na+, and the increase in the neuron's electrical potential collectively are referred to as an **action potential**. The action potential is a very brief event (less than 2 msec), because the positive potential inside the neuron triggers the opening of gates that allow K+ to exit the cell. The K+ ions are driven out of the neuron, because they are repelled by the positive charge inside the neuron and attracted to the low concentration of K+ outside of the cell. Additionally, when an action potential occurs, the Na+ gates temporarily close, preventing the further influx of Na+ ions (see Figure 3–24). This temporary period in which Na+ cannot enter into the cell and the neuron's electrical potential cannot increase in positivity is referred to as the **refractory period**. When a neuron's electrical potential becomes more positive than its resting potential, it is said to be depolarized. When a neuron becomes more negative than its resting potential, it is said to be hyperpolarized. Hyperpolarization temporarily occurs after an action potential, because the combination of the Na+ gates closing and the K+ rushing out of the neuron results in a momentary reduction in the electrical potential of the neuron.

The stimulus that elicits an action potential can be received at any location of a neuron. However, the stimulus is usually received at the dendrites, because of their relatively large surface area due to the extensive branching or to the cell body. The action potential is transmitted to the axon hillock, and from there, it is propagated down the axon. The propagation of an action potential typically occurs in a direction from the hillock toward the telodendria, because temporary closure of Na+ gates (i.e., the refractory period) prevents the Na+ ions from entering behind the action potential. The axon can be a relatively long structure, and as a result, the propagation of the action potential down the length of the axon would be time consuming if it had to continuously travel down the entire length of the axon. The function of the myelin sheath is to expedite the propagation of the axon potential as it travels down the axon. The insulation of the myelin sheath prevents ionic transfer across the membrane of the axon. However, ions can cross the axon membrane at the nodes of Ranvier (Figure 3–25). Consequently, action potential "hops" from one node of Ranvier to the next in a process called salutatory conduction. Injuries to the myelin sheath (like what occur with multiple sclerosis) reduce the efficiency of neural transmission.

When the action potential arrives at the synaptic knob, the spike in positivity opens Ca²⁺ gates, and Ca²⁺ ions rush into the neuron. The entry of calcium ions causes the synaptic vesicles located in the synaptic knob to fuse with the membrane at the tip of the

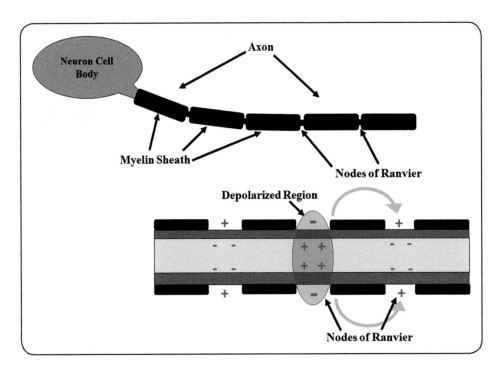

FIGURE 3–25. A visual representation of the nodes of Ranvier that exist in a myelinated axon.

axon via exocytosis and release a neurotransmitter substance into the synaptic cleft (Campbell, 1990). The neurotransmitter varies across neurons and sensory cells. In the auditory system, glutamate is the neurotransmitter released by the inner hair cells onto the dendritic fibers of the cochlear nerve.

Neurotransmitters bind to the receptors of neighboring neurons and influence the behavior of gates that are associated with the receptors (Figure 3–26). For instance, glutamate released by the inner hair cell binds to a receptor that opens a gate that allows Na+ ions to rush into the neuron, which increases the neuron's electrical potential and pushes it toward its action potential threshold. In this example, glutamate is an excitatory neurotransmitter, because it increases the likelihood that an action potential will be produced in the receiving neuron. It is worth noting that a neurotransmitter is a chemical substance, and consequently, stimulation of a neuron by a neu-

rotransmitter is an example of a neural response that is facilitated by a chemical stimulus. Other neurotransmitters may act as inhibitory neurotransmitters. For example, an inhibitory neuron may bind with a receptor that opens a CL– gate, allowing negatively charged chloride ions to enter and make the neuron's electrical potential more negative.

Most neurons form synapses with a large number of other neurons. Some of these connections may provide excitatory signals, whereas others provide inhibitory signals. The sum of these excitatory and inhibitory stimuli are integrated by the receiving neuron. If the stimulation is dominated by excitatory neurons, then it is likely that the action potential threshold will be exceeded and the neuron will fire (i.e., produce an action potential). If an action potential is indeed elicited, then it will likely propagate to the tip of the axon of the receiving neuron, and a neurotransmitter will be released from its axon into

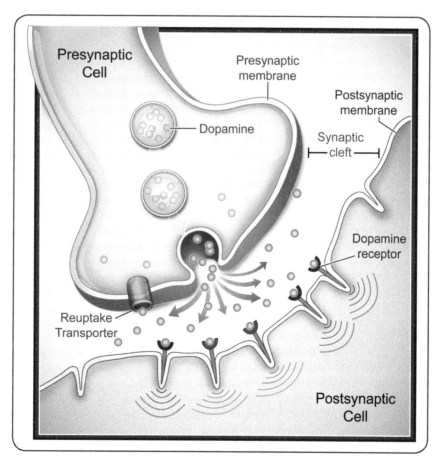

FIGURE 3–26. A visual representation of a neural synapse. Reprinted with permission from Hoit and Weismer, *Foundations of Speech and Hearing: Anatomy and Physiology* (2018). Copyright © Plural Publishing, Inc.

the synaptic cleft adjacent to the dendrite of a neighboring neuron. This wave of positivity (i.e., action potentials) will conceivably propagate from one set of auditory neurons to another from the peripheral auditory system (i.e., cochlear nerve) to the auditory cortex (Figure 3–27).

Response Properties of the Cochlear Nerve

The aforementioned discussion of neuronal physiology provides an explanation for how auditory neurons respond to stimulation. It is also important to note that the cochlear nerve possesses a spontaneous firing rate, which refers to random firing of the neuron in the absence of any stimulation. About 60% of the cochlear nerve fibers possess a relatively fast spontaneous firing rate (80 discharges per second or higher). Almost 25% of cochlear nerve fibers possess moderate spontaneous rates, and the remaining 15% have slow spontaneous rates (approximately 20 discharges per second) (Musiek & Baran, 2007). Neu-

rons with fast spontaneous firing rates typically are sensitive to low-level stimuli (i.e., down to the levels consistent with normal hearing) and have relatively narrow dynamic ranges (i.e., the neurons cease to increase their firing rates at moderate to high input levels [neural saturation]), whereas neurons with slower spontaneous firing rates tend have thresholds at moderate to higher input levels and wider dynamic ranges (i.e., their firing rates increase with increases in stimulating level over a wide range of input levels). Theoretically, the nerve fibers with fast firing rates likely code low-level signals (e.g., near threshold, soft speech in quiet), while nerve fibers with slower spontaneous rates are likely to code high-level signals (e.g., speech in moderate to high-level noise).

Phase-Locked Responses of the Cochlear Nerve

Phase-locked responsiveness is an important property of cochlear nerve function in regard to cochlear implantation. Phase-locked responsiveness refers to

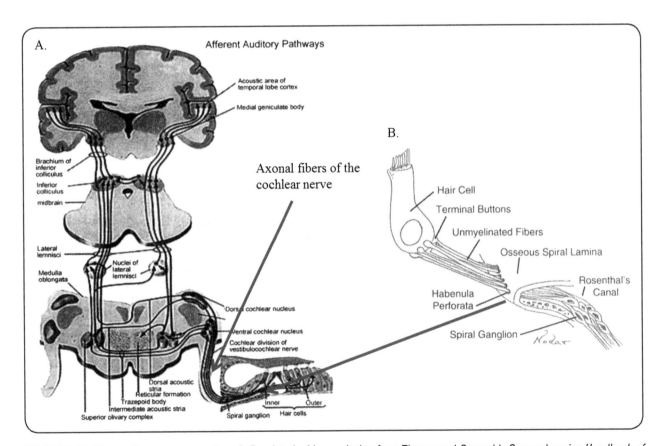

FIGURE 3–27. The auditory nervous system. **A.** Reprinted with permission from Tharpe and Seewald, *Comprehensive Handbook of Pediatric Audiology, Second Edition* (2016). Copyright © Plural Publishing, Inc. **B.** Reprinted with permission from Musiek & Baran, *The Auditory System: Anatomy, Physiology, and Clinical Correlates* (2016). Copyright © Plural Publishing, Inc.

the fact that the cochlear nerve is time-locked to the waveform of sound so that it responds at the same phase from one cycle of the sound to the next cycle. Figure 3–28A provides an example of a phase-locked response of a single cochlear nerve fiber to a sinusoidal stimulus. As shown, the nerve fiber responds at almost the exact same point in the cycle (i.e., 90 degrees) of the periodic signal. In this example, it is important to note that the individual cochlear nerve fiber did not produce a neural discharge to every cycle of the signal. This is likely attributed to the inability to fire at such a fast rate due to the refractory period of the nerve fiber. However, if a large number of cochlear nerve fibers within a localized area of the cochlea (remember that each inner hair cell is innervated by 10 to 20 Type I cochlear nerve fibers) responded to the signal in Figure 3–28B, some nerve fibers will respond to one cycle while neighboring fibers are in their refractory period. Then for the next cycle, the initial nerve fibers that responded will be in their refractory period, but fibers that did not respond to the preceding cycle may respond to the next cycle. The volley principle proposes that a group of neighboring cochlear nerve fibers may alternate in their response patterns so that collectively they respond on each cycle of the stimulating sound (see Figure 3–28B) (Wever, 1949). Phase-locking occurs for sounds with frequencies as high as about 4000 Hz

but is not present at higher frequencies (Palmer & Russell, 1986).

The phase-locked responsiveness of the cochlear nerve along with the volley principle are relevant because they offer another mechanism (along with the place principle) that the auditory system could use to code frequency and pitch. Specifically, the temporal property of the cochlear nerve response could be used to convey information about the frequency of the incoming sound. Most physiologic studies have concluded that a cochlear nerve fiber could not respond in phase on a cycle-by-cycle basis with a stimulus beyond no more than a few hundred Hz. However, the volley principle suggests that a group of nerve fibers may respond at an integer multiple of the frequency of the stimulating sound, and as result, the temporal response pattern of the cochlear nerve could provide information about the spectral composition of a sound up to at least several thousand Hz. Additionally, Moller (2001) has theorized that neurons in the auditory nervous system may be particularly adept at integrating and processing the temporal code provided by the phase-locked response pattern of the cochlear nerve.

It should be noted that the phase-locking observed in the cochlear nerve in response to acoustic stimulation is attributed to inner hair cell physiology. Specifically, the hair cell is stimulated and potentially

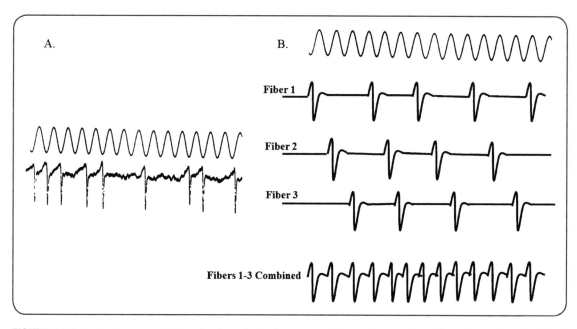

FIGURE 3–28. A visual representation of a phase-locked response of the auditory system (**A**), and the volley principle of neural conduction (**B**).

releases a neurotransmitter only when the basilar membrane is deflected toward the scala media and the stereocilia are deflected laterally. As a result, the hair cell is predisposed to stimulate the cochlear nerve at the same phase from one cycle to the next. Of course, when electrical stimulation is provided by a cochlear implant, the hair cells are typically bypassed (and are also typically non-functional), so the natural basis for phase-locking is eliminated.

Stochasticity of the Cochlear Nerve

Stochasticity of the cochlear nerve response refers to the fact that an individual cochlear nerve fiber does not perfectly respond to the mechanical response of the cochlea (Marmel et al., 2015). In other words, the cochlear nerve does not fire at a rate equal to the rate at which the stereocilia are displaced back and forth and the inner hair cells are depolarized. Instead, as shown in Figure 3–27, an individual cochlear nerve fiber follows a waveform in phase but fires in a quasi-random manner but at integer multiples of the stimulating frequency. An important aspect of stochasticity is the fact that this random variation in neural discharge is independent across cochlear nerve fibers. The random variation in neural discharge and the independence of individual cochlear nerve fibers creates a condition in which groups of neighboring nerve fibers can collectively respond to a signal and can code the temporal properties of that signal via the volley principle.

The property of stochasticity may also provide cues about the level and duration of a sound. As sound level increases above threshold, the probability of an individual cochlear nerve fiber firing increases. Also, the probability of neural discharge increases as the stimulus duration increases. Therefore, the temporal response of cochlear nerve fibers can potentially provide cues regarding the spectral, intensity, and duration properties of a stimulating sound.

Implications of Electrical Stimulation of the Cochlear Nerve on Dynamic Range, Phase-Locked Responsiveness, and Stochasticity

Cochlear implants typically stimulate the cochlear nerve with a biphasic, rectangular electrical pulse. The reader may recognize the fact that a brief duration rectangular electrical pulse (100-microsecond pulse duration) is used to generate a click-stimulus for auditory brainstem response assessment. A stimulus with a brief duration takes advantage of the fact

that the majority of auditory neurons possess what is often referred to as an onset-response property. In other words, the neuron discharges at the onset of a stimulus. Figure 3–29 provides examples of response properties of auditory neurons. A brief stimulus elicits a response from a large number of onset-responsive auditory neurons, and this collective (i.e., compound) is large enough to be detected by electrodes located on the surface of the head.

Similarly, a brief rectangular electrical pulse elicits a response from most every cochlear nerve fiber adjacent to the electrode contact from which the stimulus is delivered. Also, the rate at which the cochlear nerve's neural discharges increase is quite rapid, because the compression that occurs at the basilar membrane via the active, outer hair cell function is bypassed. As such, the cochlear nerve's discharge rate moves from threshold values to saturation very quickly. As a result, the dynamic range of the cochlear nerve to electrical stimulation is typically 10 to 20 dB (Bilger, 1977; Fourcin et al., 1979). Cochlear implant signal processing utilizes slow-acting compression to fit a wide range of acoustic inputs (e.g., 25–100 dB

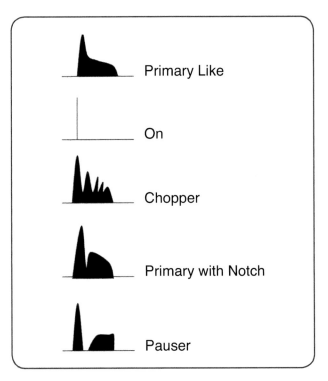

FIGURE 3–29. A visual representation of the various types of response properties of auditory neurons. Reprinted with permission from Musiek and Baran, *The Auditory System: Anatomy, Physiology, and Clinical Correlates* (2016). Copyright © Plural Publishing, Inc.

SPL) into the relatively narrow electrical dynamic range of the cochlear nerve.

Additionally, because most all of the cochlear nerve fibers respond in unison to an electrical pulse, they also all resort to a refractory state as a group. As a result, the stochasticity of the cochlear nerve is essentially eliminated. Studies have shown that the cochlear implant users can detect changes in frequency with changes in the electrical pulse rate up to about 300 pulses per second. The refractory period likely limits cochlear implant recipients from using phase-locking to process temporal changes beyond a few hundred Hz. Furthermore, the auditory system is less likely to use the volley principle to code spectral information via temporal responsiveness, because the electrical stimulation facilitates a simultaneous response from responding nerve fibers. In essence, an electrical pulse oversynchronizes the collective response of the cochlear nerve fibers, and as a result, a cochlear implant recipient is unlikely to use the temporal response pattern of the cochlear nerve to code spectral information above 300 Hz, changes in level near threshold, or changes in sound duration. Some researchers have theorized that the use of high stimulation rates (e.g., several thousand pulses per second) may promote stochasticity (Matsuoka et al., 2001; Rubinstein et al., 1999), because variability in the refractory rate of different nerve fibers would result in some nerve fibers being ready to respond to an individual pulse, whereas others do not but are available to respond to a proceeding pulse. However, it should be noted that there are no studies demonstrating improved phase-locking (i.e., temporal processing) with fast stimulation rates. In short, beyond about 300 Hz, spectral processing is likely dependent upon the place of electrical stimulation. Furthermore, cochlear implant recipients are unlikely to use changes in electrical pulse stimulation rate to code temporal information beyond a few hundred Hz; therefore, electrical stimulation is more likely to provide amplitude envelope cues (i.e., changes in sound intensity as a function of time that occur on the order of 2–50 Hz) and less likely to faithfully code fine temporal structure (i.e., rapid changes in sound intensity that occur on the order of a couple of hundred Hz to several thousand Hz).

Tonotopic Organization: Relationship of the Basilar Membrane to the Cochlear Nerve

The Greenwood function is a model that assigns a characteristic response frequency to a particular loca-

tion in the cochlea (Greenwood, 1961, 1990). It is important to note that the Greenwood function is based on stimulation at the basilar membrane. Stakhovskaya and colleagues (2007) measured the length of the cochlear duct and the spiral ganglion in nine cadavers. Stakhovskaya et al. also stained cochlear nerve fibers so that they could follow the fibers from the organ of Corti to the spiral ganglion, which allowed them to create a frequency-position map for the spiral ganglion that would correspond to a Greenwood-based tonotopic location in the cochlea. Stakhovskaya and colleagues found that the length of the spiral ganglion (12.54–14.62 mm) was considerably shorter than the length of the organ of Corti (30.5–36.87 mm when measured at the pillar cells). Additionally, they noted that the radial cochlear nerve fibers in the most apical 40% of the organ of Corti are compressed into the most apical 20% of the spiral ganglion. Considering Stakhovskaya's observations, the Greenwood function does not entirely explain the relationship between the location of a cochlear implant electrode contact and the frequency of neural stimulation.

Stakhovskaya's work has several functional implications pertaining to cochlear implantation. First, because of the compressed tonotopical organization of the apical spiral ganglion fibers relative to the organ of Corti, it may be beneficial to space low-frequency, apical electrode contacts more closely together in order to allow for frequency resolution in the apical region to be equal to what is provided in the basal region. Secondly, the position of the electrode array in the cochlea has a substantial impact on the insertion depth required to stimulate a desired frequency range. Periomodiolar electrode arrays are designed to be positioned close to the modiolus (i.e., on the medial wall of the scala tympani), whereas straight electrode arrays are more inclined to be positioned along the lateral wall of the scala tympani. Theoretically, the position of a perimodiolar electrode array should facilitate stimulation of the spiral ganglion cell bodies, while lateral wall electrode arrays would be better positioned to stimulate the dendritic fibers of the cochlear nerve. Because of the relatively short distance of the spiral ganglion, Stakhovskaya's measurements estimate that a perimodiolar electrode array must be inserted 17 mm into the cochlea to cover the entire length of the spiral ganglion. In contrast, a lateral wall electrode array must be inserted approximately 33 mm into the cochlea to entirely cover the length of the organ of Corti. Of note, research has shown that the dendritic radial nerve fibers began to degenerate relatively quickly after the onset of damage to the organ of Corti (McFadden et al., 2004; Nadol et al., 1989; Otte et al., 1978). In such an event, electrical current delivered from a lateral wall electrode array would need to travel a greater distance to facilitate stimulation in the spiral ganglion cell bodies. In contrast, the spiral ganglion cell bodies tend to survive for an extended period of time following deafness (Fayad et al., 1991; Kahn et al., 2005; Nadol, 1997).

Ascending Auditory Nervous System

The ascending auditory nervous system is composed of a hierarchy of interconnected groups of auditory nuclei that extend from the cochlear nucleus in the pons to the auditory cortex. Figure 3–20 provides an illustration of the primary structures in the ascending auditory nervous system. Of note, tonotopic organization is observed throughout these groups of nuclei.

Cochlear Nuclei

All of the afferent auditory nerve fibers from the inner hair cells innervate the cochlear nucleus, a group of auditory neurons located in the dorsolateral pons near to the juncture of the medulla oblongata (Musiek & Baran, 2007). The cochlear nucleus is the only group of neurons in the ascending auditory pathway that receives input only from the ipsilateral ear. The cochlear nucleus is composed of three divisions, the anterior ventral cochlear nucleus, the posterior ventral cochlear nucleus, and the dorsal cochlear nucleus. Although all three of the divisions of the cochlear nucleus contribute to auditory processing, the anterior ventral cochlear nucleus is most likely the section that plays the primary role in transmitting auditory information along the ascending auditory pathway. Of note, all three divisions are tonotopically organized. In general, low-frequency sounds are processed laterally and ventrally and high-frequency sounds are processed medially and dorsally. However, it should be noted that the tonotopic organization of the cochlear nucleus and the remainder of the auditory nervous system is not nearly as clearly defined as the tonotopic organization that exists within the cochlea.

Additionally, the cochlear nucleus is made up of several different types of neurons, including pyramidal, octopus, stellate, spherical, globular, and multipolar (Musiek & Baran, 2007). These different types of cells possess different response properties. For instance, the spherical cells, which are located in the anterior ventral cochlear nucleus, produce an initial spiked response followed by a steady response until the stimulus stops. Other cells produce a transient spiked response at the onset of a stimulus with no response thereafter. In contrast, pyramidal cells gradually increase their response amplitude with stimulus duration. Although the exact contribution of these different types of neurons and response properties is unclear, it is very likely that the neurons of the cochlear nucleus play a large role in maintaining the exquisite timing needed for processing timing information that is critical for speech recognition in noise and localization.

Superior Olivary Complex

The cochlear nucleus projects several fiber tracts medially and ventrally to the superior olivary complex, which is a group of neurons in the ventral, medial pons. The majority of the auditory information from the cochlear nucleus is delivered to the superior olivary complex contralateral to the stimulated ear (in fact, about 80% of the auditory information from the cochlear nucleus crosses the lower pons and travels up the contralateral ascending auditory pathway via the superior olivary complex or the lateral lemniscus) (Musiek & Baran, 2007). As a result, the superior olivary complex is the first group of neurons in the auditory system to receive input from both ears. The superior olivary complex is composed of two divisions, the medial superior olivary nucleus and the lateral olivary complex. The medial superior olivary nucleus primarily responds to low-frequency stimuli, while the lateral superior olivary body responds to a wider range of frequencies. The neurons in the medially superior olivary nucleus are sensitive to interaural timing/phase differences, which are critical for speech recognition in noise and for localizing low-frequency sounds (Moller, 2013). The neurons in the lateral superior olivary body are sensitive to interaural level differences, which are important for localizing high-frequency sounds (Moller et al., 2013).

Binaural Processing in the Auditory Nervous System

Figure 3–30 provides an example for why interaural timing-phase information is the dominant cue for

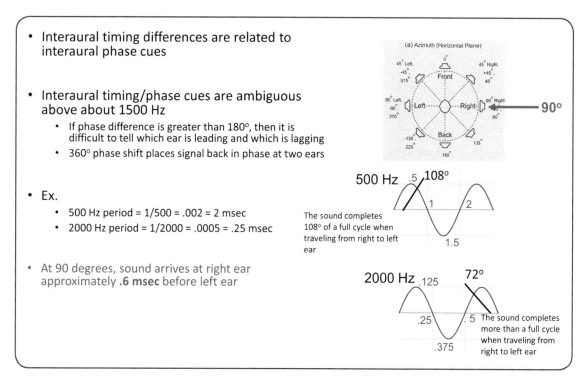

- Interaural timing differences are related to interaural phase cues

- Interaural timing/phase cues are ambiguous above about 1500 Hz
  - If phase difference is greater than 180°, then it is difficult to tell which ear is leading and which is lagging
  - 360° phase shift places signal back in phase at two ears

- Ex.
  - 500 Hz period = 1/500 = .002 = 2 msec
  - 2000 Hz period = 1/2000 = .0005 = .25 msec

- At 90 degrees, sound arrives at right ear approximately .6 msec before left ear

FIGURE 3–30. A visual representation of how the auditory system processes interaural timing/phase cues to localize sound.

processing low-frequency sounds, whereas interaural intensity differences are the dominant cue for processing high-frequency sounds. The head in Figure 3–30 has a diameter of 17.5 cm (similar to the average adult head). Based on a sound propagation velocity of 340 m/sec, a sound arising from 90 degrees azimuth will reach the right ear 0.6 msec faster than it reaches the left ear. The period of a 500 Hz pure tone is 2 msec. As a result, let's say that when a 500 Hz pure tone that originates from 90 degrees azimuth reaches the right ear, the tone is at a phase of 0 degrees. By the time it reaches the left ear, the tone will have moved through 30 percent of its cycle (0.6 msec/ 2 msec). Thirty percent of a 360 degree cycle is 108 degrees. Therefore, the 500 Hz pure tone reaching the left ear will be 108 degrees out of phase with the 500 Hz pure tone that reached the right ear at a phase 0 degrees.

Now, let's look at the same example for a 2000 Hz pure tone. A 2000 Hz pure tone has a period of 0.5 msec. If the 2000 Hz pure tone originates from 90 degrees azimuth, it will have completed a full cycle of its waveform (in 5 msec) and begin a second cycle (72° into the second cycle) before reaching the left

ear. Consequently, the interaural phase difference for the 2000 Hz pure tone is ambiguous. As may be seen from these examples, interaural timing and phase cues are related, because the phase differences are associated with the time required to complete one cycle of the waveform (i.e., the period). In short, interaural phase cues may be used to localize sounds below about 1500 Hz but are unreliable cues above 1500 Hz. Hence, it is not surprising that the low-frequency-sensitive neurons residing in the medial superior olivary body are sensitive to interaural timing/phase differences.

Furthermore, it should be noted that interaural timing/phase differences are important cues for speech recognition in noise. The **masking level difference** describes an improvement in detection that occurs in the diotic (i.e., identical stimuli presented to both ears) or dichotic (i.e., different stimuli presented to each ear) condition relative to the monotic condition (i.e., stimulus presented to only one ear). For example, the detection threshold for a speech signal presented in the presence of masking noise that is identical between two ears is about 15 dB poorer than when the same signal is presented in the presence of noise that is 180 degrees out-of-phase between the two ears. This release from masking that occurs because of the binaural auditory system's ability to capitalize uon interaural phase differences is likely attributable to processing of interaural timing/phase cues by neurons in the medial superior olivary body of the superior olivary complex. The ability to recognize a signal of interest in the presence of ongoing competing noise is often referred to as the **cocktail party effect**. The processing of interaural timing/phase cues is also likely to be important for use of **binaural squelch**, which is the ability to attend to the ear with a more favorable signal-to-noise ratio (SNR) via central processing of interaural time and intensity differences (Balkany & Zeitler, 2013).

High-frequency sounds are localized on the basis of interaural intensity cues. Let's say that a 4000 Hz tone originates from 90 degrees azimuth. A 4000 Hz pure tone has a wavelength of 8.5 cm (340 m/sec /4000 Hz = 8.5 cm). The diameter of the head (17.5 cm) is much larger than the wavelength of the 4000 Hz pure tone, and as a result, the head reflects much of the energy of the sound. The reflection of the head to high-frequency sounds is known as the **head shadow effect**, because in this example, an acoustic shadow is cast over the left ear. Consequently, the intensity at the left ear is about 10 dB lower than the intensity at the right ear (Kuhn, 1987).

Now, let's look at what happens for a 500 Hz pure tone. The wavelength of a 500 Hz pure tone is 68 cm. Thus, a 500 Hz pure tone is relatively large compared with the average diameter of the head. Consequently, a 500 Hz pure tone will "bend around" the head and arrive at the left ear with a similar intensity as what occurs for the right ear. Therefore, the interaural level difference is not a robust cue for localizing low-frequency sounds. Specifically, interaural level differences are reliable cues for the localization of sounds above about 1500 Hz but are relatively unusable for sounds below 1500 Hz.

Finally, the binaural auditory system also creates a phenomenon referred to as binaural summation, which is the sensation that a sound is louder or more perceptually salient when heard with two ears compared with just one ear alone. Binaural summation is mediated in the central auditory nervous system (i.e., the auditory brainstem and cortex). Binaural summation improves detection of low-level sounds by 2 to 6 dB (Moller, 2013; Yost, 1994). Binaural summation also contributes to an improvement in speech recognition in noise.

Implications for Processing of Interaural Cues in Implantable Hearing Technologies

Binaural processing is a matter of great interest in implantable hearing technologies. For hearing aid users, binaural interaural phase cues can be distorted but not eliminated when the external ear is occluded. Studies have shown better speech recognition in noise and localization when the external auditory meatus is open relative to the occluded condition (Winkler, Latzel, & Holube, 2016). One potential benefit of many middle ear implantable hearing devices is the potential to keep the external auditory meatus open during device use. Additionally, one of the primary benefits of electric-acoustic stimulation (e.g., hybrid cochlear implants) for people with post-operative preservation of low-frequency acoustic hearing is improvement in speech recognition in noise and localization compared with electric-only stimulation for the implanted ear.

As previously discussed, cochlear implant recipients typically struggle to code temporal information beyond 300 Hz with electrical stimulation of the auditory nerve (Clark, 1969). As a result, many cochlear implant users show limited ability to capitalize on the use of interaural timing/phase cues for speech recognition in noise (e.g., binaural squelch) and for localization of low-frequency sounds (Schafer et al., 2011). The deficiency in binaural squelch and the use of interaural phase cues have been a driving force behind the development and use of electric-acoustic stimulation. Improvements in speech recognition in noise and in localization for electric-only cochlear implant users are primarily attributed to use of the head shadow effect, binaural redundancy, and use of interaural intensity cues. More information on binaural auditory processing in children and adults with cochlear implants will be provided in Chapter 19. Binaural processing of electric-acoustic users will be discussed in greater detail in Chapter 23.

Furthermore, it should be noted that the electrode array of auditory brainstem implants is typically placed on the cochlear nucleus. Because the tonotopic organization of the cochlear nucleus is not as clearly defined as the cochlea, the desired placement of the electrode array for an auditory brainstem is not always clear. Electrically evoked auditory brainstem response assessment is often used during surgery to guide the surgeon in placing the electrode array on a location that will elicit an auditory response. Pitch matching is ideally completed during auditory brainstem implant programming in order to determine the pitch percept elicited by the different active electrodes. Finally, some have proposed a penetrating electrode array that possesses leads that may be placed at varying depths into the cochlear nucleus in an attempt to take advantage of the lateral-to-medial tonotopic organization of the cochlear nucleus.

Lateral Lemniscus and Inferior Colliculus

The lateral lemniscus is the primary ascending pathway in the brainstem and serves to transmit auditory information from the pons to the inferior colliculus. The inferior colliculus is a large group of auditory neurons on the dorsal surface of the midbrain. It is located about 3 to 3.5 cm superior to the point at which the cochlear nerve enters the brainstem. There are approximately 250,000 neurons in the inferior colliculus, a fact that underscores the increase in complexity from the peripheral auditory system (e.g., 30,000 cochlear nerve fibers) throughout the auditory nervous system (Moller, 2013; Musiek & Baran, 2007).

All auditory information from the brainstem synapses at the inferior colliculus before being transmitted to the thalamus and/or auditory cortex. The inferior colliculus is made up of a diverse contingent of neurons with different response properties. These neurons assist in the processing of temporal information in the auditory signal. There are neurons in the inferior colliculus that are sensitive to interaural timing cues and other neurons that are sensitive to interaural intensity cues. As a result, the inferior colliculus assists in localization. Of note, the superior colliculus is a group of visual neurons located immediately rostral to the inferior colliculus. Auditory and visual information are likely integrated at the levels of the inferior and superior colliculi to assist in reflexes that orient the eyes toward the direction from which a sound arrives. The brachium of the inferior colliculus is a large, myelinated fiber tract that transmits auditory information to the ipsilateral thalamus. Of note, in some cases in which severe neural atrophy exists for recipients with neurofibromatosis type 2, the stimulating electrodes of an auditory brainstem implant will be placed on the inferior colliculus rather than the cochlear nucleus.

Medial Geniculate Body of the Thalamus

The medial geniculate body of the thalamus resides in the lower dorsolateral surface of the thalamus. The medial geniculate body is composed of a group of neurons that process auditory information. The medial geniculate body is made up of three divisions, the ventral, dorsal, and medial divisions. The ventral division is the section that primarily responds to ascending auditory information.

The Cerebrum: The Auditory Cortices and Auditory Responsive Areas of the Brain

Thalamo-cortical fibers project from the medial geniculate nucleus of the thalamus to the auditory cortex. The cortex is composed of several layers of neurons that are about 3 to 4 mm thick and make up the surface of the brain. The majority of the auditory information from the thalamus arrives at the ipsilateral primary auditory cortex, which is also known as Heschl's gyrus or the transverse gyrus (e.g., Brodmann's area 41) (Figure 3–31). Heschl's gyrus is not easily observed from the outside of the brain. However, if part of the parietal and temporal lobes are removed, Heschl's gyrus is readily viewable (see Figure 3–31).

Auditory information in the primary auditory cortex projects to the secondary auditory cortex. Secondary auditory cortex has traditionally been defined as a belt that surrounds the primary auditory cortex and includes several structures, such as the supramarginal gyrus, the angular gyrus, the superior temporal gyrus, and the planum temporale (Figure 3–32). The secondary auditory cortex, which is also referred to as the association auditory area, projects auditory information throughout the rest of the cerebrum. Additionally, secondary auditory cortex delivers efferent fibers to the primary auditory cortex to modulate the response of lower levels of the auditory system. Of note, Wernicke's area (Brodmann area 42) resides in the secondary auditory cortex. A more detailed discussion of the primary and secondary auditory cortices and the role each plays in auditory and language function will be provided later in this chapter.

There are several other areas in the brain that are responsive to auditory information. Regions in the inferior frontal lobe and the inferior parietal lobe also contribute to auditory processing. Furthermore, additional areas in the temporal lobe, the insula, and the claustrum are all sensitive to sound. Of interest, several auditory areas of the cerebrum are noted to be longer/larger on the left side of the brain (Musiek & Baran, 2007). Also, research has shown the left hemisphere to be more responsive to speech stimuli, whereas the right hemisphere is more responsive

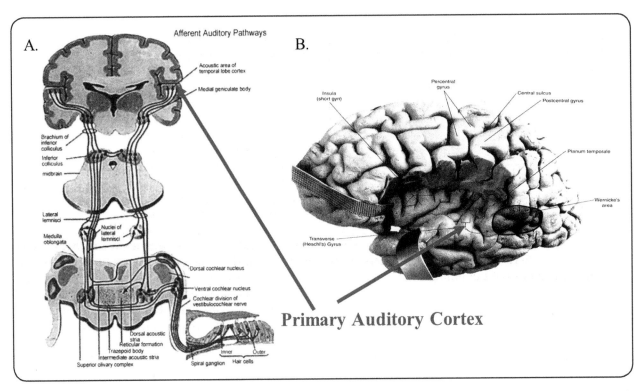

FIGURE 3–31. The primary auditory cortex. **A.** Reprinted with permission from Tharpe and Seewald, *Comprehensive Handbook of Pediatric Audiology, Second Edition* (2016). Copyright © Plural Publishing, Inc. **B.** Reprinted with permission from Bhatnagar, *Neuroscience for the Study of Communicative Disorders, Second Edition* (2002). Copyright © Lippincott Williams & Wilkins.

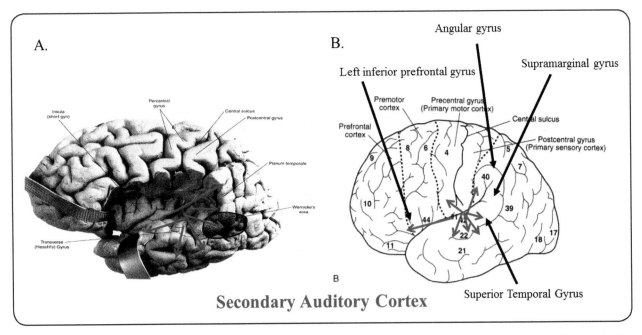

FIGURE 3–32. The secondary auditory cortex. Reprinted with permission from Bhatnagar, *Neuroscience for the Study of Communicative Disorders, Second Edition* (2002). Copyright © Lippincott Williams & Wilkins.

to music (Devlin et al., 2003). Because the majority of information (e.g., 80%) crosses at the brainstem and projects to the contralateral auditory cortex, the right ear is known to be more responsive to language than the left ear for many persons (e.g., right ear language dominant effect). The differences in anatomy and processing that exist between the two hemispheres underscore the importance of the provision of auditory information in both ears. More specifically, persons with bilateral hearing loss should typically use hearing technology (e.g., two cochlear implants, a cochlear implant and a hearing aid for the non-implanted ear) for both ears. Similarly, persons with single-sided deafness will likely experience many auditory deficits and will possibly benefit from cochlear implantation of the poorer ear.

Interhemispheric Connections

Despite the importance of bilateral hearing, it is prudent to note that the information in each hemisphere is exchanged back and forth via an interhemispheric fiber tract called the corpus callosum (Figure 3–33). The corpus callosum is a myelinated fiber tract located at the base of the longitudinal fissure. It is the longest fiber tract in the brain. The posterior portion of the corpus callosum (at the sulcus) is the region at which auditory information is exchanged between the two temporal lobes. Deficits of the corpus callosum result in a reduction in performance of higher order audi-

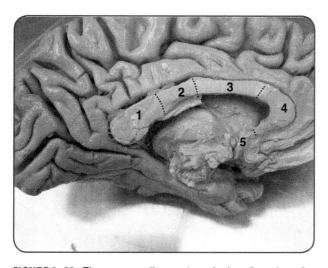

FIGURE 3–33. The corpus callosum. 1 = splenium, 2 = sulcus, 3 = trunk, 4 = genu, 5 = anterior commissure. Reprinted with permission from Musiek and Baran, *The Auditory System: Anatomy, Physiology, and Clinical Correlates* (2016). Copyright © Plural Publishing, Inc.

tory skills such as dichotic tasks, speech recognition in noise, and localization.

Development of Spoken Language in the Auditory Nervous System

Research has shown that the development of the auditory nervous system is influenced and shaped by the exposure a child has to acoustic information from the peripheral auditory system (Boothroyd, 1997; Sharma et al., 2001). If the child is exposed to a robust model of intelligible speech during the first few years of life, then the auditory part of the brain will establish rich, complex, and diverse connections with other centers of the brain, allowing for the sound to convey meaning and for the child to develop spoken language and listening abilities along with literacy skills. If a child is deprived of access to a listening-rich model of intelligible speech and diverse acoustic stimulation during the first few years of life (as may occur when a child has hearing loss), then the brain will reorganize in an attempt to improvise and become more adept at processing stimuli from other sensory systems (e.g., visual stimuli). To fully appreciate auditory brain development, particularly in the context of auditory deprivation associated hearing loss during childhood, it is helpful to provide a brief review of auditory anatomy and physiology as well as a summary of recent studies exploring auditory brain development.

Review of the Functional Auditory Anatomy and Physiology

From the brainstem to the auditory cortex, the auditory nervous system is highly complex and uses multiple mechanisms to process sound to provide the listener with an auditory signal that is meaningful. The brainstem certainly plays a vital role in several aspects of auditory processing (e.g., sound localization, the processing of speech in noise [e.g., the release from masking], in the refinement of the auditory signal to enhance processing at higher levels), but the auditory cortex will be the focus in this review of auditory brain development. The auditory cortex is the level of the auditory system that plays the most prominent role in speech recognition and spoken language development.

Figure 3–31 provides a visual depiction of the ascending auditory pathway. As shown in Figure 3–31A, all of the auditory input from the auditory brainstem and auditory thalamus arrives at the primary auditory cortex.

Many students may find it difficult to visualize the anatomical characteristics of primary auditory cortex because the primary auditory cortex is not easily viewable from a surface view of the cerebrum. However, when sections of the frontal and parietal lobes are removed, the primary auditory cortex, which is also referred to as Heschl's gyrus, can be easily seen. The primary auditory cortex is a ridge of neural tissue that courses medially and posteriorly within the sylvian fissure (see Figure 3–31B). The tonotopic organization that is first seen in the cochlea and is intact throughout the ascending auditory pathway is also present in the primary auditory cortex, where low-frequency sounds are processed toward the lateral edge of Heschl's gyrus and high-frequency sounds processed toward the medial edge.

Secondary Auditory Cortex

The secondary auditory cortex is not as clearly defined as the primary auditory cortex. The secondary cortex is comprised of multiple areas which include but are not limited to the superior temporal gyrus, the angular gyrus, the supramarginal gyrus, the planum temporale, the insula, the inferior parietal lobe, and the posterior frontal lobe (see Figure 3–32). For many years, the medical community has recognized the significant role that the secondary auditory cortex has in a listener's ability to comprehend spoken language and to derive higher-order meaning from other auditory stimuli such as music and environmental sounds. For instance, in 1874, the German physician Carl Wernicke reported that a lesion at Brodmann area 42, which is located in the secondary auditory cortex (see Figure 3–32), results in the inflicted individual being unable to understand spoken language (Wilkins & Brody, 1970).

When an individual is exposed to a robust model of intelligible speech during the first two to three years of life, the auditory areas of the brain respond vigorously when stimulated by spoken language or other meaningful sounds, an example which may be seen in research by Green and colleagues (2005). Green et al. used positron emission tomography (PET) to image the areas of the brain that were active when post-lingually deafened adults listened to intelligible speech while using a cochlear implant. Green and colleagues showed that auditory stimulation from the cochlear implant at one ear in response to running speech resulted in bilateral activation of both the primary and secondary auditory cortices for adults who had normal hearing and good access to intel-

ligible years during early infancy and childhood but lost their hearing during adulthood (Figure 3–34). It is important to stress that the auditory stimulation provided from the cochlear implant at one ear produced a broad and robust response that spanned throughout both the primary and secondary auditory cortices.

The presence of a response from the secondary auditory cortex to speech and other sounds is critically important because one of the roles of the secondary auditory cortex is to functionally couple the auditory areas of the brain to the rest of the brain. Research studies have demonstrated that the secondary auditory cortex contains a large number of connections to other areas of the brain (e.g., connections with the frontal, occipital, and parietal lobes as well as connections to deeper brain areas such as the amygdala and the hippocampus). "Intrahemispheric tract" is a term used to describe the connections between secondary auditory cortex and other areas of the brain. Most audiologists are familiar with interhemispheric tracts (in particular, the corpus callosum, which exchanges information between the right and

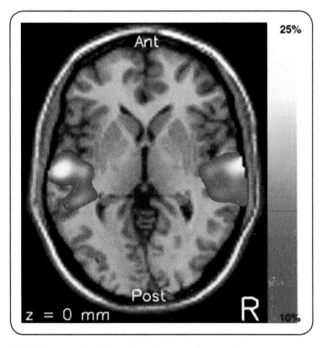

FIGURE 3–34. Activity in the primary and secondary auditory cortices in response to running speech presented to the left ear of a cochlear implant user (PET scan). Reprinted with permission from Green, Julyan, Hastings, and Ramsden, "Auditory cortical activation and speech perception in cochlear implant users: Effects of implant experience and duration of deafness," *Hearing Research* (2005), 205(1–2):184–192. Copyright © Elsevier.

left sides of the cerebrum). Intrahemispheric tracts, on the other hand, deliver information between two areas of the brain located within the same hemisphere (i.e., right or left) of the cerebrum. The arcuate fasciculus, which is pictured in Figure 3–35, is an intrahemispheric tract that delivers information from the auditory cortices of the brain to the frontal lobe for higher-order processing. There are a number of other intrahemispheric tracts that establish connections between the auditory areas of the brain and other cortical areas as well as with other areas of the auditory nervous system that are inferior to the cerebrum, such as the amygdala.

The secondary auditory cortex also sends information back to the primary auditory cortex by way of efferent tracts. The specific purpose of these efferent tracts is not entirely understood, but research suggests that the efferent connections from the secondary to primary auditory cortices modulate the response of the primary auditory cortex, which prepares the primary auditory cortex to attend to primary signals of interest. This modulation that the secondary auditory cortex provides to the primary auditory cortex may support feature extraction (also referred to as feature representation), which refers to the ability to focus on the acoustic elements that are similar to the sound the listener desires to comprehend (Allen, 1994; Kral & Eggermont, 2007; Kral & Lenarz, 2015).

Auditory Feature Extraction

Feature extraction refers to a listener's ability to attend to acoustical elements that are necessary to decode a sound of interest and that sufficiently represent a sound to enable the listener to recognize and identify an audio signal of interest. Andrej Kral and colleagues have suggested that one of the important roles of the secondary auditory cortex is to modulate the primary cortex so that the latter is able to detect relevant acoustic features that allow the listener to identify a sound (Land et al., 2016). Furthermore, Dr. Kral has proposed that the secondary auditory cortex is involved in a network with higher-order areas of the brain, and this network serves to integrate basic acoustic features into meaningful representations (i.e., auditory objects) which enable a listener to comprehend auditory information (Kral & Lenarz, 2015; Land et al., 2016).

Additionally, many neurons in the secondary auditory cortex are pluripotent, which means that

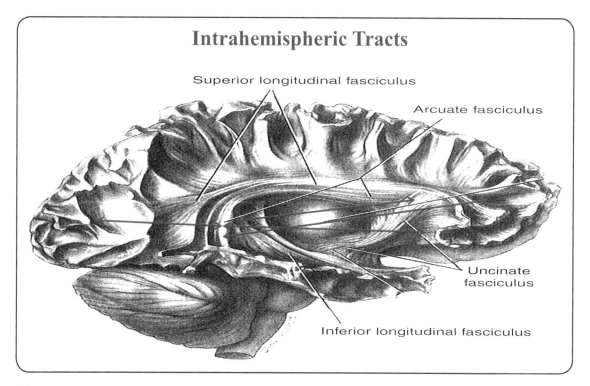

FIGURE 3–35. Intrahemispheric tracts. Reprinted with permission from Bhatnagar, *Neuroscience for the Study of Communicative Disorders, Second Edition* (2002). Copyright © Lippincott Williams & Wilkins.

they are capable of responding to multiple modes of stimulation. For instance, researchers have shown that neurons in the secondary auditory cortex are responsive to both auditory and visual stimulation, whereas other neurons in the secondary auditory cortex respond to both auditory and tactile stimulation (Schormans, Typlt, & Allman, 2017). Pluripotent neurons in secondary auditory cortex may enable multimodal integration, which combines information from multiple sensory modalities to create the holistic experiences that occur in everyday situations (e.g., the integration of auditory and visual information to allow a listener to associate a certain sound, such as an egg frying, with a visual image, such as the egg in a frying pan).

In order for auditory stimulation to elicit a meaningful experience, the secondary auditory cortex must integrate auditory information with the rest of the brain. Auditory physiologists do not fully understand the physiologic processes responsible for representing and decoding auditory objects (e.g., speech, environmental sounds, music) in the brain. However, it is well accepted that every signal received by the sensory systems is reduced to a pattern of neural activity that conveys a unique experience and meaning to the recipient. In other words, every cognitive experience of man is represented by a unique network of neurons that fire in response to input from our sensory systems, resulting in the reality that an individual perceives.

For example, let's consider the word "wet." When we hear "wet," a certain subset of neurons respond or "fire" throughout the brain, resulting in the cognitive "images" we experience. The acoustical elements of the word "wet" are represented in the primary auditory cortex in the form of the number of neurons that respond, the timing at which they respond, and the tonotopical place at which they respond. As we know from the work of Green and colleagues (see Figure 3–34), neurons in the secondary auditory cortex also respond. As previously discussed, the neurons that fire in the secondary cortex assist in modulating the response of primary auditory cortex, but also, and possibly more importantly, the responses in the secondary auditory cortex distribute the auditory stimulation to other areas of the brain, creating a complex network which may process the sound. Figure 3–36A provides an overly simplified cartoon representation of the network of neurons that may respond throughout the brain in response to the word "wet." Most of the neurons that fire are located in the primary and secondary auditory cortices, but neurons also respond in the inferior parietal and posterior frontal lobes as well as in the occipital regions and/or in multimodal regions of the secondary auditory cortex.

When the secondary auditory cortex delivers the auditory signal throughout the brain (e.g., to the inferior frontal lobe), the listener is able to derive higher-order meaning from the word "wet." For example, we may associate the word with drinking a glass of water, with getting caught in the rain, or with swimming in a lake. We may also think that we don't like to get wet if it is a cold day, or conversely, we may think that it would be nice to get wet on a hot day.

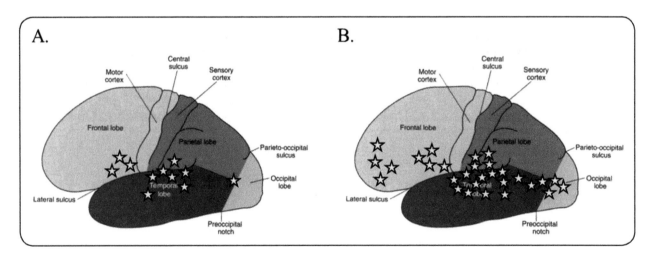

FIGURE 3–36. A cartoon representation of neural activity evoked by the word "wet" (**A**) and the listener's favorite song (**B**). Reprinted with permission from Bhatnagar, *Neuroscience for the Study of Communicative Disorders, Second Edition* (2002). Copyright © Lippincott Williams & Wilkins.

Further, engagement of neurons in the visual centers of the brain or of pluripotent neurons in the secondary auditory cortex enable a listener to form an image of "wetness" in his/her "mind's eye." For instance, the listener may associate the word "wet" with a big glass of water, a rainstorm, a dripping wet dog or child, or a wet towel. All of these perceptual images are triggered by the word "wet" because of the integration that occurs between the auditory area of the brain and other areas such as visual areas and the frontal lobe. Similarly, because of the integration that takes place between the auditory, parietal (which is involved with mediating tactile stimulation), and frontal areas of the brain, we may imagine the tactile sensation of water sprinkling on our head while in the shower. Finally, the listener can also say or produce the word "wet" because of a network established between the auditory cortices and other areas of the brain. The left inferior prefrontal cortex (i.e., Broca's region) is known to support vocal reproduction of sounds. For example, when a lesion occurs to the left inferior prefrontal cortex, the inflicted individual develops difficulty with speech production. The connection between the secondary auditory cortex and the left inferior cortex serves the anatomical and physiologic underpinning of speech production. The ability to develop the skill of speech production is compromised and is at risk when auditory information is not delivered from the secondary auditory cortex to the left inferior prefrontal cortex.

Additionally, the left inferior prefrontal cortex has been shown to possess a vital role in phonemic awareness. Phonemic awareness refers to the ability to hear, identify, and make meaningful use of the individual sounds or phonemes in words. For instance, phonemic awareness allows listeners to break the word "wet" into three phonemic units, /w/, /e/, and /t/. Phonemic awareness also allows an individual to recognize the sounds that go with the letters on the pages of a book. An example of this may be seen when watching a new reader "sound out" words. As a result, the ability to develop the literacy skills is also compromised and is at risk when auditory information is not delivered from the secondary auditory cortex to the left inferior prefrontal cortex.

Figure 3–36B provides a cartoon depiction of a more complex but similarly unique neural network or pattern of neurons that respond in the brain to the sound of a listener's favorite song. In this example, a larger and more extensive network of neurons is engaged, most likely because the listener's favorite song elicits a deeper and more complex response than the word "wet." In the elementary example of the complex network of neurons that respond to the listener's favorite song, we once again notice robust and broad activation of both the primary and secondary auditory cortices. Also, because the secondary auditory cortex serves as the launching pad that distributes the auditory information to the rest of the brain, we notice neural responses throughout other areas of the brain as well. In the listener's mind's eye, he/she may be able to see an image of two newlyweds dancing at a wedding reception as their favorite song is played by the wedding band. Once again, the visual image that is conjured in the listener's mind's eye occurs because of integration and interaction that takes place between auditory-responsive neurons in the secondary auditory cortex and visually responsive neurons. The listener may also feel a sense of happiness when he/she hears the song, because of the connection between secondary auditory cortex with the frontal lobe and other emotion-mediated areas of the brain, such as the amygdala.

The Auditory Brain and the Connectome

Every sound that arrives in our minds from our ears is represented by its own unique pattern of neural activity across the brain. In order for our auditory experiences to not just be a simple matter of detection but to also convey a higher-order meaning, auditory stimulation has to be delivered from the primary auditory cortex to the secondary auditory cortex, where it may be distributed to other areas of the brain to form a neural network or *connectome*. A connectome is a map of functional neural connections in the brain and may be thought of as the brain's wiring diagram. Figure 3–37 provides a theoretical illustration created by Andrej Kral et al. (2016) to propose a representation of the auditory component of the human brain's connectome. As previously noted, the secondary auditory cortex serves as the gateway for a connectome to be formed by the complex interaction and integration between the auditory system and other areas throughout the brain.

The typical neural connectome is formed during the first few years of a human's life through a number of processes that are dependent upon the delivery of information from the sensory systems in response to external stimuli. Through a process known as synaptogenesis (the synapse is the gap between two communicating neurons, and synaptogenesis refers to the formation of synapses), neuron-to-neuron contacts are established, which results in the formation

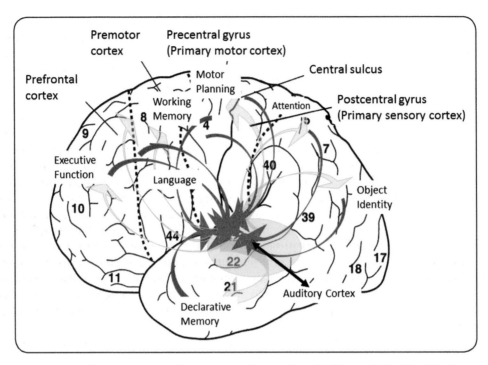

FIGURE 3–37. The auditory neural connectome. Image adapted with permission from Professor Andrej Kral based on Kral et al., 2016.

of neural pathways throughout the brain. Additionally, new synapses are developed through a process known as arborization (see the section "Neuronal Anatomy" above), which is the development, growth, and maturation of axons and dendrites and the resultant development of neural connections with neighboring neurons. The development of multiple neural connections results in the formation of neural networks. In humans, the number of synapses in the brain peaks between the first and fourth years of life, with a decline from that point forward. Functional synapses are created when neurons respond to stimulation from the peripheral sensory system. Stated differently, the development of functional synapses is reliant upon experience.

Synapses that are not used (e.g., stimulated by input from the sensory system) are eliminated by *synaptic pruning*. Synaptic pruning must happen to prevent the brain from being overwrought with synapses and inundated by an overabundance of signals from the proliferation of neural connections, many of which would not provide meaningful information about the individual's surroundings. In short, synaptic pruning eliminates synapses that do not contribute useful information relative to the individual's environment and needs; because synaptic pruning is primarily confined to synapses that do not receive

meaningful stimulation, the neural connections that do provide a person with the most useful information necessary are maintained.

Arborization, synaptogenesis, and synaptic pruning occur throughout our lives, but these neural activities are far more common during the critical period of development and maturation and diminish substantially after the first few years of life. Consequently, brain malleability, or the brain's ability to change and establish new functional connections, is greatest during the early childhood years. According to Kral and colleagues (2016), "hearing deprivation during early development prevents functional maturation, delays cortical synaptogenesis, and increases synaptic elimination, ultimately affecting central functions such as intensity coding, cortical column functioning, cochleotopic representation of auditory space, and corticocortical interactions including top-down control and auditory object formation."

Research Demonstrating the Importance of Early Auditory Stimulation

The importance of robust sensory stimulation on brain development is exemplified in numerous studies that have examined the auditory brain development in persons who were deprived of access to intelligible speech during the first few years of life. Specifically, numerous imaging studies have explored auditory brain activity in individuals with and without hearing loss. For example, Nishimura and colleagues (1999) used PET scan imaging to identify the areas of the brain that were active to a variety of different stimuli, including running speech, sign language, and meaningless hand movements. The study subjects were adults who had been deaf since birth and who had no auditory access to intelligible speech prior to receiving a cochlear implant in adulthood (i.e., the subjects communicated via sign language and were unable to receive satisfactory access to spoken language with the use of hearing aids prior to cochlear implantation).

Figure 3–38 provides an example of the areas of the subjects' brains that responded while they listened to running speech with use of their cochlear implant. As shown, running speech produced neural activity in the primary auditory cortex contralateral to the ear that was stimulated, a finding that indicates that even in the presence of a lifetime of deafness and auditory deprivation, the primary auditory cortex continues to receive auditory information from the lower auditory areas and is able to generate an auditory response (i.e., the primary auditory cortex is "hard-wired" to receive information from the lower auditory areas, regardless of whether the listener had early access to auditory information; all that is needed is a "way in," which in this case was provided through the use of a cochlear implant). This finding that the primary auditory cortex is dedicated to processing auditory signals serves to explain why congenitally deafened teenagers and adults who have no spoken language and who have never had sufficient access to auditory stimulation during their first decade or longer of life are still able to respond to warble tones presented in the soundfield at 20 to 25 dB HL after receiving a cochlear implant (assuming that the cochlear implant is adequately programmed). The primary auditory cortex is dedicated to audition and is able to support the **detection** of sound, regardless of whether the listener had early access to auditory information.

It is important to make the point that a long duration of deafness most likely results in some

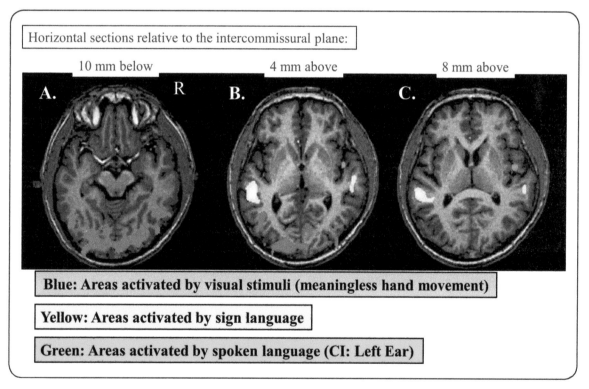

FIGURE 3–38. Neural activity evoked by visualization of meaningless hand movements (*in blue*), visualization of a story told through the use of sign language (*in yellow*), and listening to a story through audition with the use of a cochlear implant (*in green*). Reprinted with permission from Nishimura et al., "Sign language 'heard' in the auditory cortex," *Nature* (1999), *397*(6715), 116. Copyright © Springer.

reorganization of the primary auditory cortex along with at least some change and/or reduction in its responsiveness to sound (Kral & Sharma, 2012). An example of this point may be found in the research of Dietrich and colleagues, who showed that a larger area of the primary auditory cortex is dedicated to the processing of low-frequency stimuli for post-lingually deafened adults who have had a long duration of high-frequency hearing loss (Dietrich et al., 2001). However, as the research of Nishimura et al. (1999) shows, the primary auditory cortex will continue to be responsive to auditory stimuli after many years of auditory deprivation, and as a result, the primary auditory cortex can still allow for the simple detection of sound.

Quite possibly the most relevant finding of the Nishimura (1999) study was observed in the secondary auditory cortex. As shown in Figure 3–38, there was typically no response present in the secondary auditory cortex when the participants listened to running speech while using their cochlear implants. However, robust neural activity was recorded in the secondary auditory cortex when the participants observed a story being told through the use of sign language. The activity present in secondary auditory cortex while the participants followed sign language is evidence of cross-modal reorganization; in the absence of stimulation from the peripheral auditory system, the secondary auditory cortex reorganized and assisted in the processing of visual information. In essence, the secondary cortex functionally "decoupled" from primary auditory cortex and enhanced its connections to the visual centers of the brain.

The term "colonization" is used to describe the process by which one functional area of the brain (e.g., the auditory area) is transformed to respond to stimuli that are typically processed by a neighboring region. Numerous research studies have demonstrated colonization of the secondary auditory cortex by other sensory modalities (e.g., vision, tactile) in the presence of deafness (Glick & Sharma, 2017; Sharma, Campbell, & Cardon, 2015; Kral & Eggermont, 2007). Colonization of the secondary auditory cortex by other sensory modalities serves as an explanation for why persons who are born deaf and who do not have access to auditory stimulation during the first few years of life are able to develop exceptionally adept ability with other sensory modalities. For instance, Scott and colleagues have shown that persons who do not have early access to sound often develop better peripheral vision (Scott et al., 2014).

Colonization of the secondary auditory cortex may also explain the poor outcomes that are often obtained in persons who are prelingually deafened and who receive cochlear implants after the critical period of language development. When the primary and secondary auditory cortices are decoupled from one another, auditory information from the lower auditory areas cannot be adequately delivered from primary to secondary auditory cortex. If auditory information is not relayed to the secondary auditory cortex, then neural networks cannot be formed between the auditory areas of the brain and the rest of the brain to enable the higher-order processing that is required to allow a meaningful auditory experience. The auditory neural network or connectome is disrupted between the primary and secondary auditory cortex. As a result, individuals who have a congenital hearing loss, who do not have early access to auditory information (during the first few years of life), and who receive a cochlear implant after the critical period of language development are able detect sound at low presentation levels with use of the implant but frequently struggle to understand speech, derive meaning from complex sound, and develop spoken language.

When the participants watched the meaningless hand movements, neural activity was observed in the occipital lobe, but no activity was observed in the secondary auditory cortex (see Figure 3–38) (Nishimura et al., 1999), a finding that suggests that the secondary auditory cortex is predisposed to process language. Therefore, one may be tempted to conclude (although erroneously) that access to sign language during the first few years of the life of a child born with deafness is sufficient to develop the necessary synaptic connections and neural networks within and beyond secondary auditory cortex that are necessary to eventually allow for listening and spoken language development. It should be reiterated, however, that the exclusive use of visual forms of communication during the first few years of life with an absence of access to meaningful auditory information will result in colonization of the secondary auditory cortex by the visual system. Consequently, the functional neural synapses and connections are eliminated between the primary and secondary auditory cortices, and as a result, so is the delivery of auditory information to secondary auditory cortex and then on to the rest of the brain.

Critical Period of Auditory Brain Development

Andrej Kral's studies with white deaf kittens have provided insights into the exact location of the decoupling that occurs between the primary and secondary auditory cortices. Kral and colleagues have measured auditory-evoked neural responses at different layers of the auditory cortex by inserting micro-electrodes to varying depths into the auditory cortex. The auditory cortex, which is 2 to 4 mm in thickness, contains six layers of neurons (Figure 3–39). The afferent auditory nerve fibers from the auditory thalamus arrive at layer IV of the primary auditory cortex; layers I to III, which are referred to as the supragranular layers, assist in the processing of sound at the primary auditory cortex. Layers V to VI, which are known as the infragranular layers of the auditory cortex, have several functions, but most importantly, they serve as the output circuits of the primary auditory cortex. Specifically, the auditory information that is delivered from the primary auditory cortex to other areas of the brain, including to the secondary auditory cortex, is delivered from layers V and VI of the primary auditory cortex.

Kral and colleagues (2000) provided cochlear implants to their congenitally deafened cats at dif-ferent ages. For normal hearing cats and kittens who received cochlear implants during the first 3 months of life, typical neural activity was observed at all layers of the primary auditory cortex (Figure 3–40A). However, the white deaf cats who received a cochlear implant after five months of age showed typical neural activity in layers I to IV but reduced or no neural activity in the infragranular layers (V–VI) (Figure 3–40B). The results of Kral's research (2000) indicates that the decoupling that occurs between the primary and secondary auditory cortices for individuals who do not have early access to meaningful sound can be localized to the infragranular layers of primary auditory cortex. The absence of auditory responsiveness at the output circuits of the primary auditory cortex prevents the transmission of auditory information to the secondary auditory cortex. Consequently, the secondary auditory cortex cannot distribute the auditory signal to the rest of the brain, and the auditory neural network/connectome is eliminated.

Can the findings of Kral's research with cats be applied to children with hearing loss? Anu Sharma

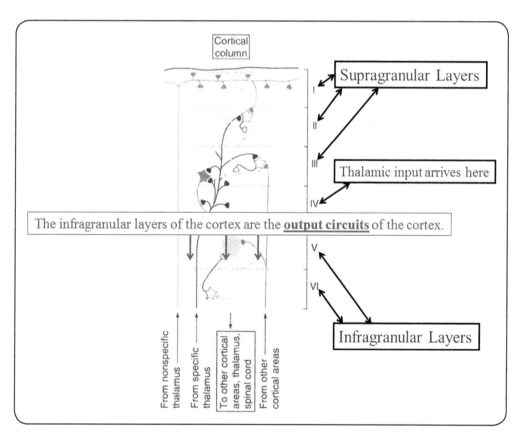

FIGURE 3–39. The six neural layers of the auditory cortex. Reprinted with permission from Møller, *Hearing: Anatomy, Physiology, and Disorders of the Auditory System, Third Edition* (2013). Copyright © Plural Publishing, Inc.

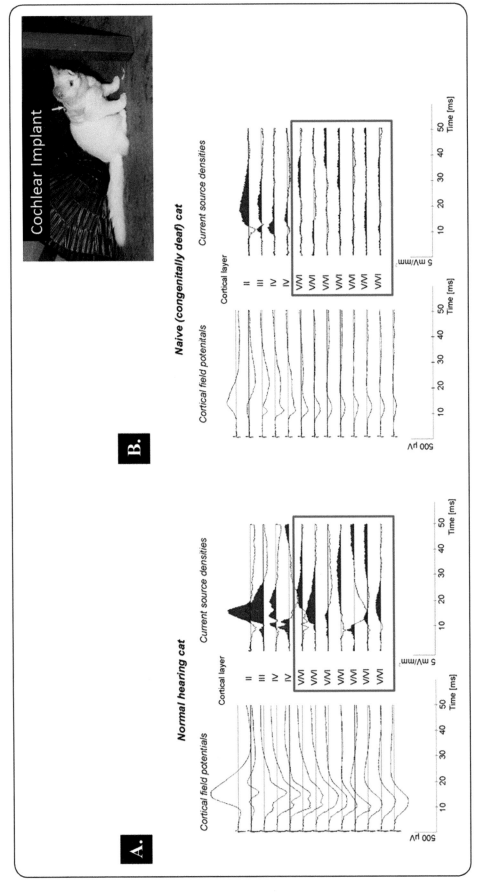

FIGURE 3–40. Auditory neural responses measured at different auditory cortical layers in a normal-hearing cat (**A**) and a late-implanted deafened cat (**B**). Images provided courtesy of Professor Andrej Kral.

measured the latency of the P1 waveform of the cortical auditory evoked potential (P1-CAEP) in children with normal hearing and in children who were born deaf and received a cochlear implant at various ages ranging from 1 year to early adulthood (Sharma et al., 2002). Children who received cochlear implants during the first three years of life had P1 latencies that were similar to the P1 latencies of children with normal hearing. In contrast, children who received their cochlear implants after 3 years of age generally had P1 latencies that fell outside of the range for children with normal hearing. Sharma proposed that the P1 latency was a biomarker of auditory brain development and that delayed P1 latencies were caused by a decoupling between primary and secondary auditory cortices.

The findings of Kral and Sharma have major implications for young children with hearing loss. Specifically, if early and extensive access to meaningful auditory stimulation is not provided during the first few years of a child's life, that child's brain and auditory brain function will be irreparably altered, and as a result, functional auditory performance and spoken language development will also be irreparably altered, at least to some extent, for the remainder of the child's life. The early provision of cochlear implants is imperative for children with severe to profound hearing loss (and many children with auditory neuropathy spectrum disorder) in order to deliver the necessary auditory stimulation to the primary auditory cortex to allow for synaptogenesis and the resultant establishment of functional connections/coupling between primary and secondary auditory cortices. Inclusion of secondary auditory cortex in the auditory system's response to auditory stimuli is necessary for the acoustic signal to be distributed throughout the brain (i.e., auditory connectome) and for sound to come to life and acquire higher order meaning.

Spoken Language Enrichment: A Necessity for Auditory Brain Development

Research has demonstrated that children who have hearing loss and are exposed to greater amounts of total intelligible speech and complex language achieve higher spoken language outcomes than their counterparts who are deprived of access to a robust model of high-level, complex language and intelligible speech (Ambrose et al., 2014, 2015; Ching & Dillon, 2013; Dettman et al., 2016; Hart & Risley, 2003; McCreery et al., 2015; Tomblin et al., 2015). Visual stimulation (e.g., sign language) does not support

typical spoken language development. The secondary auditory cortex is particularly suited to process language, but stimulation of the secondary auditory cortex with visual input does not establish the neural connections/networks required to develop listening and spoken language abilities. If a child is exposed to sign language at the expense of exposure to intelligible speech, the secondary auditory cortex will decouple from primary auditory cortex. Numerous research studies have shown poorer listening, spoken language, and literacy outcomes for children with hearing loss who use sign language or Total Communication compared with children who use listening and spoken language as their primary form of communication (Boons et al., 2012; Ching & Dillon, 2013; Dettman et al., 2016; Geers et al., 2011; Leigh, Dettman, & Dowell, 2016). It should be noted that every month of auditory deprivation during early infancy and the first few years of life is likely to result in detrimental consequences to the formation of neural networks between secondary auditory cortex and the rest of the brain.

Auditory Deprivation in Adults

Adults who were born with normal hearing and lose their hearing in adulthood typically achieve excellent outcomes with cochlear implants (see Chapter 20). As indicated in the previous section, adults who have a post-lingual onset of hearing loss are afforded with satisfactory access to meaningful sound during the early years of life, which allows for the formation of a robust auditory connectome and good auditory and spoken language abilities. It is, however, important to note that auditory deprivation secondary to severe to profound hearing loss can also have deleterious effects in the auditory areas of the brain of post-lingually deafened adults. As discussed in Chapter 20, outcomes after cochlear implantation are generally poorer for adults who have a lengthy duration of deafness, a fact that is likely attributed to changes in the auditory nervous system.

Numerous researchers have conducted imaging and auditory-evoked potential studies that have shown reduced responsiveness in the auditory areas of the brains of adults who have hearing loss (Glick & Sharma, 2017; Shiell, Champoux, & Zatorre, 2015; Strelnikov et al., 2015a, 2015b; Wolak et al., 2017). Research has shown that a larger area of the auditory cortex is devoted to the processing of low- to mid-frequency sounds in the presence of high-frequency deafness (Robertson & Irvine, 1989; Willott, Aitkin, & McFadden, 1993; Wolak et al., 2017). Additionally, numerous research studies have shown evidence of cross-modal reorganization (i.e., colonization by the visual and tactile centers of the brain) in the auditory cortices of adults with severe to profound hearing loss (Glick & Sharma, 2017; Shiell et al., 2015; Strelnikov et al., 2015a, 2015b). As a result, a period of acclimation is likely to be necessary when an adult receives a cochlear implant, especially after several years or more of deafness. A period of experience with the cochlear implant may be necessary to "reacquire" the auditory regions of the brain that may have been colonized by other sensory modalities or may have transformed to process lower-frequency auditory signals. Additionally, changes in the organization of the auditory areas of the brain are a likely explanation for why some adults experience continued difficulty after cochlear implantation. In short, some adults may be unable to "reacquire" the auditory areas of the brain if those areas have long ago been dedicated to processing visual information. The changes that occur in the auditory areas of brain secondary to hearing loss as well as after cochlear implantation underscore the importance of early intervention for hearing loss, full-time cochlear implant use for recipients, and the provision of aural rehabilitation for recipients who had a long duration of deafness prior to implantation and who continue to experience difficulty with communication after implantation.

Efferent Auditory System

The efferent auditory system is comprised oftwo divisions, the olivocochlear bundle (OCB) and the rostral efferent system (Musiek & Baran, 2007). The medial olivary complex is composed of two types of efferent nerve fibers that extend from the superior olivary complex to the cochlea (Figure 3–41). Type I efferent fibers have a relatively large diameter and are myelinated, whereas Type II efferent fibers are relatively thin and unmyelinated. Type I fibers arise from the medial superior olivary body of the superior olivary complex and traverse across the pons to innervate the base of outer hair cells of the contralateral ear. Type II efferent fibers arise from the lateral superior olivary body and innervate the afferent fibers of inner hair cells on the ipsilateral side. Although the function of the OCB is not entirely well understood, it is known to primarily have an

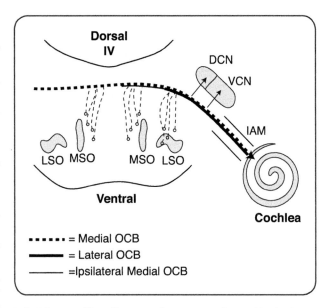

FIGURE 3–41. The efferent auditory system located in the lower brainstem. Reprinted with permission from Musiek and Baran, *The Auditory System: Anatomy, Physiology, and Clinical Correlates* (2016). Copyright © Plural Publishing, Inc.

inhibitory effect on cochlear function. Specifically, it is likely that the OCB reduces the electromotility of the outer hair cells. Conceivably, the OCB could facilitate outer hair cell saturation at higher levels. It is possible that the OCB modulates outer hair cell function in an attempt to stabilize displacement of the basilar membrane and tune the response of the peripheral auditory system in moderate- to high-level noise environments (e.g., facilitate speech recognition in noise). Although it is likely obvious, it may be worth noting that the OCB will have no effect on auditory performance of cochlear implant recipients, because the implant bypasses the structures that are innervated by the efferent nerve fibers.

The rostral efferent system is composed of efferent fibers that arise in the secondary auditory cortex and project to the primary auditory cortex. Additionally, efferent fibers project from the auditory cortex to the medial geniculate nucleus of the thalamus. From the thalamus, the efferent fibers project onward to the auditory neurons in the inferior colliculus. Of note, the rostral efferent system possesses several feedback loops in which information may be transmitted from the cortex to the thalamus and back. Feedback loops also exist between the thalamus and the inferior colliculus. Like the OCB, the function of the rostral efferent system is not clearly understood.

However, the rostral efferent system likely plays a role in integration of auditory information across lower and higher-order centers and in tuning the response of the auditory system to allow for sharper analysis of signals of interest.

changes to the auditory cortices and other areas of the auditory connectome. Appropriate hearing technology should be promptly provided to ensure consistent audibility for speech and environmental sounds in order to avoid the deleterious effects of auditory deprivation.

Key Concepts

- The auditory system is complex and elaborate, and when it functions normally, it is able to faithfully code complex acoustic signals across a wide range of intensities and frequencies.
- The external ear modifies incoming acoustic signals to provide an enhancement throughout a rather large portion of the speech frequency range and to aid in the localization of sound. These functions of the acoustic ear should be accounted for when hearing technology is designed, selected, and programmed for the user.
- The middle ear is a sophisticated system that serves to transmit an audio signal from the external auditory meatus to the cochlea and to overcome the impedance mismatch that exists between air and the cochlear fluids.
- When chronic dysfunction exists in the external and middle ear, an implantable bone conduction device may benefit the patient.
- The physical properties of the middle ear must be taken into account when designing middle ear implants.
- The cochlea serves to convert mechanical energy into neuro-electric potentials. Cochlear dysfunction can occur at several specific sites, including the cochlear hair cells and the stria vascularis.
- Cochlear implantation is usually beneficial for persons with substantial cochlear dysfunction that results in severe to profound hearing loss.
- The auditory system is tonotopically organized from the cochlea to the auditory cortex.
- The cochlear nerve is usually relatively intact in most persons with sensorineural hearing loss. If the cochlear nerve is absent or severely compromised, an auditory brainstem implant may be used to deliver stimulation directly to the cochlear nuclei of the brainstem.
- Auditory deprivation secondary to severe to profound hearing loss results in deleterious

References

Allen, J. B. (1994). How do humans process and recognize speech? *IEEE Transactions on Speech and Audio Processing, 2*(4), 567–577.

Ambrose, S. E., VanDam, M., & Moeller, M. P. (2014). Linguistic input, electronic media, and communication outcomes of toddlers with hearing loss. *Ear and Hearing, 35*(2), 139–147.

Ambrose, S. E., Walker, E. A., Unflat-Berry, L. M., Oleson, J. J., & Moeller, M. P. (2015). Quantity and quality of caregivers' linguistic input to 18-month and 3-year-old children who are hard of hearing. *Ear and Hearing, 36*(Suppl. 1), 48S–59S.

Balkany, T., & Zeitler, D. (2013). *Encyclopedia of otolaryngology, head, and neck surgery* (p. 328). Berlin, Heidelberg: Springer.

Bilger, R. C. (1977). Psychoacoustic evaluation of present prostheses. *Annals of Otology, Rhinology and Laryngology, 86*(Suppl. 38), 92–104.

Boons, T., Brokx, J. P., Dhooge, I., Frijns, J. H., Peeraer, L., Vermeulen, A. . . . van Wieringen, A. (2012). Predictors of spoken language development following pediatric cochlear implantation. *Ear and Hearing, 33*(5), 617–639.

Boothroyd, A. (1997). Auditory development of the hearing child. *Scandinavian Audiology, Supplementum, 46*, 9–16.

Brownell, W. E. (1984). Microscopic observation of cochlear hair cell motility. *Scanning Electron Microscopy,* (Pt. 3), 1401–1406.

Campbell, N. A. (1990). *Biology* (2nd ed.). Redwood City, CA: Benjamin/Cummings.

Ching, T. Y. C., & Dillon, H. (2013). Major findings of the LOCHI study on children at 3 years of age and implications for audiologic management. *International Journal of Audiology, 52* (Suppl. 2), 65S–68S.

Clark, G. M. (1969). Responses of cells in the superior olivary complex of the cat to electrical stimulation of the auditory nerve. *Experimental Neurology, 24*(1), 124–136.

Dettman, S. J., Dowell, R. C., Choo, D., Arnott, W., Abrahams, Y., Davis, A., Dornan, D., . . . Briggs, R. J. (2016). Long-term communication outcomes for children receiving cochlear implants younger than 12 months: A multicentre study. *Otology and Neurotology, 37*, e82–e95.

Devlin, J. T., Raley, J., Tunbridge, E., Lanary, K., Floyer-Lea, A., Narain, C., . . . Moore D. R. (2003). Functional asymmetry for auditory processing in human primary auditory cortex. *Journal of Neuroscience, 23*(37), 11516–11522.

Dietrich, V., Nieschalk, M., Stoll, W., Rajan, R., & Pantev, C. (2001). Cortical reorganization in patients with high frequency hearing loss. *Hearing Research, 158*(1–2), 95–101.

Flynn, M. (2004, March). Open ear fitting: Nine questions and answers. *Hearing Review.* Retrieved from http://www.hearingreview.com/2004/03/opening-ear-fittings-nine-questions-and-answers/

Fourcin, A., Rosen, S., Moore, B., Douek, E., Clarke, G., Dodson, H., & Bannister L. (1979). External electrical stimulation of the cochlea: Clinical, psychophysical, speech-perceptual and histological findings. *British Journal of Audiology*, *13*(3), 85–107.

Geers, A. E., Strube, M. J., Tobey, E. A., Pisoni, D. B., & Moog, J. S. (2011). Epilogue: Factors contributing to long-term outcomes of cochlear implantation in early childhood. *Ear and Hearing*, *32*(Suppl. 1), 84S–92S.

Glick, H., & Sharma, A. (2017). Cross-modal plasticity in developmental and age-related hearing loss: Clinical implications. *Hearing Research*, *343*, 191–201.

Green K. M. J., Julyan, P. J., Hastings, D. L., & Ramsden, R. T. (2005). Auditory cortical activation and speech perception in cochlear implant users: Effects of implant experience and duration of deafness. *Hearing Research*, *205*, 184–192.

Greenwood, D. D. (1961). Critical bandwidth and the frequency coordinates of the basilar membrane. *Journal of the Acoustical Society of America*, *33*, 1344–1356.

Greenwood, D. D. (1990). A cochlear frequency–position function for several species—29 years later. *Journal Acoustical Society of America*, *87*(6), 2592–2605.

Hall, J. W., III. (2000). *Handbook of otoacoustic emissions*. San Diego, CA: Singular.

Hart, B., & Risley, T. R. (2003, Spring). The early catastrophe: The 30 million word gap by age 3. *American Educator*, pp. 4–9. Retrieved from http://www.aft.org//sites/default/files/periodicals/TheEarlyCatastrophe.pdf

Hudspeth, A. J. (1989). Mechanoelectrical transduction by hair cells of the bullfrog's sacculus. *Progress in Brain Research*, *80*, 129–135; discussion 127–128.

Kemp, D. T. (1978). Stimulated acoustic emissions from within the human auditory system. *Journal Acoustical Society of America*, *64*(5), 1386–1391.

Kochkin, S. (2000) MarkeTrak V: "Why my hearing aids are in the drawer": The consumer's perspective. *Hearing Journal*, *53*(2), 32–42.

Kral, A., & Eggermont, J. (2007). What's to lose and what's to learn: Development under auditory deprivation, cochlear implants and limits of cortical plasticity. *Brain Research Review*, *56*(1): 259–269.

Kral, A., Hartmann, R., Tillein, J., Heid, S., & Klinke, R. (2000). Congenital auditory deprivation reduces synaptic activity within the auditory cortex in a layer-specific manner. *Cerebral Cortex*, *10*, 714–726.

Kral, A., Kronenberger, W. G., Pisoni, D. B., & O'Donoghue, G. M. (2016). Neurocognitive factors in sensory restoration of early deafness: A connectome model. *Lancet Neurology*, *15*(6), 610–621.

Kral, A., & Lenarz, T. (2015). How the brain learns to listen: Deafness and the bionic ear. *E-Neuroform*, *6*(1), 21–28.

Kral, A., & Sharma, A. (2012). Developmental neuroplasticity after cochlear implantation. *Trends in Neurosciences*, *35*(2), 111–122.

Kuhn, G. F. (1987). Physical acoustics and measurements pertaining to directional hearing. In W. Yost & G. Gourevitch (Eds.), *Directional hearing* (pp. 3–26). New York, NY: Springer-Verlag.

Land, R., Baumhoff, P., Tillein, J., Lomber, S. G., Hubka, P., & Kral, A. (2016). Cross-modal plasticity in higher-order auditory cortex of congenitally deaf cats does not limit auditory responsiveness to cochlear implants. *Journal of Neuroscience*, *36*(23), 6175–6185.

Leigh, J. R., Dettman, S. J., & Dowell, R. C. (2016). Evidence-based guidelines for recommending cochlear implantation for young children: audiological criteria and optimizing age at implantation. *International Journal of Audiology*, *55*(Suppl. 2), S9–S18.

Lipscomb D. L. (1996). The external and middle ear. In J. L. Northern (Ed.), *Hearing disorders* (3rd ed., pp. 1–13), Needham Heights, MA: Allyn & Bacon.

Liu, C., Glowatzki, E., & Fuchs, P. A. (2015). Unmyelinated type II afferent neurons report cochlear damage. *Proceedings of the National Academy of Sciences of the United States of America*, *112*(4), 14723–14727.

Lloyd, S., Meerton, L., Di Cuffa, R., Lavy, J., & Graham, J. (2007). Taste change following cochlear implantation. *Cochlear Implants International*, *8*(4), 203–210.

Marmel, F., Rodriguez-Mendoza, M. A., & Lopez-Poveda, E. A. (2015). Stochastic undersampling steepens auditory threshold/duration functions: Implications for understanding auditory deafferentation and aging. *Frontiers in Aging Neuroscience*, *7*, 63.

Matsuoka, A. J., Rubinstein, J. T., Abbas, P. J., & Miller, C. A. (2001). The effects of interpulse interval on stochastic properties of electrical stimulation: Models and measurements. *IEEE Transactions on Biomedical Engineering*, *48*(4), 416–424.

McCreery, R., Walker, E., Spratford, M., Bentler, R., Holte, L., Roush, P., . . . Moeller, M. (2015). Longitudinal predictors of aided speech audibility in infants and children. *Ear and Hearing*, *36*(Suppl. 1), 24S–37S.

Moller, A. R. (2001). Neurophysiologic basis for cochlear and auditory brainstem implants. *American Journal of Audiology*, *10*(2), 68–77.

Moller, A. R. (2013). *Hearing: Anatomy, physiology, and disorders of the auditory system* (3rd ed.). San Diego, CA: Plural.

Musiek, F. E., & Baran, J. A. (2007). *The auditory system: Anatomy, physiology, and clinical correlates*. Boston, MA: Pearson, Allyn & Bacon.

Nishimura, H., Hasikawa, K., Doi, K., Iwaki, T., Watanabe Y., Kusuoka, H., Nishimura, T., & Kubo, T. (1999). Sign language "heard" in the auditory cortex. *Nature*, *397*, 116.

Palmer A. R., & Russell, I. J. (1986). Phase-locking in the cochlear nerve of the guinea pig and its relation to the receptor potential of the inner hair cells. *Hearing Research*, *24*, 1–15.

Robertson, D., & Irvine, D. R. F. (1989). Plasticity of frequency organization in auditory cortex of guinea pigs with partial deafness. *Journal of Comparative Neurology*, *282*, 456–471.

Rubinstein, J. T., Wilson, B. S., Finley, C. C., & Abbas, P. J. (1999). Pseudospontaneous activity: Stochastic independence of auditory nerve fibers with electrical stimulation. *Hearing Research*, *127*(1–2), 108–118.

Schafer, E. C., Amlani, A. M., Paiva, D., Nozari, L., & Verret, S. (2011). A meta-analysis to compare speech recognition in noise with bilateral cochlear implants and bimodal stimulation. *International Journal of Audiology*, *50*(12), 871–880.

Sharma, A., Campbell, J., & Cardon, G. (2015). Developmental and cross-modal plasticity in deafness: Evidence from the P1 and N1 event–related potentials in cochlear implanted children. *International Journal of Psychophysiology*, *95*, 135–144.

Sharma, A., Dorman, M. F., & Spahr, A. J. (2002). A sensitive period for the development of the central auditory system in children with cochlear implants: Implications for age of implantation. *Ear and Hearing*, *23*(6), 532–539.

Schormans, A. L., Typlt, M., & Allman, B. L. (2017). Crossmodal plasticity in auditory, visual and multisensory cortical areas following noise-induced hearing loss in adulthood. *Hearing Research*, *343*, 92–107.

Scott, G. D., Karns, C. M., Dow, M. W., Stevens, C., & Neville, H. J. (2014). Enhanced peripheral visual processing in congenitally deaf humans is supported by multiple brain regions, including primary auditory cortex. *Frontiers in Human Neuroscience*, *26*(8), 177.

Shaw, E., A., G. (1966). Ear canal pressure generated by a free sound field. *Journal of the Acoustical Society of America*, *39*, 465–470.

Shaw, E. A. C. (1974). The external ear. In W. D. Keidel & W. D. Neff (Eds.), *Handbook of sensory physiology* (Vol. 1, pp. 455–490). New York, NY: Oxford University Press.

Shiell, M. M., Champoux, F., & Zatorre, R. J. (2015). Reorganization of auditory cortex in early-deaf people: Functional connectivity and relationship to hearing aid use. *Journal of Cognitive Neuroscience*, *27*(1), 150–163.

Skarzynski, H. (2017). Tonotopic organisation of the auditory cortex in sloping sensorineural hearing loss. *Hearing Research*, *355*, 81–96.

Stakhovskaya, O., Sridhar, D., Bonham, B. H., & Leake, P. A. (2007). Frequency map for the human cochlear spiral ganglion: Implications for cochlear implants. *Journal for the Association for Research in Otolaryngology*, *8*(2), 220–233.

Strelnikov, K., Marx, M., Lagleyre, S., Fraysse, B., Deguine, O., & Barone, P. (2015a). PET-imaging of brain plasticity after cochlear implantation. *Hearing Research*, *322*, 180–187.

Strelnikov, K., Rouger, J., Lagleyre, S., Fraysse, B., Demonet, J. F., Deguine, O., & Barone, P. (2015b). Increased audiovisual integration in cochlear-implanted deaf patients: Independent components analysis of longitudinal positron emission tomography data. *European Journal of Neuroscience*, *41*(5), 677–685.

Tomblin, J. B., Harrison, M., Ambrose, S. E., Walker, E. A., Oleson, J. J., & Moeller, M. P. (2015). Language outcomes in young children with mild to severe hearing loss. *Ear and Hearing*, *36*(Suppl. 1), 76S–91S.

von Békésy, G. (1941) . Über die Messung Schwingungsamplitude der Gehörknochelchen mittels einer kapazitiven Sonde [About the vibration amplitude of the ossicles measured by means of a capacitive probe]. Akust Zeits. *Experiments in Hearing*, *6*, 1–16, 95–104.

von Békésy, G. (1960). *Experiments in hearing*. New York, NY: McGraw-Hill.

Wever, E. G. (1949). *Theory of hearing*. New York, NY: John Wiley.

Wilkins, R. H., & Brody, I. A. (1970). Wernicke's sensory aphasia. *Archives of Neurology*, *22*(3), 279–280.

Willott, J. F., Aitkin, L. M., & McFadden, S. L. (1993). Plasticity of auditory cortex associated with sensorineural hearing loss in adult C57BL/6J mice. *Journal of Comparative Neurology*, *329*(3), 402–411.

Winkler, A., Latzel, M., & Holube, I. (2016). Open versus closed hearing aid fittings: A literature review of both fitting approaches. *Trends in Hearing*, *20*, 1–13.

Wolak, T., Ciesla, K., Lorens, A., Kochanek, K., Lewandowska, M., Rusiniak, M., . . . Skarzynski, H. (2017). Tonotopic organisation of the auditory cortex in sloping sensorineural hearing loss. *Hearing Research*, *355*, 81–96.

Yost, W. A. (1994). *Fundamentals of hearing* (3rd ed.). San Diego, CA: Academic Press.

Zemlin, W. R. (1998). *Speech and hearing science: Anatomy and physiology* (4th ed.). Needham Heights, MA: Allyn & Bacon.

Cochlear Implant Candidacy: Regulatory Approval

Jace Wolfe and Elizabeth Musgrave

Introduction

Several factors determine whether a patient's best interests will be served by cochlear implantation. Ultimately, the decision to recommend cochlear implantation for a patient should hinge on two basic questions:

1. Relative to the outcome possible with optimized hearing aids, will a cochlear implant improve the patient's communication abilities and/or hearing performance?
2. Relative to the outcome possible with optimized hearing aids, will a cochlear implant improve the patient's quality of life?

If the answer to one or both of those questions is yes, then the patient should be considered for cochlear implantation. However, other factors influence the cochlear implant candidacy decision. These factors include practical considerations such as:

- Do the patient and his/her family have reasonable expectations of the benefit he/she will receive from cochlear implantation?
- Are there any non-audiologic factors that will limit cochlear implant benefit (e.g., neurological deficits, severe physical disabilities making consistent device use difficult)?
- Does the patient have a support network that provides him/her with the resources needed to benefit from cochlear implantation?

All of these issues and additional factors will be discussed in Chapters 4 and 5. In this chapter, we will address the regulatory process and its influence on cochlear implant candidacy. In most places around the world, a regulatory body determines whether cochlear implants are safe for commercial, clinical use and approves guidelines or indications of use for cochlear implants for patients of different ages. These indications of use are intended to guide the clinician in identifying persons who are likely to benefit from cochlear implantation. Because each country typically has its own regulatory body that provides oversight of medical devices and drugs, the indications of use for cochlear implants vary across countries and regions. The primary focus of this chapter will be placed on the U.S. Food and Drug Administration's (FDA) role in regulating the use of cochlear implants in children and adults. However, this chapter will also provide information regarding the regulatory process in other countries around the world.

FDA Regulation of Medical Devices

The FDA is an agency that resides within the U.S. Department of Health and Human Services. The core functions of the FDA are medical products and tobacco, foods and veterinary medicine, global regulatory operations and policy, and operations. Implantable hearing technologies are medical devices that receive varying levels of oversight from the FDA. The primary role of the FDA is to safeguard the health of U.S. citizens by making certain that medical devices and drugs are safe and efficacious when approved for commercial use and by monitoring the safety and efficacy of devices and drugs across time. According to the FDA's own description of its roles, the FDA is responsible for:

Protecting the public health by assuring that foods (except for meat from livestock, poultry and some egg products which are regulated by the U.S. Department of Agriculture) are safe, wholesome, sanitary, and properly labeled; ensuring that human and veterinary drugs and vaccines and other biological products and medical devices intended for human use are safe and effective

Protecting the public from electronic product radiation

Assuring cosmetics and dietary supplements are safe and properly labeled

Regulating tobacco products

Advancing the public health by helping to speed product innovations." (FDA, 2018)

The FDA's responsibilities extend to the 50 states, the District of Columbia, Puerto Rico, Guam, the Virgin Islands, American Samoa, and other US territories and possessions (FDA, 2018). The FDA comprises seven different centers:

1. National Center for Technological Research
2. Center for Food Safety and Applied Nutrition
3. Center for Veterinary Medicine
4. Center for Biologics Evaluation and Research
5. Center for Tobacco Products
6. Center for Drug Evaluation and Research
7. Center for Devices and Radiological Health

The **Center for Devices and Radiological Health (CDRH)**, which is housed within the **Office of Medical Products and Tobacco**, is responsible for providing oversight of cochlear implants and other implantable hearing technologies. According to the FDA, the CDRH

is responsible for protecting and promoting the public health. We assure that patients and providers have timely and continued access to safe, effective, and high-quality medical devices and safe radiation-emitting products. We pro-

vide consumers, patients, their caregivers, and providers with understandable and accessible science-based information about the products we oversee. We facilitate medical device innovation by advancing regulatory science, providing industry with predictable, consistent, transparent, and efficient regulatory pathways, and assuring consumer confidence in devices marketed in the U.S. (FDA, 2017a)

There are several offices within the CDRH that regulate medical devices, including implantable hearing technologies. The **Office of Device Evaluation (ODE)** oversees the evaluation and approval of new medical devices. The **Ear, Nose, and Throat (ENT)** panel of the ODE is typically responsible for the oversight of implantable hearing technologies (FDA, 2017b). The ENT branch consists of several employees and consultants within the hearing health care field. For review of implantable hearing technologies, the ENT branch will likely call upon employees and consultants within the domains of otology, audiology, hearing science, engineering, physiology, and physics. The **Office of Science and Engineering Laboratories (OSEL)** operates as an internal support that conducts independent research and scientific analysis to provide the expertise and consultation necessary to guide the decisions, direction, and surveillance of the CDRH. The Office of Compliance (OC) safeguards and promotes public health by making certain manufacturers comply with medical device laws and FDA standards and indications for use. The **Office of Surveillance and Biometrics (OSB)** is tasked with the provision of ongoing oversight of medical devices that are approved for commercial use with the goal of ensuring the long-term safety and efficacy of the device.

The FDA categorizes medical devices into one of three regulatory classes based on the risks associated with the use of the device and the *"level of control necessary to assure the safety and effectiveness of the device"* (FDA, 2014).

I. Class I devices pose the least amount of risk to patients and are subject to the least amount of regulatory controls. Class I devices include items such as latex gloves, tongue depressors, adhesive bandages, stethoscopes, otoscopes, hospital beds, and conventional hearing aids. Class I medical devices must adhere to general FDA controls and policies which include registering the device with the FDA, use of appropriate branding and labeling, and use of approved manufacturing standards. Additionally, the manufacturer must notify the FDA prior to marketing the device and/or making it available for commercial use.

II. Class II devices pose a moderate safety risk to the patient and are subject to higher regulatory controls "to provide reasonable assurance of the device's safety and effectiveness" (FDA, 2017c). Class II devices include items such as catheters, powered wheelchairs, x-ray equipment, angioplasty, osseointegrated implantable hearing devices, and some middle ear implantable hearing devices. All of the policies that apply to Class I devices also apply to Class II devices, but the device manufacturer must also furnish the FDA with performance standards for the device. In order to receive FDA approval to market and commercially distribute Class II devices, the manufacturer must provide premarket notification of the device, which typically comes in the form of the submission of a 510(k) application.

III. Class III devices pose the highest potential risk to the patient and are subject to the highest level of regulatory control. Class III devices typically support and/or facilitate the maintenance of human life and/or prevent or limit physical impairment and disability. Class III devices include items such as pacemakers, replacement heart valves, most orthopedic implants, neurostimulators, some middle ear implantable hearing devices, cochlear implants, and auditory brainstem implants.

For Class II and III medical devices, the FDA requires the manufacturer to receive premarket approval prior to marketing and/or commercially distributing the device. For Class II devices, the premarket notification of the device comes in the form of the submission of a 510(k) application. Class II devices must possess the same intended use and similar characteristics as another Class II device or devices that have previously been approved for commercial distribution by the FDA. Because Class III devices carry a higher level of risk, the FDA provides a greater level of scrutiny before the device may be commercially distributed. Class III devices must be approved through a rigorous process referred to as a Premarket Approval (PMA) application (FDA, 2017c).

510(k)

A 510(k) submission must provide a thorough description of the device the manufacturer wishes to bring to market along with citation of predicate devices that are similar in function, design, safety, and risk (FDA, 2014b). The manufacturer must provide the FDA with performance standards for the device with a comparison to similar Class II devices already approved for commercial distribution. The manufacturer must provide information pertaining to biocompatibility, shelf life, sterility, manufacturing procedures, and so forth. Occasionally, the FDA will ask the manufacturer to provide laboratory data, animal data, or data from computer simulations. However, the FDA typically does not require the manufacturers to submit data from clinical trials with humans.

Premarket Approval and Investigational Device Exemption

Class III devices must undergo a PMA application process. The PMA consists of the provision of a variety of different forms of scientific evidence intended to support the safety and efficacy of a device while elucidating the risks associated with device use (FDA, 2017d). Because Class III devices play a significant role in supporting life and/or daily function while also possessing the greatest potential risk of all medical devices, PMAs are almost always supported by data from human clinical trials conducted with the target population for which the device is intended.

Investigational Device Exemption

The clinical data required to support a PMA for a device that is not approved for use in the United States are typically gathered in an Investigational Device Exemption (IDE) study (FDA, 2017e). The manufacturer must submit a proposal to conduct the IDE. The IDE proposal should include as much information as possible to support the manufacturer's intent to conduct a study to evaluate the safety, efficacy, and limitations of the medical device. Typically, the manufacturer will submit bench data, information from computer simulations/modeling, performance standards, and technical characteristics of the device, results from animal studies, and outcomes from human trials conducted outside of the United States. Of note, the regulatory oversight of medical devices is usually less rigorous in many countries outside the United States, and as a result, medical devices are often initially trialed outside of the United States. It is imperative that the manufacturer report on the results of all studies completed or ongoing outside of the United States.

In the IDE proposal, the device manufacturer must define the target population for the device and the indications for how the device should be used. For example, the manufacturer may indicate that a cochlear implant should be considered for adults with severe to profound hearing loss and poor aided speech recognition (e.g., monosyllabic word recognition less than or equal to 40% correct in the ear to be implanted and less than or equal to 50% correct in the best aided condition). Of course, the exact indications of use for cochlear implants will be more detailed and thorough. Of note, if the FDA approves the device for commercial distribution, the indications of use will become the labeled guidelines (i.e., indications of use), which will serve as a guide for clinicians to determine patients who are likely to benefit from the device.

Additionally, the manufacturer must clearly define the study protocol. For instance, the manufacturer must define the number of subjects that will be recruited for study participation, inclusion/exclusion criteria, study measures, number of study sessions, primary and secondary endpoints (i.e., outcome measures and when they will be completed; e.g., CNC word recognition in quiet obtained pre-implantation and at 3, 6, and 12 months post-implantation; AzBio sentence recognition in noise [+10 dB SNR] obtained pre-implantation and at 3, 6, and 12 months post-implantation).

The IDE should also include information regarding study logistics and regulation. For example, the IDE should define whether the trial will be conducted at a single site or at multiple sites. Study locations should be clearly defined. Additionally, the IDE should include a description for how the data will be stored with safeguards to protect the privacy of participants. Also, the IDE should specify how the data will be analyzed. Information regarding institutional review board (IRB) approval should be included as well, and consent forms, data collection forms, questionnaires, etc. should be submitted with the IDE. Furthermore, the manufacturer should include a plan for how monitoring will take place throughout the study to ensure that study procedures are followed closely and to identify adverse effects associated with device use.

The device manufacturer may commence with execution of the IDE study as soon as the FDA approves the IDE. The FDA's Office of Compliance will provide oversight throughout the IDE study to ensure that the examiners at each study site are adhering to the IDE study protocol. Furthermore, the

manufacturer must submit annual reports to the FDA to describe study progress, including the number of participants enrolled, data collected at endpoints, the safety and efficacy of the device as indicated by the data, and adverse events. IDE trials are conducted over several months, or more commonly, several years. Once the manufacturer believes that sufficient data have been collected to support the labeled indications of device use, the manufacturer may submit a PMA to the FDA with the intent to receive approval to commercially distribute the device per the labeled guidelines/indications of use.

Premarket Application

In the PMA, the manufacturer must provide updates on the information included in the IDE proposal (FDA, 2017d). For instance, the manufacturer must summarize the updated results of trials that have been conducted outside the United States. Also, the manufacturer must provide an update on any bench testing, animal studies, and computer modeling that have been completed since the IDE submission. Although the submission of this information is mandatory, the primary component of the manufacturer's PMA is a detailed report of the data and outcomes obtained in the IDE clinical trial. The IDE data and supporting information are reviewed by the FDA's clinicians, researchers, and statisticians to determine whether the study was conducted according to the IDE protocol and to determine whether the data support a reasonable assurance of the effectiveness and safety of the device. If the FDA decides that the data indicate that patients who met the indications for use are able to safely use the device and that the device will effectively address the purpose for which the patient is using the device, then the FDA will provide approval for the device to be commercially marketed and distributed based on the labeled indications for use (guidelines). If the FDA does not believe that the IDE study results support the safety and efficacy of a device, then the FDA may ask the manufacturer to collect additional data or revise the study protocol, or the FDA may deny the commercial distribution of the device.

In some cases, the FDA may decide that the IDE study results should be subjected to additional scrutiny. In such an event, the PMA submission is reviewed by an advisory panel of independent experts who can review IDE study data and query the manufacturer regarding concerns pertaining to the safety and efficacy of the device. The advisory panel may consist of clinicians, statisticians, researchers, physiologists, physicists, and patient representatives. Advisory panels may offer support for or against the approval to commercially distribute the device. In some cases, public commentary is solicited in the advisory process.

Additional Evaluation Following PMA Approval

Oftentimes, the FDA requires manufacturers to continue to collect data about device performance after the PMA is approved. Post-market approval studies may be required to allow for continued follow-up of subjects who participated in the IDE. For example, the FDA may ask a manufacturer to continue to evaluate the performance of hybrid cochlear implant recipients to determine whether residual hearing remains stable in both the implanted and non-implanted ears on a long-term basis following surgery and to determine whether hearing performance remains stable or improves with time. Furthermore, post-market studies are often established to compare results obtained in clinical settings to the results obtained in the well-controlled trial environments found in IDE research. Additionally, post-market registries are often established to allow for tracking of adverse events. Medical device reports (MDRs) may be submitted by patients, manufacturers, and/or health care professionals to notify the FDA of device flaws, device failures, and/or device-related adverse events (FDA, 2016a). The OSB is responsible for providing oversight of FDRs submitted for devices monitored by the FDA. Collectively, the aforementioned information gathered in post-market studies may be used to expand or limit indications for device use.

Cochlear implant manufacturers (and other Class III device manufacturers) must receive PMA approval in order to commercially market and distribute new cochlear implants and sound processors. Cochlear implant manufacturers must also submit a PMA supplement or amendment application when they make significant design changes to existing cochlear implants or sound processors. For example, the cochlear implant manufacturer would submit a PMA supplement in order to revise the indications of use for a device. The ENT branch of the ODE reviews the aforementioned PMAs. In many cases, the OSEL will conduct reviews and evaluations of the technical aspects of new devices or device changes in order to determine the safety and efficacy of new or updated technology.

If a Class III device manufacturer wishes to make changes in its manufacturing processes or quality control of a device the FDA has approved for commercial use, and the changes may influence the safety or effectiveness of the device, the manufacturer must notify the FDA's Office of Compliance (OC). The manufacturer cannot implement the proposed change until it is approved by the OC. The OC is also tasked with ensuring that manufacturers are complying with regulatory requirements for manufacturing of medical devices. Additionally, the OC provides oversight when a medical device is recalled because of safety concerns or concerns about a lack of effectiveness.

The FDA defines the process that a manufacturer must complete to make a significant change to an FDA-approved medical device as follows in the box below (FDA, 2017f; Source- FDA.gov- https://www.fda.gov/MedicalDevices/DeviceRegulationandGuidance/HowtoMarketYourDevice/PremarketSubmissions/PremarketApprovalPMA/ucm050467.htm).

Amendments (§ 814.37) or supplements (§814.39) are submitted to FDA for changes or revisions to the original PMA submission. Although a PMA supplement applies to an approved PMA, in many cases there will be amendments to the PMA or to the PMA supplement before it is approved. In addition, PMA reports may also have amendments if the applicant is requested to submit additional information on a report.

*A **PMA supplement** is the submission required for a change affecting the safety or effectiveness of the device for which the applicant has an approved PMA; additional information provided to FDA for PMA supplement under review are amendments to a supplement*

*A **PMA amendment** includes all additional submissions to a PMA or PMA supplement before approval of the PMA or PMA supplement OR all additional correspondence after PMA or PMA supplement approval.*

Changes that Require a PMA Supplement
After FDA has approved a PMA, an applicant must submit a PMA supplement for review and approval by FDA before making any change affecting the safety or effectiveness of the device unless FDA has advised that an alternate type of submission is permitted for a particular change. All changes must meet the requirements of the Quality System regulation (Good Manufacturing Practices)

under 21 CFR Part 820 including the design control requirement under §820.30. Changes for which an applicant must submit a PMA supplement include, but are not limited to, the following types of changes if they affect the safety or effectiveness of the device:

- new indication for use of the device;
- labeling changes;
- the use of a different facility or establishment to manufacture, process, sterilize, or package the device;
- changes in manufacturing facilities, methods, or quality control procedures;
- changes in sterilization procedures;
- changes in packaging;
- changes in the performance or design specifications, circuits, components, ingredients, principles of operation, or physical layout of the device; and
- extension of the expiration date of the device based on data obtained under a new or revised stability or sterility testing protocol that has not been approved by FDA. [If the protocol has been previously approved by FDA, a supplement is not submitted but the change must be reported to FDA in the postapproval periodic reports as described in the §814.39(b).]

Changes without a PMA Supplement 814.39(b)

An applicant may make a change in a device after FDA's approval of the PMA without submitting a PMA supplement if (1) the change does not affect the device's safety or effectiveness, and (2) the change is reported to FDA in a postapproval periodic report (annual report) required as a condition of approval of the device, e.g., an editorial change in labeling which does not affect the safety or effectiveness of the device. Trivial changes, such as changes in the color of a label, would not have to be included in the postapproval periodic report.

Types of PMA Supplements

The methods of notification and FDA involvement of changes to a PMA approved medical device depend on the type of change made. A summary of the types of notification and FDA involvement is outlined below.

- **PMA supplement (180 days) - §814.39(a)**
  - for significant changes that affect the safety and effectiveness of the device
  - in-depth review and approval by FDA is required before implementation of the change
  - A full PMA review including a review by an outside advisory panel may be required. The criteria for a

full PMA review includes changes in the device that may raise different types of safety and effectiveness questions or changes in which there may be no accepted test methods for evaluating the issues of safety or effectiveness.

Some 180-day PMA supplements may be reviewed using the **Real-Time Review** process. In this process the supplement is reviewed during a meeting or conference call with the applicant. FDA will fax its decision to the applicant within five working days after the meeting or call. The change must meet certain criteria to be eligible for this type of review. Supplements with detailed clinical data are generally not considered for this program. The criteria and process for the Real-Time Review program are outlined in Real-Time Premarket Approval Application (PMA) Supplements.

- **Special PMA Supplement—Changes Being Effected - §814.39(d)**
  - for any change that enhances the safety of the device or the safety in the use of the device
  - may be placed into effect by the applicant prior to the receipt of a written FDA order approving the PMA supplement.

  After FDA approves a PMA, any change described below that enhances the safety of the device or the safety in the use of the device [§814.39(d)(2)] may be placed into effect by the applicant prior to the receipt of a written FDA order approving the PMA supplement, but after the applicant receives specific acknowledgment that the application qualifies for review under §814.39(d)(2) provided that:
  - the PMA supplement and its mailing cover are plainly marked "Special PMA Supplement—Changes Being Effected";
  - the PMA supplement provides a full explanation of the basis for the changes;
  - the applicant has received acknowledgment that the application qualifies as a "Special PMA Supplement—Changes Being Effected" from FDA for the supplement;
  - the PMA supplement specifically identifies the date that such changes are being effected; and
  - the change is made according to the good manufacturing practices regulation.

  The following changes are permitted [§814.39(d)(1)]:
  - labeling changes that add or strengthen a contraindication, warning, precaution, or information about an adverse reaction;

- *labeling changes that add or strengthen an instruction that is intended to enhance the safe use of the device;*
- *labeling changes that delete misleading, false, or unsupported indications; and*
- *changes in quality controls or the manufacturing process that add a new specification or test method, or otherwise provide additional assurance of purity, identity, strength, or reliability of the device.*

The applicant is encouraged to contact the PMA Staff to assist in determining if the change meets the requirements of §814.39(b).

- **30-day Notice and 135 PMA Supplement - §814.39(f)**
  - *Used for modifications to manufacturing procedures or methods of manufacture that affect the safety and effectiveness of the device.*
  - *Changes in a manufacturing/sterilization site or to design or performance specifications do not qualify*
  - *If the change qualifies as a 30-day Notice, the change may be made 30 days after FDA receives the 30-day notice unless FDA informs the PMA holder that the 30-day Notice is not adequate and describes the additional information or action required. If the 30-day Notice was not adequate, but contained data meeting appropriate content requirements for a PMA supplement, then the 30-day Notice will become a 135-day PMA Supplement.*

Additional guidance can be found in "30-Day Notices and 135-Day PMA Supplements for Manufacturing Method or Process Changes, Guidance for Industry and CDRH."

Note: 30-day Notice is not the same as a 30-day Supplement. See below for information regarding the 30-day Supplement.

- **PMA Manufacturing Site Change Supplement**
  - *For moving the manufacturing site if certain conditions apply.*
  - *Manufacturing site must have received a Quality System/GMP inspection within the last two years.*
  - *If requirements are not met, 180-day PMA Supplement must be submitted.*

- **Annual (periodic) Report or 30-day Supplements - §814.39(e)**
  - *FDA may allow certain changes to be reported in an annual report or 30-day supplement an instead of a PMA supplement submission. (If this method*

is utilized, FDA will typically request that the information be reported in the annual report and not as a 30-day supplement.)
  - *FDA will notify applicants of this alternative through an advisory opinion to the affected industry or in correspondence with the applicant.*

FDA will identify a change to a device for which the applicant has an approved PMA and for which a PMA supplement is not required under 814.39(a). FDA will identify such a change in an advisory opinion under §10.85, if the change applies to a generic type of device. Such changes will be identified in written correspondence to each PMA holder who may be affected by FDA's decision.

FDA will require that a change, for which a PMA supplement under §814.39(a) is not required, to be reported to FDA in a periodic (annual) report or a 30-day PMA supplement. In written correspondence, FDA will identify the type of information that is to be included in the report or 30-day PMA supplement.

If FDA requires that the change be reported in a periodic report, the change may be made before it is reported to FDA. If FDA requires that the change be reported in a 30-day PMA supplement, the change may be made 30 days after FDA files the 30-day supplement, unless FDA informs the PMA holder that additional information is required, the supplement is not approvable, or the supplement is denied. The 30-day PMA supplement must follow the instructions in the correspondence or advisory opinion. Any 30-day PMA supplement that does not meet the requirements of the correspondence or advisory opinion will not be filed and, therefore, will not be deemed approved 30 days after receipt.

The applicant is encouraged to contact the PMA staff to assist in determining if the change meets the requirements of §814.39(e).

- **Document to file**
  - *for changes that do not affect the safety or effectiveness of the device*
  - *very limited or no FDA involvement prior to implementation of the change*

Minor manufacturing changes and minor quality control changes can be documented to file. Examples of changes that can be documented to file include editorial changes to a Standard Operating Procedure (SOP) to make instructions clearer and combining two SOPs into one.

- New PMA
  - Certain changes may require the submission of a complete new PMA. If any of the following changes occur, the applicant should consult the appropriate reviewing branch in the Office of Device Evaluation if:
    - the design change causes a different intended use, mode of operation, and technological basis of operation,
    - there will be a change in the patient population that will be treated with the device, or
    - the design change is so significant that a new generation of the device will be developed.

PMA Amendments (§ 814.37)
An applicant may amend a pending PMA or PMA supplement to revise existing information or provide additional information. FDA may request that the applicant amend their PMA or PMA supplement with any necessary information about the device that FDA considers necessary to complete the review of the PMA or PMA supplement.

If the applicant submits a major PMA amendment on his or her own initiative or at FDA's request, the review period may be extended up to 180 days. A major amendment is one that contains significant new data from a previously unreported study, significant updated data from a previously reported study, detailed new analyses of previously submitted data, or significant required information previously omitted.

A PMA amendment must include the PMA or PMA supplement number assigned to the original submission and the reason for submitting the amendment (FDA, 2017f).

Manufacturer's Cost of Regulatory Approval and Surveillance

Hearing aid manufacturers typically release multiple new hearing aids every year. In contrast, cochlear implant manufacturers typically develop one new cochlear implant or sound processor every several years. Because hearing aids are Class I devices, the FDA requires very little in the way of regulatory approval before a hearing aid is commercially marketed and distributed. However, the FDA regulations of Class III medical devices, such as cochlear implants and middle ear implantable devices, are quite stringent, and manufacturers are required to conduct expensive studies to collect the data necessary to support a PMA or PMA supplement. In most cases of device development, the manufacturer must employ numerous professionals to design the new device, create reports describing the device, design research studies to evaluate the safety and efficacy of the device, monitor the study and support clinicians serving as co-investigators in the study, analyzing and summarizing data and preparing a PMA for the FDA. Additionally, the FDA levies fees that the manufacturer must pay to pursue PMAs and PMA supplements. As of January 2018, the standard fee for a PMA submission, panel-track supplement, 180-day supplement, and 30-day notice were $310,764, $233,073, $46,615, and $4,972, respectively (FDA, 2017g).

Obviously, the cost associated with FDA approval of a medical device can mount quickly. Of note, the FDA has established the supplement track to approve device changes in an attempt to reduce the costs associated with approval of new technology and/or new indications. Even with the reduced charges associated with supplements rather than a full-blown PMA, the cost to bring new Class III implantable hearing technology to the market is quite expensive and laborious. As a result, cochlear implant and middle ear device manufacturers typically release new technology rather seldom relative to hearing aid manufacturers.

FDA-Approved Indications for Use for Class III Implantable Hearing Technology

Once the FDA approves a manufacturer's PMA, the device may be marketed and commercially distributed. The indications of device use that are explicitly listed in the PMA and are approved by the FDA are technically referred to as **labeled indications**. As the name implies, the labeled indications are included on or within the packaging of the medical device. The reader is familiar with FDA labeled indications, because we have all read labeled indications for prescription medications, which are also approved by the FDA prior to use in the commercial market. The labeled indications are often referred to as **guidelines**. Furthermore, many clinicians refer to the indications of use as FDA candidacy criteria.

It is important to note that the FDA-approved labeled indications/guidelines for cochlear implants and other implantable hearing devices were not developed by the FDA. Instead, the labeled indications of use/guidelines are proposed by the device manufacturer, supported by science and clinical research, and approved by the FDA once the science and clinical research demonstrates that the device is safe and effective. Stated differently, the FDA approves device indications for use but does not set device use guidelines.

It is also important to note that the implantable hearing device guidelines do not mandate how clinicians should use a device with patients. Instead, as the name implies, the FDA guidelines serve to guide the clinician in selecting patients for whom the benefit of device use are likely to outweigh the risks. The FDA provides regulation of the manufacturers of medical devices but does not govern the individual clinician or clinics. Clinicians ultimately have the responsibility to select the most appropriate intervention for their patients based on safety and effectiveness. The potential benefits of device use should be greater than the potential risks. In some cases, a clinician may recommend a medical device for a patient who does not meet the FDA-approved labeled indications of use for the device, a practice referred to as **off-label** usage (FDA, 2016b).

For example, FDA-approved labeled indications of use for a cochlear implant may state that a cochlear implant should be considered for an adult with moderate to profound sensorineural hearing loss with sentence recognition of 50% correct or poorer in the ear to be implanted and 60% or poorer in the best aided condition. A clinician may serve a patient who reports significant difficulty with speech recognition in daily listening situations. On AzBio sentence recognition in quiet assessment (60 dBA presentation level), the patient scored 60% with use of his right hearing aid, 65% with the left hearing aid, and 72% in the binaural condition. CNC word recognition (60 dBA presentation level in quiet) was 32%, 36%, and 50% in the right, left, and binaural conditions, respectively. The clinician may decide that it is likely that the patient will achieve better speech recognition and communication abilities with use of a cochlear implant for the right ear and a hearing aid for the left ear. The recommendation of a cochlear implant for the right ear is an example of off-label use of a cochlear implant. The FDA supports the off-label usage of devices and drugs when the clinician makes an evidence-based recommendation for clinical use and not for research. Of note, off-label implantation cannot be recommended for persons covered by health care plans regulated by the Centers for Medicare and Medicaid Services (CMS). Instead, when a clinician uses a device off-label, the FDA indicates certain conditions that the clinician must meet. These conditions are highlighted in the statement in the box below, found in the FDA's (2016b) *"Off-label" and Investigational Use of Marketed Drugs, Biologics, and Medical Devices – Information Sheet (https://www.fda.gov/RegulatoryInformation/Guidances/ucm126486.htm)*.

Of note, clinicians can discuss and recommend off-label use of medical devices with individual patients. However, clinicians cannot advertise off-label use of devices to the general public. Also, medical device manufacturers cannot promote off-label use of their devices. Additionally, it should be noted that the decision to make an off-label recommendation for cochlear implantation is often influenced by financial considerations. Off-label implantations are often recommended when the recipient's medical insurance company authorizes payment for the cochlear implant as well as surgical, hospital, and related fees even though the patient does not meet the FDA-approved labeled indications for use. In some cases, a patient may meet indications for cochlear implant use, but the patient's health care plan may possess criteria that are more stringent than the FDA guidelines. In such cases, the patient's only option to pursue cochlear implantation may be to pay out-of-pocket for the device and the related services.

Guidance for Institutional Review Boards and Clinical Investigators

*Good medical practice and the best interests of the patient require that physicians use legally available drugs, biologics and devices according to their best knowledge and judgement. If physicians use a product for an indication not in the approved labeling, **they have the responsibility to be well informed about the product, to base its use on firm scientific rationale and on sound medical evidence, and to maintain records of the product's use and effects.** Use of a marketed product in this manner when the intent is the "practice of medicine" does not require the submission of an Investigational New Drug Application (IND), Investigational Device Exemption (IDE) or review by an Institutional Review Board (IRB). However, the institution at which the product will be used may, under its own authority, require IRB review or other institutional oversight.*

The FDA-approved labeled indications for Advanced Bionics, Cochlear Americas, and MED-EL cochlear implants are provided in Tables 4–1, 4–2, and 4–3. The reader will notice that there are differences in the indications of use for cochlear implants marketed by each of the three cochlear implant manufacturers distributing cochlear implants in the United States. Also, the reader will notice that there are separate indications of use for children and adults. Of note, the labeled indications of use also include contraindications of use such as retrocochlear hearing loss/site-of-lesion, cochlear ossification preventing insertion of the electrode array into the cochlea, active middle ear disease and/or tympanic membrane pathology, and/or adverse reaction to device materials (e.g., silicone, titanium).

Of note, there is considerable variability in the regulation of cochlear implants in countries outside of the United States. For example, in European countries, manufacturers must receive the CE (Conformité Européene, which means European Conformity) mark in order to commercially distribute cochlear implants in the European Economic Area, which includes countries in the European Union

as well as the United Kingdom, Liechtenstein, and Norway. Switzerland is also part of the single market in which medical devices are approved with a CE mark. To receive a CE mark, a medical device must comply with European Union Directives which require manufacturers to meet detailed standards of performance, safety, efficacy, and quality. The European Union standards are typically based on those of the International Organization for Standardization (ISO). Similar to the FDA, the European Union Directive categorizes medical devices into different classes based on the risk the device places on the recipient's or user's health, safety, and well-being. The CE mark may be granted for medical devices that are similar in design, application, operation, and purpose to an existing medical device that has a CE mark. In many cases, the manufacturer must conduct a well-designed clinical trial to demonstrate the effectiveness and safety of a medical implantable device. Although the process by which a manufacturer pursues a CE mark for use in Europe is similar to the process by which FDA approval is sought for commercial distribution in the United States, the regulatory process to bring a cochlear implant to the market for

TABLE 4–1. Advanced Bionics—HiResolution Bionic Ear System

Advanced Bionics—HiResolution Bionic Ear System	
Indications for Use: The HiResolution Bionic Ear System is intended to restore a level of auditory sensation to individuals with severe to profound sensorineural hearing loss via electrical stimulation of the auditory nerve.	
Children	**Adults**

• 12 months through 17 years of age
• Profound, bilateral sensorineural deafness (≥90 dB)
• Use of appropriately fitted hearing aids for at least 6 months in children 2 through 17 years of age, or at least 3 months in children 12 through 23 months of age. The minimum duration of hearing aid use is waived if X-rays indicate ossification of the cochlea.
• Little or no benefit from appropriately fitted hearing aids, defined as:
  ○ In younger children (<4 years of age)
    • A failure to reach developmentally appropriate milestones (such as spontaneous response to name in quiet or to environmental sounds) measured using the Infant-Toddler Meaningful Auditory Integration Scale or Meaningful Auditory Integration Scale or <20% correct on a simple open-set word recognition test (Multisyllabic Lexical Neighborhood Test) administered using monitored live voice (70 dB SPL)
  ○ In older children (≥4 years of age)
    • Scoring <12% on a difficult open-set word recognition test (Phonetically Balanced-Kindergarten Test) or <30% on an open-set sentence test (Hearing in Noise Test for Children) administered using recorded materials in the soundfield (70 dB SPL)
	• 18 years of age or older
	• Severe-to-profound, bilateral sensorineural hearing loss (>70 dB)
	• Postlingual onset of severe or profound hearing loss
	• Limited benefit from appropriately fitted hearing aids, defined as scoring 50% or less on a test of open set sentence recognition (HINT Sentences)

TABLE 4–2. Cochlear Americas—Cochlear Implant System

Cochlear Americas—Cochlear Implant System	
Indications for Use: The Cochlear Nucleus Implant System is intended to restore a level of auditory sensation via the electrical stimulation of the auditory nerve.	
Children	**Adults**

• Children 12 to 24 months of age who have bilateral profound sensorineural deafness
• Children two years of age or older may demonstrate severe to profound hearing loss bilaterally
• Little benefit from appropriate binaural hearing aids, defined as:
  ○ In younger children
    ▪ Lack of progress in the development of simple auditory skills in conjunction with appropriate amplification and participation in intensive aural habilitation over a three to 6-month period. It is recommended that limited benefit be quantified on a measure such as the Meaningful Auditory Integration Scale or the Early Speech Perception test.
  ○ In older children
    ▪ ≤30% correct on the open set Multisyllabic Lexical Neighborhood Test (MLNT) or Lexical Neighborhood Test (LNT), depending upon the child's cognitive and linguistic skills. A three to six month hearing aid trial is recommended for children without previous aided experience.
	• Individuals 18 years of age or older who have bilateral, pre, peri, or postlinguistic sensorineural hearing impairment
	• Limited benefit from appropriate binaural hearing aids, as defined by test scores of 50% correct or less in the ear to be implanted (60% or less in the best-aided condition) on tape-recorded tests of open set sentence recognition
	• Moderate to profound hearing loss in the low frequencies and profound (≥90 dB HL) hearing loss in the mid to high speech frequencies

TABLE 4–3. Med-EI—Med-EI Cochlear Implant System

Med-EI—Med-EI Cochlear Implant System	
Indications for Use: The Med-EI Cochlear Implant System is intended to restore a level of auditory sensation via the electrical stimulation of the auditory nerve.	
Children	**Adults**

• 12 months of age and older who demonstrate a profound, bilateral sensorineural hearing loss with thresholds of 90 dB or greater at 1000 Hz
• Lack of hearing aid benefit is defined as:
  ○ In younger children
    ▪ Lack of progress in the development of simple auditory skills in conjunction with appropriate amplification and participation in intensive aural habilitation over a three- to six-month period
  ○ In older children
    ▪ <20% correct on the Multi-syllabic Lexical Neighborhood Test (MLNT) or Lexical Neighborhood Test (LNT), depending upon the child's cognitive ability and linguistic skills
• A three- to six-month hearing aid trial is required for children without previous experience with hearing aids. Radiological evidence of cochlear ossification may justify a shorter trial with amplification
	• 18 years of age or older who have bilateral, sensorineural hearing impairment
	• Limited benefit from appropriately fitted binaural hearing aids, defined by test scores of 40% correct or less in best aided listening condition on CD recorded tests of open-set sentence recognition (Hearing In Noise Test [HINT] sentences)
	• Bilateral severe to profound sensorineural hearing loss determined by a pure tone average of 70 dB or greater at 500 Hz, 1000 Hz, and 2000 Hz

clinical use is typically less arduous in the European Union, and as a result, cochlear implant technology is often brought to market sooner in Europe than in the United States. Additionally, the indications for use of cochlear implants are often less stringent in European counties when compared with the indications for use as approved by the FDA. For instance, in many European countries, the indications for use of the Cochlear Nucleus cochlear implant are as follows:

- Individuals aged up to 17 years who have clinically established bilateral or unilateral sensorineural hearing loss and who have compromised functional hearing with hearing aids or would receive no benefit with hearing aids. Typical preoperative hearing threshold levels in the impaired ears demonstrate a pure-tone average of moderately severe to profound degree.
- Individuals aged 18 years and older who have clinically established postlinguistic bilateral or unilateral sensorineural hearing loss and who have compromised functional hearing with hearing aids or would receive no benefit with hearing aids. Typical preoperative threshold levels in the impaired ears demonstrate a pure-tone average loss of moderately severe to profound degree.
- Prelinguistically or perilinguistically deafened individuals aged 18 years and older who have profound bilateral sensorineural hearing loss and who have compromised hearing with hearing aids.

Similar practices as implemented in the United States and Europe are used in other parts of the world for the regulation of cochlear implants for clinical use. In Australia, medical device regulation is overseen by the Advisory Committee on Medical Devices (ACMD), the Therapeutics Goods Committee, and the National Coordinating Committee on Therapeutic Goods (NCCTG). Australian regulations for medical devices are based on policies and procedures defined and articulated in the Australian "Therapeutic Goods Act 1989" (Therapeutic Goods Administration, 2011). Regulations in South America and other Latin American countries vary by country but also typically require approval based on the country's regulatory body's review of clinical trials conducted within or outside of the respective country.

Key Concepts

- The "indications of use" specify the inclusion and exclusion guidelines that clinicians should consider when determining candidacy for implantable hearing technology.

- In each country, regulatory bodies determine the indications of use for cochlear implants and other implantable hearing technologies. These regulatory bodies also oversee manufacturing processes and the safety and efficacy of implantable hearing technologies.
- In the United States of America, the Food and Drug Administration provides regulatory oversight of implantable hearing technologies. Manufacturers of implantable hearing technologies develop indications of use for their implantable devices and conduct clinical trials to generate data to warrant the indications of use and to demonstrate the safety and efficacy of their implantable technologies and manufacturing processes. The FDA reviews the indications of use and provides approval for the manufacturer to conduct clinical trials to evaluate implantable hearing technologies. The FDA also reviews the results of these clinical trials to determine whether the study data support the indications of use and approval for commercial distribution of the device.
- Countries outside of the United States have similar regulatory bodies with similar processes for determining indications of use and whether an implantable hearing device should be approved for commercial distribution.

References

FDA (2014a). *Regulatory controls.* Retrieved from https://www.fda .gov/MedicalDevices/DeviceRegulationandGuidance/Over view/GeneralandSpecialControls/default.htm

FDA (2014b). *The 510(k) program: Evaluating substantial equivalence in premarket notifications [510(k)]: Guidance for industry and food and drug administration staff.* Centers for Devices and Radiological Health, Document issued on July 28, 2014.

FDA (2016a). *Medical device reporting (MDR).* Retrieved from https://www.fda.gov/MedicalDevices/Safety/ReportaProblem/default.htm

FDA (2016b). *"Off-label" and investigational use of marketed drugs, biologics, and medical devices—information sheet.* Retrieved from https://www.fda.gov/RegulatoryInformation/Guidances/ucm126486.htm

FDA (2017a). *About the Center for Devices and Radiological Health.* Retrieved from https://www.fda.gov/AboutFDA/CentersOffices/OfficeofMedicalProductsandTobacco/CDRH/

FDA (2017b). *Ear, nose, and throat devices panel.* Retrieved from https://www.fda.gov/AdvisoryCommittees/CommitteesMeet ingMaterials/MedicalDevices/MedicalDevicesAdvisoryCom mittee/EarNoseandThroatDevicesPanel/ucm124456.htm

FDA (2017c). *Medical device overview.* Retrieved from_https:// www.fda.gov/ForIndustry/ImportProgram/ImportBasics/ RegulatedProducts/ucm510630.htm

FDA (2017d). *Premarket approval (PMA).* Retrieved from https:// www.fda.gov/MedicalDevices/DeviceRegulationandGuid ance/HowtoMarketYourDevice/PremarketSubmissions/Pre marketApprovalPMA/ucm2007514.htm

FDA (2017e). *Device advice: Investigational device exemption (IDE).* Retrieved from https://www.fda.gov/MedicalDevices/ DeviceRegulationandGuidance/HowtoMarketYourDevice/ PremarketSubmissions/PremarketApprovalPMA/ucm2007514 .htm

FDA (2017f). *PMA supplements and amendments.* Retrieved from https://www.fda.gov/MedicalDevices/DeviceRegulationand Guidance/HowtoMarketYourDevice/PremarketSubmissions/ PremarketApprovalPMA/ucm050467.htm

FDA (2017g). *FY 2018 MDUFA user fees.* Retrieved from https:// www.fda.gov/forindustry/userfees/medicaldeviceuserfee/ ucm452519.htm

FDA (2018). *What does the FDA do?* Retrieved from https://www .fda.gov/AboutFDA/Transparency/Basics/ucm194877.htm

Therapeutic Goods Administration. (2011). *Australian regulatory guidelines for medical devices, version 1.1.* May 2011, pp. 1–331. Commonwealth of Australia.

Cochlear Implant Candidacy: Adult Audiologic Assessment

Jace Wolfe

Introduction

The word **candidate** is often used to describe a person who is being considered for cochlear implantation. Assessing candidacy for cochlear implantation in adult patients is a multifaceted process which includes a variety of different types of audiologic evaluations as well as assessments by multiple professionals. At a minimum, the adult cochlear implant candidacy assessment includes evaluations by an audiologist, a cochlear implant surgeon, and an imaging specialist (e.g., a radiologist). However, other professionals may also be involved with the evaluation process, particularly when the cochlear implant candidate presents with exceptional needs. For example, a cardiologist may evaluate elderly recipients who have a history of cardiovascular disease and for whom there may be concern that surgery may place the patient's well-being at risk. Additionally, a psychologist and/or a neurologist may be involved with the assessment process if concerns exist regarding the patient's cognitive status (e.g., dementia, Alzheimer's). Furthermore, a social worker may be involved if the patient requires support related to socioeconomic, family, or transportation matters.

The primary focus of this chapter will center on the audiologist's role in the cochlear implant assessment process for adult patients. Ideally, in order to provide a thorough evaluation to identify the most appropriate hearing technology options for the patient, the audiologist should have a keen working knowledge of basic audiology diagnostics, hearing aid technology and verification, and potential advantages and limitations of all available implantable hearing technologies (e.g., cochlear implants, hybrid cochlear implants, middle ear implantable hearing devices, implantable bone conduction devices). Consequently, a variety of audiology-related topics will be highlighted in this chapter. This chapter will also briefly address non-audiologic facets of the cochlear implant candidacy assessment process. Additionally, this chapter will address prognostic factors that influence cochlear implant outcomes so that the reader can identify patients who are most likely to benefit from cochlear implantation and those who are more likely to receive limited benefit from a cochlear implant.

Case History

The cochlear implant candidacy assessment should begin with the attainment of a case history. The case history should begin by asking the potential candidate about his/her primary reason for scheduling his/her appointment as well as the objective for the appointment. It is important to understand the patient's intentions, because in some cases, he/she is unfamiliar with cochlear implant technology and is unaware of the exact objective of the appointment.

More specifically, he/she may have been informed of being referred to another hearing health care provider because hearing aids are unlikely to provide satisfactory communication. However, he/she may not have a clear understanding of the exact reason for being referred for cochlear implant candidate assessment. Quickly identifying patients who are unclear on the objective of a cochlear implant candidacy assessment allows for the expeditious provision of information that will allow the potential candidate to determine whether he/she wants to pursue cochlear implantation.

Figure 5–1 provides an example of a case history form that may be administered during an adult cochlear implant candidacy assessment. Most of the information included in this sample case history questionnaire is self-explanatory. It is important to note that the audiologist should aim to identify the duration of a potential candidate's hearing loss, hearing aid use, and duration of deafness. It is important to have an understanding of the duration of a patient's severe to profound hearing loss, because lengthy durations of severe to profound hearing loss are associated with poor speech recognition outcomes (Blamey et al., 2013; Holden et al., 2013). If possible, the audiologist should request that the patient provide serial audiograms to allow for a review of the progression of the hearing loss over time. In many cases, patients are unable to provide a long history of their audiograms. In such an event, the audiologist can gather a rough estimate of the length of a patient's duration of severe to profound hearing loss by determining how long it has been since the patient has been able to communicate over the telephone and/or understand television audio without the use of closed caption. Additionally, it is useful to know how long the patient has worn hearing aids and how long it has been since the patient has noticed that hearing aids no longer provide satisfactory communication performance.

Audiologic Assessment

The audiologic assessment should always begin with a thorough otoscopic evaluation. The audiologist should note any remarkable features of the auricle and head that may present difficulty for the patient to use a cochlear implant sound processor. For instance, if the candidate has very small, stiff auricles that adhere closely to the head, it may be difficult to comfortably wear a behind-the-ear sound processor with sufficient retention. In such a case, the audiologist may choose to recommend an off-the-ear sound processor option.

Physiologic Assessment of Auditory Function

Although physiologic measures of auditory function are not directly used to determine whether an adult meets indications of use for cochlear implantation, the audiologist should incorporate the use of physiologic measures in the battery of cochlear implant assessments. Specifically, the audiologist should routinely measure tympanometry, acoustic reflexes, and otoacoustic emissions. In fact, the audiologist should consider completing these physiologic measures at the beginning of the assessment session in order to provide a quick, objective insight into the candidate's auditory function.

Middle Ear Measurements

Obviously, middle ear measurements identify conductive disorders. In particular, the presence of acoustic reflexes suggests normal middle ear function. Estimates suggest that the acoustic reflex is not recordable in the probe ear (i.e., the ear in which the admittance probe is placed to measure for the presence of a reflex) for 80% of patients who have an air-bone gap of 10 dB (Jerger et al., 1974). The acoustic reflex is the most sensitive audiologic measure for identification of conductive hearing loss. In essence, the presence of an acoustic reflex rules out a significant conductive hearing loss in the probe ear.

Additionally, the presence of acoustic reflexes at normal levels (e.g., 75–95 dB) suggests that a moderately severe to profound hearing loss is unlikely in the ear that was stimulated to elicit the reflex. Gelfand and colleagues (1990) reported that 90% of adults with air conduction pure tone thresholds of 50 dB HL or poorer had acoustic reflex thresholds of 100 dB HL or higher when measured at the same pure-tone frequency. Furthermore, 90% of adults with air conduction threshold poorer than 70 dB HL had acoustic reflexes of 120 dB HL or higher. As a result, the presence of acoustic reflexes at lower stimulation levels suggests that a severe to profound hearing loss is unlikely. The presence of an acoustic reflex at normal to near-normal levels requires a response from a relatively sufficient number of functioning inner hair cells.

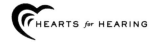

11500 N Portland Ave
Oklahoma City, OK 73120
Phone: (405)548-4300
Fax: (405)548-4350

Date: _____

Patient Name:_____ Social Security #_____

Date of Birth: _____Sex:_____ Home Phone: _____Cell:_____

Address: _____ City _____ST _____ Zip_____

County: _____ Email:_____

Primary Care Physician: _____ Phone Number:_____

Referring Physician: _____ Phone Number:_____

Otologist/ENT: _____ Phone Number: _____

Audiologist: _____ Phone Number: _____

Other Relevant Professional: _____ Phone Number: _____

Emergency Contact: _____ Phone Number: _____Relationship: _____

Insurance Company Name: _____Address:_____

Policy Number:_____ Group Number: _____ Effective Date:_____ Co-Pay: _____

Subscriber's Name:_____ Date of Birth: _____Social Security:_____

Relationship: _____ Insurance Phone _____

Secondary Insurance Company Name:_____Address:_____

Policy Number: _____ Group: _____ Effective Date:_____

Subscriber's Name:_____ Date of Birth: _____Social Security:_____

Relationship: _____ Insurance Phone:_____

I authorize my insurance benefits to be paid directly to Hearts for Hearing. I understand that I am financially responsible for any balance. I authorize Hearts for Hearing or my insurance company to release any information needed to process my claims. I give permission to you and any agent of Hearts for Hearing to contact me on any phone number/email I have provided to you, including my cell phone, for the purpose of collecting my debt, appointment reminders and changes. I am aware of this office's Notice of Privacy practices and fully understand my rights as a patient.

Signature _____Date _____

☐check here if you do not wish to receive occasional mailings from Hearts for Hearing (Newsletters, events, etc)

FIGURE 5–1. An example of an adult cochlear implant case history form. Copyright © Hearts for Hearing. *continues*

CASE HISTORY (ADULT)

Date: _____ Patient Name: _____ Date of Birth: _____

What is your primary concern regarding your hearing?

_____

_____

At what age did you first notice your hearing loss diagnosed and what caused it? -

_____

_____

Please mark "Yes" or "No" and your provider will obtain more detailed information during the appointment:

<u>HEARING HISTORY</u>

○ Yes ○ No   Exposure to loud noise?

○ Yes ○ No   Do you currently use a hearing aid or cochlear implant? ○ Right Ear ○ Left Ear ○ Both Ears

When did you start wearing hearing aids? _____

How often do you wear your hearing aids each day? _____

Do your hearing aids help you hear better?_____

Please describe any assistive listening devices that you use (Closed-captioning, amplified telephone, television device, vibrating alarm, etc.):

_____

○ Yes ○ No   Does you have a better hearing ear? ○ Right Ear ○ Left Ear

○ Yes ○ No   Do you know the magnitude of your hearing loss (e.g., mild, moderate, severe, profound, decibel level):

_____

_____

_____

○ Yes ○ No   Is there a family history of hearing loss?

If yes, please describe: _____

○ Yes ○ No   Can you understand speech over the telephone? ○ Right Ear ○ Left Ear ○ Both Ears
If not, then how long ago was it when you were last able to understand speech over the telephone?

_____

_____

○ Yes ○ No   Can you understand speech over the television? ○ Right Ear ○ Left Ear ○ Both Ears
If not, then how long ago was it when you were last able to understand speech over the television?

_____

_____

FIGURE 5–1. *continues*

MEDICAL HISTORY

○ Yes ○ No   Do you see an Ear, Nose, and Throat doctor?

                  If yes, why? _____

○ Yes ○ No   Does you have a history of ear infections, ear drainage, or fluid behind the eardrum?

○ Yes ○ No   Have you had PE tubes?

○ Yes ○ No   Have you had any other surgeries or hospitalizations that we should know about?

                  If yes, please describe: _____

○ Yes ○ No   Do you have vision problems?

○ Yes ○ No   Do you have any other diagnoses that we should know about?

                  If yes, please describe: _____

Has your child had any of the following health/medical problems?

○ Allergies	○ Ear Pain	○ Head trauma/injury	○ Memory Problems
○ Asthma	○ Ear Ringing (Tinnitus)	○ Heart Problems	○ Motor Problems
○ Balance Disorders	○ Genetic Disorder/Syndrome	○ Kidney Problems	○ Psychiatric Disorder
○ Cancer	○ Head trauma/injury	○ Measles/Mumps	○ Sinusitis
○ Diabetes	○ Heart Problems	○ Meningitis	○ Seizures
			○ Stroke

Please list medications: -

_____
_____
_____
_____
_____

How do you communicate (e.g., listening and spoken language, sign language, written notes, gestures, etc.): -

_____
_____
_____

Is there anything else you would like us to know about you and your hearing and communication history?

_____
_____

Please describe what you hope to learn and/or achieve from today's appointment?

_____
_____
_____
_____

FIGURE 5–1. *continues*

Please describe what you expect from a cochlear implant?

_____

_____

_____

_____

FIGURE 5–1. *continued*

Consequently, the presence of normal to near-normal acoustic reflexes at 500, 1000, and 2000 Hz suggests reasonably good cochlear transduction and should bring into question the need for a cochlear implant. Use of ipsilateral and contralateral acoustic reflexes may be helpful for differential diagnosis (the interested reader is referred to Hall and Swanepoel [2010] for more information on the use of acoustic reflexes for differential diagnosis and for estimation of hearing sensitivity).

Otoacoustic Emissions

The audiologist should also consider routinely measuring otoacoustic emissions (OAEs) during the cochlear implant candidacy. In most cases, patients referred for cochlear implant candidacy assessment will have a lengthy history of significant hearing loss and use of high-gain hearing aids, so OAEs will be absent (Attias et al., 2001; Deltenre et al., 1999). Based on a review of research examining the presence of OAEs as a function of pure tone audiometric threshold, Dhar and Hall (2012) reported on the likelihood of OAEs as a function of hearing threshold (dB HL). Dahr and Hall noted that OAEs will almost invariably be absent when hearing threshold exceeds 35 dB HL. They also noted that OAEs are only obtained at normal absolute amplitudes when hearing thresholds are better than 20 dB HL (Figure 5–2). As a result, the presence of OAEs may lead the audiologist to investigate further if hearing thresholds are elevated. Additionally, the presence of OAEs may imply a retrocochlear site of lesion. Furthermore, OAE assessment may be useful in persons with sloping hearing loss. If OAEs are present in the low-frequency range, then a short electrode array may be considered to avoid altering the mechanical characteristics and active cochlear amplifier in the apical region of the cochlea.

Additional Physiologic Measures of Auditory Function

Auditory evoked responses are not routinely administered as part of the audiologic battery of measures

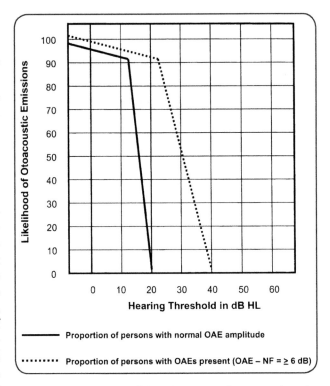

FIGURE 5–2. Likelihood of detecting a normal otoacoustic emission (OAE) (i.e., amplitude that is within normal limits) or the presence of any OAE (i.e., SNR > 6 dB) as a function of hearing threshold level. Reprinted with permission from Dhar and Hall, *Otoacoustic Emissions: Principles, Procedures, and Protocols* (2012). Copyright © Plural Publishing, Inc.

included in the cochlear implant candidacy assessment. A notable exception occurs when the audiologist has doubts about the validity of a candidate's pure tone thresholds. In such a case, the audiologist may wish to complete auditory brainstem response (ABR), auditory steady state response (ASSR), or cortical auditory evoked response (CAER) assessment to estimate the candidate's degree of hearing loss.

When cochlear implants were first introduced into clinical practice, the electrically evoked auditory brainstem response (eABR) was considered as a measure that could be used to predict a candidate's likelihood of success with a cochlear implant. Preoperative eABR assessment involves the placement of a long needle electrode through the tympanic membrane and on the promontory or niche of the round window. Electrical current is delivered through the long needle electrode and to the cochlea in an attempt to elicit the eABR. Early attempts at use of the eABR as a prognostic indicator were conducted with adults with profound sensorineural hearing loss. Published reports described the eABR as a relatively poor predictor of cochlear implant benefit (Mason, 2003; Nikolopolous et al., 2000). More recently, however, researchers have explored the use of the eABR to evaluate the potential for electrical stimulation to elicit a synchronous, auditory neural response in persons with auditory neuropathy spectrum disorder (ANSD). Gibson and colleagues (2007) have reported better speech recognition for cochlear implant recipients who had been diagnosed with ANSD and had a normal eABR relative to those who had been diagnosed with ANSD and had an abnormal eABR. Given the results of the Gibson et al. (2007) study, the eABR may harbor potential as a tool to evaluate the potential for cochlear implant benefit for persons with evidence of possible cochlear nerve dysfunction.

Pure-Tone Audiometric Assessment

A staple of the cochlear implant candidacy assessment is the pure-tone audiogram. Ideally, air conduction pure tone thresholds should be measured from 125 through 8000 Hz with stimuli delivered via insert earphones. Measurement at 125 Hz is recommended for a couple of reasons. First, the minimization of trauma to cochlear structures and preservation of residual hearing are part of the standard of care in cochlear implant surgery. Many cochlear implant candidates have an auditory response at 125 Hz, and comparison of pre- and postoperative thresholds allow for a determination of the success of hearing preservation following cochlear implant surgery. Evaluation of low-frequency hearing also assists the audiologist in planning the best strategy for providing stimulation to the cochlear implant recipient. Specifically, the audiologist can be prepared to provide acoustic amplification if low-frequency hearing is preserved post-implantation. Second, a thorough knowledge of a candidate's low-frequency hearing sensitivity enhances the audiologist's ability to counsel the candidate. For instance, it is important to inform candidates that they may lose their acoustic hearing during or after cochlear implant surgery so that they are not unpleasantly surprised if a loss of acoustic hearing does occur.

Assessment of hearing sensitivity at inter-octave frequencies is also good practice, because once again, the audiologist can determine the range over which acoustic hearing may be preserved and plan accordingly (i.e., does aidable hearing exist at 750 Hz?). Also, the audiologist will have a more thorough understanding of the candidate's hearing loss, which will help in determining whether the candidate's hearing aids are fitted appropriately during probe microphone assessment. Use of insert earphones is recommended for air-conduction pure-tone threshold assessment for several reasons. The advantages of insert earphones over supra-aural earphones are firmly established and include greater attenuation of outside ambient noise and greater inter-aural attenuation, which reduces the chances of stimulus crossover and the need for masking. Use of insert earphones is also recommended, because with the use of insert earphones, the real-ear-to-coupler difference (RECD) may be measured and the candidate's hearing loss may be precisely plotted in dB sound pressure level (SPL) for the purpose of hearing aid probe microphone measures. More specifically, insert earphones are calibrated in a 2-cc coupler, and the RECD is also measured relative to a 2-cc coupler. Because the two measures are both referenced to a 2-cc coupler, the signal level in dB SPL at the tympanic membrane may be directly determined. In contrast, supra-aural earphones are calibrated in a 6-cc coupler, so the average real-ear-to-dial difference (REDD) must be used to determine hearing thresholds in dB SPL for probe microphone measurement. As a result, the thresholds in dB SPL shown on the probe microphone display will not reflect the exact signal level present at the tympanic membrane.

As with every audiologic evaluation, the assessment of bone conduction thresholds is imperative to allow for determination of the type of hearing loss (e.g., conductive, sensorineural, mixed). Identification of an air-bone gap is often essential in determining the potential etiology of hearing loss (e.g., Carhart's notch with otosclerosis). Additionally, identification of an air-bone gap can provide further insight that corroborates a diagnosis made by the primary evaluation. For example, enlarged vestibular aqueduct syndrome, which has a cochlear site-of-lesion and commonly results in severe to profound hearing loss warranting cochlear implantation, is diagnosed via radiologic imaging (i.e., computerized tomography [CT] scan or magnetic resonance imaging [MRI]). However, a spurious air-bone gap often exists in the low frequencies because of an alteration in the mechanics of cochlear function (Merchant et al., 2007).

Audiometric Thresholds and Cochlear Implant Candidacy

As indicated in Tables 4–1 through 4–3 in Chapter 4, the pure-tone threshold criteria vary across manufacturers. For Cochlear Nucleus cochlear implants, the FDA-approved guidelines indicate that candidates with moderate to profound low-frequency hearing loss and severe to profound mid- to high-frequency loss should be considered for cochlear implantation. The reader should note the ambiguity that exists in the audiometric criterion for Cochlear Nucleus cochlear implants. Specifically, the criterion does not clearly define the frequencies that make up the low-, mid-, and high-frequency ranges. As a result, the audiologist is afforded some leeway in determining whether a candidate meets the indications of use. For instance, a candidate who has normal hearing through 500 Hz with a 45 dB HL pure-tone threshold at 750 Hz and a severe hearing loss from 3000 Hz and beyond technically meets the audiometric indications for use of a Cochlear Nucleus cochlear implant.

The audiometric guidelines for Advanced Bionics and MED-EL cochlear implants are a little more conservative than the cochlear guidelines. Advanced Bionics indications for use call for a severe to profound bilateral sensorineural hearing loss, whereas MED-EL calls for a pure-tone average (500, 1000, and 2000 Hz) of 70 dB HL or poorer. Of note, the audiometric criterion of the Centers for Medicare and Medicaid Services (CMS) calls for a bilateral moderate to profound sensorineural hearing loss. CMS guidelines typically apply to all federally regulated health care plans.

Although the audiometric criteria differ across manufacturers, most cochlear implant teams will consider a patient as a candidate for a cochlear implant of any of the three manufacturers providing cochlear implants in the United States when the patient meets indications for one of the devices. For example, if a patient has a moderate low-frequency hearing loss that slopes to a profound hearing loss in the high-frequency range but does not have a pure tone average in excess of 70 dB HL, the cochlear implant team will offer the Advanced Bionics and MED-EL cochlear implants along with the Cochlear Nucleus cochlear implant. Additionally, most cochlear implant teams

will consider a cochlear implant for candidates who do not quite meet the audiometric pure tone criterion but have speech recognition that is poor enough to meet the aided speech recognition criterion, particularly when a retrocochlear site of lesion has been ruled out. Once again, however, audiologists typically adhere to the exact criteria of CMS.

Speech Recognition Assessment

Quite possibly the most important component of the audiologic cochlear implant evaluation battery is the aided speech recognition assessment. Persons with significant hearing loss do not seek out the services of a cochlear implant team because they cannot hear low-level tones. They are interested in cochlear implantation because they are struggling to understand speech in daily listening situations. The goal of the aided speech recognition assessment is to gauge how well a potential candidate is able to understand speech with the ideal set of hearing aids appropriate for their hearing loss. As a result, it is imperative for the audiologist to not only understand how to provide an accurate evaluation of speech recognition in the soundfield but also to be able to evaluate the function and goodness of fit of the potential candidate's hearing aids. The following section briefly describes the process of hearing aid evaluation and thoroughly describes the process of aided speech recognition.

Hearing Aid Evaluation

For the purposes of determining cochlear implant candidacy, the audiologist must accomplish one basic objective when evaluating the function of a potential cochlear implant candidate's hearing aid. The audiologist must determine whether the patient's hearing aids are optimally selected and fitted to assist the patient in achieving his/her maximum aided speech recognition score for the assessment conditions. The cochlear implant assessment battery should include an evaluation of monosyllabic word recognition in quiet, sentence recognition in quiet, and sentence recognition in noise. For the purposes of candidacy assessment, word and sentence recognition in quiet are typically evaluated at a presentation level consistent with average conversational level speech (e.g., 60 dBA). Sentence recognition in noise is typically evaluated with the sentence materials presented at an average to moderately intense presentation level (e.g., 60–70 dBA) and the noise presented at a level 5 to

10 dB lower than the speech presentation level (i.e., +5 to +10 dB SNR) from the same loudspeaker used to present the speech stimuli (i.e., speech and noise both presented from a loudspeaker located at 0 degrees horizontal azimuth).

With these evaluation conditions in mind, it is important that the audiologist ensure that the gain of the potential candidate's hearing aids is sufficient to provide an appropriate output level in response to average conversational level speech. It is also important to ensure that the hearing aids do not produce internal noise or distortion that would compromise performance in the aforementioned test conditions. Because the speech and noise are presented from the same loudspeaker, the sophistication of the noise management technology in the patient's hearing aids is not critically important. Directional technology will not be beneficial for the test condition, because there is no spatial separation between the speech and competing noise (Bentler, 2005; Walden et al., 2004). Also, research has generally shown that adaptive noise reduction technology has the potential to improve comfort in noise but typically does not improve speech recognition in noise (Bentler, 2005).

It should be noted, however, that advanced signal processing strategies may improve performance in realistic listening situations. If a potential candidate does not meet indications for cochlear implant use, and the cochlear implant team decides that cochlear implantation is not in the patient's best interest, the audiologist may recommend new hearing aids if the patient is using hearing aids with inferior signal processing. For instance, advanced directional microphone technology, such as adaptive, binaural beam-forming technology, has been shown to improve speech recognition in noise (Latzel, 2013; Lee et al., 2014). Additionally, adaptive noise reduction may enhance listening comfort and effort in noisy situations. Furthermore, most modern hearing aids feature wireless hearing assistive technologies (HATs) that can significantly improve hearing performance in noise. For example, remote microphone accessory systems can improve speech recognition in noise when the user is listening to one talker (Wolfe et al., 2015a). Similarly, wireless streaming accessories can improve speech recognition for the telephone and television (Picou & Ricketts, 2013; Strelcyk et al., 2016; Wolfe et al., 2015b). In fact, the use of wireless HATs can allow for satisfactory hearing performance in many of the situations in which hearing aid users typically report the most difficulty with communication.

Electroacoustic Assessment and Biologic Listening Check

The audiologist must ensure that the potential candidate's hearing aids are not producing substantial noise or distortion that would compromise speech recognition during aided assessment. The audiologist should begin by completing a biologic listening check with a stethoscope to subjectively examine for the presence of distortion or poor sound quality. The audiologist may consider using a stethoscope with a filter to provide a modest amount of attenuation of the aided output, because the hearing aids of many cochlear implant candidates produce an output level that is high enough to potentially be uncomfortable and/or unsafe for one with normal hearing sensitivity.

In most cases, a biologic listening check performed by an audiologist with normal hearing will identify the presence of distortion or noise that would compromise aided speech recognition. However, the audiologist should be abundantly thorough in his/her hearing aid evaluation and should consider completing an electroacoustic assessment to evaluate the hearing aid performance in a 2-cc coupler to verify that the function meets the American National Standards Institute's (ANSI) tolerances relative to the manufacturer's specifications (ANSI S3.22-2009). A detailed description of the completion of electroacoustic measurement to make certain a modern hearing aid meets the manufacturer's specification re. ANSI S3.22-2009 is beyond the scope of this textbook. However, the interested reader who seeks more information on this topic is referred to the textbook *Modern Hearing Aids: Verification, Outcome Measures, and Follow-Up* (Bentler, Mueller, & Ricketts, 2016).

Real-Ear Probe Microphone Measures

In order to evaluate speech recognition in the best aided condition, the audiologist must verify that the potential candidate's hearing aids are providing optimal audibility for speech. Real-ear probe microphone measurements are the standard of care for verifying hearing aid output relative to the user's hearing loss and relative to an evidence-based prescriptive target output level (Bentler et al., 2016). Figure 5–3 provides an example of hearing aid verification via real ear probe microphone assessment. In short, real-ear probe microphone assessment involves the placement of a small silicone probe tube into the patient's external auditory meatus about 5 mm from the tympanic membrane. The probe tube is connected to a

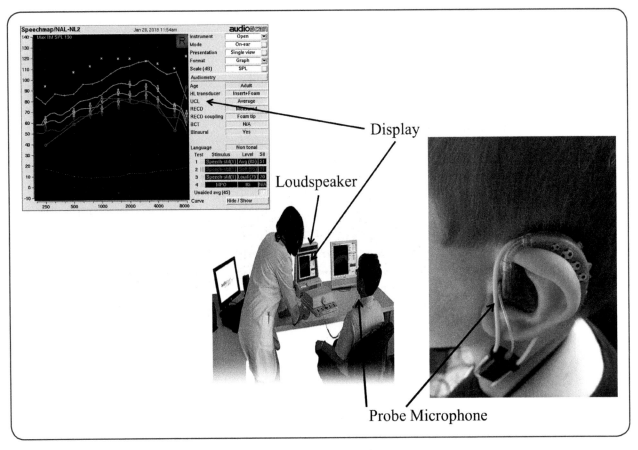

FIGURE 5–3. An example of real-ear probe microphone assessment and results.

microphone that is capable of measuring the output level of the hearing aid as the amplified acoustic signal delivered from the hearing aid enters the probe tube near the tympanic membrane. Hence, real-ear probe microphone assessment allows for a measurement of the amplified acoustic output of the hearing aid in dB SPL at the tympanic membrane while the user wears the hearing aid on/in the ear.

Ideally, the hearing aid output measured near the tympanic membrane should match (± 5 dB) evidence-based prescriptive output targets across the speech frequency range. For adults, hearing aid output is generally matched to either the National Acoustic Laboratory Non-linear 2 (NAL-NL2) or the Desired Sensation Level Version 5.0–Adult (DSL 5.0–Adult) prescriptive targets for a recorded, calibrated speech signal presented at presentation levels consistent with soft, average, and loud speech (50, 60, and 70 dB SPL, respectively). Of note, for the cochlear implant candidacy assessment, speech recognition is typically evaluated at 60 dBA, so it is appropriate to evaluate

the output of the hearing aids to a calibrated speech signal presented at 60 dB SPL from the hearing aid analyzer.

Figure 5–4 provides an example of the results of a real-ear probe microphone measurement in which the hearing aid output is appropriately matched to the NAL-NL2 prescriptive targets indicating satisfactory audibility for speech inputs. If the patient's aided speech recognition meets cochlear implant candidacy guidelines with his/her hearing aids providing a close match between output level and prescriptive targets as shown in Figure 5–4, the audiologist can conclude that the candidate has been evaluated in the best aided condition (given the hearing aid has been shown to be free of noise or distortion significant enough to impair speech recognition in the assessment conditions).

Real-ear probe microphone measurements may be completed (as previously mentioned) while the hearing aid user wears the hearing aid in his/her ear (i.e., in situ probe microphone measurement)

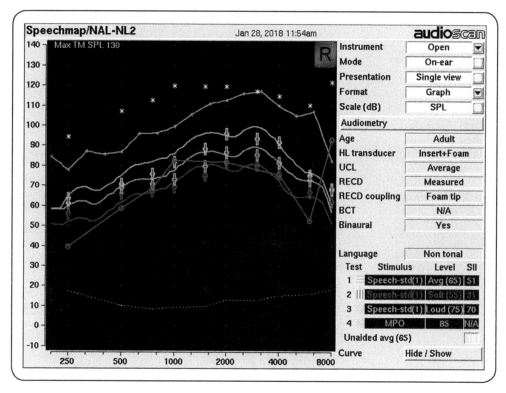

FIGURE 5–4. An example of real-ear probe microphone results with aided output set to match evidence-based prescriptive fitting targets.

or with the hearing aid connected to a 2-cc coupler (i.e., simulated measurement). Figure 5–5 provides an example of a simulated real ear probe microphone measurement completed in a 2-cc coupler. Whenever possible, the audiologist should complete in situ real-ear probe microphone measures. Because the user's hearing aid is connected to a 2-cc coupler rather than the earmold or ear dome, simulated real-ear probe microphone measures do not evaluate the individual effects of the wearer's earmold or ear dome. For example, an earmold horn effect (or a reverse horn effect) will not be captured during simulated measurement. Also, and maybe more importantly, simulated probe microphone measurements do not capture the effects of venting present in hearing aids with open-fit domes or vented earmolds.

Real-Ear-to-Coupler Difference

Prior to measurement of the hearing aid output, the audiologist should measure the patient's RECD, which is a measure of the difference in the sound pressure level measured near the patient's tympanic membrane compared with the sound pressure level measured in a 2-cc coupler. To measure the RECD, a steady-state broadband signal is delivered to a 2-cc coupler, and the level of the signal in the coupler is measured in dB SPL by a microphone connected to the coupler (see Figure 5–5). Then, the same signal is delivered through the patient's earmold or through the same insert earphone tip used for audiometric measurement, and the level of the signal is measured in the ear canal with a probe tube placed about 5 mm from the tympanic membrane (see Figure 5–5). The RECD represents the difference between the measure made near the tympanic membrane and the measure made in the 2-cc coupler (see Figure 5–5) (Bagatto et al., 2002). The RECD is generally, but not always, a positive value and is greater in the high-frequency range than it is in the low-frequency range.

So, why is it important to measure the RECD when the audiologist is going to measure the output of the patient's hearing aid while the hearing aid is worn in the ear? For purposes of real ear probe microphone verification, the RECD is used to determine the hearing aid wearer's unaided threshold in dB SPL at the tympanic membrane (i.e., the SPL-o-Gram). Because the RECD is used to determine the

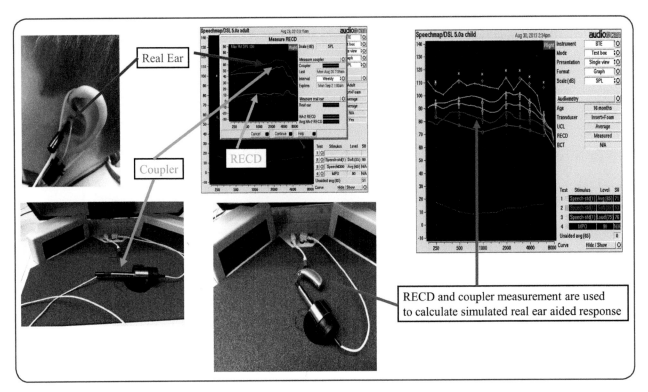

FIGURE 5–5. An example of the measurement of the real-ear-to-coupler difference (RECD).

wearer's unaided hearing thresholds, it also influences the prescriptive targets calculated from the wearer's hearing thresholds.

In the ideal world, it would be desirable to measure the exact sound pressure level of audiologic test signals (or the sound delivered from a hearing aid) at the eardrum. It is, however, not feasible to place a probe tube in the external auditory meatus to directly measure the sound pressure level of audiometric test signals as they arrive at the tympanic membrane. Instead, individualized transformation factors may be used to calculate the level of audiometric test signals at the tympanic membrane in dB SPL. Audiologic test signals are calibrated in acoustic couplers. An acoustic coupler is a cavity that provides a controlled environment in which repeatable sound level measurements may be made. Also, the dimensions of an acoustic coupler are designed to mimic the size (i.e., volume in cc) of the adult external auditory meatus from the point at which an eartip/earmold terminates to the tympanic membrane (i.e., the residual ear canal volume). The dimensions of the coupler also take into account the compliance of the tympanic membrane and the middle ear

space (i.e., the effect that the tympanic membrane and residual volume of the middle ear space have on the SPL of sounds arriving at and passing beyond the eardrum).

Insert earphones are calibrated in 2-cc couplers. The human ear is not equally sensitive to sound across the standard audiometric frequency range of 250 to 8000 Hz. If the standard audiogram were displayed in dB SPL, the level corresponding to "normal hearing" would vary as a function of frequency (Table 5–1), which would be potentially difficult for patients and other health care providers to interpret. Of course, to address this potential confusion, audiometric test signals are calibrated in 0 dB HL, which corresponds to the level at which a typical young adult is able to just detect a pure tone (or other audiologic test signal) at a given frequency. As a result, normal hearing sensitivity may be displayed on the audiogram to a common reference of 0 dB HL.

An example often helps to elucidate this concept. Consider an audiogram for an "average young adult with normal hearing" obtained using ER-3A insert earphones. Because this patient is an "average young adult with normal hearing," all of his/her thresholds

TABLE 5–1. Reference Equivalent Threshold Sound Pressure Levels (RETSPL)

Transducer	Frequency (Hz)										
	125	250	500	750	1000	1500	2000	3000	4000	6000	8000
TDH-49/50 Supra-Aural Earphones	47.5	26.6	13.5	8.5	7.5	7.5	11	9.5	10.5	13.5	13
3A Insert Earphones	26	14	5.5	2	0	2	3	3.5	5.5	2.0	0
Loudspeaker Monaural 0°	24	13	6	4	4	2.5	0.4	–4	–4.5	4.5	13.5
Loudspeaker Monaural 45°	23.5	12	3	0.5	0	–1	–2.5	–0.9	–8.5	–3	8

are obtained at 0 dB HL. Then, let's say that the insert earphones were coupled to a 2-cc coupler (insert earphones are actually calibrated in a 2-cc coupler), and the SPL is measured in the 2-cc coupler for each test frequency with the audiometric dial set at 0 dB HL. The level that we would measure would vary as a function of frequency and is referred to as the reference equivalent threshold in sound pressure level (RETSPL). RETSPLs refer to the SPLs measured in an acoustic coupler that are equal to the average hearing thresholds of otologically normal young adults. Table 5–1 provides the RETSPL for audiometric test frequencies when measuring with ER-3A insert earphones coupled to an HA-2 2-cc coupler. When the audiometer is set to 0 dB HL for a 2000 Hz pure tone presented via insert earphones, the level measured in an HA-2 2-cc coupler would be 3 dB SPL. If the audiometer attenuator was changed to 80 dB HL, then the level measured in the HA-2 2-cc coupler would be 83.0 dB SPL.

In reality, acoustic couplers do not provide a perfect approximation of the adult external and middle ear and how SPL develops at the eardrum (Dillon, 2012). As a result, the SPL measured at the eardrum for the "average young adult with normal hearing" is different from what is measured in an HA-2 2-cc coupler. The RECD is the difference in SPL measured at the eardrum compared with the SPL measured in a coupler for the same sound. Figure 5–5 provides an illustration of a measured RECD of an adult hearing aid wearer relative to the RECD of an average adult. As shown, the RECD varies as a function of frequency and is typically positive because the SPL measured at the eardrum is typically higher than what is measured in an HA-2 2-cc coupler. It should be noted that it is quite simple to measure the RECD with most clinical hearing aid analyzers.

To determine the SPL at the tympanic membrane for audiologic test stimuli delivered via insert earphones, one can simply add the RECD and RETSPL values to the audiometric dial reading (in dB HL).

Equation 5–1: SPL at Eardrum (measured with insert earphones) = Audiometric Threshold (dB HL) + 2-cc coupler RETSPL + RECD

So, let's assume a typical adult patient has an audiometric threshold of 80 dB HL at 2000 Hz when measured with an insert earphone. The SPL measured at the eardrum would be:

Equation 5–2:
80.5 dB SPL = 70 dB HL + 3 dB + 7.5 dB

Now, let's consider an example in which audiometric threshold was measured for an adult who has an external ear that is much smaller than the average adult ear. The SPL that develops at the tympanic membrane of the smaller ear for a given audiometric dial level (dB HL) is typically much higher than what would be measured at the eardrum of a typical adult; Boyle's law indicates that the SPL that is measured in a cavity is inversely proportional to the size of the cavity. Furthermore, differences in middle ear properties and mechanics also influence the SPL measured at the tympanic membrane. Because of these differences, the RECD will typically be higher than average for adults with smaller than average ears and infants and young children. Because the RECD affects the threshold measured in dB SPL at the tympanic membrane, the individual RECD must be measured to precisely determine a listener's threshold in dB SPL at the tympanic membrane.

Consider, for instance, the following example of an adult with an unusually small external ear. The 2000 Hz pure-tone threshold measured with insert earphones is 70 dB HL, and the measured RECD for this patient is 16 dB at 2000 Hz. The threshold in dB SPL at the eardrum is:

$$\text{Equation 5–3: 90 dB SPL} =$$
$$\text{70 dB HL} + \text{3 db RETSPL} + \text{17 dB RECD}$$

This example provides a compelling illustration of the fact that the eardrum SPL at a given audiometric dial level (in dB HL) for an infant or young child is typically higher than what would exist for an adult with a threshold at the same audiometric dial level. This is an important point for at least two reasons. First, as an infant grows, and his ear gets larger and his external and middle ear mechanics change, the RECD will typically decrease. As a result, even if the infant's hearing sensitivity does not change, a higher audiometric dial level will be required to reach the infant's threshold. To explain, let's refer back to the previous example provided in Equation 5–3 in which 90 dB SPL was required at the eardrum for detection of a 2000 Hz pure tone. Let's say that the infant was evaluated again at 3 years of age and an RECD of 7 dB was measured at 2000 Hz. As a result, a higher audiometric dial level is now required to reach a level of 90 dB SPL at the eardrum.

$$\text{Equation 5–4: 90 dB SPL} =$$
$$\text{80 dB HL} + \text{3 dB RETSPL} + \text{7 dB RECD}$$

Because the threshold in dB SPL at the tympanic membrane is higher for this patient than what would be measured for an adult with an average RECD, the patient's real ear probe microphone targets will also be higher. As a result, the RECD must be individually measured to ensure accurate, individualized thresholds in dB SPL at the tympanic membrane and accurate real-ear probe microphone target levels. Measurement of the individual's RECD is particularly important for many persons who are considering cochlear implants, because their aidable dynamic range of hearing is relatively narrow and must be optimized during the hearing aid fitting and verification process.

Aided Speech Recognition Assessment

During cochlear implant candidacy evaluation, the goal of the aided speech recognition assessment is to determine the patient's ability to understand speech in an open-set presentation format while wearing hearing aids that are optimally selected and fitted based on the individual's hearing impairment. For cochlear implant candidacy assessments in the United States,

speech recognition is evaluated with the Minimum Speech Test Battery (MSTB) (Nilsson, McCaw, & Soli, 1996). The MSTB was originally developed in 1996 by a committee made up of representatives from the American Academy of Audiology (AAA), the American Academy of Otolaryngology–Head and Neck Surgery (AAO-HNS), and the three cochlear implant manufacturers that commercially distribute in the United States (i.e., Advanced Bionics, Cochlear Ltd., and MED-EL). The goal of the MSTB committee was to determine a set of speech recognition measures to be used to evaluate cochlear implant candidacy in order to identify measures that are appropriate for candidacy assessment and to promote uniformity in the practices audiologists used for cochlear implant candidacy assessment. The original 1996 MSTB consisted of three measures:

1. Consonant-Nucleus-Consonant (CNC) monosyllabic word recognition test (Peterson & Lehiste, 1962) presented in quiet at a 65 dBA presentation level to evaluate open-set word recognition in quiet;
2. Hearing in Noise Test sentence recognition test (HINT) (Nilsson, Soli, & Sullivan, 1994) presented in quiet at a 65 dBA presentation level to evaluate sentence recognition in quiet; and
3. HINT presented in the presence of fixed-level, speech-spectrum noise at a +10, +5, or 0 dB SNR (the exact signal-to-noise ratio [SNR] is selected to avoid ceiling and floor effects) to evaluate sentence recognition in noise.

Because the speech recognition guidelines for cochlear implant candidacy are based on sentence recognition, the HINT test in quiet was generally used as the primary speech recognition metric cochlear implant assessment. However, Gifford and colleagues (2008) showed that ceiling effects made the HINT test an imperfect tool for evaluating both cochlear implant candidacy and postoperative cochlear implant outcomes. Gifford et al. (2008) evaluated CNC word recognition, HINT sentence recognition in quiet, AzBio sentence recognition in quiet, and the Bamford-Kowal-Bench Sentences in Noise BKB-SIN) sentence recognition test for 156 post-lingually deafened cochlear implant recipients and 50 binaural hearing aid users. The hearing aid users typically had moderate to profound hearing loss and were pursuing cochlear implantation because they had significant difficulty with communication in daily listening situations. Twenty-eight percent of the participants in the Gifford et al. (2008) study achieved scores of 100% correct on the HINT, whereas only 0.7% achieved maximum performance on the AzBio sentence recognition in quiet test. None of the subjects achieved 100% correct on the CNC word recognition test. The AzBio sentence recognition in quiet score agreed more closely with the CNC and BKB-SIN scores than the HINT score. Additionally, and most importantly for the purposes of candidacy determination, the HINT score of the vast majority of binaural hearing aid users exceeded the cochlear implant sentence recognition criterion of 60% correct in the best aided condition. Technically, they did not meet the indications for cochlear implantation even though they had moderate to profound hearing loss, reported significant difficulty with communication in the real world, and were likely to benefit from cochlear implantation. "More difficult (speech) materials are needed to assess speech perception performance of post-implantation patients—and perhaps also for determining implant candidacy" (Gifford et al., 2008).

Cochlear Implant Minimum Speech Test Battery

In recognition of the fact that the HINT in quiet sentence recognition test was no longer an appropriate measure to evaluate cochlear implant candidacy and outcomes, the MSTB committee reconvened and provided an updated recommendation of speech recognition measures to be used for cochlear implant candidacy and outcome assessment. The current MSTB (2011) may be found at:

http://www.auditorypotential.com/MSTBfiles/ MSTBManual2011-06-20%20.pdf

The MSTB (2011) comprises:

1. One full list (50 words) of CNC monosyllabic word recognition in quiet administered at a presentation level of 60 dBA,
2. One list (20 sentences) of AzBio sentences in quiet administered at a presentation level of 60 dBA (Spahr et al., 2012),
3. One list (20 sentences) of AzBio sentences in noise administered at a presentation level of 60 dBA at an SNR of +5 or +10 dB depending on what is necessary to avoid ceiling effects, and
4. One 16-sentence list-pair (8 sentences per list) of the BKB-SIN preoperatively; one 20-sentence list-pair (10 sentences per list) of the BKB-SIN postoperatively (the 20-sentence lists include SNRs down to −6 dB, rather than 0 dB, and therefore provide headroom to accommodate the expected

pre- to postoperative improvement in speech perception) (Bench, Kowal, & Bamford, 1979; Etymotic Research, Inc., 2005).

Of note, in clinical practice, many audiologists evaluate sentence recognition in quiet and in noise with the AzBio sentence recognition test, but in the interest of time, speech recognition in noise is often not evaluated a second time with the BKB-SIN test. Also of note, the MSTB specified a presentation level of 60 dBA for several reasons. The speech recognition of cochlear implant candidates and recipients was evaluated at a presentation level of 70 dB SPL in many early studies. Also, many of the FDA-approved indications of use specified a presentation level of 70 dB SPL for candidacy assessment (see Advanced Bionics HiRes 90K indications for use with young children). Research has shown that average conversational level speech occurs around 60 dB SPL (Pearson, Bennett, & Fidell, 1977). A presentation level of 70 dB SPL is representative of raised or loud speech and does not reflect the level at which we most commonly listen in everyday conversation. Additionally, researchers have evaluated pre- and postoperative speech recognition at multiple presentation levels and have concluded that cochlear implant recipients achieve similar speech recognition at 60 and 70 dBA (Firszt et al., 2004; Skinner et al., 1997). In contrast, because of limitations in gain before feedback and because of restrictions in the range of input levels that can be delivered into a restricted dynamic range of hearing, hearing aid users with severe to profound loss often achieve poorer speech recognition at 60 dBA when compared with performance at 70 dBA (Alkaf & Firszt, 2007). Consequently, evaluation of speech recognition at a 70 dBA presentation level may provide the impression that a hearing aid user is performing well when in reality, he/she encounters significant difficulty in many realistic listening situations. Furthermore, evaluating speech recognition at a raised presentation level may prevent a candidate from receiving a cochlear implant when the implant could provide substantial benefit with communication in the real world.

The MSTB committee recommended that speech recognition assessment be conducted in an audiometric sound booth that is at least 1.83 × 1.83 meters or 6 × 6 feet. The sound-treated room should meet ANSI S3.1, the American National Standard for Permissible Ambient Noise Levels for Audiometric Test Rooms (ANSI, 1999). Additionally, the speech material should be presented from a loudspeaker located one meter away from the patient at 0 degrees azimuth (i.e., directly in front of the patient). It is important to position the listener at about one meter from the loudspeaker, because if the listener is seated too close to the loudspeaker, the level of the speech signal will potentially change considerably with minor changes in body position (e.g., if the listener shifts closer to or farther away from the loudspeaker during assessment) (Walker et al., 1984). Also, the MSTB recommended that the loudspeaker be positioned approximately 86 centimeters or 39 inches from the floor. Of note, the chair in which the listener sits should be high enough to place the head of a listener of average height near the center of the cone of the loudspeaker. Ideally, an adjustable chair allows the audiologist to set the height of the chair so that all patients may be positioned with their heads at the center of the loudspeaker. From a practical perspective, it is important to ensure that the chair is comfortable for the listener and provides adequate support. The listener should be able to place both feet on the floor and sit comfortably with his/her back resting on the back of the chair. Although the provision of a comfortable chair may seem like a trivial matter, it is actually quite important, because cochlear implant candidacy assessments are rather lengthy appointments. The patient must be comfortable so that he/she may devote all of his/her attention to the assessment process.

The MSTB mentions the need for a second loudspeaker to present the competing noise signal from speech recognition in noise assessment. However, in practice, speech recognition in noise is typically evaluated with the speech and noise presented from the same loudspeaker. Most cochlear implant sound processors and hearing aids possess directional microphone technology, and the improvement offered by a directional microphone in an audiometric soundbooth with speech and noise presented from 0 and 180 degrees azimuth, respectively, overestimates the improvement the listener is likely to obtain in the real world, where the moderate- to high-level reverberation is present and the speech signal often arises from more than a meter away from the listener (Cord et al., 2004; Ricketts & Dhar, 1999; Walden et al., 2004).

Speech recognition should ideally be evaluated in the right-, left-, and binaurally aided conditions for a measure of monosyllabic word recognition in quiet, sentence recognition in quiet, and sentence recognition in noise. At the time of this writing, sentence recognition scores are typically used to determine cochlear

implant candidacy. Of note, the FDA-approved indications for cochlear implantation and the Centers for Medicare and Medicaid Services (CMS) all explicitly mention sentence recognition as the measure that is used to determine cochlear implant candidacy. However, no current guidelines explicitly state whether sentence recognition assessment should be conducted in quiet or in noise. In many social, educational, occupational, and other daily listening situations, hearing aid wearers must attempt to understand speech that is spoken in the presence of competing noise. In particular, the SNR of many daily listening situations typically occurs around 0 to 10 dB. As a result, it is logical to evaluate a potential candidate's ability to understand speech in noise in order to determine his/her ability to communicate in real world situations.

A key principle of cochlear implant candidacy and outcome evaluation is for the audiologist's assessment protocol to be consistent across patients and from session to session within patients. Specifically, it is inappropriate to evaluate sentence recognition in quiet in all patients undergoing cochlear implant candidacy assessment but to only evaluate sentence recognition in noise for persons who do not meet cochlear implant guidelines when evaluated in quiet. Choosing to only measure speech recognition in noise when it is necessary to meet cochlear implant candidacy guidelines is essentially "cherry-picking" clinical measures to achieve an outcome that satisfies an audiologist's bias regarding whether he/she believes an individual patient should receive a cochlear implant. Such a practice is potentially dangerous, because the audiologist can design a test condition that will conceivably allow for any patient to meet cochlear implant guidelines. For example, the audiologist could evaluate AzBio sentence recognition in noise at a −5 dB SNR. The hearing aid wearer is likely to perform at levels that will satisfy cochlear implant candidacy guidelines, but many persons with normal hearing will also struggle to understand speech at such an unfavorable SNR. Additionally, it is likely that the patient will continue to struggle to understand sentences at a −5 dB SNR after cochlear implantation. As a result, to avoid the temptation to manipulate test conditions to satisfy a personal, anecdotal bias, the audiologist should adopt standardized, consistent clinical practices for evaluating cochlear implant candidacy.

Furthermore, sentence recognition in quiet and in noise should both be evaluated during postoperative outcome assessment as well. Measuring sentence recognition in quiet and in noise at both the pre- and postoperative sessions allows the audiologist to determine the magnitude of the benefit patients are receiving from cochlear implantation, which is useful in guiding intervention for individual recipients (e.g., a recipient who is performing well in quiet but poorly in noise may need to be assisted in learning to use wireless HAT and/or directional microphone technology). Comprehensive pre- and postoperative speech recognition assessment is also imperative so that the audiologist may determine whether the decision to provide cochlear implantation for his/her patients is appropriate. Specifically, a knowledge of the audiologist's collective patient benefit can assist the audiologist in making candidacy decisions for future patients.

As discussed, at the time of this writing, cochlear implant candidacy speech recognition guidelines are based on sentence recognition scores. However, monosyllabic word recognition should also be completed during pre- and postoperative speech recognition assessment. Contextual and syntactic cues are available in sentences that allow listeners to accurately repeat words that they may not have necessarily understood but are able to deductively determine based on the words they do hear. Furthermore, Ching et al. (1998) showed that adult listeners with severe to profound hearing loss often primarily rely on low-frequency information (e.g., below 1500–2000 Hz) in the speech signal in order to understand sentences. As such, persons with hearing losses that slope from mild to moderate in the low-frequency range to severe to profound in the high-frequency range may perform relatively well on sentence recognition in quiet measures. In contrast, contextual and syntactic cues are sparse in monosyllabic word recognition testing. Consequently, monosyllabic word recognition assessment provides a measure of a listener's ability to extract isolated acoustic information to understand speech. In realistic situations, noise and reverberation often mask low-frequency speech information, forcing the listener to rely on mid- to high-frequency speech information. Monosyllabic word recognition provides a pure indication of the listener's ability to utilize low-, mid-, and high-frequency speech information for the purpose of speech recognition and likely provides a better indication of a listener's ability to understand speech in quiet compared with the clinical evaluation of sentence recognition in quiet.

It should be noted that a comparison of word and sentence recognition scores also allows the audiolo-

gist to determine whether a processing disorder may be responsible for a listener's difficulty to understand speech in the real world. For instance, if a potential cochlear implant candidate scores relatively well on monosyllabic in quiet but struggles to understand sentences in quiet, then the audiologist may conclude that a temporal processing and/or auditory memory deficit may be responsible for the patient's communication difficulties. Temporal processing and auditory memory deficits may not necessarily be improved by cochlear implantation, so the comparison of word and sentence recognition may very well influence the audiologist's decision to recommend cochlear implantation.

Of note, at the time of this writing, there is a trend toward the use of monosyllabic word recognition to determine cochlear implant candidacy. In particular, Cochlear Americas is conducting a clinical trial in which participants with bilateral moderate to profound sensorineural hearing loss (or poorer) qualify for unilateral cochlear implantation when best-aided CNC monosyllabic word scores are 40% or less in the ear to be implanted and 50% or less in the best aided condition. The CNC word recognition criteria used in this Cochlear Americas clinical trial are most likely to be appropriate or even conservative in identifying patients who are likely to benefit from a cochlear implant.

Gifford et al. (2010) evaluated CNC word recognition pre- and postoperatively in 22 adult cochlear implant recipients who had achieved CNC word scores of at least 30% in the best-aided (hearing aid) condition. The criterion of a minimum score of 30% correct on CNC words was selected, because it exceeded "that specified by the North American clinical trial of the Nucleus Freedom cochlear implant system." Postoperatively, CNC word recognition was evaluated in the hearing aid only, cochlear implant only, and bimodal (i.e., cochlear implant plus a hearing aid in the non-implanted ear) conditions. The mean postoperative CNC word recognition score was 82% with a mean improvement of 40 percentage points relative to the best aided condition. Furthermore, all 22 of the participants scored better than 60% correct on CNC word recognition in the bimodal condition. The impressive results of the Gifford et al. (2010) study suggest that a guideline calling for preoperative CNC word scores of 40% or less in the ear to be implanted and 50% or less in the best-aided condition will identify patients who are very likely to understand speech better with bimodal technology relative to binaural acoustic amplification. Additionally, Sladen et al. (2017) evaluated monosyllabic word recognition and sentence recognition to determine cochlear implant candidacy and long-term outcomes for a group of adult cochlear implant recipients. Sladen and colleagues reported that some of the recipients reached ceiling-level performance on sentence recognition measures, whereas none of the recipients reached ceiling-level performance on the monosyllabic word recognition test. Sladen et al. concluded that their study demonstrated that monosyllabic words were an appropriate measure to use to determine cochlear implant candidacy and for evaluating long-term post-operative hearing performance.

The speech recognition materials used outside the United States vary from country to country. In most places outside the United States, cochlear implant candidacy is assessed by evaluating word recognition. The minimum word recognition score required to satisfy cochlear implant guidelines varies across countries. However, as a general rule of thumb, a monosyllabic word recognition score of less than 40 to 50% correct in the ear to be implanted and less than 50 to 60% correct in the best-aided condition likely indicates that the patient will understand speech better with a cochlear implant.

Calibrating Speech Signals

In order to accurately administer the MSTB cochlear implant test battery (or any speech recognition test battery for that matter), it is necessary for the audiologist to ensure that speech materials are delivered in the soundfield at the desired presented level.

Recorded Speech Materials

Recorded speech signals should be directed from a computer, compact disc (CD) player, or MP3 player to the audiometer. Many clinical audiologists administer speech recognition assessment via monitored-live voice (MLV) presentation (e.g., Martin et al. [1998]) reported that 82% of clinical audiologists reported that they used monitored live voice presentation for speech recognition assessment), but for cochlear implant candidacy determination, it is imperative to use recorded speech materials. Monosyllabic word recognition depends upon the perception of low-level consonants that cannot be monitored well by the fast action of the audiometer volume unit (VU) meter. Also, use of recorded speech materials removes the

inter-audiologist and intra-audiologist variability associated with MLV presentation (Brandy, 1996; Hood & Poole, 1980). The use of MLV makes it impossible to make direct comparisons of speech recognition scores measured with an individual patient to scores obtained in clinical trials, because differences would likely exist between the acoustics of the speech signal presented via MLV versus the signals presented via recorded materials in a clinical trial. Additionally, differences in the acoustics of the voices of two different audiologists would possibly create differences in speech recognition scores obtained via MLV by the two audiologists. For example, if one audiologist had a raspy, high-pitched voice, and another audiologist had a "boomy," low-pitched voice, it is more likely that a cochlear implant candidate with a moderate sloping to profound hearing loss would meet FDA-approved cochlear implant guidelines when tested by the audiologist with the raspy, high-pitched voice. Furthermore, the use of recorded speech materials prevents speech recognition scores from being biased by audiologist delivery. For instance, during postoperative assessment, an audiologist may be tempted to over-articulate and/or speak at a moderately slow rate in order to allow the cochlear implant recipient to understand the words. Of course, pre- and postoperative speech recognition performance should not be affected by the delivery style of an individual audiologist. Finally, Roeser and Clark (2008) demonstrated that MLV speech recognition assessment is often too simple for hearing aid users and does not effectively separate hearing aid wearers who have excellent word recognition from those who may struggle. Figure 5–6 provides word recognition scores for 16 adult hearing aid wearers with noise-induced hearing loss whose monosyllabic word recognition was evaluated with MLV and recorded speech materials. As shown, most all of the patients score near ceiling on the MLV test, but over half score between 0 and approximately 70% correct on the recorded speech test. Roeser and Clark (2008) nicely illustrate the need to administer recorded speech materials in order to determine which patients are likely to experience difficulty with speech recognition and are most inclined to need a cochlear implant.

Calibrating Speech Presentation Levels

Calibration of the presentation levels of speech signals in the soundfield is a relatively straightforward and expeditious process. First, the audiologist must calibrate the level of the input signal delivered from the signal source (e.g., computer, CD/MP3 player).

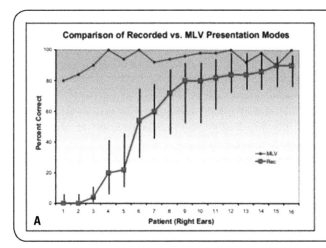
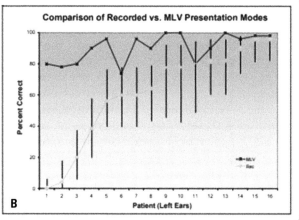

FIGURE 5–6. Comparison of word-recognition scores for the right (**A**) and left (**B**) ears between use of monitored live voice (MLV) and recorded presentation for 16 adults. The ranges shown on around the open-set scores represent the 95% confidence intervals predicted from the binomial tables published by Raffin and Thornton (1980). Image obtained from Rosier and Clark (2008), *Audiology Today*. Permission to use Figure obtained from Copyright Clearance Center.

The signal source should include a 1000 Hz calibration pure tone that may be delivered to the audiometer. The external input control dials (e.g., External A, External B, Input 1, Input 2) are adjusted so that the VU meter peaks at 0 dB during the presentation of the 1000 Hz calibration tone. The external input controls will remain in this position for the remainder of the calibration and assessment process.

Next, the signal source should allow for the presentation of a steady-state calibration signal that has a similar spectrum as the speech materials. The calibration signal is presented through the sound-field loudspeaker, and a sound level meter (SLM) is used to determine the audiometric dial setting (in dB HL) necessary to provide a presentation level of 60 dBA. The reader should note that the audiometric dial level is largely irrelevant. The audiologist must simply determine where the audiometric dial must be set to provide a presentation level of 60 dBA. To complete the calibration measurement, the SLM should be placed in the position at which the patient's head will reside during speech recognition assessment (e.g., one meter from the loudspeaker and directly in front of the center of the loudspeaker cone). The SLM should be set to A-weighted filtering with a fast response setting. Calibration of the signal level should be completed on a daily to weekly-plus basis. Every audiologist conducting cochlear implant candidacy evaluation should be aware of the computer and audiometer settings required to yield a desired presentation level for speech recognition assessment.

Additional Speech Recognition Assessment Beyond the MSTB

Completion of the MSTB is sufficient with most cochlear implant candidates. However, for candidates who cannot understand any words presented in the MSTB word and sentence recognition tasks, the audiologist should consider administering additional testing in order to establish a baseline of the candidate's speech perception capacity. Establishing a baseline of speech perception ability is important because the audiologist will eventually aim to demonstrate that the cochlear implant has improved the recipient's speech recognition relative to his/her performance with hearing aids. Most cochlear implant recipients are able to identify words presented in the MSTB open-set speech tests. However, a sparse minority of cochlear implant recipients (typically those with pre-implant histories that create a predisposition for a less favorable outcome; e.g., prelinguistically deafened with no auditory experience throughout childhood, bacterial meningitis with complete cochlear ossification) are unable to achieve open-set speech recognition with the more difficult measures included within the MSTB. As a result, it is prudent to administer easier speech recognition tests to capture the candidate's baseline speech perception capacity.

The HINT administered in quiet (Nilsson, Soli, & Sullivan, 1994), the Central Institute for the Deaf (CID) sentence test (see Davis & Silverman for details), and the Overlearned Speech Test Sentences are all examples of open-set sentence recognition tests that are typically simpler for persons with hearing loss to understand compared with AzBio sentences. Compared with AzBio sentences, the HINT, CID, and Overlearned sentences are spoken at a slower rate, only contain one talker, and contain simpler linguistic and syntactic structure. If the candidate scores less than 10% for these tests administered in quiet, then the audiologist may consider administering the tests via monitored live voice (MLV). If open-set sentence recognition is nonexistent in the MLV presentation format, the audiologist may consider administering the tests in the audio-visual mode. Specifically, the audiologist may present the sentences via live voice, and the candidate is allowed to view the audiologist's face. Of course, this mode of presentation is plagued by the same limitations previously discussed in regard to MLV assessment in this chapter. Assessment of speech perception in the audio-visual mode was commonplace in the nascent stages of cochlear implantation when developers, researchers, and audiologists hoped that cochlear implant would serve as an aid to speechreading (Eshraghi et al., 2012; Mudry & Mills, 2013). However, as cochlear implant technology improved and recipients routinely obtained open-set speech recognition in the audio-only presentation mode, audiologists abandoned the clinical assessment of speech perception in the audio-visual mode. The City University of New York (CUNY) sentence test is an example of a measure that is available in the recorded audio-visual format (Boothroyd, 2008; Boothroyd, Hanin, & Hnath, 1985). However, it is not readily available for clinical use today.

If open-set speech recognition is nonexistent, the audiologist should consider administering closed-set speech recognition tests. The Four-Choice Spondee recognition test is an example of a recorded speech test that may be presented in a closed-set mode. The audiologist may also consider closed-set tasks such as the Early Speech Perception (ESP) test (Moog & Geers, 1990), the Northwestern University–Children's Perception of Speech (NU-CHIPs) (Elliott & Katz, 1980), and the Word Intelligibility by Picture Identification (WIPI) (Ross & Lerman, 1970), all examples of recorded speech perception measures that can be administered in the closed-set format in order to establish a candidate's pre-implant baseline for speech perception.

Assessment of Functional Auditory Performance and Communication

The majority of audiologists do not use questionnaires to evaluate their patients' functional auditory

performance and communication abilities and needs (Kochkin et al., 2010). The authors' personal experience also suggests that most cochlear implant audiologists do not use questionnaires to evaluate implant candidates' perceived communication abilities and needs. There are several reasons for which cochlear implant audiologists should administer formal questionnaires to evaluate subjective communication disability and performance. First, without the use of formal questionnaires, audiologists run the risk of failing to identify a candidate's most pressing problems and the extent of those problems. Without a knowledge of the candidate's needs, the audiologist may have a difficult time adequately meeting those needs, and the patient may be disappointed with the intervention he/she receives. In essence, the needs identified through the completion of subjective questionnaires can guide the intervention process. Second, a comparison of pre- and postoperative questionnaire results allows the audiologist to determine the benefit provided by the cochlear implant. Subjective benefit is important to measure because measures of speech recognition completed in the test booth do not always correlate with subjective measures of perceived benefit/performance (Bentler et al., 2005; Wackym et al., 2007; Walden et al., 2004). Third, health care insurance companies may begin to require proof of the efficacy of an intervention to justify financial coverage of the service. In particular, health care insurance companies and the federal government may prioritize reimbursement for services that promote quality of life, occupational/social-emotional well-being, and/or disability reduction. Fourth, audiologists should administer communication needs questionnaires pre- and postoperatively to determine whether their intervention has been successful for individual recipients. Identifying a patient's primary problems and then working toward alleviating those problems is a fundamental aspect of aural rehabilitation. The hearing aid literature indicates that hearing aid wearers are more likely to be satisfied when their audiologist administers pre- and post-fitting communication needs questionnaires (Kochkin et al., 2010). It is reasonable to expect for cochlear implant recipients to also be more satisfied with their care when their audiologist takes the time and effort to identify their perceived communication/hearing needs and then determine whether cochlear implantation has met those needs. Fifth, subjective questionnaires provide a patient-endorsed validation of the need for a cochlear implant. If a patient reports little to no disability or handicap related to his/her hearing loss, then the audiologist should question the need for cochlear implantation. Additionally, if a cochlear implant recipient is dissatisfied with his/her auditory abilities after cochlear implantation and complains that cochlear implantation should not have been recommended by the audiologist, the questionnaires will corroborate the decision to pursue a cochlear implant if the recipient reported substantial hearing-related disability and handicap prior to implantation.

Questionnaires Designed to Evaluate Subjective Hearing Handicap, Communication Abilities and Needs, and Hearing Technology Benefit

There is a wide variety of questionnaires that the audiologist may choose to evaluate subjective communication abilities and needs and hearing technology benefit. The choice of which questionnaires to use is dependent upon the objective of the subjective assessment. The audiologist must determine what domains he/she would like to evaluate. The following sections describe questionnaires that probe particular domains that are of particular interest to cochlear implant audiologists.

Questionnaires Specific to Cochlear Implantation

The Nijmegen Cochlear Implant Questionnaire (NCIQ) is a comprehensive and structured Cochlear Implant Health Related Quality of Life (HRQoL) questionnaire (Hinderdink et al., 2000). It is comprised of 60 questions divided into three principal domains which are further divided into six subdomains. The three principal domains are physical, social, and psychological. The physical domain is comprised of three subdomains: basic sound perception, advanced sound perception, and speech production (e.g., Are you able to make yourself understood to strangers without using hand gestures?). Basic sound perception addresses the simple detection of speech and environmental sounds (e.g., Can you hear your own telephone or doorbell ringing?), whereas advanced sound perception addresses the patient's ability to discriminate, recognize, and/or identify complex sounds such as speech, music, and environmental sounds (e.g., Can you understand strangers without lip-reading?). The social domain is comprised of two subdomains: activity limitations (e.g., Does your hearing impairment present a serious problem during your work or studies?) and social interactions (e.g., Does your hearing impairment present a serious problem when you are with a group of persons [hobbies, sport, holi-

days]?). Self-esteem is the subdomain within the psychological domain (e.g., Do you feel anxious when talking to strangers?). Each subdomain is made up of 10 questions.

The NCIQ was designed to be administered in both the pre- and postoperative periods. For each question, the patient is asked to select from five responses on a 5-point scale. For 55 of the questions, the response categories are: (1) Never, (2) Sometimes, (3) Often, (4) Mostly, and (5) Always. For the remaining five questions, the response categories are: (1) No, (2) Poorly, (3) Moderate, (4) Adequate, and (5) Good. The answer categories (1–5; 1 = Never, 5 = Always) are transformed as follows: 1 = 0, 2 = 25, 3 = 50, 4 = 75, and 5 = 100. The average score is then calculated for each subdomain.

As can be seen in the example mentioned above, the NCIQ evaluates the effect of hearing loss and cochlear implantation from the perspectives of impairment (e.g., the hearing loss influences the detection of sound), activity limitation (e.g., unable to understand speech), and participation restriction (e.g., unable to work or reluctant to participate in social situations). Additionally, the NCIQ aims to evaluate the social/emotional/psychological effects of hearing loss and the potential benefit that cochlear implantation may offer in these domains. Hinderdink and colleagues (2000) evaluated the test-retest reliability of the NCIQ and evaluated the validity of the NCIQ by comparing pre- and postoperative NCIQ scores for a group of 45 adult cochlear implant recipients. NCIQ scores of the cochlear implant group were also compared with the NCIQ scores of 46 adults with severe to profound hearing loss who were referred for cochlear implant candidacy assessment but had yet to receive a cochlear implant. Hinderdink et al. (2000) reported that the NCIQ had good internal consistency, test-retest reliability, validity, and sensitivity to improvement offered by cochlear implantation.

The NCIQ is attractive for use in the cochlear implant assessment process because it was specifically designed for use with cochlear implant candidates and recipients. As a result, the questions are relevant to most cochlear implant recipients. Also, the NCIQ is a comprehensive instrument that measures performance and benefit in diverse domains ranging from simple sound detection to the emotional impact of hearing loss. Additionally, the NCIQ is a measure of quality of life, which may be attractive to third-party payers who require evidence of the efficacy of an intervention in order to determine whether they will provide compensation for the service, and if so, how much compensation will be provided. A limitation of the NCIQ is the fact that it is not a mainstream quality of life measure, and health care insurance companies may be unfamiliar with it and not recognize it as a credible tool to demonstrate improvement in quality of life offered by cochlear implantation. Additionally, because the NCIQ is not routinely used by many clinical audiologists, it may be unclear how the audiologist should interpret an individual recipient's questionnaire scores and determine how the NCIQ outcome should influence intervention.

The Cochlear Implant Function Index (CIFI) is another questionnaire designed specifically for the purposes of evaluating "auditory effectiveness in real world situations" (Coelho et al., 2009). The CIFI was developed to assess: (1) reliance on visual assistance, (2) telephone use, (3) communication at work, (4) hearing in noise, (5) hearing in groups, and (6) hearing in large settings. The CIFI consists of 25 items that probe the aforementioned six categories of interest. Within each category, the items are ordered so that the auditory skill becomes more complex as the participant moves through the category. For instance, within the reliance on visual assistance category, the first item states that the recipient must rely exclusively on visual assistance (e.g., sign language, closed caption), whereas the fourth and final item states that the recipient can understand speech without looking at the talker. Recipients' scores achieved within each category increase for each item they report to have mastered. For example, in the visual assistance category, recipients would receive one point if they must rely on visual cues for communication and four points if they are able to communication without visual cues. The scores within each category are summed. The authors of the test provided the following scale for gauging the recipient's CIFI outcome:

- Scores between 19 and 24: functioning at the highest level.
- Scores between 13 and 18: functioning at a high level.
- Scores between 7 and 12: functioning at a low level.
- Scores between 0 and 6: functioning at the lowest level.

The CIFI also includes three items designed to measure the recipient's tendency to avoid communication and/or social conditions because of his/her hearing loss.

Coelho and colleagues (2009) administered the CIFI to 245 recipients with one month to 19 years of cochlear implant experience. Coelho et al. (2009) found the CIFI to possess good psychometric properties. They also noted the need to correlate CIFI scores with objective measures of auditory function such as speech recognition in quiet and noise and sound detection. Like the NCIQ, the CIFI is attractive for use in the cochlear implant clinic because it was intentionally designed to evaluate cochlear implant outcomes. Also like the NCIQ, the CIFI is limited in the fact that it is not a universally recognized measure of quality of life. Additionally, because of the sparse use of the CIFI in clinical settings, it is unclear how the CIFI may be used to guide the intervention of an individual recipient.

Hearing Handicap Questionnaires

The Hearing Handicap Inventory for Adults (HHIA) (Newman et al., 1990) and the Hearing Handicap Inventory for the Elderly (HHIE) (Ventry & Weinstein, 1982) are both questionnaires that evaluate the impact that hearing loss has on an individual's daily life. The HHIA and HHIE each have 25 items which are categorized into subscales: emotional and social/situational. The items pertaining to the emotional subscale address the individual's feelings pertaining to his/her hearing loss and the psychological impact of hearing loss on both the individual and the individual's relationships with others (e.g., Does a hearing problem cause you to feel depressed? Does a hearing problem cause you to have arguments with family members?). The social/situational subscale contains items that address the individual's inability to function in daily activities (e.g., Does a hearing problem cause you to listen to the TV or the radio less often than you would like?). The HHIA is similar to the HHIE but has been modified to address listening situations that are more likely to be relevant for younger adults with hearing loss (e.g., occupational). For the HHIA and HHIE, the participant responds to each item with one of three alternatives: (1) Yes, (2) Sometimes, or (3) No. Four, two, and zero points are assigned to each "Yes," "Sometimes," and "No" response, respectively. A total score is summed for all 25 items and compared with the following response categories:

0–16 = No handicap

18–42 = Mild-moderate handicap

44 or greater = Significant handicap

A virtue of the HHIA and HHIE is that they have a lengthy history of use in audiology clinics, so many audiologists will be familiar with the measures. Additionally, the HHIA/HHIE questionnaires were intentionally designed to measure hearing loss–related activity limitation (i.e., disability) and participation restriction (i.e., handicap), so they are well suited to measure functional auditory performance in cochlear implant candidates and recipients. The HHIA/HHIE may be used pre- and postoperatively to show the benefit of cochlear implantation in the resultant reduction of communication disability and handicap. A potential limitation of the HHIA/HHIE is that neither is a universal measure of quality of life, and as a result, health care insurance companies may consider the results to be irrelevant compared with mainstream quality of life instruments. Also, the postoperative results obtained on the HHIA/HHIE may not provide the audiologist with sufficient insight to guide audiologic management.

The Communication Profile for the Hearing Impaired (CPHI) is a 145-item questionnaire designed to provide a comprehensive evaluation of a wide range of communication problems in order to determine an individual's communication strengths and limitations prior to aural rehabilitation (Demorest & Erdman, 1987). The CPHI addresses hearing-related impairments and disability and probes across five different categories: (1) Communication Performance Scales that evaluate the individual's ability to give and receive auditory information in a variety of situations, (2) Communication Environment Scales that evaluate external environmental factors and the individual's strategies and emotional adjustments used to cope with hearing loss, (3) Communication Strategies Scales that evaluate the individual's verbal and nonverbal behaviors in different situations, (4) Personal Adjustment Scales that evaluate the psycho-emotional aspects of the individual's hearing loss, and (5) Denial Scales that identify areas in which the individual may be in denial of his/her hearing loss and/or the impact that the hearing loss has on his/her life or the lives of others.

The CPHI is exceptional because not only does it evaluate the individual's perceived auditory performance, but it also evaluates the psycho-emotional consequences of the hearing loss and the favorable and unfavorable adjustments the individual has made to cope with hearing loss. The wealth of information obtained from this questionnaire may be used to develop a comprehensive aural rehabilitation program to holistically meet the unique needs of an individual. The comprehensive scope of the CPHI is also a potential limitation, because many cochlear implant audiologists may consider the CPHI to be too lengthy to administer in a busy clinical setting. Additionally, time restrictions and insufficient financial reimbursement for aural rehabilitation may prevent many clinical audiologists from applying the information acquired from the CPHI to develop an individualized aural rehabilitation program.

Questionnaires that Evaluate Hearing Aid Benefit, Satisfaction, and Performance

Numerous questionnaires are available for evaluating a patient's perceived performance, benefit, and/or satisfaction with hearing aids, including:

- Abbreviated Profile of Hearing Aid Benefit (APHAB) (Cox & Alexander, 1995)
- Client Oriented Scale of Improvement (COSI) (Dillon, James, & Ginis, 1997)
- Glasgow Hearing Aid Benefit Profile (GHABP) (Gatehouse, 1999)
- Hearing Aid Performance Inventory (HAPI) (Walden, Demorest, & Helper, 1984)
- International Outcome Inventory for Hearing Aids (IOI-HA) (Cox & Alexander, 2002)
- Satisfaction with Amplification in Daily Life (SADL) (Cox & Alexander, 1999)
- The Speech, Spatial, and Qualities of Hearing Scale (SSQ) (Gatehouse & Noble, 2004)

A description of each of these questionnaires is beyond the scope of this book. For additional information on these questionnaires, the interested reader is referred to the articles cited next to each questionnaire or to two excellent resources, *Modern Hearing Aids: Pre-Fitting Testing, and Selection Considerations* by H. G. Mueller, T. A. Ricketts, and R. Bentler and to *Modern Hearing Aids: Verification, Outcome Measures, and Follow-Up* by R. Bentler, H. G. Mueller, and T. A. Ricketts. Although the hearing aid questionnaires shown in the list above were designed to measure functional auditory performance of hearing aid users, these questionnaires do have potential application in the cochlear implant clinic. For instance, the audiologist may use these questionnaires to evaluate a potential cochlear implant candidate's perceived communication difficulty while using hearing aids. Additionally, the questionnaires may be slightly modified to assess a recipient's perceived performance with cochlear implants. For example, the audiologist could simply revise the Abbreviated Profile of Hearing Aid Benefit (APHAB) to inquire about a recipient's ability to hear with a cochlear implant rather than a hearing aid. Furthermore, the APHAB score measured after cochlear implantation could be compared with the pre-implant score to obtain an indication of the benefit of cochlear implantation. In contrast, hearing aid questionnaires are limited in that they do not provide a measure of quality of life associated with cochlear implantation. Also, most hearing aid questionnaires may not readily guide the audiologist in determining an intervention plan to manage a cochlear implant recipient's communication needs.

Client Oriented Scale of Improvement

The Client Oriented Scale of Improvement (COSI) is a questionnaire designed by researchers at the National Acoustic Laboratories (NAL) to identify an individual's communication difficulties and to determine the extent to which audiologic intervention has reduced the perceived difficulty (Dillon, James, & Ginis, 1997). The COSI is unique because it is not structured with fixed items or questions. Instead, the patient is tasked with determining up to five specific situations in which he/she is struggling to communicate because of hearing loss and would like to pursue improvement via audiologic intervention. Ideally, the patient should be specific in the description of the situation that produces communication difficulty. For example, rather than simply stating that he/she would like to hear better in noise, the patient should specify that he/she would like to better understand his/her friends while meeting for breakfast in a busy café. Next, the patient is asked to prioritize the situations he/she has identified in order of importance. After the audiologic intervention is provided, the audiologist and patient revisit the COSI to determine whether the intervention has been successful in alleviating the patient's difficulties. Figure 5–7 provides an example of the COSI form (NAL, retrieved January 28, 2018 from https://www.nal.gov.au/wp-content/uploads/sites/2/2016/11/COSI-Questionnaire.pdf). As shown, the patient notes the degree of change and final ability (with hearing aid) perceived for each of the situations previously identified. Degree of change is measured on a five-point scale with the following response options: (1) Worse, (2) No Difference, (3) Slightly Better, (4) Better, or (5) Much Better. The individual's final ability with use of hearing aids is also measured on a five-point scale with the following response options: (1) Hardly [only hears 10% of

signal of interest in the given situation], (2) Occasionally [25%], (3) Half the time [50%], (4) Most of the time [75%], or (5) Almost always [hears the signal of interest 95% of the time].

The COSI is unique for several reasons. First, it allows the patient to prioritize the communication difficulties that are most important to him/her. It is quite possible that a standardized questionnaire with fixed items may not capture the most pressing needs of a patient. The COSI assists the audiologist in identifying the unique needs of each patient. Second, the COSI essentially serves as a contract between the patient and the audiologist. Once the needs of an individual patient are identified, the audiologist and patient can set forth together to meet those needs. Identifying the patient's needs is an essential step in the determination of the specific type of hearing technology that will best meet the patient's needs. Third, the patient and audiologist revisit the patient's needs after the provision of audiologic service, and the patient directly notes the success of the intervention in improving his/her communication abilities.

The COSI can be modified to be an even more effective tool in the cochlear implant candidacy assessment and outcomes measurement battery. Table 5–2 shows an example of a modified version of the COSI originally suggested by Francis Kuk (2008). The modified COSI includes three additions. To begin, the patient indicates his/her present ability to hear in each of the situations he/she has identified. The patient's responds on the same five-point scale used to rate hearing ability in the original COSI. Then, the patient indicates his/her expected ability to hear after receiving his/her new hearing technology. Finally, the audiologist and patient determine an "agreed upon" ability for how the patient will hear after receiving his/her new hearing technology.

The modified COSI is a powerful tool for several reasons. First, inclusion of the patient's present ability to hear with hearing aids allows the COSI to be used as a tool to measure benefit obtained from cochlear implantation by comparing pre- and post-implantation scores. Second, asking the patient to indicate his/her expected ability gives the audiologist the opportunity to gauge whether the patient's expected cochlear implant outcome is realistic. Determining patient expectations is not a trivial matter. A patient with unrealistic expectations for cochlear implant benefit is likely to be disappointed with the outcome he/she achieves. The modified COSI can identify patients who have unrealistic expectations. For instance, if an adult patient who was born deaf

NAL
CLIENT ORIENTED SCALE OF IMPROVEMENT

Name : _____

Audiologist : _____

Category. _____   New _____

Date : _____
1. Needs Established _____   Return _____
2. Outcome Assessed _____

SPECIFIC NEEDS

Indicate Order of Significance

☐ _____

☐ _____

☐ _____

☐ _____

☐ _____

Categories			
1.	Conversation with 1 or 2 in quiet	5.	Television/Radio @ normal volume
2.	Conversation with 1 or 2 in noise	6.	Familiar speaker on phone
3.	Conversation with group in quiet	7.	Unfamiliar speaker on phone
4.	Conversation with group in noise	8.	Hearing phone ring from another room
		9.	Hear front door bell or knock
		10.	Hear traffic
		11.	Increased social contact
		12.	Feel embarrassed or stupid
		13.	Feeling left out
		14.	Feeling upset or angry
		15.	Church or meeting
		16.	Other

National Acoustic Laboratories
A division of Australian Hearing

Degree of Change

	Worse	No Difference	Slightly Better	Better	Much Better

CATEGORY

Final Ability (with hearing aid)

Person can hear

	Hardly Ever	Occasionally	Half the Time	Most of Time	Almost Always
	10%	25%	50%	75%	95%

FIGURE 5–7. The Client Oriented Scale of Improvement (COSI). Copyright © National Acoustics Laboratories.

141

TABLE 5–2. An Example of the Modified Client Oriented Scale of Improvement (COSI)

Areas of Improvement (Goal #)	Present Ability	Expected Ability	Agreed Ability	Final Ability	Degree of Change
Understand wife at restaurant	2	5	3	5	
Understand grandchild on phone	1	5	4	5	
Understand TV without caption	1	5	4	5	
Understand minister at church	2	5	4	5	
Hear bird songs outside	1	5	4	5	

Keys:

Ability:
1 – Hardly ever (10%)
2 – Occasionally (25%)
3 – Half the time (50%)
4 – Most of time (75%)
5 – Almost always (95%)

Degree of change:
1 – worse
2 – no difference
3 – slightly better
4 – better
5 – much better

and has never used hearing aids or a cochlear implant indicates that he expects to achieve a score of 5 for understanding his/her mother over the telephone, the audiologist must provide gentle but direct counseling to help the patient understand that the desired outcome is unlikely. Which leads us to the third benefit of a modified COSI, and that is the opportunity for the patient and audiologist to work together to determine a conservative expectation of cochlear implantation to improve performance in the situations identified by the patient.

As previously suggested, the COSI can become the contract between the audiologist and cochlear implant recipient. After the recipient has acclimated to his/her cochlear implant(s), the audiologist can revisit the COSI to determine whether cochlear implantation has provided improvement in the areas the patient has prioritized. Hence, the COSI serves as a benefit questionnaire. Additionally, the COSI may also serve as a tool to drive the aural rehabilitation process. For instance, if the recipient continues to report difficulty with understanding his/her spouse in a restaurant, the audiologist can discuss the proper use of directional microphone technology and/or wireless remote microphone technology. The audiologist may also discuss the need for the patient to try to optimize his/her listening environment. For example, the audiologist may discuss strategies for selecting a table and seating position that will optimize acoustics and the potential benefit of the noise management technology.

The primary benefit of the modified COSI is that it allows for an individualized assessment of a patient's communication difficulties. Another important benefit is that it allows the audiologist to gauge and manage patient expectations. Furthermore, the modified COSI allows the patient and audiologist to measure the benefit of cochlear implantation, and it can drive aural rehabilitation (e.g., it assists the audiologist to determine the next steps required to achieve the goals set forth in the COSI—recommend use of a remote microphone and/or communication strategies). The COSI is limited in the fact that it does not include fixed items, so the responses of individual recipients cannot be compared with group data. Also, the COSI is not a universally recognized measure of quality of life, so health care insurance companies may not view it as favorably as established measures of quality of life.

Cochlear Adult Expectations Questionnaire

Cochlear Ltd. has developed several questionnaires to evaluate a candidate's expectations of cochlear implant benefit (see the box below). These questionnaires consist of 10 declarative statements that the candidate answers as true or false. The Cochlear Adult Expectations Questionnaire is developed for two different populations, postlinguistically and prelinguistically deafened adults. The postlinguistic questionnaires contain items that address more complex and demanding listening situations, whereas

---

Postlinguistically Deafened Adult Expectations Questionnaire

(Answer TRUE or FALSE)

Name: _____   Date: _____

When I am using the Nucleus Cochlear Implant . . .

_____ 1. I will not have to use lipreading since normal hearing people do not have to use it.

_____ 2. It will be possible to tell the difference between a long and a short word.

_____ 3. It will be possible for me to hear in a limited way over the telephone.

_____ 4. Everyone who has an implant will eventually have the same hearing abilities.

_____ 5. Using listening and lipreading will make conversation easier to understand at a party.

_____ 6. The quality of the speech sound I hear will continue to improve.

_____ 7. It may be possible to understand some speech without lipreading.

_____ 8. It is OK for me to use someone else's speech processor.

_____ 9. My ability to make use of the sound I hear will improve.

_____ 10. There are things I can do to reduce the effects of background noise.

Cochlear's Adults Expectations Questionnaire. Provided courtesy of Cochlear Americas, ©2018.

---

the prelinguistic questionnaire contains a mix of rather elementary and demanding items. Example of items from the Cochlear Expectations Questionnaires include:

"It may be possible to understand some speech without lipreading."

"I will not have to use lipreading since normal hearing people to not have to use it."

The audiologist's task is to review the candidate's responses to each item and determine whether the candidate's expectations are realistic based on his/her pre-implant history.

Quality of Life Questionnaires

Numerous researchers have studied the effect of cochlear implantation on the quality of life of persons who have severe to profound hearing loss and have received a cochlear implant (DiNardo et al., 2014; Francis et al., 2002; Lassaletta et al., 2006; Sladen et al., 2017). However, most audiologists do not routinely evaluate quality of life in cochlear implant candidates and recipients in clinical settings. Incorporation of quality of life measures into the cochlear implant candidacy assessment and outcomes battery may occur if health care insurance companies demand that hearing health care providers demonstrate the efficacy of their interventions to justify reimbursement for services. Most general HRQoL measures evaluate the impact of disease and treatments on an individual's lifespan, functional states in several domains including physical, mental, emotional, and social functioning, self- and outward perceptions, satisfaction, and opportunities, ability to participate, and restrictions pertaining to academic, occupational, social, and so forth, domains.

Because quality of life is not routinely evaluated in the audiology clinic, a full discussion of generic quality of life questionnaires is beyond the scope of this chapter. The interested reader is referred to the following resources for additional information:

Sladen et al. (2017). Health-related quality of life following adult cochlear implantation: A prospective cohort study. *Cochlear Implants International*, 18(3), 130–135.

Centers for Disease Control and Prevention Health-Related Quality of Life (HRQOL) at: https://www.cdc.gov/hrqol/

Pre–Cochlear Implant Counseling

Although counseling is not necessarily a component of the audiologic cochlear implant candidacy assessment battery, a substantial amount of counseling should occur once the audiologist determines that cochlear implantation is likely in the best interest of the candidate. Cochlear implant counseling may take place at the end of the candidacy assessment session, or the patient may return for a follow-up appointment that centers around counseling. The cochlear implant candidacy assessment typically takes two to three hours to complete. As a result, some audiologists are reluctant to conduct cochlear implant counseling immediately following the assessment, because the patient may be tired and find it difficult to focus on the information that is shared. If the patient is scheduled to return on another day for cochlear implant counseling, the audiologist should send the patient home with written materials discussing cochlear implant technology and services. Additionally, the audiologist should direct the candidate to the cochlear implant manufacturer's website and online videos where additional information may be found. In some cases, it may not be convenient for the patient to return for an additional appointment (e.g., the patient lives a long distance from the clinic, finds it difficult to take time off from work, has a difficult time arranging transportation to the clinic). In these cases, the audiologist may agree to complete cochlear implant counseling at the end of the assessment session.

Once the patient is determined to be a cochlear implant candidate, the audiologist should turn his/her attention toward three general objectives:

1. The cochlear implant candidate should undergo, if he/she hasn't already, a medical evaluation by a cochlear implant surgeon who can provide a thorough otologic evaluation as well as refer the candidate for additional medical evaluation as needed (e.g., imaging, evaluation by a medical specialist such as a cardiologist). The cochlear implant medical evaluation is discussed in Chapter 12.
2. The audiologist should thoroughly inform the candidate of what to expect from cochlear implantation.
3. The audiologist should identify the candidate's unique needs (e.g., In what listening situations does the candidate covet improved hearing? Which ear(s) does the recipient prefer to have implanted?) and assist the candidate in selecting a cochlear implant system to meet those needs.

Establishing Realistic Expectations

Prior to cochlear implantation, the audiologist must establish realistic expectations for the procedure. It is perfectly reasonable for cochlear implant candidates to have the false impression that a cochlear implant will restore normal hearing. Consider the typical outcome of LASIK surgery to correct myopia (i.e., nearsightedness; inability to clearly visualize objects located at a distance). It is common for persons with myopia to undergo LASIK surgery and leave the ophthalmology clinic with normal vision. Given the success of LASIK surgery and other similarly remarkable advances in medicine, why would the cochlear implant candidate not expect to have normal auditory function after cochlear implantation? Cochlear implantation is a relatively expensive procedure (particularly compared with LASIK) that requires surgery typically performed under general anesthesia. Given the comparison to LASIK and other medical procedures, it is understandable that the lay person would assume that cochlear implantation would restore normal auditory function.

Of course, there are numerous differences in the underlying anatomy, pathophysiology, and physics of cochlear implantation and LASIK. The peripheral sensory cells of the end organ (i.e., the cochlea) are damaged in the presence of severe to profound hearing loss, whereas the sensory cells of the eye's retina are intact and functional for persons with myopia. A more appropriate analogy to draw between the auditory and visual systems would be to compare sensorineural deafness to macular degeneration, which is characterized by damage or absence of the sensory cells in the retina. Macular damage results in blindness, for which there is still no treatment as successful as cochlear implantation.

It is useful for the audiologist to clearly inform the candidate and family of the expected outcome from cochlear implantation. It is often helpful for the audiologist to provide an elementary explanation of the operation of a cochlear implant so that the candidate understands why a cochlear implant is not a replacement for normal hearing. It is also imperative that the audiologist informs the candidate of the range of outcomes that are possible with cochlear implantation. Specifically, the audiologist should inform the candidate that the spectrum of cochlear implant benefit ranges better access to sound (i.e., improved detection) with minimal improvement in open-set speech understanding to excellent open-set speech recognition without visual cues. Of course, the reasonable expectation of a given individual is influenced by his/her pre-implant history. For an adult who was born with severe to profound hearing loss and has little to no previous auditory experience, the cochlear implant is likely to only offer improvement in sound awareness with limited to no potential to allow for open-set speech recognition. On the other hand, for a middle-aged adult who had normal hearing throughout much of his/her life, has normal temporal bone anatomy, and has a short duration of deafness, substantial improvement in open-set speech recognition is expected and likely.

To aptly manage a candidate's expectations, a good rule of thumb is to "under-promise and over-deliver." The audiologist should very clearly establish the fact that there is a wide range of outcomes obtained by cochlear implant recipients and that it is impossible to unequivocally predict an individual's outcome. The first author of this chapter often aims to give the candidate enough hope of improvement so that he/she will move forward with the decision to undergo cochlear implantation while also attempting to establish a low expectation for auditory performance after cochlear implantation. Then, every effort is made to optimize the recipient's outcome in an attempt to exceed his/her expectation. When expectations are managed well and the optimal outcome is vigorously pursued, the recipient is typically satisfied. When discussing expectations, the first author typically notes that some recipients do not initially recognize the sound they perceive from implant stimulation as speech. In fact, the first author notes that some recipients report that the signal they receive sounds like high-pitched ringing, bells, or whis-

tles. Such an initial report is exaggerated and quite unlikely, but again, establishing low expectations for the initial experience with cochlear implant stimulation often facilitates a more satisfied experience for the recipient. The candidate should be informed that cochlear implantation is a marathon and not a sprint. In other words, the recipient may be dissatisfied with the sound quality and speech recognition of the sound he/she experiences during the initial stages of cochlear implant use, but sound quality and speech recognition should improve with use. The candidate should be informed that he/she will likely not reach his/her full auditory potential until 6 to 12 months after implantation. Also, the candidate should understand that persons with longer durations of deafness and/or elderly persons often require a longer period of time to reach optimal performance.

The candidate should also be informed that all cochlear implant recipients are likely to continue to struggle in some listening situations. For example, the majority of cochlear implant recipients will experience at least some difficulty with speech recognition in environments with high levels of noise and reverberation. Additionally, many cochlear implant recipients continue to experience at least some difficulty with music appreciation and aptitude. Furthermore, it is important for the audiologist to note the wide range of outcomes that exist even for persons with favorable pre-implant histories. Although many recipients with favorable pre-implant histories are able to converse over a mobile telephone, understand the dialogue on television programs or movies without closed caption, and understand speech in restaurants, there are also recipients with favorable pre-implant histories who continue to struggle in these challenging listening situations. The candidate should understand that the audiologist can make no guarantees regarding the potential of hearing in these types of listening situations but that the candidate and audiologist can work together to optimize the candidate's outcome. Of note, the audiologist should prepare the candidate that he/she may need to use wireless hearing assistive technology with the cochlear implant to achieve satisfactory performance in some difficult listening conditions.

It is often useful for the candidate to communicate with cochlear implant recipients prior to undergoing cochlear implantation. Conversing with cochlear implant recipients provides the candidate with the opportunity to gather information from a peer regarding the differences in communication and auditory function with a cochlear implant versus hearing aids. In some cases, a candidate may feel more comfortable discussing certain types of questions with a peer with hearing loss rather than with an audiologist. Ideally, the candidate should be connected with a cochlear implant recipient(s) who has a similar pre-implant history (e.g., age, duration of deafness, communication lifestyle). The audiologist may be able to pair the candidate with a recipient at his/her local cochlear implant clinic. If that is not possible or convenient, then the cochlear implant manufacturers offer support networks in which candidates may be paired with recipients who have similar pre-implant histories.

Cochlear Implant Device Counseling

The audiologist should also fully inform the candidate of the cochlear implant technology that will best meet the candidate's needs. If the audiologist believes that there is a particular cochlear implant system that will best meet the needs of the candidate, then the audiologist should inform the candidate of the characteristics and potential advantages of that system. If the audiologist believes that multiple cochlear implant systems will equally meet the needs of the candidate, then the audiologist should inform the candidate of the theoretical advantages and limitations of each cochlear implant system and assist the candidate in deciding upon the best cochlear implant system to meet his/her unique needs. Once a cochlear implant system is selected, the audiologist should assist the candidate in selecting the ideal sound processor(s), color choices for the sound processor(s), and the optimal accessory options (e.g., hearing assistive technology, batteries, wearing options). Of note, completion of the COSI may be helpful in determining the optimal cochlear implant system and accessory options for the candidate.

Finally, the audiologist should establish which ear(s) will be implanted. In some cases, a difference in anatomy may dictate which ear is implanted. The cochlear implant surgeon will be able to determine whether there is a medical reason that identifies an ear that should be selected for implantation. In other cases, the candidate's audiometric profile will determine the ear to be implanted. If one ear has a moderate hearing loss with reasonably good speech recognition capacity and the other ear has a severe to profound hearing loss with a short duration of deafness, then the audiologist would likely recommend the poorer ear for implantation. Conversely, if one ear has a long duration of deafness while the other ear has a relatively short duration of deafness with better but poor open-set speech recognition capacity, then the audiologist may choose to select the ear with a shorter duration of deafness for implantation. If there is no compelling medical or interaural audiometric difference that identifies the ear of implantation, then the audiologist should confer with the candidate to determine whether lifestyle factors may influence the ear of implantation. For example, if the patient uses the telephone frequently, he/she may want to receive the cochlear implant in the ear at which the telephone is typically used. Furthermore, if the candidate spends a great deal of time in an automobile, it may be helpful to determine whether he/she is typically the driver or passenger. A driver would likely prefer to have the cochlear implant in the right ear, whereas a passenger would likely prefer to have the cochlear implant in the left ear (assuming the candidate lives in a country where automobiles are driven on the right [not left] side of the road). If there are no compelling reasons to select a particular ear for cochlear implantation, then the first author typically recommends implantation of the right ear, because the right ear is thought to possibly have a modest advantage in speech processing (Henkin et al., 2014; Jerger & Martin, 2004; Payne et al., 2017).

Key Concepts

- The adult cochlear implant candidacy assessment should be completed by an interdisciplinary team of hearing health care professionals and should include a battery of behavioral and electrophysiologic audiology measurements.
- Aided speech recognition should be completed in the best-aided condition. The audiologist should possess a working knowledge of modern hearing aid technology and verification of hearing aid function in order to ensure that the candidate is equipped with hearing aids that are best suited to meet his/her needs.
- Ultimately, the interdisciplinary team of hearing health care professionals should determine whether a cochlear implant is likely to improve the candidate's communication abilities and quality of life.

References

Alkaf, F. M., & Firszt, J. B. (2007). Speech recognition in quiet and noise in borderline cochlear implant candidates. *Journal of the American Academy of Audiology, 18*(10), 872–882.

American National Standards Institute (ANSI). ANSI/ASA S3.1-1999, (R2013), *Maximum permissible ambient noise levels for audiometric test rooms*. Melville, NY: Acoustical Society of America.

American National Standards Institute (ANSI). ANSI S3.22-2009, *Specification of hearing aid characteristics*. Melville, NY: Acoustical Society of America.

Attias, J., Horovitz, G., El-Hatib, N., & Nageris, B. (2001). Detection and clinical diagnosis of noise-induced hearing loss by otoacoustic emissions. *Noise Health, 3*(12), 19–31.

Bagatto, M. P., Scollie, S. D., Seewald, R. C., Moodie, K. S., & Hoover, B. M. (2002). Real-ear-to-coupler difference predictions as a function of age for two coupling procedures. *Journal of the American Academy of Audiology, 13*(8), 407–415.

Bench, J., Kowal, A., & Bamford, J. (1979). The BKB (Bench-Kowal-Bamford) sentence lists for partially-hearing children. *British Journal of Audiology, 13*, 108–112.

Bentler, R. A. (2005). Effectiveness of directional microphones and noise reduction schemes in hearing aids: A systematic review of the evidence. *Journal of the American Academy of Audiology, 16*(7), 473–484.

Bentler, R., Mueller, H. G., & Ricketts, T. A. (2016). *Modern hearing aids: Verification, outcomes measures, and follow-up*. San Diego, CA: Plural.

Blamey, P., Artieres, F., Başkent, D., Bergeron, F., Beynon, A., Burke, E., Dillier, . . . Lazard, D. S. (2013). Factors affecting auditory performance of postlinguistically deaf adults using cochlear implants: An update with 2251 patients. *Audiology and Neurotology, 18*(1), 36–47.

Boothroyd, A. (2008). CasperSent: A program for computer-assisted speech perception testing and training at the sentence level. *Journal of the Academy of Rehabilitative Audiology, 41*, 31–52.

Boothroyd, A., Hanin, L., & Hnath, T. (1985). *A sentence test of speech perception: Reliability, set equivalence, and short-term learning* (Internal report RCI 10). New York, NY: City University of New York.

Brandy, W. T. (1966). Reliability of voice tests of speech discrimination. *Journal Speech Language Hearing Research, 9*, 461–465.

Ching, T. Y., Dillon, H., & Byrne, D. (1998). Speech recognition of hearing-impaired listeners: Predictions from audibility and the limited role of high-frequency amplification. *Journal of the Acoustical Society of America, 103*(2), 1128–1140.

Coelho, D. H., Hammerschlag, P. E., Bat-Chava, Y., & Kohan, D. (2009). Psychometric validity of the Cochlear Implant Function Index (CIFI): A quality of life assessment tool for adult cochlear implant users. *Cochlear Implants International, 10*(2), 70–83.

Cord, M. T., Walden, B. E., Surr, R. K., & Dittberner, A. B. (2007). Field evaluation of an asymmetric directional microphone fitting. *Journal of the American Academy of Audiology, 18*(3), 245–256.

Cox, R. M., & Alexander, G. C. (1995). The abbreviated profile of hearing aid benefit. *Ear and Hearing, 16*(2), 176–186.

Cox, R. M., & Alexander, G. C. (1999). Measuring satisfaction with amplification in daily life: The SADL scale. *Ear and Hearing, 20*(4), 306–320.

Cox, R. M., & Alexander, G. C. (2002). The International Outcome Inventory for Hearing Aids (IOI-HA): Psychometric properties of the English version. *International Journal of Audiology, 41*(1), 30–35.

Davis, H., & Silverman, S. R., (1978). *Hearing and deafness* (4th ed.). New York, NY: Holt, Rinehart & Winston.[.

Dhar, S., & Hall, J. W. III. (2012). OAE analysis. In S. Dhar & J. W. Hall III (Eds.), *Otoacoustic emissions: Principles, procedures, and protocols* (p. 99). San Diego, CA: Plural.

Deltenre, P., Mansbach, A. L., Bozet, C., Christiaens, F., Barthelemy, P., Paulissen, D., & Renglet, T. (1999). Auditory neuropathy with preserved cochlear microphonics and secondary loss of otoacoustic emissions. *Audiology, 38*(4), 187–195.

Demorest, M. E., & Erdman, S. A. (1987). Development of the communication profile for the hearing impaired. *Journal of Speech and Hearing Disorders, 52*(2), 129–143.

Dillon, H., James, A., & Ginis, J. (1997). Client Oriented Scale of Improvement (COSI) and its relationship to several other measures of benefit and satisfaction provided by hearing aids. *Journal of the American Academy of Audiology, 8*(1), 27–43.

Di Nardo, W., Anzivino, R., Giannantonio, S., Schinaia, L., & Paludetti, G. (2014). The effects of cochlear implantation on quality of life in the elderly. *European Archives of Otorhinolaryngology, 271*(1), 65–73.

Elliott, L. L., & Katz, D. (1980). *Development of a new children's test of speech discrimination* [Technical manual]. St. Louis, MO: Auditec.

Eshraghi, A. A., Gupta, C., Ozdamar, O., Balkany, T. J., Truy, E., & Nazarian, R. (2012). Biomedical engineering principles of modern cochlear implants and recent surgical innovations. *Anatomical Record (Hoboken), 295*(11), 1957–1966.

Etymotic Research, Inc. (2005). *BKB-SIN test. Speech-in-Noise Test Version 1.03, 2005*. Elk Grove Village, IL. http://www.etymotic.com

Firszt, J. B., Holden, L. K., Skinner, M. W., Tobey, E. A., Peterson, A., Gaggl, W., . . . Wackym, P. A. (2004). Recognition of speech presented at soft to loud levels by adult cochlear implant recipients of three cochlear implant systems. *Ear and Hearing, 25*(4), 375–387.

Francis, H. W., Chee, N., Yeagle, J., Cheng, A., & Niparko, J. K. (2002). Impact of cochlear implants on the functional health status of older adults. *Laryngoscope, 112*(8 Pt. 1), 1482–1488.

Gatehouse, S. (1999). A self-report outcome measure for the evaluation of hearing aid fittings and services. *Health Bulletin (Edinb), 57*(6), 424–436.

Gatehouse, S., & Noble, W. (2004). The Speech, Spatial and Qualities of Hearing Scale (SSQ). *International Journal of Audiology, 43*(2), 85–99.

Gelfand, S.A., Schwander T., & Silman, S. (1990). Acoustic reflex thresholds in normal and cochlear-impaired ears: Effects of no-response rates on 90th percentiles in a large sample. *Journal of Speech and Hearing Disorders, 55*(2), 198–205.

Gibson, W. P., & Sanli, H. (2007). Auditory neuropathy: an update. *Ear and Hearing, 31, 28*(Suppl. 2), 102S–106S.

Gifford, R., Dorman, M., Shallop, J., & Sydlowski, S. (2010) Evidence of the expansion of adult cochlear implant candidacy. *Ear and Hearing, 31*(2), 186–194.

Gifford, R. H., Shallop, J. K., & Peterson, A. M. (2008). Speech recognition materials and ceiling effects: Considerations for cochlear implant programs. *Audiology and Neurotology, 13*(3), 193–205.

Henkin, Y., Swead, R. T., Roth, D. A., Kishon-Rabin, L., Shapira, Y., Migirov, L., . . . Kaplan-Neeman, R. (2014). Evidence for a right cochlear implant advantage in simultaneous bilateral cochlear implantation. *Laryngoscope, 124*(8), 1937–1941.

Hinderink, J. B., Krabbe, P. F., & Van Den Broek, P. (2000). Development and application of a health-related quality-of-life instrument for adults with cochlear implants: The Nijmegen cochlear implant questionnaire. *Otolaryngology–Head and Neck Surgery, 123*(6), 756–765.

Holden, L. K., Finley, C. C., Firszt, J. B., Holden, T. A., Brenner, C., Potts, L. G., . . . Skinner, M. W. (2013). Factors affecting open-set word recognition in adults with cochlear implants. *Ear and Hearing, 34*(3), 342–360.

Hood J. D., & Poole J.P. (1980). Influence of the speaker and other factors affecting speech intelligibility. *Audiology, 19,* 434–455.

Jerger, J., Anthony, L., Jerger, S., & Mauldin L. (1974) Studies in impedance audiometry. 3. Middle ear disorders. *Archives of Otolaryngology, 99*(3):165–171.

Jerger, J., & Martin, J. (2004). Hemispheric asymmetry of the right ear advantage in dichotic listening. *Hearing Research, 198*(1–2), 125–136.

Kochkin, S., Beck, D., Christensen, L., Compton-Conley, C., Fligor, B. J., Kricos, P., & Turner, R. G. (2010). MarkeTrak VIII: The impact of the hearing healthcare professional on hearing aid user success. *Hearing Review, 12*(4), 12–31.

Kuk, F. (2008). *Get SET to maximize your success: Widex professional training 16, Fall 2018,* Chicago, IL.

Lassaletta, L., Castro, A., Bastarrica, M., de Sarria, M. J., & Gavilan, J. (2006). Quality of life in postlingually deaf patients following cochlear implantation. *European Archives of Otorhinolaryngology, 263*(3), 267–270.

Latzel M. (2013). Concepts for binaural processing in hearing aids. *Hearing Review,* March 28, 2013. Retrieved from http://www.hearingreview.com/2013/03/concepts-for-binaural-processing-in-hearing-aids/

Lee, J. C., Nam, K. W., Cho, K., Lee, S., Kim, D., Hong, S. H., . . . Kim, I. Y. (2014). Enhanced beam-steering-based diagonal beamforming algorithm for binaural hearing support devices. *Artificial Organs, 38*(7), 608–615.

Mason S. (2003). The electrically evoked auditory brainstem response. In H. E. Cullington (Ed.), *Cochlear implants: Objective measures.* London, UK: Whurr.

Merchant, S. N., Nakajima, H. H., Halpin, C., Nadol, J. B., Jr., Lee, D. J., Innis, W. P., . . . Rosowski, J. J. (2007). Clinical investigation and mechanism of air-bone gaps in large vestibular aqueduct syndrome. *Annals of Otology, Rhinology, and Laryngology, 116*(7), 532–541.

Minimum Speech Test Battery (MSTB). (2011). Retrieved from http://www.auditorypotential.com/MSTBfiles/MSTBManual 2011-06-20%20.pdf

Moog, J. S., & Geers, A. E. (1990). *Early speech perception test for profoundly hearing-impaired children.* St. Louis, MO: Central Institute for the Deaf.

Mudry, A., & Mills, M. (2013). The early history of the cochlear implant: A retrospective. *JAMA Otolaryngology–Head and Neck Surgery, 139*(5), 446–453.

Newman, C. W., Weinstein, B. E., Jacobson, G. P., & Hug, G. A. (1990). The Hearing Handicap Inventory for Adults: Psychometric adequacy and audiometric correlates. *Ear and Hearing, 11*(6), 430–433.

Nikolopoulos, T. P., Mason, S. M., Gibbin, K. P., & O'Donoghue, G. M. (2000). The prognostic value of promontory electric audi-

tory brainstem response in pediatric cochlear implantation. *Ear and Hearing, 21*(3), 236–241.

Nilsson, M. J., McCaw, V. M., & Soli, S. (1996). *Minimum Speech Test Battery for Adult Cochlear Implant Users.* Los Angeles, CA: House Ear Institute.

Nilsson, M., Soli, S. D., & Sullivan, J. A. (1994). Development of the Hearing in Noise Test for the measurement of speech reception thresholds in quiet and in noise. *Journal of the Acoustical Society of America, 95*(2), 1085–1099.

Payne, L., Rogers, C. S., Wingfield, A., & Sekuler, R. (2017). A right-ear bias of auditory selective attention is evident in alpha oscillations. *Psychophysiology, 54*(4), 528–535.

Pearsons, K. S., Bennett, R. L., & Fidell, S. (1977). *Speech levels in various noise environments (Report No. EPA-600/1-77-025).* Washington, DC: U.S. Environmental Protection Agency.

Peterson, G. E., & Lehiste, I. (1962). Revised CNC lists for auditory tests. *Journal of Speech and Hearing Disorders, 27,* 62–70.

Picou, E. M., & Ricketts, T. A. (2013). Efficacy of hearing-aid based telephone strategies for listeners with moderate-to-severe hearing loss. *Journal of the American Academy of Audiology, 24*(1), 59–70.

Ricketts, T., & Dhar, S. (1999). Comparison of performance across three directional hearing aids. *Journal of the American Academy of Audiology, 10*(4), 180–189.

Roeser, R., & Clark, J. (2008). Live voice speech recognition audiometry: Stop the madness. *Audiology Today, 20,* 32–33.

Ross, M., & Lerman, J. (1970). A picture identification test for hearing impaired children. *Journal of Speech and Hearing Research, 13,* 44–53.

Skinner, M. W., Holden, L. K., Holden, T. A., Demorest, M. E., & Fourakis, M. S. (1997). Speech recognition at simulated soft, conversational, and raised-to-loud vocal efforts by adults with cochlear implants. *Journal of the Acoustical Society of America, 101*(6), 3766–3782.

Sladen, D. P., Gifford, R. H., Haynes, D., Kelsall, D., Benson, A., Lewis, K., . . . Driscoll, C. L. (2017). Evaluation of a revised indication for determining adult cochlear implant candidacy. *Laryngoscope, 127*(10), 2368–2374.

Sladen, D. P., Peterson, A., Schmitt, M., Olund, A., Teece, K., Dowling, B., . . . Driscoll, C. L. (2017). Health-related quality of life outcomes following adult cochlear implantation: A prospective cohort study. *Cochlear Implants International, 18*(3), 130–135.

Spahr, A. J., Dorman, M. F., Litvak, L. M., Van Wie, S., Gifford, R. H., Loizou, P. C., . . . Cook, S. (2012). Development and validation of the AzBio sentence lists. *Ear and Hearing, 33*(1), 112–117.

Ventry, I. M., & Weinstein, B. E. (1982). The Hearing Handicap Inventory for the Elderly: A new tool. *Ear and Hearing, 3*(3), 128–134.

Wackym, P. A., Runge-Samuelson, C. L., Firszt, J. B., Alkaf, F. M., & Burg, L. S. (2007). More challenging speech-perception tasks demonstrate binaural benefit in bilateral cochlear implant users. *Ear and Hearing, 28*(Suppl. 2), 80S–85S.

Walden, B., Demorest, M., & Helper, E. L. (1984). Self-report approach to assessing benefit derived from amplification. *Journal of Speech and Hearing Research, 27,* 49–56.

Walden, B. E., Surr, R. K., Cord, M. T., & Dyrlund, O. (2004). Predicting hearing aid microphone preference in everyday listening. *Journal of the American Academy of Audiology, 15*(5), 365–396.

Walker, G., Dillon, H., & Byrne, D. (1984). Sound field audiometry: Recommended stimuli and procedures. *Ear and Hearing, 5*(1), 13–21.

Wolfe, J., Duke, M. M., Schafer, E., Jones, C., Mulder, H. E., John, A., & Hudson, M. (2015a). Evaluation of performance with an adaptive digital remote microphone system and a digital remote microphone audio-streaming accessory system. *American Journal of Audiology, 24*(3), 440–450.

Wolfe, J., Schafer, E., Mills, E., John, A., Hudson, M., & Anderson, S. (2015b). Evaluation of the benefits of binaural hearing on the telephone for children with hearing loss. *Journal of the American Academy of Audiology, 26*(1), 93–100.

6

Cochlear Implant Candidacy: Pediatric Audiologic Assessment

Jace Wolfe

Introduction

Similar to cochlear implant assessments of adults, the pediatric cochlear implant assessment aims to identify whether a cochlear implant is likely to improve the communication ability and quality of life of a child with hearing loss. However, the pediatric cochlear implant assessment process is potentially different from the adult process in many ways. For instance, the types of evaluations included in the pediatric cochlear implant assessment can vary widely, because the assessment may include children ranging in age from the newborn period to 17 years old. Audiologic assessment of infants is often centered around electrophysiologic measures of auditory function (e.g., auditory brainstem response [ABR]), whereas the audiologic assessment with a teenager is likely to primarily include behavioral measures of pure tone detection and speech recognition, very much like the adult assessment. Also, a potential objective of the pediatric cochlear implant assessment is to determine whether a cochlear implant is better able to support the development of an infant's auditory nervous system compared with what is probable with the use of hearing aids. Similarly, the decision to pursue a cochlear implant may hinge on the likelihood that the implant will facilitate optimal language and educational development relative to hearing aid use.

Furthermore, the pediatric cochlear implant assessment team is likely to include a larger number of members than the adult cochlear implant assessment team. As with the adult cochlear implant candidacy assessment, the pediatric cochlear implant assessment team will include evaluations by an audiologist, a cochlear implant surgeon, and an imaging specialist (e.g., a radiologist). However, it is also imperative for the pediatric cochlear implant team to include a speech-language pathologist who specializes in language development of children with hearing loss (e.g., a Listening and Spoken Language Specialist). The pediatric cochlear implant team should also incorporate a pediatric anesthesiologist who can ensure that the child is healthy and developmentally mature enough to undergo cochlear implant surgery under general anesthesia. Additionally, the child's pediatrician may be involved in facilitating referrals to other specialists, who may need to evaluate the child prior to implantation or who may need to provide intervention and/or support prior to and/or after cochlear implantation. Other professionals who may be involved with the pediatric cochlear implant candidacy assessment include: medical specialists (e.g., geneticist, neurologist, cardiologist), educators, a psychologist/psychometrist, a neurodevelopmental specialist, an early interventionist, a social worker, and so forth.

The primary focus of this chapter will center on the audiologist's role in the cochlear implant assessment process for pediatric patients. As with an adult cochlear implant assessment, in order to provide a thorough evaluation to identify the most appropriate hearing technology options for a child with hearing loss, the audiologist should have a keen working knowledge of basic audiology diagnostics and electrophysiologic assessment of auditory function, hearing aid technology and verification, and potential advantages and limitations of all available implantable hearing technologies (e.g., cochlear implants, hybrid cochlear implants, middle ear implantable hearing devices, implantable bone conduction devices). As a result, this chapter will address a wide variety of audiology-related topics. Also, this chapter will briefly address non-audiologic facets of the pediatric cochlear implant candidacy assessment process. This chapter will also address prognostic factors that influence cochlear implant outcomes so that the reader can identify patients who are most likely to benefit from cochlear implantation and those who are more likely to receive limited benefit from a cochlear implant.

Audiologic Assessment

For pediatric cochlear implant candidacy assessment, the audiologic evaluation battery includes several components such as a case history, subjective assessment of communication and functional auditory abilities, electrophysiologic assessment of auditory function, behavioral assessment of auditory function, hearing aid evaluation, assessment of aided auditory function, and so forth. The following sections describe the various elements of audiologic assessment of pediatric cochlear implant candidacy.

Case History

The case history should identify the family's primary concerns and their main reasons for pursuing a cochlear implant. The parents' impression of their child's needs, strengths, and limitations along with the parents' goals and expectations for their child's developmental outcomes will certainly influence the cochlear implant candidacy process. Figure 6–1 provides an example of a sample pediatric cochlear implant case history.

The case history is also an opportunity for the audiologist to gain an understanding of the support the family is able to provide for their child. Cochlear implant programming requires several appointments throughout the first year following surgery and requires quarterly or semi-annual audiology appointments throughout the child's educational years. Prior to implantation, the audiologist should identify whether the family will have difficulty attending the requisite audiology appointments (e.g., transportation issues, inability to take off time from work) so that a plan may be devised to facilitate consistent attendance.

Additionally, a child's outcome with a cochlear implant will depend on his/her access to a robust model of spoken language (Ambrose et al., 2014, 2015; Hart & Risley, 1995, 2003). The family should support the child in using the cochlear implant during all waking hours (i.e., "eyes open, ears on!"). The audiologist should take note of the child's hearing aid data log, and if hearing aid wear time is insufficient, the audiologist should discuss with the family the importance of full-time use of hearing technology and provide strategies to facilitate full-time use. Ideally, data logging should indicate at least 10 hours of hearing technology use per day.

Along with full-time hearing technology use, the family must provide their child with a rich model of abstract (higher level), intelligible spoken language. Better language outcomes are associated with the use of auditory-based habilitation and intervention (Ambrose et al., 2015; Ching & Dillon, 2013; Ching et al., 2017; Dettman et al., 2016; Geers et al., 2011). Research has also suggested that better language outcomes are associated with higher levels of maternal support and maternal education (Ambrose et al., 2015; Ching & Dillon, 2013; Ching et al., 2017; Dettman et al., 2016; Geers et al., 2011). Betty Hart and Todd Risley (1995), behavioral scientists who studied language development, estimated that normal hearing children from affluent homes heard 46 million words by their fourth birthday. Considering the importance of the provision of a vast and complex model of intelligible and meaningful speech to children with normal hearing and especially to children with hearing loss, the audiologist should seek to determine whether the family has the resources necessary to optimize the child's outcome from cochlear implantation and assist the family in providing needed supports.

Electrophysiologic Assessment of Auditory Function in Infants and Children Evaluated for Cochlear Implant Candidacy

Electrophysiologic evaluation of auditory function is typically a staple of the cochlear implant candidacy assessment of most children and should include an

CASE HISTORY (PEDIATRIC)

Date: _____ Patient Name: _____ Date of Birth: _____

What is your primary concern regarding your child's hearing and/or speech and language development?

_____

_____

Do you think your child has hearing loss?　　　○ Yes ○ No

If yes, when did it begin and what caused it? _____

_____

Please mark "Yes" or "No" and your provider will obtain more detailed information during the appointment:

HEARING HISTORY

○ Yes ○ No　　Did your child pass his/her newborn hearing screening?

○ Yes ○ No　　Has your child had any additional hearing tests before?

　　　　　　　　If yes, please describe the results: _____

○ Yes ○ No　　Is there a family history of hearing loss in childhood or early adulthood?

　　　　　　　　If yes, please describe: _____

○ Yes ○ No　　Does your child currently use a hearing aid or cochlear implant?　○ Right Ear ○ Left Ear ○ Both Ears

PREGNANCY & BIRTH HISTORY

At what hospital was your child born? _____

Length of pregnancy: _____ weeks　　　　Baby's birthweight: _____ lbs. _____ oz.

○ Yes ○ No　　Did your child spend any time in the NICU after birth?

　　　　　　　　If yes, for how long and why? _____

○ Yes ○ No　　Did mother use alcohol during the pregnancy?

○ Yes ○ No　　Did mother use tobacco during the pregnancy?

○ Yes ○ No　　Did mother use drugs during the pregnancy?

○ Yes ○ No　　Was mother Rh incompatible during the pregnancy?

○ Yes ○ No　　Did mother have any major illness during the pregnancy?

○ Yes ○ No　　Was there any infection or virus affecting mother or baby during the pregnancy?

Please check all of the following that occurred at the time of or immediately following birth:

○ Breathing/respiratory difficulties　　○ Positive for CMV　　○ Yellow/Jaundice　　○ Cleft lip/Cleft palate

○ Medications given to infant　　　　　○ Low APGAR score　　○ Blue color　　　　　○ Birth defect

○ Other　_____

FIGURE 6–1. An example of a pediatric cochlear implant case history form. Copyright © Hearts for Hearing. *continues*

MEDICAL HISTORY

○ Yes ○ No   Does your child see an Ear, Nose, and Throat doctor?

If yes, who and why? _____

○ Yes ○ No   Does your child have a history of ear infections, ear drainage, or fluid behind the eardrum?

○ Yes ○ No   Has your child had PE tubes?

○ Yes ○ No   Has your child had any other surgeries or hospitalizations that we should know about?

If yes, please describe: _____

○ Yes ○ No   Does your child have vision problems?

○ Yes ○ No   Does your child have any other diagnosis that we should know about?

If yes, please describe: _____

Has your child had any of the following health/medical problems?

○ ADD/ADHD	○ Cancer	○ Genetic Disorder	○ Meningitis
○ Allergies	○ Chicken Pox	○ Head trauma/injury	○ Motor Problems
○ Asthma	○ Ear Pain	○ Heart Problems	○ Mumps
○ Autism	○ Ear Ringing	○ Kidney Problems	○ Psychiatric Disorder
○ Balance Difficulties	○ Exposure to loud noise	○ Measles	○ Seizures

DEVELOPMENT HISTORY (complete if it applies to your child)

At what age did your child: Sit alone _____ Walk alone _____ Use first word _____ Use sentences _____

○ Yes ○ No   Do you have any concerns about your child's speech and language development?

If yes, please describe: _____

○ Yes ○ No   Is your child currently receiving speech, occupational, and/or physical therapy?

If yes, please describe: _____

○ Yes ○ No   Does your child interact well with other children?

EDUCATION HISTORY (complete if your child is enrolled in a school program)

School District: _____ Grade Level: _____

○ Yes ○ No   Does your child currently receive school-based special services?

○ Yes ○ No   Does your child have an IEP?

○ Yes ○ No   Does your child have a learning disability or difficulty in school?

If yes, please describe: _____

○ Yes ○ No   Does your child have difficulty concentrating or paying attention in school?

Is there anything else you would like us to know about your child? _____

_____

_____

FIGURE 6–1. *continued*

array of procedures. At a minimum, a child undergoing cochlear implant candidacy evaluation should have undergone assessment of middle ear function as well as otoacoustic emission and auditory brainstem response assessment. An audiologist may also consider auditory steady-state response assessment and cortical auditory evoked response assessment. The following sections provide relevant information regarding the role of electrophysiologic evaluations of auditory function in the pediatric cochlear implant candidacy assessment.

Assessment of Middle Ear Function in the Pediatric Cochlear Implant Candidacy Evaluation

Because of the frequency of middle ear dysfunction in young children, audiologists should routinely evaluate middle ear function in children who are being considered for cochlear implantation. As with the adult evaluation, assessment of middle ear function of children should minimally include tympanometry and acoustic reflex assessment. For children birth to 6 months of age, tympanometry and acoustic reflex assessment should be completed with use of a 1000 Hz probe tone. For infants with normal middle ear function, the 1000 Hz probe tone tympanogram should possess a single peak (similar to a Jerger "Type A" tympanogram [Jerger, 1970]), and the leftward tail typically deflects below baseline when pressure is swept from a positive to negative direction (Kei et al., 2003). Kei and colleagues measured 1000 Hz tympanometry in 244 ears of infants who presumably had normal middle ear function, because they passed an otoacoustic emission (OAE) screening in both ears at birth. A single-peaked tympanogram was obtained for 225 out of 240 ears. A multiple-peak tympanogram or a shallow, single-peaked tympanogram was obtained for the remaining ears in the study.

Acoustic reflex assessment is often overlooked as an important component that should be routinely included in the assessment of auditory function in infants and children. Acoustic reflex assessment provides the audiologist with valuable information regarding a child's auditory function. First, the presence of an acoustic reflex at normal presentation levels (e.g., 70–95 dB HL) usually rules out severe to profound hearing loss (Gelfand, Schwander, & Silman, 1990). The audiologist should question the appropriateness of cochlear implantation when acoustic reflexes are present at normal levels to eliciting tones at 500, 1000, and 2000 Hz. Second, the presence of an acoustic reflex rules out conductive hearing loss

in the probe ear (Jerger et al., 1974). The audiologist should be aware of whether a conductive overlay may be influencing the degree of a child's hearing loss. Third, the presence of an acoustic reflex at normal presentation levels essentially rules out auditory neuropathy spectrum disorder (ANSD) in the ear that is being stimulated to elicit the reflex (Berlin et al., 2005). Specifically, Berlin and colleagues (2005) attempted to measure acoustic reflexes in 136 children diagnosed with ANSD and found that none of the children had acoustic reflexes present at normal levels (e.g., 95 dB HL or below) for 1000 and 2000 Hz eliciting tones. Of note, a 1000 Hz probe tone should be used to measure the acoustic reflex when evaluating infants from birth to 6 months of age. Also of importance, some infants may have absent or elevated acoustic reflex thresholds to tonal stimuli but more favorable responses to a broadband noise stimulus (Bennet et al., 1982). As a result, audiologists should consider measuring the acoustic reflex to both a broadband noise signal and pure tones during the birth to 6-month period.

Otoacoustic Emission Assessment in the Pediatric Cochlear Implant Candidacy Evaluation

Otoacoustic emission (OAE) assessment is another important component of the pediatric cochlear implant candidacy evaluation. In the majority of children undergoing cochlear implant candidacy assessment, OAEs will be absent. However, the presence of OAEs will prompt the audiologist to complete additional assessment to elucidate auditory function. Present OAEs are typically associated with normal hearing sensitivity, so the audiologist will want to verify that an auditory disorder does indeed exist in a child who possesses present OAEs. The presence of otoacoustic emissions in conjunction with an abnormal ABR and/or severe to profound hearing loss is indicative of ANSD (and/or a retrocochlear hearing disorder). About 10% of children with permanent hearing loss have an etiology of ANSD. The audiologist should be aware of the presence of ANSD (or of a retrocochlear hearing loss), because audiologic and otologic management may be altered slightly. As will be discussed later in this chapter, cortical auditory evoked response (CAER) assessment should be completed with children diagnosed with ANSD. Additionally, the cochlear implant surgeon will want to closely review the magnetic resonance imaging (MRI) result of all children diagnosed with ANSD to ensure the existence of a viable cochlear nerve (Buchman et al., 2006).

Auditory Brainstem Response Assessment in the
Pediatric Cochlear Implant Candidacy Evaluation

For children born with severe to profound hearing loss, the auditory brainstem response (ABR) assessment is the gold standard procedure for estimating the type, degree, and configuration of hearing loss. In most cases, if the ABR suggests a severe to profound sensorineural hearing loss, then the child is most likely a candidate for a cochlear implant. Hang et al. (2015) reported on 1143 children who underwent click-evoked and multiple-frequency tone-burst ABR assessment over a five-year period at the University of North Carolina (UNC) Division of Audiology. A total of 105 of these children had no response present for click and tone burst ABR assessment of each ear, and follow-up information was available for 94 of the 105 children. A cochlear implant was recommended for 91 of the 94 children. Three of the 94 children were determined to have multiple comorbidities that led the UNC Division of Audiology to avoid cochlear implantation. None of the 94 children achieved satisfactory progress with hearing aid use to preclude cochlear implantation. Hang and colleagues concluded that early cochlear implantation should be considered for all children who have a bilateral no-response result on multiple frequency tone burst ABR assessment.

In many cases, audiologists who provide pediatric cochlear implant candidacy assessments and management also administer ABR assessment. However, some audiologists who specialize in cochlear implant services do not routinely complete ABR assessments. At a minimum, however, all audiologists who provide cochlear implant services should be very familiar with contemporary practices for ABR assessment. As previously mentioned, the auditory function of infants being considered for cochlear implantation is often primarily determined through the results of ABR assessment. If the audiologist conducting the cochlear implant candidacy assessment did not administer the ABR evaluation, then he/she should be able to review a child's ABR waveforms and the parameters used to stimulate and acquire the waveform to determine whether the ABR was completed in a satisfactory manner to allow for accurate estimation of auditory function as well as to estimate the degree of the child's hearing loss. Indeed, one of the areas in which audiologists are most likely to make a mistake in the assessment of auditory function in infants is in the completion and particularly in the analysis of the ABR. A detailed discussion of ABR

assessment in infants and young children is beyond the scope of this book; however, the audiologist may readily access several excellent documents that provide a detailed discussion of accurate ABR testing and analysis in infants and children:

Ontario Infant Hearing Program's Audiologic Assessment Protocol (OIHP, 2016):
https://www.mountsinai.on.ca/care/infant-hearing-program/documents/protocol-for-auditory-brainstem-response-2013-based-audiological-assessement-abra

British Columbia Early Hearing Program's Audiology Assessment Protocol (BCEHP, 2012):
http://www.phsa.ca/Documents/bcehpaudiology assessmentprotocol.pdf

England's National Health Service's Guidelines for the Auditory Brainstem Response Assessment in Infants (NHS, 2013a):
http://www.thebsa.org.uk/wp-content/uploads/2014/08/NHSP_ABRneonate_2014.pdf

England's National Health Service's Guidelines for the Assessment and Management of Auditory Neuropathy Spectrum Disorder in Young Infants (NHS, 2013b):
http://www.thebsa.org.uk/resources/

Guidelines for Identification and Management of Infants and Young Children with Auditory Neuropathy Spectrum Disorder (Guidelines Development Conference at NHS, 2008):
https://www.childrenscolorado.org/globalassets/departments/ear-nose-throat/ansd-monograph.pdf

ABR Assessment in Infants—Summary of Protocols and Standards (Wolfe, 2014a):
http://www.audiologyonline.com/articles/20q-abr-assessment-in-infants-12999

Considerations in ABR Assessment in Infants (Wolfe, 2014b):
http://www.audiologyonline.com/audiology-ceus/course/20q-abr-assessment-in-infants-25165

The first step in completing an accurate ABR assessment in infants is to begin with a set of stimulus and acquisition parameters that are evidence based and are most likely to facilitate the successful attainment of a recordable ABR in an infant or young child. Next, the audiologist must have a premeditated plan that will govern the sequence in which the ABR test will be completed. Specifically, the audiologist must have a protocol that serves as a guide to determine which ear will be tested first, which tone-burst frequency will be evaluated first, the order in which tone burst frequencies will be evaluated, the order in which air and bone conduction (if needed) stimuli will be evaluated, if and/or when click-evoked ABR testing will be completed (i.e., a click-evoked ABR is likely to add little value in the assessment of auditory function of infants with sensor hearing loss, but the click-evoked ABR is quite valuable in diagnosing ANSD when infants have absent or severely abnormal tone-burst ABR waveforms), how many "sweeps" will be completed with each waveform, the minimum noise level that must be achieved before declaration of no response, and so forth. Also, and possibly most important, the audiologist must have a protocol that facilitates accurate analysis of waveforms. Throughout the ABR assessment, the audiologist should incorporate a set of controls and safeguards to limit the potential for a mistake during ABR assessment and waveform analysis. The ABR resources listed above provide sufficient information to enable the audiologist to achieve each of the objectives discussed in this paragraph.

Auditory Steady-State Response Assessment in the Pediatric Cochlear Implant Candidacy Evaluation

Auditory steady-state response (ASSR) is an auditory evoked response facilitated by a continuous stimulus that changes rapidly (e.g., amplitude- and/or frequency-modulated tones) or a transient stimulus presented at a rapid frequency (e.g., the 40 Hz Response, which is elicited by clicks presented at a rate of 40 per second). The ASSR has several theoretical advantages over the tone burst ABR, including: (1) commercial auditory evoked response instruments routinely allow for automatic detection of the ASSR, which removes the burden of response analysis from an inexperienced audiologist, (2) multiple ASSRs may be measured simultaneously in each ear, allowing for the simultaneous assessment of auditory function at multiple frequencies in both ears, (3) the ASSR may be measured to tonal stimuli presented at the same intensities as the equipment limits of audiometers (e.g., 110–120 dB HL).

For practical intents and purposes, the theoretical attributes of the ASSR do not translate to a large advantage in the assessment of infants and young children being considered for cochlear implant candidacy. Some researchers have shown that commercial instrumentation may suggest present ASSR in persons who are actually deaf and unable to hear the ASSR stimulus (Gorga et al., 2004; Small et al., 2004).

In particular, at high stimulus intensity levels, a vestibular/myogenic response may be elicited and masquerade as an ASSR. In order to avoid these types of ambiguous results, the audiologist should manually observe tone burst ABR waveforms to conclusively determine whether an auditory response is present at high stimulus levels. Additionally, the broad cochlear excitation patterns evoked at high stimulus levels prevent the attainment of frequency-specific responses via the use of the simultaneous presentation of multiple stimuli. Furthermore, tone burst ABR assessment allows for evaluation of responses obtained to stimuli at levels of up to approximately 90 dB normal hearing level [nHL] at 500 Hz and 100 to 105 dB nHL at 2000 and 4000 Hz. As indicated by the Hang et al. (2015) study, a lack of a tone burst ABR response at equipment limits suggests a severe to profound hearing loss and identifies a child who should be considered for cochlear implantation. The additional information provided by ASSR at high intensity levels may guide the audiologist in the programming of hearing aids (e.g., should the hearing aid be programmed for an estimated behavioral threshold of 100 dB estimated hearing level [eHL] vs. 90 dB eHL), but the ASSR is unlikely to be of much additional value in identifying pediatric cochlear implant candidates compared with tone burst ABR. To conclude, tone burst and click-evoked ABR should be considered the gold standard measure for evaluating auditory function in infants and young children who cannot provide reliable behavioral responses to auditory stimuli and who are being considered for cochlear implantation. ASSR may be considered as a supplementary measure to ABR in the pediatric cochlear implant candidacy assessment battery.

Cortical Auditory Evoked Response Assessment in the Pediatric Cochlear Implant Candidacy Evaluation

The cortical auditory evoked response (CAER) may be a useful measure to include in the pediatric cochlear implant candidacy assessment. The cortical auditory evoked response represents neural activity from the auditory thalamo-cortical regions in response to speech or a frequency-specific stimulus. Recently, researchers from the National Acoustic Laboratories (NAL) in Australia have shown that the CAER measured in response to a calibrated speech token can be a valuable tool to determine whether a child may be in need of a cochlear implant. Gardner-Berry and colleagues (in press) have suggested that the absence of an aided CAER in children with ANSD implies that hearing aids are not providing sufficient stimulation to the auditory areas of the brain. Gardner-Berry et al. (in press) have reported on the provision of cochlear implants prior to one year of age in infants who have ANSD and do not have a present CAER while using hearing aids. More importantly, Gardner-Berry et al. have shown that children with ANSD achieve similar outcomes as children with cochlear hearing loss as long as the former receive appropriate audiologic intervention (e.g., either a hearing aid or a cochlear implant) at an early age (i.e., within the first few months of life).

Of note, Gardner-Berry and colleagues have also used the CAER to determine whether and how hearing aids should be fitted for infants with ANSD. Because the ABR cannot be used to estimate the hearing thresholds of children with ANSD, audiologists have typically waited to fit hearing aids when behavioral audiometric thresholds can be obtained. Many children with auditory dysfunction do not participate in behavioral audiometric threshold assessment until about 7 to 10 months of age. As a result, hearing aid fittings have often occurred at a later age for children with ANSD. Ching et al. (2017) have proposed the CAER as a tool to facilitate the early provision of hearing aids for infants with ANSD. If the CAER is present in the unaided condition, then hearing aids are not fitted. If the CAER is absent in the unaided condition or only present at high stimulus levels (i.e., 75 dB SPL), then hearing aids are fitted. Once the decision is made to fit hearing aids for a child with ANSD, the CAER is used to guide in the determination of the hearing aid gain settings (in dB). The hearing aid is initially set with gain that is appropriate for a mild hearing loss. If no aided CAER is present, the hearing aid gain is set to be appropriate for a moderate hearing loss. Hearing aid gain is increased again if the aided CAER is absent when measured with the aids set for a moderate hearing loss. The specific protocol for use of the CAER to estimate hearing aid settings for children with ANSD is detailed in an Australian Hearing protocol described by Punch and colleagues (2016). Gardner-Berry et al. (in press) have proposed that the early provision of hearing aids for children with ANSD is responsible for the favorable speech and language outcomes children with ANSD have achieved in their studies relative to children with cochlear hearing loss.

Furthermore, Punch and colleagues (2016) have suggested that the CAER may be used to determine whether hearing aids are providing sufficient benefit for children with severe cochlear hearing loss (e.g.,

70 to 80 dB HL). The finding of a present CAER suggests that a child with a severe cochlear hearing loss is receiving auditory brain stimulation with use of hearing aids. A finding of an absent CAER suggests that the child may be receiving inadequate stimulation of the auditory areas of the brain in response to speech while using hearing aids. It is prudent to note that Punch, Ching, and colleagues (2016; in press) do not make decisions to fit hearing aids or pursue cochlear implantation on the basis of CAER results alone. Instead, the CAER responses are considered in conjunction with results on subjective assessment of real world auditory function (e.g., LittlEARS, PEACH questionnaires), report from the child's caregivers and therapists, etc.

Behavioral Assessment of Auditory Function in Infants and Children Evaluated for Cochlear Implant Candidacy

Although electrophysiologic measures of auditory function are a staple in the pediatric cochlear implant assessment battery, a cochlear implant should never be recommended without also evaluating auditory function via the use of behavioral measures. The audiologist should attempt to evaluate a child's audiometric thresholds for frequency-specific stimuli and speech using approaches that research has shown to be suitable for measuring threshold-level responses in infants and young children. If possible, the audiologist should also evaluate the child's ability to understand speech with the use of hearing aids. Furthermore, the audiologist should routinely use standardized questionnaires to evaluate the child's real world auditory function. The following sections describe the components that should be included in the behavioral assessment of auditory function of infants and children being considered for cochlear implantation.

Behavioral Assessment of Audiometric Thresholds in Infants and Children Evaluated for a Cochlear Implant

Behavioral assessment of audiometric thresholds in children can be accomplished through the use of several different pediatric audiology methods, including visual reinforcement audiometry, conditioned play audiometry, and conventional audiometry. Of note, these methods may all be used to measure threshold-level responses. However, it is prudent to acknowledge that although children who have reached a developmental age of approximately 6 months can repeatedly respond near true threshold, the auditory responses of children between the ages of 6 and 24 months are often slightly suprathreshold. For instance, research has shown that infants who are 6 months of age and who have normal hearing will typically respond around 20 to 25 dB HL (Gravel & Wallace, 1998), even though their true hearing threshold is likely to be closer to 0 dB HL. Because infants and young children are inclined to respond at slightly suprathreshold levels, their near-threshold responses are often referred to as minimal response levels (MRLs), acknowledging the fact that the child's responses are not true threshold-level responses. Behavioral observation audiometry is another technique that may be used to observe auditory responsiveness but is not generally suitable to measure threshold-level responses. The following sections will provide an overview of the various techniques that may be used to evaluate audiometric thresholds in infants and young children.

Visual Reinforcement Audiometry

Audiologists should attempt to evaluate a child's behavioral audiometric thresholds prior to the recommendation and provision of a cochlear implant. Several evidence-based approaches may be used to evaluate hearing thresholds in infants and young children. The selection of the approach the audiologist employs is dependent upon the developmental age of the child. Research has established that visual reinforcement audiometry (VRA) may be used

to measure threshold-level responses in infants and children between the developmental ages of 6 and 30 months. VRA involves the use of a visual signal (a lighted/animated toy, a video, etc.) to reinforce a head-turn a child makes in response to the detection of an auditory stimulus (Figure 6–2). Many audiologists recognize the need for detailed protocols to guide the accurate completion of electrophysiologic assessment of auditory function. However, adherence to an evidence-based protocol is equally important to ensure that reliable and valid results are obtained with VRA assessment. A detailed discussion of an evidence-based VRA protocol is beyond the scope of this text. However, the interested audiologist is referred to a brief summary description of a VRA protocol in Chapter 14 of this book.

Every audiologist should ensure that he/she is adhering to evidence-based principles while conducting VRA. Use of evidence-based principles limit the likelihood that a child's false positive/invalid responses and/or the audiologist's personal biases will result in mistakes that may lead to an under- or overestimation of the child's hearing sensitivity. A departure from best practices reduces the likelihood that a comprehensive audiogram will be obtained and enhances the likelihood of an egregious mistake. Of note, children with hearing loss are often delayed in their ability to participate in the VRA task. In many cases, children with VRA will not participate with the VRA task until about 8 to 10 months of age. Also of note, the inclusion of a test assistant enhances the likelihood of the successful completion

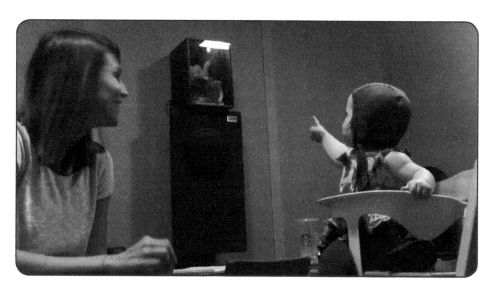

FIGURE 6–2. An example of visual reinforcement audiometry.

of VRA. A second audiologist may serve as the test assistant, but use of two audiologists is often problematic because both cannot bill insurance for their time, and audiologists are often in short supply. The child's caregiver can serve as the test assistant, but this can also be problematic because the parent is typically inexperienced with the VRA test paradigm and uncertain of the best methods to keep the child centered when stimuli are not being presented. Additionally, an inexperienced test assistant is unlikely to be aware of how to facilitate response shaping if the child does not naturally produce a head-turn. Ideally, the child's auditory-verbal therapist (AVT) can serve as the test assistant for audiologic assessment and eventually for cochlear implant programming, because the child and AVT are familiar with one another. The child will be comfortable with the AVT, and the AVT will be familiar with the child's capabilities, behavioral responses, and preferences. If AVTs are typically unavailable to assist with VRA assessment, then the audiologist should consider training a clinic employee (e.g., an audiology assistant, a nurse, an office assistant) to serve as a test assistant.

Conditioned Play Audiometry

Conditioned play audiometry (CPA) involves having the child engage in some type of fun task in which he/she performs an action in response to detecting the auditory stimulus. For example, the child may throw a ball into a bucket each time he/she hears a tone. The audiologist is only limited by his/her imagination in developing CPA tasks that may be used to engage the child's cooperation and encourage threshold-level responses. Examples of CPA tasks are shown in Figure 6–3 and include: throwing plastic fish or some other plastic toy into a bucket of water, stacking pegs, dropping a Connect 4 disk into the game grid, dropping a toy car down a poster tube, inserting birthday cake candles into playdough, dropping pennies into a bank, placing stickers onto a coloring book page, placing plastic jewels onto a royal crown, dropping candy into a cup, pushing a button to advance an image on a video screen, and so on.

CPA is typically used to evaluate audiometric responses in children between the ages of 2 and 8 years. Barr (1955) and Thompson and colleagues (1989) evaluated the feasibility of CPA in children between the ages of 2 and 6 years and 2 and 5 years, respectively. Both studies found that CPA was successfully completed greater than 95% of the time in children 3 years of age and older. For children

between 2.5 to 3 years old, Barr reported successful use of CPA in 61% of children, whereas Thompson and Weber found CPA to be successful in almost 90% of participants. For children between 2 and 2.5 years old, Barr found CPA to be used successfully in only 20% of children, whereas Thompson and Weber reported that it was successfully used in 70% of cases. Of note, Thompson and Weber used two testers in their studies, while Barr used only one tester. The higher incidence of successful completion of CPA in younger children reported by Thompson and Weber once again underscores the importance of the inclusion of a test assistant when evaluating auditory function in infants and young children.

It should be noted that some children will begin to participate in the CPA task at around 18 months old. Children are more likely to participate in the CPA task at an earlier age when they have good access to sound with the use of their hearing technology, when they use their hearing technology during all waking hours, and when they do not have additional disabilities other than hearing loss. Children are also more likely to participate in the CPA task at an early age when they are prepped outside the clinic. Ideally, the child's AVT will practice the CPA activity in the child's therapy sessions. Although practicing the CPA activity during AVT sessions does not necessarily strengthen the child's spoken language skills, it does enhance the likelihood that the child's auditory function will be accurately evaluated in the clinic. Additionally, it improves the likelihood that the audiologist will be able to establish an appropriate program during cochlear implant programming. If it is not possible to practice the CPA task during weekly therapy sessions, then the audiologist should coach the child's caregivers to practice the CPA task at home.

Establishing CPA participation at an early age (18 to 24 months old) is beneficial for multiple reasons. First, although most children in the 18- to 24-month-old range will participate in VRA assessment, children in this age range may be more likely to provide a larger number of responses before habituation/fatigue with CPA. Second, children with hearing loss typically are seen for frequent audiology appointments in which multiple measurements of sound detection are completed. For instance, unaided air and bone conduction thresholds may be evaluated along with aided sound field detection measures, and if the child has a cochlear implant, the audiologist may also measure electrical thresholds (i.e., T levels) for multiple electrodes. CPA is preferable to VRA, because the CPA task can be changed frequently in

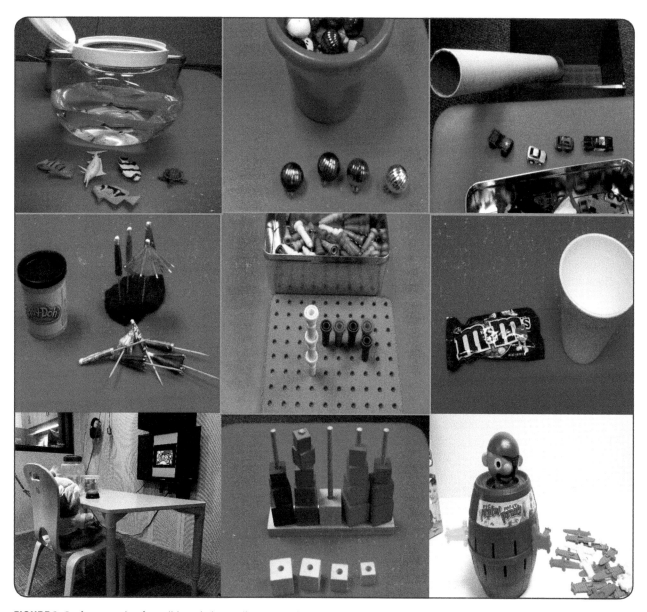

FIGURE 6–3. An example of conditioned play audiometry tasks.

an effort to maintain the child's attention over multiple test trials.

Many children are capable of cooperating with conventional audiometric practices (e.g., say "yes" or raise your hand when you hear the sound) by 4 or 5 years of age. However, out of boredom, young children will often fatigue quickly to the conventional audiometric task. The authors' anecdotal experiences indicate that some children prefer to be evaluated with CPA rather than conventional audiometry through about 10 years of age, especially when the child must participate in unaided and aided assess-

ment and with a cochlear implant program, as would be the case for a child who uses bimodal technology (i.e., a cochlear implant with a hearing aid for the non-implanted ear). The audiologist should use his/her clinical judgment to determine whether CPA or conventional audiometry should be used when children are in the 8- to 10-year-old age range.

Behavioral Observation Audiometry

With behavioral observation audiometry (BOA), the audiologist presents auditory stimuli and observes the child's behavioral responses to the test signals. The child's behavioral responses to auditory stimuli may include: a change in sucking pattern, a change in facial expression, eye widening, body movement, and so forth. Research has unequivocally demonstrated that BOA is unsuitable for the measurement of threshold-level responses in young children of any age (Thompson & Weber, 1974; Wilson & Thompson, 1984). Of note, it should also be noted that there is not one peer-reviewed publication that demonstrates that BOA may be used to acquire threshold-level responses in infants of any age, regardless of whether the BOA is characterized by high intersubjectivity (i.e., some infants respond to auditory signals at low levels [e.g., 30 dB SPL], whereas other infants with normal hearing fail to respond or only respond at moderate to high stimulus levels [e.g., 70 dB SPL]) and high intrasubjectivity (e.g., individual infants with normal hearing have been shown to respond to some test signals at low levels and other signals at moderate to high levels). Also, infants often habituate quickly to the BOA paradigm. For instance, an infant with normal hearing may initially respond one time to a test signal at 30 dB SPL and then respond at much higher levels (60–70 dB SPL) on subsequent presentations of the same test signal. Response habituation is likely because infants younger than the age in which VRA is likely to be successful (3 to 4 months) have short attention spans and simply because no reinforcement is provided to facilitate repeated responses.

Although BOA cannot be used to measure threshold-level responses, there are several reasons for why the audiologist should use BOA during the cochlear implant evaluation process. For infants in whom is diagnosed severe to profound hearing loss or ANSD at birth, the audiologist will be unable to measure threshold-level responses for at least half a year. During this period, the audiologist and parents covet additional information about the child's auditory responsiveness to sound. Although BOA does not provide threshold-level information, it may be used to evaluate the child's auditory responsiveness to sound, and as a result, BOA can provide valuable information. For instance, if BOA testing reveals that a child consistently changes his/her behavior in response to signals presented at levels consistent with moderate hearing loss, then the audiologist may choose to repeat the ABR. Also, the audiologist will be less likely to pursue early cochlear implantation for an infant who appears to be consistently responding to sounds at levels that would suggest considerable functional hearing. In contrast, if no responses are observed at audiometric limits during

BOA assessment of a 3- to 4-month-old infant, the audiologist may not necessarily conclude that the child has a profound hearing loss (because, as mentioned earlier, BOA responses of infants are quite variable). However, a finding of no BOA responses at audiometric limits corroborates a no-response ABR and is another piece in the multiple-component test battery the audiologist incorporates to determine whether early cochlear implantation is in the best interest of the infant. At the risk of being redundant, however, the authors must mention that BOA should not be used as a measure of audiometric threshold. For example, if the ABR suggests a moderate hearing loss and BOA responses are obtained in the severe hearing loss range, it is most likely that the child is responding at suprathreshold levels during BOA assessment. In such a case, the audiologist should NOT increase the gain and output of a child's hearing aids in response to the child's BOA evaluation. In short, BOA is a measure of auditory responsiveness that provides additional information to a comprehensive cochlear implant candidacy assessment, but BOA may not be used to measure audiometric thresholds.

Regardless of the type of pediatric audiometric approach (e.g., VRA, CPA, conventional) used to evaluate a child's hearing sensitivity, the audiologist should seek to acquire ear-specific and frequency-specific thresholds across the speech frequency range (e.g., 125 to 8000 Hz). Insert earphones are the preferred transducer to obtain ear-specific thresholds. The advantages of ear-specific thresholds were discussed in Chapter 5 of this textbook. The audiologist should also seek to obtain ear-specific bone conduction thresholds to determine whether a conductive hearing disorder exists. Pulsed pure tones or warbled tones (two to three presentations with a 500 msec on/off duty cycle) are the ideal stimulus for frequency-specific assessment. However, some younger children and some children with neurodevelopmental disabilities (e.g., autism) may respond more favorably to narrowband noise. Additionally, the audiologist may alternate back and forth between the use of tones and narrowband noise to maintain a child's attention over a longer period of time. With that said, the audiologists should also keep in mind the fact that narrowband noise is intended to be used for masking pure tones and not for the assessment of hearing sensitivity. In order to mask pure tones, narrowband noise is typically a few decibels higher in level than the pure tone at the same frequency. Also, narrowband noise has a wider spectrum than pure tones. The audiologist should be aware of the fact that thresholds to narrowband noise will likely be lower in level than thresholds for pure tones not only because the child may be more attentive to narrowband noise but also because narrowband noise possesses more energy than a pure tone at a corresponding frequency and audiometric dial level.

Audiometric Criteria Indicating Cochlear Implantation for Children

As discussed in Chapter 4, the FDA-approved audiometric criteria for pediatric cochlear implantation vary by age and by manufacturer. In general, the FDA-approved indications for use in children call for a bilateral profound hearing loss for children 12 to 24 months. For Nucleus devices, the indications for use are a little more lenient and specify a severe to profound hearing for children older than 24 months. Recent research suggests that existing pediatric cochlear implant guidelines may be too conservative. A number of research studies have shown better auditory, speech, and language outcomes in children who are born deaf and undergo cochlear implantation prior to 12 months of age (Bergeson, Houston, & Miyamoto, 2010; Ching & Dillon, 2013; Dettman et al., 2016; Houston, Stewart, Moberly, Hollich, & Miyamoto, 2010; Niparko et al., 2010; Moog & Geers, 2010). As a result, cochlear implantation should be considered prior to 12 months of age for children who are born with severe to profound hearing loss.

Pediatric cochlear implant guidelines are likely to be too conservative in regard to degree of hearing loss as well. Ching and Dillon (2013) found that the language outcomes of children with cochlear implants were similar to the outcomes of children who used hearing aids and had a four-frequency pure-tone average of 66 dB HL. As a result, it is likely that many children with severe sensorineural hearing loss will achieve better outcomes with a cochlear implant than they will obtain with hearing aids. For children who have severe hearing loss (e.g., pure-tone thresholds poorer than 75 dB HL) and who are making limited progress with hearing aids (as defined by scores on standardized questionnaires of real-world auditory function, caregiver and therapist report, etc.), cochlear implantation may provide better auditory and spoken language outcomes.

For children who have severe hearing loss, the audiologist must ensure that the child has consistent access to low-level speech and environmental sounds with the use of hearing aids. Real-ear probe microphone measures should indicate that hearing aid output in response to low-level speech (presented at 55 dB SPL) is audible for the child and is matched to an evidence-based prescriptive target (e.g., DSL 5.0 for children, Scollie et al., 2005). If the hearing aid output for low-level speech (55 dB SPL) is below the child's hearing thresholds, then the child's outcomes will almost undoubtedly suffer. In such a case, cochlear implantation may be warranted. Additionally, the audiologist should be concerned if the child's aided thresholds are elevated. Aided thresholds in excess of 25 to 30 dB HL suggest that the child will not hear lower-level speech components. If the hearing aid is matched to an evidence-based prescriptive target for a child with severe hearing loss, then the hearing aid output is likely optimized for the child's degree of hearing loss and limited dynamic range of hearing. As a result, the elevated aided thresholds do not necessarily suggest that the hearing aids are fitted inappropriately or are in need of an adjustment. Instead, the elevated thresholds indicate reduced audibility for low-level sounds secondary to the child's severe degree of hearing loss. Limited access to low-level sounds places a child at risk for auditory and spoken language delay. In such a case, the cochlear implant team should closely follow the child's outcomes and progress. If progress with hearing aids is limited, cochlear implantation should be considered.

Speech Recognition Assessment in Infants and Children Evaluated for Cochlear Implant Candidacy

Because the early provision of cochlear implantation (e.g., prior to 12 months of age) is necessary to optimize auditory, speech, and language outcomes, many children who are born with severe to profound sensorineural hearing loss receive cochlear implants prior to reaching an age at which speech recognition may be evaluated. However, once a child is old enough to participate in speech recognition assessment, the audiologist should routinely evaluate the child's ability to understand speech, and speech recognition assessment should be a primary component in the pediatric cochlear implant assessment battery. The following sections describe considerations for the evaluation of speech recognition of children being considered for cochlear implantation.

Hearing Aid Evaluation

According to the FDA-approved indications for cochlear implantation, aided speech recognition should be evaluated in the best-aided condition. As a result, it is imperative that the audiologist possess a thorough understanding and working knowledge of modern hearing aid technology and of how to verify the appropriate function of hearing aids. Specifically, the audiologist must be able to ensure that the hearing aid is functioning within the manufacturer's specifications, and most importantly, the audiologist should conduct probe microphone measures to ensure that the child's hearing aid output is matched to evidence-based prescriptive targets (e.g., DSL 5.0 for children) for 55, 65, and 75 dB SPL speech inputs and for a swept pure tone presented at 85 to 90 dB SPL (Figure 6–4). Probe microphone measures should ideally be conducted on the ear (i.e., in situ), but many young children will not hold still for the several minutes required for these measurements to be completed. In the cases of infants and young children (1 to 5 years old), simulated probe microphone measurements, in which the hearing aid output is measured in a 2-cc coupler and used to estimate the output that occurs when worn on the child's ear, are likely to be more convenient and to provide a more accurate representation of hearing aid function. Whether the audiologist chooses to complete in situ or simulated probe microphone measures, he/she should measure the child's real-ear-to-coupler difference (RECD) in order

to be precisely specific about the child's hearing loss in dB SPL at the tympanic membrane and to improve the accuracy of estimates calculated during simulated probe microphone measurements.

In recognition of the fact that children with hearing loss require higher sensation levels than adults for similar speech recognition abilities, the DSL 5.0 (Scollie et al., 2005) and NAL-NL2 (Dillon & Keidser, 2013) prescriptive methods prescribe greater gain and output for children compared with adults. As a result, audiologists must remember to fit and verify children's hearing aids to pediatric-based targets. Additionally, although biologic listening checks seem rather mundane and trivial relative to electroacoustic measurements, the audiologist should always use a stethoscope to listen to the hearing aids of children undergoing cochlear implant candidacy evaluation. Many infants and young children who are being considered for cochlear implantation do not possess sufficient language abilities to allow for a report to the audiologist or caregiver regarding the sound quality of the hearing aids. Consequently, the audiologist must incorporate a listening check with electroacoustic measures to evaluate the subjective sound

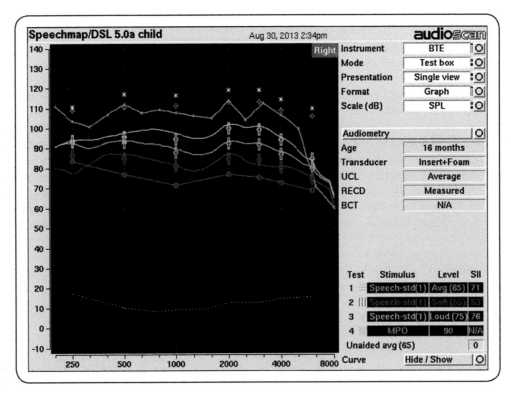

FIGURE 6–4. An example of real-ear probe microphone results with aided output set to match evidence-based prescriptive fitting targets.

quality of the child's hearing aids (e.g., identify the presence of distortion, noise, poor sound quality for speech). A thorough overview of hearing aid evaluation and verification was provided in Chapter 5, and those principles also apply when fitting and verifying hearing aids for children. The reader is referred to Chapter 5 for additional information on hearing aid evaluation and verification for the purposes of cochlear implant candidacy assessment.

Evaluating Speech Recognition in Children

There is not a universal protocol that governs the evaluation of speech recognition of children being considered for cochlear implantation. One reason for which there is no universal set of measures is the fact that the speech materials used to evaluate speech recognition in children vary widely across the age range. Closed-set speech recognition tests, such as the Early Speech Perception (ESP) test (Moog & Geers, 1990), the Northwestern University–Children's Perception of Speech (NU-CHIPS) test (Elliott & Katz, 1980), or the Mr. Potato Head test, are often used to evaluate speech recognition of young children between the ages of 2 to 5 years old. Open-set speech recognition tests, such as the Multisyllabic Neighborhood Test (MLNT) (Kirk, Pisoni, & Osberger, 1995), the Lexical Neighborhood Test (LNT) (Kirk, Pisoni, & Osberger, 1995), the Phonetically Balanced Kindergarten (PBK) (Haskins, 1949), and the Consonant-Nucleus-Consonant (CNC) (Peterson & Lehiste, 1962) tests are often used to evaluate word recognition in children between the ages of 3 to 4 years old and up. Furthermore, sentence recognition in quiet and in noise may also be assessed in older children. The following paragraphs describe considerations for the evaluation of speech recognition of children being considered for cochlear implantation.

Pediatric Minimum Speech Test Battery

Similar to the Minimum Speech Test Battery developed by cochlear implant professionals for use with adults who are being considered for cochlear implantation or whose postoperative outcomes are evaluated, a working group of academic, clinical, research, and industry professionals developed the Pediatric Minimum Speech Test Battery (PMSTB), which is a protocol for the assessment of speech recognition of children who are being considered for cochlear implantation or who are using cochlear implants (Uhler & Gifford, 2014; Uhler et al., 2017).

The PMSTB calls for the assessment of speech recognition in quiet at multiple presentation levels and in noise. Additionally, the PMSTB recommends the use of word and sentence materials. In order to include a wide variety of measures that allow for the assessment of speech recognition in children ranging in age from infancy to teenagers, the PMSTB includes a larger number of speech recognition tests than the adult MSTB. The PMSTB is arranged in a hierarchical format so that at one end of the spectrum, questionnaires completed by a child's caregivers are administered when the child is too young to participate in traditional speech recognition tasks, whereas on the other end of the spectrum, linguistically complex monosyllabic word recognition and sentence recognition in noise tests are administered with older children who have developed mature, adult-like spoken language abilities. Figure 6–5 provides an illustration of the components and implementation of the PMSTB protocol.

Auditory Skills Checklist

The PMSTB begins with the completion of the Auditory Skills Checklist and the LittlEARS questionnaire. The Auditory Skills Checklist is a criterion-referenced measure that was designed to evaluate and monitor a child's auditory abilities over time (Meinzen-Derr et al., 2007). The Auditory Skills Checklist contains 35 items that probe auditory skill development across the domains of Erber's auditory stages, detection, discrimination, identification, and comprehension (see the box below for an example of items from the Auditory Skills Checklist). The items are scored based on the feedback from the child's caregivers and the observations of the child's caregivers and audiologist. For each item, the audiologist assigns a score of 0, 1, or 2 if the child does not have the skill, has an emerging skill, or has mastered the skill, respectively. The Auditory Skills Checklist contains an item-specific guide which assists the audiologist in interpreting whether the skill is absent, emerging, or mastered. For example, within the Detection domain, an item probes whether the child can detect the Ling Six Sounds (Ling, 1976, 1989). The child does not have this skill and receives a score of 0 if he/she cannot detect any of the six sounds. The child has an emerging task and receives a score of 1 if he/she can detect at least one of the six sounds, and the child has mastered the skill and receives 2 points if he/she can detect all six sounds. The audiologist may compare an individual child's score on the Auditory

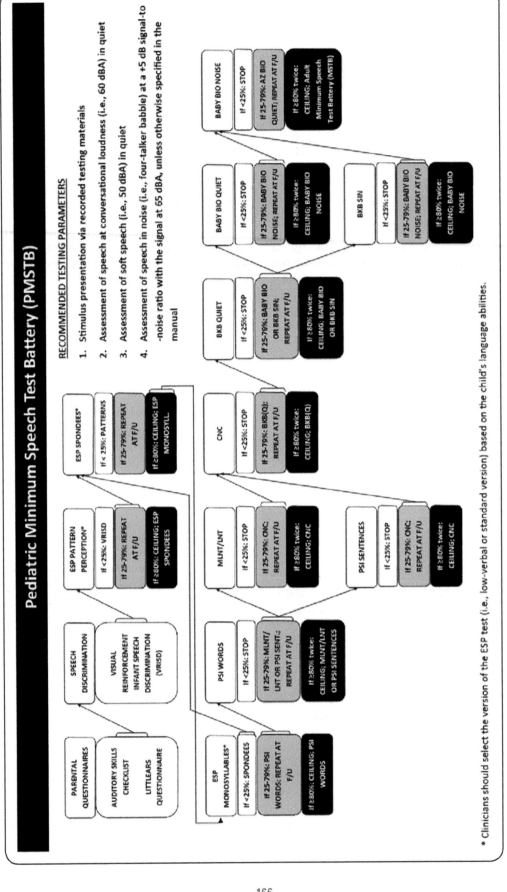

FIGURE 6–5. A flow chart describing the components and sequencing of the Pediatric Minimum Speech Test Battery (PMSTB). Copyright © Kristen Uhler.

* Clinicians should select the version of the ESP test (i.e., low-verbal or standard version) based on the child's language abilities.

Skills Checklist to normative values for children with normal hearing in order to determine whether the child is making progress commensurate with his/her normal-hearing peers (Tyberg, 2013). If the child's progress is delayed, then the audiologist may consider modifying the child's technology (e.g., adjust hearing aid settings, switch to more different hearing aids, pursue cochlear implantation). Also, the audiologist may serially administer the Auditory Skills Checklist with an individual child to determine whether the child is making sufficient progress with his/her auditory skill development. Of note, Meinzen-Darr and colleagues (2007) reported that children who received a cochlear implant at 36 months of age or earlier increased their Auditory Skills Checklist score by 8 points every three months post-implantation. If an individual child is exhibiting a slower rate of progress on the Auditory Skills Checklist while using

hearing aids, the audiologist should consider adjustments to the hearing aids settings or consideration of cochlear implantation.

LittlEARS Questionnaire

The LittlEARS questionnaire also includes 35 questions that are answered in a yes/no format by the child's caregivers (Coninx et al., 2009; Weichbold et al., 2005). Table 6–1 provides an example of items within the LittlEARS questionnaire. A score of 0 is assigned to each question receiving a "no" response, while a score of 1 is assigned to each question receiving a "yes" response. The questions describe auditory skills that become progressively more sophisticated and/or complex as the test progresses, and the audiologist is supposed to terminate the test after a "no" response is provided to six consecutive questions.

An Example of Items From the Auditory Skills Checklist

Each question has an answer characterized as D (does not have skill), E (emerging skill), and S (has skill) with the potential of 0, 1, 2 points, respectively. Performance is scored in terms of the total amount of points out of a possible 70 and by the change in scores over time. Scoring is based on the amount of time a child demonstrates specific auditory abilities as the following:

S = often

E = sometimes

D = never or rarely

Certain questions will have specified answers to help the interviewer understand what is meant by "often, sometimes, never, or rarely." For these questions, the answers are described.

Detection—the ability to determine the presence or absence of sound

Does your child . . .

1. wear the amplification device during his/her waking hours?

2. use body language to indicate when something is heard (*ex. turns head, and/or eye widening, quiets, stops action, changes facial expressions*)?

3. show awareness (*alerts or quiets in response to loud sound, turns to the sound source*) of loud environmental sounds (*ex. dog barking*)?

4. show awareness (*quiets to the sound and/or turns to the sound source*) of soft environmental sounds (*ex. microwave bell, clock ticking, etc.*)?

5. show awareness of voices (*quiets to the sound and/or turns to the sound source*), spoken at typical loudness levels (*in a regular voice*)? (*ex. gets excited when they hear their mother's voice, child playing on the floor with toy cars looks up when people are talking in the room*)?

6. detect the Ling Six Sounds (M, AH, OO, E, SH, S)?

    S = the child detects **all** of the Ling Six Sounds

    E = the child detects **at least one** of the six sounds (circle what sounds the child hears)

    D = the child **does not detect any** of the six sounds

7. detect the speaker's voice when background noise (*softer than the speaker's voice*) is present?

8. search to find out where a sound is coming from?

9. localize the correct sound source (*to the direction the sound is coming from*)?

    S = the child localizes the correct sound source most of the time

    E = the child searches to find out where a sound is coming from and/or localizes the correct sound source some of the time

    D = the child does not search or localize the sound source

TABLE 6–1. An Example of Items from the LittlEARS Questionnaire

LittlEARS Questionnaire

Date: _____

Child Name: _____

Child Birthdate: _____

	Question	Please Circle Answer!	
1	Does your child respond to a familiar voice? Example: Smiles; looks toward source; talks animatedly	YES	NO
2	Does your child listen to somebody speaking? Example: Listens; waits and listens; looks at the speaker for a longer time	YES	NO
3	When somebody is speaking, does your child turn his/her head toward the speaker?	YES	NO
4	Is your child interested in toys producing sounds or music? Example: Rattle, squeezing toy	YES	NO
5	Does your child look for a speaker he/she cannot see?	YES	NO
6	Does your child listen when the radio/CD player/tape player is turned on? Example: Listening; turns toward the sound, is attentive, laughs or sings/talks "along"	YES	NO
7	Does your child respond to distant sounds? Example: When being called from another room	YES	NO

Source: Provided courtesy of MED-EL Corporation.

The LittlEARS questionnaire is norm-reference for children with normal hearing ranging in age from birth to 24 months. A scoring chart has age plotted on the *x*-axis and the LittlEARS scores on the *y*-axis. The 95% confidence interval is also included on the scoring chart so that the audiologist may plot an individual child's score on the chart to easily determine whether the child's auditory skill development is within normal limits (Figure 6–6).

Speech Perception Assessment in the PMSTB

The PMSTB contains 12 different measures for evaluating speech perception of children. According to Uhler et al. (2017), these speech perception measures were selected to match "Kirk and colleagues' (2009) description of a comprehensive battery, which 'should permit the evaluation of a hierarchy of skills, ranging from vowel and consonant speech features through the comprehension of connected speech'" (p. 225). More specifically, the speech perception battery includes tasks appropriate for evaluating speech

discrimination in infants (e.g., visual reinforcement infant speech discrimination [VRISD]) and eventually progresses toward word recognition (e.g., Consonant-Nucleus-Consonant [CNC]) and sentence recognition (Bamford-Kowal-Bench Sentence in Noise [BKB-SIN—Bench, Kowal, & Bamford, 1979]) tests that are appropriate for assessment of speech recognition of adult recipients. The audiologist should begin with measures that match the child's ability to respond. In other words, if the child is incapable of recognizing or identifying speech, then the VRISD is a good place to start in the evaluation of speech discrimination. Once the child is able to begin to recognize words, the audiologist should progress toward the use of closed-set picture-pointing tasks. Closed-set tasks may also be most appropriate for children who have speech delay and articulation errors for whom it may be difficult to determine whether errors made on open-set tests are auditory or speech errors. The audiologist will eventually progress toward the use of open-set measures once the child is developmentally ready to do so. Once again, the audiologist

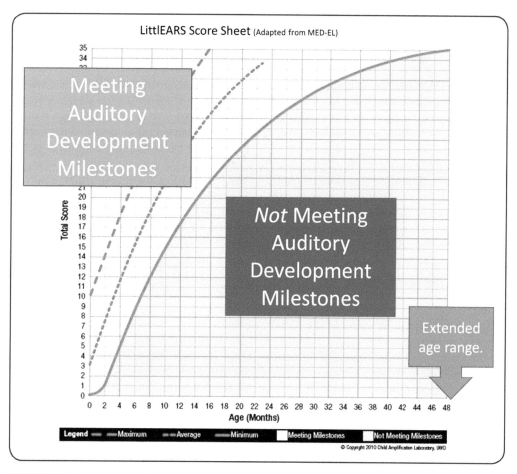

FIGURE 6–6. An example of items from the LittlEars Questionnaire scoring sheet. Image provided courtesy of MED-EL Corporation.

should take into account the child's articulation abilities when scoring open-set speech tests and exercise caution in penalizing a child for misarticulation.

The audiologist should also select measures that match the child's language age. Within the battery of open-set measures, the audiologist may select simply open-set tasks that contain words that are commensurate with the vocabulary of a pre-school child (e.g., Multisyllabic Lexical Neighborhood Test [MLNT]), or for older children, the audiologist can select the CNC word test, which contains words that are more linguistically/lexically complex. It is important to note that the audiologist should strive to select speech recognition measures that are appropriate for the child's language abilities rather than selecting tests solely on the child's chronologic age. For instance, a 7-year-old child with speech and language delays may not have a vocabulary level that is sufficient for participation with the CNC word test. In such a case, it is more appropriate for the audiologist to select a

simpler test such as the Lexical Neighborhood Test (LNT). The audiologist may choose to consult with a child's speech-language pathologist (SLP) to determine the child's speech and expressive/receptive language abilities in order to select a linguistically appropriate test. If it is not possible to obtain that information from the SLP, then the audiologist will need to use clinical judgment in selecting the most appropriate test to administer. If the child performs poorly on the selected measure, then the audiologist should reevaluate performance with a simpler measure. Likewise, if the child achieves ceiling-level performance, then the audiologist should reevaluate performance with a more difficult measure.

The PMSTB calls for assessment of speech recognition in quiet at multiple presentation levels and in noise. Specifically, the PMSTB specifies that speech perception should be evaluated in quiet at presentation levels of 50 and 60 dBA. These presentation levels were selected for multiple reasons. First, 50 and 60 dBA are consistent with soft and average conversation level speech, respectively. As a result, these presentation levels are thought to be ecologically valid and representative of how a child is able to understand soft and average speech. Secondly, the peer-reviewed literature has suggested that persons with appropriately programmed cochlear implants will perform relatively well at these levels (Baudhuin et al., 2012; Davidson, 2006; Davidson et al., 2009; Dwyer et al., 2016; Firszt et al., 2004; Geers et al., 2013; Gifford et al., 2008; Rakszwaski et al., 2016; Robinson et al., 2012; Sheffield et al., 2015). Furthermore, audiologists are accustomed to evaluating speech recognition at these levels. For assessment of speech recognition in noise, the PMSTB recommends a presentation level of 65 dBA with a +5 dB signal-to-noise ratio (SNR). The higher presentation level of 65 dBA was selected because speech levels are typically higher in noisy environments (Clark & Govett, 1995; Crukley, Scollie, & Parsa, 2011; Olsen, 1998; Pearsons et al., 1977; Smeds et al., 2015). The +5 dB SNR was recommended because it is similar to the SNR encountered in many realistic situations (Crukley et al., 2011; Pearsons et al., 1977). If a child performs poorly at a +5 dB SNR, then the audiologist should consider reevaluating performance at a more favorable SNR (e.g., +10 dB SNR).

The PMSTB provides a protocol to guide audiologists in the decision of when to transition to different measures within the battery. For instance, when a child achieves a score exceeding 75% to 80% correct, then the audiologist should administer the next most difficult test in the battery, either in the same test session or during the next test session. If the child scores below approximately 25% correct, then the audiologist should administer a simpler measure. Speech recognition in the 25% to 79% range suggests an "emergence of skills assessed in that measure, thereby suggesting the appropriateness of the measure for continued use in future test sessions" (Uhler et al., 2017). Once a child scores higher than 80% correct on the most difficult measures in the PMSTB, then the adult version of the MSTB should be used to evaluate the child's speech perception at subsequent test sessions.

Visual Reinforcement Infant Speech Discrimination (VRISD)

VRISD involves the presentation of a series of stimuli that randomly change from a "background" stimulus to a "target" stimulus (Schauwers et al., 2004; Uhler et al., 2011). For instance, the vowel /a/ may serve as

the background stimulus, whereas /i/ serves as the target stimulus. A test assistant centers the child's gaze toward the front-center and then trains/conditions the child to turn when the stimulus changes from the background to the target stimulus. The audiologist is tasked with recording the infant's hits (i.e., correct head-turn in response to a stimulus change), correct rejections (i.e., no head-turn when the stimulus does not change, false positives (i.e., a head-turn that occurs when the stimulus does not change), and misses (i.e., no head-turn when the stimulus changes). If the infant's responses are correct 75% or more of the time, then the infant is considered to have reached the criterion to indicate that he/she can correctly discriminate between the phonemes that make up the pair.

The PMSTB acknowledged the fact that the overwhelming majority of cochlear implant clinics do not administer and/or possess the resources to administer the VRISD. Nevertheless, the PMSTB recommends use of the VRISD because it is the only measure that may be used to evaluate speech discrimination in infants. Also, guidelines for the clinical administration of VRISD and normative data exist for this age group (Govaerts et al., 2006; Uhler et al., 2015). Because VRISD requires the infant to make a head-turn in response to a change in the stimulus, it is ideal for use with infants between the ages of 6 to 24 months. Of note, many infants with hearing loss may not condition to the VRISD task until 8 months or older. Also of note, infants will typically discriminate vowel contrasts prior to consonant contrasts (Boothroyd, 1984; Uhler et al., 2011).

Early Speech Perception Test

The Central Institute for the Deaf's (CID) Early Speech Perception (ESP) test is a closed-set test that may be used to measure auditory discrimination of children with a language age of 2 to 6 years old (Moog & Geers, 1990). The ESP is intended to evaluate pattern perception, spondee recognition, and monosyllabic word recognition of children who have hearing loss and limited vocabulary and linguistic abilities. The pattern perception test consists of four types of stimuli, monosyllabic words, spondees, trochees (two-syllable words with unequal emphasis on each syllable), and three-syllable words. The child is scored on whether he/she can identify the correct word. If the child cannot identify the correct word, then he/she also receives credit for selecting a word that comes from the correct category (i.e., credit for recognizing the stimulus as a three-syllable word after pointing to birthday cake when the stimulus was actually hamburger). The spondee portion of the test contains spondee words, whereas the monosyllabic portion contains single-syllable words that all begin with the letter /b/ but end with a different medial vowel and/or final consonant.

The ESP may be administered in a "low-verbal" or "standard" version. The low-verbal version involves the use of 18 different toys that may be grouped according to the three categories of the ESP test. The standard version consists of three different picture cards, each with 12 pictures that should be familiar for children ages 2 to 6 years old. The low-verbal version should be used with younger children (e.g., 2 to 3 years old), and the standard version should be used with children in the 3 to 6 years old age range. The ESP is typically administered via MLV for younger children. An MLV presentation level of 45 dB HL will approximate 60 dBA.

The authors of the PMSTB suggest that the audiologist begin with the most difficult portion of the ESP, which is the monosyllabic word list. If the child can score above 75% correct on the monosyllabic word test, then he/she is able to be evaluated with a more difficult measure in the PMSTB (e.g., Pediatric Speech Intelligibility Words). If the child scores less than 75% correct, then the audiologist should administer the spondee test. If the child scores less than 75% correct on the spondee portion of the test, then the audiologist should administer the pattern perception portion of the test.

Based on the child's responses on the test, his/her speech discrimination will be placed into one of four categories:

1. No pattern perception: Detection without the ability to discriminate syllable length (less than 75% on pattern perception test),
2. Pattern perception: Can discriminate stress/syllable length of speech but not vowel or consonant recognition (at least 75% correct on pattern perception test but less than 75% correct on spondee portion of test),
3. Some word identification: Minimal ability to discriminate words via the recognition of reduced vowel/consonant recognition (at least 75% correct on the spondee portion of the test but less than 75% correct on the monosyllabic word recognition test),
4. Consistent word identification: Ability to use spectral information to recognize words via vowel/con-

sonant recognition (at least 75% correct on the monosyllabic word portion of the test).

Pediatric Speech Intelligibility (PSI) Words and PSI Sentences

The Pediatric Speech Intelligibility (PSI) test is a closed-set test designed to measure speech recognition of children between the ages of 3 to 7 years old (Jerger, Jerger, & Abrams, 1983). The PSI was originally developed to evaluate speech recognition for the purpose of identifying auditory processing disorders, but the PSI has also been used to evaluate speech recognition of children with peripheral hearing loss (Eisenberg et al., 2006; Jerger, Jerger, & Fahad, 1985; Johnson & Winter, 2003).

The PSI word recognition test consists of 20 words that are presented in sets of 5 on one of four different picture cards. First, the audiologist should ensure that the child understands the task. The child is supposed to say each word that he/she sees on each of the cards. The audiologist may prompt the child by asking, "What is this?" The audiologist is not supposed to label the pictures for the child. Once the audiologist is certain that the child is familiar with each of the words, the audiologist should explain to the child that he/she will hear a man saying, "Show me." The child should point to the picture corresponding to the word at the end of the carrier phrase. The child may also simply repeat the word if he/she prefers that response mode. The PMSTB recommends that the PSI be presented at 60 dBA in quiet from a loudspeaker located directly in front of the child. The audiologist should ask the child to guess if he/she is uncertain of the word that was heard. The PSI word recognition test is scored on the number of words that are correctly recognized out of the total number of 20 target words. Of note, the PMSTB also suggests that the PSI word recognition test may also be presented in noise (−20, −10, 0, +10, +20 dB SNR) when the children's speech recognition approaches the test ceiling in quiet. Of note, the PMSTB authors have suggested that the PSI word test is appropriate for use with a child who has a vocabulary of at least 100 single words.

The PSI sentence test consists of 10 sentence lists comprising two closed-set pictures of five items each. Once again, the audiologist ensures that the child is familiar with the activities being described in each of the pictures. As before, the audiologist should not label the pictures for the child. Instead, the audiologist should ask the child what is happening in each picture and encourage the child to be as descriptive as possible so that it will be known that the child understands the words in the sentences associated with each picture. Then, the sentences are presented from a loudspeaker at 60 dBA. The audiologist should score the child's recognition of the target items in percent correct. The PMSTB also suggests that the PSI sentences may be used to evaluate speech recognition in noise (e.g., –20, –10. 0, +10, and +20 dB SNR).

Multisyllabic Lexical Neighborhood Test and the Lexical Neighborhood Test

The Multisyllabic Lexical Neighborhood Test (MLNT) and the Lexical Neighborhood Test (LNT) are open-set word recognition tests developed to evaluate the speech recognition of pediatric cochlear implant recipients (Kirk et al., 1995). The MLNT is composed of two- and three-syllable words, while the LNT is comprised of monosyllabic words. The MLNT is available in two "easy" and two "hard" lists of 12 words each, while the LNT is available in two "easy" and two "group" lists of 25 words each. The words included in the MLNT and LNT tests were obtained from the Child Language Data Exchange System (CHILDES), which is a database of transcribed samples of language produced by a large group of children between 3 to 5 years old (MacWhinney & Snow, 1985). The words selected from the CHILDES were categorized into "easy" and "hard" based on the frequency at which the words appear in the English language and on the lexical density of the words. Lexical density refers to the words that are phonetically similar to the target word. An indicator of lexical density is the number of words (or "neighbors") that differ only by one phoneme from the target word. For instance, the words "cheat," "please," "tease," "choose," and "cheek" are all lexical neighbors of the target word "cheese." In contrast, a word like "tiger" has very few lexical neighbors. Words that appear more frequently in the English language and that have fewer lexical neighbors are easier to recognize via audition than words that are used infrequently or that have many lexical neighbors. The MLNT and LNT are generally considered appropriate for use with children ages 3 to 6 years. According to the PMSTB, use of the MLNT and LNT is suitable for children who have a vocabulary of at least 100 single words. The MLNT and LNT are scored on the number of words that are correctly repeated (percent correct). The PMSTB also recommends scoring the number of phonemes presented correctly in an effort to identify phoneme error patterns.

Consonant-Nucleus-Consonant (CNC) Monosyllabic Word Recognition Test

The Consonant-Nucleus-Consonant (CNC) test is an open-set measure on monosyllabic word recognition (Lehiste & Peterson, 1962). The CNC test consists of ten 50-word lists that contain words that are used with at least somewhat regular frequency in everyday conversation (e.g., 192 of the words are among the 1000 most frequently used words in the English language, and only 21 words are used less than five times in one million words spoken in everyday English language). The lists are phonemically balanced (each initial and final consonant as well as each vowel is used with the same frequency within each list). For assessment of cochlear implant candidacy and outcomes, the CNC word test is usually administered from the MSTB packet. The target words of the CNC word test are spoken by a male talker and are preceded by the carrier word, "Ready . . . ." The CNC word test is scored on percentage of words repeated correctly. The audiologist may also consider scoring at the phoneme level as well to identify potential phoneme error patterns. A full list of 50 words should be administered for each condition (e.g., right ear, left ear, bilateral/bimodal/binaurally aided). The PMSTB suggests that the CNC word test may be considered for use with children who have a language age of 5 years old and up and for children who have a vocabulary of at least 100 single words. Because the CNC word test was originally developed for assessment of the word recognition of adults, many children with a language age of 5 to 6 years old will find many of the words to be unfamiliar.

Bamford-Kowal-Bench Sentences in Quiet and in Noise (BKB-SIN)

The Bamford-Kowal-Bench (BKB) sentence recognition test consists of 16 lists of 8 to 10 sentences (Bench, Kowal, & Bamford, 1979). Each list contains 50 target words. The sentences were developed on the basis of language samples obtained from 240 children who had hearing loss and were between the ages of 8 and 15 years old. The final group of 16 sentences was validated in a study with 13 children with hearing loss and 11 children with normal hearing. The sentences are presented in an open-set format, and the child is tasked with repeating every word of the sentence. The audiologist tallies the number of target words presented correctly (percent correct). The developers of the PMSTB have acknowledged that normative data do not exist for the BKB test in quiet for children between the ages of 3 and 5 years old. However, the PMSTB developers note that "several audiologists in the PMSTB working group shared that they can obtain reliable test results from children as young as 3 years" (Uhler et al., 2017). The PMSTB developers recommended the BKB sentence in quiet test for children with a language age consistent with a 3-year-old and production of at least two- to three-word sentences.

The BKB-Speech in Noise (BKB-SIN) test is comprised of the sentences described in the summary of the BKB sentences discussed above. The sentences are presented in open-set format in the presence of four-talker babble. The babble noise level increases in 3 dB steps with each sentence in each list. As a result, the SNR decreases from +21 dB for the first sentence to –6 dB for the last sentence of the list. The audiologist tallies the number of key words the child repeats correctly and subtracts that number from 23.5 to determine the SNR for 50% correct performance (SNR-50). Normative data for the BKB-SIN are provided for adults and for children in three different age groups, 5 to 6, 7 to 10, and 11 to 14 years old. The PMSTB suggests that the BKB-SIN test is appropriate for use with children who have a language age of 5 years old and up.

BabyBio Sentences in Quiet and in Noise

The BabyBio sentence recognition test (also known as the Pediatric AzBio test) is an open-set measure of sentence recognition developed for the assessment of sentence recognition of school-age children (5 years old and up) (Spahr et al., 2014). The BabyBio sentence test is comprised of 16 lists with each list possessing 20 sentences. The length of the sentences ranges from 3 to 12 words. The child's task is to repeat all of the words presented in each sentence, and the audiologist scores the number of words repeated correctly. The total score for each list is the percentage of words repeated correctly. At the time of this writing, the sentences were spoken by a female in the recorded version of the BabyBio test. The test may be presented in quiet (60 dBA presentation level) and in noise (presentation level of 65 dBA with a +5 dB SNR). The PMSTB working group suggested that the BabyBio sentence test is appropriate for use with children who have a second-grade language level.

Additional Considerations Regarding the PMSTB

As with the adult MSTB, the audiologist should try to evaluate speech recognition with the use of recorded speech materials whenever possible. Use of recorded materials allows for consistency in talker intensity and acoustic characteristics, and it avoids the artificial enhancement of speech recognition scores known to exist with monitored live voice (MLV) presentation. However, at young ages (18 months to 3 years) some children are more inclined to respond to speech presented via MLV than they are to recorded materials. Additionally, some measures developed to evaluate the speech recognition of young children are unavailable in recorded format.

The PMSTB also calls for the presentation of a full list of words or sentences whenever possible. Presentation of a full list of words or sentences increases the sensitivity of the test to detect differences in performance across conditions (e.g., unilateral vs. bilateral; different types of programs, across test sessions over time). Of note, the PMSTB recommends the use of statistical measures to determine whether a significant difference exists across conditions. In particular, the PMSTB suggested use of the Speech Recognition INTerpretation (SPRINT) charts for 25-word and 50-word lists to identify the extent of difference required to represent a statistically significant change (Thibodeau, 2006).

It should be noted that some measures included within the PMSTB contain a limited number of word lists. For example, the LNT only contains two lists of "easy" monosyllabic words and two lists of "hard" words. As a result, it is not possible to evaluate performance in each unilateral and in the bilateral conditions or at multiple levels without repeating the use of the same list or without the use of lists of differing difficulties. Additionally, many of the materials included in the PMSTB do not possess normative data for children with normal hearing, children who have hearing loss and use cochlear implants and/ or hearing aids. Consequently, many of these measures cannot be used to compare an individual child's performance to typically developing, normal-hearing peers or to children with different degrees of hearing loss and/or with different types of hearing technologies (e.g., cochlear implants, hearing aids).

The researchers, audiologists, and industry representatives who authored the PMSTB suggested that normative data could be developed if pediatric audiologists would universally adopt the PMSTB into their clinical practices and compile a multiple-center database to house the results of children with normal hearing and with different degrees of hearing loss and hearing technologies. Furthermore, the authors suggested that the availability of normative data would assist audiologists in determining cochlear implant candidacy, in counseling regarding realistic expectations and prognosis, in predicting progress over time, and in determining whether a child is making satisfactory progress. The PMSTB authors also encouraged the development of new speech recognition materials and/or new lists for existing measures so that ample assessments are available to allow for thorough evaluations of children's ability to understand speech.

Additional Consideration for Pediatric Speech Recognition

Because closed-set tasks are relatively simple and prone to ceiling effects, the audiologist should strive to measure open-set speech recognition, particularly when the child is able to articulate clearly, allowing the audiologist to score responses without the concern that errors are attributed to speech production. Younger children may be hesitant to repeat words that are presented from a loudspeaker, especially when the words are presented via recorded format and/or without a carrier phrase (e.g., MLNT and LNT). The authors have found that children as young as 30 months will repeat recorded words presented in an open-set format when they are allowed to speak into a microphone (Figure 6–7). The open-set speech recognition task may be informally modeled by the audiologist and test assistant. Specifically, the audiologist says a word into the microphone (e.g., "juice") and then holds the microphone in front of the test assistant's mouth and the test assistant says the same word. Typically, this modeling task is repeated two or three times, and then the audiologist says a word (e.g., "three") and holds the microphone in front of the child's mouth. In many instances, the child will repeat the word that the audiologist said. Once the child is conditioned to the task, then the audiologist can move to the control room and present the words from the soundfield loudspeaker. The assistant should hold the microphone in front of the cone of the loudspeaker when a word is presented and move the microphone to the child's mouth following the presentation of the target word. Usually, placing the microphone in front of the child's mouth will prompt him/her to say the word that he/she heard. It should be noted that the microphone does not have to be functional. This approach has proven to be successful with actual microphones (e.g., pass-around microphones designed for use with classroom audio distribution systems [CADS; i.e., sound-field systems] as well as with plastic play microphones.

Audiologists may also choose speech recognition measures other than those included in the PMSTB

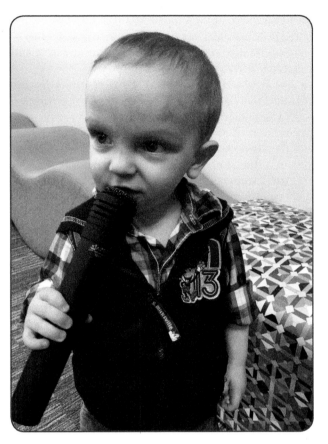

FIGURE 6–7. An example of the use of a microphone to facilitate open-set speech recognition assessment.

to evaluate the speech perception of children. For example, the Phonetically Balanced Kindergarten 50-word (PBK-50) monosyllabic word recognition test is an open-set measure developed to evaluate speech perception of children in the early elementary years (e.g., language age of 5 to 7 years old). As the name implies, the PBK-50 is composed of 50-word lists, and each list is phonemically balanced (each initial and final as well as each vowel is used with the same frequency within each list). The PBK-50 monosyllabic word recognition test is more difficult than the MLNT and LNT; it does possess four different lists that are equally difficult, allowing for assessment across the right and left ear conditions as well as in the bilateral/bimodal/binaurally aided condition.

Role of the Speech-Language Pathologist in the Pediatric Cochlear Implant Candidacy Assessment

The speech-language pathologist (SLP) is a vital member of the cochlear implant assessment team. The SLP on a cochlear implant assessment team should be familiar with typical auditory, speech, and language development as well as with facilitating speech and language development of children with hearing loss. Because about 95% of children with hearing loss are born to parents who have normal hearing and communicate via spoken language, the majority of parents of children with hearing loss desire for their child to also communicate via spoken language. As a result, the SLP ideally should be a Listening and Spoken Language Specialist (LSLS) Auditory-Verbal therapist (AVT). An LSLS-AVT works one-on-one with families of children with hearing loss to emphasize the child's exclusive use of auditory and spoken language skills (AG Bell, 2018). Numerous studies have shown that the auditory, speech, and language outcomes of children with hearing loss are optimized when the child receives auditory-based intervention services (Ambrose et al., 2015; Ching & Dillon, 2013; Dettman et al., 2016; Geers et al., 2011).

With regard to cochlear implant candidacy assessment, the SLP provides a critical item of diagnostic information. FDA-approved pediatric cochlear implant guidelines for every cochlear implant manufacturer state that a young child is a candidate for a cochlear implant when he/she fails to reach developmentally appropriate auditory milestones. The SLP is uniquely equipped to evaluate a child's functional auditory, speech, and language outcomes. Evaluation of functional auditory performance may occur through the use of parent questionnaires (e.g., LittlEARS, Infant Toddler Meaningful Auditory Integration Scale [IT-MAIS—Zimmerman, Robbins, & Osberger, 2000], the PEACH), informal parent interview inquiring about the status of a child's everyday auditory abilities, and therapist observation of the child's auditory responses during weekly AVT sessions.

Just as importantly, the SLP can provide diagnostic information regarding the child's speech and language development through the provision of norm-referenced, standardized speech and language assessments. Norm-referenced, standardized speech and language assessment quantifies a child's speech and language abilities in the form of a standard score which may be used to associate an individual child's abilities to that of the typical, normal-hearing child of a particular age. For instance, a 24-month-old child with speech and language abilities that are equivalent to other typical, normal-hearing 24-month-old children will have a standard score near 100. The child's speech and language abilities are age appropriate and equivalent to his/her chronologic age. In contrast, a 24-month-old child who has significantly

delayed speech and language scores will have a standard score that is far below the mean value of 100. Consequently, the child's speech and language abilities may be equivalent to that of typical, normal-hearing children who are much younger in age (e.g., 12 months). In this example, **the child's speech and language equivalent age is 12 months and is substantially delayed.** If this child has a severe hearing loss and has been a full-time user of appropriately fitted hearing aids, then the cochlear implant team should consider a recommendation of cochlear implantation. Such a case demonstrates the important role of the SLP in pediatric cochlear implant candidacy. In particular, **cochlear implant teams should strive to provide intervention to allow the child to achieve age-appropriate auditory, speech, and language abilities**.

Of note, research suggests that up to 40% of children with hearing loss also have additional disabilities (Gallaudet Research Institute, 2008; Picard, 2004). Often, these additional disabilities may include cognitive/neurological disabilities. With this in mind, the SLP should also evaluate a child's non-verbal intelligence quotient (IQ), because a delay in speech and language may be attributed to disabilities other than hearing loss. For example, a child who has flat, moderate hearing loss, who wears appropriately fitted hearing aids during all waking hours, but who has significant neurological disability and a delay in speech and language aptitude may more likely be inflicted by factors other than the hearing loss and hearing technology. In this case example, let's say that the child has a non-verbal IQ standard score of 70 and speech and language standard scores that are around 75 to 80. In short, the child's speech and language abilities are commensurate with his cognitive aptitude and likely indicate that the child's auditory abilities are responsible for the delay in spoken language abilities. Such an example highlights the importance of the cochlear implant team to holistically evaluate a child's functional abilities to determine the most appropriate interventions. If the members of the cochlear implant team are concerned about the potential impact of a cognitive/neurological disability on a child's spoken language progress but do not feel comfortable evaluating a child's non-verbal IQ, then the team should consider referring the child to a specialist for neurodevelopmental evaluation.

Through the provision of serial speech and language assessment across time, a SLP can also ensure that a child is making adequate speech and language progress. Ideally, a child with hearing loss should make at least one year of speech and language progress in one calendar year. For instance, if two separate formal speech and language assessments conducted 12 months apart only indicate that a child has made six months of progress, then the cochlear implant team should question why the child's progress has been stalled. In such a case, the cochlear implant team should determine whether cochlear implantation is likely to allow for faster progress. Again, however, the cochlear implant team must rule out other factors that may also be responsible for the delay in progress (e.g., inappropriately fitted hearing aids, a decrease in hearing sensitivity, inadequate hearing aid wear time, inadequate exposure to intelligible speech at home, additional disabilities, etc.).

Through the provision of modern audiology services and appropriate hearing technology, children born with any degree of hearing loss can typically develop age-appropriate speech and language skills and make one year of speech and language progress for every calendar year. When formal speech and language assessment indicates that a child's speech and language aptitude is delayed relative to the child's chronological age, the audiologist must determine whether the child's present hearing technology is appropriately provided. For example, for children with moderate hearing loss, it may be necessary to adjust the gain and output of the hearing aids to allow for better performance. Alternatively, for children who have severe to profound hearing loss and use appropriately fitted high-power hearing aids but are continuing to make inadequate progress relative to their hearing peers, the audiologist may want to consider recommendation of a cochlear implant.

Additionally, the SLP can play a valuable role in facilitating accurate audiologic assessment. As previously mentioned in this chapter, the SLP will likely see a child for assessment and therapy on at least a weekly basis, and as a result, the child is likely to be very comfortable with the SLP. Likewise, the SLP is very familiar with the child's behaviors and preferences. As a result, the SLP is the ideal test assistant for audiologic assessment (i.e., VRA and CPA). Furthermore, the SLP can work in weekly therapy sessions to establish a child's conditioned play audiometry response.

Role of the Social Worker in the Pediatric Cochlear Implant Candidacy Assessment

Numerous research studies have found that pediatric cochlear implant outcomes are poorer for children who come from families with lower socioeconomic means, lower levels of maternal education, and lower levels of caregiver support (Ching & Dillon, 2013; Geers, 2011; Niparko et al., 2010). Considering these discouraging facts, the cochlear implant team should strive to equip families with the resources they will need to optimize their children's development after cochlear implantation. During the cochlear implant assessment, the cochlear implant team should seek to identify whether the family will struggle to provide the support needed to facilitate the child's success with a cochlear implant. A social worker can provide counseling and support for families who might not have the resources needed to support the child's postoperative cochlear implant care. A social worker can identify resources to assist the family in obtaining transportation to and from audiology and therapy appointments. A social worker can also assist the family in identifying the ideal daycare setting for a child whose parents both work throughout the business day. For example, the social worker can assist the family in the completion of paperwork to apply for funding for daycare assistance as well as in locating a daycare that may be equipped to serve children with disabilities. Additionally, a social worker may be able to identify state resources that would provide supplemental income to offset time away from work while the family is bringing the child to hearing health care appointments. Furthermore, the social worker may be able to help the family to coordinate medical and therapy appointments to ensure that the child is able to receive efficient and effective care from multiple providers. Also, the social worker may be able to identify telehealth options (e.g., tele-AV therapy) for families who have difficulty traveling to a facility for care.

Role of the Psychologist in the Pediatric Cochlear Implant Candidacy Assessment

As previously mentioned, a psychologist may be able to assist in the evaluation of a child's non-verbal IQ to determine whether delays are attributed to auditory or cognitive/neurological factors. A neurodevelopmental psychologist can provide a holistic evaluation to determine a child's specific and global strengths and limitations to elucidate whether a cochlear implant may be beneficial in facilitating communication development.

Furthermore, a psychologist may be valuable in assisting families who are struggling to cope with accepting a child's hearing loss and possibly with additional disabilities. A psychologist can also assist a family that is struggling with interpersonal dynamics. A psychologist can aim to bring a family onto same page in an attempt to provide the unified support the child will need to optimize his/her outcome. Additionally, a psychologist can assist the cochlear implant team in identifying strategies to facilitate adherence to recommendations made by the hearing health care professionals that make up the cochlear implant team. For instance, a psychologist can work to identify reasons for why a family may not be adhering to the recommendation to use hearing aids and/or cochlear implant technology during all waking hours.

The Role of the Medical Evaluation in the Pediatric Cochlear Implant Candidacy Assessment

Chapter 12, which is authored by an otologist who surgically implants most of the implantable hearing technologies discussed in this book, provides a detailed review of the components included in the medical evaluation of a child being considered for cochlear implantation. Additionally, Chapter 13, which is authored by a physician who has earned a specialty in neurotology and in radiology, provides a detailed review of the components included in the radiologic imaging assessment of persons being considered for cochlear implantation. In particular, the reader is referred to the aforementioned chapters for information related to the basic otologic assessment as well as for information pertaining to the medical evaluation that is necessary to ensure that the child is healthy enough to undergo cochlear implant surgery under general anesthesia. Although these chapters provide the reader with a detailed and authoritative account of the cochlear implant medical assessment, the following paragraphs also briefly summarize some of the general highlights pertaining to the medical evaluation of pediatric cochlear implant candidates.

Medical Management to Prevent Bacterial Meningitis in Cochlear Implant Candidates and Recipients

Research has suggested that cochlear implant recipients are more likely to contract bacterial meningitis than the general population (Josefson, 2002). Indeed, recipients of the Advanced Bionics positioner, a component that was inserted into the cochlea along with the electrode array to facilitate close proximity of the array to the modiolus, were at a significantly higher risk to contract bacterial meningitis. Of note, the Advanced Bionics positioner served as a conduit for bacteria to spread from the temporal bone to the meninges of the brain, and consequently, it was removed from the commercial market in 2002. The extent of an increase in the incidence of bacterial meningitis in cochlear implant recipients who do not have positioners is not entirely clear. Although cochlear implant recipients do possess a higher incidence of bacterial meningitis, it is quite possible that the incidence of bacterial meningitis in the population of cochlear implant recipients is similar to the incidence in the population of persons who have severe to profound hearing loss but who have not undergone cochlear implantation. In short, the increased incidence of bacterial meningitis may be associated with temporal bone anomalies inherent in many persons with severe to profound hearing loss and not with the presence of a cochlear implant. To mitigate the risk of bacterial meningitis, the United States Centers for Disease Control and Prevention (CDC) recommends that all cochlear implant recipients receive vaccinations for bacterial meningitis prior to implantation and periodically thereafter. Because of the serious consequences associated with bacterial meningitis, the CDC position on vaccinations for cochlear implant recipients is provided verbatim in the box below.

Imaging of the Auditory System in Pediatric Cochlear Implant Candidates

Once again, the reader is referred to Chapter 13 for a detailed account of diagnostic imaging assessment of cochlear implant candidates. Imaging of the auditory system is imperative for all children being considered for cochlear implantation. Over the past decade, there has been a trend away from the routine use of the computed tomography (CT) scan toward the use of magnetic resonance imaging (MRI). CT scan is uniquely suited to evaluate the bony anatomy of the temporal bone, whereas MRI is better suited to evaluate soft tissue. However, many of the most common temporal bone abnormalities, such as enlarged vestibular aqueduct, cochlear aplasia, patency of the cochlear scalae, etc., may be adequately identified via MRI (Adunka, Jewells, & Buchman, 2007). If the MRI suggests a bony abnormality but better resolution is desired to clarify the extent of the disorder, then a CT scan may be ordered as a backup assessment.

The United States Centers for Disease Control and Prevention (CDC) guidelines for the use of vaccines to prevent bacterial meningitis in persons with cochlear implants (CDC, 2017).

- *Children with cochlear implants are more likely to get bacterial meningitis than children without cochlear implants. In addition, some children who are candidates for cochlear implants have anatomic factors that may increase their risk for meningitis.*
- *The bacteria Streptococcus pneumoniae (pneumococcus) causes most cases of the meningitis in people with cochlear implants.*
- *Due to their increased risk, CDC recommends pneumococcal vaccination for children who have or are candidates for cochlear implants. Audiologists should follow the pneumococcal vaccine recommendations that apply to other groups at increased risk.*
- *Recommendations for the timing and type of pneumococcal vaccination vary with age and vaccination history. See ACIP recommendations highlighted in the box to the right for details.*

Pneumococcal Recommendations by Age and Vaccination History

CDC recommends pneumococcal conjugate (PCV13) and polysaccharide (PPSV23) vaccines for children who have or are candidates for cochlear implants. Administer all recommended doses of PCV13 first. Administer PPSV23 at least 8 weeks after the most recent dose of PCV13. If PCV13 is indicated and a child has already received PPSV23, administer PCV13 at least 8 weeks after the PPSV23 dose.

Children younger than 24 months old
- *Should receive PCV13 per the childhood immunization schedule*

Children aged 24 through 71 months
- *Should receive 2 doses of PCV13 if*
  - *They have not received any doses of PCV13*
  - *They received any incomplete schedule (according to the Catch-up Immunization Schedule) with fewer than 3 doses of PCV13 before age 24 months*
- *Should receive 1 dose of PCV13 if they received any incomplete schedules with at least 3 doses of PCV13*
- *Should receive 1 dose of PPSV23 at least 8 weeks after the most recent PCV13 dose*

Children 6 through 18 years of age
- *Should receive 1 dose of PCV13 if they have not received PCV13 before regardless of whether they have already received PCV7 or PPSV23*
- *Should receive 1 dose of PPSV23 at least 8 weeks after the most recent PCV13 dose if they have not received PPSV23 before*

Other Vaccines Can Help Protect against Meningitis
- *Vaccines are available in the United States that can help protect against most of the bacteria that cause meningitis:*
  - *13-valent pneumococcal conjugate (PCV13) (Prevnar 13®)*
  - *23-valent pneumococcal polysaccharide (PPSV23) (Pneumovax®)*
  - *Haemophilus influenzae type b conjugate (Hib) (ActHIB®, Hiberix®, PedvaxHIB®, and Pentacel®)*
  - *Meningococcal conjugate (Menactra® and Menveo®)*
  - *Serogroup B meningococcal (Bexsero® and Trumenba®)*
- *There is no evidence that children with cochlear implants are more likely to get meningococcal meningitis than children without cochlear implants. The bacteria Neisseria meningitidis cause meningococcal meningitis.*

The MRI is the preferred imaging modality of choice for several reasons. First, the MRI allows for evaluation of the anatomical integrity of the cochlear nerve. Cochlear nerve assessment is of particular importance for children in whom has been diagnosed ANSD, anacusis (i.e., total profound deafness), and single-sided deafness. Several researchers have shown that these conditions are often attributed to an absent or severely underdeveloped cochlear nerve (Buchman et al., 2006; Teagle et al., 2010). Identification of cochlear nerve deficiency can assist the team in identifying children who may receive limited benefit from cochlear implantation. In a case in which a child has bilateral severe to profound hearing loss but cochlear nerve deficiency in only one ear, MRI can identify the ear that is most likely to benefit from cochlear implantation (Buchman et al., 2006). For children with bilateral cochlear nerve deficiency, the MRI identifies children who may be in need of an auditory brainstem implant. Secondly, the MRI allows for the assessment of the central nervous system, which may be of potential value if lesions are discovered that may explain cognitive/neurological disorders. Finally, a CT scan exposes the child to radiation, whereas the MRI essentially does not.

Preparing the Family for Cochlear Implantation

Numerous research studies have shown that children achieve better outcomes with cochlear implants when their caregivers are more attentive to and supportive of their needs (Ambrose et al., 2015; Chu et al., 2016; Quittner et al., 2013). Because of the importance of caregiver involvement in the outcome of children with cochlear implants, the audiologist must ensure that the child's family is fully engaged and aware of what is necessary to facilitate the child's success. If data logging has suggested insufficient hearing aid use and/or if the family has sporadically attended audiology and therapy appointments, the audiologist should strive to inform the family that their child's auditory, speech, and language development after cochlear implantation will be dependent on the adherence to full-time cochlear implant use, regular attendance to frequent audiology and therapy appointments, and the provision of a language-rich listening environment filled with robust, intelligible speech that provides a model that is conducive to language learning (Ambrose et al., 2015; Chu et al., 2016; Walker et al., 2015). An audiologist must remember that many families are not aware of the critical period of language development, and as a result, they may not be aware of the irreparable, detrimental consequences of sporadic use of hearing technology and of an environment that provides a sparse model of intelligible speech. With that in mind, the audiologist must inform the family of the critical period of language development, of the importance of full-time use of hearing technology, and how to develop a language-rich listening environment.

Selecting the Ear of Implantation

One important task of the assessment process is to determine the ear or ears to be implanted. In the case of bilateral profound hearing loss, it is highly likely that the child will achieve better hearing performance and auditory speech and language outcomes with two cochlear implants relative to the use of one cochlear implant alone or bimodal use (i.e., a cochlear implant and a hearing aid for the non-implanted ear). When compared with unilateral and bimodal

cochlear implant use, research has generally shown that bilateral cochlear implantation provides better speech recognition in noise and localization for children with bilateral profound hearing loss (Litovsky, Johnstone, & Godar, 2006; Litovsky et al., 2004; Zeitler et al., 2008). Additionally, relative to unilateral cochlear implant use, bilateral cochlear implantation has been shown to provide better language and academic outcomes (Galvin, 2015). For children with bilateral profound hearing loss, research has suggested that hearing performance and development of the bilateral auditory system are optimized when cochlear implantation is provided at an early age (i.e., 12 months or earlier) (Bauer et al., 2006; Gordon & Papsin, 2009; Peters et al., 2007; Sharma et al., 2005; Wolfe et al., 2007) and when cochlear implants are provided to each ear simultaneously (i.e., during the same surgical procedure) or sequentially (i.e., during two separate surgical procedures) with minimal delay between surgeries (e.g., 6 months or less) (Gordon & Papsin, 2009; Peters et al., 2007).

There may be some cases in which only one cochlear implant is provided, and the audiologist must weigh in on which ear is to be implanted. In some of these cases, there may be an overwhelmingly compelling medical reason to select a particular ear for implantation. For example, an MRI may indicate that one ear has a normal cochlear nerve while the other ear has a deficient cochlear nerve. Also, imaging may indicate that one ear has normal cochlear anatomy that would be conducive to a complete insertion of the electrode array while the other ear has a dysplastic or obstructed cochlea that would complicate electrode array insertion. Imaging may also indicate the presence of a unilateral middle ear and/or facial nerve anomaly that may complicate cochlear implant surgery on the affected side. Additionally, a child may have had a vascular stroke in the auditory area of one side of the brain; in that case, the cochlear implant team would typically choose to implant the ear that is on the same side as the stroke because that ear will deliver the majority of its information to the contralateral hemisphere, which is unaffected by the vascular event. Furthermore, the child may have a cerebral shunt on one side of the head that would complicate the presence of a cochlear implant and/or sound processor.

If there are no medical reasons to select a particular ear, then audiological factors may influence the decision of which ear to implant. Nittrouer and Chapman (2009) have suggested that a period of acoustic hearing in at least one ear can allow for better auditory and language outcomes for children with cochlear implants. Nittrouer and Chapman have hypothesized that fine temporal structure cues available in the aided acoustic signal provide access to prosody and pitch as well as allow for better speech recognition in noise. If the audiologist believes that the child can receive sufficient benefit from use of a hearing aid in the non-implanted ear, then it may be wise to select the poorer hearing ear for implantation so that the better ear may benefit from hearing aid use.

On the other hand, some research studies have found better outcomes when the ear with better audiometric thresholds is implanted (Boisvert et al., 2012). The audiologist will have to weigh the potential pros and cons of implanting the better versus poorer ear for each individual child. In the absence of convincing evidence on this topic, the authors have adopted the general rule of selecting the ear with better hearing thresholds for implantation if neither ear is likely to yield open-set speech recognition with the use of a hearing aid alone (i.e., both ears have profound hearing loss). However, if usable open-set speech recognition (e.g., 30–50% correct performance on open-set word recognition testing) is expected with a hearing aid alone, then the authors will select the ear with the poorer audiometric thresholds as the ear for implantation. Most infants and young children are unable to complete speech recognition assessment, and as a result, audiologists must make decisions on the ear of implantation and whether to pursue bilateral or bimodal cochlear implantation based primarily on the audiogram. Again, there is no peer-reviewed research indicating a clear method for selecting the ear of implantation or whether bilateral or bimodal use is ideal for a child. In the absence of evidence-based guidance, the audiologist must rely on clinical intuition. The authors tentatively propose the following suggestions for determining ear of implantation and bimodal versus bilateral use:

- **Tentative** suggestion (low-frequency = 125–750 Hz; high-frequency = 1500 Hz and up):
  - When better ear thresholds are flat and better than 75 dB HL, consider bimodal and implant the ear with poorer hearing thresholds.
  - When low-frequency thresholds are better than 65 dB HL with severe to profound high-frequency hearing loss, consider cochlear implantation with hearing preservation (e.g., lateral wall electrode array with shallow

insertion) for at least one ear. If unilateral cochlear implantation is initially pursued, then bilateral cochlear implantation should be pursued once benefit is demonstrated with cochlear implantation. The audiologist should be concerned about the potential deleterious effects associated with auditory deprivation due to severe to profound hearing loss in the high-frequency portion of the speech-frequency range.
  - When hearing loss is flat and in the 75 to 85 dB HL range, preference should likely be given to bimodal until evidence of bilateral disruption or poor progress exists. If performance of the implanted ear greatly exceeds performance of the aided ear, then bilateral cochlear implantation should be considered.
  - When hearing loss exceeds 85 dB HL for both ears, consider bilateral cochlear implantation.

Reviewing the Logistics of Cochlear Implantation

The audiologist should also inform the family of the cochlear implant process. Specifically, the audiologist should discuss the schedule of audiologic, medical, and habilitative/rehabilitative appointments that will be necessary for the child before and following cochlear implantation. This discussion is necessary to prepare the family for the time and financial commitments associated with the care the child will receive prior to and after cochlear implantation. The requisite appointments occur rather frequently throughout the first few months following cochlear implant surgery. Following the initial period of cochlear implant use, the family will likely need to return for medical appointments on an annual basis, audiologic appointments every two to three months, and therapy on a weekly basis throughout the first year or two and less frequently thereafter.

Reviewing Cochlear Implant Hardware

Once a child is determined to be a good candidate for cochlear implantation, the audiologist should take time to inform the family of hardware included in modern cochlear implant systems. In many cases, the family will have little to no knowledge of cochlear implant equipment. In fact, from the authors' anecdotal experience, the term cochlear *implant* leads some patients and families to erroneously believe that all of the components of the cochlear implant system will be implanted under the skin so that no external components are required. The audiologist should spend time demonstrating the various components of a cochlear implant to the family along with a clear and simple description of how each component functions. During the process of reviewing cochlear implant hardware, it is most useful to show the family the demo devices provided by the different cochlear implant manufacturers. A review of the demo hardware allows the family to fully conceptualize the physical appearance and function of each component of a cochlear implant system. Modern cochlear implant systems are available in a number of different styles (e.g., behind-the-ear [BTE], body-worn, single-unit, off-the-ear), so the prudent audiologist should demonstrate the different styles to the family to determine if a preference exists to meet the individual needs of that child and family.

The audiologist should also assist the family in determining the most appropriate make and model of cochlear implant system for the child. At some cochlear implant clinics, the audiologists determine what they believe is the best make (i.e., Advanced Bionics, Cochlear, MED-EL, Oticon, etc.) of cochlear implant system for a candidate. An audiologist may select a particular make of cochlear implant for a variety of reasons, including his/her belief that one implant will provide superior performance for the child relative to the other available implants, his/her familiarity and comfort with a particular implant and/or sound processor, the electrode array of a particular implant may be theoretically optimal for the candidate, he/she believes one implant system will be more durable or easier to use, etc. In some cases, a contractual obligation may dictate the manufacturer of the cochlear implant system a patient receives. For instance, one cochlear implant manufacturer may have established a volume contract with the surgery center so that the implants may be purchased in bulk orders at a reduced price. As a result, the specific cochlear implant system included in the bulk pricing is recommended for the candidate so that the medical center may meet its quota necessary to receive the discounted pricing. In other cases, families (and older candidates) will arrive at the clinic with preconceived notions about the cochlear implant system they prefer. In some instances, the audiologist may feel strongly that another cochlear implant system is more appropriate for the needs of the child. In such a case, the audiologist should objectively explain the rationale underlying his/her recommendation for a cochlear implant other than the system originally preferred by the family. If the audiologist and family have no strong, preceding preference for a particular cochlear implant system and if the medical center does not require use of a particular cochlear implant system, then the audiologist should inform the family of the attributes and limitations of each cochlear implant system. The family should also be provided with or directed to the informational materials provided by each cochlear implant manufacturer. The cochlear implant manufacturers' websites contain a substantial amount of information (although some of the information and claims are likely to be influenced by the manufacturer's marketing department and consequently may be biased or not fully supported by research). The manufacturers also have created videos that describe their cochlear implant systems and that may be found online (e.g., YouTube). After digesting the information describing the various cochlear implant systems, the audiologist and family can then work together to identify the cochlear implant system that best meets the needs of the child and family.

Regardless of the manufacturer of the cochlear implant selected for the candidate, the audiologist must acquaint the family with the various hardware options offered by the manufacturer. Again, the audiologist should use the demonstration kits provided by the manufacturers to show the different sound processor styles to the candidate's family. For children, it is often important to discuss various wearing options to facilitate retention, because the ears of infants and young children are often too small to support a BTE sound processor with standard-sized batteries. Figure 6–8 shows a variety of wearing configurations designed to facilitate device retention. The audiologist should discuss the advantages and limitations of various sound processors and retention options.

Furthermore, cochlear implant manufacturers have produced a variety of different accessory items that can accompany the cochlear implant. Additional accessory items include wireless remote microphone technology, wireless telephone/television devices, water-proofing covers/boxes, extra batteries, retention options, and so forth. Generally, the patient is not provided with every accessory item available for the cochlear implant system he/she receives. Instead, the recipient/family must select a subset of accessory items deemed to be most likely to be beneficial. The audiologist should inform the family of the accessory items that are available and assist the family in selecting the accessory items that are most likely to meet the recipient's needs.

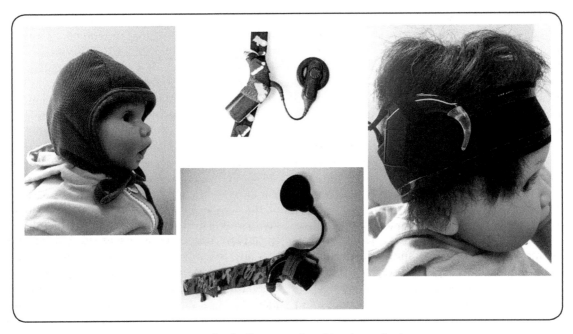

FIGURE 6–8. An example of strategies used to facilitate retention of hearing technology.

Establishing Realistic Expectations

In order to optimize the opportunity for the child's success with cochlear implants, the audiologist must strive to establish realistic expectation for cochlear implantation with the family. Helping the family to establish realistic expectations of cochlear implant benefit and performance is an important objective that is considered to be part of the candidacy assessment process. A cochlear implant offers an auditory experience that is quite different from a hearing aid. The cochlear nerve is stimulated via electrical current rather than an acoustic signal. Furthermore, many implants deliver the lowest frequency components through electrode contacts that are located in a place differing from the location for acoustic stimulation (i.e., several hundred Hz higher than the frequency of the input signal). As a result, the pitch of the human voice often is much higher than that to which the recipient is accustomed. Additionally, electrical pulsatile stimulation elicits an auditory nerve response that is much more synchronous than what is typical for acoustic stimuli. Although the signal coding strategies used in contemporary implants are quite sophisticated and are the product of countless hours of research and development, the signal processing available within cochlear implants results in a stimulating signal that is markedly different than the signal received from a normal peripheral auditory system

in response to acoustic stimulation. As a result of the aforementioned differences, speech and environmental sounds will likely possess a different sound quality and impression.

It is also important to note that many children who are being considered for a cochlear implant have severe to profound hearing loss and have had limited access to sound, even with the use of high-power hearing aids. These recipients require intensive exposure to speech and environmental sounds in order to lay a foundation within the auditory nervous system to allow processing of complex acoustic inputs. Thus, a period of auditory-focused speech and language therapy (e.g., Auditory Verbal therapy) normally is required before conversational, spoken-language skills emerge. The cochlear implant should provide access to sound across the entire speech frequency range. Additionally, a cochlear implant should provide access to low-level sounds that may have been inaudible with the use of hearing aids. However, the child will likely require several days and quite possibly several weeks to begin to associate meaning and objects with the auditory stimulation received from the cochlear implant. Also, the child will almost undoubtedly require weeks or months before developing the ability to understand speech with the cochlear implant (an exception is an older child who has lost his/her hearing after the development of spoken language and receives a cochlear implant shortly after the onset of deafness; in such a case, the child will most likely understand at least some speech with his/her cochlear implant within days of use). For example, Warner-Czyz and Davis (2008) have shown that an infant who receives a cochlear implant at 12 months of age may not speak his/her first word until 5 to 10 months post-activation, which corresponds to a chronologic age of 17 to 22 months. A 21-month-old child with normal hearing and typical development has a lexicon of almost 200 words, whereas a 21-month-old child implanted at 12 months will likely have a few spoken words (<5th percentile) (Fenson et al., 2007).

Many parents may not understand the need for the child with a cochlear implant to be exposed to a robust model of intelligible speech over several months before he/she begins to say his/her own words. In fact, many parents believe (or hope) that their child will be able to immediately understand speech once the cochlear implant is activated. Prior to implantation, the audiologist should explain that the child's auditory system will essentially be akin to that of a newborn on the day of activation. For infants who are born with profound deafness, activation of the cochlear implant represents the first day that the child has heard sound across the entire speech frequency range, and as a result, activation day may be considered as the child's "hearing birthday." The audiologist should explain that the child's auditory responses on activation day may be very similar to that of a newborn. Just as with a newborn baby, the newly activated child will be unlikely to understand speech and may not readily respond to speech and/or environmental sounds. To avoid a situation in which the families of young children with congenital deafness are disappointed on activation day because the implant does not provide hearing at "normal levels," the audiologist should fully explain the process involved with learning to listen with a new cochlear implant.

Regardless of the history, counseling will help the patient understand that implant benefit will take time to manifest. Using a conservative counseling approach, audiologists should prepare the family for the possibility that speech and environmental sounds most likely will initially possess a strange and poor sound quality. For pre-implant counseling, the authors of this chapter subscribe to the approach of attempting to "underpromise and then overdeliver." In other words, we tend to conservatively counsel the family with a deliberate intent to suggest that the recipient will require several weeks or months to adjust to the cochlear implant. The authors of this book believe that it is important to inform families that they may even initially second-guess the decision to pursue a cochlear implant for their child. Most specifically, it is imperative to stress that time is required to adjust to the implant and to realize its full benefit. The authors of this book often inform families that their children's experience with a cochlear implant will be similar to a marathon and not a sprint.

Additionally, the authors describe, in general terms, the differences in electric and acoustic hearing as well as the physiology and pathophysiology of the normal and impaired peripheral and central auditory systems. The relevance of this information to implant outcomes is discussed. We believe that this discussion is especially important in light of the impressive advances that exist in other areas of medicine and health care. For example, ophthalmologists may use laser surgery to restore 20/20 (i.e., normal) vision for patients who are near-sighted. The general public is generally very aware of this medical treatment, and many patients erroneously assume that cochlear implantation should provide a similarly expeditious and effective correction for hearing loss. It is helpful to discuss the anatomical and physiological differences between common visual and hearing impairment to aid the candidate in understanding the differences experienced in outcomes received with a cochlear implant versus laser eye surgery. At this point, we often stress that a cochlear implant is not a substitute for normal hearing.

Furthermore, the authors of this book note that there are no guarantees associated with cochlear implantation. We note that although many recipients are able to converse over the mobile telephone, follow speech on television without closed captioning, and converse in real world situations (i.e., restaurants), there are some recipients who never acquire these abilities, in spite of the best intentions and efforts of everyone involved in the process. This discussion is important because we have previously served recipients who have expressed that they understood that an adjustment process was necessary following cochlear implantation but that they also were under the impression that they would eventually regain the ability to converse on the telephone, understand speech in noisy restaurants, and/or watch TV without closed captioning. Again, most post-lingually deafened adult recipients and pre-lingually deafened children who receive implants at an early age do succeed in the aforementioned situations. It is simply important to note that these situations tend to be the most challenging for implant users and may continue to be problematic for the candidate under counsel.

Furthermore, the authors of this book often take the opportunity to discuss the use of hearing assistance technology (HAT) (e.g., personal digital RF/FM system) with cochlear implant sound processors. We have found that cochlear implant recipients are generally much more receptive to the use of HAT if the topic is discussed prior to implantation. Doing so also implicitly reiterates the fact that the cochlear implant alone may not sufficiently address the candidate's communication difficulties across every conceivable situation.

The authors of this book also review the various risks and potential negative consequences associated with cochlear implantation. Although medical risks will be covered by the cochlear implant surgeon, it is also important for the audiologist to discuss the surgical risks and considerations associated with implantation. We also discuss the increased risk of bacterial meningitis associated with cochlear implantation and the need to stay current with vaccinations for pneumococcal meningitis.

In short, the goal of pre-implant counseling is to establish a relatively conservative or limited outlook pertaining to the benefit and performance a recipient will receive with the cochlear implant, while still convincing the candidate that cochlear implantation is in his/her best interests. In addition to the verbal counseling that is provided for the cochlear implant candidate and his/her family, the audiologist should also provide written materials to the family so that they may review a tangible description of the information that has been provided. It should be noted that the implant manufacturers provide written materials that discuss some of the aforementioned information pertaining to cochlear implantation, and this information may also be found on the manufacturers' websites.

When counseling families of pediatric recipients, parents and caregivers must understand that experience with the implant is required before substantial gains are seen in a young child's communicative abilities. For example, it may take more than a year for young children without additional disabilities to develop spoken language vocabulary of even a few words. Unfortunately, approximately 40% of children with hearing loss have additional disabilities that may hinder speech and language development (Gallaudet Research Institute, 2008; Picard, 2004). Furthermore, children who are implanted at an early age (i.e., ≤1 year) may have cognitive or neurological impairments that have not been identified yet but will influence spoken language outcomes.

To prepare families of pediatric recipients and put them at ease, audiologists need to discuss all of the potential responses following activation, including sound awareness, anxiety, happiness, fear, and indifference. Most children do not display a strong aversion to their initial experience of hearing with their cochlear implant, particularly when the audiologist introduces stimulation appropriately. In fact, some are very happy with the new sound and will smile and point to their ear when they hear programming stimuli or external sounds. However, in some cases, children do become upset and cry and seek comfort from caregivers. To prevent this negative reaction, the audiologist should make every attempt to avoid overstimulation. Even with careful programming, however, a few children, especially those with minimal experience with sound, still become upset when they first hear through the implant. This is most likely due to the child being startled by the new signal he/she receives.

Finally, some children initially may be ambivalent to the sound they receive. This response will often be concerning to the child's family because they question whether the device is working. Typically, the audiologist can conduct measures, such as the electrically evoked compound action potential, that indicate that the auditory system is responding to the stimulation from the implant. Of course, this information can be conveyed to the child's caregivers to alleviate their concerns. All of the aforementioned responses are possible for a young child receiving a cochlear implant, even when he or she eventually develops considerable conversational and auditory skills. It is important that the family is prepared for each of these responses so they are not overly alarmed or disappointed on activation day.

Prior to implantation, it is beneficial to provide materials that help pre-school and elementary age children to understand the cochlear implant process. Manufacturers offer books for young children that describe the process from surgery to activation in kid-friendly language (Figure 6–9). Also, some families create photo albums depicting their own experiences and share them with other families beginning the journey of cochlear implantation.

Additionally, it is imperative that the cochlear implant team counsel a child's family about the importance of full-time cochlear implant use and intensive therapy focused on the development of auditory and spoken language abilities. Numerous studies have shown that optimal cochlear implant outcomes are dependent upon the family's commitment to full-time

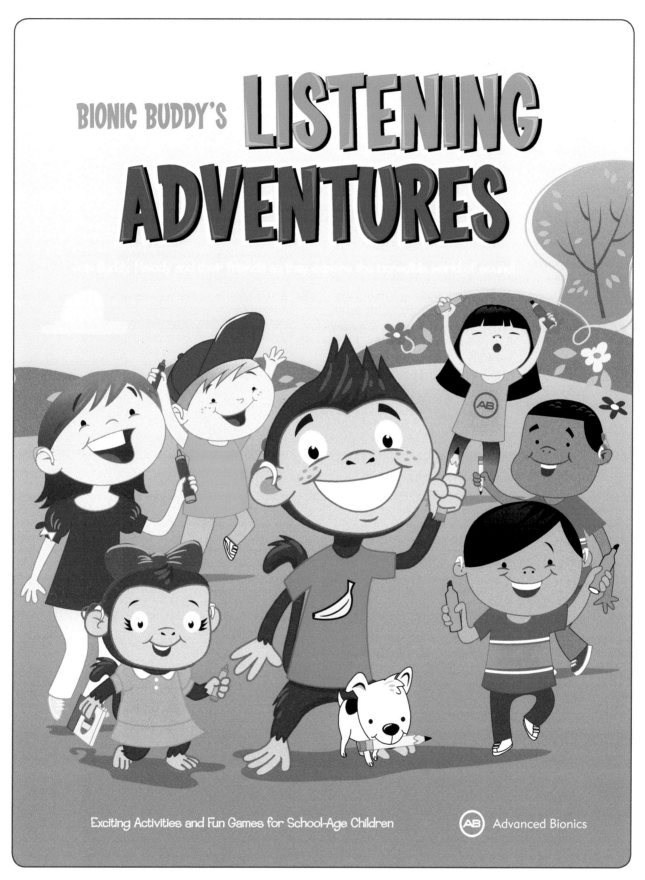

FIGURE 6–9. An example of a book that describes the cochlear implant process. Image provided courtesy of Advanced Bionics, LLC.

implant use and audition-based therapy (Ching & Dillon, 2013; Chu et al., 2016; Geers & Moog, 2011; Quittner et al., 2013). Of course, the mode of communication a family uses after cochlear implantation is entirely the choice of the family. The audiologist should assist the family in ensuring that sufficient habilitative therapy is in place to support the child's development after implantation. However, it is also the audiologist's responsibility to adequately educate the family about the different factors that influence the outcomes children achieve with their cochlear implants. Research has established that better auditory and spoken language outcome are achieved when families commit to Auditory Verbal/auditory oral based therapy compared with a Total Communication or manual based approach (Chu et al., 2016; Dettman et al., 2016; Geers, Nicholas, & Sedey, 2003; Geers et al., 2011, 2017). Families should be aware of this research when determining the type of intervention that is best for their family and child.

Key Concepts

- The pediatric cochlear implant candidacy assessment should be completed by an interdisciplinary team of hearing health care professionals and should include a battery of behavioral and electrophysiologic audiology measurements.

- Aided speech recognition should be completed in the best-aided condition. The audiologist should possess a working knowledge of modern hearing aid technology and verification of hearing aid function in order to ensure that the candidate is equipped with hearing aids that are best suited to meet his/her needs.

- Ultimately, the interdisciplinary team of hearing health care professionals should determine whether a cochlear implant is likely to improve the child's communication abilities and quality of life and to optimize the child's educational, social, and psycho-emotional development.

References

Adunka, O. F., Jewells, V., & Buchman, C. A. (2007). Value of computed tomography in the evaluation of children with cochlear nerve deficiency. *Otology and Neurotology, 28*(5), 597–604.

Ambrose, S. E., VanDam, M., & Moeller, M. P. (2014). Linguistic input, electronic media, and communication outcomes of toddlers with hearing loss. *Ear and Hearing, 35*(2), 139–147.

Ambrose, S. E., Walker, E. A., Unflat-Berry, L. M., & Oleson, J. J., & Moeller, M. P. (2015). Quantity and quality of caregivers' linguistic input to 18-month and 3-year-old children who are hard of hearing. *Ear and Hearing, 36*(Suppl. 1), 48S–59S.

Barr, B. (1955). Pure-tone audiometry for preschool children: A clinical study with particular reference to children with severely impaired hearing. *Acta Otolaryngologica, Supplement, 121*, 1–84.

Baudhuin, J., Cadieux, J., Firszt, J. B., Reeder, R. M., & Maxson, J. L. (2012). Optimization of programming parameters in children with the advanced bionics cochlear implant. *Journal of the American Academy of Audiology, 23*(5), 302–312.

Bauer, P. W., Sharma, A., Martin, K., & Dorman, M. (2006). Central auditory development in children with bilateral cochlear implants. *Archives of Otolaryngology-Head and Neck Surgery, 132*(10), 1133–1136.

Bell, A. G. (2018). A. G. Bell Association for the Deaf and Hard of Hearing, *Delivery of services by listening and spoken language specialists.* Retrieved from http://www.agbell.org/Speak/Delivery-of-Services-by-Listening-and-Spoken-Language-Specialists

Bench, J., Kowal, A., & Bamford, J. (1979). The BKB (Bamford-Kowal-Bench) sentence lists for partially-hearing children. *British Journal of Audiology, 13*, 108–112.

Bennett, M. J., & Weatherby, L. A. (1982). Newborn acoustic reflexes to noise and pure-tone signals. *Journal of Speech and Hearing Research, 25*(3), 383–387.

Berlin, C., Hood, L., Morlet, T., Wilensky, D., St. John, P., Montgomery, E., & Thibodaux, M. (2005). Absent or elevated middle ear muscle reflexes in the presence of normal otoacoustic emissions: A universal finding in 136 cases of auditory neuropathy/dys-synchrony. *Journal of the American Academy of Audiology, 16*(8), 546–553.

Boisvert, I., Lyxell, B., Maki-Torkko, E., McMahon, C. M., & Dowell, R. C. (2012). Choice of ear for cochlear implantation in adults with monaural sound-deprivation and unilateral hearing aid. *Otology and Neurotology, 33*(4), 572–579.

Boothroyd, A. (1984). Auditory perception of speech contrasts by subjects with sensorineural hearing loss. *Journal of Speech and Hearing Research, 27*, 134–144.

British Columbia Early Hearing Program (BCEHP), (2012). *Audiology Assessment Protocol, Version 4.1.* Retrieved from http://www.phsa.ca/Documents/bcehpaudiologyassessmentprotocol.pdf

Buchman, C. A., Roush, P. A., Teagle, H. F., Brown, C. J., Zdanski, C. J., & Grose, J. H. (2006). Auditory neuropathy characteristics in children with cochlear nerve deficiency. *Ear and Hearing, 27*(4), 399–408.

Centers for Disease Control and Prevention (CDC). (2017). *Use of vaccines to prevent meningitis in persons with cochlear implants.* Retrieved from https://www.cdc.gov/vaccines/vpd/mening/hcp/dis-cochlear-gen.html

Ching, T. Y. C., & Dillon, H. (2013). Major findings of the LOCHI study on children at 3 years of age and implications for audiologic management. *International Journal of Audiology, 52*(Suppl. 2), 65S–68S.

Ching, T. Y. C., Dillon, H., Leigh, G., & Cupples, L. (2017). Learning from the Longitudinal Outcomes of Children with Hearing Impairment (LOCHI) study: Summary of 5-year findings and implications. *International Journal of Audiology,* 1–7. doi:10.1080/14992027.2017.138586

Clark W., & Govett, S. (1995). *School-related noise exposure in children*. Paper presented at the Association for Research in in Otolaryngology Mid-Winter Meeting. St. Petersburg, FL.

Chu, C., Choo, D., Dettman, S., Leigh, J., Traeger, G., Lettieri, G., . . . Dowell, R. (2016, May). *Early intervention and communication development in children using cochlear implants: The impact of service delivery practices and family factors.* Presented at Audiology Australia National Conference 2016, Melbourne, Australia.

Coninx, F., Weichbold, V., Tsiakpini, L., Autrique, E., Bescond, G., & Tamas, L. (2009). Validation of the LittlEARS Auditory Questionnaire in children with normal hearing. *International Journal of Pediatric Otorhinology, 73,* 1761–1768.

Crukley, J., Scollie, S., & Parsa V. (2011). An exploration of non-quiet listening at school. *Journal of Educational Audiology, 17,* 23–35.

Davidson, L. S. (2006). Effects of stimulus level on the speech perception abilities of children using cochlear implants or digital hearing aids. *American Journal of Audiology, 15*(2), 141–153.

Davidson, L. S., Skinner, M. W., Holstad, B. A., Fears, B. T., Richter, M. K., Matusofsky, M., . . . Scollie, S. (2009). The effect of instantaneous input dynamic range setting on the speech perception of children with the Nucleus-24 implant. *Ear and Hearing, 30*(3), 340–349.

Dettman, S. J., Dowell, R. C., Choo, D., Arnott, W., Abrahams, Y., Davis, A., Dornan, D., . . . Briggs, R. J. (2016). Long-term communication outcomes for children receiving cochlear implants younger than 12 months: A multicentre study. *Otology and Neurotology, 37,* e82–e95.

Dillon, H., & Keidser, G. (2013). Siemens Expert Series: NAL-NL2 —Principles, background data, and comparison to other procedures. *AudiologyOnline.* Retrieved from http://www.audiologyonline.com/articles/siemens-expert-series-nal-nl2-11355.

Dwyer, R., Spahr, T., Agrawal, S., Hetlinger, C., Holder, J., & Gifford, R. (2016). Participant-generated cochlear implant programs: Speech recognition, sound quality, and satisfaction. *Otology and Neurotology, 37*(7), e209–e216.

Elliott, L. L., & Katz, D. (1980). *Development of a new children's test of speech discrimination* [Technical manual]. St. Louis, MO: Auditec.

Fenson L., Marchman V. A., Thal D. J., Dale P. S., Reznick J. S., & Bates E. (2007). *MacArthur-Bates Communicative Development inventories: User's guide and technical manual.* Baltimore, MD: Brookes.

Firszt, J., Holden, L., Skinner, M., Tobey, E., Peterson, A., Gaggl W., Runge-Samuelson, C., & Wackym, P. (2004). Recognition of speech presented at soft to loud levels by adult cochlear implant recipients of three cochlear implant systems. *Ear and Hearing, 25*(4), 375–387.

Gallaudet Research Institute. (2008). *Regional and national summary report of data from the 2007–08 Annual Survey of Deaf and Hard of Hearing Children and Youth.* Retrieved from http://research.gallaudet.edu/Demographics/2008_National_Summary.pdf

Galvin, K. L. (2015). Achievement of early clinical milestones and long-term functional outcomes for children and young adults with bilateral cochlear implants. *Cochlear Implants International, 16*(Suppl. 1), S16–S18.

Gardner-Berry, K., Hou, S. Y. L., & Ching, T. Y. C. (in press). Managing infants and children with auditory neuropathy spectrum disorder (ANSD). In J. R. Madell, C. Flexer, J. Wolfe, & E. Schafer (Eds.), *Pediatric audiology: Diagnosis, technology, and management* (3rd ed.), New York, NY: Thieme.

Geers, A., Davidson, L., Uchanski, R., & Nicholas, J. (2013). Interdependence of linguistic and indexical speech perception skills in school-age children with early cochlear implantation. *Ear and Hearing, 34*(5), 562–574.

Geers, A. E., Mitchell, C. M., Warner-Czyz, A., Wang, N. Y., Eisenberg, L. S., & Team, C. DaCI Investigative. (2017). Early sign language exposure and cochlear implantation benefits. *Pediatrics, 140*(1), e20163489.

Geers, A. E., Nicholas, J. G., & Sedey, A. L. (2003). Language skills of children with early cochlear implantation. *Ear and Hearing, 24*(Suppl. 1), 46S–58S.

Geers, A. E., Strube, M. J., Tobey, E. A., Pisoni, D. B., & Moog, J. S. (2011). Epilogue: Factors contributing to long-term outcomes of cochlear implantation in early childhood. *Ear and Hearing, 32*(Suppl. 1), 84S–92S.

Gelfand, S. A., Shwander, T., & Silman, S. (1990). Acoustic reflex thresholds in normal and cochlear-impaired ears: Effects of no-response rates on 90th percentiles in a large sample. *Journal of Speech and Hearing Disorders, 55,* 198–205.

Gifford, R., Shallop, J., & Peterson, A. (2008). Speech recognition materials and ceiling effects: Considerations for cochlear implant programs. *Audiology and Neurotology, 13*(3), 193–205.

Gordon, K. A., & Papsin, B. C. (2009). Benefits of short interimplant delays in children receiving bilateral cochlear implants. *Otology and Neurotology, 30*(3), 319–331.

Gorga, M. P., Neely, S. T., Hoover, B. M., Dierking, D. M., Beauchaine, K. L., & Manning, C. (2004). Determining the upper limits of stimulation for auditory steady-state response measurements. *Ear and Hearing, 25*(3), 302–307.

Govaerts, P., Daemers, K., Yperman M., De Beukelaer, C., De Saegher, G., & De Ceulaer, G. (2006). Auditory speech sounds evaluation (A(section)E): A new test to assess detection, discrimination and identification in hearing impairment. *Cochlear Implants International, 7*(2), 92–106.

Gravel, J. S., & Wallace, I. F. (1998). Audiologic management of otitis media. In F. H. Bess (Ed.), *Children with hearing impairment: Contemporary trends* (pp. 215–230). Nashville, TN: Vanderbilt Bill Wilkerson Center Press.

Guidelines Development Conference at NHS. (2008). *Guidelines for identification and management of infants and young children with auditory neuropathy spectrum disorder.* Retrieved from https://www.childrenscolorado.org/globalassets/departments/ear-nose-throat/ansd-monograph.pdf

Hang, A. X., Roush, P. A., Teagle, H. F., Zdanski, C., Pillsbury, H. C., Adunka, O. F., & Buchman, C. A. (2015). Is "no response" on diagnostic auditory brainstem response testing an indication for cochlear implantation in children? *Ear and Hearing, 36*(1), 8–13.

Hart, B., & Risley, T. R. (1995). *Meaningful differences in the everyday experience of young American children.* Baltimore, MD: . Brookes.

Hart, B., & Risley, T. R. (2003. Spring). The early catastrophe: The 30 million word gap by age 3. *American Educator,* pp. 4–9. http://www.aft.org//sites/default/files/periodicals/TheEarlyCatastrophe.pdf

Haskins, H. A. (1949). *A phonetically balanced test of speech discrimination for children* (Unpublished master's thesis). Northwestern University, Evanston, IL.

Houston, D. M., Stewart, J., Moberly, A., Hollich, G., & Miyamoto, R. T. (2012). Word learning in deaf children with cochlear implants: Effects of early auditory experience. *Developmental Science, 15*(3), 448–461.

Jerger, J. F. (1970). Clinical experience with impedence audiometry. *Archives of Otolaryngology, 92*, 311–324.

Jerger, J., Anthony, L., Jerger, S., & Mauldin, L. (1974). Studies in impedance audiometry. 3. Middle ear disorders. *Archives of Otolaryngology, 99*(3), 165–171.

Jerger, S., Jerger, J., & Abrams, S. (1983). Speech audiometry in the young child. *Ear and Hearing, 4*, 56–66.

Jerger, S., Jerger, J., & Fahad, R. (1985). Pediatric hearing aid evaluation: Case reports. *Ear and Hearing, 6*, 240–244.

Johnson, K., & Winter, M. (2003). Assessment of infants and toddlers with hearing loss. *Volta Review (Monograph)*, 221–251.

Josefson, D. (2002). Cochlear implants carry risk of meningitis, agencies warn. *British Medical Journal, 325*(7359), 298.

Kei, J., Allison-Levick, J., Dockray, J., Harrys, R., Kirkegard, C., Wong, J., Maurer, M., Hegarty, J., Young, J., & Tudehope, D. (2003). High-frequency (1000 Hz) tympanometry in normal neonates. *Journal of the American Academy of Audiology, 14*(1), 20–28.

Kirk, K., French, B., & Choi S. (2009). Assessing spoken word recognition in children with cochlear implants. In L. Eisenberg (Ed.), *Clinical management of children with cochlear implants*. San Diego, CA: Plural.

Kirk, K. I., Pisoni, D. B., & Osberger, M. J. (1995). Lexical effects on spoken word recognition by pediatric cochlear implant users. *Ear and Hearing, 16*, 470–481.

Ling, D. (1976). *Speech and the hearing-impaired child: Theory and practice*. Washington, DC: Alexander Graham Bell Association for the Deaf.

Ling, D. (1989). *Foundations of spoken language for the hearing-impaired child*. Washington, DC: Alexander Graham Bell Association for the Deaf.

Litovsky, R. Y., Johnstone, P. M., & Godar, S. P. (2006). Benefits of bilateral cochlear implants and/or hearing aids in children. *International Journal of Audiology, 45*(Suppl. 1), S78–S91.

Litovsky, R. Y., Parkinson, A., Arcaroli, J., Peters, R., Lake, J., Johnstone, P., & Yu, G. (2004). Bilateral cochlear implants in adults and children. *Archives of Otolaryngology–Head and Neck Surgery, 130*(5), 648–655.

MacWhinney, B., & Snow, C. (1985). The child language data exchange system. *Journal of Child Language, 12*, 271–295.

Meinzen-Derr, J., Wiley, S., Creighton, J., & Choo, D. (2007). Auditory Skills Checklist: Clinical tool for monitoring functional auditory skill development in young children with cochlear implants. *Annals of Otology, Rhinology, and Laryngology, 116*(11), 812–818.

Miyamoto, R. T., Houston, D. M., & Bergeson, T. (2005). Cochlear implantation in deaf infants. *Laryngoscope, 115*(8), 1376–1380.

Moog, J. S., & Geers, A. E. (1990). *Early speech perception test for profoundly hearing-impaired children*. St. Louis, MO: Central Institute for the Deaf.

Moog, J. S., & Geers, A. E. (2010). Early educational placement and later language outcomes for children with cochlear implants. *Otology and Neurotology, 31*(8), 1315–1319.

National Health Service (NHS). (2013a). *Guidance for auditory brainstem response testing in babies, version 2.1*. Retrieved from http://www.thebsa.org.uk/wp-content/uploads/2014/08/NHSP_ABRneonate_2014.pdf

National Health Service (NHS). (2013b). *Guidelines for the assessment and management of auditory neuropathy spectrum disorder in young infant, version 2.2*. Retrieved from http://www.thebsa.org.uk/wp-content/uploads/2015/02/ANSD_Guidelines_v_2-2_0608131.pdf

Niparko, J. K., Tobey, E. A., Thal, D. J., Eisenberg, L. S., Wang, N. Y., Quittner, A. L., . . . Team, C. DaCI Investigative. (2010). Spoken language development in children following cochlear implantation. *Journal of the American Medical Association (JAMA), 303*(15), 1498–1506.

Nittrouer, S., & Chapman, C. (2009). The effects of bilateral electric and bimodal electric–acoustic stimulation on language development. *Trends in Hearing, 13*(3), 190-205.

Olsen, W. O. (1998). Average speech levels and spectra in various speaking/listening conditions: A summary of the Pearson, Bennett, and Fidell (1977) report. *American Journal of Audiology, 7*(2), 21–25.

Ontario Infant Hearing Program (OIHP). (2016). *Protocol for auditory brainstem response-based audiological assessment (ABRA), version 2016.02*. Retrieved from https://www.mountsinai.on.ca/care/infant-hearing-program/documents/protocol-for-auditory-brainstem-response-2013-based-audiological-assessement-abra

Pearsons, K., Bennett, R., & Fidell, S. (1977). *Speech levels in various environments*. Washington, DC: Office of Health and Ecological Effects, Office of Research and Development, US EPA.

Peters, B., Litovsky, R., Parkinson, A., & Lake, J. (2007). Importance of age and post-implantation experience on speech perception measures in children with sequential bilateral cochlear implants. *Otology and Neurotology, 28*, 649–657.

Peterson, G. E., & Lehiste, I. (1962). Revised CNC lists for auditory tests. *Journal of Speech and Hearing Disorders, 27*, 62–70.

Picard, M. (2004). Children with permanent hearing loss and associated disabilities: Revisiting current epidemiological data and causes of deafness. *Volta Review, 104*, 221–236.

Punch, S., Van Dun, B., King, A., Carter, L., & Pearce, W. (2016). Clinical experience of using cortical auditory evoked potentials in the treatment of infant hearing loss in Australia. *Seminars in Hearing, 37*(1), 36–52.

Quittner, A. L., Cruz, I., Barker, D. H., Tobey, E., Eisenberg, L. S., Niparko, J. K., & Childhood Development after Cochlear Implantation Investigative, Team. (2013). Effects of maternal sensitivity and cognitive and linguistic stimulation on cochlear implant users' language development over four years. *Journal of Pediatrics, 162*(2), 343–348.

Rakszawski, B., Wright, R., Cadieux, J., Davidson, L., & Brenner, C. (2016). The effects of preprocessing strategies for pediatric cochlear implant recipients. *Journal of the American Academy of Audiology, 27*(2), 85–102.

Robinson, E., Davidson, L., Uchanski, R., Brenner, C., & Geers, A. (2012). A longitudinal study of speech perception skills and device characteristics of adolescent cochlear implant users. *Journal of the American Academy of Audiology, 23*(5), 341–349.

Schauwers, K., Gillis, S., Daemers, K., Beukelaer, C., & Govaerts, P. (2004). Cochlear implantation between 5 and 20 months of age: The onset of babbling and the audiologic outcome. *Otology and Neurotology, 25*, 263–270.

Scollie, S., Seewald, R., Cornelisse, L., Moodie, S., Bagatto, M., Laurnagaray, D., . . . Pumford, J. (2005). The Desired Sensation Level multistage input/output algorithm. *Trends in Amplification, 9*(4), 159–197.

Sharma, A., Dorman, M. F., & Kral, A. (2005). The influence of a sensitive period on central auditory development in children with unilateral and bilateral cochlear implants. *Hearing Research, 203*(1–2), 134–143.

Sheffield, S., Haynes, D., Wanna, G., Labadie, R., & Gifford, R. (2015). Availability of binaural cues for pediatric bilateral cochlear implant recipients. *Journal of the American Academy of Audiology, 26*(3), 289–298.

Small, S. A., & Stapells, D. R. (2004). Artifactual responses when recording auditory steady-state responses. *Ear and Hearing, 25*(6), 611–623.

Smeds, K., Wolters, F., & Rung, M. (2015). Estimation of signal-to-noise ratio in realistic sound scenarios. *Journal of the American Academy of Audiology, 26*(2), 183–196.

Spahr, A. J., Dorman, M. F., Cook, S. J., Loiselle, L. M., DeJong, M. D., Hedley-Williams, A., Sunderhaus, L. S., & Hayes, C. (2014). Development and validation of the pediatric AzBio sentence test. *Ear and Hearing, 35*, 418–422.

Teagle, H. F., Roush, P. A., Woodard, J. S., Hatch, D. R., Zdanski, C. J., Buss, E., & Buchman, C. A. (2010). Cochlear implantation in children with auditory neuropathy spectrum disorder. *Ear and Hearing, 31*(3), 325–335.

Thibodeau, L. M. (2006). Speech audiometry. In R. Roeser, M. Valente, & H. Hosford-Dunn (Eds.), *Audiology: Diagnostics* (pp. 288–313). New York, NY: Thieme Medical.

Thompson, M., Thompson, G., & Vethivelu S. (1989). A comparison of audiometric test methods for 2-year-old children. *Journal of Speech and Hearing Disorders, 54*(2), 174–179.

Thompson, G., & Weber, B. A. (1974). Responses of infants and young children to behavior observation audiometry (BOA). *Journal of Speech and Hearing Disorders, 39*(2), 140–147.

Tyberg, L. (2013). *Auditory skill development of children with normal hearing (ages birth to three years), as determined by responses to the Cincinnati Auditory Skills Checklist.* Unpublished manuscript.

Uhler, K., & Gifford, R. (2014). Current trends in pediatric cochlear implant candidate selection and postoperative follow-up. *American Journal of Audiology, 23*, 309–325.

Uhler, K., Baca, R., Dudas, E., & Fredrickson, T. (2015). Refining stimulus parameters in assessing infant speech perception using visual reinforcement infant speech discrimination: Sensation level. *Journal of the American Academy of Audiology, 26*, 807–814.

Uhler, K., Warner-Czyz, A., Gifford, R., & Working Group, P. (2017). Pediatric Minimum Speech Test Battery. *Journal of the American Academy of Audiology, 28*(3), 232–247.

Uhler K., Yoshinaga-Itano, C., Gabbard, S., Rothpletz, A., & Jenkins, H. (2011b). Longitudinal infant speech perception in young cochlear implant users. *Journal of the American Academy of Audiology, 22*, 129–142.

Walker, E. A., Holte, L., McCreery, R. W., Spratford, M., Page, T., & Moeller, M. P. (2015). The influence of hearing aid use on outcomes of children with mild hearing loss. *Journal of Speech, Language, and Hearing Research, 58*(5), 1611–1625.

Warner-Czyz, A. D., & Davis, B. L. (2008). The emergence of segmental accuracy in young cochlear implant recipients. *Cochlear Implants International, 9*(3), 143–166.

Weichbold, V., Tsiakpini, L., Coninx, F., & D'Haese, P. (2005). Development of a parent questionnaire for assessment of auditory behaviour of infants up to two years of age. *Laryngo-rhino-otology, 84*(5).

Wolfe, J. (2014b). 20Q: ABR assessment in infants—getting it right when it matters the most. *Audiology Online.* Retrieved from http://www.audiologyonline.com/audiology-ceus/course/20q-abr-assessment-in-infants-25165

Wolfe, J. (2014a). 20Q: ABR assessment in infants—summary of protocols and standards. *Audiology Online.* Retrieved from https://www.audiologyonline.com/articles/20q-abr-assessment-in-infants-12999

Wolfe, J., Baker, S., Caraway, T., Kasulis, H., Mears, A., Smith, J., . . . Wood, M. (2007). 1-year postactivation results for sequentially implanted bilateral cochlear implant users. *Otology and Neurotology, 28*(5), 589–596.

Zeitler, D. M., Kessler, M. A., Terushkin, V., Roland, T. J., Jr., Svirsky, M. A., Lalwani, A. K., & Waltzman, S. B. (2008). Speech perception benefits of sequential bilateral cochlear implantation in children and adults: A retrospective analysis. *Otology and Neurotology, 29*(3), 314–325.

Zimmerman-Phillips, S., Robbins, A. M., & Osberger, M. J. (2000). Assessing cochlear implant benefit in very young children. *Annals of Otology, Rhinology, and Laryngology Supplement, 109*(12), 42–43.

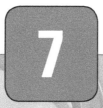

7

Basic Terminology of Cochlear Implant Programming

Jace Wolfe and Erin C. Schafer

In order to optimize the clinical service provided to cochlear implant recipients, audiologists must possess a thorough understanding of the terminology associated with cochlear implant technology and programming. With that in mind, the objective of this chapter is to familiarize the reader with the fundamental terms and concepts affiliated with cochlear implants. The first part of this chapter addresses terminology and parameters that correspond to electrical stimulation of the cochlear nerve and how acoustic signals are coded into electrical signals in each of three domains: (1) intensity, (2) frequency, and (3) time. The second part of this chapter discusses terminology associated with cochlear implant programming.

Transforming Acoustic Signals into Electrical Current to Elicit an Auditory Response

Cochlear implants directly stimulate the cochlear nerve with electrical current. In modern-day commercial systems, the electrical current is delivered in the form of a biphasic, rectangular electrical pulse (Figure 7–1 provides an example). A primary goal of cochlear implant programming and stimulation is to restore audibility for low-level (e.g., 50 dB SPL) and conversational-level (e.g., 60–65 dB SPL) speech across the entire speech frequency range, which is typically stated to span from approximately 100 to 8000 Hz (Boothroyd, 2014). Additionally, stimulation levels

should be set to optimize speech recognition. Also, stimulation levels should be selected to normalize loudness. Specifically, sounds that are perceived as being soft in loudness to persons with normal hearing should also be perceived as soft to the cochlear implant user. Furthermore, sounds that are loud to persons with normal hearing should be loud but not uncomfortable to the cochlear implant recipient.

Factors That Influence the Electrical Coding of Intensity and Loudness

Adjusting Stimulus Intensity and Loudness with Current Amplitude and Pulse Width

The intensity/loudness of an acoustic signal is represented by adjusting the intensity of the biphasic electrical pulse, which may be altered in one of two ways. The intensity pulse may be increased by increasing the **current amplitude** (i.e., height) of each phase of the biphasic electrical pulse. The intensity may also be increased by increasing the **pulse width** (i.e.,

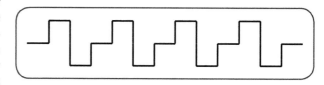

FIGURE 7–1. An illustration of biphasic electrical pulses.

duration, width) of each phase of the biphasic electrical pulse. The pulse width is the amount of time required to complete one phase of a biphasic pulse. As shown in Figure 7–2, the biphasic pulse in Figure 7–2B is twice as intense as the biphasic pulse in Figure 7–2A because the current amplitude of each phase of the signal shown in Figure 7–2B is twice the size of the current amplitude of the signal shown in Figure 7–2A. Likewise, the biphasic pulse in Figure 7–2C is twice as intense as the biphasic pulse in Figure 7–2A because the pulse width of each phase of the signal shown in Figure 7–2C is twice as long in duration as the pulse width of the signal shown in Figure 7–2A.

The intensity of an electrical signal is often described in units of **charge**, which is the product of current amplitude and pulse width.

Total charge (in nanocoulombs
[the coulomb is the unit of charge]) =
Current amplitude * pulse width

The signals in Figures 7–2B and 7–2C have twice the charge as the signal in Figure 7–2A. However, the signals in Figures 7–2B and 7–2C have equal charge.

In summary, it is important to note that the <u>intensity</u> of stimulation from a cochlear implant and the <u>loudness</u> of the signal provided by the cochlear implant may be increased by increasing the current amplitude and/or the pulse width (i.e., duration) of the electrical pulse.

Parameters of Biphasic Electrical Pulses

Figure 7–2 provides a visual illustration of other important parameters associated with electrical pulses. As shown, each half of the biphasic pulse is referred to as a phase. As a result, a biphasic pulse possesses a phase with a positive polarity and a phase with a negative polarity. Once again, the duration of each phase defines the pulse width. For biphasic pulses used with modern cochlear implant systems, each phase typically has a pulse width measured in microseconds (e.g., approximately 10 to 100 microseconds). Remember that a microsecond is one-millionth of a second, so these signals are very short in duration. The amount of time that elapses between each phase is referred to as the **interphase gap**, and the amount of time that elapses between each biphasic pulse is

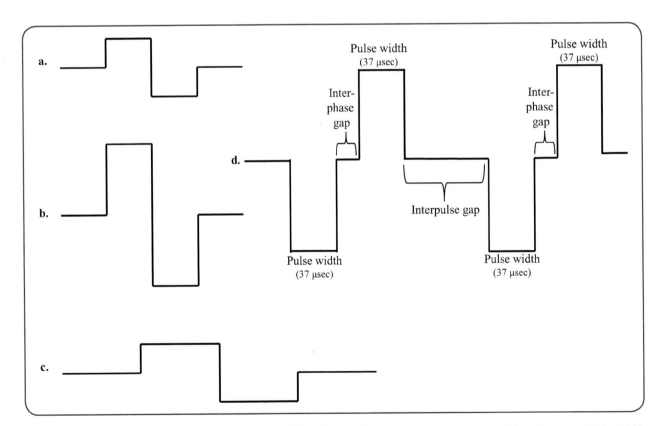

FIGURE 7–2. Increase in intensity from an original signal (**A**) achieved with increase current amplitude (**B**) and increased pulse width (**C**) and a description of how pulse width is measured (**D**).

referred to as the **interpulse gap**. As the reader may deduce from Figure 7–2, a larger number of biphasic pulses may be delivered during a given time frame when the pulse width, interphase gap, and/or interpulse gap are short in duration. In other words, to maximize the number of biphasic electrical pulses presented in one second, the pulse width, interphase gap, and/or interpulse gap must be relatively short in duration. The current amplitude, which is the height of each phase of the biphasic pulse, is also shown in Figure 7–2. In modern cochlear implant systems, current amplitude is usually measured in microamperes or milliamperes.

Ohm's Law and Voltage Compliance

As discussed in Chapter 2, cochlear implant systems possess a limit for the amount of current amplitude that may be provided to each electrode contact. This limit is determined by the voltage capacity of the sound processor battery and the resistance (i.e., impedance) at the electrode contact/tissue interface. As discussed in Chapter 2, Ohm's law states that voltage = current * resistance. As a result, the maximum

current available at each electrode contact is determined by the equation:

$$\text{Current} = \text{Voltage}/\text{Resistance}$$

The voltage capacity of the sound processor battery is fixed, whereas the resistance (i.e., impedance) at each electrode contact may vary. A lower amount of current amplitude will be available at electrode contacts with higher resistances. The maximum amount of electrical current is reached when the battery can no longer provide further power (i.e., voltage) to allow for further increases in current amplitude. The **voltage compliance limit** refers to the maximum amount of electrical current amplitude that may be delivered to an electrode contact given the voltage capacity of the battery. The "hash marks" indicated by the arrows in Figure 7–3 indicate the maximum amount of electrical current amplitude available at each electrode contact. As the reader may see from Figure 7–3, the voltage compliance limits vary across the electrode contacts. Electrode contacts with lower resistance values at the electrode/tissue interface possess lower voltage compliance limits.

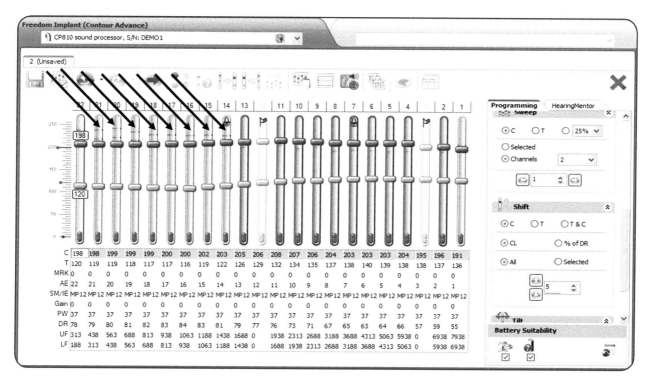

FIGURE 7–3. An example of voltage compliance levels for a cochlear implant recipient. The arrows are pointing to dashes that represent the maximum amount of electrical current that can be provided on each channel. The channels that are highlighted (i.e., channels 2–13) provide examples in which the current levels for a particular channel exceed to maximum current that may be provided by the voltage limits of the system. Image provided courtesy of Cochlear Americas, ©2018.

In some cases, an audiologist may increase stimulation levels to the point of voltage compliance limits without achieving an auditory sensation that is considered to be loud to the cochlear implant recipient. In such a case, loudness growth is insufficient. It should be noted that once voltage compliance limits are encountered, further increases in current amplitude provided in the cochlear implant programming software will not result in an increase in signal intensity or loudness. The lack of an increase in stimulus intensity and loudness that occurs when voltage compliance limits are reached is due to the fact that the sound processor battery voltage limit has been met and further increases in current amplitude are not possible because no additional voltage (i.e., power) is available. If voltage compliance limits are encountered prior to achieving a desired loudness goal, additional signal intensity may be achieved by increasing the pulse width of the biphasic electrical pulse. Of note, an increase in the pulse width may require a decrease in stimulation rate, a topic that will be covered later in this chapter.

Electrode Array Terminology

As shown in Figure 7–4, all cochlear implants possess a group of wires that project from the body of

the cochlear implant and terminate in a tip which is inserted into the cochlea. Although there is no universally accepted term to collectively describe the component that extends from the body of the cochlear implant and eventually into the cochlea, many professionals refer to it as the **electrode**. Figure 7–4 depicts the portion of the cochlear implant that is sometimes referred to as the electrode. The electrode contains electrode leads (i.e., wires), an electrode array of intracochlear electrode contacts, and extracochlear ground electrodes. The electrode may also include stiffening rings, insertion depth markers, a fan tail/wing, and/or a stopper.

As mentioned in Chapter 2, electrical pulses are generated within the body of the cochlear implant and delivered down metal alloy wires called **electrode leads**. The term "electrode lead" can be ambiguous because it can refer to each individual wire or to the collective group of wires. For the purpose of this book, the term "electrode lead" refers to an individual wire, whereas the group of wires is referred to as electrode leads. Electrode leads may be configured as straight wires or in a wave shape. Figure 7–5 shows an example of the wave-shaped electrode leads found in the MED-EL FLEX electrode. The wave-shaped configuration is designed to reduce the rigidity of the electrode, which results in a more flexible lead that may reduce trauma to cochlear structures

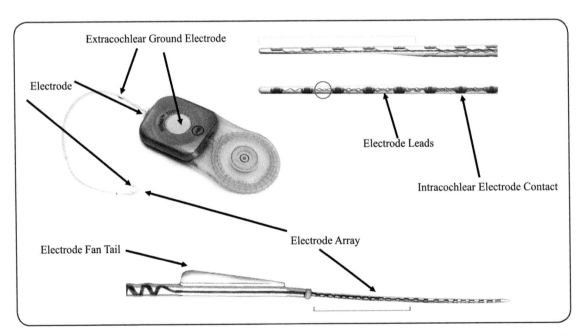

FIGURE 7–4. An example of cochlear implant electrode terminology. Images provided courtesy of Advanced Bionics, LLC, Cochlear, Ltd, and MED-EL Corporation.

during insertion into the cochlea. Each electrode lead is insulated in silicone to prevent electrical current from spreading from one lead to another. Also, the entire group of leads is encased in a silicone carrier.

An example of a fantail or wing is shown in Figure 7–4. A fantail/wing is designed to enhance the surgeon's ease of handling by providing a stiff structure that can be grasped during the insertion process. Some electrodes also possess stiffening rings, which, as the name implies, increases the rigidity of the section of the electrode. This increase in rigidity also improves the ease of handling for the surgeon. An example of stiffening rings is shown in Figure 7–6.

Intracochlear Electrode Contacts

Each electrode lead (e.g., wire) terminates at an individual **intracochlear electrode contact**. Electrical signals are sent along each wire and to each contact and are then delivered to the cochlear nerve, and each lead and intracochlear electrode contact is responsible for carrying one channel of sound.

Multiple channel cochlear implants possess multiple leads and electrode contacts, with low-frequency signals being delivered to intracochlear electrode contacts located in the apical end of the cochlea and high-frequency signals located in the basal end of the cochlea. Intracochlear electrode contacts consist of metal alloy (e.g., platinum-iridium) plates. Intracochlear electrode contacts are sometimes referred to as the **active** or the **stimulating** electrodes.

Intracochlear electrode contacts come in many shapes. For example, the Nucleus CI532 electrode shown in Figure 7–7 possesses half-banded (i.e., half-ring) electrode contacts. In contrast, the Nucleus 24 Straight electrode possesses full-banded (i.e., full-ring) electrode contacts (see Figure 7–7). Half-banded electrode contacts are designed to deliver electrical current toward the modiolus (for focused stimulation of the cochlear nerve), whereas full-banded electrode contacts emanate electrical current in all directions. A full-banded electrode contact may be appropriate for persons with common cavity cochleae, because the neural innervation may not be located in one

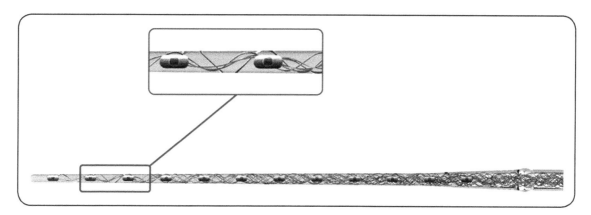

FIGURE 7–5. An example of intracochlear electrode contacts and electrode leads (i.e., wires). Image provided courtesy of MED-EL Corporation.

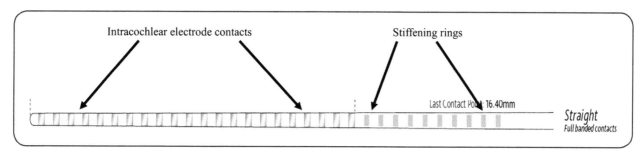

FIGURE 7–6. An example of intracochlear electrode contacts and stiffening rings. Image provided courtesy of Cochlear Americas, ©2018.

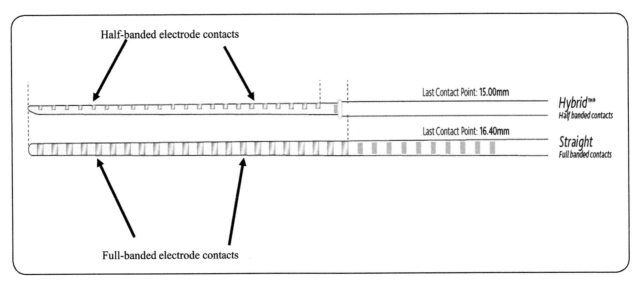

FIGURE 7–7. An example of half-banded and full-banded intracochlear electrode contacts. Image provided courtesy of Cochlear Americas, ©2018.

particular direction throughout the insertion of the different intracochlear electrode contacts. Figure 7–8 shows an example of planar-shaped (i.e., flat plates or discs) electrode contacts found in modern Advanced Bionics cochlear implants. MED-EL cochlear implants possess oval-shaped electrode contacts located on the side of the electrode carrier. The seven most basal stimulating sites of the MED-EL FLEX electrode consist of two oval-shaped electrode contacts, whereas the five most apical stimulating sites consist of one oval-shaped contact (Figure 7–9).

Cochlear Implant Electrode Arrays

The term **electrode array** is used to describe the group of intracochlear electrode contacts that are arranged at the tip of the electrode. As with electrode contacts, electrode arrays also come in different shapes and sizes. Electrode arrays are designed with two general configurations, lateral wall and perimodiolar (Figure 7–10). As the name implies, a **lateral wall electrode array** is designed to be inserted along the lateral wall of the scala tympani. Figure 7–11 provides a visual example of a lateral wall electrode array. The primary design objective of a lateral wall electrode is to avoid the delicate structures of the scala media, resulting in an atraumatic insertion. Prevention of damage to the sensory and supporting structures of the organ of Corti potentially allows for preservation of native acoustic hearing. Atraumatic insertions may also prevent retrograde degeneration of cochlear

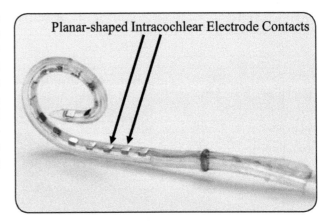

FIGURE 7–8. An example of planar-shaped intracochlear electrode contacts. Image provided courtesy of Advanced Bionics, LLC.

dendrites that may occur when cochlear hair cells and supporting cells are damaged. As a result, atraumatic insertions may be useful even for persons who do not have useful acoustic hearing prior to cochlear implant surgery, because preservation of the integrity of cochlear structures may facilitate a more favorable response of the cochlear nerve to electrical stimulation. Lateral wall electrode arrays typically have a "straight" shape or configuration. Because lateral wall electrodes do not have a pre-curved shape, it is possible to achieve a relatively deep insertion (i.e., beyond the second turn of the cochlea), particularly if the tip of the electrode array is thin and flexible.

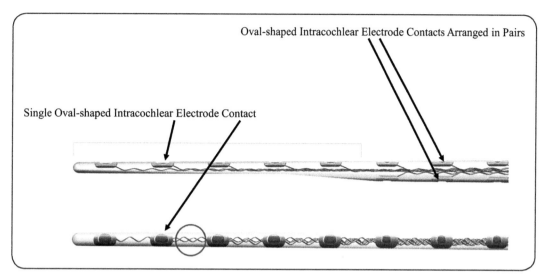

FIGURE 7–9. An example of oval-shaped intracochlear electrode contacts arranged in pairs and in single units. Image provided courtesy of MED-EL Corporation.

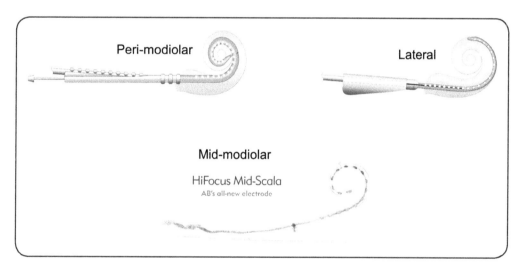

FIGURE 7–10. An example of perimodiolar, lateral wall, and mid-modiolar electrode arrays. Image provided courtesy of Cochlear, Ltd and Advanced Bionics, LLC.

Perimodiolar electrode arrays are designed to be positioned along the medial side of the scala tympani in an attempt to be positioned closely to the modiolus so as to provide proximal stimulation of the cochlear nerve. An example of a perimodiolar electrode array is shown in Figure 7–11. Perimodiolar electrode arrays are pre-curved to match the shape of the cochlea and facilitate "hugging" of the modiolus. Perimodiolar electrode arrays are often loaded in a tool called a stylet, which straightens the electrode array prior to insertion. The stylet, with the electrode array loaded inside, is inserted into the cochlea until the tip reaches the first turn of the cochlea. At that point, the electrode array is pushed forward off the stylet, while the stylet is simultaneously withdrawn from the cochlea. As the pre-curved electrode array is pushed away from the stylet, it conforms to its natural curvature and wraps toward the modiolus. The primary design objective of a perimodiolar electrode array is to achieve close proximity to the modiolus in order to *reduce the amount of electrical current required to elicit an auditory sensation/loudness* as well as to

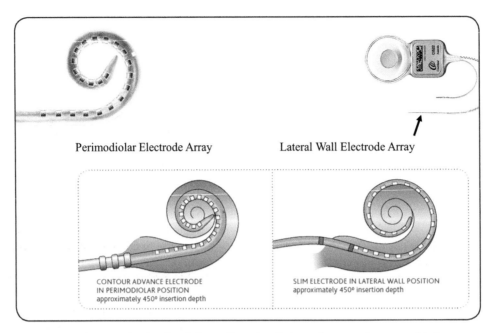

FIGURE 7–11. An example of perimodiolar and lateral wall electrode arrays. Image provided courtesy of Cochlear Americas, ©2018.

reduce the spread of electrical excitation so that a discrete group of cochlear nerve fibers is stimulated by each intracochlear electrode contact. The reduction in electrical stimulation associated with perimodiolar electrode arrays has been shown to result in lower stimulation levels for adequate loudness growth and enhanced power efficiency (i.e., reduced battery life) (Cohen, Saunders, & Clark, 2001; Gordin et al., 2009; Jeong et al., 2015; Muller, Hocke, & Mir-Salim, 2015; Runge-Samuelson et al., 2009). Additionally, Holden et al. (2013) found better speech recognition outcomes in persons who had closer proximity of the electrode array to the modiolus. As such, relative to lateral wall electrode arrays, perimodiolar electrode arrays may allow for better performance in persons who have severe to profound hearing loss prior to surgery and are unlikely to benefit from the preservation of their native acoustic hearing. However, it is important to note that poorer speech recognition outcomes are often obtained in persons for whom the electrode array dislocates from the scala tympani and partially resides in the scala media or scala tympani (Finley et al., 2008; Holden et al., 2013; Wanna et al., 2014). Dislocation of the electrode array from the desired location of the scala tympani has been shown to occur more frequently with perimodiolar electrode arrays than with lateral wall electrode arrays. Careful implementation of surgical techniques recommended

for perimodiolar electrode arrays should ensure that the perimodiolar electrode array is inserted into and remains in the scala tympani throughout the entire insertion. Aschendorff et al. (2017) reported that the Nucleus Slim Modiolar perimodiolar electrode array was inserted entirely within the scala tympani in 44 out of 44 recipients (100%) after the surgeons were trained in proper insertion techniques for the perimodiolar electrode array.

Figure 7–10 shows the Advanced Bionics Mid-Scala electrode array. The Mid-Scala electrode array is designed to reside in the center of the scala tympani (i.e., "mid-modiolar"). The design objective of the Mid-Scala electrode array is to allow for an atraumatic insertion by avoiding the delicate structures of the scala media while also allowing for closer proximity to the modiolus than a lateral wall electrode array. At the time of this writing, there were no peer-reviewed publications supporting the potential merits (e.g., hearing preservation, lower stimulation levels) of the Mid-Scala electrode array relative to perimodiolar or lateral wall electrode arrays.

Electrode arrays also differ in length. MED-EL's STANDARD and FLEXSOFT™ electrode arrays are the longest on the market at a length of 31.5 mm from the cochleostomy marker to the apical tip (MED-EL, 2017). Note that the FLEXSOFT is a lateral wall electrode array, and a full insertion to the cochleostomy typically results in an angular insertion depth of approximately 630 degrees. In contrast, the Cochlear Nucleus CI522 Slim Straight electrode array has a length of approximately 25 mm from the cochleostomy marker to the apical tip and designed for a typical angular between 450 to 540 degrees (see Figure 7–11). The difference in electrode array length and angular insertion depth between these two lateral wall electrode arrays is primarily due to philosophical differences between the manufacturers regarding the importance of achieving an insertion depth beyond the second turn of the cochlea. In short, however, a full electrode array insertion is typically considered to occur at an angular insertion depth of 450 to 630 degrees.

The Cochlear Nucleus CI532 perimodiolar electrode array spans approximately 18 mm from the cochleostomy marker to the apical tip. However, the insertion depth, as measured in angular degrees, of the Nucleus 532 electrode array is similar to what is achieved with a full insertion of the Nucleus 522 Slim Straight array. In short, a perimodiolar electrode array does not have to possess as long of a length as a lateral wall electrode array to achieve a similar angular insertion depth, because the perimodiolar electrode array is placed along the "inside track" of the cochlea. To understand this concept, it is helpful to consider the staggered starting blocks used in track and field

races in which the runners race around the curves of the track. Runners who race in the inside lanes start behind the runners who race in the outside lanes, because the distance around the track within an inside lane is shorter than the distance around the track in an outside lane (Figure 7–12). The reader is referred to Chapter 2 for a discussion of differences in cochlear nerve innervation that exist for perimodiolar versus lateral electrode arrays.

It should also be noted that cochlear implant manufacturers also produce shorter electrode arrays with the objective of avoiding the most apical regions of the cochlea in order to preserve low-frequency acoustic hearing. The Cochlear Nucleus Hybrid L24 electrode array is almost 16 mm in length from the stopper to the apical tip (Figure 7–13). In contrast, the MED-EL FLEX20 is 20 mm in length from the cochleostomy marker to the apical tip (Figure 7–14). The Cochlear Hybrid L24 is designed for a typical angular insertion depth of approximately 240 to 250 degrees, whereas the typical angular insertion depth of the MED-EL FLEX20 is approximately 360 degrees. Of note, the aforementioned Nucleus CI522 Slim Straight electrode array has a secondary marker at 20 mm to allow for a more shallow insertion depth (360 degrees) than the standard 25 mm insertion (approximately 450–540 degrees). The 20-mm insertion depth is typically intended for Nucleus 522 recipients who

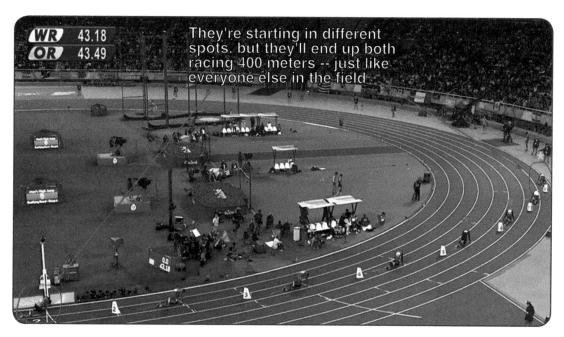

FIGURE 7–12. A visual analogy to demonstrate that a shorter distance is traveled making a loop around the inside lane of the track compared with the outside of the track.

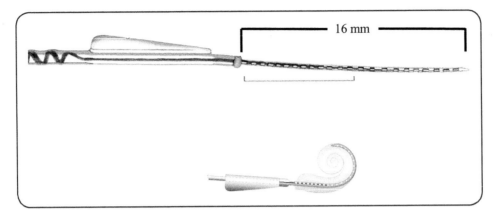

FIGURE 7–13. An example of short hybrid electrode array intended for hearing preservation. Image provided courtesy of Cochlear Americas, ©2018.

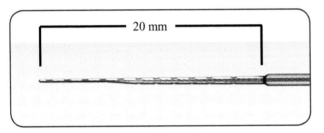

FIGURE 7–14. An example of hybrid electrode array intended for hearing preservation. Image provided courtesy of MED-EL Corporation.

have functional low-frequency acoustic hearing that is theoretically desirable to preserve.

Electrode arrays also differ across manufacturers in regard to the number of intracochlear electrode contacts contained within the array. All commercially available Cochlear Nucleus electrode arrays possess 22 intracochlear electrode contacts. Advanced Bionics cochlear implants possess 16 intracochlear electrode contacts, and MED-EL cochlear implants possess 12 different stimulating sites. Again, the differences in the number of intracochlear electrode contacts across manufacturers are largely based on philosophical differences of each company. Cochlear has sought to maximize the number of physical intracochlear electrode contacts that may be housed within the cochlea. In doing so, the 22 intracochlear electrode contacts within the Nucleus electrode arrays are typically spaced about 1 mm apart. In contrast, MED-EL's 12 stimulating sites are spaced a little over 2 mm apart with the retention of reducing the channel interaction that occurs when there is overlap in the electrical stimulation fields from neighboring electrode contacts. Of note, Cochlear contends that channel interaction is less of a concern for perimodiolar electrode arrays compared with lateral wall electrode arrays, because less electrical stimulation is required with the proximally located electrode contacts of a perimodiolar array.

Extracochlear Ground Electrode Contacts

All cochlear implant systems also contain ground electrode contacts, which serve as an **electrical ground** for stimulation and allow for the completion of an electrical circuit during stimulation. In the case of contemporary, commercially available cochlear implants, ground electrodes are **extracochlear electrodes,** which refers to the fact that they are located outside of the cochlea. A ground electrode may also be referred to as a **reference, return,** or **indifferent** electrode. During stimulation, electrical current is delivered from the current generator of the implant stimulator and then on to the intracochlear contact. As with all electrical circuits, after traveling to the intracochlear electrode contact, the current must travel to a return or ground (see Chapter 2 [p. ##] for a discussion on current flow through electrical circuits). Ground electrodes are also used as reference points for telemetry measurements such as electrode impedance assessment and the electrically evoked compound action potential (ECAP). Figure 7–15 shows an example of extracochlear ground electrodes. As shown, extracochlear ground electrodes may be housed on the body of the cochlear implant, as a ring located around the electrode leads, or at the tip of a separate lead.

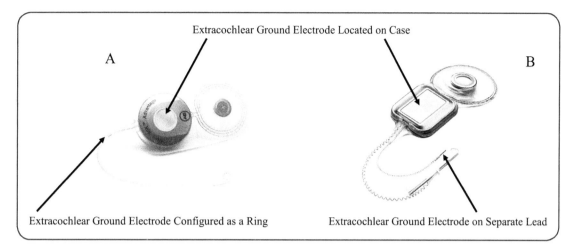

A

Extracochlear Ground Electrode Located on Case

B

Extracochlear Ground Electrode Configured as a Ring

Extracochlear Ground Electrode on Separate Lead

FIGURE 7–15. An example of extracochlear ground electrode contacts. Image provided courtesy of Cochlear, Ltd and Advanced Bionics, LLC.

Electrode Coupling Strategy/Stimulation Mode

The electrode coupling strategy, which is also referred to as the stimulation mode, indicates how channels are electrically connected to form a circuit through which current can be delivered to the cochlear nerve. As discussed in Chapter 2, in a complete electrical circuit, current travels from the power source to a resistive component and then to a return location. Cochlear implant stimulation must also be delivered through a complete circuit.

The "electrical circuit" in a cochlear implant consists of: (1) the signal/pulse generator in the internal processor (i.e., current source/output circuit/current generator), (2) the active electrode lead which travels from the signal generator to the intracochlear electrode contact, and (3) the return/ground electrode(s). Depending on the application, the audiologist's preferred terminology, and the manufacturer, the return electrodes also may be referred to as ground, indifferent, or reference electrodes. The electrode contact, cochlear fluids, and other tissues adjacent to the active electrode contact serve as the resistive elements in this circuit. The active electrode is always an intracochlear electrode and is ideally located in the scala tympani. In modern cochlear implants, the return electrode(s) usually is an extracochlear electrode (i.e., located outside of the cochlea). The return electrode is often located on the body of the cochlear implant (i.e., case of the internal stimulator). Alternatively, it may be located on the electrode lead, such as the ring electrode in the Advanced Bionics 90K

Advantage implant (see Figure 7–15A), or within a separate lead that terminates in an electrode contact that resides at a location remote from the cochlea, such as the MP2 reference electrode located at the end of the secondary lead of contemporary Cochlear Nucleus cochlear implants (see Figure 7–15B).

Types of Electrode Coupling/Stimulation Modes

Monopolar and Bipolar Electrode Coupling

Monopolar stimulation is a form of electrode coupling in which stimulation is provided to an active intracochlear electrode and an extracochlear electrode serves as the return (Figure 7–16). Monopolar stimulation is the default stimulation mode in all modern, commercially available cochlear implants. An alternative approach is *bipolar stimulation*, in which bipolar electrode coupling is employed so that electrical current is delivered to an active intracochlear electrode and a neighboring intracochlear electrode serves as the return (Figure 7–17). Specifically, bipolar stimulation (BP) occurs when the return electrode is positioned immediately adjacent to the active electrode. When the return and active electrodes are separated by one electrode contact, the bipolar stimulation is referred to as bipolar +1 (BP+1) (see Figure 7–17). BP+2 refers to bipolar coupling in which two electrode contacts separate the active and return electrodes; BP+3 refers to three electrode contacts separating the active and return electrodes; and so forth.

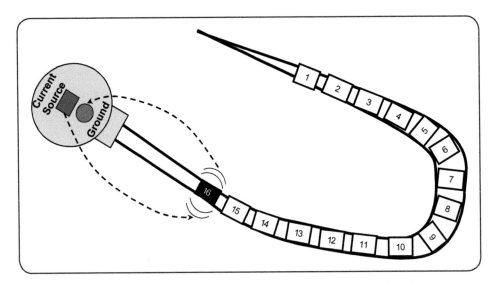

FIGURE 7–16. An illustration of monopolar electrode coupling where the single reference/ground electrode contact is located outside the cochlea and at a distance for the active (stimulating) intra-cochlear electrode contacts.

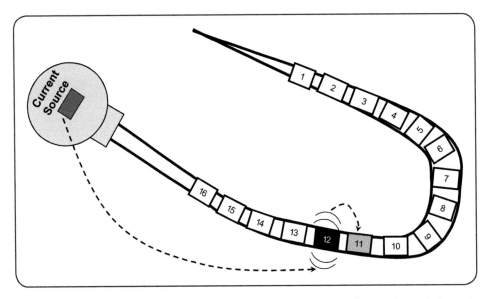

FIGURE 7–17. An illustration of bipolar electrode coupling where the reference/ground electrode contact is located inside the cochlea and in relatively close proximity to the active (stimulating) intra-cochlear electrode contacts.

Relative to monopolar stimulation, the electrical field of stimulation is narrower or more focused with bipolar stimulation, because the return electrode is located in close proximity to the active electrode. Theoretically, the narrower field of electrical stimulation associated with bipolar stimulation should result in less channel interaction compared with monopolar stimulation. However, the relatively narrow spread of electrical current that occurs with bipolar stimulation requires higher current levels (i.e., higher threshold and upper stimulation levels) to reach a given sound percept or loudness compared with monopolar stimulation. Thus, the higher current levels required for bipolar stimulation may offset the theoretical reduction in channel interaction that occurs with a narrower field of electrical stimulation. It should be specifically noted that the broader field of stimulation provided by monopolar coupling recruits a greater number of cochlear nerve fibers, which increases the *loudness* of the stimulation. Also, the higher current levels required for bipolar stimulation result in a reduction in battery life compared with monopolar stimulation. Furthermore, the broader stimulation pattern provided by monopolar stimulation results in a relatively gradual change in stimulation levels from one electrode to the next (i.e., electrical threshold [T levels] and upper stimulation [C/M/MCL] levels), so interpolation is a viable option in the monopolar mode (see explanation of interpolation later in this chapter). In contrast, stimulation requirements may change considerably from one electrode to the next with bipolar stimulation; therefore, the audiologist must measure electrical threshold and upper stimulation levels for all active electrodes. Although one may assume that the narrower field of stimulation associated with bipolar stimulation may provide better frequency resolution, it should be noted that monopolar stimulation allows for the provision of a tonotopic signal across the cochlea. Research has generally shown equivalent or better hearing performance outcomes with monopolar stimulation relative to bipolar (Pfingst et al., 2001; Zhu et al., 2012). Given the established advantages of monopolar stimulation over bipolar stimulation (e.g., lower current levels,

improvement in battery life, availability of interpolation), monopolar stimulation is the primary mode used with modern cochlear implants.

Common Ground Electrode Coupling

Common ground coupling is another electrode coupling mode used for diagnostic purposes, but it is not used for stimulation in commercially available signal coding strategies. In common ground coupling, electrical current is delivered to an active intracochlear electrode, and all of the remaining intracochlear electrodes serve as the collective return (Figure 7–18). Because all of the electrodes are coupled to one another electrically and because electrical resistance across these electrodes can be referenced to an extracochlear electrode serving as the ground (defined as zero voltage potential/reference potential), common ground coupling is the most sensitive mode to detect shorted electrodes during electrode impedance assessment.

Advanced Electrode Coupling Modes

Finally, cochlear implant researchers and manufacturers are exploring more advanced electrode coupling strategies, such as **tripolar coupling** and other higher-order coupling modes. The potential advantage of higher order coupling modes is to provide more focused stimulation to spiral ganglion dendrites

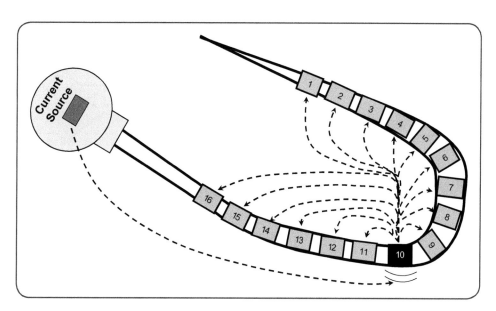

FIGURE 7–18. An illustration of common ground electrode coupling where every intracochlear electrode contact except for the stimulated electrode contact serves as a reference/ground electrode contact.

and cell bodies relative to monopolar or bipolar stimulation (Bierer & Middlebrooks, 2002; Bonham & Litvak, 2008). The primary theoretical appeal of tripolar stimulation is to reduce channel interaction and enhance frequency resolution. An example of tripolar stimulation is shown in Figure 7–19. With tripolar stimulation, current is delivered to one intracochlear electrode, and its two neighboring electrodes serve as the return electrodes. Each of these return electrodes receives half of the return current. At the time of this writing, however, no commercially available cochlear implant systems allow for these advanced methods of electrode coupling.

Electrode Impedance

Impedance refers to the resistance to the flow of energy through the medium of transmission. **Electrode impedance** is a measure of the opposition to electrical current flow through an electrode lead and across an electrode contact. It is important to note that electrode impedance is influenced not only by the physical properties of the electrode lead and contact but also by the medium surrounding the electrode lead and contact. The medium surrounding the electrode contact consists of cochlear fluids, cochlear tissues (fibrous, bony, etc.), electrolytes, macrophages, proteins, etc. The electrode impedance

measurement should be conducted at the beginning of every programming session. During the electrode impedance measurement, a relatively small electrical current, which is typically but not always inaudible to the recipient, is delivered sequentially to each active intracochlear electrode. Ohm's law is used to determine the impedance measured at each electrode contact.

Voltage (V) = Current (I) * Resistance (R)

The voltage used to deliver the electrical current to an electrode contact for the impedance measurement is a known and set value. Additionally, the electrical current that passes through the electrode contact and travels to the return electrode may be measured. As a result, two of the variables in the Ohm's law equation are known (i.e., voltage and current measured at the return electrode). As such, the electrode impedance may be calculated from Ohm's law. The actual impedance measure results are indicated by the current that returns to a reference electrode (also referred to as a ground or indifferent electrode) and how voltage is distributed to the stimulated electrode contact (and in some cases, the remaining intracochlear electrode contacts) relative to a reference electrode.

Electrode impedances should typically be greater than 1 kohm and less than 15 kohms. An electrode with an excessively low impedance (e.g., <1 kohm)

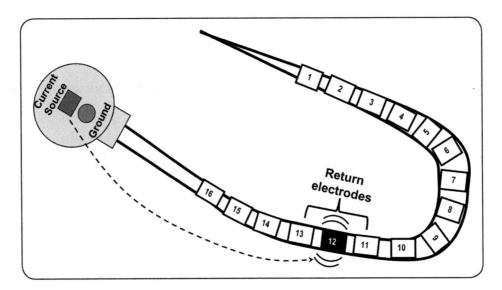

FIGURE 7–19. An illustration of tripolar electrode where electrical current is delivered to one intracochlear electrode contact and its two neighboring intracochlear electrode contacts serve as the reference/ground electrodes.

may indicate a **short circuit**. A short circuit refers to an establishment of relatively low resistance between two points in a circuit, which typically are separated by a much higher electrical resistance. Essentially, the term "short" means that two electrode leads/contacts are electrically coupled to one another in an unintended manner or through an unintended path. As a result, a shorted electrode is identified as two electrodes that are electrically connected, and consequently, an identical voltage is distributed to each electrode when only one is stimulated. Short circuits may be caused by physical contact between two electrode contacts or electrode leads, an electrical fault within the electrode lead/contact, an electrical fault within the circuit of the cochlear implant stimulator, or excessive distortion or tension on the array. Additionally, partial shorting may occur when fluid ingresses into the electrode leads or implant body and serves as a conductor to allow electrical current to travel in an unintended path. Fluid ingress may occur when the silicone insulation covering the electrode leads and/or implant body is torn. Fluid ingress may also occur if the hermetic (air-tight) seal of the implant case or feed-through channels (the ports through which the electrode leads leave the implant body and travel toward the electrode contacts) is compromised. Short circuits should be considered as persistent abnormalities, and consequently, short-circuited electrode contacts should be permanently disabled.

An electrode with an excessively high impedance (e.g., >30 kohms) is called an **open circuit**. Open circuits may be caused by anomalies (e.g., ossification) or by an air bubble or protein buildup in the electrode–tissue interface. Electrode impedances are often relatively high when the electrode contacts have not been stimulated for quite some time (i.e., at initial activation of the cochlear implant or after a long period of non-use by the recipient). This is most likely due to the presence of proteins/macrophages that have accumulated on the electrode contact and/or to the organization of the fibrous tissue surrounding the electrode contact. In most cases, electrode impedances will decrease substantially after electrical stimulation is delivered to the electrode contacts. As a result, the audiologist should not disable electrode contacts with modestly high electrode impedance values (e.g., 15 to 25 kohms) because these values will likely decrease with implant use.

Furthermore, open circuits may be caused by broken electrode leads or faulty electrode contacts. In this case, the electrode impedance will likely be measured at an infinitely high value. From a practical standpoint, the most recent version of each manufacturer's software identifies the presence of abnormal electrodes and "flags" them for management by the programming audiologist. Electrodes marked as open circuits should also be disabled but re-evaluated after a period of implant use.

Along with the absolute impedance value of each electrode, audiologists also may observe the morphology of electrode impedances (i.e., shape or change of impedances across the electrode array) and changes in impedance values across time. Ideally, electrode impedance values should be relatively similar across the electrode array or vary gradually (see Figure 7–20 for an example). Erratic electrode impedance patterns should be evaluated more closely.

It should be noted that electrode impedance is typically quite low at surgery because the electrode contacts are surrounded by cochlear fluid (e.g., perilymph). Electrode impedance often increases in the first few weeks following surgery due primarily to the buildup of proteins and macrophages on the electrode contacts as well as possibly to fibrous tissue growth in the cochlea following surgery (Hughes et al., 2001; Newbold et al., 2004). As previously discussed, it is normal for electrode impedances to be relatively high (e.g., 10 to 20 kohms) after periods of non-use. In these cases, a significant decrease in electrode impedance should occur within the first few days or even minutes of implant use. Electrode impedances will eventually stabilize during the first few weeks of electrical stimulation (Hughes et al., 2001; Newbold et al., 2004). If electrode impedance values continue to fluctuate after several months of use, the programming audiologist should monitor recipient performance closely and consider a referral to an otologist for medical evaluation. In this case, a representative of the manufacturer also should be notified. Persistently fluctuating electrode impedances may be attributed to changes within the cochlea (e.g., fibrous tissue growth), a change in the integrity and/or the electrochemical properties of the recipient's cochlear fluids and tissues (i.e., inflammation, hormonal changes, auto-immune reaction, etc.) (Wolfe et al., 2013), or a fault in the cochlear implant. The reader is encouraged to refer to Chapters 15, 16, and 17 for important and clinically relevant information pertaining to electrode impedance measurement specific to each cochlear implant manufacturer.

Electrode conditioning is a feature available in some implant systems that allows for the presenta-

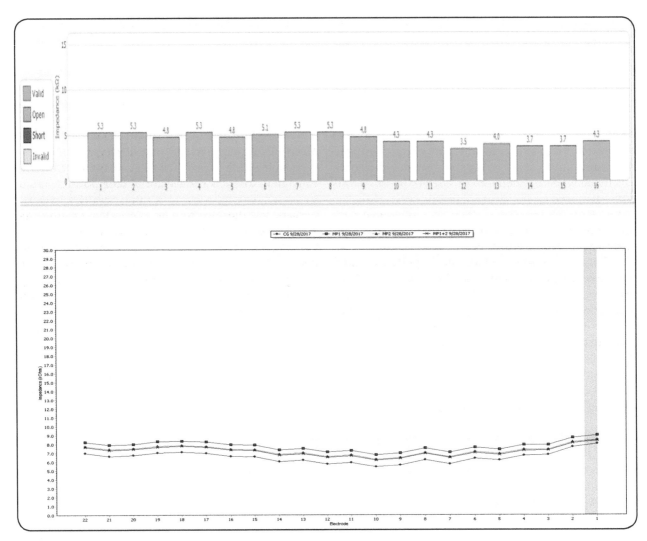

FIGURE 7–20. A visual example of electrode impedance test results.

tion of low-level current to each electrode to remove air bubbles, protein buildup, and so forth. Electrode conditioning is typically only needed prior to testing in the operating room, at initial activation, at a programming session preceded by a prolonged period of non-use, or when activating and stimulating electrodes that were previously disabled.

Abnormal electrode impedance values may compromise sound quality or produce non-auditory sensations, such as facial nerve stimulation. Other detrimental effects associated with the use of abnormal electrodes include poor speech recognition performance, inadequate loudness growth, sudden changes in loudness, and potential discomfort. Of note, electrode contacts with higher electrode impedance values generally possess relatively lower volt-

age compliance levels and higher stimulation current levels (as predicted by Ohm's law). In other words, *electrode contacts with higher impedance values require higher current levels to achieve a satisfactory loudness percept.*

Numerous reasons for changes or fluctuations in impedance exist. For instance, the electrode array may become displaced or may be moved over time. If the electrode array retracts and partially pulls into the middle ear space, the electrode contacts that move outside of the cochlea will likely possess higher electrode impedance values because they are surrounded by air rather than cochlear fluid. Also, ossification or fibrous tissue may arise in the cochlea after implantation and alter the electrode–neural tissue interface, resulting in a change in electrode impedance. A

Stenver's x-ray or a computed tomography (CT) scan (conventional or ideally a 64-slice three-dimensional image) may be useful in evaluating changes in electrode locations or anatomy of the cochlea. In general, imaging to evaluate the position of the electrode array should be considered if unexplained abnormal electrode results exist or if a sudden unexplained change in electrode impedance occurs. Additionally, changes in a recipient's hormonal levels, which may occur during adolescence, pregnancy, menopause, or hormonal therapy (e.g., testosterone supplementation), may result in a change in electrode impedances (Wolfe et al., 2013). The audiologist should consider these conditions in light of fluctuating or changing electrode impedance results.

Finally, a "normal" electrode impedance value does not necessarily imply that all is well. Figure 7–21 provides an example of an electrode impedance assessment in which the absolute values are within normal limits but the morphology is unusual and indicative of a potential problem. Specifically, all of the odd-numbered electrode contacts possess lower impedance values than the even-numbered values, creating a sawtooth pattern. Most likely, fluid has ingressed into the cochlear implant case and has caused partial shorting across all of the odd-numbered electrode leads, which are all wired on the same side of the case but on the opposite side of the case as the even-numbered electrodes.

Furthermore, it should be noted that an absolute electrode impedance value that is within normal limits does not even indicate that the electrode contact is within the cochlea. The audiologist should remember that the electrode impedance indicates how electrical current flows across an electrode contact to surrounding tissues or fluid. A "normal" electrode impedance value may be obtained when an electrode is in contact with middle ear tissue or fluids or body tissue remote from the cochlea. Again, it is important for the programming audiologist to review the cochlear implant surgeon's postoperative report and/or postoperative x-ray to determine whether all of the stimulating electrode contacts are inserted into the cochlea. Indeed, the authors of this book have encountered recipients who have had normal electrode impedance values across the array but have had electrode contacts residing in the middle ear space or even, in one exceptional case, in the cerebellopontine angle. In cases in which the recipient reports unusual or undesirable effects associated with stimulation of certain electrodes (e.g., no auditory sensation, signs of facial nerve stimulation, tactile sensation) the audiologist

should refer the recipient for imaging to evaluate the placement of the electrode array.

Telemetry

Telemetry refers to the process of using special equipment to make measurements of a certain property and send the data from the measurement to another place by radio signal (Merriam-Webster, 2018). Within the realm of implantable hearing technology, telemetry refers to the transmission of data through radio frequency communication to and from the internal implant via the electromagnetic induction link. As mentioned in Chapters 1 and 3, cochlear implants transmit signals across the scalp via near-field magnetic induction at a given **radio frequency (RF)**. The term RF is used to express the carrier frequency of the electromagnetic induction (radio) signal on which the signal of interest is modulated. Some cochlear implant systems use a single RF to transmit signals both to and from the internal device, but the Advanced Bionics Corporation uses one RF for forward transmission and a second RF for backward transmission. It is very important to also remember that the electromagnetic (RF) signal is also used to power the cochlear implant, which does not possess its own power source.

Telemetry is not only used to send the signal of interest to the internal device for eventual stimulation, but additionally, telemetry is used during the programming session to deliver signals (i.e., T level stimuli) to the implant. Finally, backward telemetry may be used to transmit signals from the internal device to the external coil, sound processor, and programming computer. Backward telemetry allows the audiologist to evaluate the integrity of the internal device (e.g., electrode impedance measurement) and to measure responses from the cochlear nerve (e.g., electrically evoked compound action potentials such as neural response telemetry [NRT], neural response imaging [NRI], and Auditory Response Telemetry [ART]). Telemetry may also be used to determine the amount of power required for the external sound processor to deliver to the internal device to allow for satisfactory operation. Similarly, telemetry allows for an estimation of battery life during typical daily use.

The terms "lock" and "link" are often used to specify successful radio communication (i.e., telemetry) between the internal and external processors. "Failure to obtain lock/link" happens when the signal cannot be transmitted from the external processor to the internal processor or vice versa.

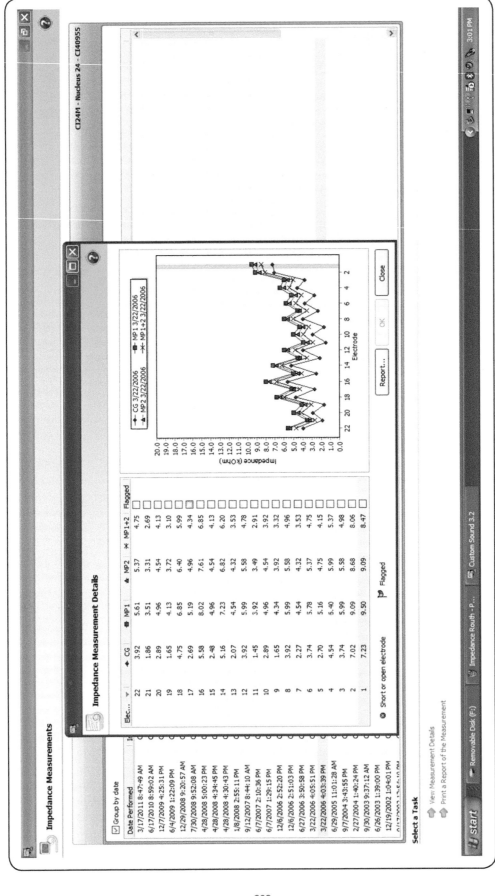

FIGURE 7–21. A visual example of electrode impedance test results. An abnormal pattern of electrode impedances is observed in this example.

208

Factors That Influence the Electrical Coding of Frequency and Pitch

Electrode Contact Versus Channel

As previously discussed, the term *intracochlear electrode contact* describes a physical contact where electrical current stimulation is delivered to stimulate the cochlear nerve. Frequency information in the incoming acoustic signal is primarily conveyed by the place of stimulation within the cochlea. Cochlear implant signal coding strategies take advantage of the tonotopic organization of the typically functioning cochlea by delivering low-frequency inputs to electrode contacts located in the apical end of the cochlea and high-frequency inputs to electrode contacts located in the basal end of the cochlea. As a result, **the primary mechanism used to code the frequency of the acoustic signal and to convey pitch is the location (i.e., place of stimulation) of the intracochlear electrode contact that is stimulated.** Stimulation of apically located electrode contacts typically elicits a low-pitch sensation, whereas stimulation of basally located electrode contacts typically elicits a high-pitch sensation.

A **channel** describes a discrete frequency range over which sound is analyzed for eventual delivery to an electrode contact. Channels are defined by analysis bands or bandpass filters with a relatively steep roll-off (although some overlap does exist between neighboring channels). In many cases, electrode contacts and stimulation are similar. For example, inputs that are processed through channel 1 are delivered to electrode contact number 1. In other rare cases, the channel number and electrode number may be different. For example, inputs processed through channel 1 may actually be delivered to electrode 2, and inputs processed through channel 2 are delivered to electrode 1. In the latter case, adjustments were made to improve the patient's tonotopic organization. The subject's pitch percept did not transition in the expected low-to-high manner when stimulation was swept across the electrodes. Therefore, switching the channel to electrode assignment restored the desired tonotopic organization. **Double channel mapping** is another example in which the inputs from two channels are delivered to one electrode (Figure 7–22); again, however, the need for double channel mapping is more the exception rather than the rule.

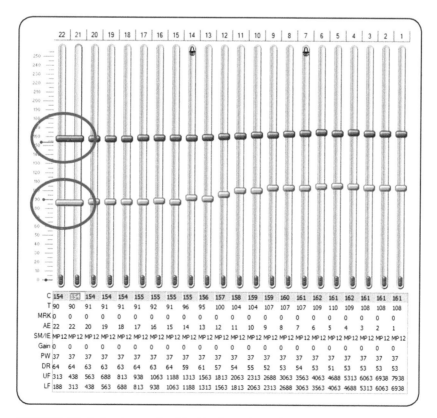

FIGURE 7–22. A visual example of double channel mapping.

Virtual Electrodes (Current Steering)

In an attempt to provide a greater number of sites of stimulation across the cochlea, Advanced Bionics and MED-EL promote the use of an alternative approach known as virtual electrodes or current steering. In the Advanced Bionics **current-steering** approach, two neighboring physical intracochlear electrode contacts are stimulated simultaneously, resulting in a focal provision of stimulation between the two contacts. As shown in Figure 7–23A, when two neighboring electrodes are stimulated simultaneously with equal magnitude of electrical current, the locus of stimulation falls within the middle of the two electrode contacts. If the magnitude of electrical stimulation is greater at one of the electrode contacts, then the locus of stimulation will occur closer to that electrode (Figure 7–23B). Steering current by delivering electrical pulses to two neighboring electrode contacts in order to generate a locus of stimulation that calls between the two physical contacts is sometimes referred to as the creation of **virtual channels**.

Intermediate pitches also can be created using sequential stimulation, as implemented in the current MED-EL approach, and require the use of bell-shaped overlapping bandpass filters to elicit pitch percepts that shift gradually within and across channels along the electrode array. In essence, the shifting of the locus of stimulation when two neighboring intracochlear electrode contacts are stimulated very closely in time creates a virtual channel that falls within the two physical electrode contacts. Additionally, it should be noted that the Cochlear Nucleus implant has the capability of applying current steering through sequential stimulation, but at this point, the approach is not used in commercially available signal coding strategies.

The primary objective of the virtual electrode/ current-steering approach is to increase the spectral-resolution abilities of recipients. As discussed in Chapter 2, the normal cochlea contains about 3,500 inner hair cells, each of which is tonotopically tuned to one individual frequency and one corresponding afferent cochlear nerve fiber. This exquisite design of the normal peripheral auditory system allows for discrimination between acoustic components that differ by approximately 1 to 2 Hz (Wier, Jesteadt, & Green, 1977). Adept spectral resolution is critical for discrimination of the different phones of speech (e.g., consonants that differ on the basis of place cues), optimal recognition of melodies and enjoyment of

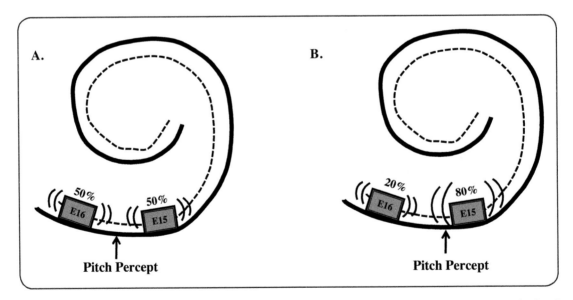

FIGURE 7–23. Illustration of current steering. **A.** Two neighboring intracochlear electrode contacts are stimulated simultaneously with equal magnitude, resulting in the primary locus of stimulation occurs in the middle of the two stimulating electrode contacts. **B.** Two neighboring intracochlear electrode contacts are stimulated simultaneously but the more apical electrode contact of the two receives a greater magnitude of electrical current resulting in the primary locus of stimulation occurring closer to electrode contact receiving the greater amount of electrical current.

music, pitch perception, and speech recognition in the presence of competing noise. Given the fact that cochlear implants provide far fewer physical stimulation sites than the number of transduction sites in normal ear (12 to 22 physical electrode contacts versus 3,500 inner hair cells), the concept of virtual electrodes (current steering) is an attempt to increase the spectral fidelity of the signal delivered to the cochlear nerve. The clinical implementation of this concept in modern signal coding strategies and cochlear implant systems along with expected clinical benefit is discussed in Chapter 8.

Frequency Allocation

As the name implies, the parameter **frequency allocation** determines how input sound frequencies are assigned to particular analysis bands (i.e., active channels). In the Advanced Bionics cochlear implants, frequency allocation is determined automatically by the programming software. If an electrode is disabled, the frequencies then are reallocated to existing active electrodes. In the Nucleus devices, adjustment of the frequency allocation parameter affects the higher limit (or the highest frequency to be delivered to the most basal electrode), as well as the width of analysis bands in the mid-frequency channels. In other words, high-frequency limit of the bandwidth is reduced (for example, from almost 8000 Hz to 7000 Hz), and the remaining restricted bandwidth (i.e., 188 to 7000 Hz) is allocated across the same number of channels, allowing for channels with narrower analysis bands. The potential virtue of narrower analysis bands is an enhancement in frequency resolution. Specifically, narrower analysis bands reduce the chance that sounds of two different frequencies will be processed within the same channel.

An additional parameter in the Nucleus programming software, referred to as "edit frequency boundaries," allows the audiologist to specify the exact cut-off frequencies of each channel. In the MED-EL device, audiologists may change the lower (70 to 350 Hz) and higher (3500 to 8500 Hz) frequency limits in 10 and 500 Hz intervals, respectively. Also, audiologists can select from four different frequency allocation tables that are each based on different psychoacoustically derived approaches. Additional information on the frequency allocation for the Advanced Bionics, Nucleus, and MED-EL devices is provided in Chapters 15, 16, and 17, respectively.

Factors That Influence the Electrical Coding of Duration/Time

Stimulation Rate

As previously discussed, commercially available cochlear implant systems deliver trains of biphasic electrical pulses to the intracochlear electrode contacts. The **stimulation rate** typically refers to the number of biphasic pulses that are delivered to <u>an individual electrode contact</u> within one second and is specified in **pulses per second** (pps). In other words, stimulation rate refers to the number of electrical pulses presented per channel per second. The earliest multiple channel cochlear implants had relatively slow stimulation rates (i.e., 250 pps or less), but contemporary systems allow for much higher stimulation rates (i.e., up to about 5000 pps). One of the theoretical benefits of faster stimulation rates is potential to provide fine temporal structure cues. The temporal properties of acoustic signals may be categorized into two broad classes, amplitude envelope cues and fine temporal structure cues. The amplitude envelope describes relatively slow changes or fluctuations in the intensity of an acoustic signal. Amplitude envelope cues typically occur on the order of about 2 to 50 Hz (Rosen, 1989). In contrast, fine temporal structure describes the rapid changes in the intensity fluctuations of the acoustic signal. Fine temporal structure cues occur on the order of about 100 to several thousand Hz (Rosen, 1989). The reader is directed to Figure 7–24 for a visual illustration of amplitude envelope and fine temporal structure. The amplitude envelope is likely the dominant temporal cue used to understand running speech in quiet (Smith, Delgutte, & Oxenham, 2002). In contrast, fine temporal structure is the more important temporal cue for the recognition of melody in music, for the vocal pitch, and possibly for speech recognition in noise (Smith, Delgutte, & Oxenham, 2002). Furthermore, in some cases, the amplitude envelope and spectrum of some speech sounds are similar; therefore, the listener must rely on differences in fine temporal structure to discern among sounds. The use of stimulation rates above a few hundred Hz theoretically possesses the potential to convey the fine temporal structure of an acoustic signal.

Aside from coding temporal cues, changes in stimulation rate also can result in changes in the user's pitch and intensity percepts. Specifically, faster

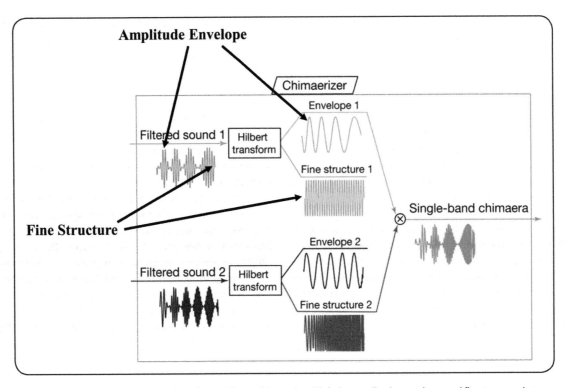

FIGURE 7–24. A visual representation of an auditory chimera in which the amplitude envelope and fine temporal structure are extracted from the original signal. Reprinted with permission from Smith, Delgutte, and Oxenham, "Chimaeric sounds reveal dichotomies in auditory perception," *Nature*, (2002), *416*(6876), 87–90. Copyright © Springer.

stimulation rates often result in a louder signal due to temporal summation and a higher pitch percept, particularly as rate is increased from 50 to 500 Hz. In fact, one of the theoretical underpinnings of the MED-EL Fine Structure Processing (FSP) signal coding strategy is the attempt to enhance both spectral/pitch and temporal resolution in the low-frequency channels by adjusting the stimulation rate to coincide with the frequency of the input signal. The reader is referred to the discussion of signal coding strategies in Chapter 8 for additional coverage of the theoretical advantages and limitations of the use of variable and/or fast (e.g., beyond 1500 pps) stimulation rates to convey fine temporal structure.

Additionally, as discussed in Chapter 3, stimulation of the cochlear nerve with electrical pulses results in a highly synchronous compound response from cochlear nerve units (i.e., individual nerve fibers/bodies) adjacent to the electrode contact. In other words, for an initial electrical pulse, all or the vast majority of the cochlear nerve units in the vicinity of the stimulating electrode contact fire in response to the stimulus, and then they all enter their refractory periods at the same time. In contrast, the normal

auditory system responds in a stochastic manner to acoustic stimulation. A stochastic response occurs when some (but not all) cochlear nerve fibers are excited in response to an individual acoustic stimulus. This stochastic response results in a refractory state for some fibers and an active state for others. As a subsequent acoustic stimulus arrives, the nerve fibers that did not initially fire will be able to respond, while the fibers that responded to the original stimulus are in their refractory or recovery periods (i.e., the so-called volley principle discussed in Chapter 3).

It has been suggested that this stochastic behavior of the cochlear nerve to acoustic stimuli allows for the coding of the pitch of a sound (Moller, 2001, 2013). The normal auditory system is capable of following changes in amplitude of an acoustic signal in a time-locked manner (Moller, 2001, 2013; Moore, 2003). This property of the normal auditory system may be beneficial because it theoretically allows the system to follow high-frequency stimuli in a per-cycle manner and provides for the acquisition of fine temporal structure. Moller (2001, 2013) also contends that the temporal response of the cochlear nerve plays a critical role in the processing of pitch and frequency. He notes that a cochlear nerve unit cannot respond to each individual cycle of a stimulus because some fibers are still in a refractory state. Fibers likely respond to multiples of the incoming stimulus rate. However, the cochlear nerve units collectively are able to follow the stimulus on a cycle-by-cycle rate. This phenomenon has previously been referred to as the "volley approach."

When using electrical stimulation rates below 2000 pps, the cochlear nerve fires in a highly synchronous manner. Because the cochlear nerve fibers are firing in unison, and subsequently possess a simultaneous refractory period, the auditory system is unable to follow rapid changes in a stimulus (i.e., fine temporal structure). Some researchers have suggested that at stimulation rates above 2000 pps, the cochlear nerve is more likely to assume stochastic firing, and as a result, a higher probability exists that the nerve units will respond in a volley-type fashion to follow fine temporal structure cues (Rubinstein et al., 2001).

In reality, a paucity of research demonstrates consistent improvements in patient performance when stimulation rates exceed 1500 pps. There are only a handful of published studies that suggest that rates exceeding 1500 pps provide improvement in speech recognition. For instance, two groups of researchers reported that subjects who converted from slower (800–1600 pps) to faster (5000 pps) coding strategies achieved better speech recognition (Dunn, Tyler, Witt, & Gantz, 2006; Koch, Osberger, Segel, & Kessler, 2004). However, the subjects in the Koch et al. study had a longer duration of experience with the higher rate coding strategy; therefore, the improvement may be attributed to learning effects. Also, in both studies, the faster strategy provided twice as many stimulation sites (i.e., intracochlear electrode contacts) and had a more sophisticated automatic gain control (AGC). As a result, other signal processing variables may have been responsible for performance gains.

Most researchers who have explored performance changes as a function of stimulation rate have concluded that the optimal stimulation rate varies on an individual basis, but in general, stimulation rates above approximately 1500 pps do not provide improvements in speech recognition in quiet or in noise (Arora, Dawson, Dowell, & Vandali, 2009; Balkany et al., 2007; Buchner, Frohne-Buchner, Battmer, & Lenarz, 2004; Vandali, Whitford, Plant, & Clark, 2000; Verschuur, 2005; Weber et al., 2007). Verschuur (2005) evaluated speech recognition at stimulation rates of 400, 800, and approximately 1500 pps for a group of MED-EL recipients. He reported that speech recognition generally improved as stimulation rate was increased from 400 to 800 pps, but no additional improvement in mean group performance was typically observed with an increase from 800 to 1500 pps. However, Verschuur did note that two subjects did show evidence of better performance with the faster stimulation rate (1500 pps). He concluded that individualized optimization of rate may be helpful to achieve the best outcomes for cochlear implant recipients.

The largest and most well-controlled study on the effect of stimulation rate on speech recognition and user preference was conducted with 71 Nucleus Freedom recipients. In this study, Balkany et al. (2007) evaluated speech recognition in quiet and in noise as well as subjective preference obtained with a wide variety of stimulation rates ranging from 500 to 3500 pps. There was not a significant difference in speech recognition obtained between the different stimulation rates. Furthermore, recipients tended to prefer the slower rates (500 Hz to 1800 pps) over the faster stimulation rates (2400 pps to 3500 pps).

Also, Weber et al. (2007) compared speech recognition at three different stimulation rates (500, 1200, and 3500 pps) with 13 recipients who used a prototype of the Nucleus 5 sound processor. Similar to the Balkany (2007) study, Weber and colleagues (2007) reported that no improvement in speech recognition was observed with rate increases from 500 to 1200 pps and from 1200 to 3500 pps. Plant et al. (2007) also evaluated speech recognition at different stimulation rates for 15 adult recipients using a prototype of the Nucleus 5 sound processor. These subjects typically preferred slower stimulation rates, but certain exceptions did exist in which a faster stimulation rate was used (2400 to approximately 3000 pps). The researchers concluded that faster stimulation rates did not improve the speech recognition of Nucleus users. Like Verschuur (2005), Balkany et al. (2007), Weber et al. (2007), and Plant (2007) concluded that differences in optimal stimulation rate are likely to exist across recipients, but in most cases, optimal performance is achieved with stimulation rates of 1200 pps and lower.

Buechner and colleagues (2010) also evaluated speech recognition as a function of stimulation rate for 13 users of the Advanced Bionics HiResolution cochlear implant system. Performance was assessed at 1500, 2500, 3000, and 5000 pps. These authors also reported limited to no mean improvement in speech recognition as stimulation rate was increased from

1500 to 5000 pps. Additionally, speech recognition tended to decrease when rate was increased from 2500 to 5000 pps. Buechner and colleagues did note that considerable intersubject variability existed in regard to the stimulation rate that yielded the best performance, which suggested that the optimal stimulation may vary on a recipient-by-recipient basis.

Likewise, Firjns et al. (2003) also assessed speech recognition in a group of Advanced Bionics CII recipients and concluded that increases in stimulation rates up to 1500 pps produced improvements in speech recognition for most subjects, but as a group, further increases typically resulted in no further improvement. Again, there were some subjects who did show modest improvement at higher rates.

Nie, Barco, and Zeng (2006) evaluated speech recognition as a function of stimulation rate (ranging from 1000–4000 Hz) for five MED-EL implant recipients. They reported a mean improvement on word recognition and sentence recognition in noise with the faster stimulation rates. The authors also noted that there was variability in the benefit of faster stimulation rates obtained across the five subjects.

In summary, a review of peer-reviewed published research suggests that stimulation rates up to several hundred pulses per second seem to be beneficial for all cochlear implant users. Research suggests that the optimal rate varies by recipient, with some individuals achieving maximum performance with and reporting a preference for rates of a few hundred pps, whereas others prefer and perform optimally with rates of up to 5000 pps (Buchner et al., 2004). Again, most recipients do not show improvements in performance with rates exceeding 1500 pps. In short, most cochlear implant users are likely to achieve satisfactory performance with stimulation rates between 500 and 1500 pps. For example, most recipients of Nucleus implants perform very well at the Nucleus default stimulation rate of 900 pps. Additionally, most Advanced Bionics and MED-EL recipients perform quite well with stimulation rates between 1000 and 1500 pps. If, however, a recipient is struggling to make progress with a stimulation rate in the 500 to 1500 pps range, the audiologist should explore whether slower or faster stimulation rates will improve performance.

Of note, the relationship between stimulation rate and recipient performance may be influenced by the technical capabilities of the cochlear implant. To optimize the delivery of high-rate electrical pulses, the current sources of the implant's internal device must be able to generate electrical pulse with narrow pulse widths with high current amplitudes. It is possible that the current generator of a particular cochlear implant may be better suited to achieve this task, and if so, then it is reasonable to expect that recipients of such a system may have a greater potential to benefit from high-frequency stimulation rates. In contrast, a system that is unable to generate a high-amplitude electrical pulse with a short pulse width may be less capable to provide adequate stimulation at higher stimulation rates. It is important to note that recipients who require a wider pulse width to elicit a satisfactory loudness percept may not be able to use high stimulation rates. When the pulse width is made wider (i.e., longer in duration), it might not be possible to deliver several thousand pulses within one second of time, because the wider pulses take too much time to deliver. As a result, the stimulation rate may need to be reduced when using a wider pulse width.

Also, the spacing between electrode contacts may influence a recipient's performance with higher stimulation rates, as closer spacing may increase the likelihood of temporal channel interaction. More specifically, a faster stimulation rate may cause undesirable electrical interaction between two neighboring channels, because the faster rate coupled with the close proximity of the neighboring electrode contacts increases the likelihood that two pulses will overlap in both space and time. Indeed, one study found an increase in speech recognition when very fast stimulation rates (e.g., 5000 pps) were used (relative to slower stimulation rates) on an 8-channel program (every other electrode contact disabled) but no improvement was observed when very fast stimulation rates were used with a 16-channel program in which all active electrode contacts are enabled (Buchner et al., 2004).

Furthermore, the sampling rate of the digital signal processor within the external sound processor must be fast enough to capture the fast fluctuations occurring in the input signal (i.e., per the Nyquist theorem, the sampling rate must be at least twice as high as the highest frequency of interest in the incoming sound). If the sampling rate is not fast enough to capture the fine temporal structure cues in the acoustic signal, then a faster stimulation rate will obviously not provide any benefit in the recognition of those fast temporal structure cues. For example, if the digital signal processor samples the incoming acoustic signal at a sampling rate of 400 Hz, then the Nyquist theorem indicates that the processor will only be able to faithfully capture intensity fluctuations up to 200 Hz (Nyquist, 1928). As a result, the cochlear implant will not be able to convey fine temporal structure information in the acoustic signal beyond 200 Hz, regardless of how fast the stimulation rate is. More research is needed to explore the potential benefits and limitations of high stimulation rates across the variety of cochlear implant systems available on the commercial market. The optimal stimulation rate may vary not only across recipients but also by device characteristics.

It should be noted that fast stimulation rates (e.g., several thousand pps) may occasionally be associated with undesirable results. Vandali et al. (2000) evaluated speech recognition in quiet and in noise at stimulation rates of 250, 807, and 1615 pps. They reported that speech recognition actually decreased as the stimulation rate was increased from 807 to 1615 pps. Additionally, they reported that higher stimulation rates were associated with a harsher sound quality for some subjects. Furthermore, one subject developed severe tinnitus at the highest stimulation rate.

Anecdotally, the authors of this text have encountered some recipients who experience similar negative effects with faster stimulation rates. For example, some recipients have reported the impression of an echo, vibration, harshness, a tinny quality, and/or distortion when rates of several thousand pps are employed. A common belief among cochlear implant programming audiologists is that faster stimulation rates are more likely to be detrimental for the very elderly, recipients with an aplastic/deficient auditory nerve, recipients with neural dysfunction (e.g., auditory neuropathy neuropathy spectrum disorder [ANSD]), and those with long (greater than 30 years) duration of deafness. Although there is some evidence to suggest that slower stimulation rates may be beneficial for recipients with the aforementioned characteristics (Pelosi et al., 2012), there are no large, well-designed published studies that conclusively corroborate this hypothesis.

In summary, the authors of this book tend to select stimulation rates between 900 and 1500 pps. Specific recommendations pertaining to stimulation rate for cochlear implant systems of different manufacturers are provided in Chapters 15 to 17. For recipients who experience difficulties with stimulation rates within a range of 900 to 1500 pps (or the stimulation rate recommended by the manufacturer), the authors will attempt to determine the optimal stimulation rate to maximize the recipients' performance. In cases in which stimulation rates are individually optimized, the authors will typically allow

the recipient to listen to programs with a variety of stimulation rates (e.g., 250 pps, 500 pps, 900–1000 pps, 1500 pps, 2000 pps, 3000 pps) to determine the rate that yields the best sound quality and speech recognition. In cases in which the recipient is uncertain of which stimulation rate is the best, the authors will provide multiple programs (each with a different stimulation rate) to allow the recipient to trial/experiment with a variety of stimulation rates in real world settings. Finally, despite the presence of conclusive evidence supporting the tactic, the authors do tend to gravitate toward slower stimulation rates for recipients who have evidence of auditory nerve dysfunction (e.g., ANSD, auditory nerve dysplasia) as well as for recipients who are very elderly or who have a long duration of deafness and are struggling to make satisfactory progress with stimulation rates in the range of 900 to 1500 pps.

It should be noted that manufacturers also frequently refer to an implant's **total stimulation rate**, or the overall maximum rate of stimulation possible, across all active electrodes within one second. Total stimulation rate usually is calculated by determining the product of the per-channel stimulation rate and the number of active channels stimulated for an incoming stimulus (per-channel stimulation rate * number of active channels stimulated = total stimulation rate). For example, if an incoming sound is delivered to 10 channels, and the per-channel stimulation rate is 900 pps, the total stimulation rate is 9000 pps.

The maximum total stimulation rate is sometimes determined by the number of pulses per second the implant is capable of delivering. For example, the total stimulation rate for the Advanced Bionics 90K implant is just over 80,000 pps (i.e., approximately 5000 pps for each channel * 16 channels = approximately 80,000 pps total stimulation rate). There are, however, exceptions to this rule. For instance, the Nucleus Freedom and CI512 devices are capable of a total stimulation rate of 32,000 pps. However, when the default Advanced Combination Encoder (ACE) signal coding strategy is selected, the total stimulation rate is 7200 pps (900 pps for each channel * 8 channels selected on each stimulation cycle). This limited total stimulation rate for ACE is historically based. When ACE was developed for commercial use, the Nucleus 24 implant was the internal device available at the time, and it was capable of a total stimulation rate of only 14,400 pps. The audiologist may access higher total stimulation rates in modern Nucleus cochlear implants (up to 3500 pps for each channel).

Basic Terminology of Cochlear Implant Programming and Processing

The following pages in this chapter introduce and discuss several terms and concepts associated with cochlear implant programming and processing. Many of these terms may be unfamiliar to the reader, because the clinical practices and technology surrounding cochlear implants vary from other audiology clinical practices and hearing technologies. The audiologist must have a thorough understanding of these terms and technologies in order to provide optimal service to cochlear implant recipients.

Stimulation Levels and the Electrical Dynamic Range

In most cases, the most important parameters an audiologist determines when programming a recipient's cochlear implant are the stimulation levels provided from the implant to the cochlear nerve. The fundamental goal of programming is to restore audibility for a range of speech sounds extending from soft speech to loud speech as well as for low- to high-level environmental sounds. Ideally, stimulation levels also are set to optimize the identification of speech sounds. Typically, speech recognition and sound quality are optimized when the maximum stimulation levels provided at each electrode contact are balanced in loudness across the electrode array. Finally, it is desirable to set stimulation levels so that normal loudness percepts are restored for speech in addition to environmental sounds. Sounds that are perceived as soft to a person with normal-hearing sensitivity also should sound soft to a cochlear implant user, while sounds that are perceived as loud for a person with normal-hearing sensitivity also should be loud, but not uncomfortable to the user.

Achieving the aforementioned goals is not an easy task because the intensity range spanning from the lowest level sounds heard by persons with normal hearing to the highest level sounds encountered in everyday situations is approximately 100 dB. This wide range of acoustic intensities must be coded into the relatively narrow **electrical dynamic range (EDR)** of the cochlear implant recipient. The EDR is defined as the difference between the cochlear implant user's perceptual threshold and most comfortable level (i.e., loud but not uncomfortable) for electrical stimulation. The EDR may be converted to decibels. The reader should note that the acoustic decibel customarily represents the log of the ratio between a measured sound pressure level (in dynes or pascals, which are units of measurement for sound pressure) and a reference value (e.g., 20 micropascals). Decibels may also be calculated by measuring the electrical voltage output of a microphone relative to a reference voltage value (e.g., 0.775 volts). In a similar way, the EDR may be converted to a decibel value. Research has suggested that the typical EDR is often around 10 to 25 dB when converted from electrical stimulation levels to decibels (Nelson, Schmitz, Donaldson, Viemeister, & Javel, 1996; Zeng & Galvin, 1999). Cochlear implant manufacturers use various types of audio compression to code the acoustical inputs of interest into the recipient's individual EDR. The following section introduces programming parameters related to the electrical dynamic range, while the next section discusses parameters associated with the acoustic input dynamic range.

Threshold of Stimulation

The **threshold of electrical stimulation** refers to the least amount of stimulation a recipient can detect when electrical signals (typically biphasic electrical pulses) are delivered to individual electrode contacts. In practice, the exact definition and name of the electrical threshold of stimulation vary across cochlear implant manufacturers. For Advanced Bionics cochlear implants, the electrical threshold is comparable to the audiometric threshold and is best defined as the lowest amount of electrical stimulation a user can detect with 50% accuracy. For the Cochlear Nucleus cochlear implant (henceforth referred to as the Nucleus cochlear implant), the electrical threshold is defined as the minimum amount of electrical stimulation the recipient can detect 100% of the time. In contrast, MED-EL defines electrical threshold as the highest level of electrical stimulation at which a response is not obtained (i.e., the amount of electrical stimulation just below that which elicits an audible percept). The electrical threshold is referred to as "**T level**" for Advanced Bionics and Nucleus and "THR" or "threshold" level in MED-EL devices.

In adults and older children, the measurement of electrical threshold is relatively straightforward and involves psychophysical measures frequently used in diagnostic audiology. The signal used to measure stimulation levels is typically a "train" of biphasic, rectangular electrical pulses occurring at the same stimulation rate used for stimulation by the cochlear implant during everyday use. The train of electrical pulses usually is presented with an on/off duty cycle of 300 to 500 milliseconds (e.g., the electrical pulse train is presented with a duration of one-half second and off for one-half of a second) with a presentation of two to three pulse trains per signal delivery (Figure 7–25). Most commonly, recipients are instructed to raise their hands or say "yes" when they hear the pulsed programming signal. To a cochlear implant user, this signal is usually perceptually similar to a beep or tone used in pure-tone audiometric assessment (i.e., they perceive two to three "beeps" during each signal presentation), although in relatively rare cases, the recipient may describe the signal as possessing a different characteristic, such as a scratchy/static noise-like percept or a buzzing sound. A persistent (i.e., throughout the several weeks of implant use) report that the programming possesses a static noise-like quality may suggest that stimulation is being delivered to an area of the cochlea with substantial neural degeneration or that is void of neural innervation. Additionally, it may be possible that stimulation is eliciting a response in an area of the auditory nervous system that has long been deprived of auditory stimulation.

The audiologist usually employs a **modified Hughson-Westlake** ascending/descending adaptive procedure to determine threshold (Carhart & Jerger, 1959). The ideal step size for testing likely varies by manufacturer because stimulation scales are different. Larger step sizes may be used for young children who have limited attention spans so that the audiologist may quickly determine a broad estimate of a stimulation level that approximates electrical threshold. For older children and adults, the attention span will be longer, and smaller step sizes may be used to more precisely determine the electrical threshold. For some recipients with tinnitus, determination of threshold may be difficult because the signal tends to "blend" with the ongoing tinnitus. This problem is especially prevalent in newly implanted users.

An alternative approach to the measurement of electrical threshold is to ask recipients to **count the number of beeps** they hear. When using the procedure, the audiologist randomly alters the number of signals presented at each trial (typically between two and five beeps at a time), and the user's task is to accurately report the number of beeps that are heard. This method assists recipients in focusing on a pulsed signal rather than the continuous tinnitus and enhances their likelihood of responding to the signal rather than the tinnitus. Furthermore, it assists the audiologist in obtaining valid T level responses for recipients who provide numerous false positive responses because of difficulty with distinguishing between the programming stimulus and their tinnitus. Use of a count-the-beeps approach often results in higher thresholds than thresholds based on conventional audiometric threshold procedures (Skinner, Holden, Holden, & Demorest, 1995). According to research, a higher threshold level may improve the salience of soft speech and environmental sounds (Holden et al., 2011; Skinner, Holden, Holden, & Demorest, 1999). However, if electrical threshold levels are set substantially higher than the recipient's true threshold of detection, the recipient may experience a constant buzzing, humming, or frying sound, or low-level ambient noise may be too noticeable and annoying. The threat of a consistently audible noise associated with excessively high electrical threshold levels is particularly a problem for recipients using Continuous Interleaved Sampling (CIS)–based signal coding strategies, because electrical stimulation is constantly present at all times on at least one channel.

Psychophysical loudness scaling is an alternative approach that is used to set the threshold of electrical stimulation. With this method, the audiologist typically begins by presenting the electrical programming signal at a sub-threshold level and then gradually increases the presentation level over time (i.e., ascending approach). Recipients are asked to acknowledge their loudness percept of the signal by pointing to categories on a loudness scale similar to the scale pictured in Figure 7–26. Electrical threshold typically is set at a level that corresponds to "barely audible" or "very soft" on the scale. Similar to the count-the-beeps approach, this method likely results in higher threshold levels than what is obtained with conventional audiometric procedures. In addition, it

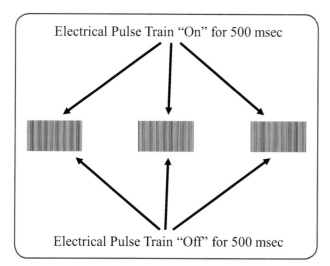

FIGURE 7–25. A visual example of electrical pulses trains with a 500-msec on/off duty cycle.

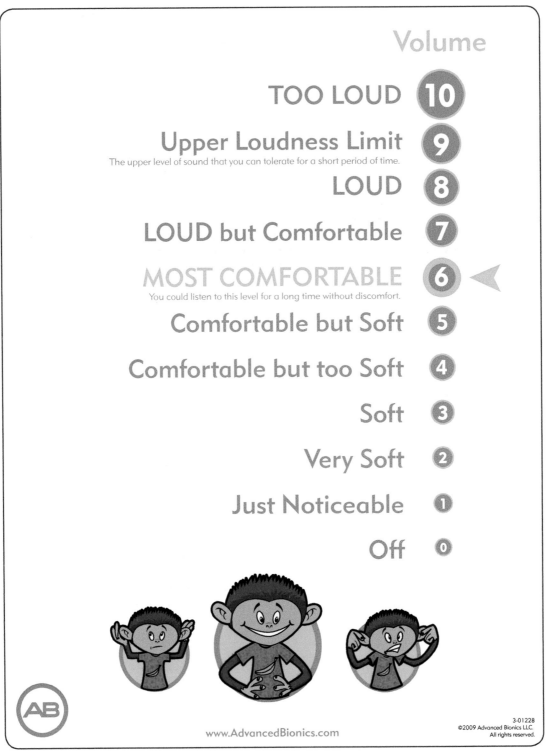

FIGURE 7–26. A visual representation psychophysical loudness scaling chart. Image provided courtesy of Advanced Bionics, LLC.

results in better detection for low-level speech and environmental sounds (Skinner et al., 1999), but also poses the risk that low-level ambient sounds may be bothersome or that the electrical stimulation may create a consistently audible signal (e.g., buzz, hum, hiss, "bacon frying").

Obtaining threshold levels may be difficult in young children with cochlear implants. The techniques for establishing threshold levels vary by age and are similar to behavioral testing approaches used by pediatric audiologists to evaluate hearing sensitivity. A detailed discussion on the measurement of thresholds in children is provided in Chapters 6 and 14.

In an effort to expedite the programming process and eliminate an audible noise that may occur when T levels are set too high in CIS-type signal coding strategies, Advanced Bionics and MED-EL have introduced programming strategies that do not require the measurement of electrical threshold. Instead, the electrical threshold is set at 0 units of stimulation or a certain percentage (e.g., 10%) of the maximum stimulation level. The magnitude of stimulation provided for low-level inputs is estimated (i.e., **estimated T levels**) by knowledge of the typical EDR associated with a particular upper stimulation level, compression processing, logarithmic mapping functions, which place the acoustic input range into the upper portion of the typical recipient's electrical dynamic range. Some research has suggested that speech recognition and audibility for soft sounds are similar when using maps with measured threshold levels versus estimated threshold levels (Spahr & Dorman, 2005). In contrast, Holden et al. (2011) found that detection thresholds for warble-tone stimuli presented in the soundfield were often lower (i.e., better) and recognition of low-level speech was often better when subjects used programs with measured threshold levels. As a result, in many cases, it may be beneficial to measure electrical-threshold levels rather than rely on the programming software to estimate threshold levels, particularly for children who require excellent audibility of low-level speech sounds for speech recognition and for speech and language development. At the very least, audiologists should evaluate a recipient's sound-field detection thresholds for warble tones to determine whether sufficient stimulation is being provided for low-level sounds. The electrical threshold should be increased or electrical logarithmic mapping functions should be adjusted (e.g., MED-EL recommends adjusting parameters other than electrical threshold, such as the Maplaw mapping function, to improve audibility

for low-level sounds; see Chapter 17 for more detail) when behavioral hearing thresholds exceed 30 dB HL for adults or 25 dB HL for children.

Upper Stimulation Levels

Upper stimulation level essentially refers to the maximum amount of electrical stimulation the cochlear implant will provide to the recipient. The upper stimulation level should be set so that high-level sounds are loud but not uncomfortable to the cochlear implant user. The terminology and definitions used to define upper stimulation level also vary across implant manufacturers. In the Advanced Bionics system, the upper limit of electrical stimulation is set at a level the user perceives as being "most comfortable." This parameter is similar to the most comfortable listening level (which is often referred to as "MCL") frequently measured in hearing aid evaluations. In Advanced Bionics cochlear implants, the upper stimulation level is known as the "M level." In the MED-EL system, upper stimulation levels are known as "maximum comfort levels" (i.e., *MCL*) and are defined as the amount of electrical stimulation considered to be "loud, but not uncomfortable." The reader should note that the MED-EL MCL is different from the MCL (i.e., most comfortable listening level) often used in hearing aid evaluations. For Nucleus implants, upper stimulation levels are known as "C levels" and are set to a level of stimulation the user considers to be "loud, but comfortable."

A cochlear implant user's upper stimulation levels are critically important because they influence speech recognition, sound quality, and the ability to monitor one's own voice and produce intelligible speech, which is of particular importance for children who are prelingually deafened. If upper stimulation levels are set inappropriately, the recipient will likely experience poor outcomes. Audiologists typically set upper stimulation levels via psychophysical loudness scaling methods or through behavioral observation. Additionally, several researchers report that the electrically evoked stapedial reflex threshold (ESRT) serves as a useful guide for determining upper stimulation levels (Brickley et al., 2005; Buckler & Overstreet, 2003; Wolfe & Kasulis, 2008). A detailed discussion of setting upper stimulation levels is provided in Chapter 14.

The reader should note that electrical threshold and upper stimulation levels may be adjusted by altering the current amplitude, pulse width, or both (i.e., electrical charge) of the electrical signal.

Increasing the current amplitude and/or pulse width will increase the magnitude of the electrical stimulus. Increasing electrical threshold should provide better access to low-level sounds, because a greater amount of stimulation is provided for low-level inputs. However, setting electrical threshold too high (i.e., substantially higher than the recipient's true detection threshold) may result in soft sounds being too loud, ambient noise being annoying/bothersome, and possibly in the electrical stimulation and/or elevated ambient noise interfering with the recipient's ability to hear meaningful low-level sounds. If electrical threshold is set well below the recipient's true detection threshold, then it is likely that audibility for low-level sounds will be poor. If upper stimulation levels are set too high, the stimulation may be uncomfortable or even painful for the recipient, speech may be distorted, and sound quality will probably be poor. If upper stimulation levels are set too low, then loudness normalization will not be achieved (i.e., moderate sounds will be too soft and high-level sounds will not be loud), and speech recognition and sound quality will likely suffer.

Mapping Acoustical Inputs into the Electrical Dynamic Range

The various cochlear implant manufacturers take different approaches to determine how a relatively wide range of desirable acoustic inputs are delivered into

the recipient's narrow electrical dynamic range. The following parameters influence how acoustical inputs are delivered into the recipient's electrical dynamic range: input dynamic range, sensitivity, compression, channel gain, and volume control. All of these parameters, as described here, influence the way the signal is coded in the intensity domain. A more detailed explanation of how these parameters are used during signal coding and programming is provided in Chapters 8, 15, 16, and 17, which describe manufacturer-specific technology and sound processor programming.

Input Dynamic Range (IDR)

The **input dynamic range** (IDR) of a sound processor is an audiologist-adjustable parameter that, along with microphone (input) sensitivity, determines the range of acoustic inputs that are mapped into the recipient's electrical dynamic range. As shown in Figure 7–27, the default IDR of contemporary cochlear implant systems ranges from 40 to 60 dB. The lower end of the IDR determines the acoustic input level that is mapped near the threshold of electrical stimulation, while the upper end of the IDR determines the acoustic input level that is mapped near the maximum electrical stimulation level (i.e., M level, MCL, or C level).

In current cochlear implants, the lower end of the IDR usually is set between 20 and 35 dB SPL, while the upper end of the IDR is set between 65 and

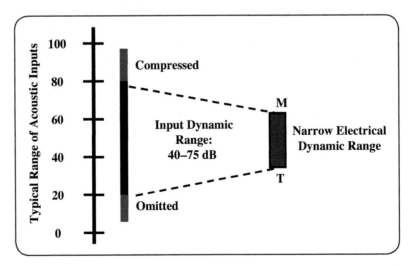

FIGURE 7–27. An illustration of a wide range of acoustic inputs (20 to 80 dB SPL) being delivered to the cochlear implant recipient's electrical dynamic range. *Note.* T = Electrical Threshold; M = Most comfortable stimulation level.

90 dB SPL depending on the manufacturer. Acoustic inputs that fall below the lower end of the IDR are mapped below the recipient's electrical threshold (i.e., below the lower end of the EDR) and are inaudible to the user of electrical threshold that has been set appropriately. Acoustic inputs that exceed the IDR are subjected to high-level **compression** (i.e., audio compression with a high compression ratio). It should be noted that the implementation of IDR in signal coding is a bit more complicated than what has been previously described. For example, Nucleus also uses a parameter known as ***instantaneous input dynamic range*** (IIDR), which refers to the range of short-term fluctuations that are mapped without compression (or other types of attenuation, such as Autosensitivity Control [ASC]) into the recipient's electrical dynamic range. The IIDR is typically set to 40 dB SPL in order to capture the range of ongoing speech amplitudes, from peaks to valleys, at a given input level.

Cochlear defines IDR as the total range of input levels the processor can analyze without clipping or significant distortion. In Nucleus processors, a change (either manually or automatically with ASC) in another parameter, known as **sensitivity**, results in a shift of the 40 dB IIDR window. As a result, the range of inputs that are mapped into the Nucleus recipient's electrical dynamic range is actually much wider than 40 dB IIDR. This concept will be discussed in detail in Chapter 16 of this book.

Sensitivity

The parameter known as **sensitivity** controls the gain provided by the sound processor microphone or some other audio input source (e.g., direct auditory input, wireless audio input). For some sound processors (e.g., Nucleus Freedom), the sensitivity parameter only adjusts the gain for the signal received by the sound processor microphone, whereas for other processors (e.g., Nucleus 7) the sensitivity parameter affects the gain of signals from the microphone and the direct auditory input source. The numerical value and effect of the sensitivity parameter varies by manufacturer and is discussed more thoroughly in Chapters 15 to 17, which discuss manufacturer-specific technology and programming.

Sensitivity interacts with the IDR/IIDR parameter to determine how acoustic inputs are mapped into the recipient's electrical dynamic range. In essence, a reduction in microphone sensitivity adjusts the IDR in a predictable manner. As shown in Figure 7–28, when the sensitivity of the Nucleus 7 sound processor is reduced from a default setting of 12 to a lower setting (e.g., closer to zero), the acoustic input level required to engage the high-level compressor (Automatic Gain Control, AGC) increases. Also, the floor of the IDR/IIDR increases to reduce the audibility of low-level sounds. Conversely, if the microphone sensitivity is increased above the default setting, audibility for low-level sounds is improved and acoustic

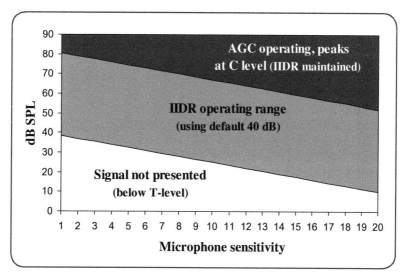

FIGURE 7–28. A representation of the instantaneous input dynamic range (IIDR) as a function of the microphone sensitivity control setting. Image provided courtesy of Cochlear Americas, ©2018.

inputs below the default ceiling of the IDR/IIDR are subjected to high-level compression (e.g., compression with a high compression ratio). Overall, the sensitivity control makes adjustments to the input signal prior to frequency analysis; therefore, its effect is similar across the frequency range of the processor.

Compression

All contemporary cochlear implant systems use audio **compression** to direct a wide range of acoustic inputs into the implant user's narrow electrical dynamic range. In essence, the compression acts as an automatic gain control, but the gain adjustment as a function of input level and the time constants that govern the responsiveness of the compression vary widely across manufacturers. For example, Advanced Bionics, Cochlear, and MED-EL all include a feature known as AGC within their input signal processing, but the manner in which AGC is implemented is very different among the three systems. Certain characteristics of the AGC may be adjusted by the audiologist (see Chapters 15–17).

Channel Gain

Adjustments to **channel gain** controls the amplification provided to the signal in a channel-specific and, therefore, frequency-specific manner. Similar to the other parameters, the effect of changing the channel gain varies by manufacturer. In cochlear implant systems using CIS-type strategies, an increase of the channel gain results in a frequency-specific increase to the input signal. An increase in channel gain should enhance the detectability and loudness of the signal in a frequency-specific manner without the need for increases in the upper stimulation level, because the incoming signal is positioned at a higher location in the recipient's EDR. This may be appealing when increases in the upper stimulation level produce undesirable effects, such as poor sound quality, facial nerve stimulation, discomfort, etc. In CIS-type signal coding strategies, adjusting the channel gain is essentially akin to making frequency-specific adjustments to the input sensitivity parameter.

For Nucleus devices, adjustment of the channel gain affects the channels that are selected for stimulation during a given stimulation cycle. Decreasing the channel gain results in a channel being less likely to be selected for stimulation, while increasing channel gain enhances the likelihood that a channel will be selected for stimulation. As a result, adjustments to channel gain should typically only be made as a last

resort. The effect of channel gain is discussed further in Chapters 15 and 16.

Volume Control

In general, the volume control parameter is fairly straightforward. Adjusting the **volume control** results in a change in the upper level of stimulation the recipient receives from the implant (i.e., C levels, M levels, or MCL). As a result, adjustments to the volume control affect the user's perception of signal loudness. Adjustment of the volume control may also affect speech recognition and sound quality. Depending on how the audiologist programs the operation of the volume control, adjusting the volume control from the maximum or default position to the minimal position may result in little to no sound percept for the patient, or this action may result in a minimal change in overall stimulation relative to what is provided with the volume control at the maximum position. Furthermore, changing the volume control setting to the maximum position may result in only a small change to stimulation levels, or this action may result in a dramatic increase in the upper stimulation level. Therefore, it is very important that the audiologist and recipient share a thorough understanding of the effect of the volume control on the stimulation provided to the user. The exact effect of the volume control setting varies by cochlear implant manufacturer, and as a result, the volume control parameter will be discussed in detail when manufacturer-specific information is discussed in Chapters 15 to 17.

Additional Programming Parameters

Sequential Versus Simultaneous Stimulation

Most contemporary cochlear implant systems deliver electrical biphasic pulses in a **sequential** fashion, in which each biphasic pulse occurs one right after another. In other words, a simultaneous presentation of two pulses never occurs. This approach is designed to reduce or prevent channel interaction, which may result in distortion or smearing of speech sounds. In contrast to sequential stimulation, **simultaneous** stimulation refers to the presentation of an electrical signal to multiple electrodes at one time. An early signal coding strategy called Simultaneous analog stimulation (SAS) used simultaneous stimulation. In the SAS signal coding strategy, the input sound was filtered into multiple channels and the acoustic output of each channel was converted into a continuous electrical analog, which was delivered simultaneously in time to all of the intracochlear electrode contacts based on the frequency of the respective channel and the position of the contact within the cochlea. Zwolan et al. (2001) showed that Advanced Bionics users with low stimulation level needs (i.e., low T and M levels) frequently performed well and preferred the SAS strategy, while recipients with higher stimulation level needs preferred sequential stimulation. Simultaneous stimulation typically is implemented with bipolar electrode coupling in an attempt to reduce channel interaction. Current signal coding strategies do not use totally simultaneous stimulation, primarily to avoid channel interaction.

Advanced Bionics cochlear implants are also capable of using an approach that is best referred to as **partially simultaneous stimulation**, which is essentially a combination of the two aforementioned approaches. With this approach, biphasic electrical pulses are provided simultaneously to two different electrode contacts, but these electrode contacts are separated by a relatively large physical distance (Figure 7–29). The objective of this approach is to allow for faster rates of stimulation per channel (because two channels are stimulated at the same time) while

limiting channel interaction (by ensuring that two electrodes that are simultaneously stimulated are separated by a relatively great physical distance) historically associated with simultaneous stimulation.

It should be noted that the previously mentioned concept of virtual channels does provide simultaneous stimulation on two neighboring channels. However, this simultaneous stimulation on two neighboring channels is intended to elicit one percept or "channel" of stimulation at one moment in time. As a result, virtual channel stimulation differs from the traditional concept of simultaneous stimulation, which sought to stimulate across several channels at one time to create multiple percepts. Advanced Bionics implements virtual channel stimulation in a sequential mode (in which two neighboring electrode contacts are simultaneously stimulated to create one channel of stimulation at one moment in time) and in a partially simultaneous mode (in which two neighboring electrode contacts in the apical end of the cochlea are stimulated simultaneously to create one channel of stimulation, while at the same time, two neighboring channels in the basal end of the cochlea are also stimulated simultaneously to create another distally located channel of stimulation at the same point in time).

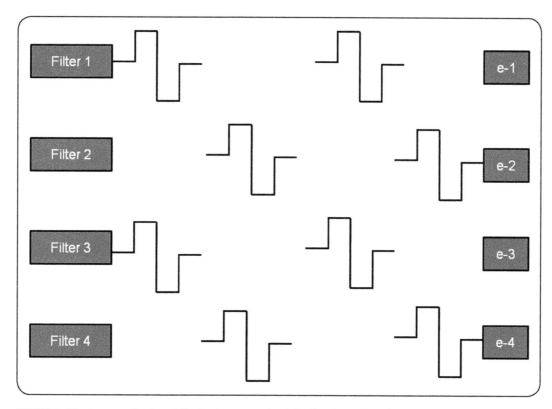

FIGURE 7–29. An example of partially simultaneous stimulation in a four-channel system.

Interpolation

As the number of cochlear implant recipients has grown, cochlear implant audiologists have struggled to manage their expanding patient caseloads. In response, manufacturers have developed streamlined programming strategies to expedite the programming process. A streamlined strategy is basically one that is designed to allow for a program that may be created quickly without sacrificing sound quality or performance. **Interpolation** refers to the estimation of stimulation levels on the basis of measured values from neighboring channels. For instance, if the measured T levels for electrodes 6 and 8 were 70 and 90, respectively, the estimated T level for electrode 7 would be 80.

In practice, interpolation often is used to estimate the stimulation levels for several electrodes that are between two measured electrodes (e.g., stimulation levels of electrodes 21 through 17 are estimated on the basis of measured values at electrodes 22 and 16). The measured values are sometimes referred to as "**anchor channels**." In the aforementioned example, the stimulation levels of channels 21 through 17 are estimated based on the stimulation levels measured on the anchor channels, 22 and 16. Research demonstrates that, on average, user performance for a large group of recipients did not decline when programs were based on interpolated versus individual channel measures (Plant et al., 2005). However, because of individual subject variation, the authors recommend that audiologists measure stimulation levels on most active channels when time allows (i.e., all even-numbered electrodes and any odd electrodes that are adjacent to two even electrodes with stimulation levels that differ substantially). In particular, the audiologist should consider measuring stimulation levels when a large difference exists in the measured values of two anchor channels. Also, because the quantity and integrity of auditory nerve elements can vary considerably in the more basal region of the cochlea, the authors recommend measurement of stimulation levels for the last three electrode contacts within the electrode array. It should be noted again that interpolation is appropriate for use when stimulation is provided with monopolar electrode coupling, because the relatively broad field of electrical stimulation provided by monopolar stimulation reduces the likelihood that large differences in stimulation levels will exist between two intracochlear electrode contacts located close to each other. In contrast, interpolation is generally considered to be inappropriate

when stimulation is provided with bipolar electrode coupling, because the electrical field is narrower and consequently stimulation levels may vary considerably from one intracochlear electrode contact to another.

Sweeping

Sweeping refers to the sequential presentation of the programming stimulus across the active electrodes at a given stimulation level. In other words, the pulsed programming stimulus (one to two "beeps") is delivered to the most apical channel (e.g., channel 22), then to the next channel (e.g., channel 21), then to the next channel (e.g., channel 20), and so on. Sweeping often is performed at the upper stimulation level (i.e., C/M/MCL level) to ensure that none of the electrodes provide maximal stimulation that is too loud or that results in an unfavorable sound quality. Sweeping, however, may be performed at lower stimulation levels (i.e., 50% of the dynamic range) to ensure equal loudness for lower-level inputs, particularly when the recipient complains that certain soft sounds are too loud or that soft speech is difficult to understand. Additionally, the perceived pitch should become progressively higher if sweeping is performed from the apical to basal direction. As such, the prudent audiologist may choose to sweep at the upper stimulation level and ensure that the pitch changes in the expected tonotopic manner. Sweeping may also be conducted to determine whether there are any channels that possess undesirable sound quality or to confirm that there are no channels that produce unwanted non-auditory side effects (e.g., facial nerve stimulation, tactile sensation, pain). Finally, sweeping may be performed across all active electrodes in succession or just across two or a few (e.g., three or four) electrodes at a time to allow for more precise responses.

Loudness Balancing

Loudness balancing refers to the successive presentation of a programming stimulus to two or more active electrodes to ensure that the subject perceives the stimuli to be equally loud when each is presented at a specified percentage of the dynamic range. Researchers have reported that the provision of stimulation resulting in equal loudness percepts across the electrode array results in optimal sound quality, and speech recognition (Dawson, Skok, & Clark, 1997; Sainz, de la Torre, Roldan, Ruiz, & Vargas, 2003). The authors of this book contend that the provision of upper stimulation levels that are equally loud across the electrode array is one of the most important facets of establishing a program that will optimize sound quality and speech recognition. If stimulation is not balanced in loudness across the electrode array, then the natural differences in intensity that exist between different speech sounds will not be conveyed to the user. For instance, in natural speech, the vowels and low-frequency consonants are higher in level than the high-frequency consonants. Also, the voiceless sibilants (/s/, /sh/) are typically higher in level than many of the other voiceless, high-frequency consonants (e.g., /h/, /f/, /θ/). These natural differences that exist in intensity across different phonemes are important cues used by the listener for speech recognition. Loudness balancing is necessary to preserve these important intensity cues. Also, if one channel provides stimulation that is substantially louder than the stimulation provided from remaining channels, then the loudest channel may dominate the recipient's overall loudness percept. When listening to broadband sounds, such as speech and environmental sounds, the user may adjust the global stimulation levels so that the stimulation present at the loudest channel is not uncomfortable. As a result, the remaining channels may provide insufficient stimulation/loudness. Loudness balancing is necessary to ensure that appropriate stimulation is provided across all channels.

Most commonly in clinical practice, two or more electrodes are stimulated at the upper stimulation level (i.e., C/M/MCL level), and the subject reports whether the stimuli are equally loud or whether one electrode possesses a louder percept. If the latter is the case, the audiologist makes an adjustment to achieve balanced loudness between the electrodes. Typically, the audiologist begins with presentation to an active electrode at the most apical location in the electrode array and progresses across electrodes in a basal direction. The number of electrodes that are balanced in a given trial often varies across audiologists (i.e., balancing two, three, four, or more at a time), but the authors prefer to balance loudness across two electrodes at a time. For example, if the audiologist begins by asking the recipient to judge loudness at C level for electrodes 22 and 21, and electrode 21 is louder than 22, then the stimulation level for electrode 21 would be decreased slightly. The loudness of the two then would be reevaluated. After the recipient reports that the loudness is balanced between the electrodes, the audiologist compares loudness at C level between electrodes 21 and 20 and eventually for the rest of the electrode array.

The adjustment to the stimulation level always should be made to the second electrode in the pair, because the first electrode is balanced to the preceding electrodes in the array.

Mixing Ratio

The **mixing-ratio** parameter controls the relative strength of the signal from the speech processor microphone and the direct auditory input (DAI) source. All contemporary cochlear implant sound processors have a DAI port (or a special battery case which facilitates a DAI connection) in order to allow for the direct delivery of an external input, such as a signal from a personal FM/RF system or MP3 player, to the sound processor. In some instances, the user may desire to listen only to the signal from the DAI source (e.g., listening to music from an MP3 player). In many situations, however, a cochlear implant user will want to hear the signals from both the DAI source and sound processor microphone. For example, children using a personal digital RF/FM system in a classroom should hear the teacher's voice from the digital RF/FM transmitter, but also their own voice and the voices of other children in the room.

Typically, the mixing-ratio parameter allows the audiologist to choose from a variety of ratios ranging in a graded manner from an equal emphasis on signals from the sound processor microphone and DAI (i.e., no attenuation of signal from sound processor microphone) to DAI only (i.e., complete attenuation of signal from sound processor microphone). The mixing-ratio parameter also may include the telecoil-mixing ratio, which controls the strength of the signals from the telecoil and sound processor microphone. It also ranges from equal emphasis between the telecoil and microphone signals to telecoil-only emphasis. Additional information on adjustment of the mixing ratio is provided in Chapters 15 and 16.

Key Concepts

- Cochlear implant technology features several terms that are not used frequently in other areas of audiology.
- The audiologist should be intimately familiar with cochlear implant terminology in order to best serve cochlear implant recipients.
- Basic cochlear implant terminology is fairly similar across the different cochlear implant

manufacturers, but each manufacturer also uses terminology that is specific to its cochlear implant system.

References

Arora, K., Dawson. P., Dowell, R., & Vandali. A. (2009). Electrical stimulation rate effects on speech perception in cochlear implants. *International Journal of Audiology*, *48*(8), 561–567.

Aschendorff, A., Briggs, R., Brademann, G., Helbig, S., Hornung, J., Lenarz, T., . . . James, C. J. (2017). Clinical investigation of the Nucleus Slim Modiolar Electrode. *Audiology and Neurotology*, *22*(3), 169–179.

Balkany, T., Hodges, A., Menapace, C., Hazard, L., Driscoll, C., Gantz, B., . . . Payne, S. (2007). Nucleus Freedom North American clinical trial. *Otolaryngology-Head and Neck Surgery*, *136*(5), 757–762.

Boothroyd, A. (2014). The acoustic speech signal. In J. R. Madell & C. Flexer (Eds.), *Pediatric audiology: Diagnosis, technology, and management* (2nd ed., pp. 201–208). New York, NY: Thieme Medical.

Brickley, G., Boyd, P., Wyllie, F., O'Driscoll, M., Webster, D., & Nopp, P. (2005). Investigations into electrically evoked stapedius reflex measures and subjective loudness percepts in the MED-EL COMBI 40+ cochlear implant. *Cochlear Implants International*, *6*(1), 31–42.

Buchner A., Frohne-Buchner, C., Battmer, R., & Lenarz, T. (2004) Two years of experience using stimulation rates between 800 and 5,000 pps with the Clarion CI implant. *International Congress Series*, *1273*, 48–51.

Buechner, A., Brendel, M., Saalfeld, H., Litvak, L., Frohne-Buechner, C., & Lenarz, T. (2010). Results of a pilot study with a signal enhancement algorithm for HiRes 120 cochlear implant users. *Otology and Neurotology*, *31*(9), 1386–1390.

Buckler, L., & Overstreet, E. (2003). *Relationship between electrical stapedial reflex thresholds and Hi-Res program settings: Potential tool for pediatric cochlear-implant fitting*. Valencia, CA: Advanced Bionics.

Carhart, R., & Jerger, J. F. (1959). Preferred method for clinical determination of pure-tone thresholds. *Journal of Speech and Hearing Disorders*, *24*, 330–345.

Cohen, L. T., Saunders, E., & Clark, G. M. (2001). Psychophysics of a prototype peri-modiolar cochlear implant electrode array. *Hearing Research*, *155*(1–2), 63–81.

Dawson, P., Skok, M., & Clark, G. (1997). The effect of loudness imbalance between electrodes in cochlear implant users. *Ear and Hearing*, *18*, 156–165.

Dunn, C., Tyler, R., Witt, S., & Gantz, B. (2006). Effects of converting bilateral cochlear implant subjects to a strategy with increased rate and number of channels. *Annals of Otology, Rhinology, and Laryngology*, *115*(6), 425–432.

Finley, C. C., Holden, T. A., Holden, L. K., Whiting, B. R., Chole, R. A., Neely, G. J., . . . Skinner, M. W. (2008). Role of electrode placement as a contributor to variability in cochlear implant outcomes. *Otology and Neurotology*, *29*(7), 920–928.

Frijns, J. H., Klop, W. M., Bonnet, R. M., & Briaire, J. J. (2003). Optimizing the number of electrodes with high-rate stimulation of the Clarion CII cochlear implant. *Acta Otolaryngologica*, *123*, 138–142.

Gordin, A., Papsin, B., James, A., & Gordon, K. (2009). Evolution of cochlear implant arrays result in changes in behavioral and physiological responses in children. *Otology and Neurotology*, *30*(7), 908–915.

Holden, L. K., Finley, C. C., Firszt, J. B., Holden, T. A., Brenner, C., Potts, L. G., . . . Skinner, M. W. (2013). Factors affecting open-set word recognition in adults with cochlear implants. *Ear and Hearing*, *34*(3), 342–360.

Holden, L. K., Reeder, R. M., Firszt, J. B., & Finley, C. C. (2011). Optimizing the perception of soft speech and speech in noise with the Advanced Bionics cochlear implant system. *International Journal of Audiology*, *50*(4), 255–269.

Hughes, M. L., Vander Werff, K. R., Brown, C. J., Abbas, P. J., Kelsay, D. M., Teagle, H., . . . Lowder, M. W. (2001). A longitudinal study of electrode impedance, the electrically evoked compound action potential, and behavioral measures in Nucleus 24 cochlear implant users. *Ear and Hearing*, *22*(6), 471–486.

Jeong, J., Kim, M., Heo, J. H., Bang, M. Y., Bae, M. R., Kim, J., & Choi, J. Y. (2015). Intraindividual comparison of psychophysical parameters between perimodiolar and lateral-type electrode arrays in patients with bilateral cochlear implants. *Otology and Neurotology*, *36*(2), 228–234.

Koch, D. B., Osberger, M. J., Segel, P., & Kessler, D. K. (2004). HiResolution and conventional sound processing in the HiResolution Bionic Ear: Using appropriate outcome measures to assess speech recognition ability. *Audiology and Neurotology*, *9*, 214–223.

MED-EL. (2017). *Mi1000 CONCERTO Surgical Guideline*. Retrieved from http://s3.medel.com/documents/AW/AW7617_50_CONCERTO%20Surgical%20Guideline%20-%20EN%20English.pdf

Merriam-Webster. (2018). Retrieved from https://www.merriam-webster.com/dictionary/telemetry

Moller, A. R. (2001). Neurophysiologic basis for cochlear and auditory brainstem implants. *American Journal of Audiology*, *10*(2), 68–77.

Moller, A. R. (2013). *Hearing: Anatomy, physiology, and disorders of the auditory system* (3rd ed.). San Diego, CA: Plural.

Moore, B. C. (2003). Coding of sounds in the auditory system and its relevance in signal processing and coding in cochlear implants. *Otology and Neurotology*, *24*(2), 243–254.

Muller, A., Hocke, T., & Mir-Salim, P. (2015). Intraoperative findings on ECAP-measurement: Normal or special case? *International Journal of Audiology*, *54*(4), 257–264.

Nelson, D., Schmitz, J., Donaldson, G., Viemeister, N., & Javel, E. (1996). Intensity discrimination as a function of stimulus level with electric stimulation. *Journal of the Acoustical Society of America*, *100*(4 Pt. 1), 2393–2414.

Newbold, C., Richardson, R., Huang, C. Q., Milojevic, D., Cowan, R., & Shepherd, R. (2004). An in vitro model for investigating impedance changes with cell growth and electrical stimulation: Implications for cochlear implants. *Journal of Neural Engineering*, *1*(4), 218–227.

Nie, K., Barco, A., & Zeng, F. G. (2006). Spectral and temporal cues in cochlear implant speech perception. *Ear and Hearing*, *27*(2), 208–217.

Nyquist, H. (1928). Certain topics in telegraph transmission theory. *Trans American Institute of Electrical Engineers (AIEE)*, *47*, 617–644.

Pelosi, S., Rivas, A., Haynes, D. S., Bennett, M. L., Labadie, R. F., Hedley-Williams, A., . . . Wanna, G. (2012). Stimulation rate reduction and auditory development in poorly performing cochlear implant users with auditory neuropathy. *Otology and Neurotology*, *33*(9), 1502–1506.

Pfingst, B. E., Franck, K. H., Xu, L., Bauer, E. M., & Zwolan, T. A. (2001). Effects of electrode configuration and place of stimulation on speech perception with cochlear prostheses. *Journal of the Association for Research in Otolaryngology, 2*, 87–103.

Plant, K., Law, M. A., Whitford, L., Knight, M., Tari, S., Leigh, J., . . . Nel, E. (2005). Evaluation of streamlined programming procedures for the Nucleus cochlear implant with the Contour electrode array. *Ear and Hearing, 26*(6), 651–668.

Rubinstein, J. T., Wilson, B. S., Finley, C. C., & Abbas, P. J. (1999). Pseudospontaneous activity: Stochastic independence of auditory nerve fibers with electrical stimulation. *Hearing Research, 127*(1–2), 108–118.

Runge-Samuelson, C., Firszt, J. B., Gaggl, W., & Wackym, P. A. (2009). Electrically evoked auditory brainstem responses in adults and children: Effects of lateral to medial placement of the Nucleus 24 contour electrode array. *Otology and Neurotology, 30*(4), 464–470.

Sainz, M., de la Torre, A., Roldan, C., Ruiz, J., & Vargas, J. (2003). Analysis of programming maps and its application for balancing multichannel cochlear implants. *International Journal of Audiology, 42*(1), 43–51.

Skinner, M. W., Holden, L. K., Holden, T. A., & Demorest, M. E. (1995). Comparison of procedures for obtaining thresholds and maximum acceptable loudness levels with the Nucleus cochlear implant system. *Journal of Speech and Hearing Research, 38*, 677–689.

Skinner, M. W., Holden, L. K., Holden, T. A., & Demorest, M. E. (1999). Comparison of two methods for selecting minimum stimulation levels used in programming the Nucleus 22 cochlear implant. *Journal of Speech, Language, and Hearing Research, 42*(4), 814–828.

Smith, Z. M., Delgutte, B., & Oxenham, A. J. (2002). Chimaeric sounds reveal dichotomies in auditory perception. *Nature, 416*(6876), 87–90.

Spahr, A. J., & Dorman, M. F. (2005). Effects of minimum stimulation settings for the Med El Tempo+ speech processor on speech understanding. *Ear and Hearing, 26*(Suppl. 4), 2S–6S.

Vandali, A., Whitford, L., Plant, K., & Clark, G. (2000). Speech perception as a function of electrical stimulation rate: Using the Nucleus 24 cochlear implant system. *Ear and Hearing, 21*, 608–624.

Verschuur, C. A. (2005). Effect of stimulation rate on speech perception in adult users of the Med-El CIS speech processing strategy. *International Journal of Audiology, 44*(1), 58–63.

Wanna, G. B., Noble, J. H., Carlson, M. L., Gifford, R. H., Dietrich, M. S., Haynes, D. S., . . . Labadie, R. F. (2014). Impact of electrode design and surgical approach on scalar location and cochlear implant outcomes. *Laryngoscope, 124*(Suppl. 6), S1–S7.

Weber, B. P., Lai, W. K., Dillier, N., von Wallenberg, E. L., Killian, M. J., Pesch, J., . . . Lenarz, T. (2007). Performance and preference for ACE stimulation rates obtained with Nucleus RP 8 and Freedom system. *Ear and Hearing, 28*(Suppl. 2), 46S–48S.

Wier, C., Jesteadt, W., & Green, D. M. (1977). Frequency discrimination as a function of frequency and sensation level. *Journal of the Acoustical Society of America, 61*, 178–184.

Wolfe, J., Baker, R. S., & Wood, M. (2013). Clinical case study review: Steroid-responsive change in electrode impedance. *Otology and Neurotology, 34*(2), 227–232.

Wolfe, J., & Kasulis, H. (2008). Relationships among objective measures and speech perception in adult users of the HiResolution Bionic Ear. *Cochlear Implants International, 9*(2), 70–81.

Zeng, F., & Galvin, J. (1999). Amplitude mapping and phoneme recognition in cochlear implant listeners. *Ear and Hearing, 20*(1), 60–74.

Zhu, Z., Tang, Q., Zeng, F. G., Guan, T., & Ye, D. (2012). Cochlear-implant spatial selectivity with monopolar, bipolar and tripolar stimulation. *Hearing Research, 283*(1–2), 45–58.

Zwolan, T., Kileny, P., Smith, S., Mills, D., Koch, D., & Osberger, M. (2001). Adult cochlear implant performance with evolving electrode technology. *Otology and Neurotology, 22*(6), 844–849.

Cochlear Implant Signal Coding Strategies

Jace Wolfe and Erin C. Schafer

Basic Cochlear Implant Signal Coding Strategies

A signal coding strategy describes the algorithm used to transform the important features of the incoming acoustical signal (i.e., amplitude, frequency, and temporal cues) into an electrical code. Ideally, this code will represent the relevant acoustic features in a meaningful manner to the cochlear nerve. Although relatively large differences exist in the default signal coding strategies used by recent cochlear implant systems, clinical trials demonstrate comparable performance across the systems of the three different cochlear implant manufacturers and indicate that all modern signal coding strategies are capable to allow for impressive open-set speech recognition abilities (e.g., mean monosyllabic word recognition performance of 60% to 70% correct, with many recipients scoring near ceiling level on clinical tests of sentence and word recognition) (Gifford et al., 2010; Gifford, Shallop, & Peterson, 2008). The following section describes contemporary cochlear implant signal coding strategies.

For several reasons, the development of signal coding strategies is a complex task. For example, speech, which is generally considered to be the most important sound coded by a cochlear implant, is a complex acoustic signal which contains a broad range of levels, a broad spectrum, and a number of different temporal cues that contribute to intelligibility. Additionally, there are often similarities and

overlap in the acoustics of dissimilar phonemes. Likewise, the acoustics of speech differ from one talker to the next. Furthermore, speech is often embedded in competing noise and is present in environments that create significant reverberation. Also, most cochlear implant recipients are not only interested in speech but would also like to listen to other sounds such as music, which may possess complex acoustics which differ from speech. Moreover, limits exist in the amount of information that may be delivered in distinct channels via electrical stimulation. Finally, there are also limits in the way in which the cochlear nerve can receive and process acoustical information when delivered via an electrical code.

This chapter provides a review of signal coding strategies used in commercially available cochlear implant systems. The first portion of this chapter provides a brief summary of many of the aforementioned challenges that exist when acoustical signals are coded into electrical signals to stimulate the peripheral auditory system. The second portion of this chapter provides a description of the signal coding strategies that have been used or are used in commercially available cochlear implant systems.

Factors That Complicate the Electrical Coding of Speech and Other Acoustic Signals

Numerous factors complicate the process of representing acoustic signals in an electrical code that stimulates the cochlear nerve. The following paragraphs summarize these factors.

The Complexities of Speech Acoustics

Speech, whether it is associated with a Western language or an Asian tonal language, is a complex signal. The recognition of speech is dependent on the processing of acoustical cues in the intensity, spectral, and temporal domains. Figure 8–1 shows a spectrogram of the AzBio sentence, "The pool was filled with dirt and leaves." In the spectrogram, intensity is depicted by the color of shading. The brightly colored regions are associated with a higher intensity, whereas the lighter shading depicts lower-level components. The bands associated with voiced speech sounds represent the **harmonics** of the **fundamental frequency** associated with the voicing. Voiceless speech sounds are characterized as being **aperiodic**, meaning they lack the harmonics seen in the voiced sounds. The spectrogram also shows that voiceless speech sounds generally possess a lower intensity than the voiced speech sounds. The spectral characteristics of each speech sound are represented by where the shading falls in the vertical plane, with low-frequency energy represented at the bottom of the graph and high-frequency sound represented at the top. The

slower changes in intensity (e.g., pauses preceding stop consonants such as with the /d/ in "dirt") can also be observed in the graph. Figure 8–1 provides an excellent visual representation of the complexities of running speech, but it does not capture all of the relevant cues necessary for speech recognition.

Vowel recognition is largely based on the listener's ability to process the first two formants of the vowel. **Formants** are spectral concentrations of acoustic energy that occur for voiced speech sounds and are created by resonances in the vocal tract (Hamill & Price, 2008). Figure 8–2 provides a visual illustration of typical formant frequencies of a sample of the English vowel /i/ (i.e., "ee" as in see). It should be noted that the spectral analysis conducted in Figure 8–1 above clearly shows voiced harmonics but not the formant frequencies that are seen in Figure 8–2. A narrowband spectral analysis was conducted to create the spectrogram shown in Figure 8–1. With narrowband spectrograms, the analysis bandwidth is typically around 45 to 50 Hz, which provides sufficient spectral resolution to allow for visualization of harmonics (MacKay, 2014). However, the presence of the individual harmonics present with the narrower analysis bands obscure the presence of the broader formant frequencies. In contrast, Figure 8–2 depicts a wideband spectrogram, which typically possesses

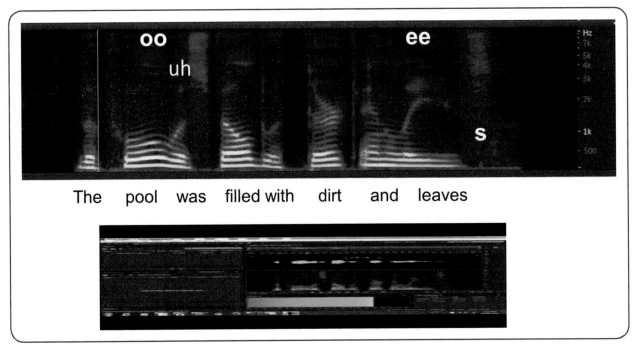

FIGURE 8–1. A spectrogram of the sentence, "The pool was filled with dirt and leaves."

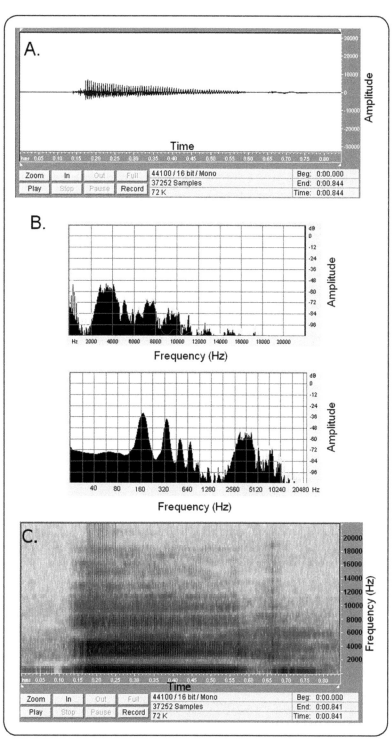

FIGURE 8–2. Analysis of the acoustics of the vowel /i/. Reprinted with permission from Hamill and Price, *The Hearing Sciences, Third Edition* (2019). Copyright © Plural Publishing, Inc.

an analysis bandwidth of 300 to 500 Hz (MacKay, 2014). This wider analysis bandwidth does not capture individual harmonics but does readily allow for visualization of the formant frequencies.

The formant frequencies of voiced speech sounds are determined by the physical dimensions of the vocal tract. The first formant (F_1) is determined by the volume of the pharyngeal cavity and how tightly the vocal tract is constricted (MacKay, 2014). The speech mechanism is depicted in Figure 8–3. A larger pharyngeal cavity during the production of the voiced speech sound is associated with a lower frequency F_1, whereas conversely, a smaller pharyngeal cavity will result in a higher frequency F_1. The pharyngeal cavity is determined by the position of the tongue and velum as well as the constriction of the pharynx. Raising the tongue and pushing it toward the lips results in a larger pharyngeal cavity, as does dilating the pharynx and elevating the velum. The second formant frequency is determined by the length and size

of the oral cavity. Once again, large oral cavities are associated with lower frequency F_2, whereas smaller oral cavities are associated with higher-frequency F_2. Placing the tongue toward the back of the mouth creates a larger oral cavity with a lower F_2, whereas placing the tongue toward the front of the mouth creates a smaller oral cavity with a higher F_2. Additionally, the position of the lips affects the dimensions of the oral cavity. Retracting the lips creates a smaller oral cavity, whereas protruding the lips outward creates a larger oral cavity. The typical formant frequencies for several English vowels are shown in Table 8–1.

As shown in Table 8–1, the vowel /u/, as in "who'd," possesses a relatively low-frequency F_1 and F_2, because the tongue is raised, which enlarges the pharyngeal cavity, and the tongue is also positioned toward the back of the mouth, which creates a relatively large oral cavity. In contrast, the vowel /i/, as in "beet," possesses a relatively low-frequency F_1 but high-frequency F_2, because the tongue is raised

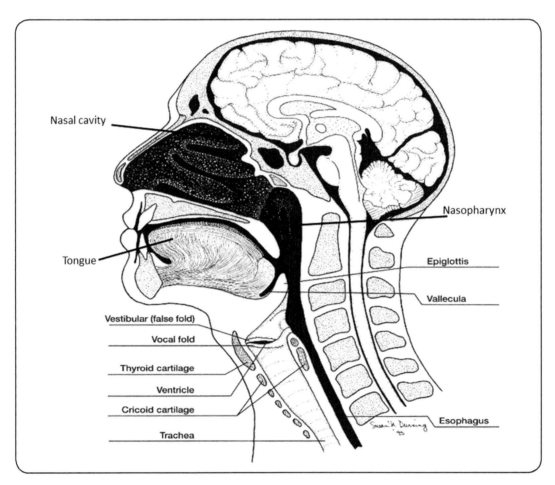

FIGURE 8–3. A visual illustration of the vocal tract. Reprinted with permission from Culbertson, Christensen, & Tanner, *Anatomy and Physiology Study Guide for Speech and Hearing, Second Edition* (2013). Copyright © Plural Publishing, Inc.

TABLE 8–1. Average Formant Frequencies for Vowels Spoken by Female Speakers

Vowel		Tongue Height	Tongue Position	1st Formant (Hz)	2nd Formant (Hz)
/i/	Feed	High	Front	429	2588
/u/	Food	High	Back	430	1755
/ɪ/	Sit	Mid-high	Front	522	2161
/ʌ/	Nut	Mid-high	Mid	767	1751
/ʊ/	Wood	Mid-high	Back	516	1685
/ɛ/	Bed	Mid-low	Front	586	2144
/ɔ/	Sawed	Mid-low	Back	816	1203
/æ/	Sad	Low	Front	836	2051
/ɑ/	Sought	Low	Back	688	1273

Source: Adapted from Assmann, P., & Katz, W. F. (2000). Time-varying spectral change in the vowels of children and adults. *Journal of the Acoustical Society of America, 108,* 1856–1866.

but pushed toward the front of the mouth with the lips retracted. As one would expect, the formant frequencies of voiced speech sounds vary by speaker and are influenced by the physical properties (mass, stiffness, and volume) of the vocal folds, pharyngeal cavity, and oral cavity. Men generally have lower frequency formants than women, and women typically have lower frequency formants than young children. One may wonder how the auditory system recognizes vowels when the formant frequencies vary rather considerably across talkers. Although the recognition of vowel sounds is determined by multiple processes, the most robust cue is likely to be the proportional difference or ratio between F_1 and F_2. The ratio between F_1 and F_2 for a given speech sound remains relatively constant across talkers. Figure 8–4 shows an example of formant ellipses, which illustrates the range of frequencies over which F_1 and F_2 can span for various speech sounds produced by different talkers. The most important point to take away from Figure 8–4 is the fact that vowel formant frequencies can vary across talkers, but the proportional relationship between F_1 and F_2 is rather stable across talkers. In general, vowel recognition is supported relatively well via electrical stimulation from a cochlear implant, because the widely spaced areas of spectral energy associated with F_1 and F_2 can be faithfully captured and conveyed with multiple-channel

systems (i.e., the spectral and intensity properties of F_1 and F_2 are represented by the magnitude of stimulation delivered to two separate intracochlear electrode contacts). However, it should also be noted that difficulties in discrimination of two different speech sounds do arise due to the similarities in the acoustic properties of the sounds.

Another example of the complexity of speech and speech recognition is shown in the samples of an array of consonants showed in Figure 8–5, which shows an example of two bilabial, plosive (i.e., stop) consonants, the voiceless /p/ and the voiced /b/. As shown in Figure 8–5, periodicity (i.e., formants) may be seen in the voiced /b/ sound, whereas the /p/ sound only possesses aperiodic energy. Also, the spectral characteristics (including the bandwidth) are different between the two sounds. Figure 8–6 shows the spectral characteristics of a variety of fricative consonants. One can see that the /s/ sound possesses more high-frequency energy (as indicated by the darker shading at the top of the graph) than the other fricatives. One can also see that in general, there are intensity differences between the four fricatives. In short, the recognition of these phonemes is dependent not only on the ability to recognize a spectral "fingerprint" of each sound but also on the ability to recognize differences in intensity that exist between the sounds. Modern cochlear implants are generally fairly adept at being able to capture and convey the range of intensities that encompasses conversational speech (roughly 25 to 65 dB SPL) as well as at capturing the spectral properties of speech through multiple-channel processing and (tonotopic) stimulation.

Speech recognition is further complicated by the fact that the acoustical properties of individual speech sounds (phonemes) change when produced with other speech sounds. **Co-articulation cues** describe the change in the acoustic properties of speech that occurs when two speech sounds are produced in conjunction with one another compared with the acoustic properties that exist when each speech sound is spoken in isolation. Figure 8–7 provides an example of co-articulation cues. As shown, the F_1 and F_2 of the vowel /ɑ/ (an in "pot") possesses a "leading tail" that rises or falls dependent on the preceding consonant. This tail and the direction in which it traverses (i.e., up or down) provides another cue of the consonant that precedes the vowel /ɑ/.

So far, this discussion on the complexities of speech has largely focused on the spectral and intensity properties of speech. However, the temporal properties of speech (and of other sounds as well) also provide valuable cues that aid in recognition.

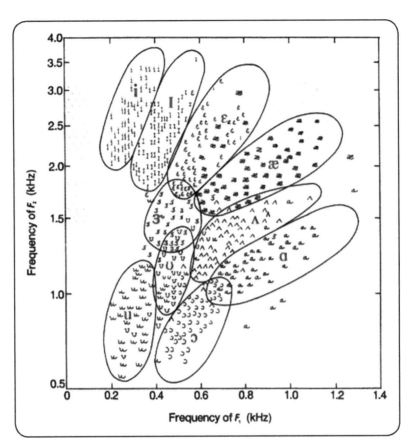

FIGURE 8–4. An example of vowel formant ellipses. Reproduced from Peterson and Barney, "Control methods used in a study of the vowels," *Journal of the Acoustical Society of America*, (1952), *24*(175), with permission of the Acoustical Society of America.

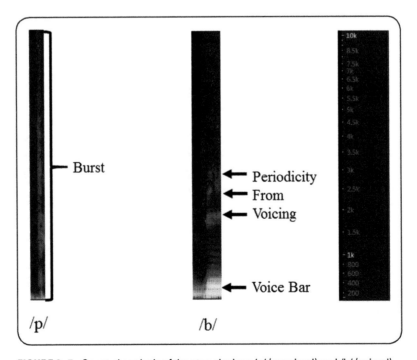

FIGURE 8–5. Spectral analysis of the stop plosives /p/ (unvoiced) and /b/ (voiced).

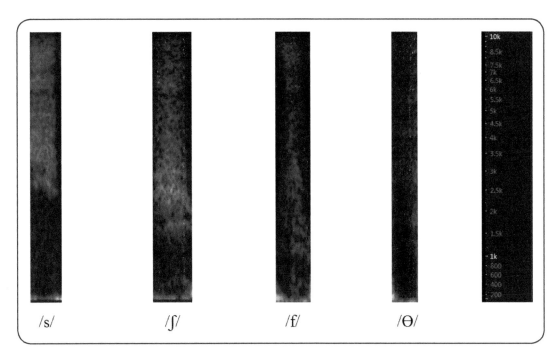

FIGURE 8–6. Spectral analysis of fricative consonants.

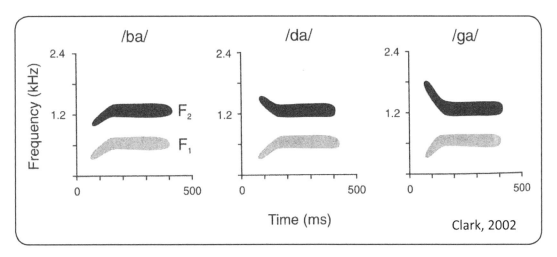

FIGURE 8–7. An example of co-articulation effects; the tail of the formant frequency of the vowel rises or falls depending on the preceding consonant. Image provided courtesy of Graeme Clark.

Temporal properties may be broadly categorized into two classes, amplitude envelope cues and fine temporal structure cues. **Amplitude envelope** cues are relatively slow changes in the intensity fluctuations of speech (or other sounds) that occur on the order of around 2 to 50 Hz. **Fine temporal structure** cues are faster changes in intensity fluctuations that occur on the order of about 150 to several thousand Hz. Amplitude envelope and fine temporal structure are shown in Figure 8–8. Smith, Delgutte, and Oxenham (2002) conducted a study in which the amplitude envelope and fine temporal structure were extracted from two different speech sounds or nursery musicals to create an auditory chimera, which included the amplitude envelope of one sound (e.g., sentence #1, melody #1) and the fine temporal structure of another sound (e.g., sentence #2, melody #2). Via this experiment, they discovered that the amplitude envelope was the

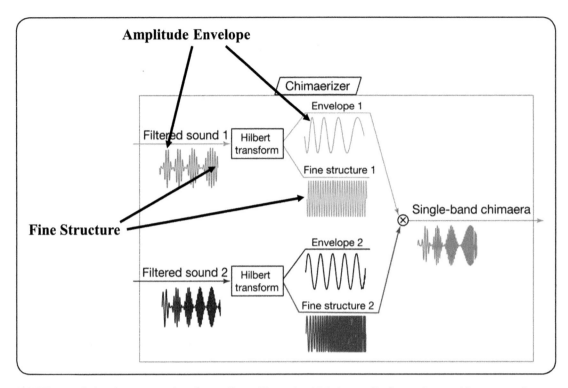

FIGURE 8–8. A visual representation of an auditory chimera in which the amplitude envelope and fine temporal structure are extracted from the original signal. Reprinted with permission from Smith, Delgutte, and Oxenham, "Chimaeric sounds reveal dichotomies in auditory perception," *Nature*, (2002), *416*(6876), 87–90. Copyright © Springer.

dominant cue used to recognize open-set sentences presented in quiet, whereas the fine temporal structure was the dominant cue used to recognize melody.

Figure 8–9 shows another example of the potential importance of temporal cues. As shown in Figure 8–9, the amplitude envelopes of the two speech tokens, /ba/ ("bah") and /bi/ ("bee"), are fairly dissimilar and could potentially serve as temporal cues that could be used to discriminate/recognize these two speech tokens. In contrast, Figure 8–10 shows an example in which the amplitude is very similar for the speech sounds, /ba/ ("bah") and /wa/ ("wah"). In this example, however, the fine temporal structure of /ba/ and /wa/ is quite different and is most likely the cue that the listener will need to use to distinguish between the two speech tokens. Of note, cochlear implant sound processors are capable of capturing both amplitude envelope and fine temporal structure cues. Additionally, modern cochlear implants are capable of varying the stimulation rate to convey these two temporal cues while stimulating the cochlear nerve. However, the cochlear nerve is unable to respond to biphasic electrical pulses quickly enough to process fine temporal structure cues beyond a few hundred

Hz (Clark, 1969). The reader is referred to Chapter 3 for a detailed discussion of cochlear nerve physiology and the limitations of electrical stimulation to convey fine temporal structure.

The aforementioned discussion of the complexities of speech has centered around speech recognition in quiet. In the real world, however, listeners are frequently forced to process speech that is embedded in competing noise and/or that is subjected to reverberation. The term "redundancy of speech" is often used to convey the fact that speech possesses multiple cues that the listener may use for the purposes of speech recognition. In noisy environments, however, many of these cues may be masked by the competing noise. For normal-hearing listeners, the auditory filters are relatively narrow (presumably due to tuning from the outer hair cells), and as a result, a sufficient amount of resolution exists to allow for the separation of the target signal of interest and the competing noise signal. Because of the relatively broad fields of stimulation that occur when the cochlear nerve is stimulated via electrical current delivered from intracochlear electrode contacts and the subsequent interaction that exists across channels of stimulation,

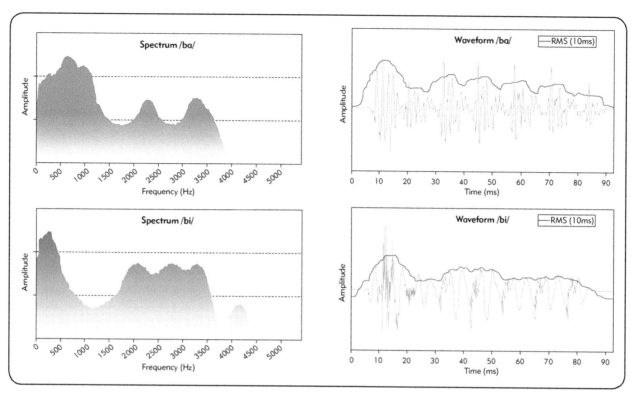

FIGURE 8–9. A visual example of the amplitude envelope and fine temporal structure of the sounds /ba/ and /bi/. Image provided courtesy of Advanced Bionics, LLC.

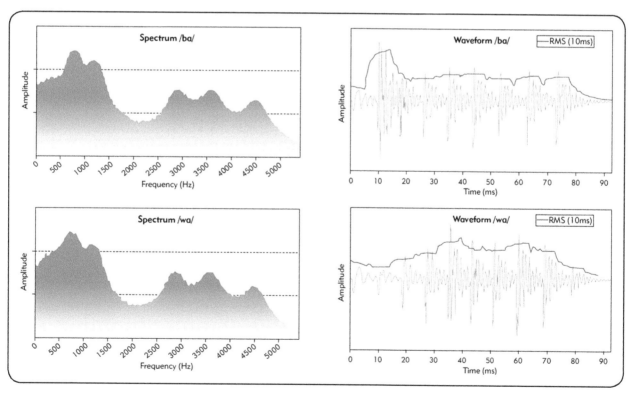

FIGURE 8–10. A visual example of the amplitude envelope and fine temporal structure of the sounds /ba/ and /wa/. Image provided courtesy of Advanced Bionics, LLC.

cochlear implant recipients are typically less adept at resolving a target signal of interest embedded in a competing noise masker.

Complexities of Music and Environmental Sounds

As implied in the earlier discussion of auditory chimeras, the cues used to recognize and process music differ from the way in which speech is processed. Figure 8–11 describes another way in which music and speech differ acoustically and in the way in which they are processed. The piano keyboard depicted in Figure 8–11 illustrates the fact that musical notes are separated very closely in the spectral domain. Also, musical notes possess a discrete spectral component. These attributes are in stark contrast to the broad spectral characteristics of vowel ellipses shown in Figure 8–4. As the reader likely surmises from Figures 8–4 and 8–11, greater frequency resolution is needed to recognize the distinct differences that exist in musical notes relative to the frequency resolution required for satisfactory speech recognition. Indeed, a number of different research studies have shown that even many high-performing cochlear implant recipients experience difficulty with the recognition

of melody and timbre of music (Gfeller et al., 2002, 2007, 2008; Limb & Rubinstein, 2012). In contrast, most cochlear implant recipients can recognize the rhythm of music relatively well, because rhythmic cues occur more slowly (Gfeller et al., 2002, 2007, 2008; Limb & Rubinstein, 2012).

In a similar manner, environmental sounds, such as a door slamming, rain, wind, a clock ticking, a human coughing, and so forth often possess complex acoustics. The recognition of many complex sounds often requires adept processing of spectral and fine temporal structure cues. Inverso and Limb (2010) developed the Non-Linguistic Sound Test (NLST) to evaluate cochlear implant recipients' ability to perceive environmental sounds other than speech. Inverso and Limb administered the NLST to 22 adult cochlear implant users and found a mean identification score of 49% correct. Inverso and Limb noted that sounds with "harmonic structure" or "repetitive temporal structure" were easier for the cochlear implant users to identify. In general, however, they noted that cochlear implant users often experienced difficulty identifying non-linguistic sounds. In recognition of the fact that cochlear implant users often struggle to accurately perceive non-linguistic sounds, many mod-

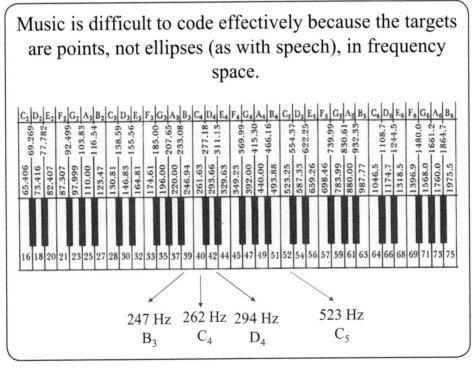

FIGURE 8–11. A visual example of spectral composition of musical notes on a piano keyboard. Image provided courtesy of Advanced Bionics, LLC.

ern cochlear implant signal coding strategies have been developed in an attempt to enhance spectral and temporal resolution so that recipients will be better able to recognize music and complex environmental sounds. There is, however, a paucity of research demonstrating substantial improvement in music and non-linguistic environmental sound perception with the use of new signal coding strategies designed to capture acoustical cues to improve recognition of these complex sounds (Adams et al., 2014; Filipo et al., 2008; Magnusson, 2011; Osberger et al., 2010; Roy et al., 2015.

Cochlear Implant Signal Coding Strategies

Cochlear implant signal coding strategies have evolved considerably over the past four-plus decades. As noted in Chapter 1, the earliest cochlear implants were single-channel devices that converted the acoustic input signal to an electrical analog and delivered that electrical signal to a single intracochlear electrode contact located in the cochlea. Because stimulation to a single intracochlear electrode contact did not access a broad range of the cochlea, it failed to deliver stimulation throughout the tonotopically organized cochlea spiral. Consequently, stimulation could not be delivered in a frequency-specific manner. Furthermore, and as previously stated, the cochlear nerve was unable to follow the rapid fluctuations in the signal when stimulated electrically. Many recipients of single-channel cochlear implants using analog electrical stimulation achieved improvement in speech recognition, but most were unable to understand speech in open-set format. The move to multiple-channel cochlear implants provided an opportunity to take advantage of the tonotopic organization of the cochlea and enhance the processing of spectral cues present in speech and non-linguistic sounds. Even with multiple-channel hardware, however, the recipient's ultimate performance is dependent on the ability of the cochlear implant system to faithfully analyze the input audio signal, code it into an electrical signal, and stimulate the cochlear nerve with a signal that may be processed to provide meaningful information to the auditory nervous system. Since the advent of the first cochlear implant systems developed in the 1960s and 1970s, a host of researchers, scientists, engineers, physicists, physiologists, and clinicians have continually worked to develop better signal coding technology in an effort to improve the outcomes of cochlear implant recipients. As a result of these improvements in technology, open-set speech recognition scores have improved considerably over the course of the past 40-plus years.

The earliest attempts at multiple-channel stimulation fell in two categories, multiple-channel analog stimulation and multiple-channel feature extraction strategies. Some researchers and scientists theorized that the first attempts with analog stimulation were largely unsuccessful because they were attempted with single-channel stimulation. As a result, attempts were made to create signal coding strategies with multiple-channel analog stimulation. Simultaneous analog stimulation (SAS) is an example of multiple-channel analog stimulation used with commercially approved Advanced Bionics cochlear implants.

Simultaneous Analog Stimulation (SAS)

Simultaneous analog stimulation (SAS) is unique compared with the aforementioned signal coding strategies. As the name implies, SAS is an analog signal coding strategy that stimulates electrode contacts with continuous electrical waveforms (rather than biphasic pulses) that are analogous to the acoustical inputs to each channel (Figure 8–12). The microphone converts the acoustic input into an electrical signal, and similar to most signal coding strategies, this signal is subjected to a bank of bandpass filters. The filters separate complex electrical signals into relatively narrow frequency bands. The electrical output from each channel is subjected to compression based on a logarithmic mapping function, and then the compressed signal from each channel is sent to a dedicated electrode. Each electrode contact is stimulated at the same time (i.e., fully simultaneous stimulation) on each cycle of stimulation.

SAS has been used commercially only in Advanced Bionics cochlear implants, but it is no longer available in the current version of programming software. The typical SAS user will be an Advanced Bionics' recipient who received an Advanced Bionics "C1" cochlear implant prior to 2002. In its clinical implementation, SAS used seven to eight active electrode contacts with bipolar electrode coupling. To counter initial difficulties of avoiding voltage compliance issues, Advanced Bionics developed an internal device/electrode array that featured bipolar electrode pairs that were spaced at a greater distance than the original C1 device. The configuration of the new C1.2 device was referred to as enhanced bipolar electrode coupling.

The primary theoretical advantage of SAS is that it preserves most all of the cues present in the original

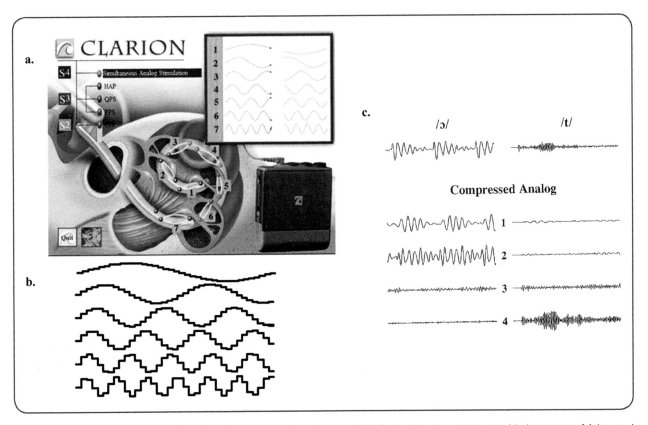

FIGURE 8–12. A visual representation of simultaneous analog stimulation (SAS) signal coding. Image provided courtesy of Advanced Bionics, LLC. Reprinted with permission from Wilson and Dorman, *Better Hearing with Cochlear Implants: Studies at the Research Triangle Institute* (2012). Copyright © Plural Publishing, Inc.

input signal. The primary disadvantage is the fact that fully simultaneous stimulation likely results in a great deal of channel interaction, which may lead to distortion. Research studies examining performance differences between SAS and Continuous Interleaved Sampling (CIS) produced mixed results (Zwolan et al., 2001). In short, this study showed that some recipients preferred and achieved at least similar performance with SAS compared with CIS. Subjects who performed well with SAS typically had favorable pre-implant histories and lower stimulation needs. Interestingly, Zwolan et al. found that recipients with the HiFocus electrode array and electrode positioner, a special component inserted along with the electrode array to facilitate proximity of the electrode contacts to the modiolus, were more likely to perform well with SAS. This finding may be attributed to the lower stimulation needs and subsequent reduction in channel interaction due to the shorter distance between the stimulating contacts and target neural elements. The electrode positioner was removed vol-

untarily from the market by the manufacturer in 2002 because it was associated with a higher incidence of bacterial meningitis.

Feature Extraction Strategies

In recognition of the limitations of analog stimulation, many researchers turned their interests to the use of biphasic electrical pulse stimulation and to **feature extraction** signal coding strategies that extracted a subset of acoustical cues from the incoming audio signal in an attempt to provide the most information thought to be most critical for speech recognition. The use of biphasic electrical pulses and feature extraction was intended to avoid the channel interaction that was identified as the most likely culprit that limited speech recognition with analog stimulation.

A block schematic for the implementation of $F_0/F_1/F_2$, which is an example of a feature extraction signal coding strategy, is depicted in Figure 8–13. The audio input signal is subjected to automatic

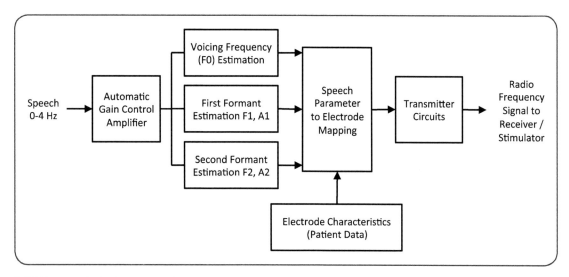

FIGURE 8–13. A block schematic for the implementation of the $F_0/F_1/F_2$ signal coding strategy.

gain control compression in order to deliver a wide range of intensities that are of potential interest to the recipient into the relatively narrow electrical dynamic range. Then, the signal is divided into different analysis bands for spectral analysis. The primary frequency present in the lowest frequency channel (i.e., the fundamental frequency) is used to modulate the stimulation rate that is delivered to the most apical intracochlear electrode contact. Modulating the low-frequency stimulation rate to coincide with the frequency in the lowest frequency channel is intended to capture the fundamental frequency of the talker's voice. Next, the sound processor attempts to identify and extract the first and second formant frequencies. F_1 and F_2 are coded by delivering biphasic electrical pulses to intracochlear electrode contacts based on the frequency of each formant and the corresponding electrode contact per the place principle (i.e., tonotopic organization; Greenwood function; see discussion on cochlear physiology in Chapter 3). The magnitude of electrical stimulation provided to each intracochlear electrode contact is determined by the intensity of the input signal and the stimulation needs of the recipient as determined by the audiologist in an implant programming session. Open-set speech recognition of the $F_0/F_1/F_2$ signal coding strategy was typically limited because information pertaining to high-frequency phonemes was not coded and delivered to the cochlear nerve. For instance, Dowell and colleagues (1987) found a mean CID-sentence recognition score of 35% correct in nine recipients using the MPEAK signal coding strategy.

The MULTIPEAK, or **MPEAK**, was an extension of the earliest feature extraction strategies. The MPEAK signal coding strategy includes the same processing that is present in the $F_0/F_1/F_2$ strategy, but MPEAK also analyzes the energy present in each of three high-frequency channels (i.e., from 2000 to 6000 Hz) and delivers electrical pulses to each of the basally located intracochlear electrode contacts that correspond to the frequency content in the high-frequency band analysis. Once again, the magnitude of electrical stimulation provided to each intracochlear electrode contact is determined by the intensity of the input signal in the corresponding analysis band (i.e., channel) and the requisite stimulation the recipient needs for that intracochlear electrode contact as determined during the cochlear implant programming session. Mean speech recognition with MPEAK was typically better than what was obtained with $F_0/F_1/F_2$ (Cohen et al., 1993; Dowell et al., 1990; Hollow et al., 1995; Parkinson et al., 1996; Skinner et al., 1991), and many recipients were able to obtain modest open-set speech recognition abilities with use of MPEAK (Cohen et al., 1993; Dowell et al., 1990; Hollow et al., 1995; Parkinson et al., 1996; Skinner et al., 1991). For instance, Dowell and colleagues (1990) reported mean Bamford-Kowal-Bench (BKB) sentence in quiet scores of 88% correct for a group of four adults using MPEAK. Furthermore, Skinner and colleagues (1991) reported mean monosyllabic word recognition scores of 29% correct for a group of seven adults using the MPEAK strategy. The improvement recipients experienced with MPEAK relative to $F_0/$

F_1/F_2 and to analog signal coding strategies showed the importance of multiple-channel stimulation, the provision of high-frequency speech information, and the attempt to limit channel interaction.

Continuous Interleaved Sampling (CIS)

A watershed accomplishment in the evolution of signal coding strategies occurred with the development of the **Continuous Interleaved Sampling (CIS)** strategy (Wilson et al., 1989). CIS utilizes biphasic electrical pulses to stimulate the cochlear nerve but is unique in feature extraction strategies because CIS does not attempt to focus on conveying a particular subset of information in the audio signal. Instead, CIS analyzes the audio signal available across several channels (typically at least eight) and comprehensively delivers that information to the cochlear nerve via electrical stimulation in an attempt to capture the amplitude envelope of the incoming acoustic signal. CIS is available in the cochlear implant systems for all three manufacturers, and it served as a precursor for most of the current signal coding strategies. As illustrated in Figure 8–14, the acoustic signal is sent through a bank of bandpass filters that separates the input signal into discrete frequency bands. (Note: In contemporary systems, filtering is accomplished through digital signal processing rather than physical analog filtering.) The tonotopic organization created by the filtering is preserved throughout signal processing and eventually represented to the auditory system via presentation to electrodes located in different positions in the cochlea (i.e., low-frequency filter outputs are eventually delivered to electrode contacts located in the apical end of the cochlea, whereas high-frequency filter outputs are delivered to electrode contacts located at the basal end of the cochlea).

The bandwidth of the filters used in CIS varies across the three different manufacturers. The output from these filters is directed to a rectifier that converts the alternating current into a direct current signal. Following the rectifier, the signal is sent through

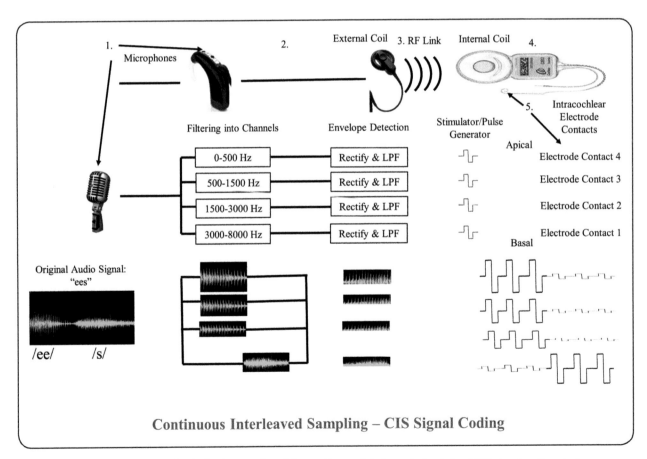

Continuous Interleaved Sampling – CIS Signal Coding

FIGURE 8–14. A block schematic for the implementation of the continuous interleaved stimulation (CIS) signal coding strategy.

a low-pass filter, where it is transformed into a temporal envelope. This envelope is analogous to the amplitude envelope of the acoustic input.

The CIS pulse rate must ideally be four to five times higher than the output from the low-pass filters to prevent aliasing errors. Because early versions of CIS-type strategies used pulse rates that were less than 2000 pps, the cutoff frequency of the low-pass filter usually is set between 200 and 400 Hz. A cutoff frequency up to 400 Hz encompasses the frequency at which the nerve can code changes in electrical pulse rate. This cutoff frequency also includes the fundamental frequency of the human voice, which is as low as 125 Hz for males and up to 400 Hz for young children.

The output of the low-pass filters is sent to a compressor that uses a logarithmic function to map the input signal into the patient's electrical dynamic range. This output from the compressor then is sent to a pulse generator, which is set to a fixed frequency (e.g., often between 800 and 1600 pps). The amplitude of the pulse train from the generator is modulated on the basis of the input received from the

compressor. Thus, the amplitude of the signal within each band is represented by the amplitude of the pulses within that same band. Finally, the modulated pulse trains in each channel are delivered to their respective electrode contacts.

Therefore, in the typical case, the intense low-frequency components of a speech signal are represented by high-amplitude pulses delivered to apical electrodes, whereas the relatively low-level, high-frequency components are represented by low-amplitude pulses delivered to the basal electrodes. All electrodes are stimulated sequentially during each stimulation cycle, and the amplitude of stimulation during each cycle corresponds to the energy present in the respective channel (Figure 8–15). Again, the frequency of the pulse trains is fixed, and stimulation occurs continuously at that stimulation frequency. Typical CIS pulse rates range from about 800 to 1600 pps and usually are implemented with 8 to 16 channels.

Blake Wilson and colleagues with the Research Triangle Institute initially evaluated CIS outcomes in a group of seven subjects who used the Symbion/Ineraid percutaneous cochlear implant system

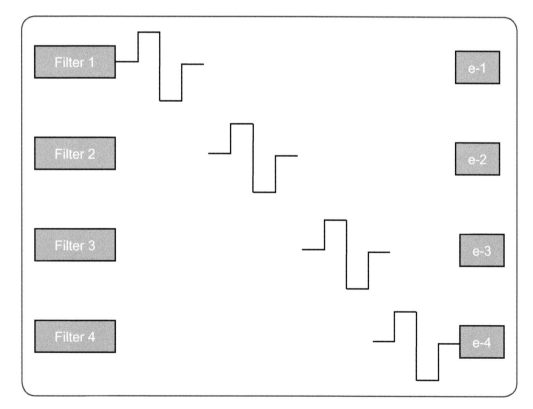

FIGURE 8–15. An example of interleaved presentation of electrical pulses of the continuous interleaved stimulation (CIS) signal coding strategy.

(Wilson & Dorman, 2012). The speech recognition of these subjects was evaluated with use of both a multiple-channel analog signal coding strategy (i.e., Compressed Analog) and CIS. Mean monosyllabic word recognition and sentence recognition in noise improved by almost 20 and 40 percentage points, respectively, with CIS compared to performance with the multiple-channel analog processor. This improvement in performance observed with the use of CIS led Wilson's team at RTI to focus on developing refinements of the strategy to allow for even greater levels of speech recognition. CIS serves as the foundation for most modern cochlear implant signal coding strategies in use today (e.g., HiRes, HiRes Fidelity 120, HiRes Optima, FSP, FS4, FS4-p).

Multiple Pulsatile Sampler (MPS)

Advanced Bionics offers a variation of CIS known as *Multiple Pulsatile Sampler* (MPS). MPS provides partially simultaneous stimulation. Specifically, two electrodes that are remotely spaced from one another are stimulated at the same time (i.e., electrodes 1 and 5; then 2 and 6; then 3 and 7; then 4 and 8). Figure 8–16 provides an elementary illustration of

MPS implemented in a 4-channel processor. The MPS strategy (with partially simultaneous stimulation) allows for a doubling in the stimulation rate (e.g., the stimulation rate increases from almost 800 pps to about 1600 pps), which should theoretically improve speech recognition (Wilson, Wolford, & Lawson, 2000). However, Wilson noted that the partially simultaneous stimulation provided by MPS increased channel interaction between the simultaneously stimulated channels, which at best may offset any benefit obtained by a faster stimulation rate, and at worst would possibly degrade performance. It should be noted that there is limited evidence suggesting better performance with MPS compared with CIS. Loizou et al. (2003) compared speech recognition obtained for nine subjects who switched between CIS (800 pps stimulation rate) and an MPS-type signal coding strategy (1600 pps stimulation rate). Four of the nine subjects showed no difference in performance with the two signal coding strategies, two obtained better performance with CIS, and two obtained better performance with MPS. Frohne-Buchner and colleagues (2003) compared a CIS-type strategy (2800 pps stimulation rate) with an MPS-type strategy (5600 pps stimulation rate) for a group of adult cochlear implant

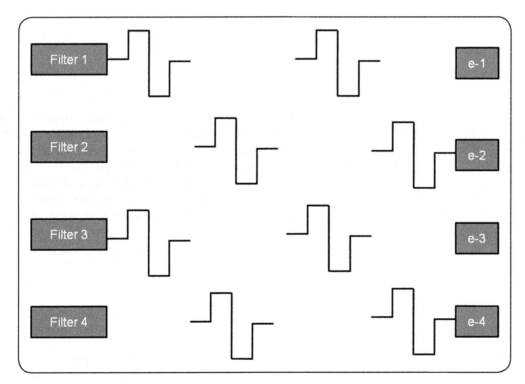

FIGURE 8–16. An example of partially simultaneous stimulation that occurs in the multiple pulsatile sampler (MPS) signal coding strategy.

users and found a statistically significant reduction with the use of partially simultaneous stimulation. It is possible that the faster stimulation rates used in the Frohne-Buchner study increased the negative effects of channel interaction that are possible during partially simultaneous stimulation.

Additional Variants of CIS

The MED-EL Corporation offers additional variations of CIS known as CIS+ and High Definition CIS (HDCIS). **CIS+** operates similarly to conventional CIS, but a Hilbert transformation is used in place of the conventional wave rectification and low-pass filtering that is used with traditional CIS. The use of a Hilbert transformation is intended to allow for a more accurate estimate of the input signal and to capture the fine temporal structure cues. In **HDCIS**, a wider frequency range is available over which to implement the CIS strategy (i.e., 250 to 8000 Hz with the option to set the lower end of the bandwidth to 70 Hz). Also, the total stimulation rate available for HDCIS is 50,704 pps. Of note, the Hilbert transformation used to create the analysis bands (i.e., channels) used in CIS+ and HDCIS creates overlapping filter bands between channels. As a result, when two neighboring channels are sequentially stimulated (with the electrical pulses falling very closely in time to one another), the locus of stimulation occurs somewhere between the center frequency of the two channels, creating intermediate pitch percepts. The exact locus of stimulation depends on the frequency of the input signal and its relation to the frequencies that make up the neighboring analysis bands. This approach at creating intermediate pitch percepts is used in an attempt to provide better spectral resolution and, in a patient with a full complement of electrodes activated, creates 250 distinct spectral bands along the electrode array. Of note, the recipient is unlikely to hear 250 different pitches because of the reduced spectral resolution of the peripheral auditory system as it responds to electrical stimulation. The number of different pitches perceived by the recipient is dependent on several factors, including cochlear nerve survival, the spread of electrical current in the cochlea, and so forth.

HiResolution Sound Processing

HiResolution (HiRes) sound processing, developed by Advanced Bionics and commercially released in the United States in 2003, is another variation of CIS processing. The primary differences between HiReso-

lution and conventional CIS include: (1) the provision of 16 active electrodes in HiRes rather than the typical 8 in CIS, (2) considerably higher maximum stimulation rates (e.g., up to 5156 pps), (3) higher cutoff frequencies for low-pass filters (e.g., 2800 Hz), and (4) a more sophisticated automatic gain control (AGC) system. Theoretically, the combination of the higher stimulation rates and filter cutoffs will improve the provision of fine temporal structure. An additional advantage may be the facilitation of stochastic firing in the auditory nerve that would more closely represent normal auditory nerve function.

HiResolution sound processing is available in two commercial forms, **HiResS** and **HiResP**. HiResS provides completely sequential stimulation, whereas HiResP provides partial simultaneous stimulation similar to the MPS strategy. In other words, HiResP provides simultaneous stimulation at 1 and 9, 2 and 10, 3 and 11, 4 and 12, 5 and 13, 6 and 14, 7 and 15, as well as 8 and 16. HiResS can deliver pulse trains with rates up to 2900 pps, whereas HiResP has a maximum stimulation rate of 5156 pps. In a clinical trial, speech-recognition performance of adult recipients was significantly better with the HiRes processing compared with conventional strategies (Koch et al., 2004). In addition, the HiRes processing was preferred by the majority of subjects.

In 2006, Advanced Bionics released a new version of HiRes known as **HiRes Fidelity 120**, which incorporates current steering. Current steering attempts to increase the number of perceptual channels in the frequency domain by simultaneously stimulating on two neighboring electrode contacts to create a locus of stimulation that falls somewhere between those two contacts (see Figure 8–17 for a visual illustration of current steering). Through the use of current steering, HiRes Fidelity 120 creates up to 120 virtual channels. Additional channels may increase the number of frequency percepts and spectral resolution and, therefore, should improve speech recognition in noise, sound quality, and music appreciation. Koch and colleagues (2007) examined the number of individual pitch percepts that could be detected between two physical intracochlear electrode contacts via the use of current steering. Data from 57 implanted ears indicated that an average of 5.4 pitch percepts were distinguished between basal electrode contacts, 8.7 between mid-array contacts, and 7.2 between apical electrode contacts. Results of a clinical trial conducted by Advanced Bionics showed that the study participants' ($n = 50$) mean word recognition and sentence recognition in quiet and in noise were essentially similar

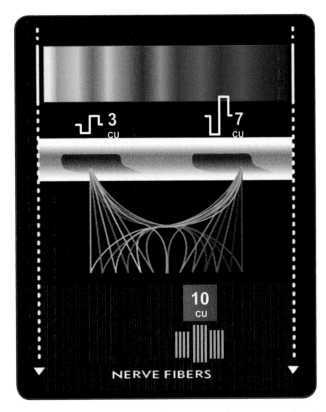

FIGURE 8–17. An illustration of current steering to create virtual electrodes. Image provided courtesy of Advanced Bionics, LLC.

HiRes Optima is the newest strategy in the HiResolution sound processing family. The primary objective of HiRes Optima is to reduce the power requirements for the processor. As previously stated, the Naída CI external sound processor is substantially smaller than its predecessor, the Harmony sound processor. The reduction in processor size required a reduction in battery size. Specifically, the zinc-air battery module must operate from two 675P zinc-air batteries.

HiRes Optima incorporates a couple of changes from HiRes Fidelity 120 that are all designed to reduce battery consumption while preserving recipient performance. HiRes Optima reduces power requirements by reducing the compliance voltage of the implant from 8 volts to 4 volts, by modifying the current steering paradigm so that stimulation is delivered only via virtual electrodes, and by modifying the pulse width management scheme to maintain the 4-volt compliance limit. In all other aspects (front-end options, frequency analysis, ClearVoice), HiRes Optima is identical to HiRes Fidelity 120 sound processing. A clinical trial conducted in 2012 showed that speech perception benefit was comparable between HiRes Optima and HiRes Fidelity 120 and that average battery life was improved by 53% (Advanced Bionics, 2012). It should be noted that for some recipients with high impedance levels, the pulse width required to achieve adequate loudness may increase and cause a subsequent reduction in the stimulation rate. However, a stimulation rate of 1000 to 1500 pps is typically achievable with HiRes Optima, so a reduction in stimulation rate that occurs with an increase in pulse width is unlikely to result in a significant decrease in speech recognition. HiRes Optima is available for the Naída CI, Neptune, and Harmony sound processors.

n-of-m *Strategies*

The common denominator among all of the aforementioned CIS-type strategies is that all active electrode contacts are stimulated (either in a sequential or partially simultaneous manner) for each cycle of stimulation. The *n-of-m* signal coding strategies, which are also sometimes referred to as "peak-picker" strategies, utilize a different approach (Wilson & Dorman, 2012). For a given input sound, the acoustic energy present in each of the m channels is determined, and stimulation is administered to only the n channels with the highest amplitude inputs (Figure 8–18). The n is typically referred to as **maxima** in these types of

between conventional HiRes and HiRes Fidelity 120 (Advanced Bionics, 2009). Superior sound quality ratings and higher music appreciation were reported with the HiRes Fidelity 120 strategy compared with the HiRes strategy. However, it should be noted that the subjects were not blinded to the signal processing strategy they were using. Donaldson, Dawson, and Borden (2011) also studied speech recognition obtained for a group of adult subjects who used HiRes and HiRes Fidelity 120 and reported no significant differences in performance obtained with the two signal coding strategies. Firszt and colleagues (2009) also found similar speech recognition scores between HiRes and HiRes Fidelity 120 for a group of seven adult participants. However, these participants did report that music quality was significantly better with use of Fidelity 120. It should be noted that as with the Advanced Bionics clinical trial (Advanced Bionics, 2009), the subjects in the Firszt et al. (2009) study were not blinded to the programming they were using. As a result, it is possible that their judgments regarding music perception and sound quality were biased.

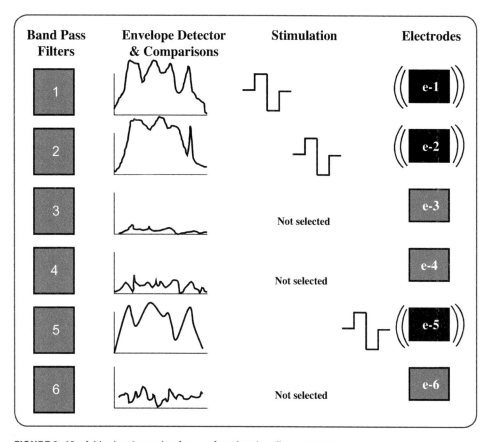

FIGURE 8–18. A block schematic of an *n*-of-*m* signal coding strategy.

signal coding strategies. The *n* (or maxima) typically varies from 8 to 12. Therefore, a program with 22 channels and a maxima of 10 will result in a train of biphasic pulses delivered to the 10 channels with the highest amplitude. The remaining 12 channels are not stimulated during that specific cycle.

The *n*-of-*m* strategies are designed to capture the prominent components present in a speech signal while discarding the relatively low fluctuations in amplitude, which are more likely to be noise. The reduction in the number of active electrodes during each cycle allows for: (1) faster stimulation rates, (2) a reduction in channel interaction and masking, and (3) an increase in battery life. The potential limitation of *n*-of-*m* approaches is that desirable information in some channels may not possess the necessary amplitude to be selected. As a result, the user will not have access to this acoustic information. However, research studies conducted with Cochlear Nucleus users indicate that they do as well or better with an *n*-of-*m* strategy (i.e., ACE) compared with CIS strat-

egies (Kiefer, Hohl, Sturzebecher, Pfennigdorff, & Gstöettner, 2001; Skinner et al., 2002).

Spectral Peak (SPEAK)

SPEAK was one of the first clinically available signal coding strategies that used the *n*-of-*m* approach. The initial components are similar to those of CIS strategies. Inputs are sent through a bank of bandpass filters, in which the complex broadband sounds are divided into narrower frequency bands. The amplitude of the inputs in each channel is determined, and the *n* channels with the highest amplitudes are selected for processing (i.e., if a maxima of 8 is selected, then 8 of the 22 active electrodes are stimulated). The outputs from those filters then are rectified and low-pass filtered with the cutoff frequency of 200 Hz. Finally, those outputs are used to modulate a train of biphasic pulses that are fixed in frequency (typically 250 pps) and are delivered to corresponding electrodes. In practice, the SPEAK strategy is implemented with bipolar electrode coupling in the previous generation Nucleus 22 implant and either bipolar or monopolar coupling in the Nucleus 24 and later implants. A maximum of 20 active channels are available, and the typical maxima is set at 8.

Advanced Combination Encoder (ACE)

ACE is also an *n*-of-*m* strategy that provides the option of using stimulation rates that are faster than those used with SPEAK. ACE is the current default signal coding strategy used with Cochlear Ltd. implants. The first version of ACE allowed for a total stimulation rate of 14,400 pps. Consequently, the per-channel stimulation rate is dependent upon the number of maxima selected. If 8 maxima is selected, then a per-channel rate of 1800 pps can be achieved (8 × 1800 = 14,400). In practice, ACE uses monopolar electrode coupling. A maximum of 22 channels are available, and the typical maxima ranges from 8 to 12. In the current version of Custom Sound programming software, the ACE signal coding strategy is implemented with a

default stimulation rate of 900 pps and 8 maxima. The authors of this book routinely use the ACE signal coding strategy with Nucleus recipients, but the maxima is typically increased to 10 (see Figure 8–19 for a visual depiction of ACE).

Research studies have shown that most recipients perform better with ACE than SPEAK (Kiefer et al., 2001; Skinner et al., 2002). ACE likely allows for better performance because of the provision of fine temporal structure cues via the higher stimulation rates of ACE. As a result, an overwhelming number of Nucleus recipients use ACE. The audiologist may wish to switch to the SPEAK signal coding strategy if the recipient experiences undesirable effects with monopolar stimulation (e.g., facial nerve stimulation), and bipolar or pseudomonopolar stimulation is required.

Cochlear also offers a variation of ACE known as **ACE(RE)** or HighACE. ACE(RE) operates exactly like ACE, but the maximum total stimulation rate is 32,000 pps rather than 14,400 pps. The advantages of ACE(RE) over ACE may be negligible for many

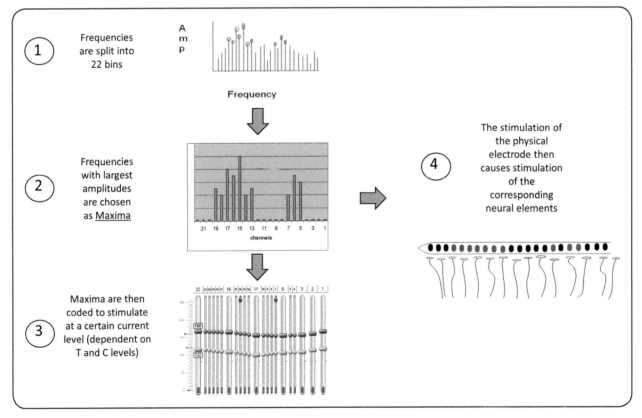

FIGURE 8–19. A visual representation of the advanced combination encoder (ACE) signal coding strategy. Image provided courtesy of Cochlear Americas, © 2018.

users because, as mentioned earlier, most recipients do not perform better with stimulation rates exceeding approximately 1500 to 2000 pps. In fact, in a large clinical trial, many subjects preferred and performed better with programs using rates at or below 900 pps (Arora et al., 2009; Balkany et al., 2007). Additionally, it should be noted that the higher stimulation rates associated with ACE(RE) (particularly with the 3500 pps stimulation rate) require a very narrow pulse width, and as a result, voltage compliance limits are often reached before an adequate loudness percept is obtained.

MP3000 is yet another Cochlear Nucleus variation of an *n*-of-*m* strategy. Similar to the approach used in modern MP3 recreational audio players, unimportant information in the input signal (i.e., low-level components that will be masked by adjacent higher level and more important components) is discarded. As a result, the signal is conveyed in a more efficient manner and without a significant compromise in quality or clarity.

Figure 8–20 provides a simplified illustration of the MP3000 strategy in operation. Across these six

channels, only channels 1 and 5 will be audible for the user because the neighboring channels will be masked. As a result, stimulation is provided to only these two channels.

The primary advantage of the MP3000 strategy is an improvement in signal efficiency, which allows (proportional to the number in maxima reduction) for longer battery life, reduction in battery size, and ultimately, smaller sound processors. Preliminary research findings suggest that speech recognition with the MP3000 strategy is better than that obtained with the ACE strategy (Buchner, Nogueira, Edler, Battmer, & Lenarz, 2008). The MP3000 signal coding strategy has been used in Europe but has yet to receive FDA approval for use in the United States.

Fine Structure Processing (FSP)

MED-EL also offers another novel CIS-type signal coding strategy, referred to as FSP, which has two important differences from the original CIS strategy. As with CIS+ and HDCIS, MED-EL FSP signal coding

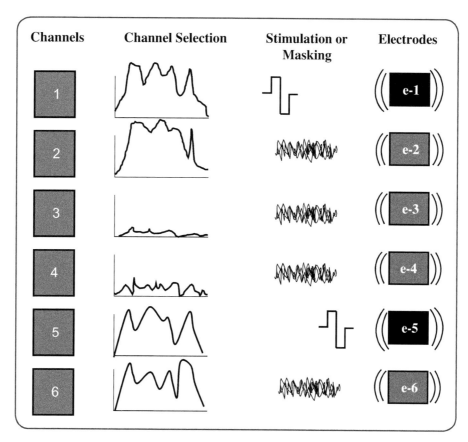

FIGURE 8–20. An elementary visual example of the MP3000 signal coding strategy.

strategies use a Hilbert transformation to analyze the audio input signal and extract the spectral, amplitude envelope, and fine temporal structure information. Also, intermediate pitches may be generated using bell-shaped, overlapping bandpass filters to provide better spectral resolution, which is important for the recognition of high-frequency phonemes, including consonants identified on the basis of place cues (i.e., /s/, /f/, /t/). The use of a CIS-based signal coding strategy with the provision of intermediate pitches fine temporal structure (described below) may improve sound quality, speech recognition in noise, music appreciation, and music recognition.

A major difference from both the traditional CIS strategy and CIS+/HDICS is that the **FSP strategy** modulates the timing of channel-specific sampling sequences (CSSS), or pulse bursts, in the lowest frequency channels, depending on the input frequency within those channels (see Figure 8–21 for a visual depiction of CSSS). In other words, the stimulation frequency used in the low-frequency, fine structure channels is determined by the frequency of the input signal within each fine structure channel. Yet another way to explain the CSSS concept is to state that the series of stimulation pulses (i.e., the stimulation rate) is triggered by the zero crossings in a channel's bandpass filter output. A zero crossing is a point in time at which an audio waveform "crosses the *x*-axis" between the condensation (i.e., peak; positive polarity) and rarefaction (i.e., trough; negative polarity) por-

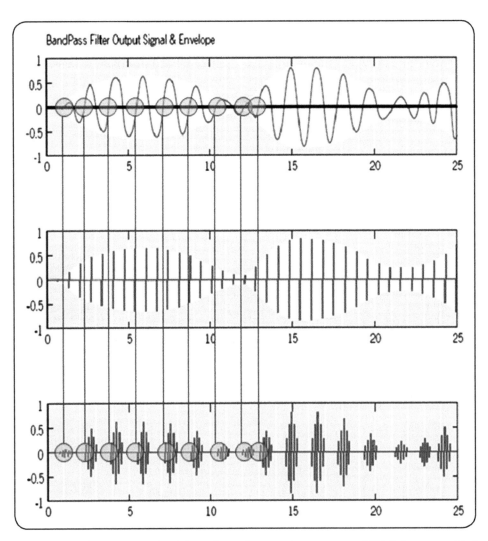

FIGURE 8–21. A visual example of channel-specific sampling sequences (CSSS). Image provided courtesy of MED-EL Corporation.

tions of the waveform. Figure 8–22 provides a visual illustration of a block-schematic of FSP signal coding.

The potential advantage of FSP signal coding/CSSS stimulation in the low-frequency channels is to provide better access to fine temporal structure by stimulating low-frequency auditory nerve fibers at the same rate as the low-frequency input signal. An improved provision of fine temporal structure may improve speech recognition, sound quality, recognition of vocal pitch, music appreciation, music recognition, and possibly even access to interaural timing cues for localization. The FSP coding (i.e., CSSS analysis and adaptive provision of stimulation rate) is typically administered up to approximately 350 Hz, which often spans the one to two most apical channels.

MED-EL has introduced two variations of the FSP strategy referred to as FS4 and FS4-p. As previously discussed, the FSP strategy usually incorporates the CSSS analysis and adaptive provision of stimulation rate up to 350 Hz, over one or two of the most apical channels. **FS4** provides the fine structure processing (CSSS) in the channels extending up to 1000 Hz (i.e., the three or four most apical channels). The primary objective is to provide enhanced fine structure processing throughout the low-frequency range.

FS4-p is a variation of the FS4 signal coding strategy. With FS4-p, fine structure processing is provided up to 1000 Hz, and parallel stimulation (simultaneous stimulation) is used to simultaneously stimulate two of the four most apical channels at the same point in time in order to provide fine temporal structure on two channels in the event that two channels each experienced a zero crossing during a stimulation frame. As a result, the stimulation rate on two of the four most apical channels may be different at any given point in time. Figure 8–23 provides a visual example of the implementation of FSP, FS4, and FS4-p. Parallel stimulation is possible because the MED-EL cochlear implant includes multiple (i.e., 24) current sources to independently stimulate each of the 12 intracochlear electrode contacts.

The FS4-p strategy possesses a novel algorithm referred to as **channel interaction compensation (CIC)**, which ensures that undesirable spatial channel interaction does not occur during the implementation of the parallel stimulation. In short, the CIC algorithm uses a patented modeling algorithm to predict when undesirable channel interaction may occur when simultaneous stimulation is provided to neighboring intracochlear electrode contacts. When channel interaction is anticipated, the magnitude of electrical

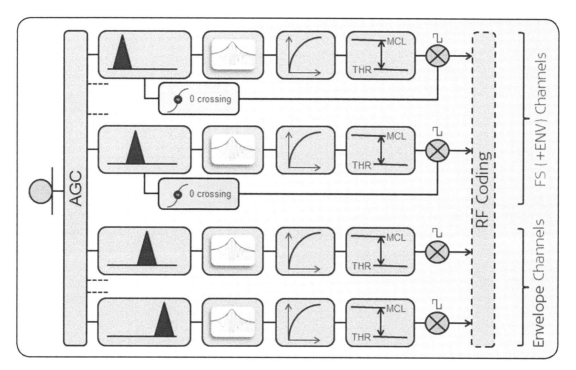

FIGURE 8–22. A visual illustration of a block-schematic of FSP signal coding. Image provided courtesy of MED-EL Corporation.

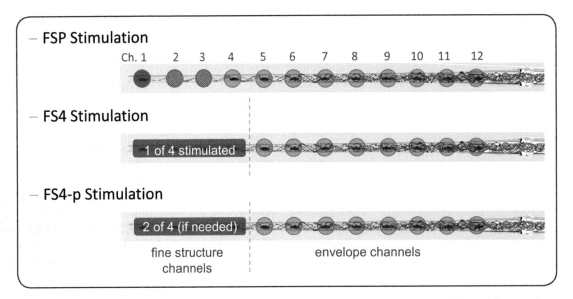

FIGURE 8–23. A visual example of FSP, FS4, and FS4-p stimulation. Image provided courtesy of MED-EL Corporation.

stimulation delivered to neighboring electrode contacts is reduced in an attempt to minimize channel interaction. Figure 8–24 provides a visual example of the implementation of CIC.

At the time of this writing, published studies examining the improvement in hearing performance offered by FSP, FS4, and FS4-p relative to CIS have produced mixed results but have shown that use of the FSP strategies does provide the potential for improved hearing performance. Seebens and Diller (2012) compared monosyllabic word and sentence recognition in quiet and in noise of 45 adults (54 ears as some participants used bilateral implants) who converted from the TEMPO+ processor with CIS+ to the OPUS 2 processor with FSP. Mean word recognition in quiet with use of FSP (77.8% correct) was significantly better than mean word recognition with use of CIS+ (62% correct). Mean word recognition in noise was also significantly better with FSP (52.1%) compared with CIS+ (27.3%). Mean sentence recognition in quiet (77.9%) and in noise (58%) with FSP were also significantly better than what was obtained with CIS+ (69.9% in quiet and 40.4% in noise). Furthermore, Muller et al. (2012) compared performance obtained with FSP versus CIS+ and HDCIS for 46 adult cochlear implant recipients and reported improvement in vowel and monosyllabic word recognition with use of FSP over the CIS strategies. They also reported that the study participants had a preference for FSP over CIS when listening to speech and music.

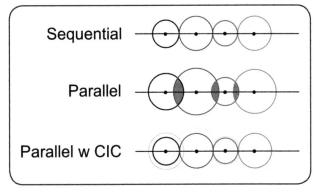

FIGURE 8–24. A visual representation of channel interaction compensation (CIC). Image provided courtesy of MED-EL Corporation.

However, sentence recognition was similar with use of FSP and the CIS strategies. Additionally, Arnoldner and colleagues (2007) compared word recognition in quiet and sentence recognition in noise obtained with CIS versus FSP for 14 adults. They found no difference in word recognition in quiet between the two signal coding strategies, but there was a statistically significant improvement in sentence recognition in noise with use of the FSP strategy. Also, subjects reported better music appreciation with FSP and an overall preference for FSP. In another study of interest, Kleine Punte, De Bodt, and Van de Heyning (2014) compared sentence recognition at several points for MED-EL users who upgraded from the

TEMPO+ to the OPUS 2 sound processor. Thirty-two participants were divided into two groups, one that used HDCIS for two years and another that used FSP for two years. Kleine Punte and colleagues reported that sentence recognition in noise improved across the two-year period for the FSP users but did not for the HDCIS users. The results of this study suggested that a period of time may be necessary for users to acclimate to FSP and realize benefit from the signal coding strategy. Furthermore, Lorens et al. (2010) reported a small but statistically significant improvement in speech recognition obtained with FSP versus CIS+ and HDCIS for a group of 60 children using the MED-EL OPUS 2 sound processor. Also of note, Roy et al. (2015) reported better bass frequency (i.e., low-frequency musical note perception) with use of FSP over HDCIS.

In contrast to the aforementioned studies that showed at least some improvement in performance with FSP compared with CIS, several studies have failed to show a statistically significant improvement with the use of FSP. Magnusson (2011) evaluated speech recognition in quiet and in noise and evaluated sound quality for speech and music for 20 experienced adult cochlear implant recipients using FSP and CIS. No difference was found between performance with FSP vs. any of the MED-EL CIS strategies (CIS+ or HDCIS). Likewise, Riss and colleagues (2011) compared word recognition in quiet, sentence recognition in noise, and melody recognition obtained between use of CIS+ and FSP for a group of 31 adult MED-EL cochlear implant users and found no difference in performance between the two signal coding strategies for any of the measures. Riss (2008) also compared speech recognition in quiet and in noise for a smaller group of 10 MED-EL adult recipients using both FSP and CIS and found no difference in performance obtained with each of the two signal coding strategies. Dillon et al. (2016) evaluated word recognition in quiet and sentence recognition in noise for 22 MED-EL adult recipients divided into two groups, one that used HDCIS for six months and another that used FSP for six months. They found no difference in speech recognition in quiet or noise between the two groups.

Of note, several studies have evaluated the use of FSP and CIS for tonal languages. Chen et al. (2013) found an improvement in Mandarin speech recognition with the use of FSP versus CIS strategies. However, Qi et al. (2017) found no differences in speech recognition obtained with FSP versus CIS+ for

a group of Mandarin-speaking adult participants. In spite of the lack of an improvement in speech recognition, Qi and colleagues did report that participants rated the FSP strategy as having better sound quality than CIS+. Tone perception also improved with use of FSP. Additionally, Schatzer and colleagues (2010) compared speech recognition obtained with CIS and FSP for Cantonese-speaking participants and found no difference in performance obtained with the two different signal coding strategies.

Riss and colleagues (2014) compared monosyllabic word recognition in quiet, sentence recognition in noise, and sound quality obtained by 33 adults with FSP compared with FS4 and FS4-p. In general, there were no statistically significant differences obtained with FS4 and FS4-p compared with FSP for any of the speech recognition measures or for any of the sound quality measures. However, 20 of the 33 subjects did choose FS4 or FS4-p over FSP, which was the signal coding strategy they used prior to the start of the study. Riss and colleagues (2016) compared word recognition in quiet and subjective sound quality obtained with HDCIS versus FS4 for 26 adult participants. Performance was evaluated with each signal coding strategy at a "low" rate of 750 pps/channel and a "fast" rate of 1376 pps/channel. They found similar word recognition with the two signal coding strategies, with a small improvement with FS4 at the faster stimulation rate. Better sound quality was reported with use of FS4 at the higher stimulation rate.

It should be noted that a unique characteristic of the MED-EL implant is the fact that the Standard and FLEXSOFT electrode arrays are 31.5 mm in length and designed to be inserted to an angular insertion depth of approximately 630 degrees, which is much deeper than the electrode arrays of other cochlear implant manufacturers. The deep insertion of these MED-EL electrode arrays is intended to position the most apical intracochlear electrode contact at a location in which the lowest frequencies in the speech-frequency range (i.e., 100 to 300 Hz) are typically coded in the cochlea. Some research studies have suggested that the stimulating intracochlear electrode contact must be positioned at the location intended to process a particular frequency range in order for the cochlear nerve and the auditory nervous system to process the fine temporal structure cues present in the signal. For instance, Prentiss et al. (2014) evaluated an individual cochlear implant recipient's ability to match pitch between acoustic and electric stimulation in an implanted ear in which a significant amount of residual low-frequency natural hearing existed after implantation. Specifically, pitch-matching was evaluated with electrical pulses delivered at stimulation rates varying from 100 to 1100 pps on electrode contacts located at apical, middle, and basal locations of the cochlea. A change in stimulation rate did not result in a change in pitch percept when electrical stimulation was delivered to the electrode contacts located in the middle and basal portions of the electrode array. However, there was a systematic decrease in pitch as the stimulation rate was decreased from 1100 to 100 pps on the apically located electrodes. Additionally, an almost one-to-one pitch match was achieved between acoustic and electric stimulation when a low-frequency stimulation rate was used on the most apically located electrode contact. Figure 8–25 displays the results obtained in the Prentiss (2014) study. In summary, theoretically, the provision of fine structure is further facilitated by the deep placement of the MED-EL Standard electrode array into the apical area of the cochlea. This deep placement allows for stimulation of auditory nerve fibers that naturally possess a low-frequency characteristic frequency.

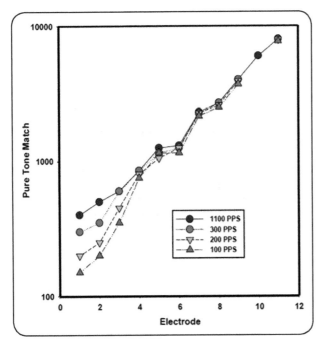

FIGURE 8–25. A visual representation pitch matching that occurs as a function of intracochlear electrode contact (depth) and stimulation rate (in pps). Image provided courtesy of Sandra Prentiss.

Key Concepts

- The evolution of cochlear implant signal coding strategy has resulted in substantial improvements in hearing performance.
- There are several differences in the modern signal coding strategies of each of the major cochlear implant manufacturers. However, impressive levels of open-set speech recognition and hearing performance may be achieved with all modern signal coding strategies.

References

Adams, D., Ajimsha, K. M., Barbera, M. T., Gazibegovic, D., Gisbert, J., Gomez, J., . . . Zarowski, A. (2014). Multicentre evaluation of music perception in adult users of Advanced Bionics cochlear implants. *Cochlear Implants International, 15*(1), 20–26.

Advanced Bionics Corporation. (2009, March). *HiRes with Fidelity 120® clinical results.* Retrieved from http://www.advanced bionics.com/UserFiles/File/3-01009-A_HiRes120_Clinical%20 Results%28Mar_05%29.pdf

Advanced Bionics. (2012). *HiRes Optima clinical results.* Valencia, CA: Author.

Arnolder, C., Riss, D., Brunner, M., Durisin, M., Baumgartner, W. D., & Hamzavi, J. S. (2007). Speech and music perception with the new fine structure speech coding strategy: Preliminary results. *Acta Otolaryngologica, 127*(12), 1298–1303.

Arora, K., Dawson. P., Dowell, R., & Vandali, A. (2009). Electrical stimulation rate effects on speech perception in cochlear implants. *International Journal of Audiology, 48*(8), 561–567.

Balkany, T., Hodges, A., Menapace, C., Hazard, L., Driscoll, C., Gantz, B., . . . Payne, S. (2007). Nucleus Freedom North American clinical trial. *Otolaryngology-Head and Neck Surgery, 136*(5), 757–762.

Buchner, A., Nogueira, W., Edler, B., Battmer, R., & Lenarz, T. (2008). Results from a psychoacoustic model-based strategy for the Nucleus-24 and Freedom cochlear implants. *Otology and Neurotology, 29*, 189–192.

Chen, X., Liu, B., Liu, S., Mo, L., Li, Y., Kong, Y., . . . Han, D. (2013). Cochlear implants with fine structure processing improve speech and tone perception in Mandarin-speaking adults. *Acta Otolaryngologica, 133*(7), 733–738.

Clark, G. M. (1969). Responses of cells in the superior olivary complex of the cat to electrical stimulation of the auditory nerve. *Experimental Neurology, 24*(1), 124–136.

Cohen, N. L., Waltzman, S. B., & Fisher, S. G. (1993). A prospective, randomized study of cochlear implants. The Department of Veterans Affairs Cochlear Implant Study Group. *New England Journal of Medicine, 328*(4), 233–237.

Dillon, M. T., Buss, E., King, E. R., Deres, E. J., Obarowski, S. N., Anderson, M. L., & Adunka, M. C. (2016). Comparison of two cochlear implant coding strategies on speech perception. *Cochlear Implants International, 17*(6), 263–270.

Donaldson, G. S., Dawson, P. K., & Borden, L. Z. (2011). Within-subjects comparison of the HiRes and Fidelity120 speech processing strategies: Speech perception and its relation to place-pitch sensitivity. *Ear and Hearing, 32*(2), 238–250.

Dowell, R. C., Seligman, P. M., Blamey, P. J., & Clark, G. M. (1987). Speech perception using a two-formant 22-electrode cochlear prosthesis in quiet and in noise. *Acta Otolaryngologica, 104*(5–6), 439–446.

Dowell, R. C., Whitford, L. A., Seligman P. M., Franz, B. K. H., & Clark, G. M. (1990). Preliminary results with a miniature speech processor for the 22-electrode/Cochlear hearing prosthesis. In T. Sacristan (Ed.), *Oto-rhinlaryngology, head and neck surgery.* Amsterdam, Netherlands: Kugler and Ghedini.

Filipo, R., Ballantyne, D., Mancini, P., & D'Elia, C. (2008). Music perception in cochlear implant recipients: Comparison of findings between HiRes90 and HiRes120. *Acta Otolaryngologica128*(4), 378–381.

Firszt, J. B., Holden, L. K., Reeder, R. M., & Skinner, M. W. (2009). Speech recognition in cochlear implant recipients: Comparison of standard HiRes and HiRes 120 sound processing. *Otology and Neurotology, 30*(2), 146–152.

Frohne-Buchner, C., Battmer, R. D., Buchner, A., et al., (2003). *The Clarion CII high-resolution mode: Paired or sequential stimulation paradigm?* Presented at the 2003 Conference on implantable auditory prostheses. Pacific Grove, CA: Conference Abstract Book, (p. 117).

Gfeller, K., Oleson, J., Knutson, J. F., Breheny, P., Driscoll, V., & Olszewski, C. (2008). Multivariate predictors of music perception and appraisal by adult cochlear implant users. *Journal of the American Academy of Audiology, 19*(2), 120–134.

Gfeller, K., Turner, C., Mehr, M., Woodworth, G., Fearn, R., Knutson, J. F., . . . Stordahl, J. (2002). Recognition of familiar melodies by adult cochlear implant recipients and normal-hearing adults. *Cochlear Implants International, 3*(1), 29–53.

Gfeller, K., Turner, C., Oleson, J., Zhang, X., Gantz, B., Froman, R., & Olszewski, C. (2007). Accuracy of cochlear implant recipients on pitch perception, melody recognition, and speech reception in noise. *Ear and Hearing, 28*(3), 412–423.

Gifford, R. H., Dorman, M.F., Shallop, J. K., & Sydlowski, S.A. (2010). Evidence of the expansion of adult cochlear implant candidacy. *Ear and Hearing, 31*(2), 186–194.

Gifford, R. H., Shallop, J. K., & Peterson, A. M. (2008). Speech recognition materials and ceiling effects: Considerations for cochlear implant programs. *Audiology and Neurotology, 13*(3), 193–205.

Hamill, T. A., & Price, L. L. (2008). Acoustics of speech. In *The hearing sciences* (pp. 137–152). San Diego, CA: Plural.

Hollow, R. D., Dowell, R. C., Cowan, R. S., Skok, M. C., Pyman, B. C., & Clark, G. M. (1995). Continuing improvements in speech processing for adult cochlear implant patients. *Annals of Otology, Rhinology, and Laryngology, Supplement, 166,* 292–294.

Inverso, Y., & Limb, C. J. (2010). Cochlear implant-mediated perception of nonlinguistic sounds. *Ear and Hearing, 31*(4), 505–514.

Kiefer, J., Hohl, S., Sturzebecher, E., Pfennigdorff, T., & Gstöettner, W. (2001). Comparison of speech recognition with different speech coding strategies (SPEAK, CIS, and ACE) and their relationship to telemetric measures of compound action potentials in the Nucleus CI 24M cochlear implant system. *Audiology, 40*(1), 32–42.

Kleine Punte, A., De Bodt, M., & Van de Heyning, P. (2014). Long-term improvement of speech perception with the fine structure processing coding strategy in cochlear implants. *ORL Journal of Oto-Rhino-Laryngology and Its Related Specialties, 76*(1), 36–43.

Koch, D. B., Downing, M., Osberger, M. J., & Litvak, L. (2007). Using current steering to increase spectral resolution in CII and HiRes 90K users. *Ear and Hearing, 28*(2), 38S–41S.

Koch, D. B., Osberger, M. J., Segel, P., & Kessler, D. K. (2004). HiResolution and conventional sound processing in the HiResolution Bionic Ear: Using appropriate outcome measures to assess speech recognition ability. *Audiology and Neurotology, 9,* 214–223.

Limb, C. J., & Rubinstein, J. T. (2012). Current research on music perception in cochlear implant users. *Otolaryngology Clinics of North America, 45*(1), 129–140.

Loizou, P. C., Stickney, G., Mishra, L., & Assmann, P. (2003). Comparison of speech processing strategies used in the Clarion implant processor. *Ear and Hearing, 24*(1), 12–19.

Lorens, A., Zgoda, M., Obrycka, A., & Skarzynski, H. (2010). Fine structure processing improves speech perception as well as objective and subjective benefits in pediatric MED-EL COMBI 40+ users. *International Journal of Pediatric Otorhinolaryngology, 74*(12), 1372–1378.

MacKay, I. R. A. (2014). *Acoustics in hearing, speech, and language sciences: An introduction.* Upper Saddle River, NJ: Pearson Education.

Magnusson, L. (2011). Comparison of the fine structure processing (FSP) strategy and the CIS strategy used in the MED-EL cochlear implant system: speech intelligibility and music sound quality. *International Journal of Audiology, 50*(4), 279–287.

Muller, J., Brill, S., Hagen, R., Moeltner, A., Brockmeier, S. J., Stark, T., . . . Anderson, I. (2012). Clinical trial results with the MED-EL fine structure processing coding strategy in experienced cochlear implant users. *ORL Journal of Oto-Rhino-Laryngology and Its Related Specialties, 74*(4), 185–198.

Osberger, M. J., Quick, A., Arnold, L., & Boyle, P. (2010). Music benefits with HiRes Fidelity 120(R) sound processing. *Cochlear Implants International, 11*(Suppl. 1), 351–354.

Parkinson, A. J., Tyler, R. S., Woodworth, G. G., Lowder, M. W., & Gantz, B. J. (1996). A within-subject comparison of adult patients using the Nucleus *F0F1F2* and *F0F1F2B3B4B5* speech processing strategies. *Journal of Speech and Hearing Research, 39*(2), 261–277.

Prentiss, S., Staecker, H., & Wolford, B. (2014). Ipsilateral acoustic electric pitch matching: A case study of cochlear implantation in an up-sloping hearing loss with preserved hearing across multiple frequencies. *Cochlear Implants International, 15*(3), 161–165.

Qi, B., Liu, Z., Gu, X., & Liu, B. (2017). Speech recognition outcomes in Mandarin-speaking cochlear implant users with fine structure processing. *Acta Otolaryngologica, 137*(3), 286–292.

Riss, D., Arnoldner, C., Baumgartner, W. D., Kaider, A., & Hamzavi, J. S. (2008). A new fine structure speech coding strategy: Speech perception at a reduced number of channels. *Otology and Neurotology, 29*(6), 784–788.

Riss, D., Hamzavi, J. S., Blineder, M., Flak, S., Baumgartner, W. D., Kaider, A., & Arnoldner, C. (2016). Effects of stimulation rate with the FS4 and HDCIS coding strategies in cochlear implant recipients. *Otology and Neurotology, 37*(7), 882–888.

Riss, D., Hamzavi, J. S., Blineder, M., Honeder, C., Ehrenreich, I., Kaider, A., . . . Arnoldner, C. (2014). FS4, FS4-p, and FSP: A 4-month crossover study of 3 fine structure sound-coding strategies. *Ear and Hearing, 35*(6), e272–e281.

Riss, D., Hamzavi, J. S., Selberherr, A., Kaider, A., Blineder, M., Starlinger, V., . . . Arnoldner, C. (2011). Envelope versus fine structure speech coding strategy: A crossover study. *Otology and Neurotology, 32*(7), 1094–1101.

Roy, A. T., Carver, C., Jiradejvong, P., & Limb, C. J. (2015). Musical sound quality in cochlear implant users: A comparison in bass frequency perception between fine structure processing and high-definition continuous interleaved sampling strategies. *Ear and Hearing, 36*(5), 582–590.

Schatzer, R., Krenmayr, A., Au, D. K., Kals, M., & Zierhofer, C. (2010). Temporal fine structure in cochlear implants: Preliminary speech perception results in Cantonese-speaking implant users. *Acta Otolaryngologica, 130*(9), 1031–1039.

Skinner, M. W., Holden, L. K., Holden, T. A., Dowell, R. C., Seligman, P. M., Brimacombe, J. A., & Beiter, A. L. (1991). Performance of postlinguistically deaf adults with the Wearable Speech Processor (WSP III) and Mini Speech Processor (MSP) of the Nucleus multi-electrode cochlear implant. *Ear and Hearing, 12*(1), 3–22.

Skinner, M. W., Holden, L. K., Whitford, L. A., Plant, K.L., Psarros, C., & Holden, T. A. (2002). Speech recognition with the Nucleus 24 SPEAK, ACE, and CIS speech coding strategies in newly implanted adults. *Ear and Hearing, 23*(3), 207–223.

Wilson, B. S., & Dorman, M. (2012). *Better hearing with cochlear implants: Studies at the research triangle institute*. San Diego, CA: Plural.

Wilson, B., Wolford, R., & Lawson, D. (2000). *Speech processors for auditory prostheses* (pp. 1–61). Research Triangle Park, NC: Center for Auditory Prosthesis Research.

Zwolan, T., Kileny, P., Smith, S., Mills, D., Koch, D., & Osberger, M. (2001). Adult cochlear implant performance with evolving electrode technology. *Otology and Neurotology, 22*(6), 844–849.

9

Advanced Bionics Cochlear Implants and Sound Processors

Jace Wolfe and Erin C. Schafer

Introduction

This chapter will provide a review of Advanced Bionics cochlear implants and sound processors. The programming of Advanced Bionics cochlear implants will be discussed in Chapter 15.

Advanced Bionics Sound Processors

Naída CI Q Series Sound Processors

At the time of this writing, the newest Advanced Bionics sound processor is the Naída CI Q90 sound processor (Figure 9–1). The Naída CI Q-series sound processors (Q30, Q70, and Q90) possess a number of features that are unique among commercially available cochlear implant sound processors, including four different microphone options, interaural audio streaming and data exchange, up to five different listening programs per ear, the ability for a single sound processor to be used interchangeably between ears, a tri-color light emitting diode (LED) light, compatibility with a hearing aid (the Naída Link hearing aid; Figure 9–2) and a contralateral routing of signal (CROS) device (the Naída Link CROS; Figure 9–3). The interaural audio streaming capability allows communication between two Naída CI sound processors for bilateral recipients, between a Naída CI sound processor and a Naída Link hearing aid for bimodal

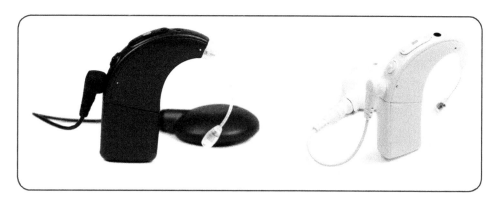

FIGURE 9–1. A visual example of the Advanced Bionics Naída CI Q series sound processor. Image provided courtesy of Advanced Bionics, LLC.

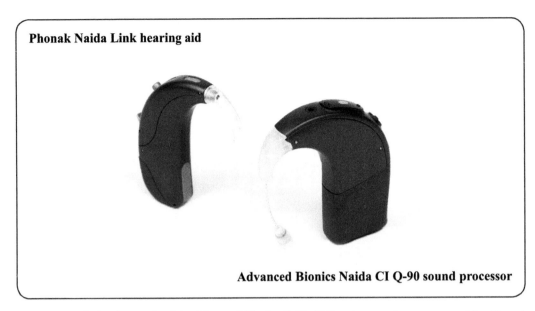

FIGURE 9–2. A visual example of the Advanced Bionics Naída CI Q series sound processor and the Phonak Naída Link hearing aid. Image provided courtesy of Advanced Bionics, LLC.

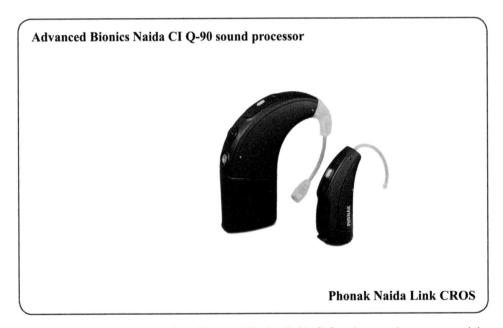

FIGURE 9–3. A visual example of the Advanced Bionics Naída CI Q series sound processor and the Phonak Naída Link CROS. Image provided courtesy of Advanced Bionics, LLC.

listeners, and between a Naída CI sound processor and a Naída Link CROS device for use on the non-implanted ear in unilaterally implanted recipients. Many of these unique features of the Advanced Bionics Naída CI Q sound processor have been a result of Sonova Holding AG's acquisition of the Advanced Bionics Corporation in 2009. Sonova is a manufacturer of hearing instruments, with brands including Phonak and Unitron. In particular, many Phonak hearing aid technologies and features have been integrated into the Advanced Bionics cochlear implant system. In fact, Naída is the name of the high-powered line of Phonak hearing aids. The Naída CI Q70 sound processor was commercially approved by the U.S. Food and Drug Administration (FDA) in September 2013. In the summer of 2015, Advanced Bionics announced FDA approval for the commercial distribution of the Naída CI Q30 and Q90 sound processors. The Naída CI Q30, Q70, and Q90 are identical in size and appearance but differ in technological features, with the Q90 possessing the most sophisticated technologies. The availability of these devices may vary globally (e.g., the Q30 device is not available in the U.S.). The Naída CI sound processors must be programmed in the Advanced Bionics SoundWave software platform, via the Computer Programming Interface 3 (CPI-3) (Figure 9–4).

The Naída CI Q processor is significantly smaller (40%) than its ear-level predecessor, the Harmony processor. In fact, the width of a Naída CI Q70 sound processor is similar to a Phonak Naída power behind-the-ear (BTE) hearing aid, which is commonly used by persons with severe to profound hearing loss prior to cochlear implantation. Of note, the Naída CI Q sound processor may be used by recipients of the Advanced Bionics CII (C2), HiRes 90K, HiRes 90K Advantage, and HiRes Ultra cochlear implants. The Naída CI Q sound processor is not compatible with the Advanced Bionics C1 cochlear implant. Recipients of the C1 implant must use the Advanced Bionics Harmony or the Platinum Series sound processor.

When worn in the standard wear configuration, the Naída CI Q possesses four components (Figure 9–5):

(1) the sound processor, (2) the power source (the PowerCel lithium-ion rechargeable battery), (3) the T-Mic™ 2, and (4) the headpiece, which is composed of a cable and an external transmitting coil. The head piece is available in two forms, the conventional Universal Headpiece and the AquaMic Headpiece, which is waterproof and must be used when the recipient is involved in water play (Figure 9–6). The microphone of the AquaMic Headpiece possesses a special nanotechnology covering that protects it from moisture. The AquaMic headpiece and cable have an Ingress Protection (IP) 68 rating, which indicates that it is safe for swimming and full exposure to and submersion in water. Of note, the underneath side of the Universal Headpiece is black, whereas the underneath side of the AquaMic Headpiece is gray (Remember, "gray for water play!").

Sound Processor Microphones

The variety of available microphone options is an exceptional feature of the Naída CI Q sound processor. In the standard wearing configuration, there are four microphone options: (1) the T-Mic™ 2, (2) two omnidirectional microphones that may be used to provide omnidirectional and (3) adaptive directional beamforming, and (4) an integrated microphone within the headpiece (Figure 9–7). The T-Mic 2 is an updated version of the original T-Mic, and provides better aesthetics and comfort than its predecessor. The T-Mic 2 consists of a cable that extends from the

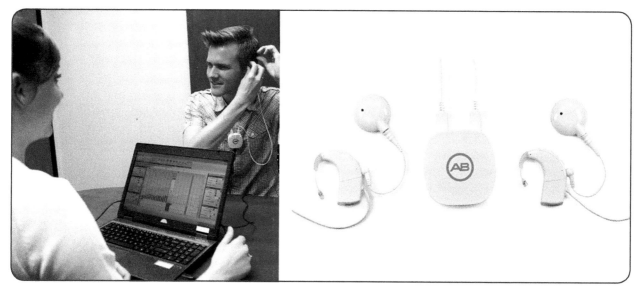

FIGURE 9–4. A visual example of the Advanced Bionics CPI-3 programming interface. Image provided courtesy of Advanced Bionics, LLC.

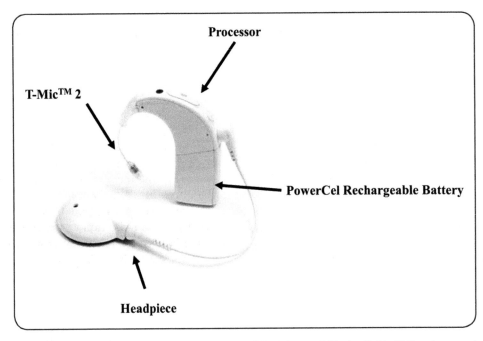

FIGURE 9–5. A visual example of the components of the Advanced Bionics Naída CI Q series sound processor. Image provided courtesy of Advanced Bionics, LLC.

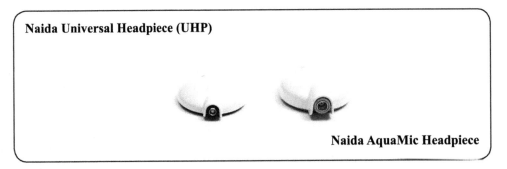

FIGURE 9–6. A visual example of the Advanced Bionics Naída Universal Headpiece and the Naída Aqua-Mic Headpiece. Image provided courtesy of Advanced Bionics, LLC.

earhook of the sound processor and terminates at a microphone that is positioned at the opening of the external auditory meatus.

The original objective of the T-Mic, first introduced in 2003 for use with the CII BTE sound processor, was to allow for more natural and effective telephone use by placing the microphone at the same location where the telephone receiver is placed during conversations. Additionally, the T-Mic provides for a more natural location of sound direction compared with the typical microphone placement at the top of the auricle with a standard BTE sound proces-

sor. Specifically, the location of the T-Mic takes advantage of the "pinna effect," which is known to enhance high-frequency sounds and funnel sounds arriving from in front of the listener toward the external auditory meatus while providing modest attenuation for high-frequency sounds arriving from behind the listener (i.e., the T-Mic provides a small directional effect). It is known that use of an omnidirectional microphone located at the top of the ear results in a negative directivity index, which may degrade speech recognition in noise. Indeed, research has shown that use of the T-Mic provides an improvement in speech recognition in noise compared with use of the sound processor's omnidirectional microphone located at the top of the auricle (Gifford & Revit, 2010; Kolberg et al., 2015). Furthermore, many recipients report that they like the fact that the T-Mic may be used with circumaural (over the ear) earphones, which are popular consumer electronic devices.

The T-Mic 2 comes in three sizes (small, medium, and large) to accommodate different ear sizes and shapes. The T-Mic 2 also includes a design-integrated microphone cover to protect against dirt or debris. This cover may be replaced every three to four months or if plugged by debris. Furthermore, the T-Mic 2 may be removed and replaced by a conventional behind-the-ear processor earhook that only serves the purpose of maintaining retention of the processor on the recipient's ear. The conventional earhook is also available in multiple sizes to fit different ears (Fig-

ure 9–8). The T-Mic 2 and conventional earhooks are both tamperproof and must be removed by using a small tool to remove a retention pin.

The Naída CI Q sound processor is also unique in the way in which it can utilize two omnidirectional electret condenser microphones for directional listening. The audiologist may program the Naída CI Q to operate in omnidirectional mode in which only the front microphone of the sound processor is active. Both of the sound processor microphones may be enabled to allow for a variety of directional options. For example, the "UltraZoom" mode is an adaptive beamformer based on Phonak hearing aid technology that positions the null of the directional pattern to coincide with the direction from which the most intense noise is arriving. The auto UltraZoom feature uses a complex algorithm that considers 46 different input parameters to differentiate speech from noise and automatically switches between omnidirectional and adaptive directional mode when the recipient moves from a quiet to a noisy environment.

StereoZoom is another Phonak directional hearing aid technology that uses Phonak interaural audio streaming to combine the directional response of the dual-microphone directional system of each sound processor of bilateral cochlear implant recipients to achieve a four-microphone beam-former that possesses greater focus on sounds arriving from the front and more attenuation of sounds arriving from the rear. The directivity index (i.e., the degree to which the microphone system focuses on sounds from 0 degrees azimuth while attenuating sounds from other directions) is larger for bilateral beamformers compared with dual-microphone directional systems (Figure 9–9). Research has shown significantly better speech recognition in noise with StereoZoom relative to UltraZoom for bilateral hearing aid, bilateral CI, and bimodal as well as unilateral+CROS listening configurations (Buchner et al., 2016; Cardenas et al., 2017).

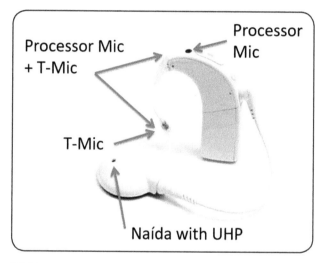

FIGURE 9–7. A visual example of the microphone inputs of the Advanced Bionics Naída CI Q series sound processor. Image provided courtesy of Advanced Bionics, LLC.

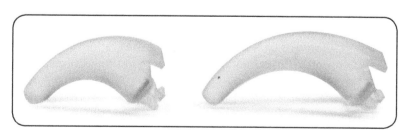

FIGURE 9–8. A visual example of the earhooks of the Advanced Bionics Naída CI Q series sound processor. Image provided courtesy of Advanced Bionics, LLC.

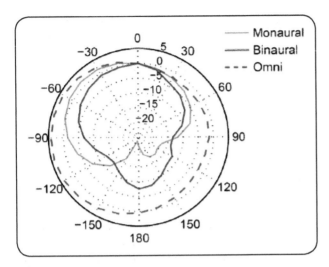

FIGURE 9–9. An illustration of the polar plot pattern of UltraZoom and StereoZoom. Polar plots for an omnidirectional microphone, monaural beam-former (UltraZoom), and binaural beam-former (StereoZoom) obtained using a single noise source from varying angles. Circles indicate the gain in decibels (dB) relative to the 0-degree response. Image provided courtesy of Advanced Bionics, LLC.

ZoomControl is another Phonak hearing aid technology that is exclusively available to Advanced Bionics cochlear implant recipients. ZoomControl is a fixed microphone mode that directs the primary axis of sensitivity of the microphone mode toward the right or left or behind the user. ZoomControl is typically included in a secondary program that the recipient may access for special listening situations. For instance, when driving a car, the recipient may wish to use ZoomControl so that the microphone polar plot pattern is most sensitive to sounds arriving from the right, which is the direction from which the front-seat passenger may be sitting. For bilateral users, ZoomControl will also stream the audio signal captured at the right ear over to the left ear. Alternatively, if the passenger is riding in the backseat, a ZoomControl program may be created so that the microphones are most sensitive for sounds arriving from behind the recipient.

Advanced Bionics is the only cochlear implant manufacturer that provides the option of the use of a microphone within the external transmitting coil (i.e., headpiece) for use with a BTE or body-worn sound processor. The Universal and AquaMic headpieces both include an integrated electret condenser omnidirectional microphone, which may be activated when an ear-level microphone is not being used (e.g.,

for infants with small ears that do not accommodate a BTE processor or for adults who use the Neptune for sports). However, the authors strongly recommend use of the ear-level microphones when possible in order to take advantage of interaural timing cues and directionality that are more likely to be available if binaural hearing technology is worn on or at the ears rather than on the head or body.

Digital Signal Processing (DSP)

The Naída CI Q possesses a sophisticated digital signal processor, which has a 16-bit analog-to-digital converter which allows for a front-end DSP dynamic range of 96 dB. The sampling rate of the digital signal processor is 17.4 kHz, which allows for accurate representation of the input spectrum beyond 8000 Hz via complex digital analysis (e.g., Hilbert transformation). The input dynamic range (IDR) of the processor (which is determined by a host of factors, including but not limited to the DSP dynamic range, the noise floor of the microphone, and the maximum limit of the microphone) ranges from 20 to 80 dB, with the range of audio input levels captured without overload or compression limiting spanning from approximately 25 to 105 dB SPL. The DSP chip of the Naída CI Q features the same technologies available in the Phonak Quest hearing aid chip. This chip enables access to many of the advanced signal processing features available in the Phonak Quest hearing aid line, including adaptive directionality (UltraZoom), bilateral beam-forming (StereoZoom), and adaptive signal processing that attempts to automatically adjust processor settings to meet recipient needs across a wide variety of acoustic settings. Additionally, the Naída CI Q processing chip allows for the use of a technology known as HiBAN, which stands for Hearing instrument Body-Area Network. HiBAN is a system designed to transmit audio and control data over a short distance (typically 20 cm or 8″). HiBAN technology is used for several purposes, including: (1) the wireless delivery of an audio signal from a neck-worn interface known as the ComPilot, which receives audio signals from personal electronic devices (e.g., mobile telephone, MP3 player, television) via Bluetooth, (2) for bilateral or bimodal Naída CI Q 70/90 users with a Naida Link HA, HiBAN allows for the delivery of control data from one sound processor to another, and (3) for bilateral Naída CI Q users (and bimodal Naída Link users), HiBAN allows for the delivery of an audio signal from one sound processor to another.

The HiBAN network allows for the wireless streaming of control and audio signals by transmitting digital data at a carrier frequency of 10.6 MHz via a digital magnetic induction link from one sound processor to another or from the ComPilot neckloop to a receiving antenna located within the sound processor. The induction link and the 10.6 MHz transmission frequency substantially reduces power consumption relative to long-range radio frequency transmission at a 2.4 GHz carrier frequency (e.g., Bluetooth). Additionally, the 10.6 MHz carrier frequency allows for audio streaming between ears without distortion or absorption by the head (i.e., auricle, noise, head, etc.). Interaural audio streaming via a 2.4 GHz carrier frequency is technically challenging because the short wavelength of the 2.4 GHz signal is distorted and/or absorbed by the head. However, it is likely that future advances in technology will overcome this challenge.

The HiBAN system possesses a codec (i.e., digital coder and decoder) program which allows for the compression of the audio signal prior to transmission. This process removes unnecessary components (i.e., acoustic components that do not contribute to the intelligibility or sound quality of the signal) from the audio signal to reduce the size of the signal being transferred and is similar to the process used with MP3 files. The codec program allows for audio signals with a bandwidth up to 8000 Hz to be streamed between ears with minimal transmission delay (2 msec or less).

Binaural VoiceStream Technology™ is a type of signal processing that is made possible by the HiBAN technology. Binaural VoiceStream Technology allows for binaural processing and audio streaming for recipients of bilateral Advanced Bionics cochlear implants (with CII/HiRes 90K, HiRes Ultra, or later cochlear implants). Binaural VoiceStream Technology allows for the use of several unique and potentially beneficial signal processing features, including binaural directionality (e.g., StereoZoom, ZoomControl) and binaural telephone use (DuoPhone). Of note, the HiBAN technology also allows for bilateral processor adjustments (i.e., QuickSync—when a recipient makes an adjustment to the program button or volume control of one processor, that adjustment is automatically made to the sound processor on the opposite ear). Figure 9–10 provides a list of signal processing features that are included in the Naída CI Q30, Q70, and Q90 sound processors.

Furthermore, a wide range of signal coding strategies may be used with the the Naída CI Q sound pro-cessors, including continuous interleaved sampling (CIS), HiRes, HiRes Fidelity 120, HiRes Optima, and ClearVoice strategy. Detailed information pertaining to the management, programming, and signal processing capabilities of the Naída CI Q sound processors may be found in Chapters 8 and 15.

Processor Controls

The Naída CI Q sound processor possesses two user controls, a dedicated push-button volume control and a program button (Figure 9–11). Pressing the top half of the volume control button increases stimulation level, whereas pressing the bottom half of the volume control results in a decrease in stimulation level. The range over which the volume control may adjust stimulation levels may be adjusted by the programming audiologist. Also, the volume control may be disabled.

The Naída CI Q sound also has a program button, which may be pressed to access up to five programs per ear (i.e., separate programs for typical listening situations such as noisy environments, music, telephone, hearing assistance technology). It should be noted that the Naída CI Q may be safely programmed for both the right and left ears for bilateral cochlear implant recipients. In other words, the user may use the processor interchangeably between ears, and the sound processor will use the program with stimulation created for the ear with which it is being used. As a result, up to five programs for each ear may be loaded onto one sound processor for a total of ten programs within the processor. Advanced Bionics cochlear implants (CII and later) possess bidirectional telemetry, which means one inductive link carrier frequency is used to deliver information and power from the sound processor to the cochlear implant and another inductive link carrier frequency is used to deliver information from the cochlear implant to the sound processor. This bi-telemetry communication between the Naída CI Q processor and the cochlear implant internal device allows for automatic determination of which ear the processor is stimulating. The Harmony, Neptune, and Naída CI Q sound processors are the industry's only sound processors that possess this feature. With the Harmony, however, each program slot must be dedicated to one ear. The Harmony sound processor possesses three program slots, so program #1 may be loaded with a map for one implanted ear, and program #2 or #3 may be loaded with a map for the opposite ear. Additionally, it should be noted that the program button can be disabled by the audiologist within the programming software.

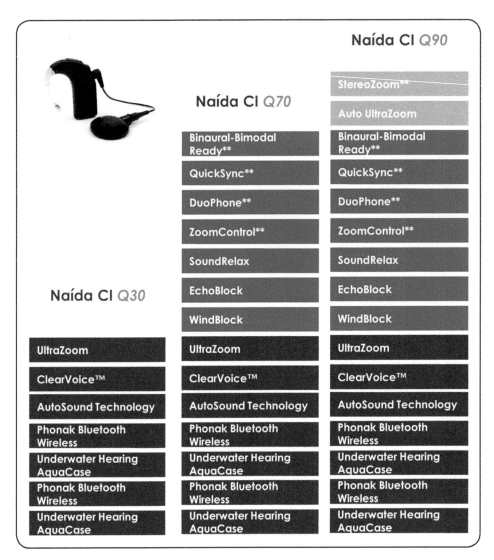

FIGURE 9–10. The features of the Advanced Bionics Naída CI Q series sound processors. Image provided courtesy of Advanced Bionics, LLC.

The program button may also be used to place the processor in standby mode, a low power state in which no stimulation is provided from the processor. This may be desirable if the recipient wants to refrain from receiving an audio signal from the device but does not want to remove the processor from the ear or the power source from the processor. Examples include a recipient who is concentrating on a task and does not want to be distracted by outside noises or a recipient who is subjected to unwanted, annoying noise. To actively enable standby mode, the user must press on the program button for 4 seconds and then release it. Additionally, the processor passively enters standby mode if the processor

does not achieve lock with the internal device (i.e., communication between the external sound processor and internal cochlear implant) for more than a 5 minute period. The recipient must simply press the program button to return to the settings used prior to the initiation of standby mode. Standby mode is a programmable feature within the fitting software.

Processor Water Resistance and Alerting Lights

The Naída CI Q sound processor possesses water-resistant covers over both microphones in order to provide resistance to moisture damage from perspiration, rain, and so forth. Additionally, the Naída sound

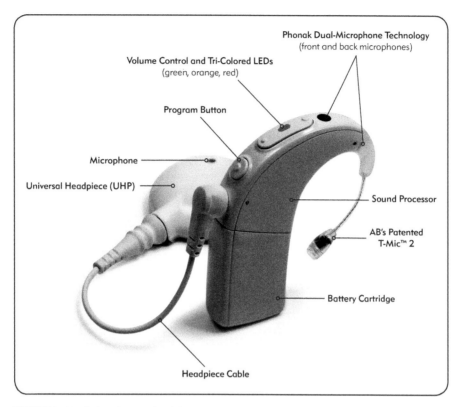

Phonak Dual-Microphone Technology
(front and back microphones)

Volume Control and Tri-Colored LEDs
(green, orange, red)

Program Button

Microphone

Universal Headpiece (UHP)

Sound Processor

AB's Patented
T-Mic™ 2

Battery Cartridge

Headpiece Cable

FIGURE 9–11. A visual example of the components of the Advanced Bionics Naída CI Q series sound processor. Image provided courtesy of Advanced Bionics, LLC.

processor's buttons and points of connection to the headpiece cable and battery are hermetically sealed to enhance water resistance, and as a result, the Naída CI Q possesses an Ingress Protection (IP) rating of 57. The IP rating system classifies devices in relation to their degree of resistance to the intrusion of water and other foreign objects. It is a two-digit number, with the first number referring to the resistance to the intrusion from solid objects and the second number referring to the intrusion of liquid. The Naída CI Q's IP rating of 57 indicates that it is protected against penetration of solid foreign objects equal to or greater than 1.0 mm in diameter and may be left in a meter tall bucket of water for 30 minutes and still function to the manufacturer's specification. Tables 9–1 and 9–2 provide a complete description of the IP rating scale.

It should be noted that the IP57 rating of the Naída CI Q sound processor is only valid when the T-Mic 2 is removed and substituted with the conventional earhook (i.e., the T-Mic 2 is not water resistant). It should also be noted that the on-board microphones of the Naída CI Q are protected by

microphone covers that the recipient or audiologist should periodically replace (typically every three to six months). It is also important to mention that an IP57 rating does not indicate that a device is fully waterproof. For example, the user should not swim with the sound processor or use it while showering.

Advanced Bionics has offered a waterproof solution for the Naída CI Q sound processor to allow for its use while swimming and during other activities in which the Naída CI Q would be subjected to water (or other liquids) being forcefully directed toward the processor or when the processor may be submerged frequently and/or for longer periods of time. The AquaCase is a small, waterproof box in which the Naída CI Q may be placed for protection against water (Figure 9–12). The AquaCase contains O-ring seals around the openings and creases of the case to prevent the ingress of liquid. It also contains a lock and latch so that the case is not accidentally opened during use. The AquaCase also contains a clip that may be attached to the user's shirt, bathing suit, or armband. Additionally, the AquaCase contains a

TABLE 9–1. Ingress Protection (IP) Rating System for Solid Objects (first number in rating)

Rating	Object Size	Description
0	Not Applicable	No protection against ingress of solid objects
1	>50 mm	Protection against ingress of any large surface of the body (e.g., back of the hand) but not against deliberate contact with a body part
2	>12.5 mm	Protection against ingress of smaller body parts (e.g., finger) or similar objects
3	>2.5 mm	Protection against ingress of small tools (e.g., screwdriver) or thick wires
4	>1 mm	Protection against ingress of thin wires, screws, etc.
5	Dust Protected	Ingress of dust is not prevented in entirety, but dust ingress will not affect operation of the device
6	Dust Tight	Complete resistance to the ingress of dust; complete protection against ingress of solid objects

Note. IEC 60529—Degrees of Protection Provided by Enclosures (IP Code). Located at http://www.maximintegrated.com/app-notes/index.mvp/id/4126

Source: Provided courtesy of Advanced Bionics, LLC.

TABLE 9–2. Ingress Protection (IP) Rating System for Liquid Objects (second number in rating)

Rating	Liquid/Application	Details
0	Not applicable	Not protected against liquid ingress
1	Dripping water (vertically falling drops) shall have no effect	10-minute exposure duration. Liquid equivalent to 1 mm of rainfall/minute
2	Vertically dripping water causes no harmful effect when device is oriented at an angle up to 15° from its typical use position	10-minute exposure duration. Liquid equivalent to 3 mm of rainfall/minute
3	Protection against vertical spraying water falling from an angle of 60° above the device	5-minute exposure duration. Water volume: 0.7 liters/min. Pressure: 80–100 kPa
4	Water splashing against the device from any angle does not harm the device	5-minute exposure duration. Water volume: 10 liters/min. Pressure: 80–100 kPa
5	Water projected from a nozzle (6.5-mm) will not harm the device	3-minute exposure duration. Water volume: 12.5 liters/min. Pressure: 30 kPa at 3-m distance
6	Water projected in powerful jets (12.5-mm nozzle) will not harm the device	3-minute exposure duration. Water volume: 100 liters/min. Pressure: 100 kPa at 3-m distance
7	Ingress of water is not harmful when device is completely immersed in water	30-minute exposure duration. Bottom of device immersed in ≥1 m of water with the top of the device immersed in ≥15 mm of water
8	Continuous immersion in water at a depth of more than 1 meter under typical use conditions without harmful effect	Continuous immersion. Depth specified by manufacturer. Waterproof for typical use

Source: Provided courtesy of Advanced Bionics, LLC.

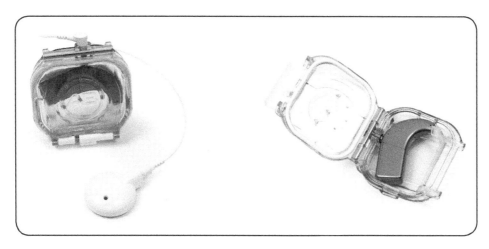

FIGURE 9–12. A visual example of the components of the AquaCase for the Advanced Bionics Naída CI Q series sound processor. Image provided courtesy of Advanced Bionics, LLC.

waterproof connector port into which the Aqua cable may be plugged on the outside of the case and the sound processor cable port may be connected on the inside of the case. The Aqua cable is then connected to the AquaMic headpiece. Use of the Naída CI Q in the AquaCase with the Aqua cable and AquaMic headpiece provides an IP68 protection rating.

The Naída CI Q70 sound processor also features a light-emitting diode (LED) that is designed to provide information pertaining to a variety of different functions and operations of the processor. The LED can signify the remaining life of a battery, the program the recipient is using, the status of the communication between the external and internal devices (i.e., lock), and whether the processor is receiving an audio input of moderate level or greater. The LED illuminates in three different colors including green, red, and orange. The reader is referred to Table 9–3 for more information on the function indicated by the color and blinking pattern of the LED.

All Advanced Bionics Naída CI Q sound processors may be used with two different remote accessories: (1) the AB Phonak myPilot remote control pictured in Figure 9–13, and (2) the Phonak ComPilot shown in Figure 9–14. The Phonak ComPilot is a wireless streaming device that is worn around the neck. The ComPilot contains a Bluetooth receiver that allows connectivity to consumer electronics, including Bluetooth-enabled mobile telephones, laptop computers, remote microphones, televisions, and so forth. The audio signal obtained by the ComPilot from the consumer electronic device is delivered to the Naída

CI Q sound processor via digital near field magnetic induction from the loop worn around the recipient's neck. Of note, the ComPilot may also receive audio signals from the Phonak Remote Mic and the Phonak TV LinkS streamer (Figure 9–15). The ComPilot may also be plugged into the TV LinkS device to allow for charging of the ComPilot battery. Research suggests that use of these accessories allows for better speech recognition in noise and when the signal of interest arrives from a distance (Johnstone, 2016). Furthermore, direct audio streaming via a television listening device is likely to improve the user's ability to understand the audio signal of the television, particularly in noisy and reverberant situations and/or when the user sits more than a few feet away from the television loudspeakers. Moreover, the ComPilot may be programmed by the audiologist so that the recipient may use it as a remote control to adjust the volume control and program setting of the Naída CI Q sound processor.

Connecting Processor to External Sources

The Naída CI Q sound processor is equipped with multiple options that allow the recipient to connect to external electronic devices. Aside from connecting to external devices via the ComPilot Bluetooth device, the Naída CI Q sound processor possesses a programmable internal telecoil that the recipient may access via a separate telecoil program created by the programming audiologist. Additionally, the Phonak Roger 17 digital radio receiver may be coupled to

TABLE 9–3. Naída CI Q90 Sound Processor LED Indications

Color	Behavior	Programmable	Indication
Orange	Blinks at start-up	No. Battery indicator is only available with use of the rechargeable PowerCels and AAA PowerPak. Battery life indicators are not available with use of Zn-Air batteries.	• 4 quick blinks indicate that the battery is fully charged • 2–3 quick blinks indicate that the battery is sufficiently charged to power the Naída CI Q90 • 1 quick blink indicates that the battery is nearly depleted • No blinking indicates depleted battery; replace with charged or new battery
	Solid	Yes	The battery is almost depleted
	Blinks twice every three seconds	Yes	The battery is almost depleted and cannot support stimulation (Sleep Mode)
	Fades out	No	The Naída CI Q90 is entering Sleep Mode
Red	Blinks once per second	Yes	Loss of lock with the implant
	Blinks rapidly (more than once per second)	No	Intellilink™ enabled and the Naída CI Q90 is connected to the wrong implant
	Solid	No	Sound processor error condition. Fully remove and re-insert the battery to reset processor
	Blinks 5 times	No. If using AB myPilot this pattern is the default.	Response to AB myPilot's request to "Find Paired Devices." The Right paired device will identify itself with this LED pattern.
Green	Flickers in response to loud inputs	Yes	The sound processor and microphone are responding to sound
	Blinks at start-up, after battery status, and upon program change	No	• 1 blink indicates program one • 2 blinks indicate program two • 3 blinks indicate program three • 4 blinks indicate program four • 5 blinks indicate program five
	Solid	No	A processor that is not yet programmed
	Blinks 4 times	No. If using AB myPilot this pattern is the default.	Response to AB myPilot's request to "Find Paired Devices." The Left paired device will identify itself with this LED pattern.

Note. Use of some Naída CI accessories may obscure the processor LED.

Source: Provided courtesy of Advanced Bionics, LLC.

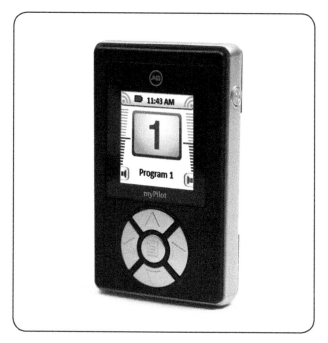

FIGURE 9–13. The Advanced Bionics myPilot remote control. Image provided courtesy of Advanced Bionics, LLC.

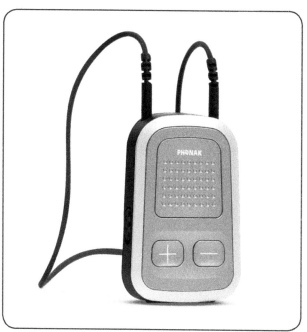

FIGURE 9–14. The Phonak ComPilot. Image provided courtesy of Advanced Bionics, LLC.

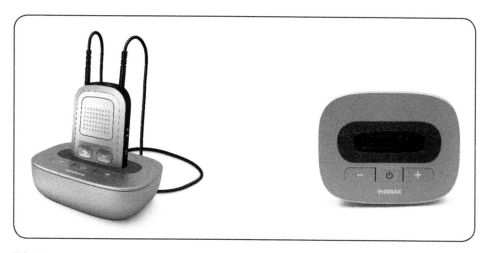

FIGURE 9–15. The Phonak ComPilot with TV LinkS Streamer. Image provided courtesy of Advanced Bionics, LLC.

a Roger-dedicated direct auditory input (DAI) connector at the base of the 170 mAh PowerCel battery (Figure 9–16).

The Naída CI Listening Check is another accessory item developed for use with the Naída CI Q processor. The Naída CI Listening Check device (Figure 9–17) allows an audiologist, caregiver, or significant other with normal hearing to listen to the signal that is delivered from the microphones or accessory input of the Naída processor. Commercial earphones (that do not have an integrated microphone) with a 3.5-mm mini-audio plug must be plugged into the audio port of the Listening Check. It is important to note that the signal that the listener perceives from the Listening Check device is not identical to the signal the cochlear implant user receives. Instead, the

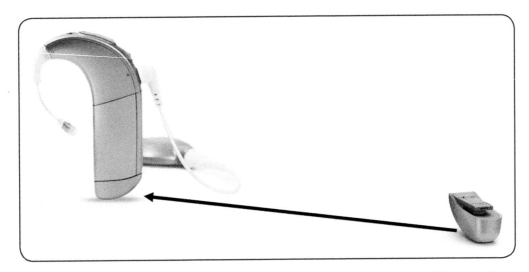

FIGURE 9–16. The Phonak Roger 17 radio receiver. Image provided courtesy of Advanced Bionics, LLC.

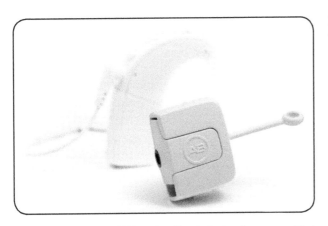

FIGURE 9–17. Naída CI Listening Check device. Image provided courtesy of Advanced Bionics, LLC.

signal from the Listening Check is simply the signal that is delivered from the Naída CI Q microphones or accessory audio input. There is no way for any listening device to allow for an examiner to listen to the signal after it has been fully processed by the sound processor and delivered to the cochlear nerve via the cochlear implant. Simply put, the Listening Check allows an audiologist or caregiver to evaluate the integrity of the microphone or the signal received from an accessory input such as the telecoil or Roger remote microphone. The Naída CI Listening Check is powered by the PowerCel of the Naída processor.

Programming audiologists, parents, daycare workers, auditory-verbal therapists, speech-language pathologists, and early childhood educators should have access to the Listening Check device and should use it routinely (e.g., audiologists should use it at every clinical visit, parents should use it on a daily basis, educators should use it to evaluate the sound processor microphone and the integrity of the signal from the Phonak Roger remote microphone system).

Advanced Bionics Universal and AquaMic Headpieces

The Universal Headpiece (UHP) was introduced with the Neptune sound processor and is now compatible with all Advanced Bionics sound processors. The headpiece is composed of a transmitting coil and magnet, and an integrated electret, condenser, omnidirectional microphone, which may be activated when an ear-level microphone is not being used (e.g., for infants with small ears that cannot allow for sufficient retention of a BTE processor; for active children and adults who must wear the processor in their hair or in a special case attached to their clothing or body during sports or other vigorous activities). As previously mentioned, the AquaMic headpiece is recommended for use with the AquaCase. When the AquaMic headpiece is used during water activities, the user should switch to a second program that disables sound processor microphones and activates the microphone of the AquaMic headpiece. The programming audiologist may determine the active microphone for each listening program during the programming session.

The UHP and AquaMic headpieces are held to the head by magnets that are housed under the removal cover of the headpiece. A special removal

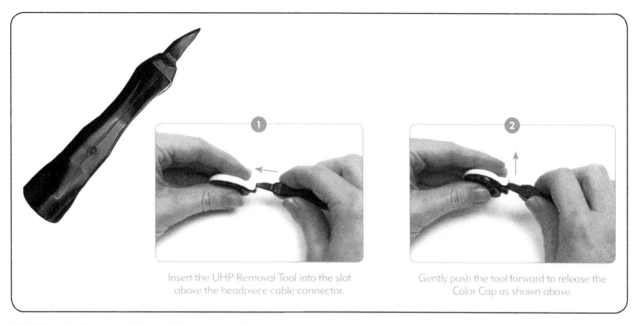

FIGURE 9–18. Removal of the headpiece cover with removal tool. Image provided courtesy of Advanced Bionics, LLC.

tool (Figure 9–18) is provided to separate the head-piece cover from the headpiece. Up to four magnets may be placed in a small "well" that resides in the transmitting coil underneath the headpiece cover. If less than four magnets are required to facilitate satisfactory headpiece retention, then a small foam "spacer" may be placed in the well to prevent the magnets from moving in the well and producing a rattling sound. A small circular cover patch resides at the center of the underneath side of the headpiece. This patch may be removed to add one thin, external UHP magnet to the external well created by the removal of the patch. The thin, external magnet may be included if sufficient retention cannot be achieved with use of four magnets in the internal well. The audiologist must determine the appropriate number and configuration (i.e., magnets placed in the upper well, the shallow underneath well, or both) for each individual in order to achieve consistent headpiece retention without unnecessary pressure and/or irritation of the skin underneath the headpiece site. Figures 9–19 and 9–20 provide information for determining appropriate magnet strength for the Advanced Bionics headpiece. The reader is referred to Chapters 14 and 23 for general guidance on determining appropriate transmitting coil/headpiece strength.

The UHP may be used with a variety of cable lengths depending on the processor type and wearing configuration/preference. The headpiece cables are available in four different color options (beige, dark brown, black, and white). Finally, the Naída headpiece cable rotates 360 degrees in the headpiece connector to allow for a more comfortable fit, to facilitate better retention to a wide variety of head sizes and shapes, and to improve durability of the headpiece cable and sound processor cable port.

Battery Module

The Naída CI Q may be powered by a variety of different battery options, including a lithium-ion rechargeable battery that is available in multiple sizes (Figure 9–21), a zinc-air battery cartridge that uses two 675P (power) zinc-air batteries (Figure 9–22), and an AAA *PowerPak* designed to provide longer battery life from a case that is worn off of the ear (e.g., clipped to the shirt at the shoulder, clipped to an armband, clipped to the hair), which provides power to the processor from three AAA alkaline batteries and is connected to the processor by a long cable (Figure 9–23).

The rechargeable PowerCel battery is available in five different sizes (110 Mini, 170 Mini, 170, and 230). The number (e.g., 110, 170, 230) refers to the capacity of each battery in milliamperes per hour (i.e., 230 refers to a capacity of 230 milliamperes per hour).

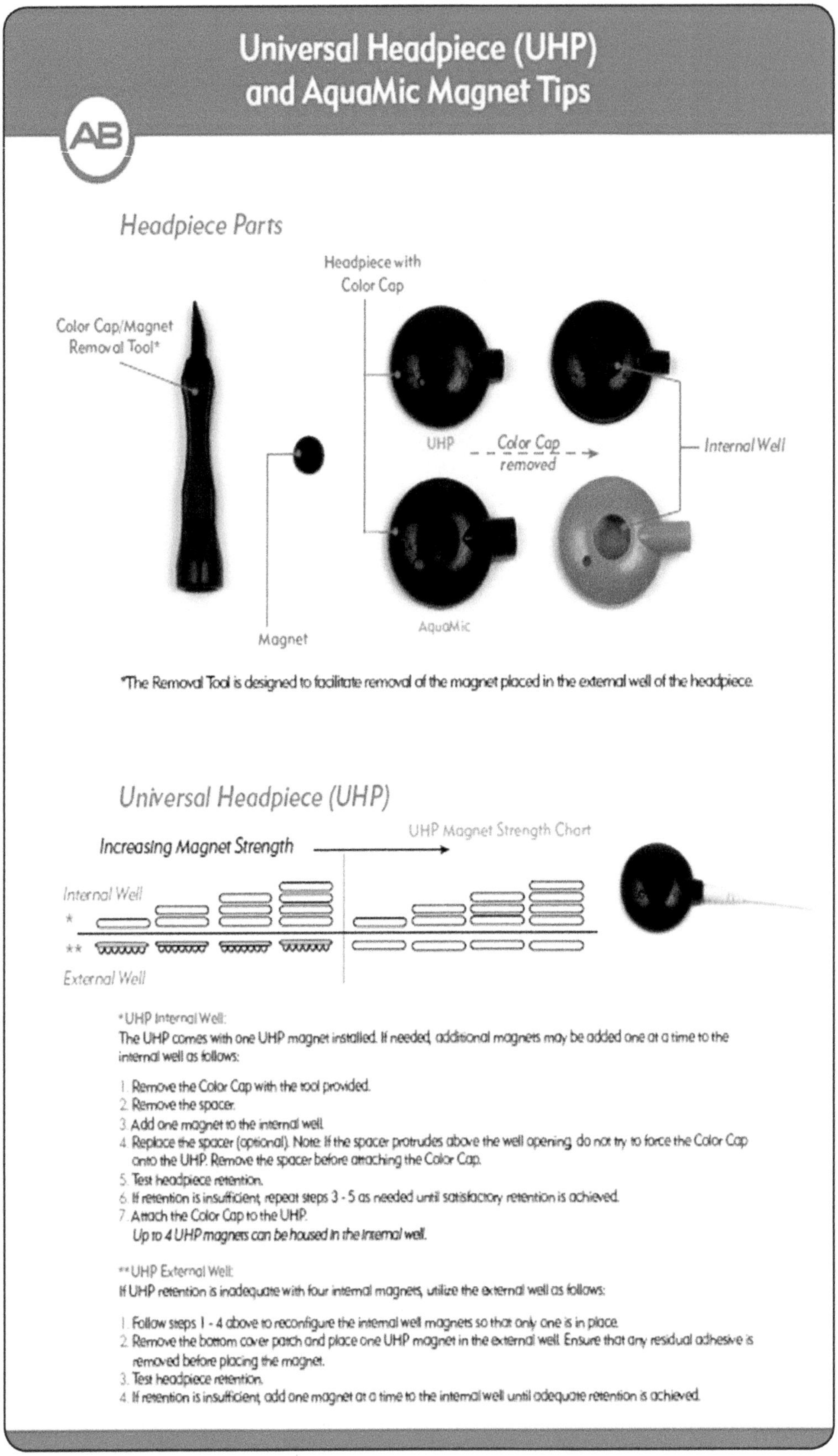
Universal Headpiece (UHP)
and AquaMic Magnet Tips
Headpiece Parts
Headpiece with
Color Cap
Color Cap/Magnet
Removal Tool*
UHP
Color Cap
removed
Internal Well
Magnet
AquaMic
*The Removal Tool is designed to facilitate removal of the magnet placed in the external well of the headpiece.
Universal Headpiece (UHP)
UHP Magnet Strength Chart
Increasing Magnet Strength
Internal Well
*
**
External Well
*UHP Internal Well:
The UHP comes with one UHP magnet installed. If needed, additional magnets may be added one at a time to the internal well as follows:
1. Remove the Color Cap with the tool provided.
2. Remove the spacer.
3. Add one magnet to the internal well.
4. Replace the spacer (optional). Note: If the spacer protrudes above the well opening, do not try to force the Color Cap onto the UHP. Remove the spacer before attaching the Color Cap.
5. Test headpiece retention.
6. If retention is insufficient, repeat steps 3 - 5 as needed until satisfactory retention is achieved.
7. Attach the Color Cap to the UHP.
Up to 4 UHP magnets can be housed in the internal well.
**UHP External Well:
If UHP retention is inadequate with four internal magnets, utilize the external well as follows:
1. Follow steps 1 - 4 above to reconfigure the internal well magnets so that only one is in place.
2. Remove the bottom cover patch and place one UHP magnet in the external well. Ensure that any residual adhesive is removed before placing the magnet.
3. Test headpiece retention.
4. If retention is insufficient, add one magnet at a time to the internal well until adequate retention is achieved.

FIGURE 9–19. Naída Universal Headpiece magnet information. Image provided courtesy of Advanced Bionics, LLC.

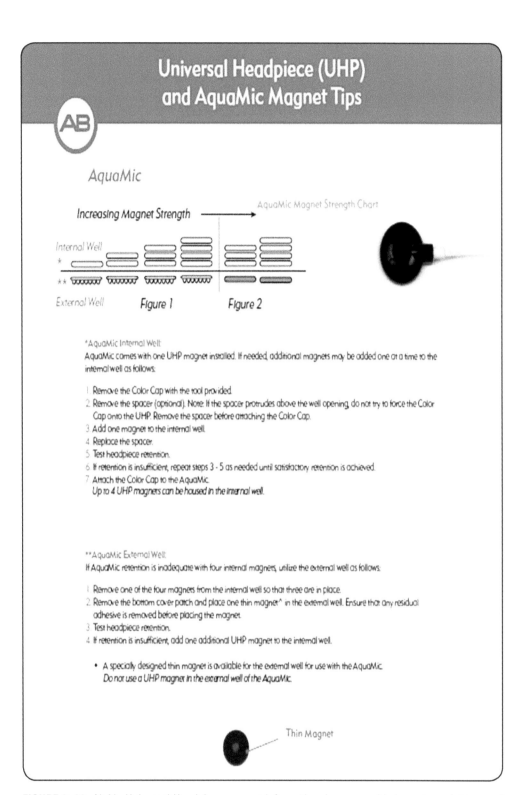

FIGURE 9–20. Naída Universal Headpiece magnet information. Image provided courtesy of Advanced Bionics, LLC.

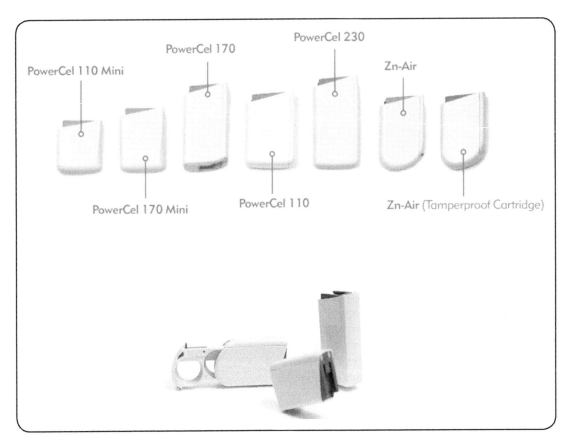

FIGURE 9–21. Battery options for the Advanced Bionics Naída CI Q series sound processor. Image provided courtesy of Advanced Bionics, LLC.

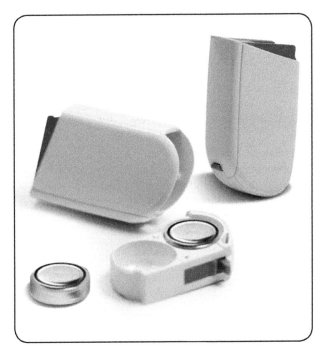

FIGURE 9–22. Zinc-air 675 battery module for the Advanced Bionics Naída CI Q series sound processor. Image provided courtesy of Advanced Bionics, LLC.

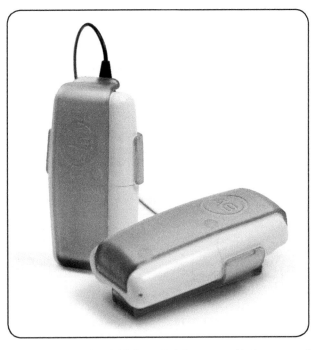

FIGURE 9–23. Naída *AAA PowerPak*. Image provided courtesy of Advanced Bionics, LLC.

Each of the different rechargeable batteries provides the same voltage to power the processor, with the only functional difference between the three being the fact that the smaller batteries have a shorter use time between charges. The PowerCel 170 Mini battery is smaller than the standard PowerCel 170 battery, but there is no difference in battery power or operating life between the standard and Mini versions. As a result, the Mini versions are particularly attractive for use with small ears. Advanced Bionics reports that after a full charge, the typical (mean) operating hours are 12 (and up to 17 hours), 18 (up to as many as 25 hours), and 25 hours (up to 36 hours) for the 100, 170, and 230 PowerCels, respectively (actual usage time can depend on the user's power requirements, programmed parameters, and device use).

In addition, the PowerCel 170 battery contains a track at its base to allow for connection to a Phonak Roger 17 receiver, which was designed exclusively for the Advanced Bionics Naída Q cochlear implant. It is important to note that the PowerCel 170 Mini does not possess an input for the Roger 17 receiver.

The Zinc-Air Battery Pak has a removable cover so that the user may insert two 675P zinc-airs into the cartridge (when placing devices in dry aid kit overnight, it is advisable to remove the batteries to keep them from discharging completely). The Zn-Air Battery Pak allows for an average operating life of 31 hours (up to 56 hours) with the use of high-powered (made for cochlear implant) 675 zinc-air batteries. The zinc-air cartridge contains two vent holes on each side of the case to allow air to power the batteries. The presence of these vent holes makes the zinc-air battery module less water-resistant than the rechargeable PowerCel batteries. The zinc-air cartridge is available in a tamperproof option to prevent a young recipient from removing and ingesting the disposable batteries.

Finally, the Naída CI Q sound processor may be powered by a module referred to as the AAA PowerPak, which uses three AAA rechargeable or disposable alkaline batteries. The AAA PowerPak is designed to be clipped onto the user's clothes or worn in a pocket. It is coupled to the Naída CI sound processor by a special cable (available in lengths of 5, 11, 22, and 32 inches/13, 28, 56, and 81 cm) and the "Naída CI Power Adapter." Advanced Bionics reports that the AAA PowerPak possesses an average operating life of 129 hours (up to 183 hours) when powered by three alkaline AAA batteries.

The PowerCel batteries are charged in a special charger referred to as the Naída PowerCel Battery Charger (Figure 9–24). The PowerCel charger's USB

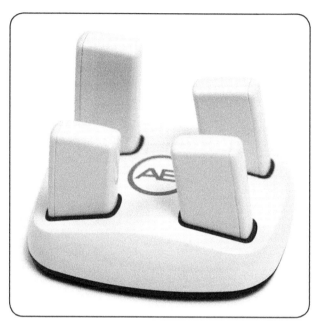

FIGURE 9–24. Naída PowerCel Battery Charger. Image provided courtesy of Advanced Bionics, LLC.

power cord may be plugged into any USB port (i.e., USB port on a computer) and may also be connected to a power supply adapter provided by Advanced Bionics. Power supply adapters include plugs for outlets of a variety of different countries as well as a special car charger adapter. The PowerCel charger possesses an LED that illuminates a green color when the PowerCel charger is receiving sufficient power to charge the batteries.

The PowerCel charger possesses four charging stations so that four PowerCel batteries may be charged simultaneously. Each charging station has an LED to indicate the charging status of the battery. A blue light denotes that the PowerCel is charging, whereas a green light indicates that the PowerCel is fully charged. A red light (or no light) indicates that the battery or the charging station is faulty. A fully depleted PowerCel battery requires 2 to 3 hours of charging to acquire a full charge. Finally, no damage will occur to the charger or to the battery cartridge if a zinc-air battery cartridge is inadvertently placed on the PowerCel charger.

Neptune Sound Processor

In January 2012, Advanced Bionics received FDA approval for the Neptune sound processor (Figure 9–25).

The Neptune processor was revolutionary in several ways. First, for almost 15 years, the cochlear implant industry had transitioned away from the use of body-worn processors and toward the use of progressively smaller and more sophisticated ear-level processors. The Neptune sound processor was counter to this trend because it was designed to be worn off the ear as a body-worn or head-worn (clipped to a swim cap or to the hair of women) processor.

Another unique design feature of the Neptune sound processor is the fact that it is the industry's first fully waterproof, swimmable sound processor. With an IP (ingress protection) rating of 68, the Neptune can resist moisture damage even when the recipient wears it while swimming vigorously or diving into pool, lake, or ocean water. This feature is important to many recipients and their families, because it allows the recipient to hear during water recreation activities and in situations in which the user perspires heavily without concern for damage to the sound processor. Historically, many implant recipients have reported that they have had to remove their processor to prevent damage in these types of activities, and consequently, they have been unable to enjoy listening during important social and/or occupation settings (in the case of a job that requires vigorous manual labor).

Yet another unique design objective of the Neptune processor was the fact that it was developed to possess a similar appearance to modern personal consumer electronic devices. Specifically, it resembles many small, portable MP3 players, which are commonly used by persons with normal hearing (Figure 9–26). Furthermore, the Neptune sound processor offers all of the same signal coding strategies as

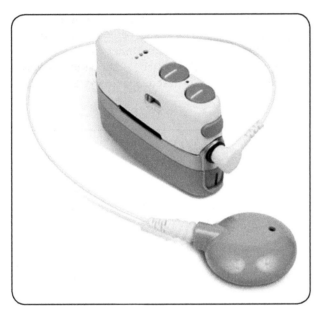

FIGURE 9–25. Advanced Bionics Neptune sound processor. Image provided courtesy of Advanced Bionics, LLC.

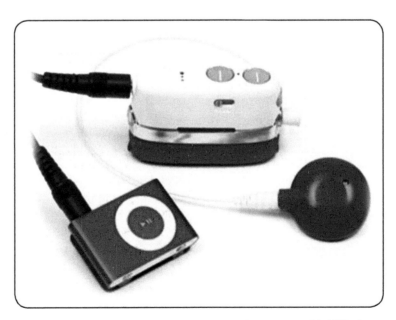

FIGURE 9–26. Advanced Bionics Neptune sound processor with MP3 player. Image provided courtesy of Advanced Bionics, LLC.

the Naída CI Q and Harmony sound processors (discussed later in this chapter), including HiRes Optima and Fidelity 120. Also, the ClearVoice input processing technology, which has been proven to improve speech recognition in noise (Koch et al., 2014; Wolfe et al., 2015), may be used with the Neptune sound processor. Of note, many of the Phonak input processing technologies available in the Naída CI Q sound processor (e.g., UltraZoom, StereoZoom, ZoomControl, DuoPhone, Quick Sync, Wind Block, EchoBlock) are unavailable in the Neptune. Programs created for the Naída CI Q and Harmony sound processors may simply be converted to the Neptune processor with use of the SoundWave programming software, but certain input processing technologies may not transfer, which may alter performance obtained between the Neptune and Naída CI Q sound processors. Also, if the recipient uses the microphone on the Neptune's headpiece, differences in microphone placement between the Neptune and ear-level sound processors may result in differences in sound quality and/or hearing performance between the two types of sound processors, even when the same program is used. It should be noted that a special T-Mic adapter, called T-Comm, may be ordered for use with the Neptune processor to allow for T-Mic placement on the ear with use of the Neptune (Figure 9–27).

One other novel aspect of the Neptune processor, shown in Figure 9–28, is the fact that it may be used in two configurations: (1) the Neptune Connect mode with an array of user controls and (2) the more

streamlined, waterproof mode, in which the controls are fully removable to allow for the smallest wearing configuration. The Neptune Connect configuration is the mode of operation intended for daily use and is intended for use with the UHP described in the Naída CI Q section of this chapter.

The Neptune Connect offers user-adjustable dials that allow the recipient to change the volume and sensitivity of his/her processor (if the audiologist has programmed these controls to be enabled for use by the recipient). The Neptune Connect also provides a slider-program switch (Figure 9–29), which provides the user with three different programs as well as a

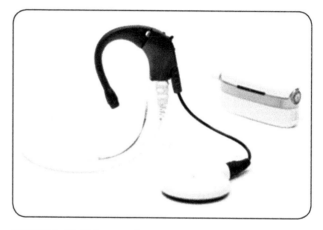

FIGURE 9–27. T-Comm w/Neptune. Image provided courtesy of Advanced Bionics, LLC.

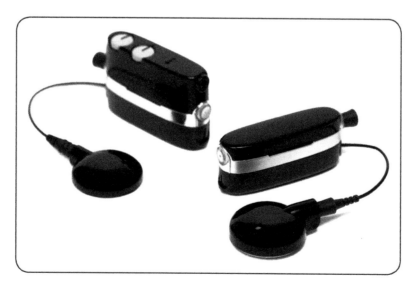

FIGURE 9–28. Different use options of the Neptune sound processor. Image provided courtesy of Advanced Bionics, LLC.

special setting (depicted as a triangle) referred to as the "monitor" mode. This mode allows a caregiver or audiologist with normal auditory function to listen to the input from the microphone or Euro Port Connector with a set of conventional earphones plugged into the 3.5-mm auxiliary connector of the Neptune Connect. Furthermore, the Neptune Connect has a Euro Port (Figure 9–30) that allows for the connection of a typical Euro Port FM/Roger receiver. Finally, the Neptune Connect has an audio input port to allow the user to connect personal audio devices (e.g., MP3 players, tablets, notebook computers) with an aux-

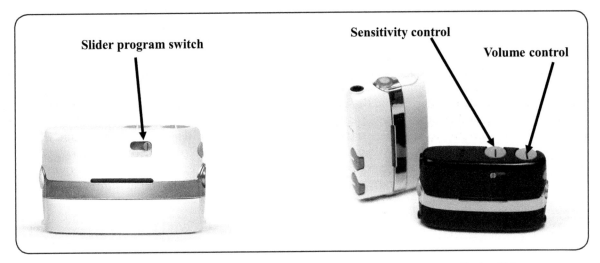

FIGURE 9–29. Controls of the Neptune sound processor. Image provided courtesy of Advanced Bionics, LLC.

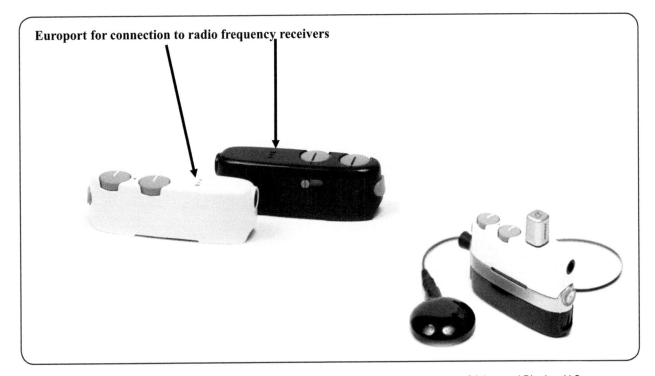

FIGURE 9–30. Euro Port connection of the Neptune sound processor. Image provided courtesy of Advanced Bionics, LLC.

iliary cable with a 3.5-mm phono plug. Advanced Bionics advises the audiologist to create a program with a mixing ratio with 10 dB of attenuation for use of the auxiliary input of the Neptune (programming of the mixing ratio of Advanced Bionics sound processors will be discussed in Chapter 15). It should be noted, once again, that the Neptune processor is not waterproof when the Neptune Connect configuration is used.

To use the Neptune as a waterproof processor, the recipient must remove the Neptune Connect cover, which makes the Neptune controls inaccessible, and replace it with a solid cover. Management of Neptune controls for both the Connect and swimmable options will be discussed later during the discussion of programming of Advanced Bionics devices. To waterproof the Neptune, the recipient must also switch from the UHP to the AquaMic waterproof headpiece. In order to achieve the IP68 water resistance, the AquaMic headpiece must also be used with the AquaMic cable. Once again, the underneath side of the UHP is black, whereas the underneath side of the AquaMic is gray ("gray for water play" to indicate the gray headpiece as the AquaMic). Many recipients prefer to use the Neptune in the swimmable configuration, particularly in active situations, because it is significantly smaller than the Connect configuration.

Pediatric-Friendly Features

The Neptune sound processor possesses a number of other pediatric-friendly options and features. For example, the Neptune possesses an LED within the power button (Figure 9–31) to alert the user or caregiver of the status of operation of the device as well as to program changes. Table 9–4 provides an illustration of a handout from Advanced Bionics that explains the information provided by the LED light. Furthermore, the Neptune features an audible alarm that can be programmed to alert the caregiver when the headpiece has fallen from the child's head (i.e., lock is lost between the external sound processor and the cochlear implant internal device) or when the battery is nearly depleted. Additionally, the covers of the Neptune case are difficult to remove without a specific hand movement in order to tamperproof the processor for young children (Figure 9–32). Finally, Advanced Bionics has provided a number of different configurations in which the Neptune sound processor may be worn for a variety of different situations (e.g., swimming, exercise, daily use for adults, daily use for infants and young children) (Figure 9–33).

Neptune Battery Options

Another user-friendly feature of the Neptune processor is the fact that it is powered by one AAA battery. Recipients may use a rechargeable NiMH AAA battery or AAA alkaline battery, which may be particularly beneficial in instances in which a power source is unavailable to charge rechargeable batteries (e.g., during a power outage, while on vacation, on an outdoor camping trip). Advanced Bionics reports that the typical user will receive about 13 hours of operating

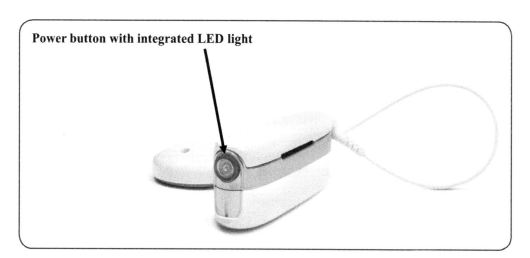

Power button with integrated LED light

FIGURE 9–31. Neptune power button with integrated LED light. Image provided courtesy of Advanced Bionics, LLC.

TABLE 9–4. Information Describing Neptune LED Light Function

Color	Behavior	Programmable	Indication
Orange	Blinks at start-up	No	• 4 quick blinks indicate that battery is fully charged • 2–3 quick blinks indicate that the battery is sufficiently charged to power the system • 1 quick blink indicates that the battery is nearly depleted • No blinking indicates depleted battery; replace with charged or new battery
	Solid	Yes	The battery is almost depleted
	Blinks twice every three seconds	Yes	The battery is depleted and cannot support stimulation
	Fades out	No	The sound processor is powering down
Red	Blinks once per second	Yes	Loss of lock with the implant
	Blinks rapidly (more than once per second)	No	Wrong implant connected
	Solid	No	Sound processor error condition. Fully remove and re-insert battery to reset processor
Green	Flickers in response to loud inputs	Yes	The sound processor and microphone are responding to sound
	Solid	No	Indicates an empty program slot or monitor (Δ) position
	Blinks at start-up, after battery status, and upon program change	No	• 1 blink indicates program one • 2 blinks indicate program two • 3 blinks indicate program three

Note. Use of some Neptune accessories may obscure the processor LED; therefore, audible alarms may be desirable for use with very young children to ensure caregiver notification of loss or lock or low battery status.

Source: Provided courtesy of Advanced Bionics, LLC.

time from a AAA NiMH rechargeable battery, 20 hours of operating time from a lithium battery, and 12 hours of use with a AAA alkaline battery. There are at least two benefits of using AAA batteries to power the Neptune. First, AAA batteries are readily available at most every department store, pharmacy, and convenience store around the world, so the recipient does not need to order specialized batteries from the implant manufacturer. Second, because of the widespread commercial application and availability of AAA batteries, they are much more affordable than the batteries that are specifically developed for use with implant sound processors.

Harmony Sound Processor

The Naída CI Q sound processor is incompatible with the Advanced Bionics C1 cochlear implant. As a result, recipients of the C1 cochlear implant (the CII was commercially approved in 2002, so C1 recipients are likely to have received their implant in early 2002 or earlier) must use the Harmony sound processor (shown in Figure 9–34), which is the ear-level predecessor of the Naída CI Q sound processor. It should be noted that the Harmony processor is no longer available to or serviced for recipients of CII, HiRes 90K, or HiRes Ultra cochlear implants. The Harmony

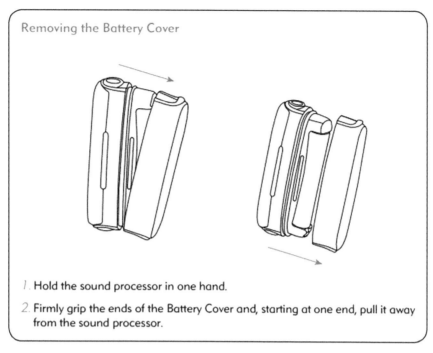

Removing the Battery Cover

1. Hold the sound processor in one hand.

2. Firmly grip the ends of the Battery Cover and, starting at one end, pull it away from the sound processor.

FIGURE 9–32. Removal of Neptune battery cover. Image provided courtesy of Advanced Bionics, LLC.

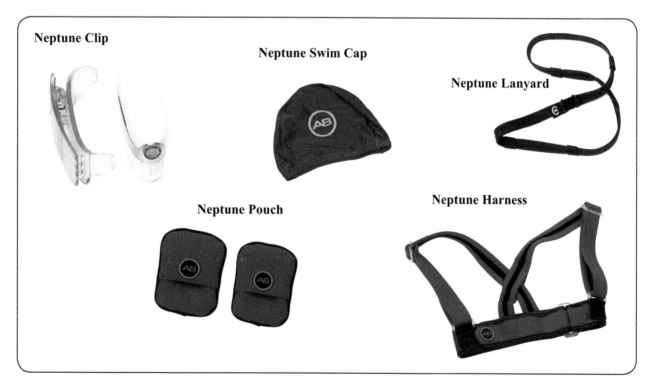

Neptune Clip

Neptune Swim Cap

Neptune Lanyard

Neptune Pouch

Neptune Harness

FIGURE 9–33. Neptune wearing options. Image provided courtesy of Advanced Bionics, LLC.

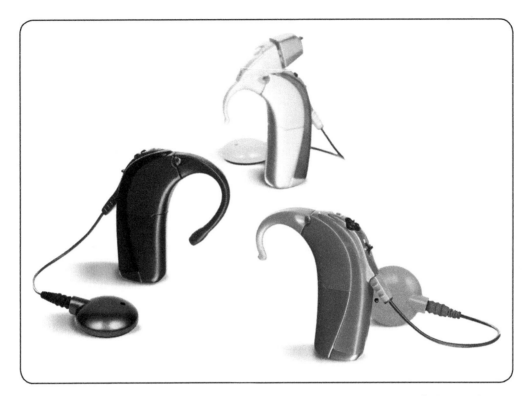

FIGURE 9–34. Advanced Bionics Harmony sound processor. Image provided courtesy of Advanced Bionics, LLC.

sound processor possesses a digital signal 16 bit (96 dB) front end processor, sampling rate of 17.4 kHz, maximum input dynamic range of 96 dB (i.e., maximum range of sound inputs handled without distortion), and a built-in, manually accessible telecoil. The Harmony sound processor has two user controls: (1) a rotary volume control located toward the top of the anterior spine of the processor and (2) a three-position slider switch that is located just below the volume control and that allows for use of three distinct user programs. An LED (light emitting diode) light on the upper spine of the processor allows for troubleshooting and for indication of device status (e.g., whether lock is obtained, program number that recipient is using, audio input is exceeding 65 dB SPL). A metal post at the top of the sound processor is used for coupling to specialized earhooks, such as the T-Mic. The primary microphone (an omnidirectional electret microphone) of the sound processor is located just below the post to where the earhook is connected.

Several different earhooks may be connected to the post at the top of the Harmony, including the conventional earhook, the T-mic, the iConnect (to allow a remote microphone receiver with a Europort to be connected to the Europort connector of the iConnect), and the Direct Connect earhooks to which specialized cables made by Advanced Bionics may be connected to consumer electronic devices such as a personal audio device (e.g., MP3 player). The conventional earhook does not deliver an auxiliary signal to the sound processor and serves only to retain the device over the ear.

The Harmony features a socket for the headpiece cable. The term "headpiece" has historically been used to describe the Advanced Bionics transmitting cable, the transmitting coil, and the external magnet. The UHP is the primary headpiece available for use with the Harmony sound processor, but a different cable (e.g., the Harmony UHP cable) is required than what is used for the Naída CI Q and Neptune processors. Previously, the Harmony processor was used with the same headpiece that was designed for its predecessor, the Auria sound processor. That headpiece, which is no longer distributed, was available in two shapes, a flat shape (designed for use with the CII internal device) and a concave shape (designed for use with the HiRes 90K internal device) that conforms to the curvature of the head and improves retention. All UHP headpieces possess a flat underneath side. It should be noted that the cable of the older model Auria/Harmony headpiece was hard-wired into the headpiece, so when the cable failed, the entire product had to be replaced. This was one of the primary reasons the headpiece was replaced with a separate Harmony cable and the UHP coil.

The Harmony sound processor is powered by a lithium-ion rechargeable battery (i.e., Harmony PowerCel). It is available in two different sizes, a compact version (PowerCel Slim) and a larger version (PowerCel Plus). For recipients of the CII and later-developed cochlear implants, the PowerCel version should allow for a full day of use on a single charge for many users; however, the PowerCel Plus may be selected for recipients who have atypically high power needs such as those with thick skin flaps, exceptionally high stimulation levels, or unusually high electrode impedances. The PowerCel Plus is especially useful for C1 recipients, because the C1 is less efficient than later Advanced Bionics cochlear implants, and its operation requires a greater magnitude of power from the external sound processor. As a result, the PowerCel Plus will provide a more reasonable operating time per charge.

Phonak Naída Link Hearing Aid

The Phonak Naída Link (see Figure 9–2) is another example of the benefit of the association between Advanced Bionics and the Phonak hearing aid company, both of which are subsidiaries of the Sonova Group. The Phonak Naída Link hearing aid is essentially a variation of the conventional Phonak Naída hearing aid, which is a high-gain and output hearing aid that was originally introduced for commercial use in 2008 for persons with severe to profound hearing loss. Since 2008, the Naída hearing aid has undergone many different transformations to allow for upgrades in hearing aid hardware and signal processing, such as frequency-lowering processing, directional microphone technology, acoustic feedback cancellation, and so forth. The Phonak Naída Link was commercially released in 2016 and is the first hearing aid that has been deliberately designed for bimodal users (persons who use a cochlear implant and a hearing aid for the non-implanted ear) to function optimally with a Naída CI Q70 or Q90 cochlear implant sound processor.

A collaboration between Phonak and Advanced Bionics resulted in the development of a new Phonak prescriptive formula, the Adaptive Phonak Digital Bimodal (APDB) fitting target, which aims to align the frequency response, loudness growth functions, and automatic gain control (AGC; compression) characteristics between the Naída CI sound processor and the Naída link hearing aid. Specifically, the bandwidth of the Naída Link hearing aid is adjusted to theoretically optimize the gain prescription based on the National Acoustic Laboratory's model of effective audibility (Ching et al., 2001). In cases of sloping hearing loss, the low-frequency gain will be increased in an attempt to capitalize on the cues for which the listener is most likely to be able to effectively process, whereas the high-frequency gain and output are substantially attenuated (refer to Figure 9–35 for an example) to avoid amplification in frequency ranges likely to include dead regions. A wider frequency response is employed for flat moderate hearing losses and reverse slope hearing losses. Additionally, the gain model is set in an effort to provide audibility for low-level inputs (i.e., 55 dB SPL) while ensuring comfort for moderate-level (65 dB SPL) to higher-level inputs (≥75 dB SPL and higher).

Furthermore, an attempt is made to align the interaural loudness growth functions by using the same compression parameters (compression kneepoint = 63 dB SPL; compression ratio = 12:1). Also, the slow-acting (attack/release times >1 sec) dual-loop AGC (which essentially acts as an automatic volume control) of the Naída CI Q is incorporated into the Naída Link hearing aid so that the compression time constants are similar between ears. The conventional Phonak Naída hearing aid uses syllabic compression (attack/release time <50 msec), which operates much faster in the time domain than the compression used in Advanced Bionics cochlear implants. Although there is a paucity of research examining the potential benefits of a hearing aid designed to function with a cochlear implant sound processor, early reports do suggest that better speech recognition in noise is obtained by bimodal users who are provided with matched automatic gain control compression characteristics between the hearing aid and cochlear implant sound processor (Veugen et al., 2016). An Advanced Bionics white paper provides a summary of the results of three experiments of speech recognition in noise obtained with the Naída Link programmed with APDB compared with performance obtained with a conventional hearing aid. In general, a significant improvement in speech recognition in noise was observed with use of the Naída Link relative to performance with other hear-

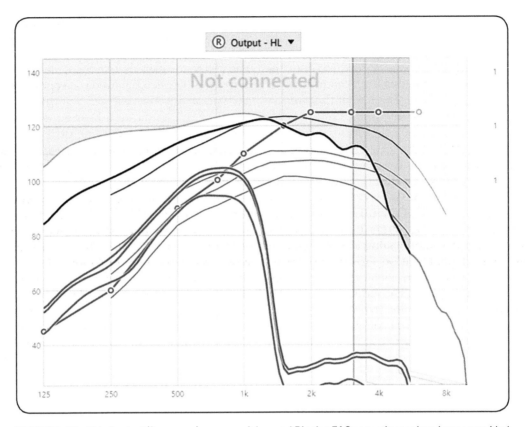

FIGURE 9–35. Aided output (frequency) response Advanced Bionics EAS acoustic receiver. Image provided courtesy of Advanced Bionics, LLC.

ing aids programmed with traditional gain-frequency responses, particularly when the study participants possessed normal temporal fine structure capabilities (Advanced Bionics White Paper, 2016).

Another benefit of the Phonak Naída Link hearing aid is that bimodal users may potentially benefit from the Phonak Binaural VoiceStream technologies. StereoZoom (binaural beamforming), DuoPhone (interaural telephone streaming), and ZoomControl are all available to users of the Phonak Naída Link hearing aid and the Advanced Bionics Naída CI Q70 or Q90 sound processor. Also, wireless accessories, such as the Phonak ComPilot and the Phonak Roger system, may be used to stream audio to both ears of bimodal users. The Phonak Naída Link is available in two models, the RIC (receiver-in-the-canal) and UP (Ultra Power). The RIC model may be used with a variety of different receivers, with smaller receivers allowing for an extended high-frequency response (up to 8900 Hz) with moderate maximum gain (45 dB SPL in a 2 cc coupler) and output (109 dB SPL in a 2 cc coupler) and larger receivers allowing for limited

high-frequency bandwidth (5100 Hz) high maximum gain (65 dB SPL in a 2-cc coupler) and output (130 dB SPL in a 2-cc coupler). The Phonak UP behind-the-ear hearing aid has an upper frequency bandwidth of 4900 Hz with a maximum 2-cc coupler gain and output of 82 and 139 dB SPL, respectively. Of note, the Phonak Naída Link hearing aid is programmed with the audiologist in the Phonak Target hearing aid fitting software. Additionally, during the cochlear implant programming session, the audiologist must initialize the Naída CI Q sound processor to be used in the bimodal mode with the Phonak Naída Link hearing aid.

Phonak Naída Link CROS

Another product of the collaborative relationship between Advanced Bionics and Phonak is the Phonak Naída Link CROS device (see Figure 9–3). The contralateral routing of signal (CROS) hearing aid has been available for decades as a potential solution for persons with single-sided deafness. The CROS device consists of an ear-level microphone that captures the sound present at the poorer ear and transfers it to the better-hearing, opposite ear by way of short-range radio transmission. The Phonak CROS aid uses the proprietary Hearing instrument Body Area Network (HiBAN) with Binaural VoiceStream technology. The Binaural VoiceStream Technology utilizes near-field magnetic induction (NFMI) to stream full speech bandwidth audio from a device on one ear to the device on the opposite ear. According to the Advanced Bionics recipient database, 78% of Advanced Bionics cochlear implant recipients are unilateral implant users (Naída Link CROS Training Materials, 2017). Reasons that persons with bilateral profound hearing loss may choose unilateral cochlear implantation include: (1) insurance does not cover bilateral cochlear implantation, (2) medical issues prevent a second surgery, (3) the recipient does not want to undergo a second surgery, (4) the recipient wishes to wait on new technology or inner ear medical therapies (e.g., hair cell regeneration), and so forth. It is well known that cochlear implant recipients who have bilateral profound hearing loss may continue to struggle with understanding speech in noise and speech that originates from the side of the non-implanted ear. The Phonak Naída Link CROS is intended to address these limitations.

In short, the Phonak CROS hearing aid is worn on the non-implanted ear and delivers the audio signal at that ear to the Naída CI Q70 or Q90 sound processor (the Naída CI Q30 sound processor is not compatible with the Naída Link CROS). The Naída CROS features a dual-microphone directional system and a mute button. The mute button may be pushed to mute the microphone of the CROS device by the user in situations in which the non-implanted ear is primarily exposed to noise (e.g., when the recipient is driving a car and the non-implanted ear is next to the window). It is powered by a PowerOne zinc-air size 13 battery, which should last three to five days. Advanced Bionics recommends that the Phonak Naída Link CROS be worn with the CROS SlimTube to facilitate adequate retention.

There is no need for the audiologist to program the Phonak Naída Link CROS. However, the audiologist must initialize the Naída CI Q70 or Q90 sound processor as a CROS device. When configured as a CROS device, the Naída CI Q sound processor will continuously monitor for the presence of a signal from the Naída Link CROS device. When the CROS microphone is active and the CROS delivers a signal to the Naída CI Q processor, the recipient will hear equal input from the Naída CI and the Naída Link CROS. When the CROS is not detected, the recipient will hear only the Naída CI Q input.

The Naída Link CROS automatically matches the microphone mode of the Naída CI Q sound processor. For instance, if the Naída CI Q is in omnidirectional mode, then the CROS will also be in omnidirectional mode. If the Naída CI Q is in directional mode (UltraZoom or StereoZoom), then the CROS will automatically switch to the same microphone mode. As previously noted, the StereoZoom binaural beamformer provides significantly better speech recognition in noise compared with conventional adaptive directional microphone systems. As a result, the use of StereoZoom with the CROS device may offer a substantial improvement in speech recognition in noise. Additionally, the Naída CI Q sound processor may also simultaneously receive audio signals from the Naída Link CROS and the Phonak Roger system. If a HiBAN accessory device is used (e.g., ComPilot, TVLink II, RemoteMic), then the HiBAN accessory audio input will take priority over the CROS.

Advanced Bionics Cochlear Implants

HiRes Ultra Cochlear Implant

In July 2016, Advanced Bionics received FDA approval for the commercial distribution of the HiRes Ultra cochlear implant (Figure 9–36). The HiRes Ultra contains what Advanced Bionics refers to as the Implant-

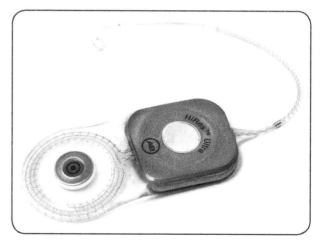

FIGURE 9–36. Advanced Bionics HiRes Ultra cochlear implant. Image provided courtesy of Advanced Bionics, LLC.

able Cochlear Stimulator (ICS), which contains the electronics of the implant. The electronics of the HiRes Ultra are similar to the electronics contained in the Advanced Bionics CII, HiRes 90K, and HiRes 90K Advantage cochlear implants. The HiRes Ultra also contains a telemetry coil, a removable magnet, and an electrode lead and array. The entire internal device package is hermetically encased in a biocompatible silicone covering to prevent rejection by the human body and to limit the ingress of bodily fluids into the internal device and electrode leads. The electronics package is housed in a titanium case, which is considerably thinner than its predecessor, the HiRes 90K cochlear implant. Specifically, the titanium case of the HiRes Ultra has a thickness of 4.5 mm and a weight of 10 grams, compared with a thickness of 5.5 mm and a weight of 12 grams for the HiRes 90K cochlear implant.

The HiRes Ultra electronics possess several characteristics that are unique and sophisticated relative to modern cochlear implant systems. The ICS includes a DSP that performs complex digital analyses on the signal received from the external sound processor and determines the magnitude of electrical stimulation needed for each electrode contact to elicit a desired auditory percept based on the program created by the audiologist. The DSP of the HiRes Ultra includes an information update rate of 90,000 updates/second and a stimulation rate of 83,000 pulses/second, both of which are faster than what is available in other commercially available cochlear implants. The analog-to-digital converter of the ICS contains a resolution of 9 bits and a sampling rate of 25 kHz. Additionally, the HiRes Ultra contains 16 independent output circuits (each with its own capacitor), which are each linked to one of the 16 individual intracochlear electrode contacts. In short, the 16 independent output circuits allow for independent stimulation of each intracochlear electrode contact and for a high level of precise control over the stimulation provided to the user. The HiRes Ultra ICS device also contains a bidirectional telemetry system, which enables continuous transmission of information from the external sound processor to the internal device and vice versa. The signal from the external processor is transmitted at a carrier frequency of 49 MHz, whereas the signal from the internal device is transmitted at 10.7 MHz. The bidirectional telemetry system is unique to Advanced Bionics cochlear implants (CII implants and later) and allows for several beneficial features such as real-time determination of the power needed from

the external sound processor to operate the ICS. The HiRes Ultra also contains the IntelliLink technology, which is a system in which the ICS communicates with the external sound processor to establish an association between the implant and sound processor. IntelliLink allows an external sound processor to be loaded with programs for the right and left ear, and the communication between the sound processor and ICS determines which program to use to stimulate the ear on which the sound processor is being worn. IntelliLink also prevents the sound processor of one recipient from being used to stimulate the cochlear implant of another recipient.

The HiRes Ultra internal receiving/telemetry coil is shown in Figure 9–37 with the internal magnet positioned within a Silastic sleeve in the center of the coil. The silastic sleeve permits temporary removal of the internal magnet so that the patient may undergo magnetic resonance imaging (MRI) with a strength of 3.0 tesla (T). For MRI with 1.5T strength, imaging can be done with the magnet in place and the recipient's head tightly bandaged following a protocol published by Advanced Bionics. In either case, the recipient's surgeon should ideally be consulted prior to the procedure. As can be seen in Figures 9–36 and 9–37, the durable, biocompatible titanium case, which houses the ICS, is positioned just below the telemetry coil. Also, the primary extracochlear ground electrode (i.e., return or reference contact) is located in the center of the casing of the internal stimulator.

Advanced Bionics uses the term "electrode" to collectively describe the electrode lead and the electrode array. The electrode array houses the intracochlear electrode contacts that ultimately provide electrical stimulation to the cochlea. The electrode array exits the internal stimulator through a component called feedthrough. The electrode lead possesses a fantail shape as it exits the internal stimulator. This fantail shape provides flexibility and durability to the lead, which is particularly useful because the ICS case is typically placed within a recessed bed (created by the surgeon) in the skull bone. The electrode lead contains 16 small wires that carry the electrical signal from each of the 16 independent output circuits in the ICS to the corresponding 16 individual intracochlear electrode contacts. Just beyond the fantail is a secondary extracochlear ground electrode contact (i.e., return/reference) referred to as the ring electrode. In rare cases, the audiologist may switch the extracochlear ground electrode contact used for stimulation from the case ground electrode to the

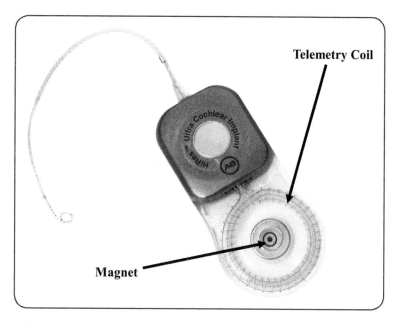

FIGURE 9–37. Advanced Bionics HiRes Ultra cochlear implant. Image provided courtesy of Advanced Bionics, LLC.

ring electrode. The ring electrode is also used as the reference electrode for the measurement of neural responses from the cochlear nerve using the Neural Response Imaging (NRI) assessment module. The NRI module is the platform in the Advanced Bionics system used for measurement of the electrically evoked compound action potential.

At the time of this writing, Advanced Bionics also introduced the development of a new cochlear implant, the HiRes Ultra 3D implant, but this device was not yet approved for commercial distribution in the North America, Europe, or other parts of the world. The HiRes Ultra 3D is similar to the HiRes Ultra except for the fact that the former contains a magnet that orients itself in three dimensions with the magnetic lines of flux of an external magnetic field. As a result, the implant and magnet may be left in place with minimal to no torque provided by the magnetic field on the implant. Consequently, the recipient may undergo MRI with a strength of up to 3.0 tesla without the feeling of pain or discomfort, without the concern of the magnet being extracted from the implant, without the need to orient the head in a special position, and without the need for head bandaging. However, as with conventional dipole magnets, the magnet within the HiRes Ultra 3D implant the will still produce a "shadow artifact" in the temporal lobe area near the implant site.

Mid-Scala Electrode Array

In May 2013, Advanced Bionics commercially released the HiFocus Mid-Scala Electrode in the United States (Figure 9–38). The HiFocus Mid-Scala Electrode is the electrode array that is available with the HiRes Ultra cochlear implant. Over the past several years, cochlear implant manufacturers and researchers have explored and are continuing to explore the theoretical advantages and limitations of perimodiolar or "modiolar-hugging" (i.e., near the modiolus, which is on the medial wall of the cochlea and is in close proximity to the cochlear nerve fibers) versus lateral wall electrode arrays (which lie away from the medial wall, under the basilar membrane). Although research has failed to show either type of electrode array to be unequivocally better than the other, each electrode array does possess its own attributes that are theoretically advantageous. Specifically, by avoiding the organ of Corti, lateral wall electrode arrays may cause less trauma to the delicate cochlear structures in the scala media, and consequently, may be ideal for preserving residual hearing and for preserving the cochlea for future medical interventions (e.g., hair cell regeneration). In contrast, compared with a lateral wall array, a perimodiolar array should require less electrical current to facilitate a response from the cochlear nerve and thereby require less

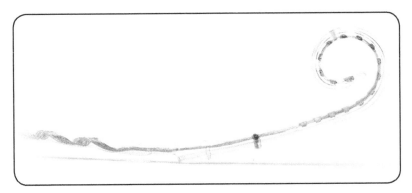

FIGURE 9–38. Advanced Bionics Mid-Scala electrode. Image provided courtesy of Advanced Bionics, LLC.

power to achieve a given loudness percept. In addition, perimodiolar placement may result in reduced channel interaction (channel interaction is the spread of electrical current from the cochlear nerve fibers and/or cell bodies most proximal to the electrode contact being stimulated to the cochlear nerve fibers and cell bodies that are more proximal to neighboring electrode contacts). Indeed, research has demonstrated that recipients of perimodiolar electrode arrays require lower levels of electrical stimulation to achieve a given level of loudness and performance (Cohen, Saunders, & Clark, 2001; Tykocinski et al., 2001) and that channel interaction may be lower in recipients of perimodiolar electrode arrays (Hughes & Abbas, 2006).

Although studies have shown that some recipients of lateral wall electrodes do achieve almost full preservation of low-frequency residual hearing (Gantz & Turner, 2004; von Ilberg, Baumann, Kiefer, Tillein, & Adunka, 2011; Wanna et al., 2015, 2018), there are also certainly instances in which hearing preservation has been achieved with perimodiolar electrodes, particularly with thin perimodiolar arrays (e.g., Nucleus 532 electrode array). Furthermore, to the authors' knowledge, there is no published research available at this time to indicate that lateral wall electrode arrays enhance the likelihood that a recipient will be able to pursue inner ear pharmacological treatments that may arise in the future, particularly when both perimodiolar and lateral wall electrode arrays are located in the scala tympani.

In the midst of these conflicting design attributes and theoretical advantages and limitations of lateral wall and perimodiolar electrode arrays, the HiFocus Mid-Scala Electrode was developed in an attempt to capitalize on the theoretical advantages of both a

perimodiolar and a lateral wall electrode array. As the name implies, the Hi-Focus Mid-Scala Electrode is designed to lie in the center of the scala tympani in order to remain reasonably proximal to the modiolus (and cochlear neural elements) while also not making physical contact with the delicate cochlear structures necessary to maintain residual hearing. Early reports do indicate that hearing preservation is possible with the Mid-Scala electrode array. Hunter et al. (2016) reported on outcomes of 39 ears in which the Mid-Scala electrode array was inserted for recipients who had functional preoperative low-frequency acoustic hearing (i.e., defined as an air conduction threshold of 85 dB HL or better at 250 Hz in the ear to be implanted). At one year post-activation, 38.5% of these recipients had partial hearing preservation.

It is also important to note that the HiFocus Mid-Scala Electrode is much thinner than other curved Advanced Bionics electrode arrays. The HiFocus Mid-Scala Electrode has a cross-sectional diameter of 0.5 × 0.5 mm at the apical end (intracochlear electrode contact 1) and 0.7 × 0.7 mm at the basal end (intracochlear electrode contact 16). A thinner diameter is important, because the array is less likely to come in contact with delicate cochlear structures, and the array is more likely to be successfully inserted through the round window. Some surgeons and researchers believe that round window insertion provides a higher likelihood of hearing preservation and cochlear atraumaticity than insertion of the array into a cochleostomy. Additionally, inserting the electrode array into the round window ensures that the insertion will begin in the scala tympani. However, it is important to note that conclusive data do not exist to clearly indicate one entry point (round window versus cochleostomy) to be superior over another. At any rate, with a thinner electrode array, the surgeon is able to make a smaller cochleostomy, which may be beneficial.

The HiFocus Mid-Scala Electrode possesses two blue markers, a distal marker between intracochlear electrode contacts 5 and 6 and a proximal marker that is located lateral to the most basal electrode contact (i.e., intracochlear electrode contact 16; see Figure 9–38). The HiFocus Mid-Scala Electrode is loaded on a sty-

let, which straightens the pre-curved electrode array prior to insertion (Figure 9–39). It should be noted that it is possible to reload the array onto the stylet if the surgeon needs to do so. The surgeon may insert the HiFocus Mid-Scala by a free-hand approach or with the use of the HiFocus Mid-Scala Insertion Tool (Figure 9–40). The electrode array is inserted into the cochlea until the proximal marker is adjacent to the

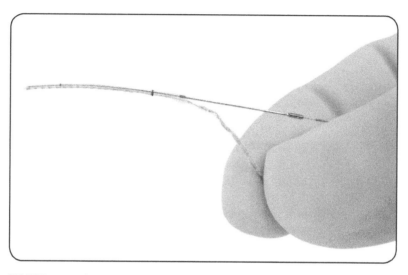

FIGURE 9–39. Advanced Bionics Mid-Scala electrode in stylet. Image provided courtesy of Advanced Bionics, LLC.

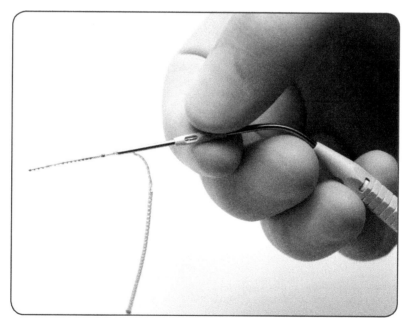

FIGURE 9–40. Advanced Bionics Mid-Scala electrode in stylet with insertion tool. Image provided courtesy of Advanced Bionics, LLC.

cochleostomy/round window opening. At that point, the surgeon uses a pair of forceps to grasp the stylet and hold it in place while the electrode array is advanced off the stylet and into the cochlea. After following these steps, the electrode array should curve around the basal turn of the cochlea as it is advanced away from the stylet. The surgeon should continue to insert the electrode array into the cochlea until the distal marker is positioned in the cochleostomy. Of note, a protective sleeve/stop exists at the neck of the electrode array to prevent further insertion into the cochlea.

The HiFocus Mid-Scala Electrode possesses planar (flat, plate-like) intracochlear electrode contacts; the surgeon must ensure that the intracochlear electrode contacts face superiorly (toward the modiolus) in order to provide direct stimulation toward the modiolus and hence the neural elements. The length of the electrode lead from the fantail to the neck of the electrode array is 18.5 mm. The length of the electrode array from the apical tip to the proximal blue marker is 18.5 mm with the intracochlear electrode contacts spaced across a distance of 15 mm, which results in approximately 1 mm of separation between electrode contacts. The HiFocus Mid-Scala Electrode is intended to be inserted to an angular depth of approximately 420 to 450 degrees.

HiFocus™ SlimJ Electrode Array

The Advanced Bionics HiFocus SlimJ electrode array is a thin lateral wall electrode array designed to cover the majority of the spiral ganglion population while also allowing for preservation of cochlear structures (Advanced Bionics, 2017). The SlimJ electrode also contains characteristics that are intended to allow for ease of handling and insertion by the surgeon. The SlimJ electrode is 23 mm in length from the insertion depth marker (i.e., the blue marker that the surgeon

should position at the cochleostomy or entrance of the round window) to the tip of the array (Figure 9–41). The SlimJ electrode array is 0.55 × 0.26 mm at the tip of the array and 0.79 × 0.61 mm at the insertion depth marker (i.e., the lateral end of the electrode array). The thin diameter of the SlimJ allows for insertion into the round window, an extended round window, or a cochleostomy. The SlimJ electrode array contains 16 planar-shaped, platinum intracochlear electrode contacts that span across a distance of 20 mm. The intracochlear electrode contacts are evenly spaced with 1.3 mm between contacts. When fully inserted to a linear depth of 23 mm, the SlimJ electrode array is inserted to an angular insertion depth of approximately 420 degrees in the typical cochlea. The implant surgeon uses forceps to grasp the SlimJ electrode array at "wing." The surgeon uses a "free-hand" approach with forceps to insert the SlimJ into the cochleostomy until the blue marker of the electrode array lies at the cochleostomy. The surgeon must make certain to position the planar-shaped electrode contacts toward the modiolus so that electrical stimulation is directed toward the cochlear nerve.

HiRes 90K Advantage Cochlear Implant

In September 2012, Advanced Bionics received FDA approval for the HiRes 90K Advantage implant (Figure 9–42). The HiRes 90K Advantage essentially contains the same electronics as the HiRes Ultra and HiRes 90K implants. The case of the ICS of the HiRes 90K Advantage implant is thicker than the HiRes Ultra cochlear implant. The thinner profile of the HiRes Ultra makes it especially attractive for infants, young children, and elderly persons (these three groups typically have thinner bone density and skin flaps) because the HiRes Ultra's lower profile requires less removal of skull bone to make a recessed bed to

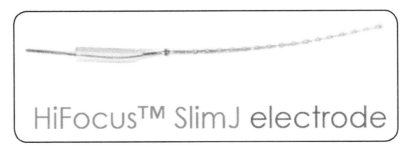

FIGURE 9–41. Advanced Bionics HiFocus SlimJ electrode. Image provided courtesy of Advanced Bionics, LLC.

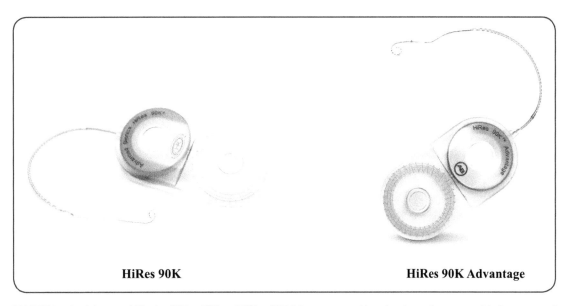

FIGURE 9–42. Advanced Bionics HiRes 90K and HiRes 90K Advantage cochlear implants. Image provided courtesy of Advanced Bionics, LLC.

accommodate the implant. Also, the HiRes Ultra is less prominent when positioned underneath the skin.

The primary difference between the HiRes 90K Advantage and the original HiRes 90K cochlear implant is an improvement in the mechanical design of the antenna coil. For the Advantage implant, the antenna coil is reinforced with a high-density polymer fiber component to address a small number of previous failures in which the coil had failed. The fiber, positioned adjacent to the braided gold coil wire in the antenna, offers resistance to any movement in the silastic carrier that would otherwise induce a tensional force in the gold wire. Moreover, the case of the HiRes 90K Advantage was designed to withstand high impact forces (i.e., blow to the head, automobile accident, fall), safely enduring an impact of up to 6 joules, which exceeds the cochlear implant industry's impact resistance standards.

The HiFocus 1j Electrode has also been available for use with the HiRes 90K implant. The HiFocus 1j electrode has a gently curved shape. The diameter of the HiFocus 1j electrode is 0.4 mm at the apical end and 0.8 mm at the basal end. Therefore, the 1j electrode permits a relatively small cochleostomy for insertion. The total length of the HiFocus 1j electrode array is 25 mm (from tip to neck) with the intracochlear electrode contacts spaced across a distance of 17 mm. It is intended to be inserted to an angular insertion depth of 400 to 500 degrees. The HiFocus 1j is loaded into an insertion tube and may be inserted

with the use of the HiFocus 1j Electrode Insertion Tool. The surgeon must position the opening of the insertion tube toward the modiolus so that the 16 planar intracochlear electrode contacts of the 1j electrode are oriented toward the cochlear neural elements.

HiRes 90K Implantable Cochlear Implant

The HiRes 90K possesses the same electronics as the HiRes 90K Advantage and the HiRes Ultra cochlear implants. Also, the case of the HiRes 90K is essentially identical to the HiRes 90K Advantage implant. As previously discussed, the antenna of the original HiRes 90K implant was slightly less durable than the reinforced antenna of the HiRes 90K Advantage. As a result, the HiRes 90K Advantage has replaced the HiRes 90K implant. The Advanced Bionics HiRes 90K internal device featured three electrode array choices, the HiFocus Helix electrode array, the HiFocus 1j electrode array, and the Mid-Scala array. The Helix electrode array has a subtly coiled shape, which is intended to facilitate close proximity of the electrode contacts to the modiolus and peripheral auditory neural elements (Figure 9–43). The Helix electrode array is tapered so that the apical end is much thinner than the basal end to allow the surgeon better visualization of the cochleostomy during electrode array insertion. The Helix electrode array is 0.6 mm in diameter at the apical end and 1.1 mm at the basal end. The Helix electrode array is a perimodiolar ("peri" refers to near or around the modiolus) electrode array and is intended to be inserted to an angular insertion depth of 360 to 420 degrees. The Helix electrode array has been replaced by the HiFocus Mid-Scala Electrode.

Advanced Bionics CII Cochlear Implant

The Advanced Bionics CII cochlear implant is shown in Figure 9–44. The CII cochlear implant possesses essentially the same electronics as the HiRes 90K and HiRes Ultra cochlear implants. The CII cochlear implant was the last Advanced Bionics cochlear implant to house the ICS within a ceramic case. All of the modern Advanced Bionics signal coding strategies, signal processing, telemetry measures (e.g.,

electrode impedance measures, Neural Response Imaging, IntelliLink), and external sound processors may be used with the CII cochlear implant. The CII implant was discontinued because the titanium case of later Advanced Bionics cochlear implants has proven to be more durable and resistant to impact than the ceramic case of the CII implant.

Key Concepts

- Advanced Bionics offers a variety of sound processors to meet the unique needs of children and adults who have received Advanced Bionics

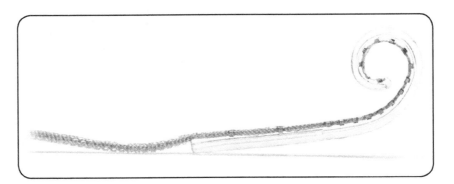

FIGURE 9–43. Advanced Bionics Helix electrode. Image provided courtesy of Advanced Bionics, LLC.

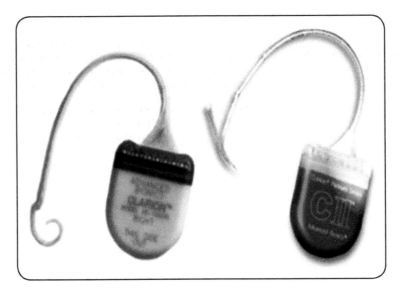

FIGURE 9–44. Advanced Bionics CII cochlear implant. Image provided courtesy of Advanced Bionics, LLC

cochlear implants. Advanced Bionics recipients may choose from ear-level or body-worn sound processors.

- Advanced Bionics sound processors are equipped with adaptive signal processing designed to improve hearing performance in challenging listening situations.
- Advanced Bionics sound processors are also equipped with interaural streaming and may be used with a variety of different wireless hearing assistive technologies.
- Advanced Bionics cochlear implants may also be used with a hearing aid designed for bimodal use and with a CROS.
- Advanced Bionics offers a variety of different cochlear implants and electrode arrays to meet the unique needs of recipients. Surgeons may select from perimodiolar, mid-modiolar, and lateral wall electrode arrays.

References

Advanced Bionics. (2016). *Optimizing hearing for listeners with a cochlear implant and a contralateral hearing aid.* Retrieved from https://4f9f43c1b16d77fd5a81-7c32520033e6d1a7ac50 ad01318c27e4.ssl.cf2.rackcdn.com/content/19000/19063/ resource2apdbimodalfittingformulawhitepaper.pdf

Advanced Bionics. (2017). *The foundation of better hearing: AB implantable technology.* Retrieved from https://www.advanced bionics.com/content/dam/advancedbionics/Documents/Glo bal/en_ce/Products/HiRes-Ultra/HiRes-Ultra-Brochure.pdf

Büchner, A., Heeren, W., Klawitter, S., & Lenarz, T. (2016). *Benefit of advanced directional microphones for bilateral cochlear implant users.* Presented at Fourteenth International Conference on Cochlear Implants and Other Implantable Technologies (CI2016), Toronto, ON, Canada.

Cardenas, E., Downing, S., Oexmann, J., & Crew, J. (2017). *Beyond one ear: Benefits of CROS, bimodal, and bilateral for speech understanding in complex environments.* Manuscript submitted for publication.

Cohen, L. T., Saunders, E., & Clark, G. M. (2001). Psychophysics of a prototype peri-modiolar cochlear implant electrode array. *Hearing Research, 155*(1–2), 63–81.

Gantz, B. J., & Turner, C. (2004). Combining acoustic and electrical speech processing: Iowa/Nucleus hybrid implant. *Acta Oto-Laryngologica, 124*, 344–347.

Gifford, R. H., & Revit, L. R. (2010). Speech perception for adult cochlear implant recipients a realistic background noise: Effectiveness of preprocessing strategies and external options for improving speech recognition in noise. *Journal of the American Academy of Audiology, 21*(7), 441–451.

Hughes, M. L., & Abbas, P. J. (2006). Electrophysiologic channel interaction, electrode pitch ranking, and behavioral threshold in straight versus perimodiolar cochlear implant electrode arrays. *Journal of the Acoustical Society of America, 119*, 1538–1547.

Hunter, J. B., Gifford, R. H., Wanna, G. B., Labadie, R. F., Bennett, M. L., Haynes, D. S., & Rivas, A. (2016). Hearing preservation outcomes with a mid-scala electrode in cochlear implantation. *Otology and Neurotology, 37*(3), 235–240.

Johnstone, P. M. (2016). *Use of microphone technology to improve speech perception in background noise in pediatric CI users.* Presented at Fourteenth International Conference on Cochlear Implants and Other Implantable Technologies (CI2016), Toronto, ON, Canada.

Koch, D. B., Quick, A., Osberger, M. J., Saoji, A., & Litvak, L. (2014). Enhanced hearing in noise for cochlear implant recipients: Clinical trial results for a commercially available speech-enhancement strategy. *Otology and Neurotology, 35*(5), 803–809.

Kolberg, E. R., Sheffield, S. W., Davis, T. J., Sunderhaus, L. W., & Gifford, R. H. (2015). Cochlear implant microphone location affects speech recognition in diffuse noise. *Journal of the American Academy of Audiology, 26*(1), 51–58.

Naída Link CROS Training Materials. (2017). Valencia, CA: Advanced Bionics.

Tykocinski, M., Saunders, E., Cohen, L. T., Treaba, C., Briggs, R. J., Gibson, P., . . . Cowan, R. S. (2001). The contour electrode array: Safety study and initial patient trials of a new perimodiolar design. *Otology and Neurotology, 22*(1), 33–41.

Veugen, L. C., Chalupper, J., Snik, A. F., Opstal, A. J., & Mens, L. H. (2016). Matching automatic gain control across devices in bimodal cochlear implant users. *Ear and Hearing, 37*(3), 260–270.

von Ilberg, C. A., Baumann, U., Kiefer, J., Tillein, J., & Adunka, O. F. (2011). Electric-acoustic stimulation of the auditory system: A review of the first decade. *Audiology and Neurotology, 16*(Suppl. 2), 1–30.

Wanna, G. B., Noble, J. H., Gifford, R. H., Dietrich, M. S., Sweeney, A. D., Zhang, D., . . . Labadie, R. F. (2015). Impact of intrascalar electrode location, electrode type, and angular insertion depth on residual hearing in cochlear implant patients: Preliminary results. *Otology and Neurotology, 36*(8), 1343–1348.

Wanna, G. B., O'Connell, B. P., Francis, D. O., Gifford, R. H., Hunter, J. B., Holder, J. T., . . . Haynes, D. S. (2018). Predictive factors for short- and long-term hearing preservation in cochlear implantation with conventional-length electrodes. *Laryngoscope, 128*(2), 482–489.

Wolfe, J., Morais, M., Schafer, E., Agrawal, S., & Koch, D. (2015). Evaluation of speech recognition of cochlear implant recipients using adaptive, digital remote microphone technology and a speech enhancement sound processing algorithm. *Journal of the American Academy of Audiology, 26*(5), 502–508.

10

Cochlear Nucleus Cochlear Implants and Sound Processors

Jace Wolfe and Erin C. Schafer

Introduction

This chapter will provide a review of Cochlear Nucleus cochlear implants and sound processors. The programming of Nucleus cochlear implants will be discussed in Chapter 16. Cochlear Ltd. manufactures the Nucleus cochlear implant series, which includes a number of different cochlear implants which are primarily distinguished by a certain type of electrode array. All Nucleus recipients may use the Nucleus 7 or Nucleus 6 behind-the-ear sound processors. Also, most Nucleus recipients may use the Kanso™ single-unit, off-the-ear sound processor. Cochlear Nucleus cochlear implant systems will be described in the following section.

Nucleus Sound Processors

Nucleus 7 Sound Processor

In the summer of 2017, Cochlear received Food and Drug Administration (FDA) approval to commercially distribute the Nucleus 7 cochlear implant sound processor, which is also known as the CP1000 sound processor (Figure 10–1). Of note, the letters "CP" in the model name refer to "Cochlear Processor," and the "10" refers to the tenth generation of Cochlear sound processors. The two zeros at the end of the

"1000" specify a particular model within the tenth generation. If another variation of the Nucleus 7 processor is brought to the commercial market, it will likely be referred to as the CP1010. The Nucleus 7 is composed of three major components: (1) a sound processor with the digital signal processor and user controls, (2) a battery module, and (3) a cable/coil with a removable magnet. Of note, the Nucleus 7 cable/coil is referred to as the SlimLine Coil Cable. It is thinner (i.e., lower profile) than the coil used for the Nucleus 6 sound processor, which is the predecessor to the Nucleus 7. Additionally, the SlimLine Coil Cable is a one-piece unit with the cable permanently fixed into the coil (i.e., non-removable). The SlimLine is available in four lengths: 6, 9, 11, and 25 cm. Furthermore, the removable magnet is available in seven different strengths (1/2, 1, 2, 3, 4, 5, and 6). At the time of this writing, the Nucleus 7 sound processor may be used with all Nucleus cochlear implants except for the Nucleus 22 .

Nucleus 7 Features

The Nucleus 7 sound processor possesses several unique features, including the fact that it is the first cochlear implant sound processor made for use with the Apple iPhone smartphone (Apple iPhone 5 and later generations). The made-for-iPhone (MiFi) technology is a product of a collaborative partnership that Cochlear Ltd. has formed with the GN ReSound hearing aid company, which has developed and

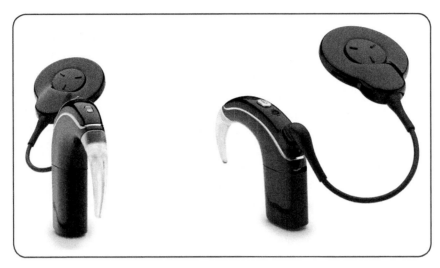

FIGURE 10–1. Nucleus 7 (CP1000) sound processor. Image provided courtesy of Cochlear Americas, ©2018.

incorporated a number of 2.4 GHz wireless audio streaming technologies for its line of hearing aids. The Nucleus 7 sound processor can receive telephone and media (e.g., video, music, games) audio signals directly from an Apple iPhone without the need of a streaming interface accessory device. Additionally, the new *Nucleus Smart* app may be downloaded on a smartphone and used to control the settings of the sound processor (e.g., volume/sensitivity adjustment, program change, audio sources [wireless accessories] and mixing), to evaluate the function and operation of the sound processor (e.g., battery life, hours of use per day, link/lock status) and to locate the sound processor when it is misplaced (Figure 10–2). Also, the Nucleus Smart App features the Hearing Tracker, which logs the time in speech and the number of times the coil loses link on a daily basis. The information provided by the Hearing Tracker may be of particular benefit to the families of children, because the data will allow the family to pursue a goal of a certain amount of implant use per day (e.g., at least 10 hours per day). Moreover, the iPhone may be used as a remote microphone accessory that streams the audio captured at the microphone of the smartphone directly to the Nucleus 7 sound processor. Of note, the following Apple devices are compatible with the Nucleus 7 sound processor:

- iPhone 4s and later
- iPad Pro and later
- iPad Air and later
- iPad 4th generation and later

- iPad Mini and later
- iPod Touch 5th generation and later

Up to five of the aforementioned Apple products may be paired to a Nucleus 7 sound processor, but the Nucleus 7 sound processor may only be actively connected to one compatible Apple device at any given moment in time. To switch from one Apple device to another, the Bluetooth must be switched off of the active device, and the Bluetooth connection may then be established with the desired Apple product. Additionally, compatible Apple products may be paired to two Nucleus 7 sound processors to allow for bilateral audio streaming for bilateral Nucleus recipients and may also be paired with the ReSound Lynx 3D and ReSound Enzo 3D and later-generation wireless ReSound hearing aids to allow bimodal users to steam audio to both ears simultaneously. Only one Nucleus 7 recipient may be connected to a particular Apple product. As a result, siblings, spouses, friends, or colleagues who have Nucleus 7 sound processors will each need their own compatible Apple device to allow for audio streaming.

It should also be noted that the Nucleus Smart App may be used with Android devices and the Nucleus 7 sound processor. Among other functions, the Nucleus Smart App allows Android users to adjust the settings of their sound processor (e.g., volume control, sensitivity, program, etc.), enable/disable wireless accessories, and locate their processor when it is missing. However, telephone audio and music may not be streamed from Android devices directly

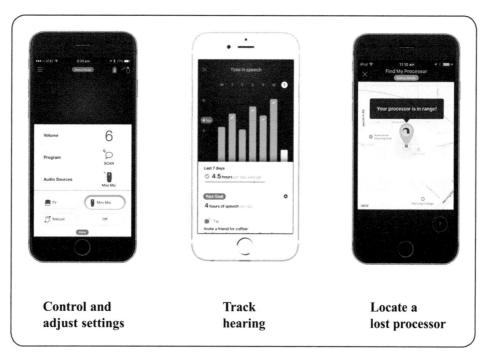

FIGURE 10–2. Nucleus 7 Nucleus Smart App. Image provided courtesy of Cochlear Americas, ©2018.

to the Nucleus 7. Instead, Android users need the Cochlear Phone Clip to stream audio from their Android device to the Nucleus 7 processor.

Furthermore, the Nucleus 7 sound processor is smaller than its predecessor, the Nucleus 6 sound processor. Technical specifications associated with the Nucleus 7 sound processor are shown in Table 10–1. With use of the compact rechargeable battery, the Nucleus 7 sound processor is the lightest sound processor (at 7.9 grams) available on the commercial market at the time of this writing. Of note, three battery options are available to power the Nucleus 7. The recipient may choose from two lithium-ion rechargeable batteries, the small *Compact* battery or the *Standard* battery, or the recipient may use the zinc-air module, which uses two disposable 675 high-powered zinc-air batteries (Figure 10–3). Tamperproof locks are available to prevent young children from removing each of the different types of battery modules from the processor as well as the cover case from the disposable battery module. When using the standard, zinc-air battery module, the Nucleus 7 sound processor has a water resistance rating of IP44. It may be splashed with water and still maintain normal function. When used with the rechargeable battery modules, the Nucleus 7 has an IP57 rating, which means it will retain normal function after being

submerged in 3 feet of water for up to 30 minutes. Cochlear developed the rechargeable batteries with the objective that they will provide the typical recipient with one full day of use per charge. Cochlear estimates that the typical user will receive an average of approximately 60 hours of operation from the zinc-air battery module and an average of approximately 10 to 14 hours and 20 to 24 hours from the *Compact* and *Standard* modules, respectively. It should be noted that the Nucleus 7 rechargeable batteries continue to function at 80% or greater capacity after 400 charging cycles. Also of note, the Nucleus 7 rechargeable batteries contain a technology referred to as a Protection Circuit Module (PCM), which serves to prevent the battery from overcharging and from discharging an unsafe amount of current. The rechargeable batteries may be charged on the Nucleus Y-Charger (which plugs into an adapter that allows it to be connected to an AC electrical outlet or into a standard 2.0 (or higher) USB port, or by the USB charger, which may also be plugged into a 2.0 or higher USB port (Figure 10–4).

The Nucleus 7 sound processor features titanium connectors to couple the battery module to the sound processor. These titanium connectors allow for a sturdier sound processor that is resistant to damage when accidentally dropped to the floor. Additionally, the

TABLE 10–1. Dimensions (Weight, Length, Width, etc.) of the CP1000

Technical Specifications						
Model number	CP1000					
Wireless frequency	Proprietary 2.4 GHz low power bidirectional wireless link					
Wireless communication range	Remote control: At least 2 m		Made for iPhone control: At least 2 m		Made for iPhone streaming: At least 7 m	
Coil operating frequency	5.0 MHz					
Operating voltage	2.0 V–4.25 V (processing unit) 2.0 V-2.6 V (coil)					
Power consumption	20 mW–100 mW					
Button functions	Turn processor on and off, turn audio streaming on and off, change program					
Capacity / Voltage range	Compact rechargeable battery module 91 mAh/3.7 V					
	Standard rechargeable battery module 183 mAh/3.7 V					
	Disposable battery module 2 PR44 (zinc-air) batteries 1.45 V (nominal each)					
Charge cycles	≥80% capacity after 400 charge/discharge cycles at room temperature					
Device dimensions		**Length**	**Width**	**Depth**	**Weight**	**Diameter**
	CP1000 with medium earhook with compact rechargeable battery	36.5 mm	9.0 mm	45.0 mm	7.9 g	N/A
	CP1000 with medium earhook with standard rechargeable battery	43.3 mm	9.0 mm	45.4 mm	9.8 g	N/A
	CP1000 with medium earhook with disposable batteries (including two 675 zinc-air)	43.7 mm	9.0 mm	45.1 mm	10.1 g	N/A
	Compact rechargeable battery module	18.0 mm	9.0 mm	17.8 mm		N/A
	Standard rechargeable battery module	24.8 mm	9.0 mm	17.8 mm		N/A
	Standard battery module	29.4 mm	9.0 mm	17.3 mm		N/A
	Coil and cable (without coil magnet)			5.8 mm	3.9 g	30.3 mm

Source: Provided courtesy of Cochlear Americas, ©2018.

Nucleus 7 sound processor contains a nano-coating, which is intended to enhance the reliability of the processor. Nano-coating technology is commonly used in commercial electronics to improve water resistance, particularly in humid environments or other situations (e.g., sports, strenuous occupational settings) in which a gas may convert into a liquid (i.e., condensation).

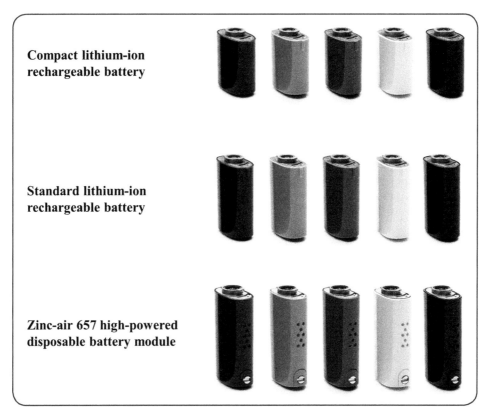

FIGURE 10–3. Compact and Standard Nucleus 7 rechargeable batteries. Image provided courtesy of Cochlear Americas, ©2018.

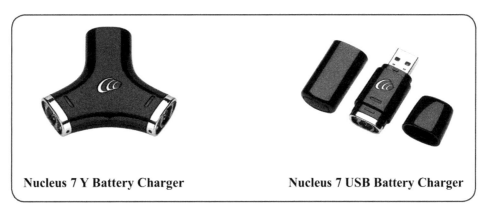

FIGURE 10–4. Nucleus 7 rechargeable battery charger. Image provided courtesy of Cochlear Americas, ©2018.

Nucleus 7 Microphone Technology

The Nucleus 7 sound processor possesses two omni-directional microphones that are used to form a dual-microphone directional beam-former. The dual-microphone system allows for a number of different microphone modes including: (1) Standard: a modest degree of directionality is created to mimic the directivity index of the unaided ear, (2) Zoom: a directional mode with a fixed polar plot pattern that provides a relatively large directivity index and attenuation for sounds arriving from the rear hemisphere, (3) Focus: an adaptive directional mode that automatically positions the directional null toward the direction from which the most intense noise is arriving, and (4) Scan: an automatic scene classifier which monitors the acoustics of the user's listening environment and attempts to select the microphone mode designed to optimize hearing performance for the specific situation. Of note, the microphones are protected by a microphone cover that should be replaced every two to three months in order to preserve the directional properties of the dual-microphone beam-former (Figure 10–5).

Nucleus 7 Electronics

Cochlear reports that the digital signal processor (DSP) chip of the Nucleus 7 sound processor is five times smaller than the DSP chip of its predecessor, the Nucleus 6 sound processor. Despite its smaller size, the DSP chip of the Nucleus 7 sound processor is more sophisticated and power efficient than the Nucleus 6 sound processor DSP chip. For example, the Nucleus 7 sound processor DSP chip allows for up to a 50% increase in battery life compared with what is attainable with the Nucleus 6 sound processor DSP chip. The DSP chip of the Nucleus 7 sound processor contains a 16-bit microcontroller that controls six DSP cores. The multiple cores within the processor allow for multiple operations to be executed simultaneously (e.g., directional processing, scene analysis, compression), whereas the microcontroller serves to integrate the functions of the different cores

to ensure efficient and effective signal processing and stimulus delivery. Additionally, the Nucleus 7 sound processor has a hardware accelerator, which allows for audio streaming. This was an essential inclusion in order to allow the Nucleus 7 sound processor to receive the 2.4-GHz digital radio frequency (RF) signal that is streamed from the wireless accessories developed by the GN ReSound hearing aid company as well as the proprietary 2.4-GHz signal from compatible Apple mobile devices.

Nucleus 7 User Options

The Nucleus 7 contains a telecoil that may be manually or automatically enabled. Moreover, the Nucleus 7 sound processor contains a push button on the spine of the processor to allow the user to switch the program and/or to activate auxiliary audio sources, and an LED light to alert caregivers and the user of the function of the processor. Figure 10–6 provides information regarding the function of the LED light. The Nucleus 7 may be powered on and off by simply connecting and disconnecting the battery, respectively. When the battery is connected, the Nucleus 7 may also be powered on or off by pressing on the push button until the LED light illuminates or turns to a steady orange, respectively. Once the Nucleus 7 is powered on, a short press of the button will change the program. A two-second press will activate the telecoil (if enabled by the audiologist) and/or wireless accessories that are paired to the processor. If the telecoil is enabled by the audiologist, a two-second press will initially activate the telecoil and subsequent two-second presses will activate the wireless accessories.

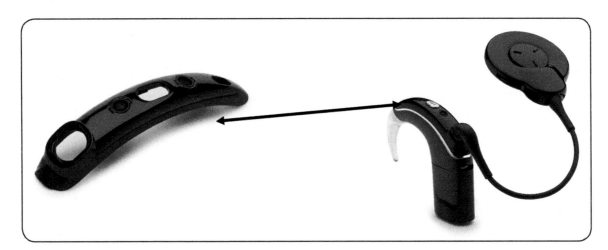

FIGURE 10–5. Nucleus 7 microphone covers. Image provided courtesy of Cochlear Americas, ©2018.

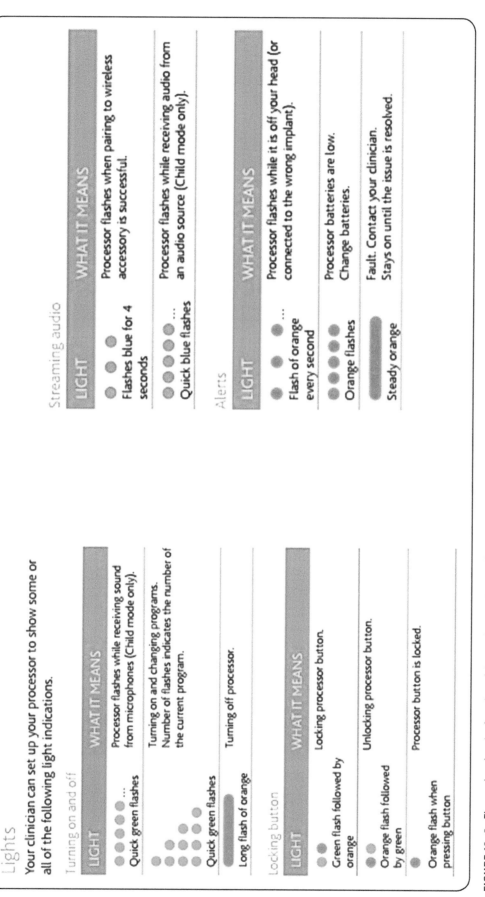

Lights

Your clinician can set up your processor to show some or all of the following light indications.

Turning on and off

LIGHT	WHAT IT MEANS
Quick green flashes	Processor flashes while receiving sound from microphones (Child mode only).
	Turning on and changing programs. Number of flashes indicates the number of the current program.
Quick green flashes	
Long flash of orange	Turning off processor.

Locking button

LIGHT	WHAT IT MEANS
	Locking processor button.
Green flash followed by orange	
	Unlocking processor button.
Orange flash followed by green	
	Processor button is locked.
Orange flash when pressing button	

Streaming audio

LIGHT	WHAT IT MEANS
Flashes blue for 4 seconds	Processor flashes when pairing to wireless accessory is successful.
Quick blue flashes	Processor flashes while receiving audio from an audio source (Child mode only).

Alerts

LIGHT	WHAT IT MEANS
Flash of orange every second	Processor flashes while it is off your head (or connected to the wrong implant).
Orange flashes	Processor batteries are low. Change batteries.
Steady orange	Fault. Contact your clinician. Stays on until the issue is resolved.

FIGURE 10–6. Figure showing the function of the nucleus 7 LED light (shown in Cochlear user manual). Image provided courtesy of Cochlear Americas, ©2018.

Furthermore, the Nucleus 7 possesses an acoustic driver to which the cable of a receiver-in-canal (RIC)–style receiver may be coupled (Figure 10–7). The RIC receivers are available with a variety of different cable lengths and with three different power levels. Specifically, the receivers are available in 60, 85, and 100 dB models, which are intended to provide sufficient gain and output for hearing thresholds up to 60, 86, and 100 dB HL, respectively. The receivers may be coupled to custom ear shells or to domes which are available in different sizes and in open and closed configurations.

Nucleus 7 Accessories

Several accessory items are available for use with the Nucleus 7 sound processor. The CR310 Remote Control may be used to adjust the volume/sensitivity settings, change the program, and activate/deactivate auxiliary audio sources (e.g., Nucleus Mini Mic 2 remote microphone) (Figure 10–8). Of note, the Nucleus 7 CP1000 does not possess a direct auditory input (DAI) port. However, the recipient may use a special adapter to achieve some DAI functionalities. For instance, the Roger 20 receiver may be connected between the battery module and Nucleus 7 sound processor (Figure 10–9). Also, a Monitor Earphone Adapter may be connected between the processor and battery module to allow a listener to plug a pair of earphones into a standard 3.5 phono port and perform a listening check of the signal delivered from the sound processor microphone or auxiliary audio source.

A variety of different wireless streaming digital hearing assistance technology accessories are available for use with the Nucleus 7 sound processor.

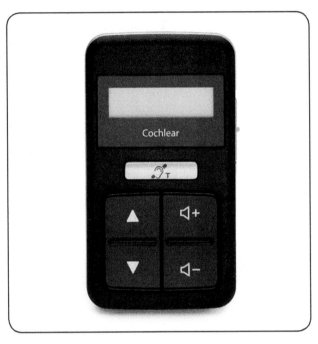

FIGURE 10–8. Nucleus 7 Remote Control (CR310). Image provided courtesy of Cochlear Americas, ©2018.

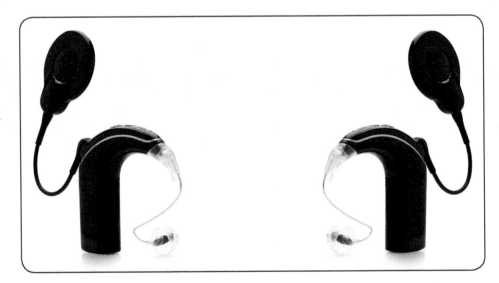

FIGURE 10–7. Nucleus 7 (CP1000) with acoustic receiver for electric-acoustic stimulation. Image provided courtesy of Cochlear Americas, ©2018.

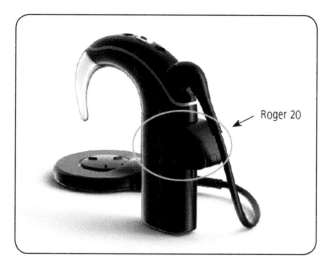

FIGURE 10–9. Phonak Roger 20 receiver coupled to Nucleus 7 CP1000 sound processor.

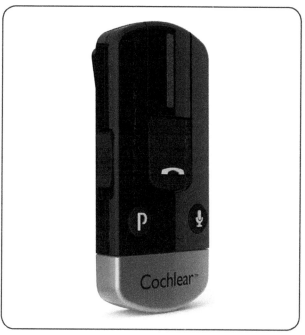

FIGURE 10–10. Cochlear Phone Clip for wireless audio streaming from Bluetooth-enabled devices to Nucleus 6 and Nucleus 7 sound processors. Image provided courtesy of Cochlear Americas, ©2018.

These wireless accessories include the Cochlear Mini Microphone 2+ remote microphone, the Cochlear Phone Clip, and the Cochlear TV Streamer. Of note, each of these wireless accessories may also be used with the Nucleus 6 and Kanso sound processors, and the information pertaining to these accessories also applies to the Nucleus 6 and Kanso sound processors. In the following paragraphs, the wireless accessories will be described for use with the Nucleus 7, but the reader should know that these accessories may be used with the Nucleus 6 and Kanso in a similar fashion.

The Nucleus wireless accessories stream audio signals directly to a receiver (i.e., antenna) housed within the Nucleus 7 sound processor via GN ReSound's proprietary digital RF transmission at the 2.4 GHz ISM (Industry, Science, Medical) band, which is globally license free. GN ReSound reports that its proprietary system possesses a shorter delay (approximately 20 msec) from the transmitter to the receiver compared with Bluetooth devices, and it also reports that the power requirements are significantly lower than Bluetooth transmission. These advantages are attributed to the fact that the system is proprietary and dedicated for use with GN ReSound hearing aids or Cochlear Nucleus sound processors, whereas Bluetooth is an open platform used with a variety of commercial electronics. As a result, the proprietary system may be designed to be more efficient in its operation.

The Cochlear Phone Clip (Figure 10–10) allows for audio streaming from a Bluetooth-enabled mobile telephone to the Phone Clip via Bluetooth and then from the Phone Clip to the Nucleus 7 sound processor via GN ReSound's proprietary wireless transmission. The Phone Clip has a lithium-ion rechargeable battery that provides up to 6 hours of talk time and 80 hours of standby use (with ReSound hearing aids equipped for wireless streaming) on a full charge. The Phone Clip must be paired to the user's mobile telephone (or other Bluetooth-enabled device) and to the user's Nucleus 7 sound processor. Pairing to the telephone is accomplished by pressing a small blue button under the case at the base of the Phone Clip and then activating the Bluetooth pairing process of the telephone. Once the telephone identifies the Phone Clip, the user must enter the code "0000," and pairing to the telephone is complete. The user then presses the white button at the base of the Phone Clip and places the battery onto the Nucleus 7 sound processor. When the Nucleus 7 processor powers on, it enables pairing mode and will connect to the Phone Clip.

After pairing is complete, the user should clip the Phone Clip next to his/her collar to allow for capture of the user's voice and delivery to the mobile telephone. Likewise, the audio signal from the telephone is also sent from the Phone Clip to the mobile telephone, allowing for hands-free telephone use. The user may remain connected between the Phone Clip and two Bluetooth-enabled devices at the same time. In order to switch between streaming devices, the recipient simply presses the button on the front center of the Phone Clip (shaped like a phone handset). The same button also is used to answer and end telephone calls.

The Cochlear Mini Microphone 2+ (Figure 10–11) is designed to be clipped onto the shirt collar of a person whom the Nucleus 7 user wishes to hear. Because of the close proximity to the talker's mouth, the Mini Microphone 2+ captures the speech signal of interest and wirelessly streams it to the Nucleus 7 sound processor via ReSound's proprietary digital wireless transmission. Of note, the Mini Microphone 2+ contains two omnidirectional microphones that are used to create a beam-former that focuses on the speech of the talker when the microphones are oriented toward the talker's mouth. Wolfe (2016) showed that speech recognition in noise is significantly better with the Mini Microphone 2+ compared with its predecessor, the Mini Microphone, which only contained an omnidirectional microphone. The Mini Microphone 2+ also possesses a 3.5 mm audio input phone port allowing for a hard-wired connection to the headphone jack of any audio device (e.g., MP3 player, handheld video game, notebook computer). The audio signal may then be streamed to the Nucleus 7 sound processor. Additionally, the

Mini Microphone 2+ contains a three-prong Euro port to which a three-prong remote microphone radio receiver (e.g., Phonak Roger X receiver) may be connected. Moreover, the Mini Microphone 2+ contains a telecoil, which may be used to capture audio signals from neckloop or room induction loops. The signal from the induction loop is captured by the telecoil and then transmitted to the Nucleus 7 by way of wireless digital audio streaming. The user may manually activate the desired microphone mode and/ or telecoil. The Mini Microphone 2+ also contains a volume control to increase/decrease the intensity of the signal delivered to the sound processor.

Furthermore, the Mini Microphone 2+ contains an accelerometer and gyroscope that can sense the orientation of the remote microphone. If the Mini Microphone 2+ is laid flat on a table, it will automatically go into "conference mode" and use an omnidirectional microphone pattern. In contrast, if it is oriented vertically, as it would be if it were worn around the neck or on the collar, then the beam-former will automatically transform into a directional mode.

The Mini Microphone 2+ possesses a lithium-ion rechargeable battery, which lasts up to 11 hours on a full charge (charging time is approximately 2 to 3 hours). It has a reported range of 82 feet depending on the characteristics of the environment and situation of use. Like the Phone Clip, the Mini Microphone 2+ must be connected to the Nucleus 7 sound processor. This is accomplished by removing the silver cover from the base of the device and pressing the connecting button. Then, the Nucleus 7 sound processor

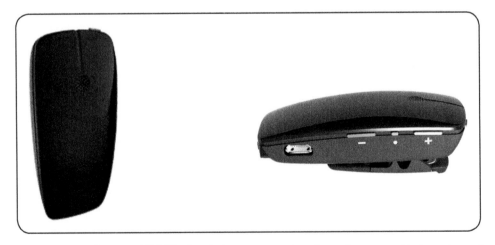

FIGURE 10–11. Cochlear Mini Mic 2+ wireless remote microphone. Image provided courtesy of Cochlear Americas, ©2018.

is powered on and the connecting process should automatically complete. It should be noted that the Mini Microphone has a volume control to allow the user to find a comfortable listening loudness.

Cochlear also offers the Mini Microphone 2 remote microphone. It is similar to the Mini Microphone 2+ but is smaller and does not contain adaptive directional microphone responses (the Mini Microphone always remains in directional mode), a Euro Port connector, a telecoil, or 3.5-mm phone plug socket. Additionally, the Mini Microphone 2 lithium-ion rechargeable battery provides 10 hours of operation.

The Cochlear TV Streamer 2 (Figure 10–12) allows for wireless streaming (ReSound's proprietary digital radio transmission at 2.4 GHz) from the accessory device directly to the Nucleus 7 sound processor. As with the aforementioned wireless accessories, the Nucleus 7 sound processor must be connected to the TV Streamer. This is accomplished by pressing the pairing button on the TV Streamer and then powering on the Nucleus 7 sound processor. The pairing process should occur automatically. One Nucleus 7 sound processor may be connected to as many as three TV Streamer devices, and each TV Streamer may be connected to multiple sets of Nucleus sound processors. The range of transmission of the united TV Streamer is up to approximately 21 feet. If the user leaves the area of transmission for less than 5 minutes, then the TV Streamer will automatically reconnect to the recipient's Nucleus 7 sound processor when the user returns to the room. The TV Streamer also possesses a volume control, which allows the user to adjust the volume of the signal he/she receives independently of the volume setting on the television. Again, these wireless accessories may also be used with the Nucleus 6 and Kanso sound processors.

Nucleus 7 Wearing Options

A variety of different wearing configurations are available for the Nucleus 7 sound processor. The Hugfit is a small, soft, flexible (silicone) loop/tube that spans from base of the earhook and connects to the tip of the earhook (Figure 10–13). It is designed to secure the sound processor on the ear. The Snugfit is a pliable hook that extends from the base of the earhook and conforms around the backside of the auricle and underneath the earlobe (Figure 10–14). The Snugfit is also designed to facilitate retention. The Koala Clip may be coupled to the Nucleus 7 to allow for attachment of the processor to the recipient's clothing (Figure 10–15). The earmold adapter allows for simple connection of the Nucleus 7 earhook to a custom earmold (Figure 10–16). Also, the HeadWorn adapter may be used to allow for the processor to

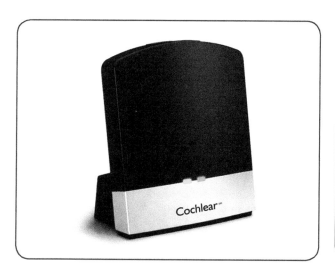

FIGURE 10–12. Cochlear TV Streamer for audio streaming from television to Nucleus 6 and Nucleus 7 sound processors. Image provided courtesy of Cochlear Americas, ©2018.

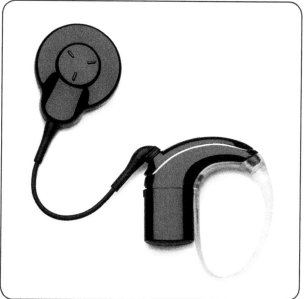

FIGURE 10–13. Hugfit for retention of Nucleus 7 sound processor. Image provided courtesy of Cochlear Americas, ©2018.

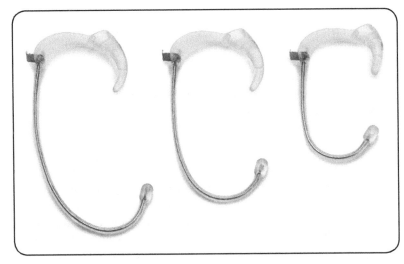

FIGURE 10–14. Snugfit for Nucleus 7 sound processor. Image provided courtesy of Cochlear Americas, ©2018.

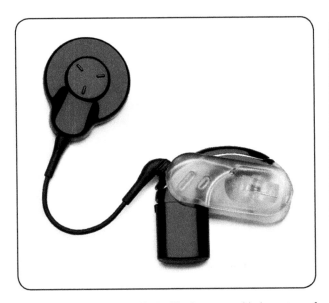

FIGURE 10–15. Nucleus 7 Koala Clip. Image provided courtesy of Cochlear Americas, ©2018.

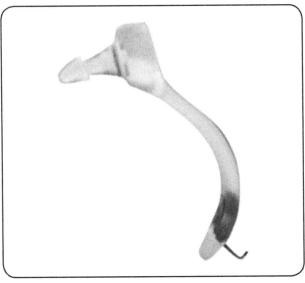

FIGURE 10–16. Nucleus 7 Earmold Adapter. Image provided courtesy of Cochlear Americas, ©2018.

be worn on the head (off the ear) (Figure 10–17). Of note, the Headworn Adapter is available in right and left side models and must be positioned so that the processor faces the same way that it does when worn on the ear. Additionally, Cochlear offers the Nucleus 7 Aqua+ water accessory and Aqua+ cable, which may be used to fully waterproof (i.e., IP68) the Nucleus 7 sound processor (Figure 10–18).

Nucleus Kanso Sound Processor

In September 2016, Cochlear announced that it had received FDA approval to commercially distribute the Nucleus Kanso, Cochlear's first single-unit, off-the-ear sound processor (Figure 10–19). As of the time of this writing, the Kanso is the smallest and lightest-weight off-the-ear sound processor on the commercial market. The Kanso comprises five primary components: (1) two omnidirectional microphones that allow for a directional beam-former, (2) a sophisticated digital signal processor that analyzes the input audio signal and determines the level of stimulation required to deliver an electromagnetic signal to the cochlear implant, (3) a transmitting coil that creates and delivers the electromagnetic signal to the cochlear implant, (4) a magnet that is housed inside the processor and that facilitates adherence to the cochlear implant, and

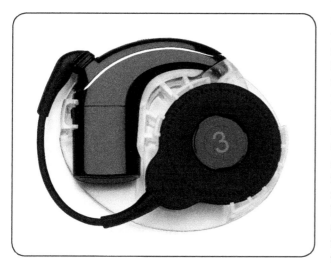

FIGURE 10–17. Nucleus 7 Headworn Adapter. Image provided courtesy of Cochlear Americas, ©2018.

(5) two high-powered, zinc-air 675 batteries to power the system for up to 16 hours of operation.

Furthermore, the Kanso contains a 2.4 GHz wireless digital radio receiver, and as a result, it is compatible for use with all of the wireless streaming accessories that may be used with the Nucleus 6 sound processor (i.e., Mini Mic 2+, Phone Clip, TV Streamer). Moreover, the Kanso contains a telecoil that may be used to capture signals from the telephone, induction neckloops, and induction room loops. Additionally, the Kanso contains an LED light that alerts the user and/or caregivers of the function of the device and a push button that may be used to power the device on and off, to change the program, and to activate/deactivate the telecoil and/or wireless streaming. The button may be held down until the LED light illuminates to power on the processor. Likewise, the button may be pressed until the LED light turns to a steady orange to power the processor off. Once the Kanso is powered on, a quick press of the button will change the program. The number of flashes of the LED light (e.g., one through four flashes) and/or a private audible alarm will alert the recipient and/or caregiver of the program number that is being used. Pressing the button for two seconds will enable the wireless streaming and/or telecoil. If the telecoil is disabled by the audiologist, then each two-second button press will simply scroll through the wireless accessories that are paired to the Kanso. If the telecoil is enabled, the first two-second

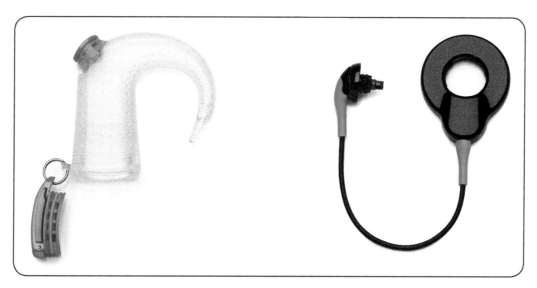

FIGURE 10–18. Nucleus Aqua+ water accessory and Aqua+ cable. Image provided courtesy of Cochlear Americas, ©2018.

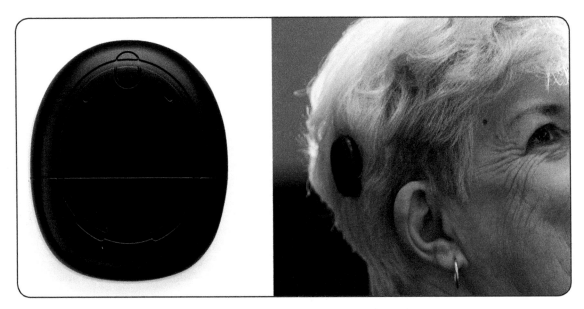

FIGURE 10–19. Nucleus Kanso sound processor. Image provided courtesy of Cochlear Americas, ©2018.

button push will activate the telecoil, and subsequent button presses will activate the wireless accessories paired to the Kanso.

Nucleus Kanso Microphones

The dual-microphone directional system allows for the same microphone modes as are available with the Nucleus 6 and 7 sound processors (e.g., Standard, Zoom, Focus). In the "Standard" microphone mode, the beamformer provides a slightly positive directivity index that mimics that of the unaided auricle. However, in order for the processor to achieve a directional response similar to the unaided ear, the microphones must be oriented along the horizontal axis. As a result, it is important to inform the user to place the sound processor on the head so that the LED light is located in the "12:00 position" (Figure 10–20). Of note, the microphones are protected by removable covers that should be replaced every two or three months to preserve the directional properties of the dual-mic directional system.

Nucleus Kanso Electronics

The electronics package of the Kanso sound processor is essentially identical to the electronics of the Nucleus 6 processor. Consequently, all signal processing (e.g., Scan, Wind Noise Reduction, SNR-NR) and

FIGURE 10–20. Image showing the proper orientation of the Nucleus Kanso sound processor when worn on the head. Image provided courtesy of Cochlear Americas, ©2018.

signal coding strategies (e.g., ACE, ACE(RE), SPEAK, CIS) that are available with the Nucleus 6 are also available with the Kanso. Research examining speech recognition in quiet and in noise obtained with the

Kanso and Nucleus 6 found similar performance between the two conditions (Mauger et al., 2017). Of note, the Kanso may also be used with the CR210 and CR230 Remote Assistants to allow for convenient access to various signal processing schemes available in multiple programs and to access wireless streaming and/or the telecoil.

Nucleus Kanso Wearing Options

The removable magnet of the Kanso is available in seven different strengths (1/2, 1, 2, 3, 4, 5, and 6) (Figure 10–21). If the Kanso causes discomfort or redness at the implant site, a SoftWear pad may be placed on the underneath side to facilitate comfort. To ensure that the device is not damaged if it becomes dislodged from the recipient's head, a Safety Line may be attached to the Kanso and clipped to the recipient's hair (Figure 10–22). The Safety Line prevents the Kanso from falling to the floor if it falls from the head. For recipients who are involved with physical activities or for children, the Headband assists with retention of the Kanso (Figure 10–23). Additionally,

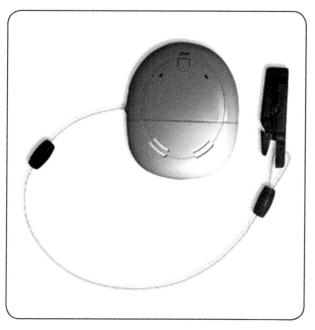

FIGURE 10–22. Nucleus Kanso Safety Line to prevent Kanso sound processor from falling to the floor if dislodged from the head. Image provided courtesy of Cochlear Americas, ©2018.

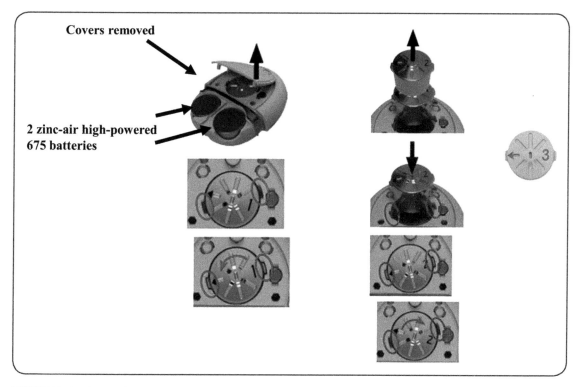

FIGURE 10–21. Image showing Nucleus Kanso magnets and magnet installation. Image provided courtesy of Cochlear Americas, ©2018.

the Aqua+ for Kanso allows for IP68 waterproof protection. Of note, the Kanso is available in a large range of colors to match the recipient's hair and/or skin color.

Nucleus 6 Sound Processor

In August 2013, Cochlear Americas received FDA approval to commercially distribute the Nucleus 6 cochlear implant system, which includes the CP910 and CP920 external sound processors (Figure 10–24) and the CR210 and CR230 wireless remote assistants (Figure 10–25). Of note, the Nucleus 6 sound processor is compatible with all Nucleus cochlear implants, including the Nucleus 22 implant.

The Nucleus 6 sound processor is available in two different models, the Nucleus CP910 and Nucleus CP920 (see Figure 10–24). The primary difference between the two models is that the CP920 possesses

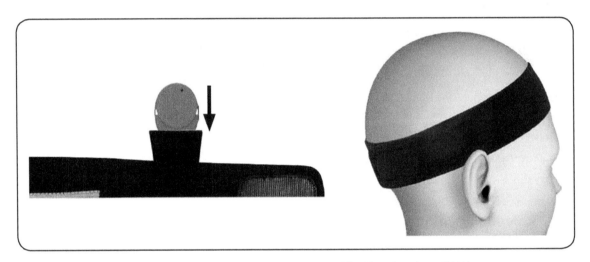

FIGURE 10–23. Nucleus Kanso Headband. Image provided courtesy of Cochlear Americas, ©2018.

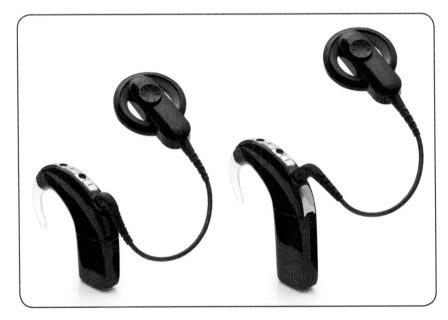

FIGURE 10–24. Nucleus 6 sound processors (CP910 and CP920). Image provided courtesy of Cochlear Americas, ©2018.

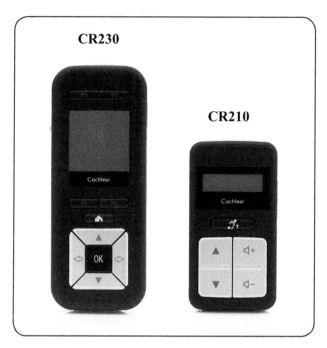

FIGURE 10–25. Nucleus 6 remote controls (CR210 and CR230). Image provided courtesy of Cochlear Americas, ©2018.

a direct auditory input (DAI) port, whereas the CP910 does not. As a result, the recipient may couple a personal remote microphone radio receiver or a personal audio device, such as an MP3 player or mobile telephone (by way of the audio accessory cable), to the CP920 sound processor but not to the CP910. In contrast, the CP910 sound processor is 6% smaller than the CP920 and Nucleus 5 sound processors. Again, it should be noted that both the CP910 and CP920 sound processors contain a 2.4 GHz digital radio receiver and are compatible with Cochlear's proprietary wireless hearing assistance technologies (this portfolio of wireless accessories, which were designed by the GN ReSound hearing aid company, will be described in detail later in this chapter).

The remaining electronic characteristics of the CP910 and CP920 are identical, and as a result, the processors will be referred to collectively as the Nucleus 6 sound processor for the remainder of this text unless a distinction must be made regarding the DAI functionality or size difference between the two devices. The Nucleus 6 sound processor contains three major components: (1) a sound processor with a DSP and user controls, (2) a battery module, and (3) a coil with a removable magnet and a removable cable. Of note, a special coil is used for Nucleus 22 recipients, because Nucleus 22 implants

use a 2.5 MHz carrier frequency to deliver the signal from the sound processor to the implant. All Nucleus cochlear implants manufactured after the Nucleus 22 use a 5 MHz carrier frequency for signal transmission between the sound processor and cochlear implant. The N6 coil for Nucleus 22 recipients contains a green ring inside the port to which the cable is connected.

As with the Nucleus 7 sound processor, the Nucleus 6 sound processor includes two omnidirectional microphones to allow for a dual-microphone beamformer with the same directional capabilities as the Nucleus 7. Microphone covers protect the Nucleus 6 microphones and should be replaced every two to three months to ensure the directional response properties of the dual-microphone beamformer. The Nucleus 6 sound processor also contains an automatically activated telecoil to allow for improved hearing on the telephone and with induction loop hearing assistance technology (HAT). Furthermore, the Nucleus 6 sound processor possesses an acoustic driver and the capability to replace the conventional earhook with a RIC acoustic component for recipients who have usable low-frequency hearing after implantation (Figure 10–26). Finally, the Nucleus 6 sound processor also features a 2.4 GHz radio frequency receiver to allow for audio streaming from a remote microphone or a mobile telephone or television via

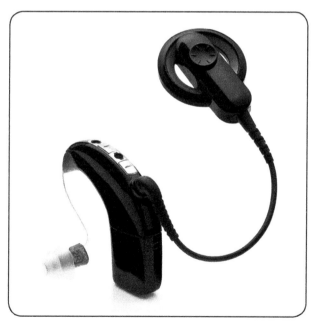

FIGURE 10–26. Nucleus 6 with acoustic receiver for electric-acoustic stimulation. Image provided courtesy of Cochlear Americas, ©2018.

an accessory transmitter designed specifically for the Nucleus 6 via a partnership between Cochlear and the GN ReSound hearing aid company.

Additionally, Cochlear reports that the DSP chip of the Nucleus 6 processor is five times more powerful than the DSP of its predecessor, the Nucleus 5 sound processor. The Nucleus 6 has several upgraded signal processing features compared with the Nucleus 5, and as a result, it was imperative to design the DSP chip that could support these features while also not using more electrical power. The DSP chip of the Nucleus 6 features six DSP cores controlled by a 16-bit microcontroller. In comparison, the Nucleus 5 sound processor (with the CHAMP-L ASIC chip) possesses four separate digital cores, which are controlled by an 8-bit microcontroller. The six different cores present within the processor allow for multiple operations to be executed simultaneously (e.g., directional processing, scene analysis, compression), whereas the microcontroller serves to integrate the functions of the six digital cores to ensure efficient and effective signal processing and stimulus delivery. Furthermore, the DSP of the Nucleus 6 sound processor features a processing speed that is twice as fast as the DSP of the Nucleus 5 sound processor. Furthermore, the Nucleus 6 DSP is a 16-bit processor with a 16,000-Hz input sampling rate. The overall input dynamic range for broadband sounds delivered to the Nucleus 6 sound processor is just shy of 80 dB SPL (i.e., a low end of approximately 23 dBA for broadband inputs with an upper range of just over 100 dBA). Additionally, the Nucleus 6 sound processor has a hardware accelerator, which allows for audio streaming. This was an essential inclusion in order to allow the N6

processor to receive the 2.4-GHz digital RF signal that is streamed from the wireless accessories developed by the GN ReSound hearing aid company. Finally, the DSP of the Nucleus 6 possesses a substantially larger memory relative to the Nucleus 5 sound processor in order to allow for the comprehensive data-logging feature available within the Nucleus 6 processor.

Wearing Options

The CP910 and CP920 sound processors are designed to be worn at ear level with a standard battery module, but there are several wearing options designed to facilitate use on the ear for a variety of different use applications. Multiple earhook sizes are available. The "small" earhook is often used by children and adults with small ears. The small earhook may also be configured with a small pin, which must be inserted through a hole at the base of the earhook where it attaches to the processor. This pin is intended to allow a young child's caregiver to "lock" the earhook to the processor to prevent it from becoming accidentally dislodged. Earhooks in "standard" and "large" sizes are also available for adults and older children for whom the "small" earhook is too small.

Nucleus 6 users may also use the "Snugfit" device, which was described earlier for the N7 processor. The Snugfit device is also available in various sizes to accommodate different ear sizes, and a tamperproof Snugfit option is available. The recipient may also use the "Mic Lock," which is comprised of a small loop that couples to the processor and is attached to a piece of tubing that may be connected to the earhook of the processor (Figure 10–27).

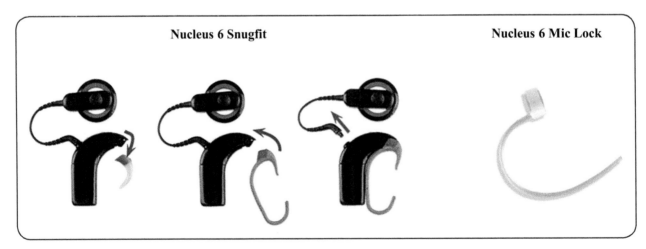

Nucleus 6 Snugfit   **Nucleus 6 Mic Lock**

FIGURE 10–27. Nucleus 6 sound processor with Mic Lock. Image provided courtesy of Cochlear Americas, ©2018.

Furthermore, "off-the-ear" wearing options also exist. The battery module may be attached to the sound processor via a long cable and clipped to the user's clothing via a specialized holder. This "body-worn" option, which is referred to as "Litewear," may be selected for very young children (Figure 10–28) and recipients involved in sports because it minimizes the size of the unit worn on the ear. Of course,

the Nucleus 6 sound processor may also be attached to a standard earmold to facilitate retention. Finally, the Aqua+ accessory is available for use with the Nucleus 6, providing waterproof protection (IP68).

For recipients who use the acoustic component, the Nucleus 6 sound processor will be attached to the acoustic receiver, which is coupled to either a generic dome or to a custom-fit earmold. More specifically, the earhook of the Nucleus 6 sound processor may be removed and replaced with a receiver-in-the-canal (RIC) acoustic component (see Figure 10–26). The Nucleus 6 sound processor possesses an acoustic driver to operate the acoustic component, which may be used to amplify low-frequency sounds for recipients who have preservation of low-frequency hearing following implant surgery. The open dome is likely to be more appropriate for recipients who have normal hearing up to a mild hearing loss at 500 Hz and below, while the closed dome and custom shell options are likely to be more appropriate for recipients who have more significant amounts of low-frequency hearing loss. In particular, the custom shell will probably be imperative for recipients who have moderate to severe low-frequency hearing loss.

Battery Options

As with the Nucleus 7, the Nucleus 6 battery is available in three configurations: (1) a smaller, compact rechargeable battery module, (2) a standard rechargeable battery module using a built-in lithium-ion battery, and (3) a standard, zinc-air battery module with two #675 zinc-air batteries (Figure 10–29). Tamper-proof locks are available to prevent young children from removing each of the different types of battery modules from the processor as well as the cover case from the disposable battery module. The rechargeable batteries should be used for maximum water resistance (IP57 without Aqua+ accessory and IP68 with Aqua+). Recipients are able to obtain up to 30 hours of use with the standard rechargeable battery of the Nucleus 6 and up to 18 hours of use with the Nucleus 6 compact battery (80% of Nucleus 6 users will obtain at least 8 hours of use from the compact rechargeable battery). The Nucleus 6 rechargeable batteries have a lifespan of at least 365 charge cycles.

Like the Nucleus 7, the Nucleus 6 features titanium connectors to couple the battery module to the sound processor, a feature which enhances the sturdiness of the processor. Additionally, the Nucleus 6 sound processor contains a nano-coating to improve water resistance.

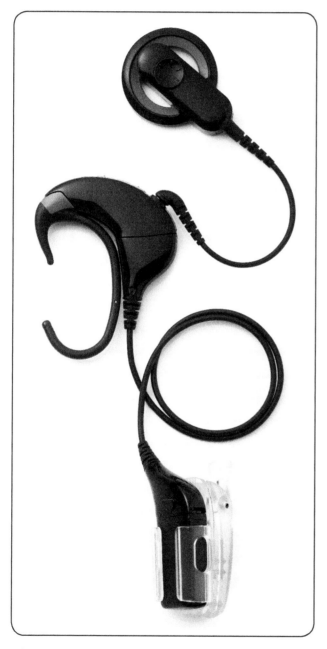

FIGURE 10–28. Nucleus 6 Litewear option. Image provided courtesy of Cochlear Americas, ©2018.

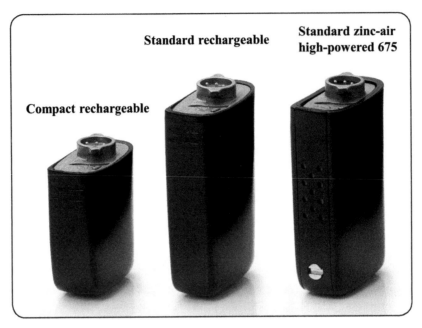

FIGURE 10–29. Nucleus 6 battery options. Image provided courtesy of Cochlear Americas, ©2018.

Processor Buttons and Lights

The Nucleus 6 sound processor has two push buttons for adjustments of various parameters by the recipient. In the default "Basic" mode, the bottom button allows the recipient to change to one of four programs with a short press. The top button may be used to manually activate or deactivate the built-in telecoil. The audiologist may also program the processor in the "Advanced" mode, which enables the recipient to make adjustments to the volume or the microphone sensitivity. In the "Advanced" mode, a short press of the bottom or top buttons decreases and increases the volume or sensitivity (depending on whether the audiologist has programmed the processor buttons to function as a volume or sensitivity control), respectively. A long press of the bottom button changes the program, and a long press of the top button activates and deactivates the telecoil. It should be noted that the "Advanced Mode" is rarely used by adults or children. Finally, the buttons may be locked for young children to disallow changes to the controls.

Additionally, the Nucleus 6 sound processor has a bicolor LED light at the apex of the processor adjacent to the removable earhook. The LED light indicates the status of the processor as well as the status of the signal delivered to the internal device. The light may be deactivated, programmed to indicate the function of each button push, or programmed to alert caregivers to the status of the processor during routine use (e.g., battery life, sound detection, transmission to internal device). Figure 10–30 provides detailed information pertaining to the function of the LED light.

Processor DAI Port

A DAI accessory port is located on the spine of the CP910 sound processor just below the cable (Figure 10–31). This port allows for coupling to a personal remote microphone radio receiver and external accessories, such as an external microphone, MP3 player, or smartphone via the personal audio cable, mains isolation cable, and monitoring earphones. The sound processor is designed to automatically recognize the connection of a DAI (and mix the signal appropriately). Monitoring earphones may also be plugged into the accessory port. It is important to remember that the monitoring earphones do not allow one to listen to the signal the implant user ultimately receives, but instead, the normal-hearing listener is able to evaluate the signal after it has been subjected to input processing but prior to delivery to the recipient.

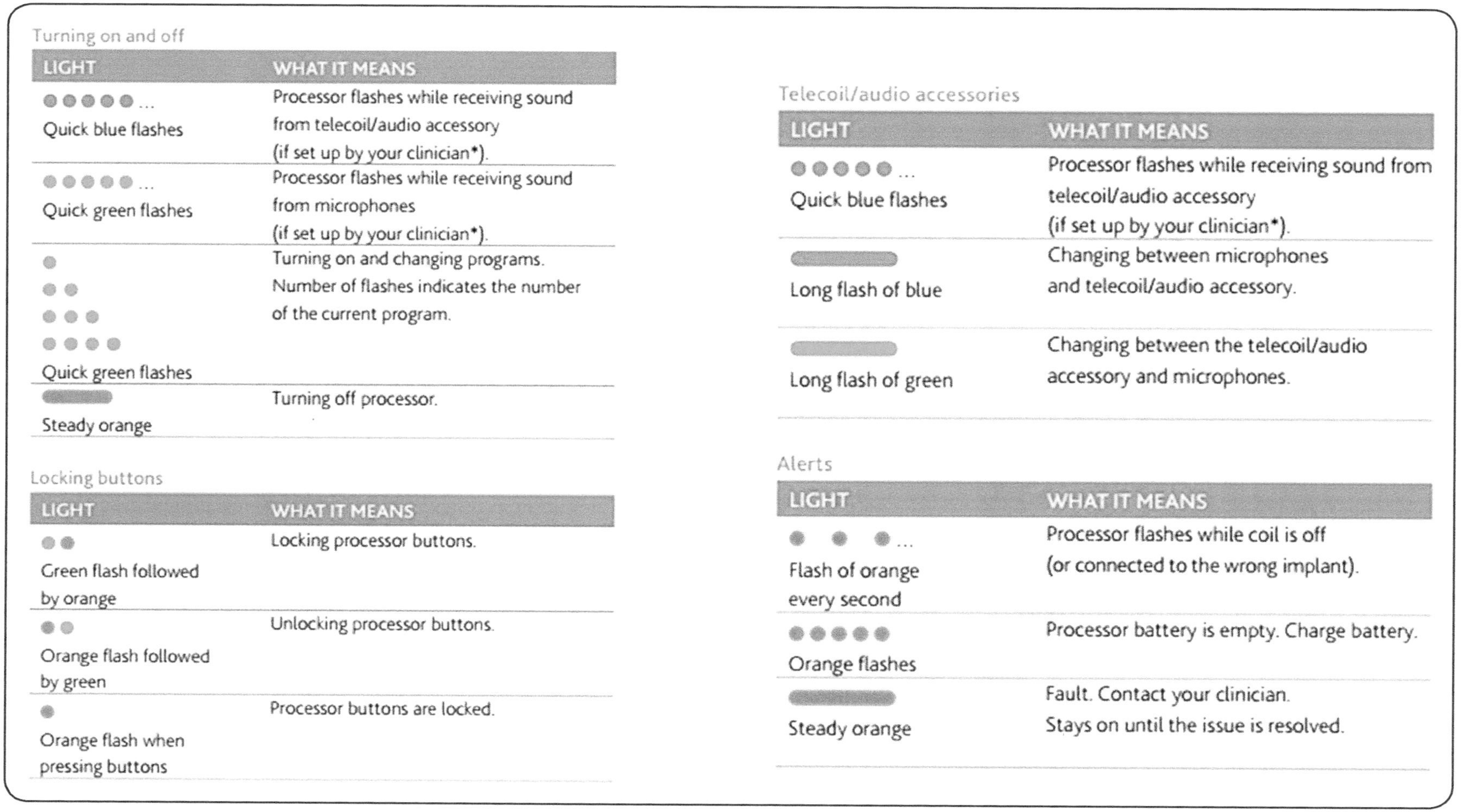

Turning on and off

LIGHT	WHAT IT MEANS
● ● ● ● ... Quick blue flashes	Processor flashes while receiving sound from telecoil/audio accessory (if set up by your clinician*).
● ● ● ● ... Quick green flashes	Processor flashes while receiving sound from microphones (if set up by your clinician*).
● ● ● ●	Turning on and changing programs. Number of flashes indicates the number of the current program.
Quick green flashes	Turning off processor.
Steady orange	

Locking buttons

LIGHT	WHAT IT MEANS
● ● Green flash followed by orange	Locking processor buttons.
● ● Orange flash followed by green	Unlocking processor buttons.
● Orange flash when pressing buttons	Processor buttons are locked.

Telecoil/audio accessories

LIGHT	WHAT IT MEANS
● ● ● ● ... Quick blue flashes	Processor flashes while receiving sound from telecoil/audio accessory (if set up by your clinician*).
Long flash of blue	Changing between microphones and telecoil/audio accessory.
Long flash of green	Changing between the telecoil/audio accessory and microphones.

Alerts

LIGHT	WHAT IT MEANS
● ● ... Flash of orange every second	Processor flashes while coil is off (or connected to the wrong implant).
● ● ● ● ● Orange flashes	Processor battery is empty. Charge battery.
Steady orange	Fault. Contact your clinician. Stays on until the issue is resolved.

FIGURE 10–30. Figure showing function of the Nucleus 6 LED light. Image provided courtesy of Cochlear Americas, ©2018.

Wireless Remote Assistants

The Nucleus 6 processor is designed for use with either the CR210 or CR230 wireless remote assistant (see Figure 10–25). The CR230 features two-way communication between the cochlear implant system and the diagnostic interface of the remote assistant, which allows the user access to a wide range of system controls and diagnostic capabilities. The CR230 remote must be paired to a Nucleus 6 sound processor by placing the processor transmitting coil on the back of the CR230 remote assistant. Not only does the CR230 allow the user to have control over a number of processor settings, but it also provides comprehensive information pertaining to processor function to the user via a full-color LED screen and an audible alarm (Figure 10–32).

The CR230 allows for control over a wide array of Nucleus 6 sound processor settings, including, volume, sensitivity, program, audio accessory mixing ratio, telecoil mixing ratio, the LED and audible alarm settings, and locking of the processor settings. The CR230 remote also may be used to evaluate the status of Nucleus 6 sound processors. The recipient or caregiver may check the battery life, the integrity of the processor, cable/coil, microphone, and RF coupling (i.e., Link/lock) between the external and internal components. If a problem is identified, the CR230 remote will offer a series of suggestions to the user to attempt to mitigate the problem. Additionally, the CR230 remote assistant has a rechargeable battery. Finally, the CR230 remote assistant has an audible alarm that provides an audible warning when the status of the processor is compromised (e.g., battery is low, transmitting coil falls off the head). With the provision of control over a wide range of processor settings along with the diagnostic and troubleshooting features, the authors consider the CR230 remote

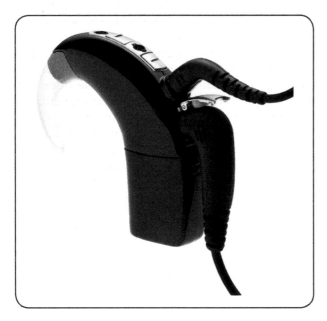

FIGURE 10–31. Direct Auditory Input port of the Nucleus 6 (CP910) sound processor. Image provided courtesy of Cochlear Americas, ©2018.

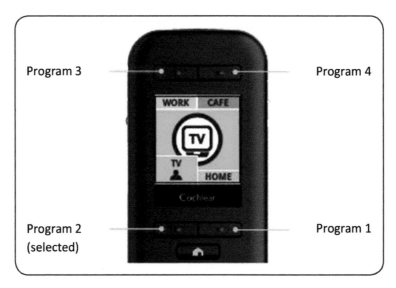

FIGURE 10–32. Close-up view of the Nucleus CR230 LED screen with diagnostic indicator. Image provided courtesy of Cochlear Americas, ©2018.

assistant to be the preferred remote for use with infants and young children.

The CR210 remote assistant is significantly smaller than the CR230 remote, as well as possessing fewer capabilities. It provides a simple user interface that allows for the adjustment of the program, volume or sensitivity (but not both), and telecoil (enable/disable). The aforementioned settings are displayed on a liquid-crystal display (LCD) screen. Additional settings (accessory mixing ratio, processor button lock, LED light, etc.) cannot be controlled by the CR210 remote. The CR210 also does not allow for diagnostic assessment of cochlear implant function, and it does not possess a troubleshooting guide. It has a disposable CR2032 or a 5004LC 3V standard lithium coin cell battery, which is estimated to have a life of about three months if the CR210 is used about 15 times a day. The CR210 also possesses an attachable ring that allows the CR210 to be carried on a keychain. The authors consider the CR210 remote assistant to be a good choice for adult recipients and older children (particularly elderly adults who may become confused with new technology) because it is small, simple to use, and provides control over most settings an adult would prefer to adjust.

Nucleus Cochlear Implants

The Nucleus Profile Cochlear Implant

In the summer of 2015, The FDA approved the Cochlear Nucleus Profile cochlear implant for com-

mercial distribution in the United States. At the time of this writing, the Nucleus Profile cochlear implant is the thinnest cochlear implant on the commercial market and is 40% thinner than its predecessor, the Nucleus Freedom cochlear implant (see Figure 10–33 for a visual of the Nucleus Profile cochlear implant). The Nucleus Profile is composed of: (1) a sophisticated, digitally driven stimulator that is housed in a hermetically sealed titanium case, (2) a platinum-iridium coil used for signal transmission between the sound processor and implant, (3) a removable magnet positioned in a Silastic sleeve located in the center of the coil, (4) an electrode with platinum-iridium electrode leads and 22 intracochlear electrode contacts, and (5) two extracochlear electrode contacts (one on the case and another on a separate lead) that are used for different electrode coupling/stimulation modes. Of note, the Nucleus Profile cochlear implant is encased in a biocompatible silicone insulation. Also of note, the titanium case of the Nucleus Profile is 2.5 times stronger than that of the Freedom implant.

The Nucleus Profile implant has a similar electronics package as the Nucleus Freedom cochlear implant. The Profile has a maximum stimulation rate of 31,500 pulses per second and a DSP featuring an asynchronous architecture. This asynchronous architecture allows, among other things, the Freedom implant to produce stimulus pulses at any point in time rather than confining stimuli to a fixed pulse grid. This capability will allow the Profile to execute peak-derived timing signal coding strategies, which aim to stimulate at rates consistent with the temporal fluctuations in the input signal and harbor potential for improvement of speech recognition. The current

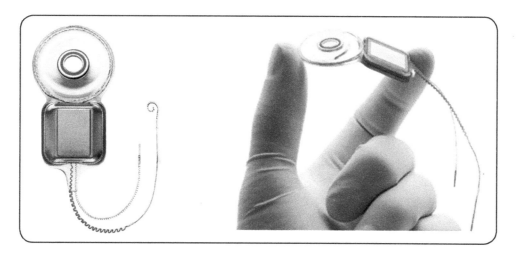

FIGURE 10–33. Nucleus Profile cochlear implant. Image provided courtesy of Cochlear Americas, ©2018.

generator of the Nucleus Profile is capable of delivering electrical pulses with an amplitude of 10 microamperes to 1.75 milliamperes at a pulse width ranging from 12 to 400 microseconds.

Additionally, the Nucleus Profile implant has a telemetry system that facilitates two-way transmission of information from the external and internal devices. A carrier frequency of 5 MHz is used to transmit the signal in both directions. The amplifier used to record responses from the auditory nerve for diagnostic purposes (i.e., the amplifier used to record Neural Response Telemetry [NRT]) has a low noise floor (less than 1 microvolt) and, as a result, enables acquisition of robust neural responses at relatively low stimulation levels. Furthermore, although it is not currently available for clinical use, the Nucleus Profile implant offers dual-electrode stimulation, which allows for fast, sequential stimulation of neighboring electrodes to elicit a maximum point of stimulation between two physical electrode contacts (with significantly improved battery life due to impedance drop).

The internal magnet that is positioned within a silastic sleeve in the center of the internal receiving (telemetry) coil may be removed if the patient needs an MRI. It should be noted that the Physician's Packet included with Nucleus Profile implants distributed in the United States indicates that an MRI may be conducted with the magnet in place so long as the physician has followed the manufacturer's protocol for bandaging the recipient's head and the strength of the MRI is 1.5 tesla (T) or less. Of note, it is likely that the magnet will cast a "shadow" on the MRI in the area around the implant. Additionally, an MRI scan of up to 3.0T strength may be conducted when the magnet is removed. The internal magnet contains a black circle on the side that should be facing up when inserted into the Silastic sleeve (i.e., the black ring should face away from the skull).

One unique characteristic of the Nucleus Profile implant is a reference/return electrode (known as the "Monopolar 1" or "MP1") located at the tip of a separate lead (i.e., separate from the intracochlear electrode array). This arrangement permits broader stimulation fields and a reduction in the amount of current needed for a given level of stimulation. The surgeon typically places the MP1 electrode contact in the temporalis muscle adjacent to the implanted ear. The Nucleus Profile also has an extracochlear return electrode located on the case of the stimulator (referred to as the "Monopolar 2" or "MP2"). A wide variety of stimulation modes are available and include the use of both return electrodes in isolation and in tandem, along with a special mode known as common ground stimulation (see Chapters 7 and 16).

Nucleus Freedom Internal Device

The Nucleus Freedom internal device (CI24RE) (Figure 10–34) was introduced into the market in the United States in April 2005. Like the Nucleus Profile, the Nucleus Freedom is composed of: (1) a sophisticated, digitally driven stimulator housed in a hermetically sealed titanium case, (2) a platinum-iridium coil used for signal transmission between the sound processor and implant, (3) a removable magnet positioned in a Silastic sleeve located in the center of the coil, (4) an electrode with platinum-iridium electrode leads and 22 intracochlear electrode contacts, and (5) two extracochlear electrode contacts (one on the case and another on a separate lead) that are used for different electrode coupling/stimulation modes. The electronics/stimulator package of the Freedom implant is essentially identical to the electronics/stimulator of the Nucleus Profile, and as a result, the information pertaining to the Profile that was described in the previous section also applies to the Freedom implant. The primary difference between the Freedom and Profile implants is that the former

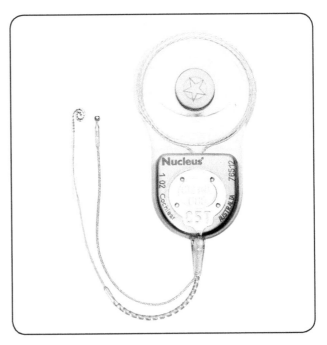

FIGURE 10–34. Nucleus Freedom cochlear implant. Image provided courtesy of Cochlear Americas, ©2018.

possesses a thicker titanium case. Of significance, over 170,000 recipients have received the Nucleus Freedom cochlear implant worldwide, and the reliability rating (i.e., the cumulative survival rate) is 99.0% after 12 years of use.

Also as with the Profile, the Nucleus Freedom contains two reference/return electrodes, the MP1 electrode that is on a separate lead and placed in the temporalis muscle, and MP2 which is located on the titanium case. The Nucleus Freedom is also approved for MRI, which may be conducted at 3.0T with the magnet removed and at 1.5T with the magnet in place and the head bandaged. Of note, the Nucleus CI422 cochlear implant uses the Freedom case and electronics.

Nucleus Electrode Arrays

Cochlear offers a choice of several different electrode arrays (Figures 10–35 and 10–36), including the: (1) Slim Modiolar Electrode, (2) Contour Advance Electrode, (3) Slim Straight Electrode, (4) Hybrid L24 Electrode, (5) Full-Band Straight Electrode, and (6) the Auditory Brainstem Implant (ABI) array. Each

of these cochlear implant electrode arrays will be described in the following sections. The Nucleus ABI will be discussed in Chapter 25.

Nucleus Slim Modiolar Electrode

In 2016, Cochlear announced the commercial launch of the Slim Modiolar Electrode (Figure 10–37). The Slim Modiolar Electrode is the thinnest perimodiolar electrode array in the cochlear implant industry. It occupies 60% less volume in the scala tympani compared with the size of its predecessor, the Contour Advance electrode array. The thin diameter of the Slim Modiolar Electrode is intended to allow for round window insertion into the scala tympani and to avoid the delicate structures of the organ of Corti. The perimodiolar shape of the Slim Modiolar Electrode is designed to position the array next to the modiolus to facilitate close proximity to the cochlear nerve, resulting in a reduction in electrical stimulation required to facilitate an auditory response as well as to reduce channel interaction. Indeed, research has shown lower stimulation levels and neural response thresholds with Nucleus perimodiolar electrode arrays relative to straight electrode arrays (Cohen et al., 2003;

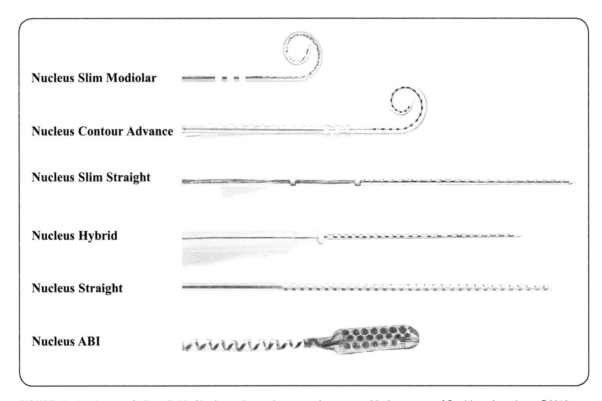

FIGURE 10–35. Image of all available Nucleus electrode arrays. Image provided courtesy of Cochlear Americas, ©2018.

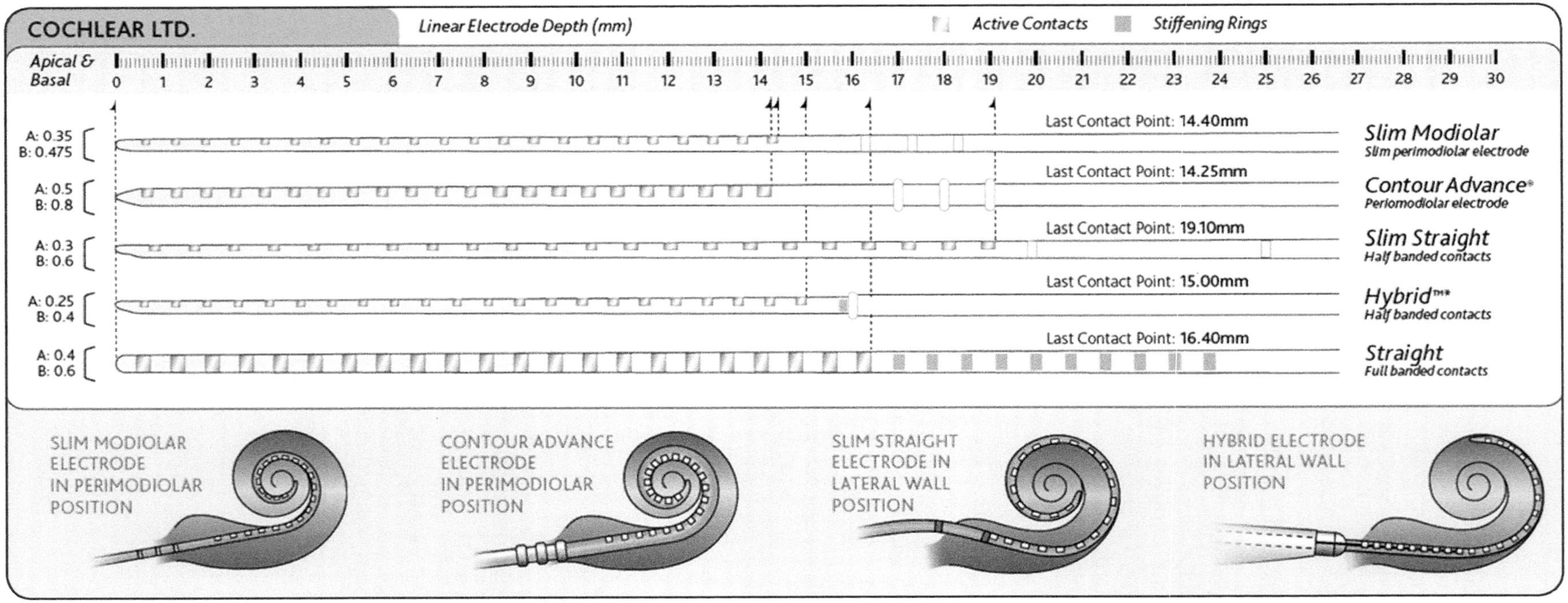

FIGURE 10–36. Image of all available Nucleus electrode arrays. Image provided courtesy of Cochlear Americas, ©2018.

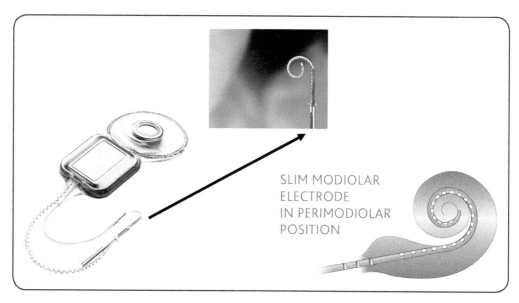

FIGURE 10–37. Nucleus Slim Modiolar Electrode. Image provided courtesy of Cochlear Americas, ©2018.

Dowell, 2012; Esquia et al., 2013; Holden et al., 2013; van der Beek et al., 2005).

The Slim Modiolar Electrode array contains 22 platinum-iridium stimulating leads and 22 intracochlear platinum, half-banded electrode contacts, which are positioned toward the modiolus in order to direct electrical current toward the cochlear nerve. The 22 intracochlear stimulating electrode contacts (i.e., physical stimulation sites) provide a greater number of physical stimulation sites than are offered by competing implant manufacturers. The Slim Modiolar Electrode contains a "Softip," which is designed to reduce trauma to delicate cochlear structures during insertion. Insertion of the device using the Advanced Off-Stylet technique, along with a consistent method for identification of the cochleostomy site (i.e., the round window, an extended round window, or a cochleostomy drilled just anterior and inferior to the round window), is recommended by Cochlear Ltd. The Softip and insertion technique reduce lateral wall force and increase the likelihood that the electrode array not only is inserted in the scala tympani, but also remains in the scala tympani throughout insertion. Of note, temporal bone studies have shown near zero insertion force with preservation of the delicate structures of the cochlea and no intracochlear trauma in 98% of specimens (Cochlear, 2014, 2015; Roland, 2005). It should be noted that the Stylet contains a fan-tail that facilitates ease of handling and insertion by allowing the surgeon to grasp the fan-tail with a pair of forceps. Moreover, the surgeon may reload the electrode array into the Stylet if needed.

The Slim Modiolar electrode array, which is inserted approximately 18 to 20 mm into the cochlea, is intended to be inserted to an angular insertion depth of 420 to 450 degrees. The distance between the tip of the electrode array and the most basal electrode is 15 mm. The cross-sectional diameter of the Slim Modiolar Electrode is 0.35 mm at the tip of the array and 0.475 mm at the base. Additionally, the Slim Modiolar electrode possesses a marker to guide the surgeon in achieving the proper insertion depth (approximately 18 mm). The electrode contacts in the Slim Modiolar Electrode array are spaced in a nonlinear manner to maximize the uniformity of spectral coverage for a given number of electrodes and to promote a higher probability of good speech perception. It should be noted that less than 1 mm typically exists between electrode contacts.

Nucleus Contour Advance Electrode

The Nucleus Contour Advance array was approved by the FDA for commercial distribution in the United States in 2005. The Contour Advance is also a perimodiolar electrode array with a "Softip" (Figure 10–38). The same advantages of a perimodiolar array mentioned in the discussion of the Slim Modiolar Electrode also apply to the Contour Advance. As with the Slim Modiolar Array, the Contour Advance is designed to be inserted with use of the Advanced Off-Stylet technique into a cochleostomy that is drilled just anterior and inferior to the round window. The

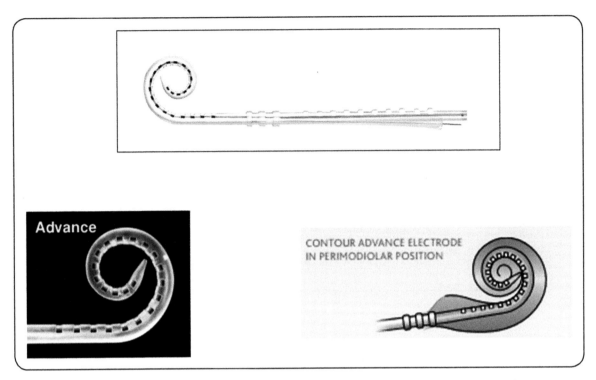

FIGURE 10–38. Nucleus Contour Advance electrode array. Image provided courtesy of Cochlear Americas, ©2018.

primary difference between the Contour Advance and the Slim Modiolar Electrode is that the former has a larger cross-sectional diameter of the Contour Advance (5 mm at the tip of the array and 0.8 mm at the base), which typically prevents a round window insertion and results in the Contour Advance occupying a larger space within the scala tympani. However, when the cochleostomy is drilled in the appropriate location and the Advanced Off-Stylet procedure is used, research has shown that the Contour Advance is inserted into and remains within the scala tympani throughout the entire insertion and results in minimal trauma to the cochlear structures (Aschedorff et al., 2007, 2017; Finley et al., 2008, Wanna et al., 2015). The Contour Advance possesses 22 half-banded platinum intracochlear electrode contacts. Furthermore, the Contour Advance electrode array is inserted to approximately the same insertion depth as the Slim Modiolar Electrode (18–20 mm into the cochlea, an angular insertion depth of 420–450 degrees). The distance between the tip of the electrode array and the most basal electrode is 15 mm. Moreover, the Contour Advance electrode also possesses a marker to guide the surgeon in achieving the proper insertion depth (approximately 18 mm). Of note, the Contour Advance electrode array is available with both the Nucleus Profile and Freedom cochlear implants. The Nucleus Profile with the Contour Advance is referred to as the Nucleus CI512 implant, whereas the nucleus Freedom with Contour Advance is referred to as the CI24RE(CA).

Nucleus Slim Straight Electrode

The Nucleus Slim Straight Electrode array was commercially released in the United States in 2012. The Slim Straight is a thin, lateral wall ("straight") electrode array (Figure 10–39). Specifically, the cross-sectional diameter of the Slim Straight Electrode is 0.3 mm at the tip of the array and 0.6 mm at the base of the array. The Slim Straight contains 22 half-banded platinum intracochlear electrode contacts positioned over 20 mm, resulting in a little less than 1 mm between electrode contacts (with essentially linear spacing between contacts). The Slim Straight Electrode was developed with several design objectives in mind. First, the thin diameter was intended to allow for a round window or extended round window insertion into the scala tympani. Second, the thin cross-sectional diameter is also intended to occupy a small

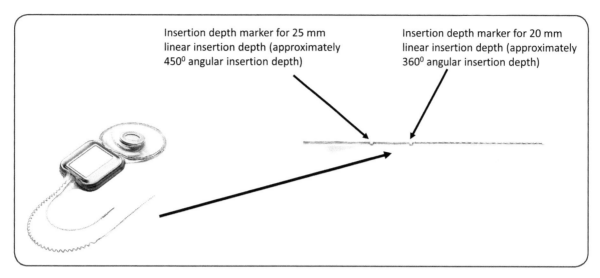

Insertion depth marker for 25 mm linear insertion depth (approximately 450⁰ angular insertion depth)

Insertion depth marker for 20 mm linear insertion depth (approximately 360⁰ angular insertion depth)

FIGURE 10–39. Nucleus Slim Straight electrode array Nucleus Straight array. Image provided courtesy of Cochlear Americas, ©2018.

proportion of the scala tympani and consequently avoid the delicate structures of the scala media. Third, and likewise, the straight orientation and lateral wall placement is also intended to avoid the delicate structures of the cochlea. Collectively, these properties are intended to facilitate an atraumatic insertion and potentially preserve the recipient's native acoustic hearing, particularly in the low-frequency range (i.e., below 1000 Hz). Moreover, the Slim Straight Electrode may be appealing to a recipient who is interested in pursuing inner ear medical treatments that may be made available in the future (e.g., hair cell regeneration). However, it is important to note that there is no evidence that a recipient will be more or less able to benefit from future advances in inner ear medical treatments after receiving a particular type of cochlear implant electrode array.

The Slim Straight Electrode possesses two depth markers, one at 25 mm from the tip of the electrode array and another at 20 mm from the tip of the array. Inserting a lateral wall electrode array to a depth of 25 mm results in an angular insertion depth of approximately 420 to 450 degrees in the typical recipient, which is similar to the angular insertion depth of the Slim Modiolar and Contour Advance electrode arrays. Achieving an angular insertion depth of 420 to 450 degrees is desirable for recipients who have severe to profound hearing loss and for whom there is a remote likelihood that benefit will be achieved from low-frequency acoustic stimulation. Inserting a

lateral wall electrode array 20 mm into the scala tympani results in an angular insertion depth of about 360 degrees in the typical recipient, which roughly corresponds to the location at which a 1000 Hz sound is coded in the cochlea (Greenwood, 1961, 1990; Stakhovskaya et al., 2007). As a result, the electrode array is not inserted into the apical region of the cochlea where low-frequency sound is coded, which may enhance the possibility of preserving low-frequency acoustic hearing. Consequently, the shallower insertion depth of 20 mm is intended for recipients who have better preoperative low-frequency hearing in order to enhance the likelihood of electric-acoustic use after surgery. As shown in Figure 10–39, the Slim Straight Electrode has a surgical handle that is designed to facilitate ease of use and handling for the surgeon. Also, the surgical handle serves as a guide for the surgeon so that the half-banded intra-cochlear electrode contacts are positioned toward the modiolus. Moreover, the Slim Straight contains a tapered basal stiffener between the surgical handle and the 20-mm marker that is intended to provide a smooth, single-motion insertion and minimize the possibility of the electrode buckling during insertion. Also, the Slim Straight possesses a soft silicone tip which is intended to promote an atraumatic surgery. The Slim Straight may be inserted by "free hand" or with the Advanced Off-Stylet forceps. When the Nucleus Profile implant and Slim Straight Electrode are paired together, the total package is referred to as the Nucleus CI522. When the Slim Straight is paired with the Nucleus Freedom implant, the total package is referred to as the Nucleus CI422.

Nucleus Straight Electrode Array

The Straight electrode array is only available with the Freedom implant (CI24RE[ST]; see Figures 10–35 and 10–36). The Straight Array is the predecessor to the Contour Advance and is not a perimodiolar electrode (i.e., it is a lateral wall electrode array). With a cross-sectional diameter of 0.4 mm at the apical end and 0.6 at the basal end, it is thinner than the Contour Advance but not quite as thin as the Slim Straight and Modiolar Slim Electrodes. Further, the Straight Array features 22 intracochlear, full-band electrode contacts and 10 inactive stiffening rings that aid in the insertion of the array. Furthermore, the Straight Array is almost 17 mm, and because it is typically inserted along the lateral wall of the cochlea, the angular insertion depth approaches 360 degrees. The Straight Array is recommended for patients who may have a common cavity deformity of the cochlea; the full-banded electrodes deliver electrical stimulation in all directions, which is a useful feature for common cavity cochleae because the location of neural innervation is not precisely known as it is with the modiolus of the typical cochlea. Additionally, because it is more rigid, the Straight Array may be considered for recipients with fibrous tissue growth in the cochlea (i.e., bacterial meningitis), because its increased rigidity compared with the Nucleus perimodiolar and Slim Straight arrays enhances the likelihood that it will pass through soft fibrous tissue.

Nucleus Double Array

It should be noted that Cochlear used to offer the Double Array electrode array with the Nucleus 24 cochlear implant (Figure 10–40). The Nucleus Double Array possesses two electrode leads to be placed in two different cochleostomies, one in the traditional basal location and another at a more apical locale. The Double Array is intended for postmeningitic recipients who have significant cochlear ossification preventing a full insertion of a conventional, single electrode array. At the time of this writing, the Double Array was not being offered.

Nucleus L24 Hybrid Cochlear Implant

In November 2013, Cochlear received FDA approval to commercially market the Cochlear Nucleus L24 Hybrid cochlear implant in the United States (Figure 10–41). The Nucleus L24 Hybrid cochlear implant was designed with the primary intent of preserving low-frequency hearing and is intended for use with recipients who have significant low-frequency hearing preoperatively (better than 60 dB HL at 500 Hz). The Nucleus Hybrid implant possesses a similar electronics and housing package as the Nucleus Profile and Freedom implants. The primary difference between the Nucleus Hybrid and other Nucleus cochlear implants lies in the electrode array. The Nucleus L24 Hybrid electrode lead possesses a relatively large fantail, which is intended to facilitate ease of handling while the surgeon inserts the electrode array into the cochlea. Additionally, the section of

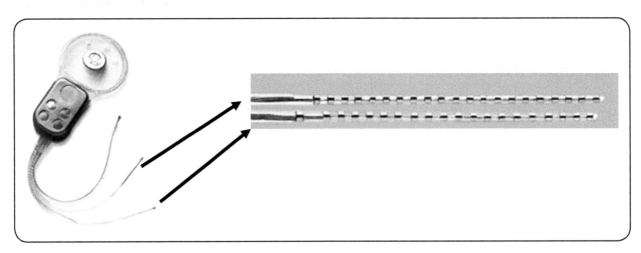

FIGURE 10–40. Nucleus Double Array (no longer commercially available). Image provided courtesy of Cochlear Americas, ©2018.

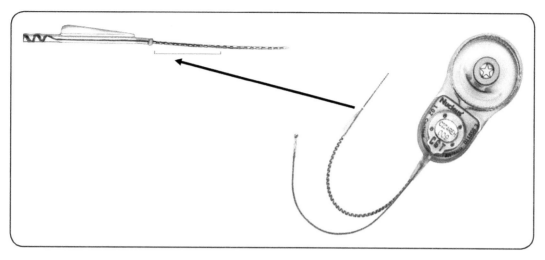

FIGURE 10–41. Nucleus L24 Hybrid cochlear implant. Image provided courtesy of Cochlear Americas, ©2018.

the electrode lead adjacent to the fantail is rather stiff, which also enhances the ease of handling during the insertion process. Furthermore, the electrode lead possesses a "stopper," which serves as a clear guide to how deeply the electrode array should be inserted. Also, the electrode array itself is designed to be inserted to a depth of approximately 230 degrees (about 16–17 mm), and the cross-sectional diameter of the Nucleus L24 Hybrid electrode array is 0.25 by 0.35 mm at the apical end of the array and 0.4 by 0.55 mm at the basal end of the array. The array is thin enough to be inserted into the round window or into an extended round window cochleostomy (the choice is typically dependent on surgeon's preference and recipient anatomy). Finally, the Nucleus L24 Hybrid electrode array is intended to be inserted with the use of a "soft" surgical insertion procedure, which is designed to protect the cochlea from injury during insertion. Research exploring the advantages and limitations of the Nucleus L24 Hybrid cochlear implant has generally found favorable speech recognition outcomes and low-frequency hearing preservation (Lenarz et al., 209, 2013; Roland et al., 2016).

Key Concepts

- Cochlear Ltd. offers a variety of sound processors to meet the unique needs of children and adults who have received Nucleus cochlear implants. Nucleus recipients may choose from ear-level or head-worn sound processors.

- Nucleus sound processors are equipped with adaptive signal processing designed to improve hearing performance in challenging listening situations.
- Nucleus sound processors are also equipped with wireless digital radio frequency technology that allows the recipient to stream audio to and from personal electronic devices using a variety of different wireless hearing assistive technologies.
- Cochlear Ltd. offers a variety of different cochlear implants and electrode arrays to meet the unique needs of recipients. Surgeons may select from perimodiolar and lateral wall electrode arrays, short and conventional-length electrode arrays, flexible and stiff electrode arrays, electrode arrays with half-band and full-band electrode contacts, and electrode arrays with thin and conventional cross-sectional diameters.

References

Aschendorff, A., Briggs, R., Brademann, G., Helbig, S., Hornung, J., Lenarz, T., . . . James, C. J. (2017). Clinical investigation of the Nucleus Slim Modiolar Electrode. *Audiology and Neurotology*, *22*(3), 169–179.

Aschendorff, A., Kromeier, J., Klenzner, T., & Laszig, R. (2007). Quality control after insertion of the nucleus contour and contour advance electrode in adults. *Ear and Hearing, 28*(Suppl. 2), 75S–79S.

Cochlear. (2014). Data on file—CI532 Temporal Bone Usability Test Report, 2014—Windchill 588021.

Cochlear. (2015). Data on file—EA32 Electrode Insertion Safety and Performance Study, 2015—Windchill 415680.

Cohen, L., Richardson, L., Saunders, E., & Cowan, R. (2003). Spatial spread of neural excitation in cochlear implant recipients: Comparison of improved ECAP method and psychophysical forward masking. *Hearing Research, 179*, 72–87.

Dowell, R. (2012). Evidence about the effectiveness of cochlear implants for adults. In L. Wong & L. Hickson (Eds.), *Evidence based practice in audiology: Evaluating interventions for children and adults with hearing impairment* (pp. 141–166). San Diego, CA: Plural.

Esquia-Medina, G. N., Borel, S., Nguyen, Y., Ambert-Dahan, E., Ferrary, E., Sterkers, O., & Bozorg Grayeli, A. (2013). Is electrode-modiolus distance a prognostic factor for hearing performances after cochlear implant surgery? *Audiology and Neurotology, 18*, 406–413.

Finley, C. C., Holden, T. A., Holden, L. K., Whiting, B. R., Chole, R. A., Neely, G. J., . . . Skinner, M. W. (2008). Role of electrode placement as a contributor to variability in cochlear implant outcomes. *Otology and Neurotology, 29*(7), 920–928.

Holden, L. K., Finley, C. C., Firszt, J. B., Holden, T. A., Brenner, C., Potts, L. G., Gotter, B. D., . . . Skinner, M. W. (2013). Factors affecting open-set word recognition in adults with cochlear implants. *Ear and Hearing, 34*(3), 342–60

Lenarz, T., James, C., Cuda, D., Fitzgerald O'Connor, A., Frachet, B., Frijns, J. H., . . . Uziel, A. (2013). European multi-centre study of the Nucleus Hybrid L24 cochlear implant. *International Journal of Audiology, 52*(12), 838–848.

Lenarz, T., Stover, T., Buechner, A., Lesinski-Schiedat, A., Patrick, J., & Pesch, J. (2009). Hearing conservation surgery using the Hybrid-L electrode. Results from the first clinical trial at the Medical University of Hannover. *Audiology and Neurotology, 14*(Suppl. 1), 22–31.

Mauger, S. J., Jones, M., Nel, E., & Del Dot, J. (2017). Clinical outcomes with the Kanso off-the-ear cochlear implant sound processor. *International Journal of Audiology, 56*(4), 267–276.

Roland, J. T. (2005). A model for cochlear implant electrode insertion and force evaluation: Results with a new electrode design and insertion technique. *Laryngoscope, 115*(8), 1325–1339.

Roland, J. T., Jr., Gantz, B. J., Waltzman, S. B., Parkinson, A. J., & Multicenter Clinical Trial, G. (2016). United States multicenter clinical trial of the cochlear nucleus hybrid implant system. *Laryngoscope, 126*(1), 175–181.

van der Beek, F. B., Boermans, P. P., Verbist, B. M., Briaire, J. J., & Frijns, J. H. (2005). Clinical evaluation of the Clarion CII HiFocus 1 with and without positioner. *Ear and Hearing, 26*(6), 577–592.

Wanna, G. B., Noble, J. H., Gifford, R. H., Dietrich, M. S., Sweeney, A. D., Zhang, D., . . . Labadie, R. F. (2015). Impact of intrascalar electrode location, electrode type, and angular insertion depth on residual hearing in cochlear implant patients: Preliminary results. *Otology and Neurotology, 36*(8), 1343–1348.

Wolfe, J. (2016, May). *Cochlear Mini Mic 2+*. Presented at American Cochlear Implant Alliance 2016 Conference, Toronto, Canada.

MED-EL Cochlear Implants and Sound Processors

Jace Wolfe

Introduction

This chapter will provide a review of MED-EL cochlear implants and sound processors. The programming of MED-EL cochlear implants will be discussed in Chapter 17.

MED-EL Corporation

The MED-EL Corporation manufactures the SYN-CHRONY cochlear implant, which may be used with the SONNET and OPUS 2 behind-the-ear sound processors as well as with the RONDO™ single-unit, off-the-ear sound processor. MED-EL cochlear implant systems possess several features and technologies that are unique to the cochlear implant industry. The MED-EL cochlear implant systems will be described in the following section.

SONNET Sound Processor

The SONNET sound processor is designed to be light-weight (i.e., 8.1 grams with Micro rechargeable battery), comfortable, and simple to use across a variety of listening (Figure 11–1). The SONNET is compatible for use with all models of MED-EL cochlear implants. The digital signal processor of the SONNET proces-

sor performs a Hilbert transformation on the input audio signal to extract the spectral and temporal cues (both amplitude envelope and fine temporal structure). The digital signal processor (DSP) of the SONNET also allows for implementation of an "automatic volume control" with a dual-loop automatic gain control (AGC) compression circuit (i.e., two compression thresholds, one with a lower kneepoint and slow time constants and another with a higher kneepoint

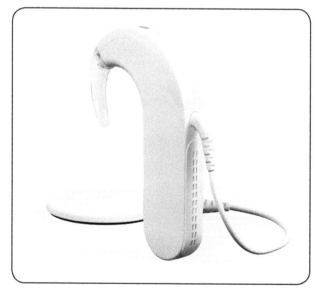

FIGURE 11–1. MED-EL SONNET sound processor. Image provided courtesy of MED-EL Corporation.

and faster time constants) to deliver a wide range of acoustic input intensities into the relatively narrow electrical dynamic range (EDR). Furthermore, the SONNET contains a 2.4 GHz antenna for future digital radio applications and a telecoil. An "FM battery cover" may also be coupled to the SONNET to allow for use of a radio frequency receiver with a 3-prong Euro connector.

Additionally, The SONNET sound processor allows for use of Automatic Sound Management 2.0 (ASM 2.0) sound processing, which includes several new processing features. For instance, the SONNET contains two omnidirectional microphones to provide a dual-microphone, advanced directional beamformer. The audiologist may select from four different microphone modes, (1) Omnidirectional, (2) Adaptive directional, which adaptively positions to null of the microphone response to coincide with the direction from which the most intense noise is arriving, (3) Natural, which implements a polar plot pattern that mimics the modest positive directivity of the natural ear, and (4) Automatic, which automatically switches between the aforementioned modes. More-

over, the ASM 2.0 features wind noise reduction and an automatic volume control, and the SONNET processor possesses data logging.

The SONNET sound processor possesses a new transmitting cable that connects to the DL Coil. The new transmitting cable possesses reinforced plugs so that it is more durable than the cable used with the OPUS 2 sound processor, which is the predecessor of the SONNET. The DL Coil is a very low-profile external transmitting/receiving coil that transmits the signal of interest and power required to operate the implant at a carrier frequency of 12 MHz. An integrated bi-color LED light housed at the base of the DL Coil serves as an indicator to monitor implant coupling and signal caregivers of any problems. The cover of the DL Coil may be removed so that the coil magnet may be replaced. The magnet is available in nine different strengths (five different magnets [i.e., 1–5] with adjustable strengths; a paperclip or ballpoint pen may be used to rotate the magnet between a "+" position, which provides stronger attraction, and a "–" position, which provides weaker position) (Figure 11–2).

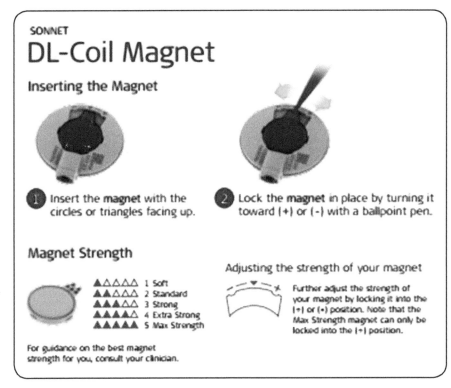

FIGURE 11–2. Various magnet strengths available for DL-Coil with adjustment in strength of a specific magnet by rotating position of the magnet between the "+" and "–" positions. Image provided courtesy of MED-EL Corporation.

The SONNET processor has a 54 ingress protection (IP) rating and is advertised as being water resistant and splashproof, although a waterproof cover is available that results in a 68 IP rating. Also, the SONNET does not contain any control switches (power button, program switch, etc.); these adjustments are made through the accompanying Fine Tuner remote control. It is powered on and off by connecting and disconnecting the battery cover to and from the processor, respectively. The SONNET may be powered by rechargeable batteries or by two 675 high-powered zinc-air batteries. The battery cover, which has a tamperproof locking mechanism, may be removed from the base of the processor to change the batteries. The rechargeable battery simply and easily snaps into and out of the battery connector. The frame of the rechargeable battery module and of the 675 battery module may also be removed from the SONNET by pushing a lever at the base of the SONNET processor. This configuration allows the SONNET processor to be modular in design. Two rechargeable batteries are available for use with the SONNET, the SONNET Rechargeable Battery (MED-EL reports up to 10 hours of operating time per charge) and the SONNET Rechargeable Battery Micro (up to 7 hours of operating time per charge). According to MED-EL, each battery requires 3 to 4 hours of charging time. The SONNET allows reportedly up to 60 hours of use time with two 675 zinc-air batteries. The SONNET rechargeable batteries are charged on the SONNET Charging System (Figure 11–3).

Finally, in the SONNET electric-acoustic stimulation (EAS) variant of the sound processor, an acoustic receiver is present at the apex of the SONNET EAS processor. The conventional earhook may be removed and replaced with an acoustic earhook that may be coupled to any standard earmold (Figure 11–4). The acoustic receiver of the SONNET EAS is capable of an overall gain of 48 dB SPL and a maximum power output of 118 dB SPL. It also possesses six channels to allow for flexible programming of the low-frequency acoustic signal up to 2000 Hz. Of note, the SONNET is actually available in two variations, an electric only version (i.e., SONNET) and an electric-acoustic version (i.e., SONNET EAS), which contains the acoustic receiver within the processor.

SONNET Wearing Options

A number of different wearing options are available for the SONNET sound processor. Figure 11–5 shows several of these alternatives. The BabyWear option consists of a long DL Coil cable and a clip that allows the SONNET to be attached to the child's clothing. The BabyWear option is designed to completely remove the processor from small ears. The ActiveWear option consists of a cable that couples the sound processor to the battery, which is coupled to a clip that is attached to the wearer's clothes. The ActiveWear option is designed for adults and children who participate in sports, exercise, and dance but is also an excellent alternative for infants as well because the sound processor may be worn on the ear. Additionally, MED-EL offers the BTE (behind-the-ear) Headband, which may be used to hold the SONNET in a small loop on the headband. The Mini Battery Pack allows the SONNET to be connected to a

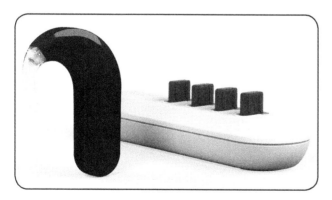

FIGURE 11–3. SONNET Charging System. Image provided courtesy of MED-EL Corporation.

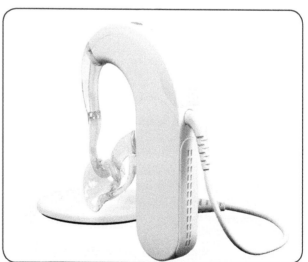

FIGURE 11–4. SONNET with acoustic earhook for electric-acoustic stimulation. Image provided courtesy of MED-EL Corporation.

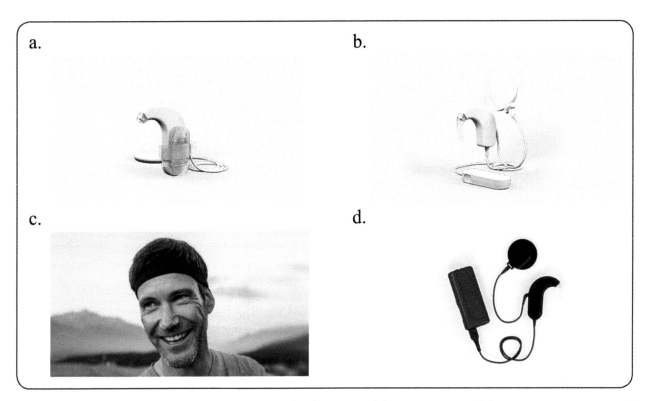

FIGURE 11–5. BabyWear option (**A**); ActiveWear Option (**B**); BTE Headband (**C**); Mini Battery Pack (**D**). Images provided courtesy of MED-EL Corporation.

cartridge that holds a single AAA battery. The AAA battery allows an average of 37 hours of continuous use. The Mini Battery Pack may also be powered with a rechargeable DaCapo PowerPack battery, which provides an average of 16 hours of operation. Finally, the WaterWear cover may be placed over the SONNET to allow for fully waterproof use (IP68 rating) (Figure 11–6).

OPUS 2 Sound Processor

The OPUS 2 external sound processor, introduced in 2008, is typically used as a BTE sound processor (Figure 11–7). It is a small, lightweight processor that has several enhanced features compared with the previous generation of processors (i.e., TEMPO+ and OPUS 1). The OPUS 2 has a fully digital sound processor that uses a Hilbert transformation to analyze incoming acoustic inputs. The input frequency range of the sound processor extends from 70 to 8500 Hz, and the sound processor can accommodate up to four user programs. It has an omnidirectional micro-

phone located at the top of the processor just behind the earhook. It should be noted that the TEMPO+ and OPUS 1 sound processors feature the same input frequency range as the OPUS 2 and utilize a Hilbert transformation in the analysis of the input signal.

Additionally, a light-emitting diode (LED) light can be used to alert the user or caregiver of the processor status, and there is a manually accessible telecoil. The earhook of the OPUS 2 sound processor is attached to the apex of the processor by a small pin. The purpose of this pin is to prevent young children from removing and ingesting the earhook. The earhook is available in multiple sizes to accommodate different ear sizes. The OPUS 2 sound processor does not include any user controls (other than an on/off switch). Instead, the user may adjust processor settings via a remote control, which will be discussed later.

MED-EL offers a full portfolio of wearing options for the OPUS 2 (which will be discussed below) to facilitate excellent retention and comfort for recipients with varying ear anatomies, developmental needs, and communication lifestyles. In the ear-level configuration, the OPUS 2 sound processor is com-

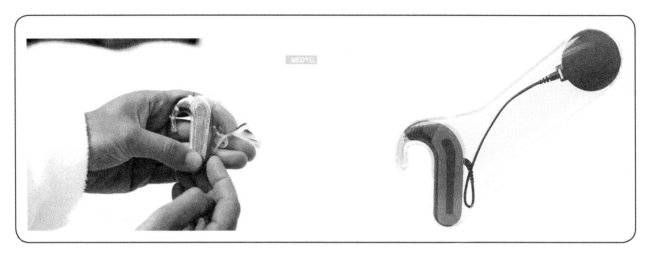

FIGURE 11–6. WaterWear. Image provided courtesy of MED-EL Corporation.

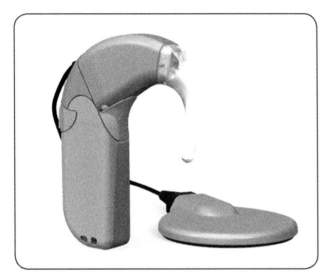

FIGURE 11–7. MED-EL OPUS 2 sound processor. Image provided courtesy of MED-EL Corporation.

posed of three primary components: (1) the sound processor (i.e., control unit), (2) the angled battery pack, and (3) the cable and coil. The OPUS 2 sound processor may be used with every MED-EL cochlear implant that has ever been introduced onto the commercial market (e.g., CONCERT, SONATA TI[100], PULSAR CI[100], COMBI 40+).

The coil was updated in 2011 with the release of the thinner and lower-profile D-coil that is engineered to be 50% more energy efficient than its predecessor. The D-coil features a removable cable, which comes in several lengths to allow for variation in head size

and wearing configurations (battery estimates with D-coil below). The magnet strength of the D-coil may be adjusted by the programming audiologist to accommodate a range of adhesive needs across recipients. This is accomplished by sliding the magnet between the "+" and "−" positions to strengthen or weaken the adhesive strength. Also, themagnet may be lifted out of the D-coil and replaced with a magnet of the desired strength. Magnet strengths are available in soft (one dot on the side of the magnet), standard (two dots), strong (three dots), and super strong models (four dots). The radio frequency (RF) used to transmit the signal from the D-coil to a MED-EL cochlear implant is 12 MHz, which is the same RF carrier frequency used with all MED-EL implants and external transmitting coils.

Battery/Wearing Options

MED-EL currently offers two battery options for use with the OPUS 2 sound processor when worn on the ear. For each ear-level option, a "connecting piece" is required to couple the battery pack to the processor.

The Standard Battery Pack (Figure 11–8) may be used with one of the DaCapo rechargeable batteries, or three disposable zinc-air 675 batteries may be used. The DaCapo rechargeable battery is 20% lighter than three zinc-air 675 batteries, and MED-EL reports that up to 16 hours of use time may be achieved with the Standard Battery Pack and the DaCapo rechargeable battery. Additionally, up to 90 hours of battery life may be achieved with the use of the Standard Battery Pack with three zinc-air 675 batteries.

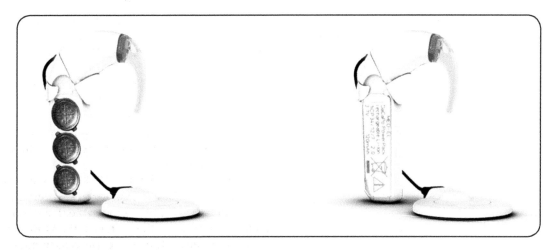

FIGURE 11–8. OPUS 2 Standard Battery Pack with 675 zinc-air and rechargeable battery options. Image provided courtesy of MED-EL Corporation.

In addition to the standard ear-level battery pack, MED-EL also offers the OPUS 2 XS Battery Pack, which was released in 2012 (Figure 11–9). The OPUS 2 XS Battery Pack uses two disposable zinc-air 675 batteries and is smaller and lighter than the Standard Battery Pack. In fact, when the OPUS 2 processor is used with the XS Battery Pack, it is one of the smallest ear-level sound processors commercially available in the cochlear implant industry at the time of this writing. The XS option may be particularly attractive for young children, as it reduces processor size and weight while allowing for BTE use. This facilitates a more favorable microphone location than can be obtained with body-worn options, such as the BabyBTE™/ActiveWear configurations mentioned below. MED-EL reports that up to 60 hours of battery life may be obtained with the XS Battery Pack.

Additional options are available to cater to unique patients' needs. Similar to the SONNET, the OPUS 2 may be used with pediatric configurations (i.e., Baby-BTE or ActiveWear). A straight battery pack, a fixation piece, and a long cable attaching the coil to the processor allows the OPUS 2 system to be clipped to a user's clothing without anything on the ear. This option may be particularly attractive for very young children or people who play sports; however, care should be taken to position the processor microphone appropriately (i.e., toward typical sound source at 0 degrees azimuth). However, this option is not ideal for bilaterally implanted children, where the intra-aural level differences need to be accurately maintained to help with localization, speech recognition

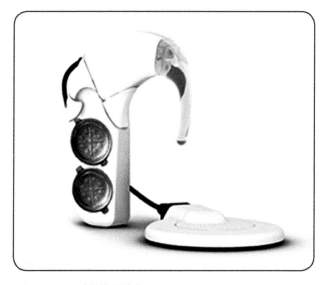

FIGURE 11–9. OPUS 2 XS Battery Pack. Image provided courtesy of MED-EL Corporation.

in noise, and other bilateral processes that require preservation of interaural cues.

MED-EL also offers a Children's Battery Pack (Figure 11–10), which possesses a long cable connecting the battery to the sound processor. This configuration allows young children to wear the processor on the ear and the battery on the body. The Children's Battery Pack is similar in size to the Standard ear-level Battery Pack and uses three disposable zinc-air 675 batteries. MED-EL reports that the Children's Battery Pack provides up to 90 hours of use with three zinc-air 675 batteries. This is an attractive option for young, bilaterally implanted children because interaural cues will be preserved more effectively than if the sound processor microphone was worn on the body. It should be noted, however, that the Children's Battery Pack does not have a DAI port for use with FM/RF systems. MED-EL suggests that the recipient use the OPUS 2 telecoil with an induction neckloop when the Children's Battery Pack is being used and use of a personal digital RF/FM system is also desired. Of note, an FM receiver may also be connected directly to the OPUS 2 sound processor with use of the FM battery cover which has a three-prong Euro Port at its base.

MED-EL also offers the Mini Battery Pack option (Figure 11–11). Like the Children's Battery Pack, the Mini Battery Pack uses a long cable that connects the sound processor to the battery unit. Again, this configuration allows the sound processor microphone to be positioned at the ear, whereas the battery, which possesses a great deal of the sound processor's bulk, may be clipped to the body. The Mini Battery Pack may be used with the DaCapo rechargeable battery (up to 16 hours of use) or with an alkaline or rechargeable AAA battery. The Mini Battery Pack does include a three-prong Euro Port to allow DAI.

The OPUS 2 rechargeable batteries are charged in the DaCapo charger, which was specifically developed by MED-EL to charge DaCapo rechargeable batteries (Figure 11–12). MED-EL recommends that the DaCapo charger be plugged into a wall outlet, not a surge protector/strip. The DaCapo charger possesses an array of LED lights that indicate the status of the charging cycle (e.g., "charging," "full"). Four hours is required to charge a dead battery to a full charge. The DaCapo rechargeable battery has a nominal voltage capacity of 3.7 volts and may be charged over 500 times before replacement is necessary.

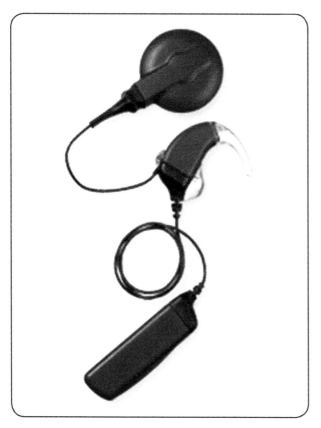

FIGURE 11–10. Children's Battery Pack. Image provided courtesy of MED-EL Corporation.

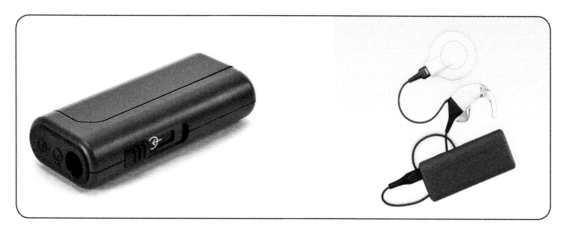

FIGURE 11–11. Mini Battery Pack. Image provided courtesy of MED-EL Corporation.

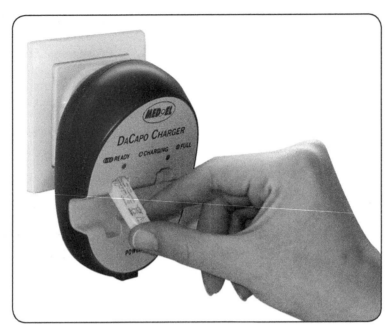

FIGURE 11–12. DaCapo Charger with rechargeable batteries. Image provided courtesy of MED-EL Corporation.

RONDO

The RONDO™, which was introduced in 2013, is the first-ever, single-unit external sound processor (Figure 11–13). The control unit, battery pack, and transmitting coil are integrated into one device. The RONDO™ was not designed to replace the OPUS 2 sound processor. It is an option that allows the recipient to wear the entire device on the head, but off of the ear. It was built on the same electronics/signal processing platform as the OPUS 2 (discussed below) and includes Automatic Sound Management and FineHearing Technology. In short, the RONDO™ can provide the same types of signal coding strategies and sound processing as the recipient uses with the OPUS 2 processor.

The RONDO™ has an omnidirectional microphone, and MED-EL recommends that the processor be placed so that the microphone is pointing straight up or straight down. That same placement is also recommended to promote optimal use of the telecoil. The RONDO™ does not contain external controls, such as a program switch or volume control. Instead, the recipient may use the FineTuner remote control to adjust the settings on the processor. Connectivity with accessories can be completed via the integrated telecoil or via direct connect (DAI) with the Mini Battery Pack and connection cable. For children, the

authors do not recommend the RONDO be used during sports or heavy activity due to the possibility of the device falling off during strenuous activity. However, MED-EL does offer a Sports Headband that has a pocket for the RONDO to improve device retention when patients are active (Figure 11–14). Increasing the magnet strength may help with retention but may be uncomfortable or cause complications to the skin flap if used for extended periods of time. The programming audiologist may adjust magnet strength by removing a cap on the RONDO processor and inserting a magnet with one of four different strengths. The RONDO also includes a protection sleeve and a place to which a retention cord may be attached to prevent the processor from being lost if it falls from the head. It should be noted that a diametric magnet is available for the RONDO for use with the SYNCHRONY implant.

Battery Options

The RONDO uses three 675 batteries that will provide up to five days or 90 hours of use. Currently, there is not a rechargeable battery option or DAI/FM receiver option unless the device is configured with an off-the-processor battery pack (mini battery pack) that uses one AAA alkaline battery or a DaCapo Rechargeable battery. Of note, the RONDO 2

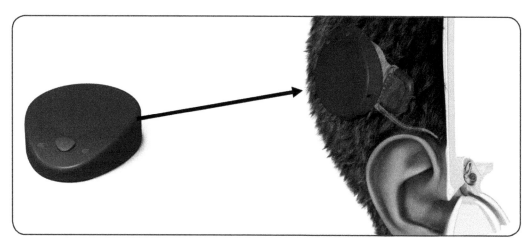

FIGURE 11–13. MED-EL RONDO sound processor. Image provided courtesy of MED-EL Corporation.

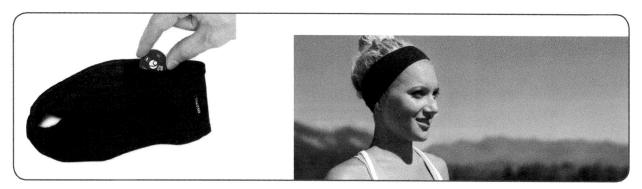

FIGURE 11–14. RONDO Sports Headband. Image provided courtesy of MED-EL Corporation.

has been announced in the global market but is not available in the United States at the time of this writing. The RONDO 2 sound processor has an integrated rechargeable battery that is charged on an induction charging platform and will offer a full day of use on one charge. The RONDO 2 rechargeable battery is anticipated to last five years.

FineTuner

MED-EL recipients may adjust their sound processor settings with a FineTuner remote control, which was the first remote control to be introduced into the cochlear implant industry. The FineTuner (Figure 11–15) allows the recipient to adjust the volume, change the microphone sensitivity, and select up to four user programs from up to approximately 2.5 feet away. The FineTuner uses near-field magnetic induction at a carrier frequency of approximately 9000 Hz to transmit information from the remote to the proces-

sor. Furthermore, the recipient may use the FineTuner to activate the integrated telecoil in a telecoil-only mode (T) or a telecoil-plus processor-microphone mode (MT). The FineTuner can be used to make unilateral or bilateral adjustments to the processor.

It is quite simple to synchronize the FineTuner to one or both of a recipient's processors. The audiologist or recipient must simply turn off the SONNET, RONDO, or OPUS 2 sound processor, place the DL Coil/D-coil/RONDO over the MT key of the FineTuner, and then turn the processor on. Two amber indicator lights will blink briefly to indicate successful synchronization.

When using the SONNET/OPUS 2, the FineTuner only needs to be synced for the first fit, when using a new processor, or when receiving a replacement FineTuner. When using the RONDO processor, the remote needs to be resynced any time a new configuration is programmed into the device. For purposes of ease of use and safety, the buttons of the FineTuner can be locked manually or programmed (within the programming software) to disable certain features/settings.

Additional features in MED-EL systems

There are several additional features in MED-EL external sound processors, such as private alerts, Sound-

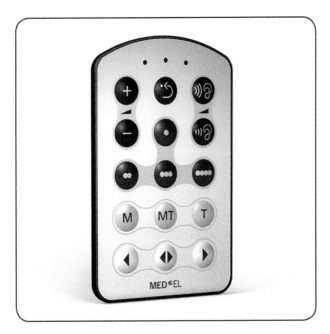

FIGURE 11–15. MED-EL FineTuner. Image provided courtesy of MED-EL Corporation.

Guard, and IRIS™. Private alerts may be enabled by the audiologist to signal that setting changes have been made or to alert the patient that the battery is low (in OPUS 2 sound processors and later). Sound-Guard monitors against electrostatic discharge (ESD) and when detected will discontinue stimulation, and the LED light will flash. The processor can be rebooted and the device will be restored to its settings, usually with no need for reprogramming. The IRIS™, which stands for Individual Recognition of Implant System, ensures that only the correct ear is stimulated. Of note IRIS is unavailable for use with COMBI 40+ cochlear implants and TEMPO+ sound processors.

Another novel aspect to this processor is the OPUS 2 FM Battery Pack Cover with a three-pin Europlug port (Figure 11–16), When this battery cover is in use, the Europort plug is located at the base of the processor. It enables wireless coupling of a personal digital RF/FM receiver (e.g., Phonak Roger X, Phonak MLxi, Oticon Amigo R2) to the processor. Additionally, the recipient may connect a specialized audio cable to the Europlug port to allow connection to personal audio devices, such as MP3 players, laptop computers, handheld video game consoles, mobile telephones, and so forth. Two different specialized audio cables are available: a yellow cable is used to obtain a 50/50 mixing ratio (50% input from processor microphone and 50% input from auxiliary device for use with an MP3 player or phone), and a red cable is used when the recipient chooses to primarily focus on the auxiliary input (90/10 mixing ratio

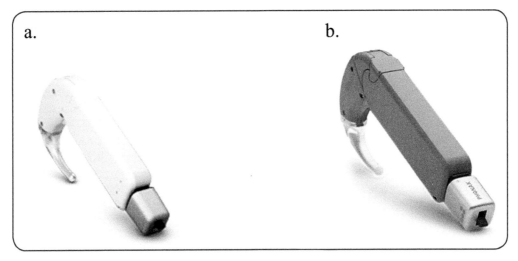

FIGURE 11–16. **A.** SONNET FM Battery Cover; **B.** OPUS 2 FM Battery Cover. Images provided courtesy of MED-EL Corporation.

with 90% input from the auxiliary device and 10% from the sound processor microphone). A bilateral audio Y-cable is available to allow bilateral recipients to connect personal audio devices to both of their implant processors.

An additional hearing assistance technology option is use of an induction neckloop via the T-coil. The recipient may use the FineTuner to select between telecoil only (T) use or a 50/50 mix of the telecoil and microphone (MT). MED-EL offers an interactive assistive listening device database on its website.

SYNCHRONY Cochlear Implant

The MED-EL SYNCHRONY (Mi1200) cochlear implant was approved for commercial use by the FDA in 2015. The SYNCHRONY is a small, low-profile cochlear implant, which makes it attractive for use with infants and other recipients with thin skull depth (Figure 11–17). The SYNCHRONY is composed of a titanium case that houses the electronics package and a gold-wired receiving/transmitting coil, which is encased in a silicone insulation. The SYNCHRONY possesses several unique features. It contains two titanium fixation pins at the base of the underneath side of the titanium case. These pins are designed to facilitate stabilization of the implant in place at the skull because they are inserted into two small holes that the surgeon drills into the bone. Additionally, the SYNCHRONY contains a magnet which is diametrically magnetized. In a typical disk-shaped magnet, the poles of the magnet are oriented axially, meaning that one pole is located at the top side of the disk (e.g., like the "heads" side of a coin), whereas the opposite pole is located at the bottom side (e.g., the "tails" side of a coin). When an axial magnet is subjected to a strong magnetic field, such as exists in an MRI, the magnet is attracted and repelled along the direction of its axis, which results in the magnet being lifted in an up and down direction. This lifting motion is referred to as magnetic torque. Movement of an axial magnet in a direction that is perpendicular to its axis places stress on the skin flap overlying the implant and is potentially painful for the recipient and damaging to the skin flap. It is worthwhile to note that all cochlear implants (not just those from MED-EL) are rated MRI Conditional, and it is vitally important that the manufacturer's instructions for MRI scanning be followed anytime a cochlear implant recipient must undergo MRI assessment. The manufacturer's recommendations for MRI assessment include factors such as patient positioning in the scanner, specific limits on specific absorption rate (SAR), no use of the audio processor near the MRI machine, and so forth. Additionally, MED-EL recommended that recipients of earlier MED-EL implants not undergo MRI assessment until six months have passed after surgery (to allow for scar tissue to form around the implant), but that requirement was removed for recipients of the SYNCHRONY implant because there isn't a concern about torque on the implant with the diametric magnet. Of note, if an audiologist is uncertain of whether the recipient has a diametric or axial magnet, he/she may use the MED-EL magnet identifier card to visualize through the skin flap which magnet type is in the implant.

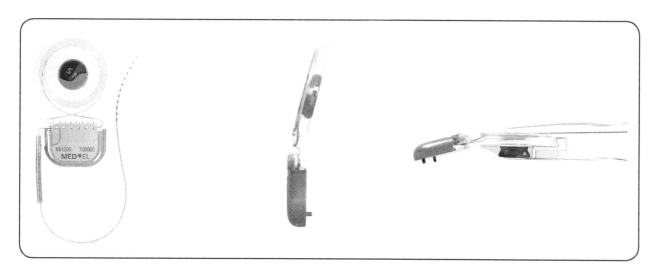

FIGURE 11–17. MED-EL SYNCHRONY (Mi1200) cochlear implant. Image provided courtesy of MED-EL Corporation.

The diametric magnetization of the SYNCHRONY magnet places the two magnetic poles on the curved surface area of the magnet and opposite one another (Figure 11–18). To envision the orientation of the magnetic poles of the SYNCHRONY magnet, the reader should think of a clock with one pole spanning from 12:00 to 6:00 and the opposite pole extending from 6:00 back to 12:00 (Stangl, 2015). When exposed to an external magnetic field, the diametrically magnetized SYNCHRONY magnet rotates within a hermetically sealed housing, with no lifting motion, which essentially eliminates torque (provided the patient is positioned in the scanner according to MRI scanning instructions from the manufacturer). As a result, an MRI may be completed with the magnet in place without patient discomfort and without the risk of damaging the implant or skin flap. The FDA has approved of the use of a 3.0 tesla (T) MRI without the need of removal of the magnet of the SYNCHRONY implant. Of note, the presence of the SYNCHRONY magnet will cast a shadow around the location of the magnet, so an MRI will not provide visualization of the cerebrum in the vicinity of the implant when the magnet is in place. If it is necessary to use MRI to minimize image distortion and to visualize the brain at a location near where the implant resides, a cochlear implant surgeon may remove the magnet from the underneath side of the SYNCHRONY. The fact that the magnet can only be removed from the underneath side of the implant makes it almost impossible for the magnet to be dislocated due to trauma.

The SYNCHRONY also features a sophisticated DSP with a powerful microchip and several electrode array options. For all MED-EL cochlear implants, a 12 MHz carrier frequency is used to transmit the signal from the sound processor to the internal device. The SYNCHRONY cochlear implant allows for a total maximum stimulation rate of 50,704 pulses per second. It has independent output circuits for each channel, enabling precise delivery of stimulation and providing the capability for simultaneous activation of channels. In addition, each channel has independent output capacitors for safety purposes. The independent output circuits allow for simultaneous presentation of stimulation on as few as 2 and as many as 12 channels. Sequential non-overlapping stimulation may also be delivered to minimize the potential for channel interaction. The SYNCHRONY utilizes a digital Hilbert transformation to extract the spectral and temporal properties of the input audio signal. The analysis bands are overlapping with bell-shaped filter skirts, which allow for the provision of a "virtual channel effect." The independent output circuits may generate electrical pulses with a current amplitude ranging from 0 to 1200 microamperes and a pulse width ranging from 2.1 to 425 microseconds. Of note, the SYNCHRONY (and all MED-EL i100 cochlear implants) is capable of delivering biphasic and triphasic electrical pulses.

MED-EL cochlear implants are made available with a number of different electrode array options, which are discussed in the section below. MED-EL cochlear implants possess two extracochlear electrode contacts, a primary return (or reference) electrode and a secondary reference electrode (i.e., ECAP/ART measures). Both of these extracochlear

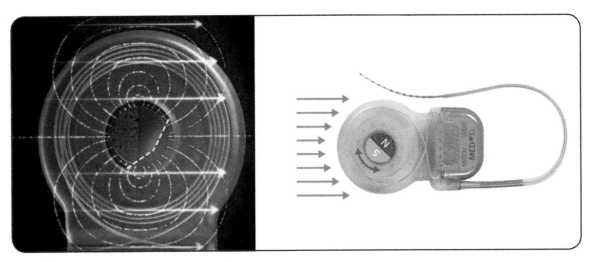

FIGURE 11–18. Image showing the orientation of the magnet poles of the diametric magnet. Image provided courtesy of MED-EL Corporation.

electrode contacts are located on the titanium casing of the implant (however, it should be noted that the reference electrode for the PULSAR CI^{100} is located on a secondary remote lead and positioned under the temporalis muscle). The reference electrode is used for recording the electrically evoked compound action potential via Auditory nerve Response Telemetry (ART). Finally, the SYNCHRONY cochlear implant contains the Unique Implant ID (Individual Recognition of Implant System [IRIS]) system, which prevents stimulation from a processor programmed for the opposite ear or for another recipient.

MED-EL Electrode Array Options

MED-EL offers the largest selection of electrode options within the implant industry, some of which are shown in Figure 11–19. These electrode options are designed to accommodate different cochlear duct lengths and to provide "complete cochlear coverage" for all recipients. The newest electrode array options include the FLEX series, released in 2012, and the FORM series, which is not commercially available in the United States at the time of this writing but is available in many countries. Also, traditional electrode array options make up the "Classic Series" and include the Standard, Medium, Compressed, and Split electrodes. All MED-EL electrode arrays contain 12 stimulating sites, which are made of oval-shaped intracochlear electrode contacts. The stimulating sites consist of two configurations: (1) one oval-shaped intracochlear electrode contact or (2) two oval-shaped intracochlear electrode contacts that are paired together to form one stimulating site. Although differences exist in the physical properties of the different MED-EL electrode arrays, two common themes of all MED-EL electrode arrays are: (1) the length of a MED-EL electrode array is generally longer than the electrode arrays of other manufacturers, and (2) all MED-EL electrode arrays are lateral wall electrode arrays.

MED-EL FLEX Series

The FLEX series includes the most modern electrodes options available for the majority of MED-EL recipients. The unique characteristics of FLEX electrode technology are as follows:

1. The seven most basal stimulating sites each consist of pairs of oval-shaped electrodes, which is similar to what is found in the MED-EL Standard Array of the Classic Series. However, the five most apical stimulating sites consist of just one electrode contact, which enhances the flaccidity and reduces the cross-sectional diameter of the apical end of the array.

2. The diameter of the FLEX Array is narrow at the apical tip of the array and increases at the basal end where the electrode array resides in the round window or cochleostomy. This tapered design, which is shown in Figure 11–20, allows for increased mechanical flexibility at the tip of the array, an increase in the potential to insert the array into the narrow lumen of the most apical region of the scala tympani, which becomes narrower as one progresses from the base to the apex, and an increase in the surgeon's ease of handling the electrode array at the basal end.

3. The wires in the FLEX series of MED-EL electrode arrays are configured in a wave-shaped pattern, which further enhances its flexibility and promotes an atraumatic insertion (see Figure 11–20).

The FLEX electrode array is offered in four variants (Figure 11–21):

1. FLEXSOFT or FLEX31: The total length from the apical tip to the marker positioned at the cochleostomy is 31.5 mm. The 12 stimulating sites are arranged across 26.4 mm, resulting in over 2 mm of spacing between stimulating sites. The cross-sectional diameter is 1.3 mm at the basal marker and 0.5 × 0.4 mm at the apical tip. The FLEXSOFT/FLEX31 is the longest electrode array in the FLEX series and is designed for a deep cochlear insertion to enable complete "cochlear coverage."

2. FLEX28: The total length from the apical tip to the marker positioned at the cochleostomy is 28 mm. The 12 stimulating sites are arranged across 23.1 mm, resulting in just under 2 mm of spacing between stimulating sites. The cross-sectional diameter is 0.8 mm at the basal marker and 0.5 × 0.4 mm at the apical tip. MED-EL notes that the FLEX28 electrode array is "suitable for 96% of normal cochlear anatomies" (Hardy, 1938; Lee, Nadol, & Eddington, 2010). It may also be beneficial for recipients who have substantial residual hearing at 500 Hz and below with severe to profound hearing loss of 750 Hz and above. In this case, the FLEX 28 may allow for a better opportunity for hearing preservation in the low frequencies.

3. FLEX24: The total length from the apical tip to the marker positioned at the cochleostomy is 24 mm.

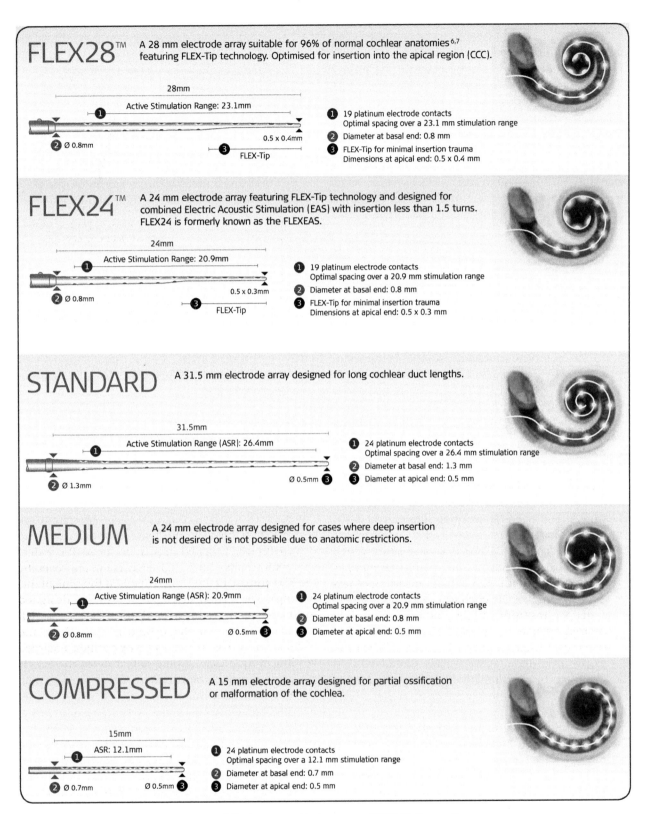

FLEX28™ A 28 mm electrode array suitable for 96% of normal cochlear anatomies[6,7] featuring FLEX-Tip technology. Optimised for insertion into the apical region (CCC).

28mm

Active Stimulation Range: 23.1mm

① ② Ø 0.8mm ③ 0.5 x 0.4mm FLEX-Tip

① 19 platinum electrode contacts
Optimal spacing over a 23.1 mm stimulation range
② Diameter at basal end: 0.8 mm
③ FLEX-Tip for minimal insertion trauma
Dimensions at apical end: 0.5 x 0.4 mm

FLEX24™ A 24 mm electrode array featuring FLEX-Tip technology and designed for combined Electric Acoustic Stimulation (EAS) with insertion less than 1.5 turns. FLEX24 is formerly known as the FLEXEAS.

24mm

Active Stimulation Range: 20.9mm

① ② Ø 0.8mm ③ 0.5 x 0.3mm FLEX-Tip

① 19 platinum electrode contacts
Optimal spacing over a 20.9 mm stimulation range
② Diameter at basal end: 0.8 mm
③ FLEX-Tip for minimal insertion trauma
Dimensions at apical end: 0.5 x 0.3 mm

STANDARD A 31.5 mm electrode array designed for long cochlear duct lengths.

31.5mm

Active Stimulation Range (ASR): 26.4mm

① ② Ø 1.3mm Ø 0.5mm ③

① 24 platinum electrode contacts
Optimal spacing over a 26.4 mm stimulation range
② Diameter at basal end: 1.3 mm
③ Diameter at apical end: 0.5 mm

MEDIUM A 24 mm electrode array designed for cases where deep insertion is not desired or is not possible due to anatomic restrictions.

24mm

Active Stimulation Range (ASR): 20.9mm

① ② Ø 0.8mm Ø 0.5mm ③

① 24 platinum electrode contacts
Optimal spacing over a 20.9 mm stimulation range
② Diameter at basal end: 0.8 mm
③ Diameter at apical end: 0.5 mm

COMPRESSED A 15 mm electrode array designed for partial ossification or malformation of the cochlea.

15mm

ASR: 12.1mm

① ② Ø 0.7mm Ø 0.5mm ③

① 24 platinum electrode contacts
Optimal spacing over a 12.1 mm stimulation range
② Diameter at basal end: 0.7 mm
③ Diameter at apical end: 0.5 mm

FIGURE 11–19. MED-EL electrode array portfolio. Image provided courtesy of MED-EL Corporation.

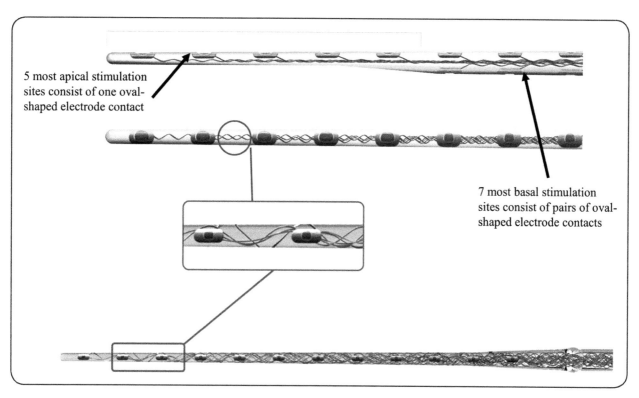

5 most apical stimulation sites consist of one oval-shaped electrode contact

7 most basal stimulation sites consist of pairs of oval-shaped electrode contacts

FIGURE 11–20. Close-up of MED-EL FLEX array showing tapered design, zig-zag leads, and electrode sites with single-electrode contacts versus paired-electrode contacts. Image provided courtesy of MED-EL Corporation.

The 12 stimulating sites are arranged across 20.9 mm, resulting in over 1.5 mm of spacing between stimulating sites. The cross-sectional diameter is 0.8 mm at the basal marker and 0.5 × 0.3 mm at the apical tip. The FLEX24 was originally referred to as the FLEXEAS array and is designed for electric-acoustic stimulation with an insertion of less than 1.5 turns of the cochlea or situations where a deeper insertion might not be achieved or desired, such as reimplantation in a patient who previously used another manufacturer's shorter electrode array.

4. FLEX20: The total length from the apical tip to the marker positioned at the cochleostomy is 20 mm. The 12 stimulating sites are arranged across 15.4 mm, resulting in just under 1.5 mm of spacing between stimulating sites. The cross-sectional diameter is 0.8 mm at the basal marker and 0.5 × 0.3 mm at the apical tip. The FLEX20 is designed for electric-acoustic stimulation for persons with considerably functional low-frequency hearing and high-frequency deafness (i.e., 1500 Hz and above).

MED-EL FORM Series

The electrode arrays in the MED-EL FORM series each contain 24 platinum, oval-shaped intracochlear electrode contacts arranged in pairs to form 12 physical stimulation sites (the FORM series is not approved by the FDA for use in the United States at the time of this writing). The FORM electrode arrays are designed for malformed cochleae and for cases in which extrusion of perilymphatic fluid is likely from the cochleostomy (e.g., common cavity cochlea, enlarged vestibular aqueduct). A unique feature of the FORM electrode arrays is the inclusion of the SEAL, which is an integrated enlargement of silicone (1.9 mm in diameter) that is just proximal to the base of the electrode array that serves as a stopper to close off the cochlear opening to prevent leakage of perilymphatic fluid and to prevent the electrode array from being inserted beyond a certain point into the cochlea. The FORM array is available in two different variants:

1. FORM24: The total length of the array is 24 mm from the base of the SEAL to the apical tip. The

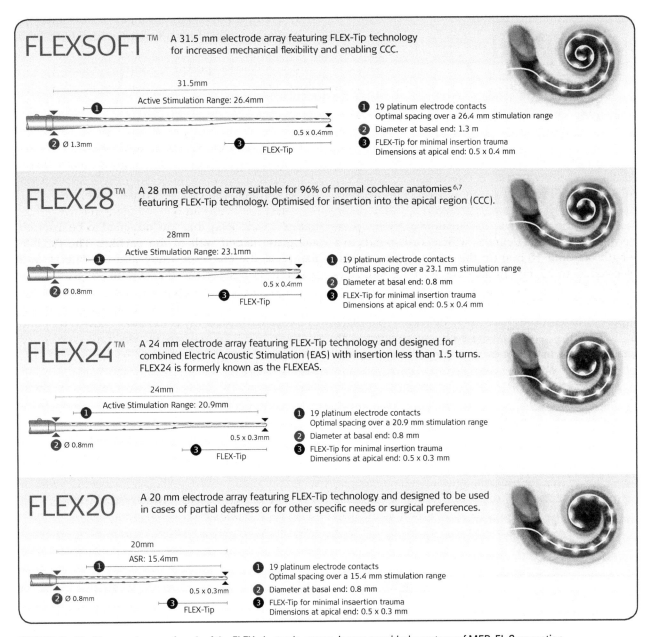

FIGURE 11–21. Close-up image of each of the FLEX electrode arrays. Image provided courtesy of MED-EL Corporation.

12 stimulating sites are arranged across 18.7 mm (Active Stimulating Range [ASR]), resulting in almost 1.5 mm of spacing between stimulating sites. The cross-sectional diameter is 0.8 mm at the base of the SEAL and 0.5 mm at the apical tip. The FORM24 is intended for use in open (i.e., no cochlear ossification or obliteration) or malformed cochleae and in cases in which perilymphatic leakage is possible.

2. FORM 19: The total length of the array is 19 mm from the base of the SEAL to the apical tip. The 12 stimulating sites are arranged across 14.3 mm (ASR), resulting in just over 1.0 mm of spacing between stimulating sites. The cross-sectional diameter is 0.8 mm at the base of the SEAL and 0.5 mm at the apical tip. The FORM19 is intended for use in malformed cochleae (e.g., Mondini's aplasia, common cavity), obstructed cochleae (e.g., ossified/obliterated cochleae), and in cases in which perilymphatic leakage is possible.

Classic Electrode Array Series

The Classic electrode array series consists of three electrode arrays, the STANDARD, the MEDIUM, and the COMPRESSED arrays. The unique and potentially beneficial aspect of the Standard MED-EL electrode array is that it is designed to be inserted much deeper than electrode arrays developed by other manufacturers. For example, the Standard Array has a 31.5-mm array length from the apical tip to the seal placed in the cochleostomy and is intended to be inserted to an angular insertion depth of about 630 degrees. Conventional electrode arrays offered by other manufacturers typically are inserted to an angular insertion depth of 420 to 540 degrees, which corresponds to a length of about 18 mm (in the case of perimodiolar electrodes) to 25 mm (in the case of lateral wall electrodes). For electrode arrays inserted to an angular insertion depth of 450 to 540 degrees, low-frequency inputs (150 to 500 Hz) are likely delivered to a place in the cochlea that is innervated by nerve fibers with characteristic frequencies that are several hundred Hz higher than the frequency of the original sound (Landsberger et al., 2015, 2016; Prentiss, Staecker, & Wolford, 2014; Schatzer et al., 2014). Deeper insertion of the electrode array (i.e., 31.5 mm/630 degree angular insertion depth) may provide more favorable access to low-frequency sounds because low-frequency stimulation will be provided to cochlear nerve fibers that have characteristic frequencies corresponding to those of the input sounds (Hochmair et al., 2015; Prentiss, Staecker, & Wolford, 2014). The longer length and deeper insertion of the STANDARD

array is one of the components of MED-EL's attempt to provide complete cochlear coverage along with fine structural cues. Of note, the FLEX 28 is similar in length (28 mm vs. the 31 mm for the STANDARD) and allows for deep cochlear coverage for most recipients. When MED-EL moved from the Classic series to the FLEX series, there was also a parallel change in surgical practice from the use of a cochleostomy to the use of the round window for electrode insertion. Use of the round window results in a slightly greater insertion depth (e.g., a few mm), so a FLEX 28 achieves full insertion in the vast majority of cochleae.

The STANDARD array is a straight, relatively flexible electrode array that was designed to be inserted along the lateral wall of the cochlea. The flexible nature of the electrode array and the lateral wall insertion is designed to facilitate hearing preservation and a reduction in trauma to the delicate structures in the scala media. The cross-sectional diameter of the STANDARD array is relatively narrow (0.5 mm at the tip and 1.3 mm where the electrode is designed to rest in the round window or cochleostomy). The narrow diameter allows for a round window insertion. In fact, MED-EL promotes the use of a round window insertion to facilitate delivery into the scala tympani and to reduce cochlear trauma. Other characteristics of the STANDARD array include 24 oval-shaped platinum electrode contacts that are arranged in pairs to form 12 stimulating sites (Figure 11–22). As stated previously, the STANDARD array is 31.5 mm in length from the apical tip of the electrode array to the seal, which resides at the round window or cochleostomy; however, the 12 stimulating sites are arranged

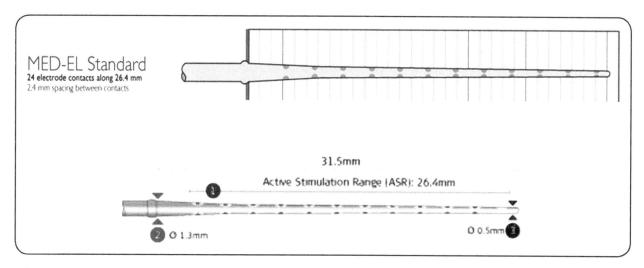

FIGURE 11–22. Close-up of the MED-EL Standard electrode array. Image provided courtesy of MED-EL Corporation.

26.4 mm across the array (beginning approximately 1 mm from the tip). This allows for 2.4 mm of spacing between each stimulating site, which is greater than what exists for other electrode arrays in the implant industry. As a result, it is quite possible that less channel interaction is present for the STANDARD array relative to other implant electrode arrays.

The MEDIUM array's intracochlear electrode contacts span 20.9 mm across the array with a 1.9 mm space between each stimulating site. The MEDIUM array may be used when a deep insertion is not possible (e.g., shorter cochlear duct length, abnormal cochlear anatomy, such as a Mondini's dysplasia, fibrous tissue growth secondary to bacterial meningitis, reimplantation after previous use of another brand). Furthermore, the electrode contacts of the COMPRESSED array are placed 12.1 mm across the array with 1.1-mm spacing between sites. The COMPRESSED array is intended for recipients who have ossification or fibrous tissue growth in the cochlea.

Additional MED-EL Electrode Arrays

MED-EL offers the SPLIT array, which is designed for cases in which significant ossification exists in the cochlea and is available when requested by a cochlear implant surgeon (Figure 11–23). The 12 contact pairs are arranged on two separate electrode arrays that use the same spacing as the compressed array; seven electrode contact pairs (stimulation sites) are on one array and five electrode pairs are on the

other. When using this array, the surgeon must make two cochleostomy sites to insert one array into the upper-basal turn of the cochlea and the other into the lower-basal region. To be precise, the two cochleostomy sites are essentially two straight "tunnel drill-outs" that the surgeon makes in an ossified cochlea. With the SPLIT array, the audiologist must reorder the tonotopic arrangement of the bandpass filters at the initial programming, depending on which of the two electrode arrays was placed in the lower-basal turn and which was place in the upper turn of the cochlea.

MED-EL ABI Array

The MED-EL ABI array is a "paddle-shaped" electrode array designed to be placed on the auditory nuclei of the brainstem (i.e., cochlear nucleus in most cases or inferior colliculus in significant neural degeneration is present at the cochlear nuclei) (Figure 11–24). As the name implies, the ABI array is intended for use as an auditory brainstem implant (ABI). The ABI contains 12 stimulating electrode contacts and one reference contact, all of which are located on the paddle, which is 5.5 mm long and 3 mm wide. The paddle is held in place on the brainstem by a polyester mesh. At the time of this writing, the MED-EL ABI array is not approved by the FDA for commercial distribution in the United States, but it has been used in off-label cases under compassionate use clearance. The MED-EL ABI is used clinically in Europe and other countries outside of the United States.

Additional MED-EL Cochlear Implants

MED-EL CONCERT Internal Device

The MED-EL CONCERT (Mi1000) internal device (referred to as CONCERTO in countries outside the US, but will be referred to here as the CONCERT) was released in 2011 (Figure 11–25). The titanium case (i.e., physical dimensions), the transmitting coil, and the electronics package of the CONCERT is identical to that of the MED-EL SYNCHRONY. Of note, the casing of the CONCERT is 25% thinner than the casing of its predecessor, the SONATA TI[100]. Similar to the SYNCHRONY, a PIN variant is available that features two small pins positioned on the back of the CONCERT case and is intended to be inserted by the surgeon into the recipient's skull to facilitate better retention and to prevent lateral rotation at the point

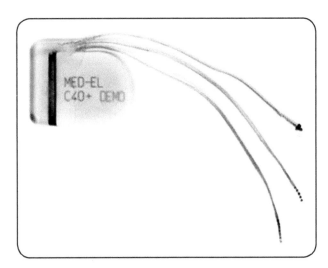

FIGURE 11–23. MED-EL Split electrode array. Image provided courtesy of MED-EL Corporation.

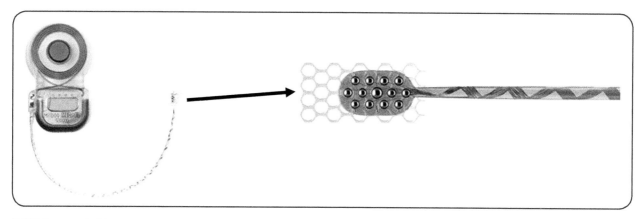

FIGURE 11–24. MED-EL ABI array. Image provided courtesy of MED-EL Corporation.

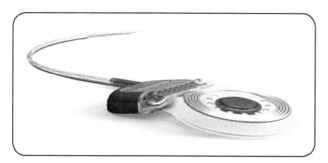

FIGURE 11–25. MED-EL CONCERT (Mi1000). Image provided courtesy of MED-EL Corporation.

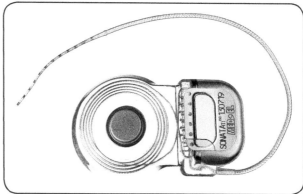

FIGURE 11–26. MED-EL SONATA TI^{100}. Image provided courtesy of MED-EL Corporation.

at which the CONCERT case contacts the skull. The CONCERT PIN is optional and selected based on the preference of the surgeon.

SONATA TI100 Internal Device

The SONATA TI^{100} was the first MED-EL internal device encased in titanium with a silicone covering over the receiving coil and case (Figure 11–26). The electronics package of the Sonata TI^{100} is identical to that of the SYNCHRONY and CONCERT. The primary difference between the CONCERT and the SONATA is that the latter is larger. Of note, the poles of magnets of the CONCERT, SONATA, and PULSAR are axially oriented and are FDA approved for 1.5T MRI scans without surgical removal of the internal magnet (MED-EL, 2013). Health care providers should follow MED-EL's recommendations for MRI scanning (i.e., tight compression bandage wrapped around the recipient's head [not required for SYNCHRONY

recipients], etc.) in order to ensure recipient safety and to uphold the manufacturer's warranty. These recommendations are available on MED-EL's website.

PULSAR CI100 Internal Device

Additionally, the MED-EL PULSAR CI^{100} has the same electronics as the SYNCHRONY, CONCERT, and SONATA implants, but the PULSAR electronics are housed in a ceramic casing (Figure 11–27). The PULSAR CI^{100} is slightly smaller than the SONATA TI^{100}. Although the titanium casing may improve durability and reduce the chance of failure due to impact trauma, the primary reason MED-EL introduced the titanium casing was to answer surgeons' requests for a housing that did not require being fully recessed in the skull. It should be noted that the MED-EL ceramic

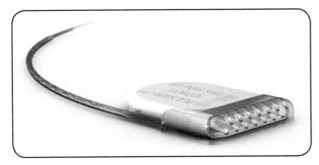

FIGURE 11–27. MED-EL PULSAR CI¹⁰⁰. Image provided courtesy of MED-EL Corporation.

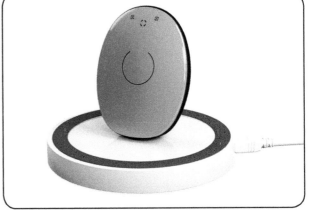

FIGURE 11–28. MED-EL RONDO 2 sound processor with RONDO 2 charging pad. Image provided courtesy of MED-EL Corporation.

case of the PULSAR CI¹⁰⁰ has a relatively low rate of failure and case fracture.

MED-EL RONDO 2 Sound Processor

At the time at which this textbook was headed to press, MED-EL announced the release of the RONDO 2, which is the second generation of MED-EL's single-unit, off-the-ear sound processor (Figure 11–28). The RONDO 2 is similar in design to its predecessor, the RONDO, but the RONDO 2 is smaller than the RONDO, and it contains an integrated rechargeable lithium-ion battery that may be charged by placing the RONDO 2 on a charging pad designed by MED-EL. According to MED-EL, a four-hour charging typically provides 18 hours of use. The rechargeable battery is expected to last more than five years. The Mini Battery Pack (with a AAA battery) may be connected to the RONDO 2 to provide a backup power option if the rechargeable battery is depleted.

The RONDO 2 contains one push button that allows the user to power on/off the sound processor. The RONDO 2 may be used with the Fine-Tuner remote control to select from up to four programs, adjust the volume and sensitivity settings, and activate/deactivate the built-in telecoil. The RONDO 2 contains an omnidirectional microphone and may be used with the MED-EL WaterWear accessory. The RONDO 2 may be used with all commercially available MED-EL signal coding strategies. Also, the RONDO 2 magnet is available in four strengths for use with both the SYNCHRONY implant and previous models of MED-EL cochlear implants. Finally, the RONDO 2 is available in multiple colors and may be used with a variety of different covers that alter the external appearance of the sound processor.

Key Concepts

- MED-EL offers a variety of sound processors to meet the unique needs of children and adults who have received MED-EL cochlear implants. MED-EL recipients may choose from ear-level or head-worn sound processors. Adapters may be used so that ear-level processors may also be worn on the head or body.
- MED-EL sound processors are equipped with adaptive signal processing designed to improve hearing performance in challenging listening situations.
- MED-EL sound processors are equipped to allow the user to connect to hearing assistive technologies via a telecoil or a special FM battery cover.
- MED-EL offers a variety of different cochlear implants and electrode arrays to meet the unique needs of recipients. Surgeons may select from lateral wall electrode arrays of different lengths, stiffness, and conventional cross-sectional diameters.

References

Franz, D. (2015). MRI trends and the MED-EL SYNCHRONY cochlear implant. *AudiologyOnline*, August 17, 2015. Retrieved from http://www.audiologyonline.com/interviews/mri-trends-and-med-el-15071

Hardy, M. (1938). The length of the organ of Corti in man. *American Journal of Anatomy, 62,* 291–311.

Hochmair, I., Hochmair, E., Nopp, P., Waller, M., & Jolly, C. (2015). Deep electrode insertion and sound coding in cochlear implants. *Hearing Research, 322,* 14–23.

Landsberger, D. M., Svrakic, M., Roland, J. T., Jr., & Svirsky, M. (2015). The relationship between insertion angles, default frequency allocations, and spiral ganglion place pitch in cochlear implants. *Ear and Hearing, 36*(5), e207–e213.

Landsberger, D. M., Vermeire, K., Claes, A., Van Rompaey, V., & Van de Heyning, P. (2016). Qualities of single electrode stimulation as a function of rate and place of stimulation with a cochlear implant. *Ear and Hearing, 37*(3), e149–e159.

Lee, J., Nadol, J.B., & Eddington, D.K. (2010). Depth of electrode insertion and postoperative performance in humans with cochlear implants: A histopathologic study. *Audiology and Neurootology, 15*(5), 323–331.

Prentiss, S., Staecker, H., & Wolford, B. (2014). Ipsilateral acoustic electric pitch matching: A case study of cochlear implantation in an up-sloping hearing loss with preserved hearing across multiple frequencies. *Cochlear Implants International, 15*(3), 161–165.

Schatzer, R., Vermeire, K., Visser, D., Krenmayr, A., Kals, M., Voormolen, M., . . . Zierhofer, C. (2014). Electric-acoustic pitch comparisons in single-sided-deaf cochlear implant users: frequency-place functions and rate pitch. *Hearing Research, 309,* 26–35.

12

Medical and Surgical Aspects of Cochlear Implantation

R. Stanley Baker

Introduction

The purpose of this chapter is to provide a basic over-view of the medical and surgical aspects related to cochlear implantation. In order to effectively under-stand the basic principles of cochlear implant surgery, a student should observe an actual cochlear implant (CI) surgery. Instead of providing still shot images of the different stages of cochlear implant surgery, a cochlear implant surgery with an adult recipient was video recorded, and the video of that surgery is available as a supplement to this chapter.

The CI Surgeon

Surgeons who perform CI surgery have a background in otolaryngology (ENT) and then advanced train-ing in otology and neurotology. The scope of the CI surgeon's role will vary from one case to the next, depending on what is needed for a given patient, and will vary from one CI program to the next, depend-ing on the experience and expertise of the other professionals on the CI team. Some CI surgeons are fortunate to have a close working relationship with experienced, compassionate, and expert audiologists and speech language therapists. In an interdisciplin-ary setting, the surgeon's role for routine cases can be limited to making the initial evaluation, monitoring

the ongoing workup, reassuring the patient/parents, reviewing scan images, and performing the surgical procedure. This type of patient- and family-centered team approach is most important for young children with hearing loss. In other practice settings, typi-cally serving only adult patients with hearing loss, the CI surgeon may work with an audiologist who does part-time CI work, as well as non-CI audiology work. In this setting, the surgeon may need to see the prospective CI patient more often and take a more active role in the evaluation process, especially in counseling the patient and family.

In addition to the medical evaluation and surgi-cal procedure, the CI surgeon should be able to antic-ipate problems and identify issues that might arise on the path to a successful CI patient outcome. These issues include initiating pneumococcal vaccinations early in the evaluation, anticipating health insur-ance coverage problems so that precertification and insurance authorizations will be successful, and coor-dinating any general anesthetics needed for tympa-nostomy tubes, auditory brainstem responses (ABRs), and scans. Identifying undermanaged general health issues may also be important. The CI surgeon's role also includes inspiring confidence and providing reassurance for patients, parents, and families, who might be emotionally challenged by the new diagno-sis of hearing loss and frightened by the prospect of surgery. The responsibility for frank and sometimes difficult discussions about surgery or challenging cases is also part of the CI surgeon's role.

Medical Evaluation

The medical evaluation may be different for patients in the various age categories, from infants to older children, adults, to elderly patients.

History

All medical evaluations begin with a good history, and the pertinent issues will be different for patients of various ages. For *infants*, pregnancy and perinatal issues that might suggest cytomegalovirus (CMV), jaundice, or undiagnosed meningitis need to be explored. The family history may need to consider issues that could suggest syndromal hearing loss, such as family members with facial features of Waardenburg's, family members with a combination of hearing and vision loss suggesting Usher's syndrome, history of family members with syncope or sudden cardiac death that might suggest Jervell and Lange–Nielsen syndrome, and so forth. It should be noted that the process and expense of consultations and testing to rule out relatively uncommon syndromal hearing loss diagnoses can become a burden on the parents of young children with hearing loss. It may be helpful to identify a geneticist who can efficiently work through the syndromal and genetic hearing loss issues at a later date. This allows the family to stay focused on the important task of fitting and maintaining a trial hearing aid fitting, so as to be ready for early cochlear implant surgery, if needed.

When *older children* develop severe-profound hearing loss, these tend to be cases of progressive hearing loss with enlarged vestibular aqueduct syndrome (EVAS), progressive CMV hearing loss, and auditory neuropathy spectrum disorder (ANSD). Occasionally, older children may present a case of delayed diagnosis of hearing loss, which creates a serious urgency for intervention.

For *adults*, the most efficient gathering of historical information may be done after reviewing the current audiogram or, ideally, serial audiograms. An informed family member may be helpful if the patient's hearing loss compromises the interview process. In this age group, a history of acute dizzy spells might lead to investigation of vestibular disorders. Smokers may need cessation counseling. If the patient is on anticoagulants, this may need to be discussed with the prescribing physician, to determine the relative risk of stopping the medication for CI surgery. It may also be helpful to note the presence or absence of "speech-reading" skills that partially compensate for a severe-profound hearing loss. The articulation features of "deaf speech" may reveal the likelihood of pre-linguistic hearing loss.

Issues to be explored with *elderly patients* (and hopefully an informed family member) include whether hearing remediation presents an opportunity to preserve independent living. If cognitive limitations are prominent, this may limit the rehabilitation potential for cochlear implantation. Estimating the duration for high-frequency hearing loss may identify a limitation for CI potential. More than 30 years of high-frequency loss can be associated with atrophic changes in the central auditory pathways that result in poor speech understanding with a CI. Securing family support for the surgery aftercare is important if the patient's mobility and dexterity are limited. The same family members may need to be involved in learning to use the external CI components. Older patients may not drive, and so transportation may need to be secured for medical and audiology appointments. General medical issues that might present perioperative risks should be explored, and consultation with the primary care physician or cardiologist may be needed. Older patients often have a cardiac pacemaker that mandates anticoagulation and excludes the possibility of an MRI scan.

Physical Exam

The CI medical examination begins in the clinic and continues with imaging procedures—CT and/or MRI. Examination of infants should include a focus on possible physical stigmata of syndromal hearing loss. Otoscopic findings of ear canal abnormalities should be noted. Middle ear disease is common in children, and it is important to use pneumatic otoscopy to find middle ear fluid that might add to the child's hearing loss or complicate CI surgery. In older children, tonsil and adenoid problems as well as allergic rhinitis tendencies may be identified. In adults and elderly patients, assessing the middle ear status with pneumatic otoscopy and otomicroscopy is also important, and anatomical signs of previous otologic surgery should be noted. In young children, the curvature of the postauricular skull may affect the space or location on the skull that is available to place a CI, and parents may need to know this. In adults, scalp lesions and possible skin cancers may need to be considered. Scars from previous otosurgery or a facelift may affect the planned location for a CI surgery incision.

Imaging studies are crucial in the medical/surgical evaluation. Otologic surgeons tend to like the bone structural information provided by CT scans that can reveal important anatomical factors, such as: the extent of mastoid bone pneumatization, large emissary veins, prominent sigmoid sinus or jugular bulb, facial recess density, and facial nerve displacement. Otic capsule anomalies and structural problems, including enlarged vestibular aqueduct (EVA), modiolar defects, cochlear duct obstruction, and cochlear otosclerosis are also seen on CT scans. CT scans require radiation, and this should be considered, especially in children. Modern CT scan techniques minimize the x-ray exposure.

MRI scans are typically more lengthy procedures and often require a general anesthetic in children. Some adults become claustrophobic inside the MRI machine and may need sedation. Nevertheless, critical diagnostic information is provided by MRI scans when cochlear nerve deficiency or tumors such as acoustic neuroma are suspected. Although post CI MRI scans are more feasible in recent years, it is still a difficult and often uncomfortable procedure. This makes a pre-op MRI evaluation seem like the last good opportunity for a scan that might yield important incidental findings or useful baseline information for the future. The reader is referred to Chapter 13 for a more detailed discussion of considerations pertaining to imaging of the auditory system for cochlear implant candidates.

The CI Operation

The CI operation is typically a one- to two-hour outpatient procedure done under general anesthetic, with a low risk of problems or complications. In comparison to some other otologic and neurotologic surgeries, the typical CI operation is a more predictable and often less stressful procedure. Nevertheless, a series of technical points must be understood and precisely executed in order to minimize the chance of problems and maximize the patient's hearing outcome.

It can be useful for other nonsurgical members of the CI team to observe a CI operation in order to have a good understanding of what happens. Prospective CI patients and families typically develop a good rapport with their CI audiologist and will inevitably ask questions about upcoming CI surgery.

In simple terms, the surgical procedure begins with a postauricular incision and making a place to seat the receiver/stimulator (R/S the main component

of the implant). Then a sequence of progressively smaller openings are made—first, an opening into the skull (the mastoidectomy), then an opening from the mastoid into the middle ear (the facial recess), then finally an opening from the middle ear into the cochlea (the cochleostomy). When the surgical dissection work is completed, the receiver/stimulator (R/S) is positioned, the electrode is inserted, and the incision is closed.

The anatomical location of the facial nerve places the facial nerve directly in the "surgical field" during CI surgery. To find the "facial recess" opening from the mastoid into the middle ear, the facial nerve is identified and it defines one side of the triangular shaped facial recess. In order to best protect the facial nerve, a facial nerve monitor is used to detect any "stimulation" of the nerve that might occur while removing bone from near the nerve or while reaching through the facial recess to work in the middle ear. The facial nerve monitor uses very small transdermal needles in the face to detect the electrical activity that would result from nerve stimulation.

Before starting the operation, the anticipated location on the head for the R/S package is determined and marked in a way that can lead to placing it in the same position on the skull, once the scalp flaps are elevated. Considerations for where the receiver/stimulator is positioned include: a relatively flat area on the skull that is close to the ear, but not so close as to cause a bulge that interferes with the external processor and eyeglasses. In the unlikely event of a post-surgery breakdown in the closure of the skin incision, keeping the R/S at least 1 cm away from the incision can protect it from exposure. Such exposure would likely require removal of the R/S and revision surgery. The "scalp flaps" are the areas of scalp on either side of the incision which are raised off the skull and later returned to cover the implant and cover over the newly emptied mastoidectomy space. Once the scalp flaps are elevated and retracted, the CI surgeon identifies "landmarks" that guide a location for opening the mastoid bone with an otologic drill. Irrigation fluid and surgical suction are used to remove the bone chips and dust and to prevent excess heating from the drilling process. The bone in and near the mastoid will have different densities and texture. Ideally, the mastoid is well "pneumatized" with spongy bone that has air containing small "sinus like" spaces lined by healthy mucosal membranes. However, the mastoid can be densely "sclerotic" if childhood ear and mastoid infections occurred, and the mucosa can be thick or inflamed. In younger children, parts of the mastoid usually contain bone marrow.

At some point in the bone-drilling work, the surgeon may also create a "trough" in the bone adjacent to the mastoid cavity. This trough will be the location for the proximal part of the electrode where it is attached to the R/S. As drilling progresses deeper in the mastoid, anatomical landmarks are identified until the facial nerve and its chorda tympani branch are visible. These two nerves define two sides of the triangular shaped "facial recess" which is the passageway from the mastoid into the middle ear. Working through the facial recess, the round window membrane is exposed. Sometimes the visibility of the membrane is improved by removing small areas of "bony overhang" using a small diamond bur on the otologic drill.

There are different techniques for making the opening from the middle ear into the cochlea. Depending on the patient's anatomy, the electrode type, and the surgeon's preference, the opening for the electrode to pass into the scala tympani of the cochlea may be in the round window membrane or through a cochleostomy that is separate from and just inferior to the round window membrane. Some surgeons prefer a compromise between these two and call it an "extended round window cochleostomy."

After all this dissection, drilling, and preparation, the R/S is placed in position and secured to prevent subsequent "migration." Like any surgical implant, after weeks to months of "healing," the R/S will be surrounded by a "capsule" of scar tissue that holds it firmly in place. Meanwhile, depending on the shape of the R/S and surgeon's preference, a tight pocket under the scalp and a "bone recess" may secure the R/S. Sometimes a "tie-down" suture is used and the suture may be anchored in the tough covering of the bone or passed through holes drilled in the bone.

Various means of passing the electrode array into the cochlea are used, depending on the type of electrode and the surgeon's preference. In recent years, more attention has been focused on minimizing "insertion trauma" that would damage the delicate parts of the cochlea and induce postoperative inflammation and fibrosis. Insertion of the active electrode into the scala tympani duct of the cochlea is usually followed by gently positioning and packing soft tissue around the electrode, at the cochleostomy, so as to result in a "tissue seal" that protects the cochlea from any infection that might subsequently occur in the middle ear. The extra length of the proximal part of the electrode is then coiled into a favorable position in the mastoidectomy space. The scalp flaps are returned to position over the mastoid and over the R/S. Then the skin closure is done.

At some point after electrode placement, electrical testing of the CI and/or an x-ray may be done to confirm the integrity of the implant and the location of the active electrode in the cochlea. If a problem is detected, the option of repositioning the electrode is available before leaving the operating room suite. A pressure bandage is typically applied before leaving the operating room. The pressure of the bandage may help keep fluid or blood from accumulating beneath the scalp flaps and absorbs any discharge from the incision.

Manufacturer/Electrode Selection

For typical CI cases, most surgeons defer to audiologist and patient preference for device selection. In certain cases, such as otic capsule anomalies, postmeningitic ossification, hearing preservation priorities, and revision surgeries, manufacturer selection and electrode options may be mandated by those considerations. These cases can be a good opportunity for collaborative discussion in cochlear implant team staffing sessions.

Hearing Preservation

As the field of CI has progressed, electrode developments and refined surgical techniques have allowed the preservation of low-frequency hearing to become a reasonable expectation. FDA approval of "hybrid cochlear implants" has made "electroacoustic hearing" a clinical reality. Preserving hair cells and neural elements in the cochlea yields better CI hearing results. Preserving low-frequency hearing opens up CI options to a broader range of hearing loss patients. Precise surgery and good patient selection based on demographic factors and audiometric data can give patients the best odds for useful hearing preservation after CI surgery. Thoughtful discussions of hearing preservation cases based on scientific data and past team experience can be among the most useful results of CI staffing conferences.

Bilateral Cochlear Implantation

The goal of maximizing CI remediation of hearing loss often leads to bilateral cochlear implantation. In children with congenital and early-onset profound hearing loss, the advisability of simultaneous bilateral cochlear implant versus sequential cochlear implant surgeries leads to interesting discussions about priorities and preferences. Some parents may understandably prefer a single surgery session for both sides. However, if the goal is to provide the earliest possible speech stimulation and the lowest chance of surgical/anesthetic complications, a sequential strategy may be preferred.

Special Considerations for Special Cases

- Post-meningitis: Soft neurological deficits and hearing loss are the most common sequelae of meningitis. Fortunately, childhood immunizations have made the need for post-meningitis cochlear implant much less common. Children (and adults) recovering from meningitis need special attention to their hearing and prompt scanning and treatment, if any hearing loss is detected. Radiologic findings of labyrinthitis ossificans can lead to urgent cochlear implant surgery, before the scalae are obstructed by fibrosis and reactive bone formation. CT scans may underestimate the extent of cochlear ossification. Although fibrotic and post inflammatory narrowing of the scalae is an expected surgical finding in post-meningitis CI cases, complete obstruction is usually limited to the most basal end of the cochlea near the round window. This allows satisfactory electrode insertion in most post-meningitis cases.
- EVAS: This radiographically defined condition can be considered a relatively mild failure of the inner ear to completely form during fetal development and is often associated with the Mondini deformity. Children (and adults) with enlarged vestibular aqueduct syndrome (EVAS) seem to be some of the best cochlear implant users, perhaps because their hearing was relatively intact earlier in life. Once the scan findings of EVA are made, parents are often advised to restrict the affected child from activity/sports that pose a risk of blows to the head and barotrauma. This is done in the hopes it will minimize further progression of the sensorineural hearing loss. "Pulsatile perilymph" is typically seen during surgery when an EVAS cochlea is opened and extra attention is devoted to definitive packing of soft tissue around the electrode, so as to isolate the otic capsule (inner ear) from any future otitis media. In a minority of these cases, the modiolus may be dehiscent and this allows free flow of cerebrospinal fluid (CSF) through the perilymphatic space and

out of the cochleostomy, into the middle ear. This makes the "sizing" and then packing of the cochleostomy especially important, so as to prevent postoperative CSF leakage. In cases of modiolar dehiscence, the use of a straight or "lateral wall" type of intracochlear electrode is advisable, to avoid the possibility of a "modiolar hugging" electrode passing through the modiolus into the internal auditory canal.
- Common Cavity Deformity: This is a more severe version of an "underdeveloped" inner ear and again it is defined by the radiographic findings. One of the anatomical features of these dysplastic cochleas is the location of the neuroepithelium along the inner surface of the outer wall of the common cavity, in contrast to the inner wall location for a more normal cochlea. This makes a straight electrode advisable, so that the electrode will curl favorably along the outer wall of the common cavity. In cases of common cavity deformity, the expectations for hearing results that a CI can provide are more limited.
- Cochlear Nerve Deficiency (CND): The MRI finding of a small or absent cochlear nerve combined with a sensorineural hearing loss can be categorized as "cochlear nerve deficiency." These cases often present with audiologic findings of auditory neuropathy spectrum disorder (ANSD), and this makes an MRI scan important in the evaluation of patients with ANSD. Although expectations for CI hearing results are more limited in cases of CND, the results may be surprisingly good if functioning cochlear nerve fibers are displaced onto the adjacent vestibular nerve or facial nerve. This is the reason that CI is always tried, before considering Auditory Brainstem Implant in cases of children with CND.

Revision Surgery

Patients and parents occasionally ask if they will need revision surgery in the future as technology advances. As life expectancy exceeds 80 years for children with cochlear implants, we can only imagine what advances may come during their lifetime. CI manufacturers have designed the implanted receiver/stimulators to be a "stable platform" compatible with future external updates and developments. Therefore, we would not want to remove an intact, functioning internal device. Revision CI surgeries are occasionally needed for "medical reasons" or "device reasons."

Medical reasons include infection, implant migration necessitating refixation, and rarely to thin the subcutaneous scalp tissue if it is too thick for adequate external magnet adherence. Cochlear implants might need to be removed (and replaced at a later date) because of intractable infection or removed and immediately replaced for internal device failures. Although it is disappointing when a revision surgery is needed, the results are typically favorable for solving the medical or device related problem, and the recovery from surgery is at least as quick as the original surgery.

Key Concepts

- Surgeons who perform cochlear implant surgery have a background in otolaryngology (ENT) and then advanced training in otology and neurotology.
- The cochlear implant surgeon should conduct a thorough medical and physical evaluation to ensure that the cochlear implant candidate is medically suitable for cochlear implant surgery and is likely to benefit from cochlear implantation.
- The CI operation is typically a one- to two-hour outpatient procedure done under general anesthetic, with a low risk of problems or complications. A series of technical points must be understood and precisely executed in order to minimize the chance of problems and maximize the recipient's hearing outcome.
- Bilateral cochlear implantation is generally the standard of care for individuals with bilateral severe to profound hearing loss. Benefit from bilateral cochlear implantation is generally greater for individuals who have a shorter duration of deafness.
- The surgeon must take special considerations into account when providing cochlear implants for recipients for whom it may be beneficial to preserve acoustic hearing as well as for individuals with enlarged vestibular aqueduct syndrome, common cavity deformity, cochlear nerve deficiency, a history of bacterial meningitis, and so forth.

13

The Role of Imaging in Implantable Hearing Devices

Anthony M. Alleman

Imaging plays an important role in the presurgical evaluation of patients being considered for implantable hearing devices. Additionally, the presence of these devices becomes relevant when patients subsequently need medical imaging. The workhorse imaging modalities for the evaluation of the auditory system include computed tomography (CT) and magnetic resonance imaging (MRI). An understanding of the basic strengths and weaknesses of these techniques is helpful in determining the appropriate imaging strategy for a given patient and clinical situation. Radiologists with subspecialty training, neuroradiologists, can be valuable consultants in complex clinical cases.

CT uses x-ray radiation to obtain three-dimensional images of the auditory system. These images can be reconstructed in multiplanar two-dimensional and three-dimensional images to best illustrate a given patient's anatomy. CT scans display the relative density of various anatomical structures. Thus, CT is an excellent tool for evaluating the temporal bone (Fruauff et al., 2015), which is largely made up of air-filled bony chambers and fluid-filled spaces surrounded by bone. MRI uses no ionizing radiation, but rather a magnetic field and radio frequency energy to create three-dimensional models of water-containing tissues with exquisite detail. Additionally, multiple pulse sequences can be used to better define specific anatomical features, including emphasis on neural and vascular structures, brain architecture, water, and lipids (Figure 13–1) (Fruauff et al., 2015). Func-

tional MRI and diffusion tensor imaging are advanced modalities that hold promise in evaluating speech and language processing and neural pathways. MRI is an inferior modality in the evaluation of bony anatomy of the temporal bone given cortical bone's lack of water.

The roles of MR and CT imaging are complementary. For the evaluation of bony anatomy, especially in the setting of pre-surgical planning, CT is often preferable (Angtuaco et al., 2017). Additionally, CT is useful in the post-implantation setting for the evaluation of complications, device integrity, electrode location, and unrelated neurological medical conditions. The desire for information gathered by CT must be balanced with the need to use ionizing radiation, the dose of which should be minimized by using modern techniques. Modern CT scanners are very fast and images can often be obtained without the use of sedation.

Soft tissue anatomy of the proximal portions of the auditory pathway are best analyzed with MRI (Fruauff et al., 2015). The contents of the internal auditory canal, the cerebellar pontine angle, brainstem, and brain are often poorly distinguishable gray structures on CT. MRI clearly demonstrates elegant, interrelated, and distinguishable nerves, blood vessels, brainstem, cerebellum, and brain (Angtuaco et al., 2017). MRI scans are obtained using expensive, claustrophobic, and noisy machines. Combined with the relatively long imaging time compared with CT, MRI frequently requires sedation in children. The risks of recurrent

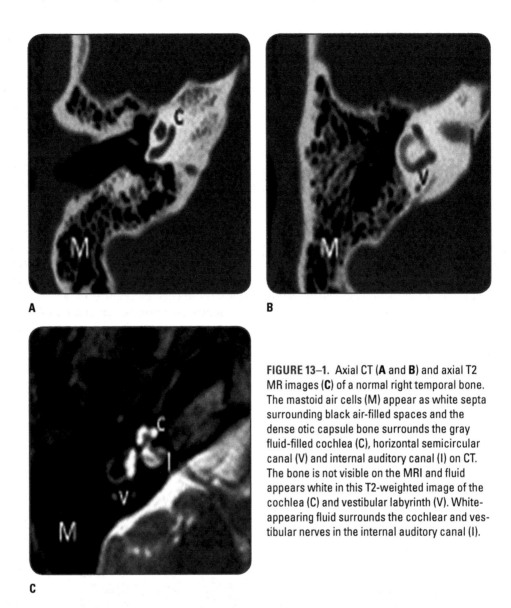

FIGURE 13–1. Axial CT (**A** and **B**) and axial T2 MR images (**C**) of a normal right temporal bone. The mastoid air cells (M) appear as white septa surrounding black air-filled spaces and the dense otic capsule bone surrounds the gray fluid-filled cochlea (C), horizontal semicircular canal (V) and internal auditory canal (I) on CT. The bone is not visible on the MRI and fluid appears white in this T2-weighted image of the cochlea (C) and vestibular labyrinth (V). White-appearing fluid surrounds the cochlear and vestibular nerves in the internal auditory canal (I).

anesthesia to developing children and individuals with complex medical problems must be weighed against the need for clinical information. Most preoperative imaging can be obtained without the use of gadolinium-based contrast agents, which may be retained in portions of the brain. Given the strong magnetic fields associated with MRI, many medical devices (such as implantable hearing devices) may be contraindicated for patients in the MRI scanning environment. When considering which device provides the best option for a given patient's needs, it is worth considering the limitations on future imaging as different manufacturers and devices impact how and if a patient can be imaged in the future. This becomes

particularly relevant in older individuals who are at risk for common medical ailments, such as stroke, and in young children, who could conceivably carry their devices for 80 years or longer.

When embarking on an imaging strategy for the evaluation of a given patient, the optimal approach is to determine the information needed to balance it against the limitation of the available imaging modalities. For the assessment of conductive hearing losses, CT is the preferred modality hands-down as the bony anatomy usually reveals the source. MRI is frequently the preferred modality for evaluation of sensorineural hearing loss in older individuals and when cochlear nerve aplasia is suspected, but many congenital anomalies are displayed adequately on CT (Jiang et al., 2014; Schwartz & Chen, 2014).

CT scanning is frequently employed in the pre-implantation setting, as it displays bony landmarks well known to the otologist/neuro-otologist, permits anticipation of anatomical variations and pitfalls, and often displays recognized patterns of developmental anomalies. From CT, it is easy to determine the extent of mastoid pneumatization, course of the facial nerve, size and aeration of the facial recess, and patency of the round window (Figure 13–2). Bony anatomical anomalies such as displaced facial nerves, aberrant blood vessels, and chronic infection processes that can complicate pre-surgical planning for cochlear implantation can be prospectively identified. Additionally, many developmental anomalies such as enlarged vestibular aqueducts, cochlear aperture stenosis, and labyrinthine malformations are readily apparent on CT scans.

MRI is helpful in documenting the anatomic integrity of the auditory nerve and in the evaluation of brainstem or auditory pathway pathology that is invisible to CT. Many developmental syndromes associated with hearing loss have central neurological abnormalities best demonstrated on MRI. Additionally, MRI obtained for neurologic conditions may allow early anticipation of future hearing compromise.

The following images demonstrate the advantages and disadvantages of CT and MRI. On CT, one can readily distinguish the dense bone of the otic capsule. The structures within the labyrinth are mostly below the resolution of these imaging modalities (except for the modiolus) and appear as a uniformly gray fluid signal. By comparison, the fluid-filled inner ear structures are readily apparent on MRI and the surrounding bony anatomy is less well defined. When it comes to determining the relationship of the facial nerve, sigmoid sinus, emissary veins, and the round window, the bony definition of CT appears superior. When determining the presence or absence of a cochlear nerve, CT can only imply its absence by demonstrating an absent cochlear aperture (Figure 13–3). MRI can display the cochlear nerve from the brainstem to the cochlea (Figure 13–4).

Many common congenital conditions, including inner ear morphological abnormalities, are well displayed on CT. This includes the spectrum from minor cochlear and vestibular labyrinthine abnormalities to common cavities and complete aplasia (Figure 13–5). Acquired bony conditions such as cochlear otosclerosis are readily imaged by CT (Figure 13–6), although isolated conductive hearing loss associated with fenestral otosclerosis does not require imaging (Angtuaco et al., 2017; Wegner et al., 2016).

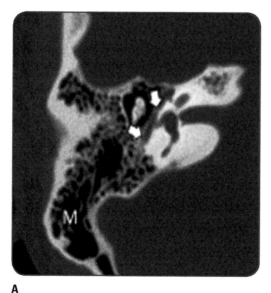
A

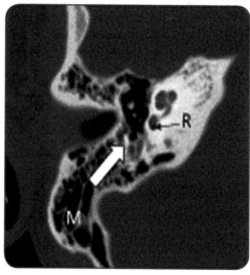
B

FIGURES 13–2. (A and **B)** Preoperative axial CT images of the right temporal bone permits evaluation of the relationships of the mastoid air cells (M), facial nerve (*short white arrows*), facial recess (*long white arrow*), and round window niche (*black arrow R*).

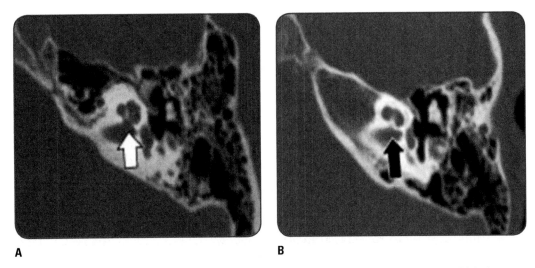

A

B

FIGURE 13–3. Axial CT scan (**A**) demonstrates a normal fluid-filled cochlear aperture through which the nerve enters the cochlea (*white arrow*). The aperture may be completely replaced by bone in the setting of cochlear nerve aplasia (*black arrow,* **B**).

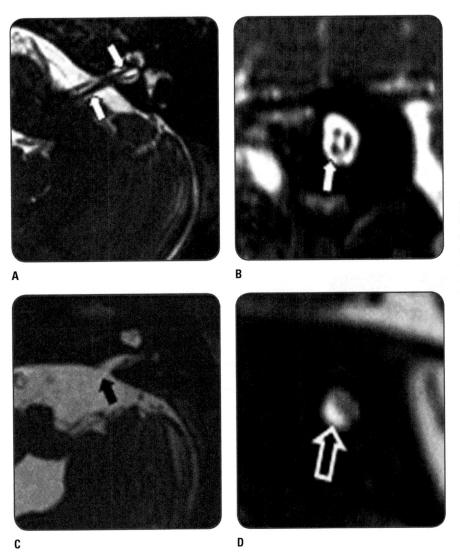

A

B

C

D

FIGURE 13–4. Axial (**A**) and sagittal (**B**) high-resolution images of the internal auditory canal demonstrating the normal black-appearing cochlear nerve (*white arrow*), which is absent in a case of cochlear nerve aplasia; space normally occupied by the nerve is replaced with spinal fluid (*black arrow,* **C** and **D**).

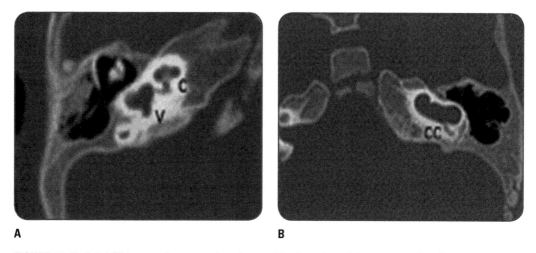

A   B

FIGURE 13–5. Axial CT images demonstrating abnormal horizontal semicircular canal (V, **A**) and cochlea. (**B**) demonstrates common cavity deformity (CC). Compare with normal structures in Figures 13–1A and 13–1B.

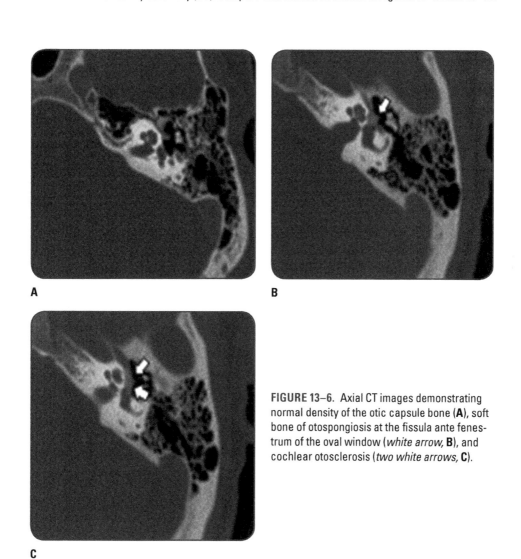

A   B

FIGURE 13–6. Axial CT images demonstrating normal density of the otic capsule bone (**A**), soft bone of otospongiosis at the fissula ante fenestrum of the oval window (*white arrow,* **B**), and cochlear otosclerosis (*two white arrows,* **C**).

C

Some pathologies can be demonstrated on both MRI and CT. Enlarged vestibular aqueduct syndrome was initially defined as enlargement of the bony portion of the vestibular aqueduct with an associated deformity of the apex of the cochlea on CT (Figure 13–7). Occasionally, enlarged vestibular aqueducts, the associated cochlear anomaly, and frequently associated enlarged endolymphatic sacs are visible on MRI, but are less reliably demonstrated.

Cochlear ossification is demonstrated on CT by bone density replacing the fluid-filled space of the cochlea and is often a progressive finding, especially in the post-meningitis setting. MRI can also demonstrate abnormal fluid signal and enhancement within the cochlea during the acute meningitis episode and identify patients at risk for developing cochlear ossification (Stone et al., 2009). In MRI, labyrinthitis ossificans is characterized by the loss of the normal fluid signal within the cochlea. Unfortunately, both modalities may underestimate the amount of ossification encountered at surgery (Figure 13–8) (Hassepass et al., 2013).

When a patient is implanted with a device, it is important to counsel him/her to carry the implant information card at all times, as the information is vital in an emergency where imaging is required. The bone anchor for bone-anchored hearing aid (BAHA) devices is generally MRI compatible when the processor is removed, but may degrade image quality (Figure 13–9). Additionally, some cochlear implants cannot enter the MRI suite, as they are affected by the strong magnetic currents (Figure 13–10). Each of the cochlear implants that can be scanned require unique safety measures, including wrapping the head or even removing the magnet. If the device is not known, imaging cannot safely proceed until the device is definitively identified. When imaging is necessary to document device and electrode positioning, high-resolution CT or rotational tomography is the preferred technique (Figure 13–11) (Gnagi et al.; Lui et al., 2013).

Imaging often plays an integral role in the assessment of hearing loss and in the preoperative planning for cochlear implantation. In select cases, imaging can assist the clinician in determining device physical integrity and position. In many cases, future medical imaging strategies are impacted by the model of device implanted.

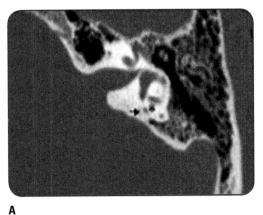

A

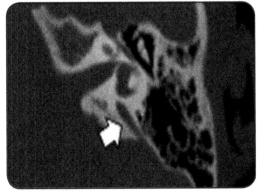

B

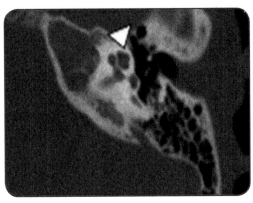

C

FIGURE 13–7. Enlarged vestibular aqueduct syndrome. Axial CT (**A**) demonstrating normal appearing fluid-filled endolymphatic duct (*black arrow*) is smaller in caliber than the adjacent posterior semicircular canal (*). (**B**) demonstrates the enlarged vestibular aqueduct (*white arrow*) and associated apical cochlear abnormality (*white arrowhead,* **C**).

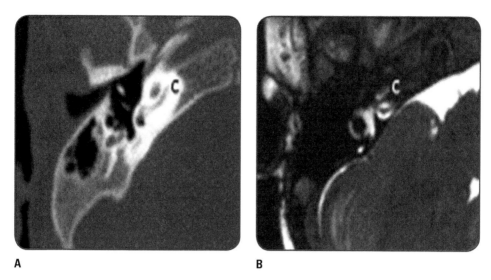

A   B

FIGURE 13–8. Labyrinthitis ossificans. The fluid-filled spaces of the cochlea seen in axial CT Figure 13–1A (normal cochlea) is replaced by bone in this case of labyrinthitis ossificans (C, **A**). The T2-weighted MRI demonstrates replacement of the white appearing fluid seen in the normal cochlea (Figure 13–1C) with black appearing bone (C, **B**).

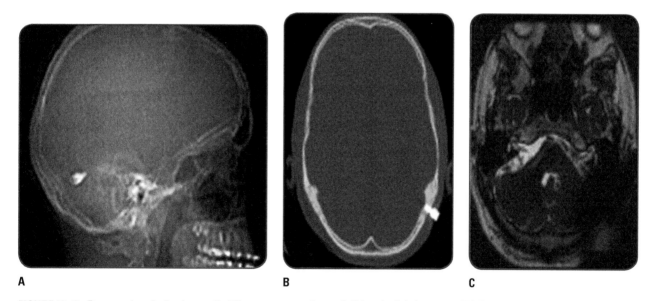

A   B   C

FIGURE 13–9. Bone anchor device imaged in CT scan-scout radiograph (**A**) and axial plane scan (**B**). Even though the device is relatively small, it creates a significant artifact on MRI imaging (*darkened area right lower corner of image in* **C**).

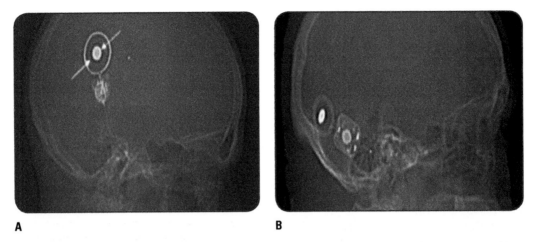

A

B

FIGURE 13–10. CT scan-scout image demonstrating the round magnet normally positioned within the cochlear implant (*arrows,* **A**). In **B**, the magnet was dislocated by an MRI scanner and is now sitting perpendicular to its seat in the implant.

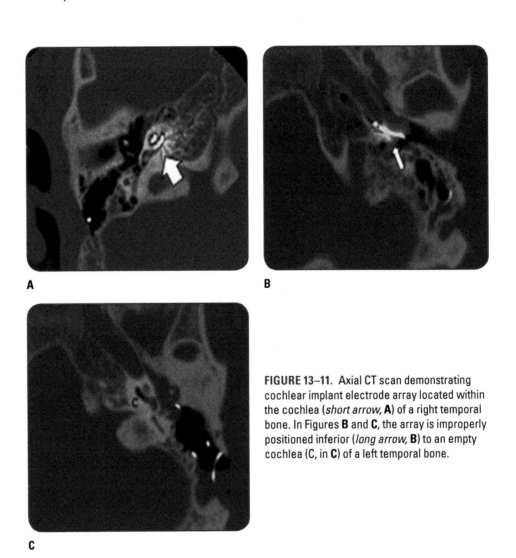

A

B

FIGURE 13–11. Axial CT scan demonstrating cochlear implant electrode array located within the cochlea (*short arrow,* **A**) of a right temporal bone. In Figures **B** and **C**, the array is improperly positioned inferior (*long arrow,* **B**) to an empty cochlea (C, in **C**) of a left temporal bone.

C

Key Concepts

- Imaging plays an important role in the presurgical evaluation of patients being considered for implantable hearing devices. Additionally, the presence of these devices become relevant when patients subsequently need medical imaging.
- The workhorse imaging modalities for the evaluation of the auditory system include computed tomography (CT) and magnetic resonance imaging (MRI).
- An understanding of the basic strengths and weaknesses of these techniques is helpful in determining the appropriate imaging strategy for a given patient and clinical situation.
- Radiologists with subspecialty training, neuroradiologists, can be valuable consultants in complex clinical cases.

References

Angtuaco, E. J., Wippold, F. J. II., Cornelius, R. S., Aiken, A. H., Berger, K. L., Broderick, D. F., Brown, D. C., . . . Vogelbaum, M. A. (2017). *Expert panel on neurologic imaging. ACR Appropriateness Criteria® hearing loss and/or vertigo.* Retrieved from https://www.guideline.gov/summaries/summary/47674

Fruauff, K., Coffey, K., Chazen, J. L., & Phillips, C. D. (2015). Temporal bone imaging. *Topics in Magnetic Resonance Imaging 24*, 39–55.

Gnagi, S. H., Baker, T. R., Pollei, T. R., & Barrs, D. M. (2015). Analysis of intraoperative radiographic electrode placement during cochlear implantation. *Otology and Neurotology, 36*, 1045–1047.

Hassepass, F., Schild, C., Aschendorff, A., Maier, W., Beck, R., Wesarg, T. & Arndt, S. (2013). Clinical outcome after cochlear implantation in patients with unilateral hearing loss due to labyrintitis ossificans. *Otology and Neurotology, 34*, 1278–1283.

Jiang, Z. Y., Odiase, E., Isaacson, B., Roland, P. S., & Kutz, J. W. (2014). Utility of MRIIs in adult cochlear implant evaluations. *Otology and Neurotology, 35*, 1533–1535.

Lui, C., Peng, J., Li, J., Yang, C. H., Chen, C. K. &Hwang, C. F. (2013). Detection of receiver location and migration after cochlear implantation using 3d rendering of computed tomography. *Otology and Neurotology, 34*, 1299–1304.

Schwartz, S. R., & Chen, B. S. (2014). The role of preoperative imaging for cochlear implantation in postlingually deafened adults. *Otology and Neurotology, 35*, 1536–1540.

Sone, M., Mizuno, T., Naganawa, S. & Nakashima, T. (2009). Imaging analysis in cases with inflammation-induced sensorineural hearing loss. *Acta Oto-laryngologica, 129*(3), 239–243.

Wegner, I., van Waes, A. M. A., Bittermann, A., Buitinck, S. H., Dekker, C. F., Kurk, S. A., . . . Grolman, W. (2016). A systematic review of the diagnostic value of CT imaging in diagnosing otosclerosis. *Otology and Neurotology, 37*, 9–15.

Fundamental Practices of Cochlear Implant Programming

Jace Wolfe

Although there are some differences in cochlear implant programming across the various manufacturers, there are also many similarities. Regardless of the make and model of the cochlear implant, there are several fundamental aspects of cochlear implant programming that serve as the foundation for creating a good map. This chapter addresses the basic principles of cochlear implant programming that are necessary to provide a map that will optimize auditory, speech, and communication abilities as well as user satisfaction.

Pre-Activation Procedures

Realistic Expectations Prior to Activation

Helping the recipient and family to establish realistic expectations is one of the most important objectives prior to activation. No matter how thoroughly expectations are discussed, recipients and families often have high expectations for the hearing performance that will be achieved and the amount of time and the effort required to optimize the individual's outcomes after cochlear implantation. Because of the inflated expectations many recipients and family members have prior to implantation, implant recipients are often discouraged with their performance during the first few days or even weeks of use. This is especially true for teenagers and adults who have

long periods of deafness prior to implantation. However, some adults with residual hearing and families of young children with congenital deafness are also disappointed that the implant does not provide the recipient with hearing at "normal levels" and that he/she still experiences difficulty with communication in certain situations. To reduce the chances that the recipient and family members are disappointed with the outcome achieved after cochlear implantation, the audiologist should consider revisiting the topic of realistic expectations prior to activating the recipient's cochlear implant. The reader should refer to Chapters 5 and 6 for information pertaining to the management of realistic expectations of cochlear implant performance and benefit.

Using a responsible counseling approach, audiologists should remind adult recipients of the possibility of limited speech recognition after implantation and for the possibility that speech and environmental sounds will most likely sound strange and have a poor sound quality immediately after implantation. Specifically, the audiologist should suggest that some recipients report that speech sounds robotic, mechanical, or cartoonish (e.g., many recipients report that speech sounds like Mickey Mouse, Donald Duck, Darth Vader, or like someone is speaking after inhaling the gas from a helium-filled balloon) or that speech may even sound like noise or ringing bells rather than speech. In reality, most adult cochlear implant recipients are able to understand speech to at least some extent during the first few days of implant use and are quickly able to acclimate and adjust to the sound quality of the signal provided by the implant. However, the recipient will be less likely to be disappointed during the early stages of activation if the audiologist provides an a priori warning that speech may sound unnatural during the early stages of implant use. The audiologist should also consider informing the implant candidate and new recipient that he/she may initially regret his/her decision to receive a cochlear implant, but after several weeks or months of implant use, he/she should adapt to the auditory signal that he/she receives from the implant and perform much better than he/she did with hearing aids. Most specifically, it is imperative to stress that time is required to adjust to the implant and to obtain the full benefit the implant can offer.

In short, the primary goal of pre-implant counseling is to establish a relatively conservative or limited outlook pertaining to the benefit and performance a recipient will receive with the cochlear implant, while still convincing the candidate that cochlear implantation is in his/her best interests. The audiologist should also inform the recipient and his/her family of basic information that will assist the recipient in adjusting to the new implant and in optimizing the satisfaction and benefit obtained with/from the cochlear implant.

When counseling families of pediatric recipients, parents and caregivers should be reminded that experience with the implant is required before substantial gains are seen in a young child's listening and spoken language abilities. As discussed in Chapter 6, it is imperative that audiologists prepare families of pediatric recipients by discussing all of the potential responses that a child might have to the initial auditory stimulation from his/her cochlear implant, including sound awareness, anxiety, happiness, fear, and indifference. Most children do not display a strong aversion to their initial experience of hearing with their cochlear implant, particularly when the audiologist introduces stimulation appropriately. In fact, some are very happy with the new sound and will smile and point to their ear when they hear programming stimuli or external sounds. However, in some cases, children do become upset, cry, and seek comfort from caregivers. To prevent this negative reaction, the audiologist should make every attempt to avoid overstimulation. Even with careful programming, however, a few children, especially those with minimal experience with sound, still become upset when they first hear through the implant. This is most likely due to the child being startled by the new signal he/she receives. On the other hand, some chil-

dren may exhibit a very limited response or even no response to the initial auditory stimulation received from the cochlear implant. The child's family is likely to become concerned when the child does not overtly respond to the new signal from the cochlear implant. Typically, the audiologist can conduct measures, such as the electrically evoked compound action potential (see Chapter 18), that indicate that the auditory system is responding to the stimulation from the implant. Of course, this information can be conveyed to the child's caregivers to alleviate their concerns. However, the caregivers are less likely to be overly concerned with their child's tempered response to stimulation from the implant if the audiologist has prepared them for the possibility ahead of activation. In short, it is important that the family is prepared for each of the different types of responses that children may provide at cochlear implant activation so that the family is not overly alarmed or disappointed on activation day.

Reviewing Logistics of Cochlear Implant Programming

The audiologist should also provide the recipient and family members with a schedule of the appointments necessary for cochlear implant programming and audiologic assessment and management. A provision of a cochlear implant audiology schedule will prepare the family for the time and financial commitments associated with postoperative appointments. The majority of audiological appointments occur during the first year (i.e., diagnostic testing, programming). After the first year, medical and audiology appointments are less frequent for most recipients. As previously discussed, auditory-based habilitative/rehabilitative appointments are essential (e.g., one hour per week) throughout the first few years of a child's implant use and are critically important for infants and young children. Because of limitations in health care insurance reimbursement, qualified personnel, and time, many adult recipients do not receive formal aural rehabilitation, but in reality, the vast majority of adults are likely to benefit substantially from at least a short-term period of post-activation aural rehabilitation. Aural rehabilitation is usually instrumental in building the confidence of the newly implanted adult. The focus of this rehabilitation should include orientation to the new recipient's cochlear implant equipment, including the appropriate use of multiple programs and hearing assistive technology (HAT) to successfully address difficult situations. Many adult recipients are reluctant to resume telephone use because it was previously very difficult with hearing aids. One of the goals of aural rehabilitation should be to facilitate the recipient's return to telephone use. Additionally, many long-term deafened cochlear implant recipients may have developed maladaptive strategies to compensate for their hearing loss. Aural rehabilitation should assist the new recipient in identifying these strategies and eliminating them. Also, consistent error patterns may be identified in the recipient's speech recognition. The programming audiologist may make programming adjustments in an attempt to ameliorate the errors that are observed during aural rehabilitation sessions. Examples of basic aural rehabilitation activities that an audiologist can conduct with new adult recipients may be found in Chapter 23.

Listening and spoken language based therapy must be provided to the families of infants and young children who receive cochlear implants. Children with hearing loss must be exposed to a listening-rich environment filled with intelligible speech in order to optimize auditory and spoken language skills. A Listening and Spoken Language specialist should coach the child's caregivers to create the listening-rich environment that the child needs to reach his/her full potential in auditory skill development. For more information on Auditory-Verbal therapy for children with cochlear implants, the interested reader is referred to *Auditory-Verbal Therapy for Young Children with Hearing Loss and Their Families, and the Practitioners Who Guide Them* by Warren Estabrooks, Karen MacIver-Lux, and Ellen A. Rhoades.

Setting the Stage for Cochlear Implant Programming

Audiologists should attempt to prepare the programming clinic in order to facilitate success on the day of cochlear implant activation and for all subsequent programming sessions. For example, the audiologist should ensure that the décor and furniture in the clinic are appropriate for the recipients who are being served; appropriate furniture and décor are especially important for infants and young children. The chair in which the recipient sits for programming should be comfortable and provide adequate support so that the recipient is able to fully participate throughout the session. The chair in which the infant sits should provide ample support for the child's torso and buttocks, so that the child is stabilized and does not

need to devote all of his/her motor skills to sitting upright in the chair. Providing an infant with a chair that offers adequate support will allow the child to devote his/her motor skills to the task of executing a head turn in response to the programming stimulus, a skill which is essential for the successful completion of visual reinforcement audiometry. For children of all ages, it is important to ensure that the child's legs and/or feet are well supported and resting on a stable surface. If the child's feet are not positioned on a stable surface, then he/she may be inclined to kick or shuffle his/her feet throughout the session, which may distract the child from the task of responding to programming stimuli. Figure 14–1 provides examples of pediatric chairs and tables that are appropriate for cochlear implant programming sessions with children. Babies and young toddlers should ideally be seated in a highchair during programming (Figure 14–2); the audiologist should be aware that high-backed highchairs may knock off the external transmitting coil from the child's head. An effective solution is to place a back support between the baby and the highchair back to provide support and keep the head away from the back. Also, some highchairs have low backs that will not displace the coil from the child's head. Highchairs with straps are helpful because they prevent the child from falling out of the chair or attempting to climb out of the chair before the programming session is completed. Some infants are reluctant to sit by themselves. In such cases, the audiologist should have a comfortable chair with armrests so that the caregiver may hold the child during the programming session. However, behavioral testing for the measurement of stimulation levels is best completed while child sits by himself/herself in a highchair. Examples of seating that is conducive for older toddlers and preschool-aged children are shown in Figures 14–1 and 14–2. A child-sized picnic table is also an option for children who are able to sit still throughout the programming session, because the table provides a surface for games used during programming (e.g., conditioned play toys, computer tablets, coloring books, playdough) used during pediatric programming sessions. Also, some children are more comfortable and at ease when provided with the opportunity to sit in furniture designed for a young child. Adults should be provided with comfortable chairs with armrests so the recipient is able to attend throughout the programming session.

For adults and children, the audiologist should be careful to avoid giving cues about the programming signals that are presented to the patient. Children, in

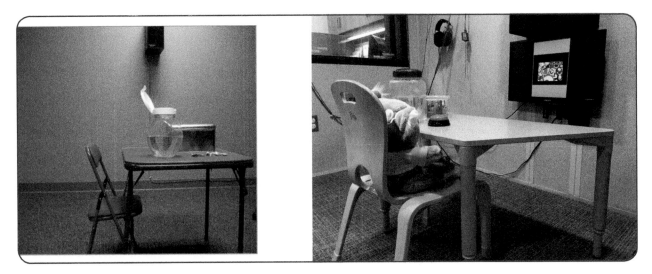

FIGURE 14–1. Examples of pediatric-friendly furniture.

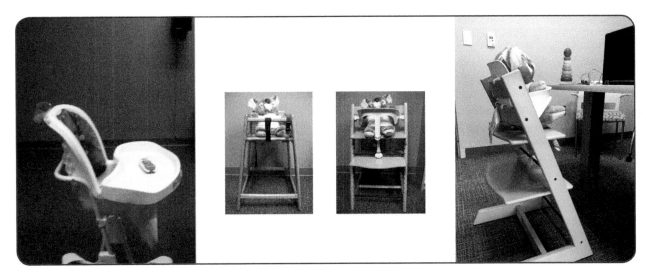

FIGURE 14–2. Examples of pediatric-friendly furniture.

particular, are very adept at watching the audiologist's computer monitor, hands, facial expressions, body language, and so on, in an attempt to determine when they should respond to programming stimuli. Older children and adults are often seated directly in front of the programming audiologist and computer so that the audiologist may observe the child's responses to the programming stimuli and the child cannot see the monitor of the programming computer. Also, the audiologist should ensure that the recipient's family members are not providing cues to the presence of the programming stimulus. It is not uncommon for the recipient's family members

to unintentionally change facial expressions or body language during the presentation of stimuli, so the programming audiologist must ensure the child is not receiving supplemental cues about the presence of the programming stimuli.

In most cases, family members and friends should be welcome to attend programming sessions. However, if the audiologist believes that the extended family and friends are preventing the recipient from focusing on the task at hand, he or she may need to request that the family members wait outside and possibly abstain from attending future appointments. Family members often wish to attend the activation of a child's cochlear implant. If the audiologist believes that the presence of a large number of family members will distract the child and prevent the attainment of responses needed to create a good cochlear implant program, then the audiologist may need to ask family members to wait outside of the programming room until the information needed for programming is acquired. Also, the audiologist may suggest that a video be obtained of the initial activation session and shared with extended family members.

The Fundamentals of Cochlear Implant Programming

Physical Evaluation

On the day of activation, the audiologist should conduct a bilateral otoscopic evaluation and should inspect the incision site for signs of irritation or infection. A middle ear effusion is likely in the first few weeks following cochlear implant surgery. If the middle ear effusion appears to be purulent, the audiologist should refer the recipient for otologic assessment. Additionally, otologic evaluation is warranted if there is a sign of infection, inflammation, or bleeding near the incision and/or implant site.

Next, the audiologist should determine the appropriate magnet strength for the external transmitting coil. Determination of the appropriate magnet strength is a subjective skill that the audiologist should develop over time. The audiologist should strive to select a magnet strength that is sufficient to prevent the transmitting coil from repeatedly falling off of the recipient's head while also avoiding a magnet strength that is overly excessive. When the audiologist places the coil on the head, there should be some attraction, but that attraction should not be so strong that it forcefully pulls the coil from the audiologist's hand to the recipient's head. Furthermore, the coil should not easily fall off when the recipient turns his/her head back and forth. However, it should most likely dislodge when the recipient brushes his/her hand against the coil. For older children and adults, the audiologist may ask the recipient to stand up on his/her toes and then drop to his/her heels. If the coil falls off the recipient's head, then the magnet strength likely needs to be increased.

If the audiologist selects a magnet that is too strong for the recipient, the pressure of the coil on the head may compromise circulation to the skin underlying the coil. If excessive adherence secondary to excessive magnet strength persists for a prolonged period of time (e.g., several weeks), it is possible that the skin under the coil may necrotize, which could result in a skin flap breakdown that would necessitate reimplantation. Cochlear implant skin flap breakdown from an excessively strong magnet is uncommon, but the audiologist should err on the side of being conservative when selecting magnet strength. Older children and adults will typically complain of a headache or a dull discomfort if the coil magnet strength is too strong. The audiologist should counsel the recipient to reduce magnet strength if discomfort or itchiness arises around the coil site. Infants and young children cannot verbalize any discomfort that they may experience from excessive magnet strength. Consequently, the audiologist should be particularly cautious when selecting the magnet strength for younger recipients. Also, audiologists should counsel the child's caregivers to routinely inspect the implant site for signs of irritation.

As a general rule of thumb, infants, young children, and elderly women are often more likely to have thin skin flaps and require a weaker magnet strength. In contrast, middle-aged males and obese recipients are more inclined to have thicker skin flaps and require a stronger magnet strength. Furthermore, recipients who have stiff wiry hair may need stronger magnets. For recipients with thick skin flaps and thick hair, it may be necessary for the audiologist to shave the hair at the coil site in order to achieve good adherence of the external coil to the cochlear implant.

It should be noted that the parents of newly implanted young children are often inclined to request excessive magnet strengths, because the coil tends to frequently fall off of the head of active toddlers. Again, the audiologist should exercise caution when considering an increase in magnet strength and counsel the child's caregivers accordingly if a stronger magnet seems unwarranted. If the magnet never falls off of the head of an active toddler, then it is likely that the magnet is too strong. It should also be mentioned that higher magnet strength may be necessary at activation, because there may be swelling at the implant site related to the surgery. When swelling resolves around the implant site, the audiologist should determine whether the magnet strength needs to be reduced. The audiologist should also counsel recipients and their family members of the likely need to reduce magnet strength after the swelling around the implant site subsides. Of note, the pressure of the coil on the implant site may also result in a reduction in the thickness of the skin flap.

Most surgeons order an x-ray to be completed in the operating room to confirm that the electrode array is properly inserted in the cochlea. The programming audiologist should confer with the cochlear implant surgeon to determine whether there were any complications related to the electrode array insertion or to any other aspect of the operation. In particular, the audiologist should be aware of any intracochlear electrode contacts that are not fully inserted into the cochlea. The surgeon should make the audiologist aware of electrode array insertions that are unusually shallow or deep. Additionally, the audiologist should be aware of any evidence of cochlear ossification or fibrous tissue growth (e.g., bacterial meningitis, fibrous scar tissue).

Selecting a Signal Coding Strategy

After the physical examination is completed, the audiologist commences creating a program for the recipient's newly implanted ear. First, the audiologist should select the signal coding strategy that will be used in the recipient's sound processor. As described in Chapter 8, each manufacturer offers several different signal coding strategies that have all been shown to support the development of open-set speech recognition. Research has shown that some recipients perform better with one signal coding strategy over another (Pasanisi et al., 2002). Most recipients will achieve satisfactory performance with use of the manufacturer's recommended signal coding strategy. As a result, during the first month of implant use, the audiologist should consider providing the manufacturer's recommended signal coding strategy to the newly implanted recipients. If the recipient does not meet the audiologist's expectations of hearing performance after several weeks of use of the manufacturer's recommended signal coding strategy, then the audiologist can consider switching to an alternative signal coding strategy. Chapters 15, 16, and 17 contain manufacturer-specific recommendations for which signal coding strategy and additional programming parameters the audiologist should select for newly implanted recipients.

It should be reiterated that most recipients will achieve satisfactory outcomes with modern signal coding strategies when the audiologist has optimized the stimulation levels that are used to stimulate the recipient's cochlear nerve. When a recipient is not making satisfactory progress with his/her cochlear implant, the audiologist should ensure that stimulation levels are optimized prior to switching to a new signal coding strategy or to adjusting secondary programming parameters such as stimulation rate, input dynamic range, and so forth.

If the recipient is performing below the audiologist's expectations after several weeks of cochlear implant use and the audiologist is certain that the stimulation levels are appropriate, then the audiologist should attempt other programming adjustments. For instance, the audiologist may create programs with stimulation rates that are slower and faster than the stimulation rate that the recipient has been using during the first few weeks of implant use. Elderly recipients and recipients with cochlear nerve pathology (e.g., auditory neuropathy, multiple sclerosis, cochlear nerve aplasia, etc.) may perform better with lower stimulation rates. The audiologist may also create new programs with alternative signal coding strategies. When stimulation rate and/or signal coding strategy is adjusted, the audiologist will need to re-measure stimulation levels. If the recipient is uncertain of which signal coding strategy (or stimulation rate) provides the best performance, then the audiologist should provide the recipient with at least two programs with different signal coding strategies (or stimulation rates) to allow the recipient the opportunity to trial the alternative settings in the real world.

Young children, in particular, are typically unable to provide reliable verbal feedback about their auditory experiences with different signal coding strategies. Therefore, as a first step, the manufacturer-recommended signal coding strategy should be used (see Chapters 15–17 for the authors' manufacturer-specific recommendations on signal coding strategies and programming parameters for use with children). If audiologic assessment and, more importantly, speech and language development are unfavorable, then the audiologist may consider trying an alternative signal coding strategy or stimulation rate. However, as previously discussed in the aforementioned paragraphs, a child's progress and performance with his/her cochlear implant is largely influenced by the stimulation levels that are programmed by the audiologist. As a result, the audiologist's primary objective should be to determine the most appropriate stimulation levels for a child rather than attempting to identify the optimal signal coding strategies or adjusting other programming parameters (e.g., stimulation rate, input dynamic range). The authors will attempt to change signal coding strategies and adjust other programming parameters (e.g., stimulation rate, input dynamic range [IDR], maxima) only after it has been determined that the stimulation levels have been optimized and the child is continuing to struggle. Of note, when a young child is making poor progress after implantation, the audiologist should schedule the child for frequent programming/ assessment appointments with the goal of ensuring that the cochlear implant MAP is optimized to meet the child's needs. The audiologist should also ensure that the child's cochlear implant sound processor is functioning appropriately and that the child is using the cochlear implant during all waking hours (i.e., review data logging at each programming session). Additionally, the audiologist should remain in close contact with the child's caregivers and therapists to determine whether changes made to the child's MAP have resulted in a favorable change in the child's hearing abilities. If concerns persist, the audiologist should continue to explore strategies to enhance the child's progress.

Streamlined Versus Comprehensive Programming

Each of the cochlear implant manufacturers have created signal coding strategies and programming platforms that expedite cochlear implant programming for two reasons. First, there is a growing number of individuals receiving cochlear implants, and improvements in the efficiency of service delivery is imperative to meet the needs of the expanding recipient population. Second, reimbursement for cochlear implant programming is typically poor, so there is a need to minimize the amount of time spent providing cochlear implant services to each recipient to minimize financial losses incurred by the cochlear implant clinic.

Historically, cochlear implant programming involved a comprehensive battery of measures to determine stimulation levels for each electrode contact in the array. Consequently, cochlear implant programming sessions were quite lengthy (e.g., two hours). In contrast, streamlined approaches reduce the number of measurements the audiologist must complete to create a cochlear implant program. In the following paragraphs, basic programming procedures will be discussed for both streamlined and comprehensive approaches.

Measuring Stimulation Levels

Researchers and clinical audiologists often give a great deal of attention to programming parameters,

including stimulation rate, input dynamic range, and frequency allocation. Although these parameters clearly can impact performance, the most important aspect of programming is the optimization of the recipient's stimulus levels. The following section discusses the various procedures used to determine appropriate stimulation levels for adults and children.

Setting Threshold Levels for Adults

The threshold of electrical stimulation (i.e., T level) is an important programming parameter because it determines the amount of stimulation necessary to ensure that a low-level sound (e.g., 25 dB SPL) is audible to the recipient. The provision of appropriate T level stimulation also serves to normalize loudness for low-level sounds (i.e., low-level audio inputs sound "soft" to the recipient just as the signal would sound "soft" to an individual with normal hearing). In general, the procedures for determining T levels are similar to those used to obtain routine audiometric thresholds and are relatively straightforward. However, as previously mentioned, research has suggested that many adults with contemporary Advanced Bionics and MED-EL cochlear implants experience good outcomes and have sufficient audibility for low-level sounds with use of streamlined programs in which T levels are set to zero or estimated on the basis of the upper-stimulation level (Spahr & Dorman, 2005). When T levels are set to a minimum amount of stimulation or at a certain percentage of the upper-stimulation level, the signal coding strategy uses a mapping function to provide a level of stimulation that should ensure audibility for low-level acoustic inputs. The mapping functions used to determine stimulation levels provided for various audio input levels are based on the typical electrical dynamic range of an implant user. As a result, they yield satisfactory results for the typical user, but the results may be less than ideal for recipients who have an electrical dynamic range that is markedly different from typical recipients. Consequently, the audiologist should consider measuring T levels to optimize audibility for the individual recipient, particularly when the recipient's soundfield warbled tone thresholds indicate insufficient audibility for low-level sounds (i.e., poorer than 25–30 dB HL).

For conventional programming sessions in which T levels are measures, T-level assessment often begins on a low-frequency channel because listeners with hearing loss are more likely to recognize a stimulus that was familiar prior to surgery (i.e., most individuals had some low-frequency hearing prior to surgery).

The audiologist should increase the level of the low-frequency programming stimulus until the signal is clearly audible to the recipient. After audibility is established, the audiologist should proceed with traditional threshold testing using an adaptive-bracketing procedure, such as the modified Hughson-Westlake (Carhart & Jerger, 1959). Recipients tend to respond to lower stimulation levels for descending presentations compared with ascending presentations (i.e., a hysteresis effect). Therefore, to ensure audibility of soft acoustic inputs, T levels should be based on recipient's responses to T-level stimuli delivered in the ascending direction.

The step-size for ascending and descending presentations varies. Assessment of precise T levels at the initial activation can be difficult for several reasons, including: (1) recipients are not accustomed to the signal delivered from the implant, (2) the recipient may have gone quite a long time without hearing an auditory signal at the frequency at which the stimulus is being delivered, and (3) the recipient experiences difficulty distinguishing the T-level stimulus from his/her tinnitus. Therefore, at initial activation, the recipient may respond at suprathreshold levels during T-level assessment. Suprathreshold responses to T-level stimuli are particularly prevalent when cochlear implants are activated for infants and young children. Because the recipient's T-level responses are likely to change over the first few weeks of cochlear implant use (due to changes in the recipient's attentiveness to the signal as well as to changes in electrode contact impedance and to changes that may occur within the cochlea), the audiologist should not be overly concerned with determining precise T levels during the first few days of implant use. As a result, the audiologist may choose to use relatively larger measurement step-sizes during the first programming appointment or two. Throughout the first month of implant use, the recipient will become more adept at responding to the programming signal, and the audiologist should measure T level with a smaller measurement step size.

To measure T levels of older children and adults, the audiologist should ask the recipient to say "yes" or raise his/her hand when he/she hears the programming signal. The exact definition of T level varies across manufacturers, but as a general rule, T level is set to 50% threshold level (or just below) for Continuous Interleaved Sampling (CIS)–type strategies and to the minimum amount of stimulation necessary for 100% detection for *n*-of-*m* strategies. T levels should be based on at least two recipient responses to the programming signal (presented on a given channel) when presented in ascending presentation mode.

After determining the T level on a given electrode (i.e., channel), the audiologist should proceed with the measurement of T levels for other electrodes across the electrode array. For young children, the audiologist should try to quickly measure T level for different frequency segments throughout the electrode array using a staggered approach. In other words, after measuring T level on an apical electrode, the audiologist should measure T level on a basal electrode next and then measure T level on an electrode in the middle of the array. From that point, another apically located electrode may be measured followed by another basally located electrode. Young children often have short attention spans and may abruptly decide that they no longer wish to participate in the T-level measurement process. If this occurs, the aforementioned staggered strategy of T-level measurement will allow for a representation of T-level measurements across the frequency range. If the recipient fatigues during the measurement of T levels, then the audiologist may estimate T levels across the rest of the electrode array by interpolating the T levels on unmeasured channels based on the T levels determined for channels at which measurements were completed (see Chapter 7 for an explanation of interpolation).

Once the first few cochlear implant programming sessions are completed with a recipient, the audiologist will most likely have identified the recipient's T levels. As a result, the audiologist may begin T-level testing at stimulation levels at which the recipient previously responded and then quickly proceed with determination of the lowest stimulation level that the recipient can detect. T levels should be measured several times during the first year of cochlear implant use. After an adult recipient has a stable cochlear implant program and is performing well, evaluation and programming should occur one to two times per year. Children should be seen for cochlear implant programming and audiologic assessment every three months until they are 7 years old. However, if audiologic and speech and language assessment indicate that the child is making satisfactory progress with his/her cochlear implant, and the child's caregivers have no concerns, then the audiologist should avoid making changes to stimulation levels merely for the sake of making a change. A suggested programming and evaluation schedule for adult and pediatric implant recipients is provided in Chapter 23.

Negative consequences may arise when T levels are not programmed appropriately. When T levels are set too low, the recipient will not have adequate audibility of low-level or soft sounds. When a recipient has insufficient audibility for low-level sounds (e.g., sound-field warbled tone detection thresholds are poorer than 25–30 dB HL, speech recognition is poor for low-level speech [50 dBA], the recipient or the recipient's caregivers report difficulty with low-level sounds), the audiologist may consider increasing the T level to improve the recipient's access to low-level sounds. However, the audiologist should also be aware of other programming parameters that may be adjusted to optimize audibility for low-level sounds (see Chapters 15–17). When T levels are set too high (i.e., above the real threshold), the subject may hear too much ambient noise, low-level sounds may elicit a loudness percept that is higher than what would be experienced with a listener with normal hearing, and the recipient's electrical dynamic range will be reduced unnecessarily. Also, when T levels are set too high in CIS-type strategies, the user may report a continuous noise that sounds like "bacon frying," "buzzing," "hissing," "humming," or "static."

In addition to traditional threshold measurement techniques (i.e., modified Hughson–Westlake), the audiologist may use methods to measure T levels, including the: (1) count-the-beeps method, (2) psychophysical loudness scaling, and (3) threshold estimation. The count-the-beeps method may be appropriate for recipients who have difficulty distinguishing between their tinnitus and a continuous programming stimulus. When using the count-the-beeps approach, the audiologist alters the number of programming stimuli that are presented during each stimulus trial, and the recipient is asked to count the number of programming stimuli that were presented (e.g., the audiologist presents one, two, three, four, or five "beeps," and the recipient must determine the correct number). With this method, the T level typically corresponds to the stimulus level that is audible to the recipient on 100% of stimulus presentations. T levels set with the counting-the-beeps method will likely be higher than T levels that are set with the Hughson–Westlake method. Skinner, Holden, Holden, and Demorest (1995) showed that use of the count-the-beeps method for setting T levels results in better access to low-level sounds compared with programs created via the audiometric-style approach (i.e., Hughson–Westlake). The count-the-beeps method may also be a successful approach to be used with recipients who provide excessive false positive responses as well as to improve audibility for low-level sounds for recipients who have less than

ideal sound-field detection thresholds when T levels are based on conventional audiometric measurement.

Psychophysical loudness scaling may also be used to set T levels at the stimulation level corresponding to a soft-loudness percept. Using a chart for assessing loudness growth, the audiologist gradually increases the presentation level starting at a point that is inaudible and eventually stopping when the stimulus level is perceived as "most comfortable" or "loud." T level is set to the stimulus level that corresponds to a psychophysical rating of "very soft" or "soft" (Figure 14–3). When comparing traditional (i.e., Hughson–Westlake) and loudness scaling methods, Skinner and colleagues (1995) concluded that programs established using loudness scaling resulted in better access to low-level sounds. Of note, the Skinner et al. (1995) study was conducted with cochlear implant technology that was not designed to provide audibility for audio inputs below 35 dB SPL when used at default settings. Modern cochlear implant systems are designed to provide ready access to low-level sounds, and as a result, audibility of low-level inputs is often sufficient with T levels set using a conventional Hughson–Westlake audiometric-style approach. However, the psychophysical loudness scaling approach may be beneficial for recipients who have abnormally slow loudness growth over the lower portion of their electrical dynamic range (EDR) (e.g., all stimuli from 125 to 155 clinical units are perceived as soft) and typical or fast growth for the upper portion of the EDR (e.g., 155 to 164 clinical units equals the percept ranging from soft to loud, but comfortable). Limited or slow loudness growth over a substantial portion of the lower end of the EDR sometimes is described as a "T-tail," which refers to the limited change in loudness percept across a wide range of stimulation levels in the lower part of the EDR. When a T-tail occurs, it often is helpful to increase T levels to the point at which loudness begins to grow with increases in stimulus level. Detection of T-tails and the point at which loudness begins to grow above threshold can only be identified by use of the psychophysical scaling method. The psychophysical loudness growth approach (i.e., setting T level to a "soft" percept) may also be used to improve sound-field detection thresholds (audibility of low-level sounds) for recipients who have elevated soundfield thresholds (e.g., 35 dB HL and higher) with programs based on conventional measurements (e.g., Hughson–Westlake). However, it should be noted that T-tails are relatively rare, and the psychophysical scaling approach is typically not required to

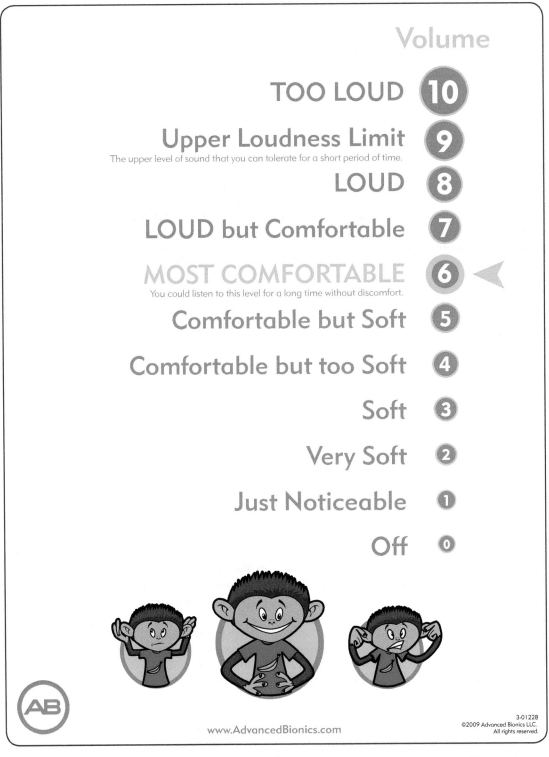

Volume

TOO LOUD ⑩

Upper Loudness Limit ⑨
The upper level of sound that you can tolerate for a short period of time.

LOUD ⑧

LOUD but Comfortable ⑦

MOST COMFORTABLE ⑥ ◄
You could listen to this level for a long time without discomfort.

Comfortable but Soft ⑤

Comfortable but too Soft ④

Soft ③

Very Soft ②

Just Noticeable ①

Off ⓪

FIGURE 14–3. An example of a chart that may be used for loudness measurements. Image provided courtesy of Advanced Bionics, LLC.

facilitate good access to low-level sounds with use of modern cochlear implant technology.

Another alternative method for determining T levels is through the use of manufacturer-developed estimation strategies in which T levels are estimated on the basis of the recipient's upper-stimulation levels. Research has shown that most recipients achieve adequate audibility for low-level sounds when T levels are estimated from upper-stimulation levels (Spahr & Dorman, 2005). However, some studies have shown that estimated T levels result in inadequate audibility of low-level sounds for some recipients (Holden et al., 2011). As a result, the audiologist should consider measuring T levels, especially when a recipient has unsatisfactory audibility for low-level sounds. Of note, unlike the count-the-beeps and psychophysical loudness scaling methods, the T-level estimation method was not developed to optimize audibility for low-level sounds. Instead, the T-level estimation method is a streamlined programming approach designed to expedite the process of programming a cochlear implant.

Special Considerations for Setting Threshold Levels for Children

Setting electrical-threshold levels for children can be challenging; however, appropriate T levels can be determined for most children by using traditional, age-appropriate audiologic methods to determine behavioral hearing thresholds of infants and young children. Techniques for measuring behavioral hearing thresholds of children include behavioral observation audiometry (BOA), visual reinforcement audiometry (VRA), conditioned play audiometry (CPA), and the standard audiometric approach used for adults. The success of a particular technique is dependent on the chronological and developmental age, mood, motivation, behavior, and listening experience of the child as well as to the conditioning/reinforcement strategies and skill level of the programming audiologist and programming assistant.

An animated, enthusiastic, and skilled programming test assistant is essential for obtaining optimal stimulation levels with children. It is almost impossible for a single audiologist to effectively program the cochlear implant sound processor of an infant or young child, manage the child's behavior, attend to any questions or concerns the child's caregivers may have, and facilitate cooperation from the child during a lengthy programming session. Many clinics designate an audiologist as the programmer and a sec-

ond audiologist or a speech-language therapist (e.g., Listening and Spoken Language Specialist [LSLS]) as the test assistant. Children will be particularly comfortable with their speech-language pathologist or LSLS whom they see on a weekly basis. Also, the LSLS is familiar with the child and will be aware of strategies that may be used to facilitate the child's cooperation with the implant programming process. Additionally, the LSLS can work with the child during weekly therapy sessions to develop listening skills needed to determine appropriate stimulation levels (e.g., CPA: drop the toy in the bucket when stimulus heard, loudness balancing, loudness scaling). When the child's LSLS or another audiologist is unavailable, an audiology assistant may serve as the programming assistant. Furthermore, the programming audiologist may coach the clinic receptionist to serve as a capable programming assistant. Of note, use of an audiology assistant is less expensive than scheduling two audiologists to program the implant of one child. The primary requirement is that the assistant is familiar with the objective of the task and the procedures required to obtain accurate responses from the child and is adept at managing the behavior of the child. The roles of the test assistant include facilitating a conditioned response from the child, attempting to keep the child from producing false positive responses when programming stimuli are not presented, keeping the child engaged with the programming task, ensuring that the transmitting coil remains on the child's head so that stimulation may be delivered, managing the child's behavior, assisting in the completion of objective measures (e.g., facilitating the child's cooperation so that electrically evoked stapedial reflex threshold test and electrically evoked compound action potential assessment may be completed), and helping to observe the child's responses to the stimuli delivered from the cochlear implant.

In pediatric audiology, BOA has long been considered an unreliable method of determining the threshold of audibility of a young child. Research has shown that infants typically respond at suprathreshold levels when the BOA procedure is used and that infants quickly fatigue to the presentation of auditory stimuli (Thompson & Weber, 1974; Wilson & Thompson, 1984). There are no peer-reviewed studies that indicate that BOA (with observation of any type of response such as a change in the child's sucking response, breathing pattern, facial expression, eye-widening, etc.) may be used to obtain threshold-level auditory responses from infants and young children.

However, BOA may be the only method available to observe auditory responsiveness to cochlear implant stimulation for some recipients (i.e., infants, recipients with neurological and/or motor disabilities). Consequently, the audiologist may have to use BOA to observe the auditory responsiveness to cochlear implant stimulation for recipients who cannot participate with other threshold-seeking procedures (e.g., VRA, CPA, traditional audiometry). When auditory responsiveness is evaluated via BOA, the audiologist should keep in mind that the recipient's responses are likely to be suprathreshold in nature. As a result, the audiologist may consider globally decreasing the T levels from the recipient's minimum response levels observed during the BOA procedure. Additionally, when BOA is being conducted, it is likely that the recipient will respond at lower stimulation levels to complex stimuli such as speech (Wilson & Thompson, 1984). As a result, the audiologist may want to evaluate the recipient's auditory responsiveness when the implant is active during live speech mode to determine whether the recipient responds to lower levels of stimulation in response to speech compared with the responses obtained to the frequency-specific programming stimuli. For example, the audiologist may decrease stimulation levels well below the levels at which the recipient responded to the frequency-specific programming stimulus. Then, the audiologist would activate the cochlear implant in live speech mode and globally increase stimulation levels while observing for signs of a response from the recipient. For children who cannot participate in traditional threshold-seeking procedures (VRA, CPA, etc.), the audiologist should use a combination of behavioral observations and objective measures to determine the stimulation levels that are appropriate for a child. For young children who have Advanced Bionics and MED-EL cochlear implants and who cannot provide threshold-level responses, the audiologist may choose to estimate T levels based on the upper-stimulation levels that are provided for the child.

Traditional VRA testing techniques are optimal for determining T levels in pediatric implant recipients with a developmental age ranging from 8 to 20 months. As a result, it is imperative that pediatric cochlear implant clinics have VRA equipment in the room in which cochlear implants are programmed. The attainment of accurate auditory thresholds with the use of VRA is dependent upon the abilities of the programming audiologist and test assistant to effectively administer the VRA procedures. The programming audiologist and test assistant must both be familiar with evidence-based procedures used to complete VRA to obtain threshold-level responses in infants and young children. A complete description of VRA technique is beyond the scope of this book. However, because of the vital importance of VRA in the creation of cochlear implant programs for infants and young children, a brief description of an evidence-based VRA protocol is provided below. The reader is referred to additional resources for a more thorough and excellent description of VRA assessment (Gravel, 2000; Gravel & Hood, 1999).

Outline of the Hearts for Hearing Protocol for Visual Reinforcement Audiometry in Children

1. Preparation
   a. The child should be seated comfortably (torso and feet supported) with reinforcing toys located at ±90° relative to the child.
   b. The reinforcing toys should be invisible prior to signal presentation.
   c. The programming assistant should ensure that the child's attention is at midline. This may be achieved by displaying a mundane toy (e.g., peg, block). The toy should be interesting enough to establish midline attention but not so distracting that it causes the child to ignore the programming stimulus.
2. Establish the Conditioned Response
   a. Present a signal below a level at which the audiologist believes a response will be audible and increase in relatively large step-sizes (e.g., 5–10 CL for Nucleus recipients) until the child makes a full (90-degree) head turn. It is important to note that in classical VRA, the procedure is initiated by a period of response shaping (i.e., conditioning). However, in clinical VRA, this period of response shaping may waste valuable attention and responses of young children. As a result, many experts suggest that VRA should be initiated by immediately searching for threshold (Gravel, 2000; Gravel & Hood, 1999). Once the audiologist and test assistant observe the child make a time-locked, volitional head turn to the test signal, the audiologist should commence with a threshold search (see point "3" ["Threshold Search"] in this outline).
   b. The audiologist should activate the VRA reinforcer (e.g., toy, video screen) immediately after the child makes a time-locked head turn (90 degrees) toward the reinforcer.

c. Type of test signal: The audiologist should begin with stimulation to an apical channel. After threshold (minimum response level [MRL]) is obtained, proceed in a staggered approach (basal electrode followed by middle electrode, etc.)

  i. Measure as many electrodes as the child's attention will allow.

  ii. Response shaping should be conducted as necessary if volitional head turn does not occur.

d. Response Shaping

  i. The audiologist should present the programming signal at a level presumed to be audible to the child, and the test assistant should orient the child to the VRA reinforcer. The audiologist can determine a level that is likely to be audible by examining the child's electrically evoked compound action potential (ECAP) threshold (see Chapter 18). The programming signal should be audible to the child when presented at levels exceeding the ECAP threshold.

  ii. As the programming assistant orients the child toward the VRA reinforcer, the audiologist should pair the signal presentation with activation of the VRA reinforcer for one or two seconds. The objective of response shaping is to cue the child that the presence of the programming signal will lead to activation of the reinforcer. The goal of response shaping is for the child to make a head turn toward the reinforcer when the programming signal is presented.

  iii. After response shaping is completed, the audiologist and programming assistant should observe for volitional head turn at the same level used for response shaping. In other words, the test assistant does not direct the child's attention to the VRA reinforcer. Instead, they wait to see if the child will turn to the VRA reinforcer without direction when the programming signal is presented.

  iv. If the child becomes captivated with the VRA reinforce and does not want to redirect his/her gaze back to midline, the test assistant should use an engaging toy (light, puppet, etc.) to bring back to midline. The toy used to bring the child's

attention back to midline should be compelling enough to get the child to turn away from the reinforcer while also not captivating the child to the point that he/she will no longer make a head turn in response to the programming stimulus.

  v. Response shaping should be attempted a second time if the child does not make a volitional head turn without direction or cueing from the programming assistant.

  vi. The VRA procedure should be abandoned if a volitional head turn does not occur after final shaping attempt.

  vii. The audiologist should then attempt to establish a VRA conditioned response with bone conduction stimulation (vibrotactile stimulation at equipment limits of audiometer at 250/500 Hz). Use of vibrotactile stimulation to establish VRA conditioned response will allow the audiologist to determine whether the child is capable of a head turn and may also facilitate the child's understanding of VRA procedure. If the child does not participate in VRA when the signal is delivered via bone conduction, then the audiologist should conclude that the child will not condition to the VRA task.

3. Threshold Search

a. After the audiologist confirms that the child is capable to producing a conditioned response in the VRA procedure, the threshold search should commence. The audiologist should decrease the signal level (e.g., by 10 CL) and present the test signal again

b. The audiologist should use up/down 10 CL bracketing steps to determine threshold (up 5/down 10 dB and eventually up 2/down 4 CL steps may be used for later tests when the audiologist can pursue threshold with a finer resolution, because she/he has a better idea of where threshold resides)

c. The electrical threshold (T level) is obtained when the child responds twice (or three times if doubts persist) to the test signal in an ascending presentation Test Order

  i. Obtain VRA thresholds to stimulation delivered to Apical, Middle, Basal, Mid-Apical, Mid-Basal, Most Basal electrodes ("hopping" from one part of the array to another to acquire thresholds across the frequency range)

4. Pearls to Keep in Mind Regarding VRA
   a. Use control trials to look for false positive responses
      i. If the false positive response rate is less than 30% during control trials, the recipient's responses are likely to be reliable. If the false positive rate is greater than 50% in control trials, then the audiologist should abandon the VRA task.
      ii. The audiologist should be certain that T levels are not set erroneously because false positives are taken as true responses. Pediatric audiologist and researcher Robert Nozza reminds us, "It's easy to teach head turn but the hard part is to prevent head turn when unneeded" (Tharpe, 2015).
   b. Audiologists should remember that one accurate threshold is better than several inaccurate thresholds. Consequently, the audiologist should ensure that the VRA task is carefully administered to ensure the validity of the responses that are observed and recorded.
   c. VRA is a test of detection, not a test of orientation. As a result, a full head turn should be reinforced regardless of whether the child turns toward the ear that is stimulated.
   d. Once a conditioned response is established, prompting/cueing should be avoided or used with extreme caution.
      i. The programming assistant should communicate with the audiologist if it appears that the test signal may be audible but the child is not producing a head turn. The audiologist and programming assistant can repeat response shaping if necessary.
      ii. The programming audiologist should communicate with programming assistant when test signal is likely to be audible but the child is not responding. Again, response shaping may be necessary.
   e. Providing reinforcement of responses other than a full head turn or a CPA response is playing with fire and is likely to increase the likelihood of obtaining false positive responses
   f. Alternate frequency (i.e., channel) of stimulation to maintain attention
   g. When in doubt, do not reinforce!
   h. The programming audiologist and assistant should communicate throughout the VRA procedure to ensure that valid responses are obtained.

Traditional CPA testing techniques are suitable for measuring T levels in children with developmental ages ranging from 2 to 8 years. Many children are able to develop a conditioned play response as young as 18 months, particularly when the child practices on the CPA task in therapy sessions and/or at home. Additionally, some older children (≥6 years) will prefer a conventional audiometric approach, whereas others will not be able to maintain attention over long periods of time; as a result, CPA may prove to be the best approach to obtain T levels for children throughout the elementary-age period (up to 11 years old). Therefore, audiologists should be flexible and use the approach that yields the most reliable and valid threshold responses for a particular child.

In order for CPA to be effective, the child must be interested in the CPA task. Because children with cochlear implants must attend multiple programming sessions and audiometric evaluations per year, the audiologist should provide a variety of exciting and entertaining CPA tasks. Figure 14–4 provides several examples of CPA games proven successful for establishing T levels. For young children or those who are inattentive and hyperactive, it may be necessary to use multiple CPA toys during the session. In fact, the author of this chapter has used as many as 10 to 15 different CPA tasks in a session to facilitate the attainment of T levels across the array for a child with a short attention span and sound field, which aided warbled tone detection thresholds in the audiometric test booth.

Although conventional toys and snacks often serve as excellent manipulatives to facilitate CPA assessment, electronic media may also be used to facilitate CPA success. For instance, a monitor may be connected to a button that the child may push when he/she detects the programming signal. When the child pushes the button, a slide is advanced within a PowerPoint slide show possessing child-friendly pictures (child-friendly images such as Disney figures, Pixar figures, comic book heroes, princesses, animals, etc.). Additionally, there are several tablet apps that may be used to obtain T levels via a CPA approach. For instance, the child can "launch an angry bird" each time he/she hears the test signal. The audiologist is encouraged to use his/her imagination to determine ways in which tablet apps may be used to measure T levels.

The same ascending/descending approach used to measure thresholds in adults also is applicable to young children. However, for young children with

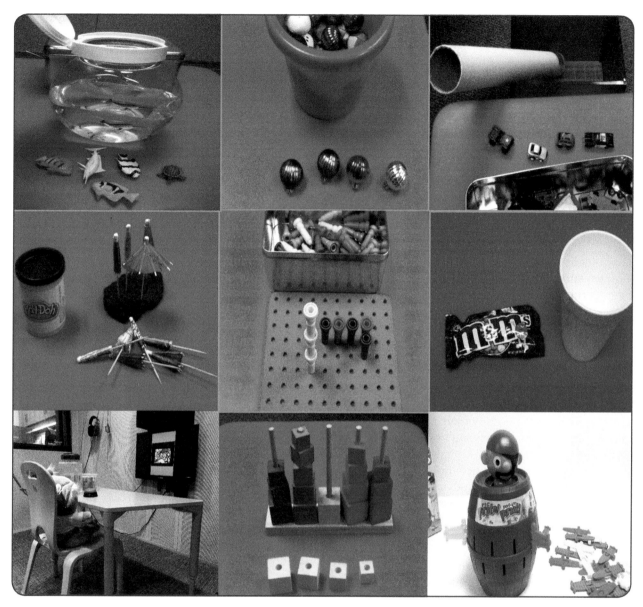

FIGURE 14–4. Examples of conditioned play audiometry activities.

shorter attention spans, larger step sizes may be used to obtain T levels. Also, similar to adult procedures, measurement of T levels should begin with a low-frequency (i.e., apical) electrode contact. When a valid threshold is obtained for a low-frequency contact, the audiologist should promptly move on to an electrode contact in the basal end of the array followed by attainment of a threshold for an electrode in the middle of the array. If the child's attention is maintained, T levels should be obtained on as many electrodes as possible. Interpolation should be used to estimate T levels on unmeasured channels.

At initial activation, the child's T levels are likely above the true threshold. Thus, it may be necessary to provide a slight decrease in the T levels used in the child's map. Children's T levels appear to increase through the first few months of implant use and stabilize by three months to one year post implantation (Henkin et al., 2006; Henkin, Kaplan-Neeman, Muchnik, Kronenberg, & Hildesheimer, 2003; Hughes et al., 2001). As a result, children should be seen frequently for mapping during the first few months of cochlear implant use, and the audiologist should re-measure T levels at these frequent programming sessions. Also, aided soundfield warbled tone thresholds should be measured to ensure that the child has satisfactory access to low-level sounds (i.e., 20–25 dB HL aided thresholds). After the first 6 months of implant use, the authors recommend that young children return for evaluation and programming on a quarterly basis until the child is 7 years old (or for up to two years post-activation for children who are older than 7 years at the time of activation) in order to ensure that T levels are appropriate.

By no later than 1-month post-activation, the audiologist should measure the child's minimal response levels in the soundfield to frequency-specific stimuli (i.e., warbled tones). Responses should be no greater than 30 dB HL in the low frequencies (250 and 500 Hz) and should not exceed 25 dB HL in the mid to high frequencies. If the child's responses do not meet these criteria, the audiologist should seek to optimize T-level stimulation through manual adjustments or consider adjusting other parameters (e.g., IDR, Maplaw) to optimize access to low-level sounds (see Chapters 15 through 17 for manufacturer-specific adjustments that may be made to optimize access to low-level audio inputs).

Manufacturer-developed, threshold-estimation procedures may be used with children only when T levels cannot be measured easily and soundfield detection thresholds indicate that the estimated T levels are providing good access to low-level sounds (i.e., soundfield detection thresholds at 25 dB HL or better). In general, manual measurement of T level should be completed with children to ensure adequate stimulation for low-level inputs.

The audiologist should be attentive for signs of insufficient access to low-level sounds. If the child's caregivers or LSLS reports that the child does not consistently respond to soft sounds, then it may be necessary to increase T levels. Finally, if sound-field detection thresholds are elevated, T levels should be increased to provide better access to low-level sounds. Prior to adjustment of T levels, the audiologist should verify that elevated soundfield thresholds are not related to a faulty microphone. If the sound processor contains microphone covers to protect against moisture and debris, then the audiologist should ensure that the covers are clean and free of obstruction and debris. It should be noted that MED-

EL recommends adjustment of the Maplaw parameter to improve access to low-level sounds instead of increasing THR (threshold) levels (Chapter 17).

Additional Measure to Ensure Adequate T Levels and Confirm Audibility

For children and adults, many audiologists ensure adequate audibility for sounds across the speech frequency range by confirming that the recipient can detect all six Ling sounds (/ah/, /oo/, /ee/, /s/, /sh/, and /m/; Ling, 1976, 1989). These six phonemes encompass the typical range of speech frequencies, so audibility for the Ling sounds should ensure audibility for most all of the sounds within the speech frequency range. During the first few days of implant use, all six Ling sounds should be audible when spoken at an average conversational level, 6 feet away from the user. By 1 month of implant use, all six Ling sounds should be audible when spoken at an average conversational level from a distance of at least 15 feet from the user. Furthermore, a goal of accurate discrimination of all six Ling sounds should be rapidly pursued, and on a daily basis, the caregivers of young children should be coached to routinely conduct the Ling six sound test to ensure that the child can detect all six sounds.

Setting Upper-Stimulation Levels for Adults

The provision of optimal upper-stimulation levels (i.e., M, most comfortable level [MCL], or C levels depending on manufacturer) is one of the most important components of the cochlear implant programming process. Even with adult recipients, it can be difficult to determine exactly where upper-stimulation levels should be set across the electrode array in order to provide optimal sound quality and speech recognition. Underestimating the upper-stimulation levels may sacrifice speech recognition, hamper sound quality, and limit the recipient's ability to monitor his/her own voice (i.e., intensity, vocal quality). Overestimating stimulation levels may cause discomfort, hinder speech recognition, adversely influence sound quality, and foster an aversive reaction to the implant.

Similar to T levels, the maximum level of stimulation that a recipient will tolerate is likely to change over the first few months of cochlear implant use. Many users are able to reach a desired level of stimulation for optimal performance after several weeks of cochlear implant use (see Chapters 21 and 22). However, some recipients will require gradual changes over several months to reach an optimal upper-stimulation level. Most importantly, recipients differ in the upper-stimulation levels that they initially will tolerate and in the upper-stimulation levels that yield the best hearing performance. There is no "one-size-fits-all" universal set of stimulation levels that may be applied across all recipients to yield optimal performance.

There are several methods used to determine a cochlear implant recipient's upper-stimulation levels, including psychophysical loudness scaling, global adjustment of stimulation levels, electrically evoked stapedial reflex threshold assessment, and loudness balancing. Psychophysical loudness scaling was previously discussed as a measure that may be used to set T levels in order to optimize audibility for low-level sounds. Similar procedures are employed when psychophysical loudness scaling is used to determine upper-stimulation levels. The programming stimulus is presented to an electrode contact or to a band of channels, and the recipient is asked to indicate the loudness level of the stimulus by pointing to a loudness scaling chart (see Figure 14–3). The audiologist gradually increases the level of the programming stimulus until the recipient reports that the signal has reached a loudness level that corresponds to the level the manufacturer recommends for upper-stimulation level (e.g., "most comfortable" for Advanced Bionics, "loud but comfortable" for Cochlear, and "loud but not uncomfortable" for MED-EL). Psychophysical loudness scaling may be repeated for many, if not all, of the electrode contacts in the array. If upper-stimulation levels are not measured for each individual electrode contact, interpolation may be used to estimate the levels of the unmeasured electrode contacts. When cochlear implants were initially made available for commercial use, psychophysical loudness scaling was routinely used to determine upper-stimulation level on an electrode-by-electrode basis. However, frequency-specific psychophysical loudness scaling is time consuming, and more importantly, it may not be entirely indicative the of upper-stimulation levels that are optimal for real world use. When recipients use their cochlear implants during real world use, they listen to broadband complex sounds, and the loudness of those everyday sounds is determined by summation that occurs when stimulation is delivered across multiple channels. As a result, the recipient's overall loudness experience when listening to broadband sounds may be quite different from the loudness experience when listening to frequency-specific

sounds (Bentler & Pavlovic, 1989; Walker et al., 1984). Furthermore, loudness scaling responses obtained via clinical measurement have been shown to have levels of intersubject and intrasubject variability as well as to be dependent upon the instructions provided to the listener (Dillon, 2012).

Another approach to setting upper-stimulation levels is to provide a global increase in upper-stimulation levels while the recipient listens to live speech and environmental sounds. The audiologist provides a gradual global increase in the upper-stimulation levels with the objective of determining upper-stimulation levels that will optimize comfort, clarity, and sound quality of speech and environmental sounds.

Setting upper stimulation via a global adjustment is an efficient and potentially effective method to identify the optimal upper-stimulation levels for a recipient. If T levels have been measured at the activation session (Figure 14–5A), then the audiologist should provide a global decrease in T levels to a point at which the T level stimulation should be inaudible to the newly activated adult recipient (Figure 14–5B). Then, upper-stimulation levels should be superimposed on the T levels (see Figure 14–5B). Next, the audiologist should inform the recipient that "the implant will be activated so that you (the recipient) will be able to hear speech and other sounds in the room. The goal will be to slowly increase the 'volume' of the sound until it is at a most comfortable level. The new sound from the implant may be unnatural at first. Don't worry. It will get better with time. For now, we just want the 'volume level' to be comfortable. The 'volume' will be increased slowly. Please let me know if the implant gets too loud, and I will decrease the 'volume level' so that it is comfortable."

After the explanation is completed, the audiologist activates the implant in live speech mode and gradually increases the upper-stimulation levels while the recipient listens to the speech of family members or the audiologist. Oftentimes, recipients will inform the audiologist that the optimal level has been reached, when in reality, an additional increase in upper-stimulation level may improve clarity and sound quality of speech and environmental sounds. Consequently, when a recipient initially reports that upper-stimulation levels are satisfactory, the audiologist should inform the recipient that a small increase in stimulation will be provided in order to determine whether sound quality and speech recognition improve. The audiologist should remind the recipient that the upper-stimulation levels will be decreased

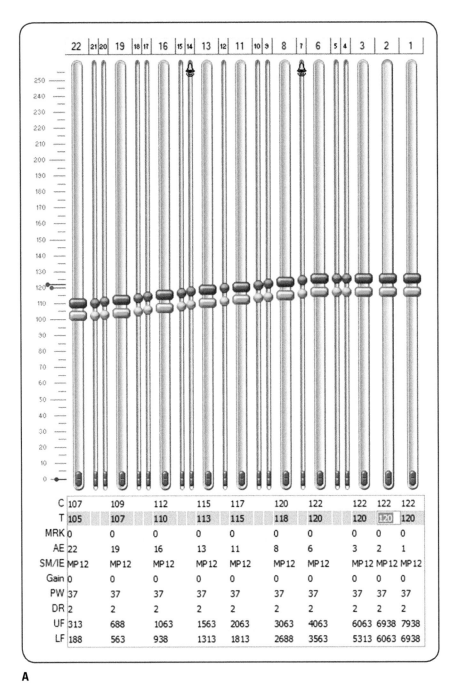

A

FIGURE 14–5. Examples of stimulation levels based on T-level measurements and global adjustment of upper stimulation levels. See the description in the text for an explanation of how the stimulation levels were determined. *continues*

if the recipient considers speech and environmental sounds to be too loud or associated with poorer sound quality. Typically, the additional increase in upper-stimulation level does improve the recipient's percept. Upper-stimulation levels are increased in small increments until the recipient reports that sound quality, speech recognition, and/or comfort begins to deteriorate. At that point, upper-stimulation levels are decreased to a point that provides optimal sound quality, speech recognition, and comfort for the recip-

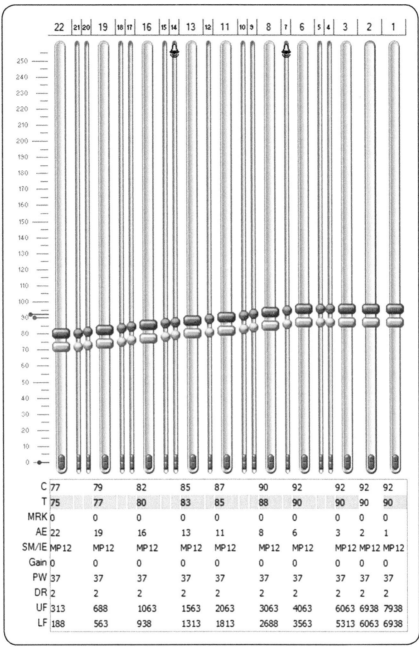

B

FIGURE 14–5. *continues*

ient (Figure 14–5C). This approach allows the recipient to fully explore his/her electrical dynamic range to ensure that upper-stimulation levels are optimized. The audiologist should closely monitor the reaction of the recipient. If the recipient exhibits overt signs that the stimulation from the implant is becoming uncomfortable or too loud, the audiologist should be prepared to decrease the upper-stimulation levels. Once upper-stimulation levels are globally increased to a comfortable level, the audiologist should increase T levels back to the levels at which they were previously measured (Figure 14–5D). A global decrease from the measured T-level values may need to be provided if the recipient complains of a static/buzz-

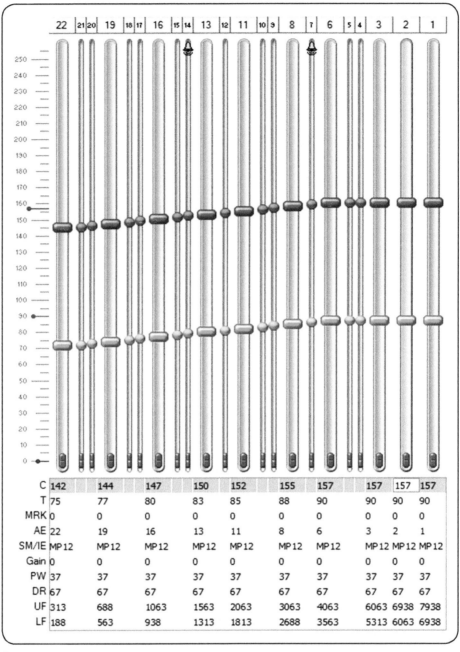

C

FIGURE 14–5. *continues*

ing noise or ambient noise being too noticeable with T levels set to the measured levels.

Research has shown that the upper-stimulation level profile (i.e., the "shape" of the upper-stimulation levels across the electrode array) is typically flatter than the T-level profile (Botros & Psarros, 2010). As such, when upper-stimulation levels are globally increased, the audiologist should consider arbitrarily flattening the upper-stimulation level profile. Of note, the upper-stimulation levels should not be set to the same level across the electrode array. Instead, the audiologist should "smooth" the upper-stimulation

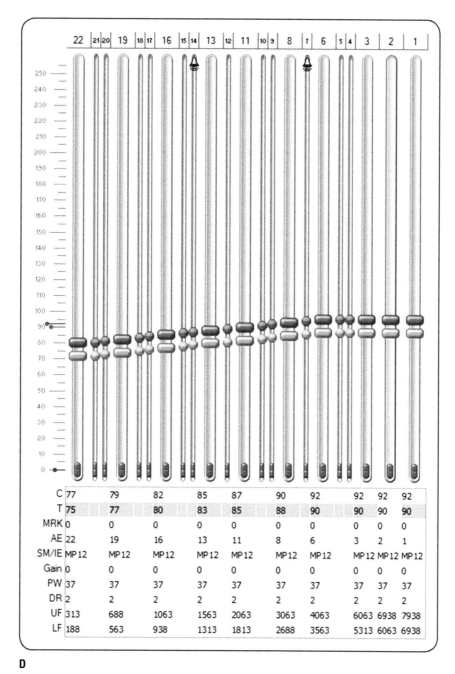

D

FIGURE 14–5. *continues*

profile so that the upper-stimulation levels do not change abruptly across the electrode array (Figure 14–5E). For example, if the T levels at the basal end of the array are substantially higher than the T levels at the apical end of the array, then the upper-stimulation levels should also likely be higher at the

basal end of the array. However, the audiologist may consider providing a slight decrease of the upper-stimulation levels so that the upper-stimulation level profile is flatter than the T-level profile. As a result, the electrical dynamic range at the basal end of the array will be narrower than the electrical dynamic

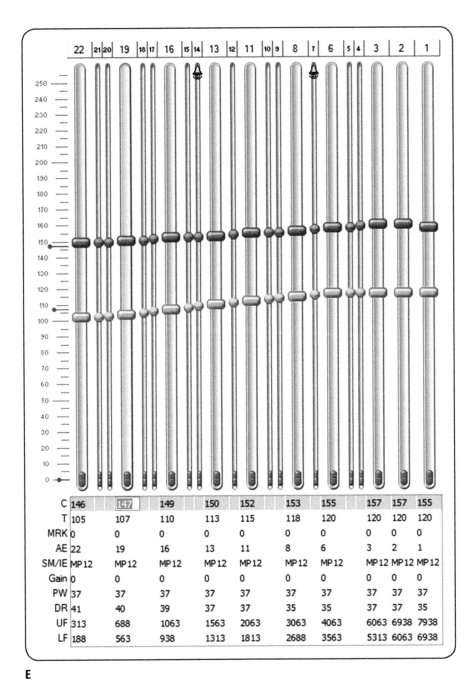

E

FIGURE 14–5. *continued*

range at the apical end. Botros and Psarros (2010) showed that the upper-stimulation level profile is more likely to be flat when the global upper-stimulation levels are high. As such, the upper-stimulation level profile is especially more likely to be flatter than the T-level profile for recipients who have wider electrical dynamic ranges.

At the activation session, some audiologists also will elect to "tilt" or provide tapered decreases or increases in the low- or high-frequency portion of the array to address the recipient's complaints or comments regarding sound quality. For instance, if the recipient reports that sounds have too much bass or are too sharp, the audiologist can taper off the upper-stimulation levels in the low or high frequencies, respectively. On the other hand, if a recipient cannot hear his or her voice very well or if speech lacks sufficient clarity, the audiologist may increase upper-stimulation levels in the low or high frequencies, respectively.

After upper-stimulation levels are globally set to a comfortable level, the audiologist should balance the loudness of upper-stimulation levels across the electrode array. Loudness balancing is typically not completed during the activation session. Within a week or two of implant use, however, the audiologist should attempt to balance the loudness at the upper-stimulation level across all channels. Ensuring equal loudness at the upper-stimulation level is likely one of the most important components in creating a program that provides optimal speech recognition and sound quality. Indeed, many evidence-based hearing aid prescriptive methods (NAL, NAL-NL2) have unequivocally demonstrated that the provision of equal loudness across the frequency range results in optimal speech recognition and sound quality (Byrne, 1986; Byrne, Parkinson, & Newall, 1990; Dillon, 2012; Dillon & Keidser, 2013). Establishing equal loudness across the electrode array assists in maintaining the typical loudness/intensity relationship that exists for different phonemes. For example, low-frequency phonemes (e.g., vowels) are typically louder and more intense than high-frequency phonemes (e.g., fricatives). If high-frequency upper-stimulation levels were considerably louder than the low-frequency upper-stimulation levels, then the recipient may perceive the fricatives to be much more intense than vowels, which would likely impair speech recognition and sound quality.

Additionally, Sainz et al. (2003) showed that loudness balancing is necessary to optimize global upper-stimulation levels. For example, if the upper-stimulation level provided on one channel (or a few channels) is significantly louder than the upper-stimulation levels on remaining channels, then global stimulation levels will be set to a point that will allow the loudness to remain comfortable on the channel (or subset of channels) that elicits the loudest percept. Consequently, the upper-stimulation levels on the remaining channels may possess suboptimal upper-stimulation levels.

Ideally, the loudness balancing measurement should be completed at the upper-stimulation level (or 80%–90% of the upper-stimulation level for MED-EL recipients) for two channels at a time. Loudness balancing typically begins with the most apical channel and progresses toward the more basal end of the array. However, for some recipients who have a difficult time tolerating high-frequency stimuli, the audiologist may consider conducting loudness balancing from the basal end toward the apical end. A visual chart should be used to facilitate the loudness balancing procedure (Figure 14–6). The audiologist must provide clear instructions to the recipient to ensure that the loudness balancing assessment is valid. The audiologist should say, "Now, you are going to hear two sounds. I want you to tell me if the first sound is louder, the second sound is louder, or if they are the same loudness. The two different sounds will likely be different in pitch. Please ignore the pitch of the two sounds and only pay attention to the loudness. The second sound may sound sharper than the first because the pitch is higher, but please focus only on the loudness difference between the two sounds."

When conducting loudness balancing, the adjustment to the stimulation level always should be to the second electrode in the pair because the first electrode is balanced to the preceding electrodes in the array. Once loudness balancing is completed, the audiologist should activate the program in live speech mode and ensure that the upper-stimulation levels are globally adjusted to optimize clarity, sound quality, and comfort. Occasionally, small changes in global upper-stimulation levels are necessary to optimize auditory performance after loudness balancing has been completed.

A third and more objective approach to setting upper-stimulation levels is the use of electrically evoked stapedial reflex threshold (ESRT). Many audiologists use ESRT as a standard component of their programming test battery because it is a straightforward and simple measure to administer. The ESRT should be measured with all cochlear implant recipients regardless of age. The ESRT has been shown to serve as a good predictor of appropriate upper-stimulation levels (Gordon, Papsin, & Harrison, 2004; Hodges et al., 1997; Spivak et al., 1994a, 1994b). Also, the ESRT may be used to identify cases in which upper-stimulation levels may be excessively high, and the ESRT provides a useful objective measure of the auditory system's responsiveness to high-level electrical stimulation. The reader is referred to Chapter 18 for a detailed description of the ESRT, including guidance for how the ESRT may be used to estimate upper-stimulation levels of cochlear implant recipients.

Once assessment of the upper-stimulation level is completed, the audiologist may consider sweeping at the upper-stimulation level. Sweeping simply

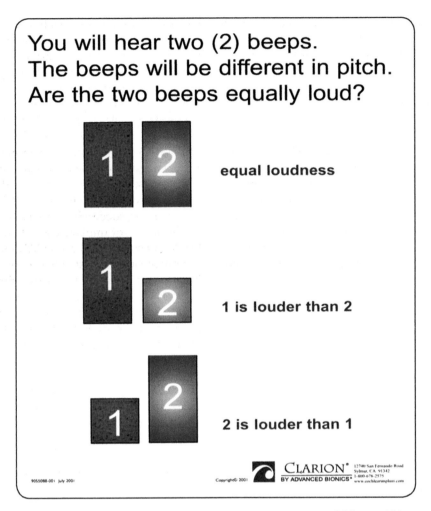

FIGURE 14–6. Loudness balancing chart. Image provided courtesy of Advanced Bionics, LLC.

involves the sequential presentation of the programming stimulus across the electrode array. Sweeping is generally not necessary when loudness balancing has been completed and upper-stimulation levels have been globally set to an optimal level. Instead, sweeping may provide useful information when the recipient is experiencing problems with sound quality or non-auditory side effects (e.g., facial nerve stimulation). Sweeping may serve to identify electrodes on which stimulation produces undesirable effects.

When implementing this procedure, the programming stimulus is presented sequentially or swept across all electrode contacts in the array (typically) beginning at the apical end and ending at the base. Three objectives are associated with electrode sweeping: (1) measuring sound quality, (2) determining appropriate pitch transitions, and (3) confirming equal loudness

across channels. Sweeping to evaluate sound-quality issues is not performed at every mapping session, but it is a good practice for newly implanted recipients for whom loudness balancing has not been completed or for recipients who are experiencing difficulties that cannot be resolved with conventional mapping techniques or troubleshooting of the external equipment. For example, the programming stimulus should typically possess a tonal percept; if the recipient reports hearing a noise-like sound (e.g., static), experiences pain or other unwanted sensations, has facial nerve stimulation, or simply reports poor sound quality, the audiologist may consider disabling or adjusting the stimulation on the contact.

The audiologist may use electrode sweeping to ensure that the recipient perceives an orderly and expected transition in pitch as stimulation is swept from the apical (i.e., low pitch) to the basal (i.e., high pitch) portion of the array. If the expected tonotopic organization is not observed, the audiologist may either disable electrodes that cause an unexpected change in pitch or reallocate the anomalous electrodes to different channels.

Finally, sweeping may be used to confirm equal loudness across the entire array rather than the traditional two to three electrodes at a time (i.e., loudness balancing). When using this procedure, the audiologist instructs the recipient to listen to all of the stimuli and raise a hand if any sounds are substantially softer or louder than the rest. This task may be performed at upper-stimulation levels or at lower portions of the electrical dynamic range. Again, sweeping is typically unnecessary for loudness balancing if the audiologist has already conducted loudness balancing on a channel-by-channel basis.

The audiologist should be familiar with the typical upper-stimulation levels and electrical dynamic ranges for a particular make, model, and electrode array of the implant under study. For example, Nucleus recipients typically possess an electrical dynamic range between 20 to 60 CL with most recipients having an electrical dynamic range around 40 to 50 CL, Advanced Bionics recipients typically possess M levels ranging between 150 to 250 charge units with M levels below 100 and above 300 charge units being relatively rare, and MED-EL recipients typically possess MCL levels between 10 and 25 charge units with MCL below 5 charge units and over 400 charge units being quite exceptional. Questions should arise when a recipient's stimulation levels and/or electrical dynamic range differ markedly from typical values. Of course, appropriate exceptions to typical values do exist (i.e., some recipients perform quite well with stimulation levels that deviate from the norm), but the audiologist should confirm through speech recognition assessment, sound-field detection thresholds, and subjective assessment that the recipient's levels are optimized, particularly when the stimulation levels deviate from what are typical for a particular make and model of implant/electrode array and for a recipient with a given pre-implant history.

Setting Upper-Stimulation Levels for Children

The ESRT is highly recommended for the estimation of ideal upper-stimulation levels of infants and children, and audiologists always should attempt to complete this measure with pediatric recipients. ESRT is a valuable measure for the determination of opti-

mal upper-stimulation levels because psychophysical loudness measures typically are not feasible for children until they are at least 4 years old (at 4 years, a child may begin to provide very basic feedback regarding whether a sound is too soft or too loud). Furthermore, precise measures of loudness scaling and loudness balancing are often not achievable until approximately 6 to 8 years of age. The ESRT can occasionally be measured at implant activation for some children. However, for many children, the programming stimulus will be too loud when presented at levels necessary to elicit the ESRT. Typically, the ESRT may be successfully measured within the first month or two of implant use. Chapter 18 provides a detailed description of the ESRT along with guidance for how the audiologist may use the ESRT to estimate the upper-stimulation levels of infants and children. Chapter 18 also provides a description of the electrically evoked compound action potential (ECAP) and the relationship of ECAP to stimulation levels. The reader is referred to Chapter 18 for information on the use of objective measures to estimate the upper-stimulation levels of children.

In the event that the ESRT cannot be recorded, the audiologist must rely on behavioral measures to determine upper-stimulation levels at the activation session. For children who are preschool-aged and younger, this almost invariably means using behavioral observation of the child's reactions following stimulation. There are numerous strategies available to estimate upper-stimulation levels from behavioral observations. First, the audiologist may globally increase upper-stimulation levels while the child listens to speech and environmental sounds. The audiologist should begin with a relatively flat upper-stimulation level profile and upper-stimulation levels that should be inaudible to the child. Initially activating at audible levels may startle and upset the child, making it difficult to complete the remainder of the programming session. If T levels were successfully measured, then the audiologist should globally decrease T to a level that is inaudible to the child and superimpose upper-stimulation levels on the T levels (see Figure 14–6).

Once the audiologist has set the stimulation levels to a level that is inaudible to the child, the sound processor should be activated in live speech mode and the upper-stimulation levels should be gradually increased in small increments while the parent or programming assistant continuously vocalizes to the child (e.g., "ba, ba, ba"; "hi, Johnny!"). The programming audiologist should note the level at which the child initially responds to speech. Upper-stimulation levels should be gradually increased in small steps until a typical electrical dynamic range (relative to the T-level measurements—i.e., 40 CL in Nucleus devices) is achieved or the upper-stimulation levels that are typical for the recipient's implant (e.g., 150–250 charge units for Advanced Bionics recipients or 10–25 charge units for MED-EL recipients; note that recommendations in a MED-EL programming guide suggest that MCL of 5 charge units is likely to be appropriate for initial activation with the goal of increasing MCLs to optimal levels at future appointments [MED-EL Fitting Guide]). Of course, the audiologist should not attempt to reach "expected" upper-stimulation levels if the child exhibits any signs that the stimulation at that stimulation level is aversive. Considerable caution should be exercised to ensure that upper-stimulation levels do not cause discomfort or other undesirable effects.

A child's responses to the stimulation he/she receives may be somewhat subtle, so the programming audiologist and programming assistant must be very adept at observing even the most subtle signs of anxiety on the part of the child. It is also helpful to have the child's caregivers watch the child's responses and provide feedback if they feel that the child is becoming anxious. Typically, the child should be engaged in a mildly entertaining task (e.g., looking at toys, watching a tablet or television) while the upper-stimulation levels are increased and all parties are observing the child's responses to auditory stimulation from the implant. When the child begins to exhibit signs that the stimulus is too loud, the audiologist should immediately decrease the stimulation level to avoid providing a signal that upsets the child. Subtle signs that the stimulation levels are reaching a point that may approach the child's upper level of loudness comfort include the child: holding his or her breath; exhibiting facial expressions of mild concern; looking to a caregiver for reassurance or reaching for the caregiver; looking with concern at the audiologist or programming assistant; tensing or stiffening the body or shoulders; playing more actively or aggressively; pushing the toy or tablet away, arching his/her back; wringing hands, clothes, or toys; and producing eye-blinks in response to the auditory stimulation (e.g., transient sounds such as clapping).

For example, it is common that a child will be happily playing with a toy (e.g., stuffed animal, ball, block, doll, toy car) while upper-stimulation levels are being gradually increased, but once the auditory signal begins to approach a point that approaches the child's upper level of comfort, then the child will stop playing with the toy, push it away, or toss it off the highchair tray. Also, if the child is seated in a highchair, he/she may reach for a parent when the signal begins to approach a point that is too loud. If the child is in his/her parent's lap, then he/she may turn to hug the parent or bury his/her face in the parent's chest. It is critically important to promptly observe these signs, as they are a possible indication of mild discomfort. When these signs are observed, the stimulation should be immediately decreased until the child appears to be at ease again. Continuing to increase the stimulation level eventually will possibly lead to overstimulation, an adverse reaction, and a negative association with the cochlear implant. If overstimulation occurs, it may be difficult to convince the child to wear the sound processor during the early stages. When the child shows signs that the upper-stimulation levels may be approaching his/her upper loudness tolerance levels, the audiologist should proceed with caution with further increases. If the upper-stimulation levels are gradually increased in small steps again, and the child once again shows signs that the level is becoming too loud, the audiologist should err on the side of being conservative and set the upper-stimulation levels at a point that ensures comfort. Again, remember that cochlear implant activation for a child should be viewed as a marathon rather than a sprint. Although it is important to provide the child with stimulation levels that will optimize auditory performance, the audiologist should first strive to facilitate the child's bonding with the implant. Upper-stimulation levels may be increased as needed throughout the first few weeks or months of use in order to reach optimal stimulation levels at a pace that is tolerated by the child.

If the child shows no signs of discomfort, then the audiologist should set upper-stimulation levels to a point providing a typical electrical dynamic range (relative to the T levels that were previously measured) or to an overall level that appears to provide audibility for speech and environmental sounds without exceeding levels that are typical for the implant and electrode array of the child. As previously mentioned, Nucleus recipients typically possess an electrical dynamic range between 20 and 60 CL with most recipients having an electrical dynamic range around 40 and 50 CL, Advanced Bionics recipients typically possess M levels ranging between 150 and 250 charge units with M levels below 100 and above 300 charge units being relatively rare, and MED-EL recipients typically possess MCL levels between 10 and 25 charge units with MCL below 5 charge units and over 400 charge units being quite exceptional. The audiologist's decision on where to set upper-stimulation levels should also be influenced by the results of objective measurements (e.g., ESRT, ECAP). For instance, upper-stimulation levels should not exceed ESRT. Furthermore, the audiologist should be leery of upper-stimulation levels that are substantially higher than the child's ECAP thresholds. Again, the reader is referred to Chapter 18 for more information on the use of objective measures for cochlear implant programming.

It should be noted that when activating the cochlear implants of infants and young children, it is particularly wise to sweep at upper-stimulation level once the levels have been set in live speech mode. This will allow the audiologist to identify any channel-specific undesirable effects, such as loudness discomfort or a non-auditory response, such as facial nerve stimulation.

When upper-stimulation levels cannot be estimated by ESRT measures and the child can only provide limited feedback about the loudness of the signal he/she receives from the implant, the audiologist should once again provide an upper-stimulation level that is relatively flat or that changes gradually across the array. Again, the upper-stimulation level profile is typically flatter than the T-level profile and becomes even more flat as upper stimulation levels are increased to levels that are substantially higher than T levels. Fine-tuning of upper-stimulation levels may be accomplished over time as the audiologist gathers information from observations during programming sessions as well as from the child's caregivers and therapists. For example, an increase in high-frequency upper-stimulation levels may be warranted if the listening and spoken language specialist (LSLS)/auditory-verbal therapist (AVT) reports that the child does not consistently respond to high-frequency phonemes (fricatives such as /s/).

Although it is the exception, some children simply do not exhibit many signs that they are detecting the programming stimulus. The audiologist should be very cautious to avoid overstimulation in these cases, particularly when objective measures, such as the ECAP and ESRT, indicate that the stimulation levels should be audible to the child. T levels and upper-stimulation levels should be gradually increased over time while seeking feedback from the child's AVT and caregivers. For instance, an increase in T levels and upper-stimulation levels would be warranted if the child's caregivers reported limited

to no responsiveness to speech and environmental sounds during everyday use. The audiologist should consistently administer evidence-based, subjective questionnaires to evaluate the auditory skill development of the child. Excellent tools to accomplish this objective include the LittlEars and PEACH questionnaires (Ching & Hill, 2005; Tsiakpini et al., 2004). The reader should also refer to the University of Western Ontario PedAMP battery for the assessment of auditory skill development (Bagatto, Moodie, & Scollie, 2010), which includes normative values that should be achieved with levels of auditory experience.

Upper-stimulation levels may also be measured to a single-channel programming stimulus. This approach provides a frequency-specific assessment of loudness judgment, which may yield helpful information regarding the child's stimulation needs across the frequency range. However, as previously mentioned in the discussion of measurement of upper stimulation levels of adults (in this chapter), channel-specific loudness measurements do not always closely associate with the loudness a recipient experiences for complex, broadband sounds. Consequently, upper stimulation levels should ultimately be based on the child's responses to live speech and environmental sounds. Indeed, the audiologist will have an indication of the child's responsiveness to stimulation on each channel if frequency-specific T level measurements were completed. Of note, channel-specific loudness measures can be useful when the child is experiencing non-auditory side effects or expressing discomfort with or aversiveness to use of the device.

If channel-specific measures are completed, the audiologist should use a similar approach as previously described for the adjustment of upper-stimulation levels to live speech. Specifically, the programming stimulus should initially be presented at a low level and then be slowly increased in small steps. The audiologist, the programming assistant, and the child's caregiver should all closely observe for any signs that the signal may be approaching an uncomfortable level for the child. Again, all parties should look for subtle signs of aversiveness on the part of the child, and every attempt should be made to avoid stimulating at a level that would cause discomfort for the child. It is worth reiterating once again that channel-specific measures may result in upper-stimulation levels that vary considerably across the electrode array. Although some recipients do require a different magnitude of stimulation across the electrode array, it should be mentioned again that upper-stimulation levels for programs using monopolar coupling are often relatively flat compared with the T-level profile (Botros & Psarros, 2010). At the very least, the audiologist should be leery of upper-stimulation levels that change markedly from one electrode to the next or from one section of the electrode array to the next. The audiologist should confirm that a valid reason exists to support the decision to set upper-stimulation levels at substantially different levels across the electrode array.

For older children (≥4 years), upper-stimulation level may be set via simplified psychophysical loudness approaches as described by Serpanos and Gravel (2002). Figure 14–7 shows an example of a basic loudness scaling card which may be used to successfully evaluate loudness with preschool and elementary-aged children. Children who are 8 to 9 years old and good readers often can participate in the traditional psychophysical loudness scaling procedures. Again, it should be noted that loudness assessment is frequently a difficult task with children who are born with severe to profound hearing loss. That is the primary reason why the ESRT is an important measure for estimating optimal upper-stimulation levels of children. Many older children are able to complete loudness balancing assessment (i.e., which of the two sounds is louder?). When ESRT cannot be obtained, loudness balancing should be attempted with children 6 years of age and older.

In summary, setting the upper-stimulation levels for young children is quite possibly one of the most challenging tasks facing the programming audiologist. The audiologist should proceed conservatively in order to prevent loudness discomfort and a subsequent reluctance on behalf of the child to use his/her cochlear implant. However, optimal progression of the child's auditory-skill development is greatly influenced by the provision of sufficient stimulation from the implant across the speech frequency range. Stimulation levels that are inappropriately low may deprive the child of the access he/she needs to develop age-appropriate speech, language, and auditory abilities. When possible, the provision of upper-stimulation levels for children should be based on the ESRT measurement. When ESRT cannot be obtained, the audiologist must rely on a combination of behavioral observation of the child's responses to speech, environmental sounds, and programming stimuli as well as on the audiologist's knowledge of what constitutes appropriate stimulation levels for a typical recipient with a particular type of cochlear implant. The audiologist should receive continuous feedback from the child's therapists and caregivers to ensure that the stimulation from the implant is not uncomfortable but that it provides sufficient access to speech sounds across the frequency and intensity ranges common for everyday use. Subjective questionnaires are often helpful to provide a formal assessment of the child's auditory skill development that may be referenced to age-appropriate norms. Although the ECAP response is not an excellent predictor of upper (or lower) stimulation levels, it may be used as a guide to determine stimulation levels that should provide audibility and to avoid excessive stimulation (see Chapter 18). The audiologist should work diligently and persistently until he/she is confident that the child's upper-stimulation levels are set appropriately.

It is prudent to comment on one more matter regarding the measurement of upper-stimulation levels in infants and young children. Numerous studies have shown that audiologists have a tendency to increase the upper-stimulation levels of infants and young children over time (Henkin et al., 2003, 2006; Hughes et al., 2001). These studies have also shown that there is a tendency for the upper-stimulation levels of children to eventually exceed the upper-stimulation levels used by adult recipients. More than likely, there is not a compelling reason for children to require significantly higher upper-stimulation levels than adult recipients. Most likely, children's upper-stimulation levels are higher than adults because young children are unable to provide verbal feedback about the sound quality, clarity, and comfort of the signal they receive from their cochlear implants. As a result, audiologists provide small increases in upper-stimulation levels at each of the child's programming sessions. Over time, the small increases provided at each session eventually result in upper-stimulation levels being higher than what are typically used by high-performing adult recipients. One may contend that a child's hearing performance may eventually suffer if stimulation levels are gradually increased to a point that is excessive. During the first few weeks or months that a child uses his/her cochlear implant, the audiologist should work hard to identify the optimal stimulation levels for the child based on the principles and procedures described in the previous sections and on the results of objective measurements of auditory function (see Chapter 18). Once optimal stimulation levels are established (and an optimal MAP has been created), the audiologist should avoid the temptation to make changes to the child's program simply for the sake of making changes. The child's auditory, speech, and language abilities should be continually

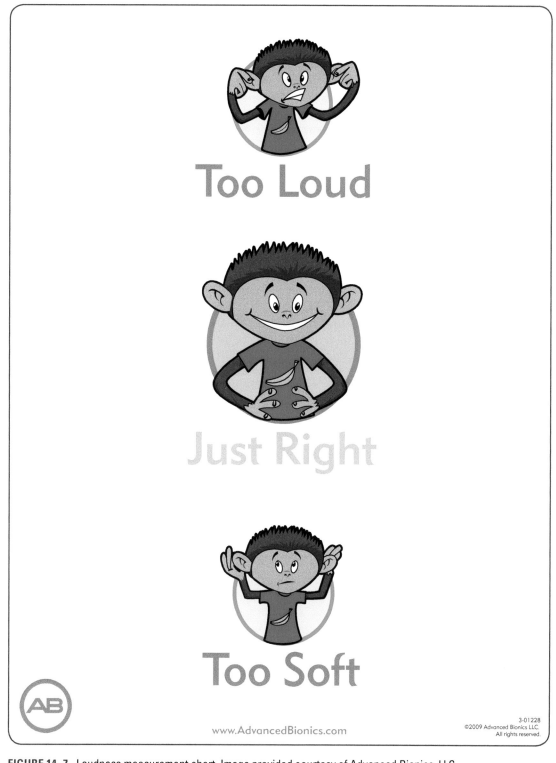

FIGURE 14–7. Loudness measurement chart. Image provided courtesy of Advanced Bionics, LLC.

evaluated by the audiologist and the child's LSLS (or speech-language pathologist) throughout the child's early elementary years. If the child's progress is satisfactory (e.g., audiologic assessment, standardized questionnaires of functional auditory performance, standardized speech and language assessment), then the child's MAP should probably not be altered. However, changes should be made to stimulation levels (or other program/MAP parameters) if deficiencies are identified in the formal assessment process.

Additional Considerations in the Measurement of Stimulation Levels

While adjusting upper-stimulation levels in live speech mode, it may be helpful for children to play with noisemakers (e.g., drum sticks, xylophones, tambourines; Figure 14–8). Typically, when upper-stimulation levels are set too low, children will play the noisemakers enthusiastically and create sounds that are excessively loud. However, when the upper-stimulation levels approach an uncomfortable level, children will stop playing vigorously with the noisemakers or will start blinking to any sharp or loud sounds the noise-

makers produce. The upper-stimulation level should be set below the level that elicits these behavioral changes and at a level that is obviously tolerable by the child. Additionally, these noisemakers may be used to evaluate the child's responsiveness to sounds occurring at different frequency ranges (low-, mid-, and high-frequency sounds).

Adjustments to Special Parameters

Stimulation Rate

As mentioned in Chapter 7, a great deal of interest exists in how stimulation rate affects performance. Numerous researchers have explored the effect of stimulation rate on speech recognition and perceptual sound quality (Balkany et al., 2007; Buechner et al., 2010; Firjns et al., 2003; Nie, Barco, & Zeng, 2006; Plant et al., 2007; Shannon, Cruz, & Galvin, 2011; Verschuur, 2005; Weber et al., 2007). The fundamental principles of stimulation rate and research on the effect of stimulation rate on recipient outcomes were described in Chapter 7 of this book. Collectively, research examining the effects of stimulation rate on

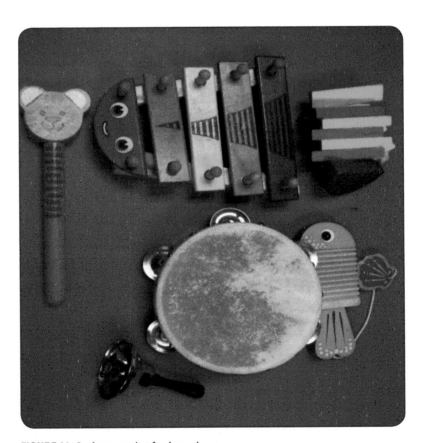

FIGURE 14–8. An example of noisemakers.

speech recognition tends to indicate that most users benefit from increase in rate from a few hundred pps to about 1500 pps, but little to no benefit occurs when stimulation rates are increased from 1000 to 1500 pps to 2000 pps and beyond (Balkany et al., 2007; Buechner et al., 2010; Firjns et al., 2003; Nie, Barco, & Zeng, 2006; Plant et al., 2007; Shannon, Cruz, & Galvin, 2011; Verschuur, 2005; Weber et al., 2007). However, it is important to note that individual exceptions do exist, and as a result, it may be helpful to allow recipients to experience a range of stimulation rates in order to select the rate that optimizes individual performance.

Because sound clinical decisions should be based on evidence-based research, an initial stimulation rate of approximately 900 to 1500 pps is typically appropriate for most implant recipients. The exact recommendation for an initial stimulation rate is specific to each cochlear implant system (i.e., make and model) and is provided in Chapters 15 through 17.

In general, most recipients perform quite well with the stimulation rates recommended in this book (i.e., 900 to 1500 pps). However, if a recipient is performing below expectations after several weeks of cochlear implant use, the audiologist should consider providing the recipient with multiple stimulation rates for trial use. Of note, elderly recipients, persons with significant cochlear malformations (e.g., common cavity), persons with an exceptionally long duration of deafness (e.g., greater than 20 years), and recipients with neural pathology (e.g., auditory neuropathy spectrum disorder, multiple sclerosis, cochlear nerve aplasia) may be more likely to benefit from slower stimulation rates.

It is often impossible for young children to provide reliable feedback about various stimulation rates. For pediatric programming, the audiologist should begin with the stimulation rate that is best supported by clinical research or the manufacturer's recommendation. Once again, stimulation rates between 900 to 1500 pps should provide satisfactory outcomes for the vast majority of children. Audiologists should experiment with adjustment of stimulation rate in young children only when expected progress is not achieved.

A few additional items pertaining to stimulation rate are worth noting:

1. Increasing stimulation rate often has the effect of decreasing T levels because of temporal summation. C levels do not change nearly as much with stimulation rate increases. As a result, the recipient's electrical dynamic range will likely increase with increases in stimulation rate (Shannon, Cruz, & Galvin, 2011).
2. Increases in stimulation rate (particularly above 2000 pps) may result in shallower loudness growth at the lower end of the electrical dynamic range, which may reduce the salience of low-level speech sounds (Kreft et al., 2004).
3. Increases in stimulation rate may enhance the likelihood of undesirable channel interaction (Middlebrooks, 2004).
4. Increases in stimulation may increase the pitch perceived by the recipient.
5. Although rare, high stimulation rates (i.e., greater than 2000 pps) may elicit tinnitus or complaints of poor sound quality (e.g., harshness, echo).

Pulse Width

When voltage compliance limitations prevent the provision of an increase in electrical current level, the pulse width should be increased (i.e., widened) to provide the increase in stimulation and loudness growth necessary to meet the recipient's auditory needs. An inverse relationship exists between pulse width and stimulation rate. Higher stimulation rates require a narrower pulse width. If a recipient requires high levels of stimulation, the pulse width may have to be increased. As a result, the stimulation rate will have to be decreased. In general, pulse widths between 20 and 40 µsec allow for sufficient current levels to be provided within the voltage compliance limits of the implant while also allowing for a suitable stimulation rate (e.g., 900 to 1500 pps). The exact manner in which stimulation rate and pulse width are managed varies slightly from one cochlear implant system to another and are discussed in detail in Chapters 15 through 17.

Channel Gain

Channel gain affects the intensity of the signal before it is processed by the external sound processor. After the audiologist ensures that stimulation levels are optimized for recipients using CIS-type strategies, adjustments to channel gain may address subtle sound quality complaints or speech recognition difficulties. For instance, if upper-stimulation levels are set as high as a patient can tolerate but he or she still complains of muffled speech, channel gains may be increased in the high frequencies. Additionally, if a recipient reports that his or her own voice is too soft and low-frequency upper-stimulation levels cannot be increased without exceeding the voltage limits of the device, the audiologist may increase low-frequency channel gains to enhance the loudness. Furthermore, to improve speech recognition and comfort in noise, the audiologist may create a program that includes decreased gains in the low-frequency channels. In reality, when stimulation levels are set appropriately, there is usually no need to adjust channel gains. It is important to note that gains should be adjusted as a last resort in *n*-of-*m* type of strategies. Channel gain affects the amplification provided to the input signal prior to processing, and as a result, decreasing the channel gain reduces the likelihood that the channel will be selected for stimulation (i.e., as a maxima) in an *n*-of-*m* strategy.

Frequency Allocation

Frequency allocation is particularly relevant when one or more electrodes must be disabled. With Advanced Bionics cochlear implants, frequency allocation is determined automatically and is not an audiologist-adjustable parameter. However, in the Cochlear Corporation and MED-EL devices, the audiologist can control how frequencies are allocated to electrodes, but significant differences exist in the way this parameter is adjusted between the two systems (see Chapters 16 and 17).

In general with contemporary cochlear implant systems, when electrodes are disabled, the bandwidth of each channel becomes wider, but the overall range of input frequencies that are coded across all channels remains the same. Wider channel bandwidths may result in the processing of sounds with two different frequencies within the same channel, which may make the two different audio inputs sound similar. As a result, narrower channel bandwidths are preferable to allow for better spectral resolution. According to research, restricting the upper end of the input frequency range from about 10,000 Hz to approximately 8000 Hz resulted in narrower channel bandwidths across the speech frequencies and improved speech recognition (Skinner, Holden, & Holden, 1995, 1997). Because disabling electrodes may influence frequency allocation and performance, it should be done only when necessary. Disabling may be necessary when an electrode has abnormal electrode impedance values, elicits undesired non-auditory side effects (e.g., facial nerve stimulation, pain), possesses a poor auditory response relative to other electrodes (e.g., stimulation on the electrode produces a static-like noise percept, poor sound quality), or requires stimulation levels that are considerably higher than the rest of the electrodes within the array.

The total range of frequencies allocated for adults should extend out to at least 6000 Hz to allow for good speech recognition and sound quality across most environments. For children, it may be desirable to allocate frequencies out to at least 7000 Hz. Children require access to a wider bandwidth (i.e., at least 8000 Hz) than adults in order to acquire optimal speech recognition and production (Pittman, 2008; Stelmachowicz, Pittman, Hoover, & Lewis, 2001).

Frequency allocation is particularly important for recipients who use electroacoustic stimulation (EAS). The reader is referred to Chapter 24 for a detailed discussion of the management of recipients who use EAS.

Key Concepts

The key information provided in this chapter should provide the reader with a basic understanding of the following basic principles for cochlear implant programming:

- The audiologist recipient will conduct a physical examination of the head and ear at every programming appointment. The audiologist should also provide adept counseling in an effort to ensure that the recipient is fully aware of the information needed to optimize benefit and satisfaction obtained with the cochlear implant.
- The provision of optimal stimulation levels is likely to be the most important parameter that the programming audiologist determines for the recipient. A variety of well-established techniques exist to determine the most appropriate stimulation levels for adult and pediatric recipients.
- The audiologist may adjust a number of other parameters (e.g., stimulation rate, pulse width, channel gain, frequency allocation, IDR, maxima) in an effort to optimize the performance and benefit of each individual.

References

Bagatto, M. P., Moodie, S. T., & Scollie, S. D. (2010). *The University of Western Ontario Pediatric Audiological Monitoring Protocol (UWO PedAMP) Version 1.0: Training manual*. London, Ontario, Canada: The University of Western Ontario.

Balkany, T., Hodges, A., Menapace, C., Hazard, L., Driscoll, C., Gantz, B., . . . Payne, S. (2007). Nucleus Freedom North American clinical trial. *Otolaryngology–Head and Neck Surgery, 136*(5), 757–762.

Bentler, R. A., & Pavlovic, C. V. (1989). Comparison of discomfort levels obtained with pure tones and multi-tone complexes. *Journal of the Acoustical Society of America, 86*(1), 126–132.

Botros, A., & Psarros, C. (2010a). Neural response telemetry reconsidered: I. The relevance of ECAP threshold profiles and scaled profiles to cochlear implant fitting. *Ear and Hearing, 31*(3), 367–379.

Buechner, A., Brendel, M., Saalfeld, H., Litvak, L., Frohne-Buechner, C., & Lenarz, T. (2010). Results of a pilot study with a signal enhancement algorithm for HiRes 120 cochlear implant users. *Otology and Neurotology, 31*(9), 1386–1390.

Byrne, D. (1986). Effects of frequency response characteristics on speech discrimination and perceived intelligibility and pleasantness of speech for hearing-impaired listeners. *Journal of the Acoustical Society of Amurica, 80*(2), 494–504.

Byrne, D., Parkinson, A., & Newall, P. (1990). Hearing aid gain and frequency response requirements for the severely/profoundly hearing impaired. *Ear and Hearing, 11*(1), 40–49.

Carhart, R., & Jerger, J. F. (1959). Preferred method for clinical determination of pure-tone thresholds. *Journal of Speech and Hearing Disorders, 24*, 330–345.

Ching, T. Y., & Hill, M. (2005) *Parents' Evaluation of Aural/Oral Performance of Children: P.E.A.C.H.* Chatswood, New South Wales, Australia: Australian Hearing.

Dillon, H. (2012). *Hearing aids* (2nd ed.). Turramurra, Australia: Boomerang Press.

Dillon, H., & Keidser, G. (2013). Siemens Expert Series: NAL-NL2—Principles, background data, and comparison to other procedures. *Audiology Online.* Retrieved from http://www.audiologyonline.com/articles/siemens-expert-series-nal-nl2-11355

Frijns, J. H., Klop, W. M., Bonnet, R. M., & Briaire, J. J. (2003). Optimizing the number of electrodes with high-rate stimulation of the Clarion CII cochlear implant. *Acta Otolaryngologica, 123*, 138–142.

Gallaudet Research Institute. (2008). *Regional and national summary report of data from the 2007–08 annual survey of deaf and hard of hearing children and youth.* Retrieved from http://research.gallaudet.edu/Demographics/2008_National_Summary.pdf

Gordon, K. A., Papsin, B. C., & Harrison, R. V. (2004). Toward a battery of behavioral and objective measures to achieve optimal cochlear implant stimulation levels in children. *Ear and Hearing, 25*(5), 447–463.

Gravel, J. S. (2000). Audiologic assessment for the fitting of hearing instruments: Big challenges from tiny ears. In R. C. Seewald (Ed.), *A sound foundation through early amplification: Proceedings from an international conference* (pp. 33–46). Chicago, IL: Phonak AG.

Gravel, J. S., & Hood, L. J. (1999). Pediatric audiologic assessment. In F. E. Musiek & W. F. Rintlemann (Eds.), *Contemporary perspectives in hearing assessment* (pp. 305–326). Needham Heights, MA: Allyn & Bacon

Henkin, Y., Kaplan-Neeman, R., Kronenberg, J., Migirov, L., Hildesheimer, M., & Muchnik, C. (2006). A longitudinal study of electrical stimulation levels and electrode impedance in children using the Clarion cochlear implant. *Acta Otolaryngologica, 126*(6), 581–586.

Henkin, Y., Kaplan-Neeman, R., Muchnik, C., Kronenberg, J., & Hildesheimer, M. (2003). Changes over time in electrical stimulation levels and electrode 24M cochlear implant. *International Journal of Pediatric Otorhinolaryngology, 67*(8), 873–880.

Hodges, A. V., Balkany, T. J., Ruth, R. A., Lambert, P. R., Dolan-Ash, S., & Schloffman, J. J. (1997). Electrical middle ear muscle reflex: Use in cochlear implant programming. *Otolaryngology–Head and Neck Surgery, 117*(3 Pt. 1), 255–261.

Holden, L. K., Reeder, R. M., Firszt, J. B., & Finley, C. C. (2011). Optimizing the perception of soft speech and speech in noise with the Advanced Bionics cochlear implant system. *International Journal of Audiology, 50*(4), 255–269.

Hughes, M. L., Vander Werff, K. R., Brown, C. J., Abbas, P. J., Kelsay, D. M., Teagle, H., . . . Lowder, M. W. (2001). A longitudinal study of electrode impedance, the electrically evoked compound action potential, and behavioral measures in Nucleus 24 cochlear implant users. *Ear and Hearing, 22*(6), 471–486.

Kreft, H. A., Donaldson, G. S., & Nelson, D. A. (2004). Effects of pulse rate and electrode array design on intensity discrimination in cochlear implant users. *Journal of the Acoustical Society of America, 116*(4), 2258–2268.

Ling, D. (1976). *Speech and the hearing-impaired child: Theory and practice.* Washington, DC: Alexander Graham Bell Association for the Deaf.

Ling, D. (1989). *Foundations of spoken language for the hearing-impaired child.* Washington, DC: Alexander Graham Bell Association for the Deaf.

MED-EL Fitting Guide for First Fitting of OPUS 1 and OPUS 2 with MAESTRO 3.0. (n.d.). Innsbruck Austria: MED-EL Worldwide Headquarters.

Middlebrooks, J. C. (2004). Effects of cochlear-implant pulse rate and inter-channel timing on channel interactions and thresholds. *Journal of the Acoustical Society of America, 116*, 452–468.

Nie, K., Barco, A., & Zeng, F. G. (2006). Spectral and temporal cues in cochlear implant speech perception. *Ear and Hearing, 27*(2), 208–217.

Pasanisi, E., Bacciu, A., Vincenti, V., Guida, M., Berghenti, M. T., Barbot, A., . . . Bacciu, S. (2002). Comparison of speech perception benefits with SPEAK and ACE coding strategies in pediatric Nucleus CI24M cochlear implant recipients. *International Journal of Pediatric Otorhinolaryngology, 64*(2), 159–163.

Picard M. (2004). Children with permanent hearing loss and associated disabilities: Revisiting current epidemiological data and causes of deafness. *Volta Review, 104*, 221–236.

Pittman, A. L. (2008). Short-term word-learning rate in children with normal hearing and children with hearing loss in limited and extended high-frequency bandwidths. *Journal of Speech, Language, and Hearing Research, 51*(3), 785–797.

Plant, K., Holden, L., Skinner, M., Arcaroli, J., Whitford, L., Law, M. A., . . . Nel, E. (2007). Clinical evaluation of higher stimulation rates in the Nucleus Research Platform 8 system. *Ear and Hearing, 28*(3), 381–393.

Serpanos, Y., & Gravel, J. (2002). Growth of loudness assessment in children using cross–modality matching (CMM). In R. Seewald & J. Gravel (Eds.), *A sound foundation through early amplification, Proceedings of the Second International Conference* (pp. 75–84). Switzerland: Phonak AG.

Shannon, R. V., Cruz, R. J., & Galvin, J. J. (2011). Effect of stimulation rate on cochlear implant users' phoneme, word and sentence recognition in quiet and in noise. *Audiology and Neurotology, 16*, 113–123.

Skinner, M. W., Holden, L. K., & Holden, T. A. (1995). Effect of frequency boundary assignment on speech recognition with the SPEAK speech-coding strategy. *Annals of Otology, Rhinology, and Laryngology, 104*(Suppl. 166), 307–311.

Skinner, M. W., Holden, L. K., & Holden, T. A. (1997). Parameter selection to optimize speech recognition with the Nucleus implant. *Otolaryngology–Head and Neck Surgery, 117*(3 Pt. 1), 188–195.

Skinner, M. W., Holden, L. K., Holden, T. A., & Demorest, M. E. (1995). Comparison of procedures for obtaining thresholds and maximum acceptable loudness levels with the Nucleus cochlear implant system. *Journal of Speech and Hearing Research, 38*, 677–689.

Spahr, A. J., & Dorman, M. F. (2005). Effects of minimum stimulation settings for the Med-El Tempo+ speech processor on speech understanding. *Ear and Hearing, 26*(Suppl. 4), 2S–6S.

Spivak, L. G., & Chute, P. M. (1994a). The relationship between electrical acoustic reflex thresholds and behavioral comfort levels in children and adult cochlear implant patients. *Ear and Hearing, 15*(2), 184–192.

Spivak, L. G., Chute, P. M., Popp, A. L., & Parisier, S. C. (1994b). Programming the cochlear implant based on electrical acoustic reflex thresholds: Patient performance. *Laryngoscope, 104*(10), 1225–1230.

Thompson, G., & Weber, B. A. (1974). Responses of infants and young children to behavior observation audiometry (BOA). *Journal of Speech and Hearing Disorders, 39*(2), 140–147.

Tsiakpini, L., Weichbold, V., Kuehn-Inacker, H., Coninx, F., D'Haese, P., & Almadin, S. (2004). *LittlEARS Auditory Questionnaire.* Innsbruck, Austria: MED-EL.

Verschuur, C. A. (2005). Effect of stimulation rate on speech perception in adult users of the Med-El CIS speech processing strategy. *International Journal of Audiology, 44*(1), 58–63.

Walker, G., Dillon, H., Byrne, D., & Christen, C. (1984). The use of loudness discomfort measures for selecting the maximum output of hearing aids. *Australian Journal of Audiology, 6*(1), 23–32.

Weber, B. P., Lai, W. K., Dillier, N., von Wallenberg, E. L., Killian, M. J., Pesch, J., . . . Lenarz, T. (2007). Performance and preference for ACE stimulation rates obtained with Nucleus RP 8 and Freedom system. *Ear and Hearing, 28*(Suppl. 2), 46S–48S.

Wilson, W. R., & Thompson, G. (1984). Behavioral audiometry. In J. Jerger (Ed.), *Pediatric audiology* (pp. 1–44). San Diego, CA: College-Hill Press.

15

Programming Advanced Bionics Cochlear Implants

Jace Wolfe and Erin C. Schafer

Introduction to Programming Advanced Bionics Cochlear Implants

This chapter will describe the principles, practices, and procedures pertaining to the programming of contemporary Advanced Bionics cochlear implants.

Advanced Bionics CPI-3 Programming Interface

An interface device is required to connect the recipient's sound processor to the programming computer. The Advanced Bionics **Computer Programming Interface 3 (CPI-3)** (Figure 15–1) is used to connect to Advanced Bionics sound processors. The CPI-3 is connected to the computer via a USB to micro-USB cable. The USB port of the programming computer powers the CPI-3, so that the CPI-3 does not need an external power source.

The CPI-3 interface allows for simultaneous connection to two sound processors for convenient programming of recipients of bilateral cochlear implants. The CPI-3 possesses three LEDs, a blue light that indicates the device is receiving power and two green lights that indicate the device is connected to the recipient's sound processor(s). The CPI-3 may be clipped to the recipient's clothing, it may be worn around the recipient's neck on a lanyard, or it may be placed on the computer desk. Advanced Bionics provides an array of specialized programming cables

that may be plugged into the micro-USB ports at the top of the CPI-3 to allow for a connection to a range of Advanced Bionics sound processors.

Programming Advanced Bionics Sound Processors

Creating an effective, base program for the Naída CI Q sound processor is fairly simple, but the new audiologist may initially be overwhelmed by the extensive array of sophisticated and unique hardware and signal processing options available in the sound processor and programming software. As a result, the audiologist should be familiar with the processor and the various signal processing features of the Naída CI Q sound processor in order to assist the user in reaching his/her full potential with the cochlear implant(s).

Advanced Bionics Programming Software

Advanced Bionics sound processors are programmed using **SoundWave** software platform. As with all software programming cochlear implant manufacturers, SoundWave is updated to allow for operation with new sound processors, signal processing, and additional developments. After SoundWave is launched, the audiologist is prompted to open the file of an existing recipient (Figure 15–2) or to create a new

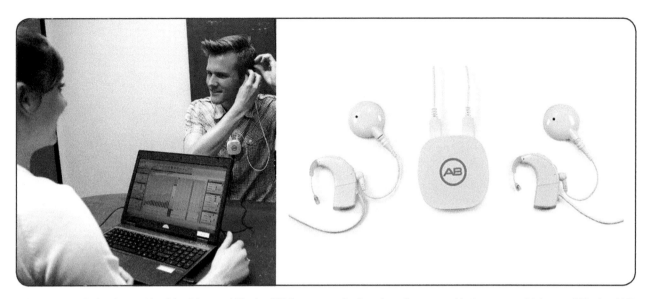

FIGURE 15–1. A visual example of the Advanced Bionics CPI-3 programming interface. Image provided courtesy of Advanced Bionics, LLC.

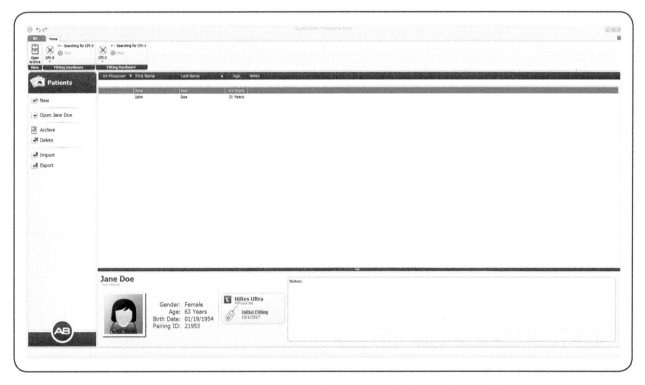

FIGURE 15–2. Patient screen of SoundWave software. Image provided courtesy of Advanced Bionics, LLC.

patient (Figure 15–3). Once a new patient's personal information (e.g., name, date of birth, sex/gender) is entered into the patient information field, SoundWave software then requires the audiologist to identify and enter the ear(s) that is(are) implanted and the model of cochlear implant and electrode array used by the recipient (Figure 15–4). It is important that the audiologist confer with the surgeon to learn the exact

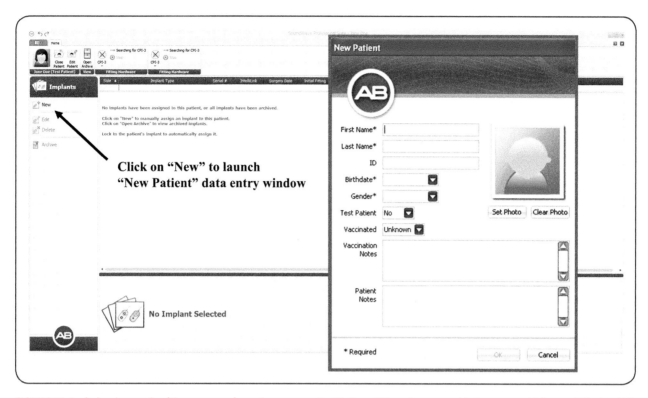

Click on "New" to launch "New Patient" data entry window

FIGURE 15–3. A visual example of the process of creating a new patient in SoundWave. Image provided courtesy of Advanced Bionics, LLC.

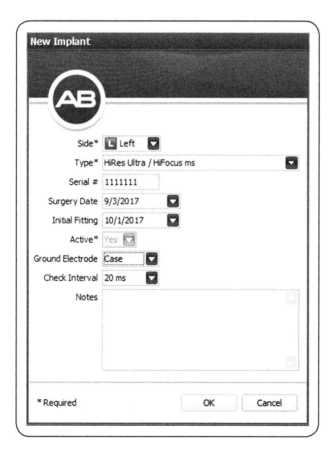

FIGURE 15–4. A visual example of the process of entering implant information for a new patient in SoundWave. Image provided courtesy of Advanced Bionics, LLC.

model of the implant and the electrode array that the recipient has received. Most new recipients will receive the latest model of cochlear implant, which at the time of this writing is the HiRes Ultra cochlear implant with the HiFocus Mid-Scala Electrode, but exceptions may possibly exist. Of note, if a recipient transfers his/her services from one clinic to another, the new clinic may connect the recipient's sound processor(s) to SoundWave, and if the audiologist chooses to add the recipient to the clinic's database, the SoundWave software will automatically upload the programs/maps that are loaded on his/her processor along with the information pertaining to the recipient's cochlear implant and electrode array.

Connecting the Sound Processor and Conducting the Electrode Impedance Measurement

When the CPI-3 interface is successfully coupled to the programming computer, a CPI-3 interface icon is displayed at the top of the SoundWave (Figure 15–5). If the computer does not successfully connect to the CPI-3, the audiologist may access a "**Fitting Hardware Configuration**" menu in the upper left corner of

the SoundWave software (Figure 15–6). Then, the audiologist may "autoconfigure" to the CPI-3 (Figure 15–7). Once the CPI-3 is connected, a sound processor may be connected to the CPI-3 by way of a cable designed for the processor. The SoundWave software will recognize the presence of the sound processor when it is connected to the CPI-3. The software may prompt the audiologist to "Prepare" the sound processor to be used for programming. Sound processor preparation will upload any available firmware upgrades to the processor.

Once the processor is connected, it should be placed on the recipient's ear (or body in the event that the processor is worn on the body rather than on the ear), and the external headpiece should be adhered to the implant site. When communication is established between the external sound processor and the cochlear implant (i.e., when "lock" is obtained), the SoundWave software will indicate that lock has been obtained by displaying an Advanced Bionics implant icon along with a textual description of the implant (see the programming ribbon at the top of Figure 15–5). At this point, the audiologist should see the CPI-3 as well as the recipient's external sound processor(s) and cochlear implant(s)

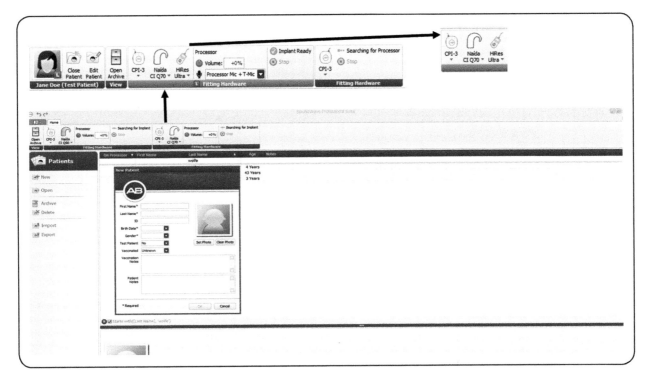

FIGURE 15–5. A visual example of the ribbon bar that shows connection of Advanced Bionics cochlear implant components. Image provided courtesy of Advanced Bionics, LLC.

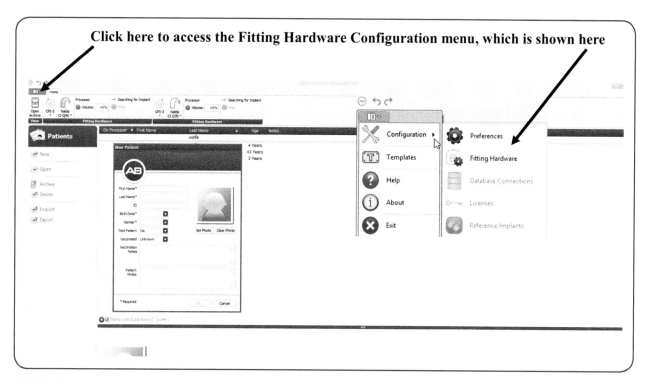

FIGURE 15–6. A visual example of the process of configuring the CPI-3 for programming in SoundWave. Image provided courtesy of Advanced Bionics, LLC.

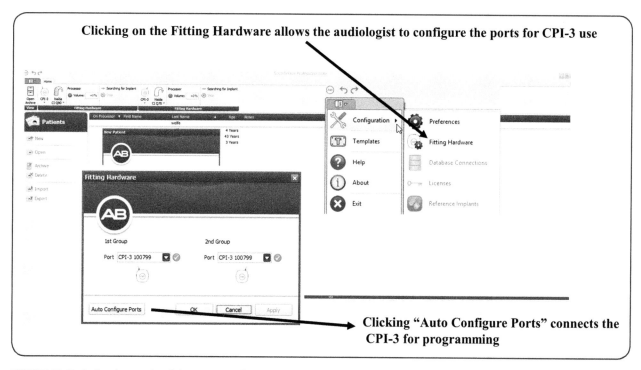

FIGURE 15–7. A visual example of the process of configuring the CPI-3 for programming in SoundWave. Image provided courtesy of Advanced Bionics, LLC.

highlighted in the ribbon at the top of the SoundWave screen. Once the lock is obtained with the recipient's cochlear implant, an electrode impedance measurement will be automatically completed (Figure 15–8). If desired, the audiologist can disable the automatic impedance measurement, which would then require the audiologist to manually initiate the impedance measurement.

When the processor icon does not display in the SoundWave software, the audiologist should ensure that the Naída CI Q processor is firmly and completely attached to the programming connector and that the programming cable is firmly plugged in to the CPI-3. If a Harmony processor does not successfully connect to the computer, the audiologist should "wiggle" the programming connector that couples to the processor. Many times, this will facilitate a connection. The audiologist may also inspect the contact points at the base of the sound processor. If the connection points are obstructed with debris or oxidation, the audiologist may attempt to remove the debris (with a brush and/or alcohol swab) and retry connecting to the processor. If the software continues

to show that no connection has been established to the processor, the audiologist should attempt to connect to the recipient's back-up sound processor or to a clinic loaner processor, or the audiologist should attempt to use a different programming cable.

Finally, when the software indicates that a connection has been established with the CPI-3 interface and sound processor, but not with the cochlear implant (e.g., internal device), the audiologist should replace the external sound processor's cable and headpiece. If the problem persists, then the audiologist may need to replace the sound processor, as it is possible that the cable port on the sound processor is faulty. If the problem continues to persist, then the audiologist should contact the manufacturer for assistance in troubleshooting a possible fault with the cochlear implant.

The automatic measurement of electrode impedance is a unique feature of the Advanced Bionics SoundWave software, whereas the other implant manufacturers require the audiologist to manually start the impedance measurement. The audiologist may review the results of the impedance measurement

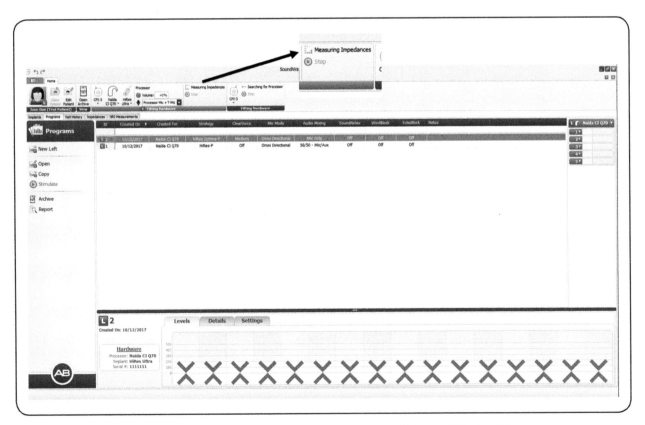

FIGURE 15–8. Impedance measurement in SoundWave. Image provided courtesy of Advanced Bionics, LLC.

and/or repeat the electrode impedance assessment by selecting the "Impedances" tab (Figure 15–9). Of note, the results of the impedance measurement will also be displayed in a table at the base of the programming/mapping screen, which is available when the audiologist opens a new or existing program to begin the programming process.

The electrode impedances of Advanced Bionics cochlear implants are measured in the monopolar electrode coupling mode, with impedance measurements made on all 16 intracochlear electrodes, with the case ground electrode serving as the terminal

point of the return path. **The normal range of electrode impedance values obtained with Advanced Bionics C-II, HiRes 90K, and HiRes Ultra implants spans from 1.0 to 30.0 kOhms**. The normal electrode impedance range obtained with the C1 implant ranges from 1.0 to 150 kOhms. Electrode impedance results are depicted in bar graph form in the electrode impedance tab measurement field. Electrodes with normal impedances are displayed as green bars, indicating that they are serving as "valid" functioning electrodes (Figure 15–10). "Open" electrodes possess impedance values that are higher than the normal

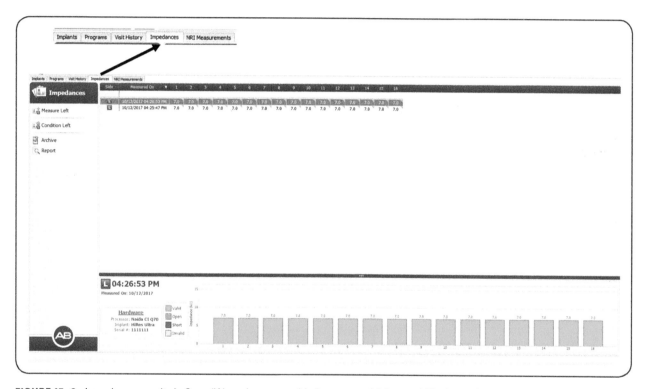

FIGURE 15–9. Impedance results in SoundWave. Image provided courtesy of Advanced Bionics, LLC.

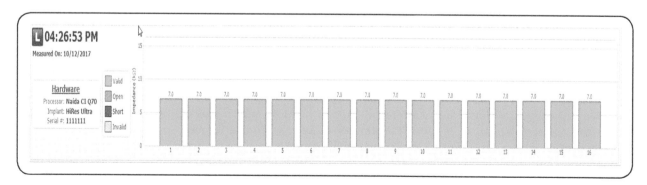

FIGURE 15–10. Impedance results in SoundWave. Image provided courtesy of Advanced Bionics, LLC.

range and are displayed in yellow on the bar graph. As mentioned before, when electrode impedances are slightly outside of the normal range (e.g., within 10 kOhm of the upper limit of normal) at implant activation or after a long period of non-use, it is recommended that the audiologist provide electrical stimulation to the electrode contacts for a few minutes and then re-administer the impedance test. Running "Conditioning" within the software can provide such low level stimulation. Of note, relatively higher charge levels will be needed for electrodes with higher impedance values (e.g., greater than 10 kOhms). "Short" electrodes are defined either as a single electrode with an impedance value between 0.5 and 1.0 kOhms or as an electrode having a significant electrical interaction with one or more other electrodes. Electrode shorts are displayed in purple in the bar graph display. Finally, electrodes with impedances below 0.5 kOhms are considered to be "invalid" and are displayed in the color gray in the bar graph display. Short electrodes should always be immediately disabled and excluded from use in the recipient's program. Open and invalid electrodes should also be disabled if they are persistently outside of the normal impedance range.

Advanced Bionics SoundWave software utilizes a form of **electrical field imaging and modeling** to identify electrode shorts. With the electrical field imaging technique, a small amount of current is sent to an electrode via monopolar electrode coupling, and the resultant voltage that is present at every other electrode in the array relative to the stimulated electrode/monopolar ground connection is measured and compared. Shorted electrodes possess abnormally low electrode impedance values, and even when it is not directly stimulated, a shorted electrode contact will show a measured value that is close to that of the stimulating electrode.

Within the impedance tab, the audiologist also may perform **electrode conditioning** to eliminate any substances present at the electrode contact (e.g., fibrous tissue, protein deposits, macrophages, air bubbles) through the application of a low-level current. The presence of these substances around the intracochlear electrode contacts typically causes elevated electrode impedances at initial activation of the implant or after a period of non-use of the implant; however, impedances almost always decrease over time with consistent stimulation. Electrical stimulation may result in reorganization of the fibrous tissue matrix surrounding the electrode contacts, which leads to a reduction in impedance. Additionally, the electrical stimulation from conditioning may eliminate the substances surrounding the intracochlear electrode contacts. The audiologist should consider conducting electrode conditioning after a prolonged period of non-use of the implant, particularly if the electrode impedances are relatively high (e.g., greater than 10 kOhms).

Creating a Program in the Advanced Bionics SoundWave Software

As shown in Figure 15–11, the audiologist must select the "Programs" tab in the SoundWave software to create a program for the recipient. A new program may be created by double-clicking on the "New Right," "New Left," or "New Bilateral" options on the left side of the screen while in the "Programs" platform. An existing program may be opened by double-clicking on a program that has been saved from a previous programming session.

Selecting a Sound Processing Strategy

After a program is opened, the audiologist is able to adjust a large number of parameters. The first step of creating a new program is to select the signal coding strategy the recipient will use. The audiologist may select from a number of signal coding strategies available within SoundWave, including: HiRes-P (HiResolution Paired), HiRes-S (Sequential), HiRes-P with Fidelity 120, HiRes-S Fidelity with Fidelity 120, HiRes Optima-S, HiRes Optima-P, CIS (Continuous Interleaved Sampler), and MPS (Multiple Pulsatile Sampler).

The software default signal processing strategy is HiRes-P. However, for recipients who use CII or later cochlear implants and Naída CI Q, Neptune, or Harmony sound processors, the authors recommend using with HiRes Optima-S signal coding strategy (Advanced Bionics, 2012), which is the newest Advanced Bionics signal coding strategy at the time of this writing (see Figure 15–12 for an example of how the audiologist may select the signal coding strategy used by the Advanced Bionics recipient). The Optima strategy incorporates current steering to create virtual channels, which may be beneficial for some recipients (Advanced Bionics Corporation, 2009). Furthermore, the Optima signal coding strategy is more power efficient than the HiRes Fidelity 120 strategy and will consequently allow for better battery life.

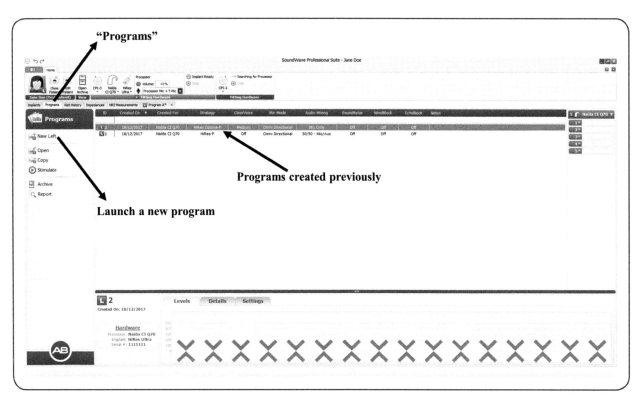

FIGURE 15–11. A visual example of the process of creating programs in SoundWave. Image provided courtesy of Advanced Bionics, LLC.

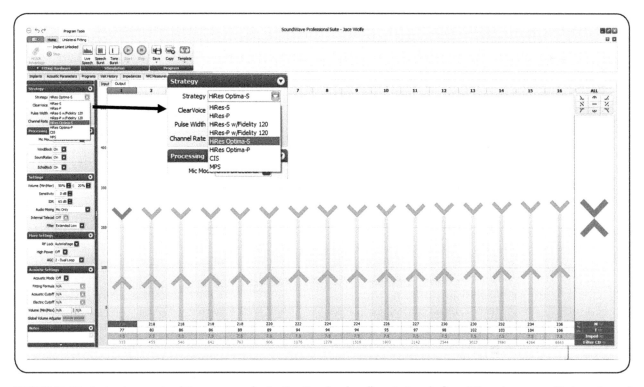

FIGURE 15–12. A visual example of the process of selecting the signal coding strategy in SoundWave. Image provided courtesy of Advanced Bionics, LLC.

The HiRes Optima-S signal coding strategy is recommended over the HiRes Optima-P strategy because the sequential nature of electrode stimulation of the HiRes-S variants theoretically reduces the chance for deleterious channel interaction compared with the partially simultaneous stimulation provided by the HiRes-P strategies. Additionally, the stimulation rate per electrode available with Optima-S should be more than sufficient for most recipients.

Moreover, the authors recommend manually setting the pulse width for the HiRes Optima-S strategy (as well as other signal coding strategies) to 37.7 microseconds. The wider pulse width of 37.7 microseconds allows for a per-electrode stimulation rate of 1500 to 2000 pps, which should be more than sufficient for most recipients. Research examining the effects of stimulation rate has shown that increases in per-electrode stimulation rates up to about 1500 pps may allow for improvement in speech recognition for many subjects (Wilson, 2006). However, increasing the per-channel stimulation rate beyond 1500 pps does not generally provide an improvement in speech recognition for most recipients, and in fact, some recipients may show deleterious effects at higher stimulation rates (Arora, Dawson, Dowell, & Vandali, 2009; Balkany et al., 2007; Buchner, Frohne-Buchner, Battmer, & Lenarz 2004; Vandali, Whitford, Plant, & Clark, 2000; Verschuur, 2005; Weber et al., 2007; Wilson, 2006; see Chapters 7 and 8 in this book for more detail). Of note, some researchers who are accustomed to a narrower pulse width may notice a change in sound quality when the pulse width is widened. If a recipient is performing well with a narrow pulse width and fast stimulation rate, then there is no reason to alter either parameter. However, if the recipient's hearing performance is unsatisfactory and/or he/she reports poor sound quality, a reduction in stimulation rate may be beneficial.

It should be noted that some recipients may require a pulse width greater than 37.7 microseconds. Some recipients perform better at slower stimulation rates (e.g., 500 to 1000 pps). Research examining the effect of stimulation rate on speech recognition and subjective preference has indicated that slower rates are beneficial and preferred by some participants (Arora, Dawson, Dowell, & Vandali, 2009; Balkany et al., 2007; Buchner, Frohne-Buchner, Battmer, & Lenarz 2004; Vandali, Whitford, Plant, & Clark, 2000; Verschuur, 2005; Weber et al., 2007). Also, recipients with evidence of neural dysfunction (e.g., cochlear nerve deficiency, auditory neuropathy spectrum dis-

order) and/or the possibility of auditory processing issues may perform better with slower stimulation rates. Furthermore, some elderly recipients may perform poorly with faster stimulation rates (Zhang, Runge-Samuelson, & Friedland, 2011). The audiologist must employ a wider pulse width to provide slower stimulation rates. Additionally, a wider pulse width may be needed to avoid exceeding the voltage compliance limits of the cochlear implant. There is a greater need for a wider pulse width to avoid voltage compliance limits when working with recipients who have requisite higher stimulation levels and/or higher electrode impedances. It should be noted that in default mode (as described in an upcoming section), the SoundWave software automatically manages the pulse width to avoid voltage compliance issues, and many users receive satisfactory outcomes while using the pulse width and stimulation that is automatically determined by the SoundWave software. Finally, at the time of this writing, the HiRes Optima and Fidelity 120 strategies are not approved by the FDA for use with children. However, many cochlear implant audiologists routinely use HiRes Optima and Fidelity 120 with infants and young children. Additionally, research has indicated that children perform well with the use of these current-steering strategies (Chang et al., 2009; Mancini et al., 2009).

Previous clinical trials show substantial variation in user preferences across the aforementioned signal coding strategies (Koch et al., 2004; Wong et al., 2009). The authors contend that most recipients achieve satisfactory performance with the HiRes Optima-S signal coding strategy. Furthermore, the authors' anecdotal experience suggests that it is preferable to focus on determining the ideal stimulation levels for a recipient during the first few weeks of implant use, as most recipients will do quite well with contemporary signal coding strategies when stimulation levels are optimized. However, for subjects who are struggling with sound quality complaints and/or poor speech recognition after at least one month of use, the audiologist should attempt to determine whether alternative signal coding strategies and/or stimulation rates may allow for an improvement in recipient performance. As previously discussed, most recipients perform quite well with the HiRes Optima and HiRes Fidelity 120 signal coding strategies, as these modes are highly sophisticated and represent the most advanced strategies currently available in the Advanced Bionics system (Advanced Bionics, 2012; Büchner et al., 2012; Dunn, Tyler, Witt, & Gantz,

2006). However, the authors do manage some recipients who seem to perform better with the legacy signal coding strategies (e.g., HiRes-S/CIS/MPS).

With the CIS and MPS signal coding strategies, every other channel is disabled (typically every even-numbered electrode). It is possible that the reduced number of channels in the older signal coding strategies may limit channel interaction, which may be beneficial for a small subset of recipients. Furthermore, it should be noted that a wider pulse width (i.e., 75 microseconds) and slower stimulation rate is employed with these legacy signal coding strategies (i.e., 829 pps for CIS), which may also be beneficial for a small proportion of recipients. Again, it should be noted that use of legacy programs (e.g., CIS, MPS) for CII and 90K recipients is the rare exception rather than the rule. Ultimately, clinical judgment should be used to determine whether alternative signal coding strategies should be introduced, and if so, to determine the appropriate time to introduce the different signal coding strategies.

It should be noted that C1 recipients using the Harmony processor may be programmed in the Sound-Wave software platform, but they may only be programmed with the Harmony sound processor. Older Advanced Bionics sound processors, such as the Platinum Speech Processor body-worn processor, have been obsolesced by Advanced Bionics. C1 recipients who still use older processors must be programmed in the SCLIN software platform along with the previous generation of computer programming interface (CPI) if the clinic still has access to that software and hardware. C1 Harmony wearers must use one of the original Advanced Bionics signal coding strategies: Simultaneous Analog Stimulation (SAS), CIS, or MPS. Most of these recipients will have used SAS, CIS, or MPS for many years, and as a result, it is not common practice to deviate from their customary signal coding strategy (i.e., it is not typically recommended to switch to CIS if the recipient has always used MPS or SAS).

ClearVoice

ClearVoice is a speech-enhancement strategy that intends to improve speech perception in noise without compromising speech understanding in quiet. It is an algorithm integrated into HiRes Fidelity 120 sound processing and makes channel-specific determinations of whether the input signal is mostly noise or contains useful information for understanding speech. ClearVoice attenuates the "noisy" channels

while leaving the information-bearing channels relatively unaffected. The result is an improvement in the overall signal-to-noise ratio (SNR).

An audiologist-selectable ClearVoice gain setting determines the maximum channel-specific attenuation that is applied in a given program—up to 6 dB of attenuation for Low, up to 12 dB of attenuation for Medium, and up to 18 dB of attenuation for High (Figure 15–13). This selection can be programmed to meet the individual requirements and personal preference of each user. The authors typically use ClearVoice for all recipients and select a "Medium" setting of ClearVoice for most. However, the "Low" or "Strong" setting may be selected for older children and adults who complain of too much or too little noise reduction, respectively.

The ClearVoice algorithm may be used with the HiRes Optima and HiRes Fidelity 120 signal coding strategies and with the Harmony, Neptune, and all Naída CI Q sound processors. For implementation of ClearVoice, the input signal is analyzed using a fast Fourier transformation (FFT), and the spectrum is divided into 15 channels across the 16 intracochlear electrode contacts. Then, a Hilbert transform is used to extract the temporal information from the speech signal. An SNR estimator is used to provide an ongoing estimate of the background noise level in each of the 15 spectral channels. Additionally, an estimate is determined of the speech and noise present in each of the 15 channels. Next, the instantaneous energy is measured in each of the 15 channels and compared with the ongoing noise level within each channel. For channels in which the instantaneous energy is similar to the ongoing noise level, a determination is made that the channel primarily contains noise, and the level (i.e., gain) of that channel is attenuated by the amount indicated by the ClearVoice setting (i.e., Low, Medium, or High). If the instantaneous energy present within a channel is higher than the ongoing noise, then the input is considered to be speech, and little to no attenuation is provided. For channels that are deemed to consist primarily of noise, the amount of attenuation is determined by the SNR within a channel as well as the ClearVoice setting selected by the audiologist. ClearVoice settings of Low, Medium, and High result in a maximum attenuation of 6, 12, and 18 dB, respectively. This selection can be programmed to meet the individual requirements and personal preference of each user. Furthermore, recipients may be equipped with multiple programs, each possessing different strength of ClearVoice. From the

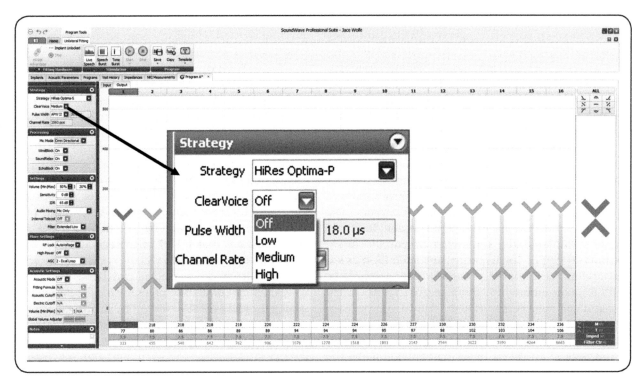

FIGURE 15–13. A visual example of the process of adjusting ClearVoice in SoundWave. Image provided courtesy of Advanced Bionics, LLC.

point in which the sound processor is activated with a ClearVoice program, approximately 1.6 seconds of signal analysis is required before ClearVoice begins to attenuate channels with an unfavorable SNR. Of note, when ClearVoice is enabled, the audiologist should ensure that the loudness of the program is still optimal to the recipient. If the recipient reports that the overall loudness is too soft, then the audiologist may globally increase M levels in live speech mode to obtain an optimal loudness for the recipient.

An FDA clinical trial showed that ClearVoice significantly improved speech understanding in speech-spectrum noise and multi-talker babble, did not compromise listening in quiet, and was preferred for everyday listening (Koch, Quick, Osberger, Saoji, & Litvak, 2014). Of historical note is that this trial represented the first time a regulatory superiority claim had been met for a new cochlear-implant sound-processing algorithm compared with existing strategies (ClinicalTrials.gov, 2012). Additionally, Wolfe et al. (2015) found that the use of ClearVoice significantly improved speech recognition in noise (compared with the no-ClearVoice condition) when participants listened with the Naída CI Q70 sound processor alone as well as when the participants used the Naída CI Q70 with the Phonak Roger remote microphone.

Setting Stimulation Levels and Stimulation Rate

In the SoundWave platform, stimulation levels are measured in charge units. Charge units are the product of the amplitude of the stimulus current, the pulse width, and an arbitrary constant (k = 0.013). This unit of stimulation represents a constant charge, and its value is always the same, regardless of the pulse width. Stated differently, if the pulse width is increased, the current is decreased to maintain the same charge value. In the software default mode, the objective is to use a short pulse width in order to allow for a fast stimulation rate. Therefore, at lower stimulation levels, an increase in charge units is achieved by increasing the current amplitude. As stimulation levels continue to increase and voltage compliance limits are approached or reached, increases in stimulus current amplitude can no longer be provided. Consequently, the pulse width is automatically increased by the software. This frees the audiologist from having to monitor the pulse width to ensure stimulation remains within voltage compliance.

The SoundWave software provides three options for adjusting the pulse width, including *APWI* (Automatic Pulse Width I), *APWII* (Automatic Pulse Width II), and *Manual*. It is important to note that only *APWII* and *Manual* are available for use with the Naída CI Q sound processors. Also, *APWII* is the default selection for the HiRes Optima, HiRes, and HiRes Fidelity 120 signal coding strategies. *APWII* automatically manages pulse width and current amplitude, with a primary goal of ensuring that stimulation on every electrode (even those with outlier impedance or upper stimulation levels) is within voltage compliance. The software seeks to maximize stimulation rate, but the automatically selected pulse width is first determined based on the goal of strictly remaining within voltage compliance limits. The *APWII* algorithm plays an important role in optimizing battery life for the Naída CI sound processor. It should be noted that the *APWII* mode is implemented somewhat differently for the Optima strategies versus other Advanced Bionics signal coding strategies. For the Optima strategy, the *APWII* mode employs a 4-volt target to manage the pulse width required to remain within voltage compliance. In contrast, for the HiRes and HiRes Fidelity 120 strategies, the *APWII* mode employs an 8-volt target to determine the pulse width required to remain within voltage compliance. The lower voltage target used with the Optima strategy is designed to improve

power efficiency, which should allow for longer battery life. This is especially important for the Naída CI sound processor, which possesses a small battery designed to enhance comfort, retention, and cosmetics. It should also be noted that the lower voltage target used for Optima strategies is one reason for why the Optima may require a longer pulse width than the HiRes and HiRes Fidelity 120 strategies.

The audiologist may also select the *Manual* pulse width mode for HiRes Optima users. In fact, as mentioned earlier, for all HiRes signal coding strategies (HiRes, HiRes with Fidelity 120, and Optima), the authors recommend manually setting the pulse width to 37.7 microseconds (or higher if the software indicates that a 37.7 microsecond pulse width is insufficient to maintain voltage compliance). When the *Manual* mode is selected, the pulse width typically must be equal to or greater than the pulse width selected by the *APWII* mode. The processor stimulation rate (Figure 15–14) is tied to the pulse width, and the wider pulse width of 37.7 microseconds allows for a per-electrode stimulation rate between 1500 and 2000 pps, which should be more than sufficient for most recipients. Again, a review of published research

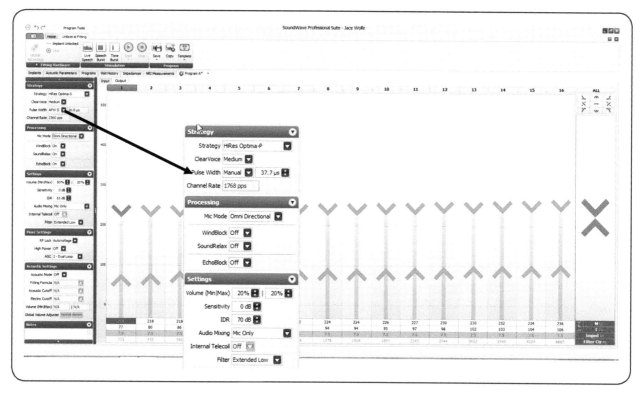

FIGURE 15–14. An example of a number of different programming parameters within SoundWave including pulse width adjustment. Image provided courtesy of Advanced Bionics, LLC.

studies examining cochlear implant stimulation rate suggests that increases in per-electrode stimulation rates up to about 1500 pps result in improvement in speech recognition for most subjects with performance becoming variable at higher stimulation rates (Wilson, 2006—see Chapter 3 for more detail). Furthermore, the wider pulse width (37.7 microseconds) allows for lower current amplitude, which may limit channel interaction and non-auditory side effects (e.g., facial nerve stimulation). The authors have found this combination of pulse width (37.7 microseconds) and stimulation rate (1500–2000 pps) to provide satisfactory performance for most recipients. However, if recipients are struggling with poor sound quality and/or speech recognition after more than 4 weeks of implant use, the authors will manually change the pulse width to trial slower and faster stimulation rates. It should be noted that the software will display a warning icon (Figure 15–15) when the selected pulse width results in stimulation levels on some electrodes being outside of voltage compliance limits. In this case, the audiologist should increase the pulse width.

The *APWI* mode also automatically determines the current amplitude and pulse width required to yield a charge unit level that is within voltage compliance for the implant. However, the primary objective of the *APWI* algorithm is to use the shortest pulse width allowed so that the fastest possible stimulation rate may be provided. The exact function of the *APWI* algorithm is proprietary, but does allow for stimulation on a small number of electrodes to be outside of voltage compliance. Typically, these electrodes will possess an electrode impedance or M level (e.g., upper-stimulation level) that is markedly higher than the rest of the electrodes in the array.

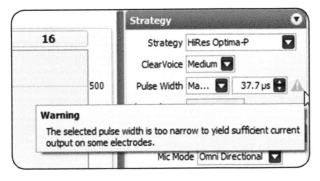

FIGURE 15–15. Warning that pulse width is too narrow to provide requested stimulation levels. Image provided courtesy of Advanced Bionics, LLC.

Finally, the default pulse width for CIS and MPS signal coding strategies is 75.4 microseconds. This wider pulse width was necessary when CIS and MPS were used with first-generation implants because the current sources of these implants were not sufficient to provide a biphasic rectangular pulse with a large enough current amplitude to yield satisfactory loudness growth. The audiologist may manually switch the pulse width from 75.4 microseconds to either 150.9 or 226.3 microseconds. It should be noted that 75.4 microseconds is more than sufficient for most CIS/MPS users. Exceptions may arise for users who have high stimulation levels secondary to auditory abnormalities, such as a cochlear deformity (e.g., Mondini's or cochlear duct ossification associated with bacterial meningitis) or an aplastic (deficient) auditory nerve.

Stimulus Units

The range of stimulation levels provided by the software is 0 to 6000 charge units, but M levels (i.e., upper-stimulation levels) for most recipients typically fall within a range of 100 to 300 charge units. Stimulus level grows linearly in the SoundWave software, so the recipient's loudness percept will typically grow at a slower rate than what is observed in the Cochlear CustomSound and MED-EL MAESTRO programming platforms, in which the stimulus increases logarithmically. For this same reason, the electrical dynamic range (e.g., the range between electrical threshold and upper level of stimulation) in Advanced Bionics charge units is typically wider than what is typically observed in Cochlear and MED-EL recipients. It should be noted that stimulation levels may vary according not only to recipient characteristics but also to differences in the cochlear implant electrode array. As a group, recipients of perimodiolar electrode arrays (e.g., HiFocus Mid-Scala, Helix) are more likely to have lower stimulation levels than recipients of HiFocus 1j electrode arrays. Additionally, Advanced Bionics recipients who were implanted with a positioner device to facilitate close proximity of the electrode array to the modiolus will be more likely to have lower stimulation levels.

Measuring T Levels

In the default programming mode, T level is automatically set to 10% of the established M-level value. In most cases, this estimation of T level allows recipients to access low-level sounds, and performance is similar between estimated and measured T levels (Holden et al., 2011). However, Holden et al. (2011) reported that measured T levels did allow for better sound-field detection thresholds in a group of 10 Advanced Bionics recipients. To optimize audibility for low-level sounds, the audiologist does have the option to set T levels manually on a single electrode basis or by adjusting T levels globally. T levels may be measured on individual electrodes by selecting the "Tone Burst" stimulus in the "Stimulation" pane at the top of the programming screen (Figure 15–16). Additionally, the audiologist may simply click and drag any individual T-level arrow icon and it will automatically "unlink" to allow T levels to be manually set. Then, the audiologist simply has to use the mouse of the programming computer to "click" on the T-level icon of the channel to be measured. Stimulation levels may be adjusted by using the up/down arrow keys of the keyboard of the programming computer or by selecting the T-level or M-level field and typing in a desired charge unit number and hitting "enter" on the keyboard. The audiologist must press the "S" key on the programming keyboard to deliver stimulation.

The audiologist may also choose to make global adjustments of T levels. This may be done by "click-ing" and "dragging" the Global T level adjuster or by clicking on the T level icon and then selecting the "All" option in the upper right corner of the programming screen. Subsequent adjustments will alter all T levels across the electrode array. Increasing T-level stimulation provides more stimulation for low-level sounds, which may be helpful if the recipient has elevated sound-field detection thresholds or if recognition of soft speech is inadequate. In contrast, T levels may need to be decreased if the recipient reports hearing a constant "frying," static, or buzzing noise. All HiRes signal coding strategies are advanced iterations of the CIS signal coding strategy, and due to the continuous delivery of electrical pulses inherent in CIS-based strategies, the recipients may hear the constant, low-level stimulation and complain of a low-level audible noise when T levels are too high. In such a case, the audiologist should ensure that the recipient is not simply hearing ambient noise in the room (i.e., the building's heating or air conditioning system). This may be determined by asking the recipient to step into an audiometric sound booth. If the low-level noise ceases, it is most likely that the recipient is hearing ambient room noise and should be encouraged to acclimate. If the sound persists, then it is likely that T levels are too high.

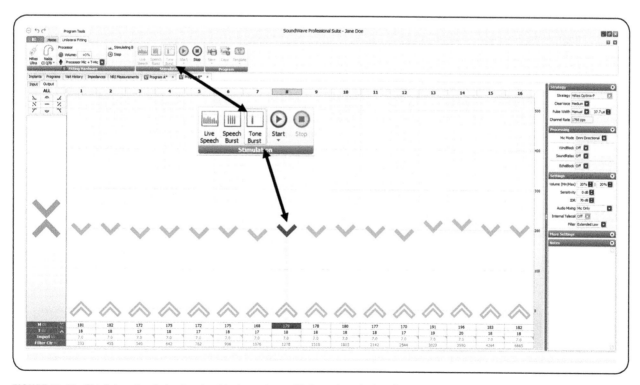

FIGURE 15–16. Obtaining stimulation levels with channel-specific (tone-burst) stimuli. Image provided courtesy of Advanced Bionics, LLC.

T levels should be measured when the implant equipment (i.e., sound processor microphone, etc.) is functioning within normal limits and sound-field detection thresholds are elevated (i.e., child ≥25 dB HL; adult ≥30 dB HL). For measuring T levels in children, the authors of this chapter suggest a 5-charge unit-down and 10-charge-unit-up approach with tone-burst stimuli. Young children are likely to provide a minimal response level instead of a true threshold; therefore, after measuring T levels, the audiologist may consider a small global reduction (the authors typically use a 10–15 charge unit reduction) to lessen the possibility of a child perceiving constant low-level electrical noise.

Measuring M-Level Stimulation

The default method of measuring M levels is unique in the Advanced Bionics programming platform. Instead of presenting biphasic pulses to individual electrode contacts, a **Speech Burst** stimulus is used. The Speech Burst consists of white noise filtered through three or four channels and is presented at the user's typical stimulation rate. There are three theoretical advantages to using Speech Burst stimuli over conventional single-channel programming stimuli. First, simultaneous presentation of the stimulus across multiple channels provides a more valid representation of the spectral characteristics of complex speech and environmental sounds (which typically possess a broadband spectrum) compared with presenting stimulation on only one channel. Second, simultaneous presentation on multiple channels more closely resembles expected summation across channels in live speech mode and accounts for loudness summation (i.e., M levels may be more accurate) that occurs when listening to complex sounds in the real world. Third, simultaneous presentation across several channels is potentially more time efficient than single-channel measurements (i.e., all 16 electrodes may be evaluated with 4 measurements instead of 16 measurements, because the signal is presented across four channels at a time). Furthermore, Advanced Bionics research studies show similar performance when using programs created using single-channel versus Speech Burst measures (Advanced Bionics, 2003a). It should be noted, however, that use of Speech Burst stimuli may underestimate M level for a given channel if the requisite level for that channel is substantially lower than the other channels that make up the Speech Burst.

In the default mode, audiologists measure M levels for each of the four Speech Burst bands

(i.e., Speech Bursts at channels 1–4, 5–8, 9–12, and 13–16) in order to evaluate across the electrode array. After M levels are measured for Speech Bursts, the audiologist should decrease M levels globally and activate the program in "Live Speech" mode, which allows the audiologist to make channel-specific or global (across all channels simultaneously) adjustments to stimulation levels. In live speech mode, the audiologist should increase M levels globally until the recipient reports that speech and environmental sounds are perceived at a most comfortable listening level (Figure 15–17). After these adjustments, the audiologist should consider balancing the loudness at M levels on a channel-by-channel basis using tone bursts across the electrode array. Loudness balancing is typically conducted from the apical end of the array toward the basal end. Again, the act of loudness balancing at M levels typically results in a program that provides satisfactory speech recognition and sound quality for the user. Balancing at M level will typically flatten or smooth the M level profile and account for any channel-specific changes that are not captured by the use of Speech Burst stimuli. If the recipient reports unsatisfactory sound quality or speech perception after the aforementioned M-level adjustments, then the audiologist may fine-tune the M levels per the recipient's report (i.e., decrease high-frequency M levels if the recipient reports that speech is too "tinny").

It should be noted that additional adjustments may be made while in live speech mode. First, as shown in Figure 15–18, the audiologist may select different microphone configurations: T-Mic2, processor microphone only, a combination of the two, headpiece microphone, omnidirectional, UltraZoom, etc. Additionally, the audiologist may select different volume control settings, the telecoil input, ComPilot streaming, ComPilot mixing, ClearVoice, and so forth. These adjustments are easily accessible to the audiologist, so a variety of program settings and sound input options may be trialed during a programming session to determine which options best meet a recipient's needs and/or to demonstrate to the recipient the proper function of various features.

Furthermore, it should be noted that M levels also may be measured with single-channel tone-burst stimuli. The audiologist simply selects the tone-burst option and obtains M level on a single channel using the same keyboard/software function as previously described for the measurement of single-channel T levels. Additionally, some audiologists (including the authors of this chapter) choose to increase

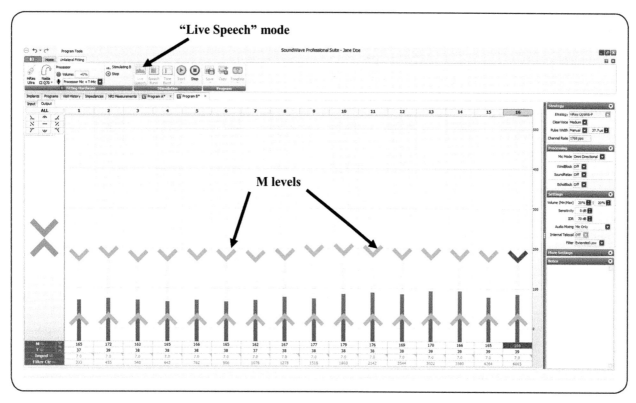

FIGURE 15–17. M level adjustment in live speech mode. Image provided courtesy of Advanced Bionics, LLC.

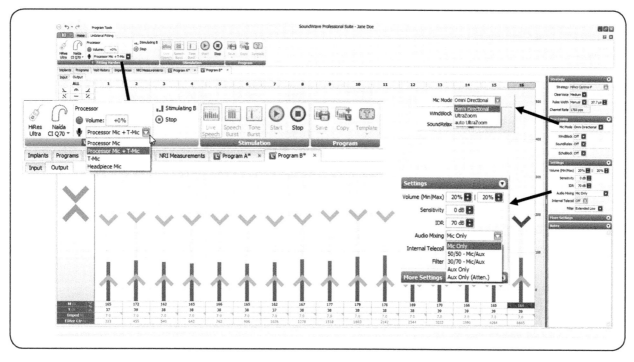

FIGURE 15–18. An example of adjustments that may be made to microphone mode and mixing ratio. Image provided courtesy of Advanced Bionics, LLC.

M levels globally (set at a flat profile) in live speech mode to the recipient's most comfortable listening level. Then, M levels are balanced in loudness across the electrode array on a channel-specific basis. Additionally, channel-specific adjustments are made to address sound quality complaints of the recipient or to improve speech clarity as needed.

Upper-stimulation levels are closely related to the electrically evoked stapedial reflex threshold (ESRT); therefore, this may be the ideal and most objective approach for setting M levels in some recipients (i.e., young children). The ESRT also is highly correlated to measured M levels when both were conducted with Speech Burst stimuli (Buckler & Overstreet, 2003). In addition, M levels based on Speech Burst ESRT may allow for better speech recognition than programs created via psychophysical loudness scaling (Wolfe & Kasulis, 2008). In many cases, recipients will prefer M levels that approach but do not reach their ESRT. To establish M levels based on ESRT, the audiologist will: (1) measure the ESRT across the electrode array (either with Speech Bursts or preferably with tone bursts on every other channel), (2) decrease the M levels globally to a level that is soft to the recipient, (3) activate the sound processor in live speech

mode, and (4) gradually increase M levels until the recipient indicates that the speech signal is most comfortable. For children who are unable to provide verbal feedback about the signal, M levels should typically be set 5% to 10% below ESRT unless the recipient shows signs of discomfort. For example, if the ESRT is measured at 200 charge units, then the estimated M levels would be set between 180 and 190 charge units unless the recipient exhibited signs that the stimulation levels were set too high at 5% to 10% of the M level. Of course, in that case, M levels should be decreased to a level that optimizes comfort, sound quality, and performance. For all recipients, it is unlikely that the M level will exceed the ESRT. Of note, most Advanced Bionics recipients have M levels ranging from 150 to 250 charge units with M levels below 100 and above 300 charge units being relatively rare.

Finally, it should be noted that stimulation levels may also be adjusted for both ears simultaneously when programming bilateral cochlear implant recipients. The audiologist simply opens a program for one ear and then "clicks" on the "Bilateral" icon in the ribbon bar at the top of the programming screen (Figure 15–19). This allows the audiologist to open an

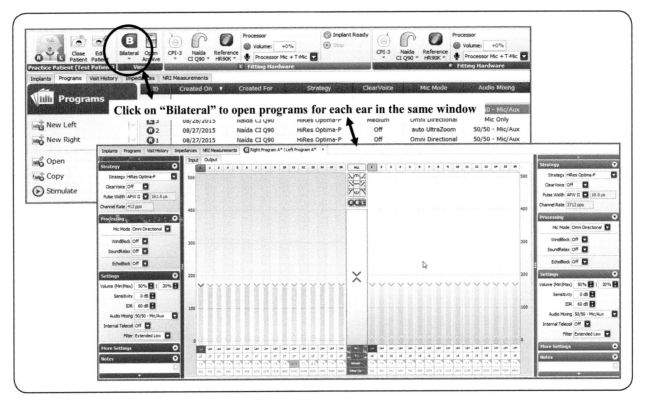

FIGURE 15–19. Bilateral programming. Image provided courtesy of Advanced Bionics, LLC.

existing program for the other ear or a new program. Using the selected programs, the audiologist may provide live speech stimulation for each ear simultaneously and make channel or global adjustments to T and M levels while in bilateral live speech mode.

Additional Programming Parameters

Microphone Sensitivity and Volume Control

The sensitivity of the sound processor can be adjusted in the SoundWave software, but typically, it should remain at the default setting. Essentially, the sensitivity controls the gain (±10 dB) applied to the signal as it is relayed from the microphone to the bandpass filters. Adjustments in sensitivity affect all frequencies equally. An increase in sensitivity will improve access to low-level sounds, but may degrade hearing in noisy environments. Conversely, a decrease in microphone sensitivity may improve comfort in noise, but also will diminish audibility for low-level sounds (e.g., 20 to 25 dB SPL). An example of an instance in which the audiologist may choose to alter the sensitivity setting would be for a recipient who does not hear low-level sounds well but for whom an increase in T levels produces an audible noise (e.g., frying or buzzing noise). In such a case, a small increase in the sensitivity setting (e.g., +3 dB) may improve access to low-level sounds without the addition of extraneous noise. The sensitivity setting within a program may

be adjusted by clicking on the up/down arrow buttons that reside to the right of the window displaying the sensitivity setting (Figure 15–20) or by inserting any whole number between –10 and +10 dB into the window next to the "Sensitivity" control and hitting the "enter" button on the keyboard. Sensitivity of the Naída CI may also be adjusted manually via the AB myPilot remote. Neptune processor users may also manually adjust the sensitivity on the processor. It should be noted that the automatic gain control featured in all Advanced Bionics processors is quite effective at adjusting to a wide range of input levels to capture the signal of interest for the user. As a result, the authors typically disable the sensitivity control. The effect of adjusting the sensitivity control will be discussed later in this chapter.

Adjustments to the volume control setting on any Advanced Bionics sound processor essentially has the effect of adjusting the M-level stimulation delivered to the recipient. The volume control parameter in SoundWave determines maximum and minimum M levels (and the range over which the M levels change) that may occur with adjustment of the volume control from the default setting. When the Naída CI Q sound processor is powered on, the volume setting is at the default control setting. If the recipient places his/her processor into standby mode, the processor will resume function at the volume control setting which was previously used prior to standby mode. Also, when the recipient changes programs,

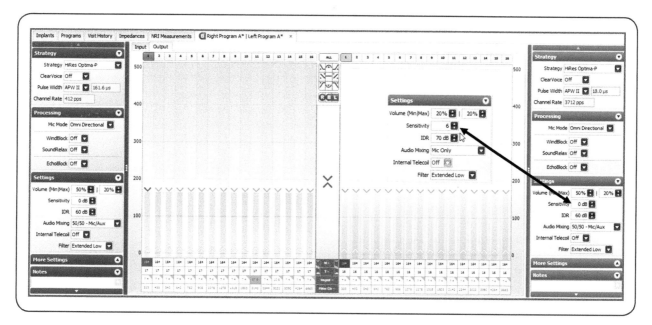

FIGURE 15–20. Adjustment of the sensitivity setting. Image provided courtesy of Advanced Bionics, LLC.

the volume setting is maintained. Therefore, if he or she increased the volume control in program 2 and then changes to program 3, the volume will remain at the same increased setting that was selected in program 2. Of note, the default volume setting of other Advanced Bionics processors (e.g., Neptune, Harmony, Auria) is at the "12:00 position" on the volume control wheel.

The extent to which the M level can be reduced ranges from 0 to ±100% and is related to a percentage of the dynamic range. For instance, at a setting of −50%, reducing the volume control from the default position to the minimum position decreases the M level by 50% of the electrical dynamic range (EDR). For this example, if T level is 10 charge units and M level is 100 charge units, then adjusting the volume control from the default setting to the minimum position will decrease the M level by 45 charge units (i.e., [100 − 10] * 0.5 = 45). As a result, at the minimum volume control setting, the recipient would receive stimulation at 55 charge units for high-level input sounds. If the minimum setting is programmed to 0, then a reduction in the volume control below the default position will not decrease the M level at all. This may be appealing for children who have no tolerance problems (i.e., they tolerate M levels during all waking hours) and like to adjust their volume controls. Finally, if the lower end of the volume control is adjusted to −100%, reduction of the volume control to the minimum setting will result in M levels corresponding to T levels. When using the sound processor at a volume control setting of −100%, the recipient may hear a low-level noise if the T levels are set to an audible level. Setting the volume control range with a lower limit of −100% may be appealing for new recipients who are acclimating to their implant or for recipients who are sensitive to auditory stimulation after a period of non-use (e.g., after awakening in the morning). The recipient or recipient's caregiver may place the volume control at a minimum setting prior to placing the processor on the head. Then, the volume control may be slowly increased to the preferred setting over the course of a few seconds. Of note, once a recipient becomes acclimated to cochlear implant use, which usually takes only a few days, or at most a few weeks, it is most common for the volume control setting to be left at the default setting at all times.

The audiologist should exercise caution when setting the upper range of the volume control (VC) parameter (e.g., +50%). Considering the example provided in the paragraph above, an upper-range value of 100% would allow the user to increase the

M-level setting from 100 charge units at the default volume control position to 190 charge units at the maximum position (i.e., M level of 100 charge units − T level of 10 charge units = an electrical dynamic range of 90 charge units; 100% of EDR = 90 charge units; M level of 100 charge unit + 90 charge units with VC range at 100% = 190 charge units when VC is set to maximum position). If M levels are set accurately with the volume control at the default setting, then a 100% increase in stimulation relative to the electrical dynamic range (or even 50%) is rarely, if ever, appropriate. When the volume control provides too much headroom for increasing M levels, the user may encounter uncomfortable stimulation levels. Additionally, when the range of the volume control is large (e.g., ±100%), then small changes of the volume control dial result in relatively large changes in stimulation and presumably the loudness the recipient experiences. Consequently, for adults, the upper end of the volume control range should be set between 10% and 25% to allow a small increase in volume as needed. Additionally, the authors typically set the lower end of the volume control range to be no greater than −50% and typically at −20% to −25%. This smaller volume control range allows the user to be more precise in selecting alterations as needed. Given the fact that M levels are set appropriately for the recipient, a recipient will be unlikely to need a larger range over which to adjust the stimulation levels, and the increase in precision in which the volume control can be adjusted will likely be beneficial. For children who have optionally programmed M levels (i.e., based on ESRT), the upper end of the volume control range should be set to 0 to prevent a further increase in M-level stimulation and potential discomfort, and the minimum range of the volume control should be set to allow for little to no adjustment of stimulation (e.g., 0% to −10%). Disabling the volume control range for infants and young children who are acclimated to their cochlear implants will eliminate the possibility of the volume control being inadvertently adjusted to provide sub-optimal stimulation levels. Of note, the software default values for the volume control range are −50% to +20%.

Channel Gains

The **channel-gain** parameter allows for frequency-specific adjustments to the gain of the signal from the microphone. The channel gain adjustment may be accessed by selecting the "Input" tab that is located just above and to the left of the "channel 1" marker in the programming screen (Figure 15–21). **When a**

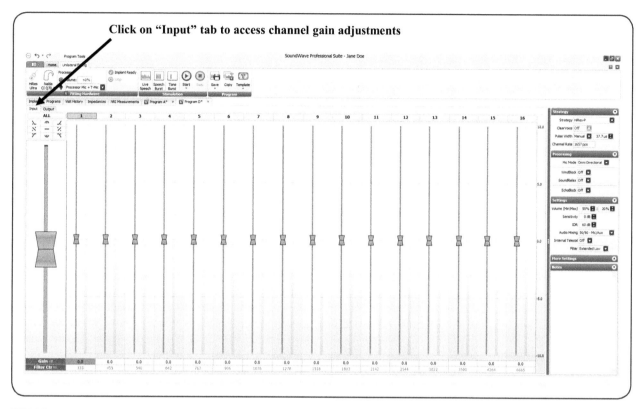

FIGURE 15–21. Adjustment of gain settings. Image provided courtesy of Advanced Bionics, LLC.

patient has appropriate stimulation levels, adjustment to channel gains is most likely unnecessary. As a result, channel gain adjustments are typically seldom made. However, it may be helpful for recipients who cannot tolerate changes in M level and have complaints about sound quality (e.g., increase channel gain to provide better access for high-frequency sounds when it is not possible to increase stimulation levels because of patient discomfort or non-auditory side effects). Reducing high-frequency channel gain may improve sound quality when the recipient reports that speech and environmental sounds are too sharp or tinny, whereas a reduction to low-frequency channel gains may improve listening comfort and performance in noisy environments. In contrast, increasing low-frequency channel gain will likely change overall loudness and may result in a sound quality that has more "fullness," whereas increasing high-frequency gain channels may enhance sound quality and/or the ability to understand speech.

Input Dynamic Range (IDR) and Automatic Gain Control

As previously discussed in Chapter 3, a wide range of acoustic input levels that are of potential inter-est to the recipient (i.e., 20 to 120 dB SPL) must be processed by a relatively narrow electrical dynamic range (EDR) of hearing (i.e., 10 to 25 dB). The two types of signal processing that are most important in accomplishing this objective in the Advanced Bionics software are the **input dynamic range** (IDR) and dual-loop **automatic gain control** (AGC) processing (Spahr, Dorman, & Loiselle, 2007). These interact closely with the electrical stimulation levels corresponding to M level (most comfortable) and T level (threshold). Inputs at the upper end of the IDR are stimulated at M level, while inputs at the lower end of the IDR are stimulated at T level. The resultant function is called a mapping function (Figure 15–22). The sensitivity and volume controls further affect how a wide range of acoustic inputs may be mapped into a relatively narrow range of electrical hearing.

The microphone of the Advanced Bionics cochlear implant possesses an overall dynamic range of about 84 dB SPL (Advanced Bionics, 2003). The dynamic range of the microphone is determined by the noise floor of the microphone and by the highest-level sound the microphone can handle without distortion, which occurs when the diaphragm of the microphone reaches the limits of its maximum displacement or

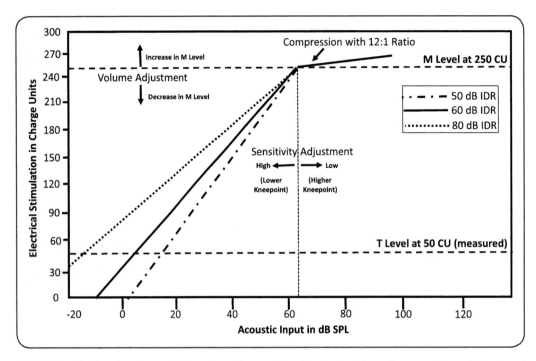

FIGURE 15–22. Mapping of acoustic input dynamic range into the electrical dynamic range with an illustration of the effect of adjustment to IDR, volume control, and sensitivity. Image provided courtesy of Advanced Bionics, LLC.

when it strikes the case of the microphone. The IDR of the cochlear implant sound processor determines the range of acoustic inputs that will be mapped within the recipient's EDR without the use of compression processing with a high compression ratio (i.e., 10:1 or greater). The default IDR of the Advanced Bionics system is 60 dB. Figure 15–22 provides an illustration of the acoustic input levels that are mapped into the EDR with the IDR set to 60 dB (solid black line in Figure 15–22), the microphone sensitivity set to "0," and the volume control set to the default condition. As shown, the recipient has an M level of 250 charge units, and T levels have been measured and set to 50 charge units. A sound with an input level of 3 dB SPL results in the provision of stimulation at T level, a sound that has an input level of 63 dB SPL results in the provision of stimulation at M level, and sounds with an input level exceeding 63 dB SPL are subjected to compression processing with a high compression ratio (similar to compression limiting processing in hearing aids), resulting in the provision of stimulation near M level. With measured T levels and an IDR of 60 dB, the CI recipient should have access to conversational level, moderate as well as soft sounds. Of note, with measured T levels, the inputs in the lower end of the 60 dB IDR likely fall within the noise floor

of the microphone. In case T levels are not measured and set at a level lower than the actual Ts, an IDR of >60 dB will improve the recipient access to softer sounds (see Figure 15–22). Of note, when T levels are estimated at 10% of M level rather than measured, the slope of the mapping function will decrease and less stimulation will be provided for very low-level sounds (compare Figures 15–22 and 15–23).

Adjusting the IDR primarily affects audibility for low-level sounds but also affects stimulation provided for moderate-level sounds. As shown in Figure 15–22, increasing the IDR to 80 dB (dotted line in Figure 15–22) results in an acoustic input of −15 dB SPL receiving T-level stimulation. Although inputs at and above 65 dB SPL are still subjected to compression processing with a high compression ratio, the entire IDR input/output function is shifted upward, resulting in an increase in stimulation levels for acoustic inputs up to 65 dB SPL. Increasing the IDR from the default of 60 dB to 80 dB will provide better audibility for low-level sounds but may also decrease speech recognition in noise, because low-level noise inputs may be mapped higher into the recipient's relatively narrow EDR (Holden et al., 2011). Additionally, the recipient will most likely perceive the 80 dB IDR to provide a louder signal because stimulation levels are

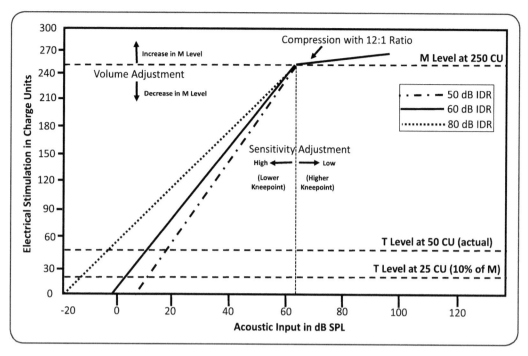

FIGURE 15–23. Mapping of acoustic input dynamic range into the electrical dynamic range with an illustration of the effect of adjustment to IDR, volume control, sensitivity, and T level. Image provided courtesy of Advanced Bionics, LLC.

higher for input levels of 65 dB SPL and below. Even for higher-level inputs (i.e., >65 dB SPL), a higher proportion of the low-level components of the audio signal will be subjected to M-level stimulation.

In contrast, the dashed line in Figure 15–22 provides an example of the effect of decreasing the IDR from 60 dB to 50 dB. As shown, acoustic inputs with a level of approximately 15 dB SPL are mapped at T level, and a relatively lower amount of electrical stimulation is provided for all acoustic inputs, with levels ranging from 0 to 65 dB SPL. Decreasing the IDR from the default setting will result in a reduction of audibility for low-level sounds. However, lower-level noise will be less likely to be mapped into the recipient's EDR. Higher-level inputs will be stimulated at lower electrical levels. Since the 40 dB dynamic range of speech is still being captured, and because less low-level noise is likely introduced to the EDR, the overall signal-to-noise ratio of the signal delivered to the relatively narrow EDR may be improved in noisy environments (see Figure 15–22). Indeed, Holden et al. (2011) evaluated speech recognition in noise of Advanced Bionics recipients using 50, 65, and 80 dB IDR and concluded that "individual scores and preferences revealed that a 50 dB IDR should be provided as an option for listening in noise." In another study,

examining the effect of IDR on the speech recognition of children, Baudhin and colleagues (2012) also concluded that the use of individualized programming and multiple IDRs may allow for optimal hearing performance across a range of listening environments.

Figure 15–22 also shows the effect of two adjustable controls on the IDR: sensitivity and volume control. At a sensitivity setting of 0 dB, the kneepoint of the AGC (slow loop) occurs, based on input frequency, at an average input level of 63 dB SPL. As shown, increasing the sensitivity essentially (up to +10 dB) has the effect of down-shifting IDR toward the left (i.e., lower-level inputs will be mapped at T level or above, and lower- to moderate-level inputs will be mapped at a higher position in the EDR). As a result, soft sounds will become more audible, which may be helpful in quiet environments but may result in poorer speech recognition in noise. Decreasing the sensitivity (up to −10 dB) shifts the IDR up and to the right, so audibility for low-level sounds will be decreased, sounds with an input level below 65 dB SPL will likely elicit a softer loudness percept, and speech recognition in noise may improve. A higher sensitivity setting may be helpful for music perception as well because it reduces the compression that is applied to music, which is known to have a wide dynamic range and a moderate to high sound pressure level.

Changing the sensitivity setting does not change the slope of the mapping function. Adjustment of volume control, on the other hand, can increase or decrease the slope of the mapping function. Increasing the volume control increases the magnitude of electrical stimulation (in charge units) provided for sounds with an input level of 65 dB SPL and higher, whereas decreasing the volume control reduces the amount of electrical stimulation provided for sounds with an input level of 65 dB SPL and higher. Because the range of electrical stimulation levels that are used to code sounds across the IDR changes with decreases and increases in the volume control setting, an adjustment of the volume control affects stimulation levels and loudness percepts elicited for sounds across the entire IDR. As the reader can likely surmise, increasing the volume will increase loudness, and decreasing the volume control will reduce loudness. The effect of the volume control setting on speech recognition will vary depending upon a number of factors, including but not limited to the stimulation levels that are most appropriate for the recipient, the input level of the sound of interest, the slope of the recipient's EDR, and so forth.

As previously discussed, real-world listening environments often possess sounds with input levels exceeding 65 dB SPL. In fact, in noisy restaurants, workplaces, school cafeterias, sporting events, social situations, and so on, the speech and competing noise almost always exceeds 70 dB SPL and may even approach 90 dB SPL or higher (Crukley, Scollie, & Parsa, 2011; Pearsons, et al., 1977). If the upper end of the IDR was fixed so that all input levels exceeding 65 dB SPL were always subjected to compression processing with a high compression ratio, Advanced Bionics recipients would struggle to understand speech in moderate- to high-level noise environments. In noisy situations, talkers typically increase their vocal level so that their speech is delivered at a positive speech-to-noise ratio. However, if all inputs exceeding 65 dB SPL were compressed significantly, then the positive speech-to-noise ratio would essentially be eliminated by the high compression ratio. Additionally, there would be little to no change in loudness with increases in input level above 65 dB SPL. Advanced Bionics has effectively addressed this issue by incorporating an automatic gain control (AGC) with its IDR.

All modern Advanced Bionics sound processors feature **AGC-II** compression processing, which is a dual-action compression developed by Brian Moore and colleagues (Moore & Glasberg, 1988; Moore, Glasberg, & Stone, 1991; Stone et al., 1999). AGC-II processing possesses two compression thresholds (i.e., gain controls), one with a relatively low compression threshold (63 dB SPL) and long attack (325 msec) and release times (1000 msec) and another with a higher compression threshold (72 dB SPL) and fast attack (less than 0.6 msec) and release times (8 msec). Typically, the slower-acting control determines the amplifier gain for most everyday sounds (e.g., speech, continuous noise, music), and the faster-acting control serves to quickly decrease amplifier gain for transient, high-level sounds (i.e., when the momentary output level increases by 8 dB above the continuous level determined by the slow-acting system; e.g., door slamming, cough/sneeze, dinner plate dropping, alarm sounding) (Advanced Bionics, 2003b).

When the recipient moves from a quiet environment with low-level speech to a noisy environment with high-level speech and noise, the slow-acting component of the AGC-II system will automatically adjust the amplifier gain to position the input signal at an appropriate location within the IDR. As a result, low-level inputs will receive a boost to ensure audibility but will also be placed at a relatively low position in the EDR, resulting in a soft loudness perception. In contrast, the gain will be decreased for higher-level inputs so as to avoid high-level compression at the top end of the AGC. In essence, the slow component of AGC-II functions as an automatic volume control that captures a wide range of acoustic input levels of interest and places the wide range of input signals within the narrow EDR. Of note, the slow compression time constants of the slow AGC-II component prevent the amplifier gain from being quickly increased/decreased during the pauses and peaks of running speech. As a result, the output does not produce a pumping effect while attempting to follow the short-term fluctuations of speech. Additionally, because the slow component of AGC-II (with its relatively slow response times) is paired with a relatively low compression threshold, a moderate compression ratio may be used to "squeeze" the wide range of acoustic inputs of interest into the recipient's narrow EDR. Moreover, the fast component of AGC-II protects the user against and maintains comfort for transient, intense sounds. Furthermore, if the increase in input level is very brief, then the gain will return to normal quickly because of the fast release time of the fast component of AGC-II. As a result, audibility will be restored for important sounds that follow high-level transient noise. In short, the 60 dB IDR and AGC-II of the Advanced Bionics cochlear implant function to provide audibility for low-level inputs, attempt to restore normal loudness percepts for a wide range of acoustic inputs, allow for the preservation of the short-term fluctuations of speech without significant compression, and allow for the coding of high-level speech in noise without significant compression.

The IDR can be adjusted from 20 to 80 dB and can be set on a program-by-program basis. Some recipients may benefit from a program with an increased IDR (e.g., 70–80 dB) to enhance sound quality for music. A wider IDR may also be useful for quiet environments in which it is useful to hear soft speech (e.g., listening to the television at home). Furthermore, research has suggested that a narrower IDR may improve listening comfort and speech recognition in noise (Holder et al., 2011). Of note, however, an IDR of 60 to 65 dB allows for excellent performance across a wide variety of listening environments because of the AGC-II. Additionally, a narrower IDR may be less important for noisy situations when the recipient has access to ClearVoice and directional microphone technology (i.e., StereoZoom, UltraZoom).

Audio-Mixing Ratio

The function of the **audio-mixing ratio** is different for the Naída CI Q processor compared with all other Advanced Bionics processors. For the Naída sound processor, the audio-mixing ratio adjusts the relative strength of the signal arriving from the microphone to the signal arriving from the telecoil or from a Phonak Roger receiver that is connected to the base of the PowerCel 170 (i.e., the telecoil and the Roger signal are the only inputs considered as an "auxiliary source"). Several audio-mixing ratio (Mic/Aux) options are available (see Figure 15–18), including: (1) Mic only—the sound processor microphone is the only input enabled for the processor, (2) 50/50—the input from the microphone and auxiliary source receive equal emphasis, but there is 6 dB of attenuation to each input to account for loudness summation that may occur when a signal is simultaneously delivered from two microphones, (3) 30/70—the input from the microphone(s) used with the sound processor is attenuated by 12 dB along with 3 dB of attenuation provided to the signal from the auxiliary source to provide a greater emphasis on the auxiliary input, (4) Aux Only—the sound processor microphone is disabled so that only the auxiliary input is active, and

(5) Aux Only (Atten.)—the sound processor microphone is disabled and the auxiliary input is active but attenuated by approximately 20 dB.

For all other Advanced Bionics sound processors (Harmony, Neptune, etc.), the audio-mixing ratio adjusts the relative strength of signals arriving from the microphone of the speech processor to the signals arriving from any other auxiliary source (e.g., FM system, iPod or other battery-operated devices, or T-Mic coupled to the direct auditory input of the processors as well as the telecoil input). Because the T-Mic is coupled to the auxiliary input post of ear-level sound processors prior to the Naída CI Q sound processor (i.e., Harmony), the audio-mixing ratio had to be set to "Aux Only" in order to select the T-Mic as the only microphone option (i.e., disable the sound processor microphone). Furthermore, when the T-Mic is used with the Harmony, a 50/50 mixing ratio results in the T-Mic and the Harmony microphone both being active.

The difference in the audio-mixing ratio parameter in the Naída CI Q sound processors as compared with all other Advanced Bionics sound processors is noteworthy. For the Naída CI Q sound processor, the audiologist should only create a program with "Aux" input for situations in which the recipient is planning on using the telecoil or Phonak Roger remote microphone (RM) system with the Roger 17 receiver. In this case, a 50/50 mixing ratio would allow the recipient to hear the signal from the telecoil or Roger system as well as the signal from the Naída CI Q microphone. The "Aux Only" option would allow the recipient to have a "telecoil-only" or "Roger digital RM only" program, which may be helpful when using a telephone or Roger RM system in a noisy environment or when the recipient wants to connect the Roger pen to an MP3 player or computer and wishes to listen to only the audio that is streamed to the sound processors. It is important to note that the recipient will not hear any microphone input when the "Aux Only" program is selected. As a result, this option is an inappropriate choice for young children because they would be deprived of access to incidental sounds and to their own voice if the sound processor was inadvertently switched to a program with "Aux Only" mixing. The 50/50 mixing ratio is recommended for use with infants and young children and for RM use in educational settings. The default audio-mixing ratio for all processors is the "50/50" option.

Of note, during the programming session, the Naída microphone input (T-Mic 2, processor microphone, Processor Mic + T-Mic2, headpiece microphone) is selected from the microphone source menu (shown in Figure 15–18). When the sound processor is programmed at the end of the programming session, the audiologist must "click" on the Naída CI Q sound processor icon to select the desired microphone configuration for each program (Figure 15–24). If the audiologist is certain that the recipient will never use the auxiliary input, then the authors recommend the "Mic Only" mixing option because no attenuation will be provided to the Mic input(s). Alternatively, the recipient may be provided with two programs, one with "Mic Only" for situations in which the telecoil is not used and another with mixing for when the telecoil is used.

It should also be noted that mixing occurs at the Naída microphone when two microphone inputs are selected from the microphone source menu. As described later in the section pertaining to loading of programs onto the Naída processor (i.e., processor configuration), the audiologist may control microphone mixing separately by choosing to enable the recipient's T-Mic2 and sound processor microphone for simultaneous use. When this option is selected, the signal from each output is attenuated

by 6 dB to account for the summation that exists when the microphone signals are combined with one another. Because of this summation and the 6 dB of attenuation at each microphone, the total output of the joint microphone signals will be similar to what was obtained if either microphone was used independently.

It is also worth noting that some Naída CI Q users may perceive incidental sounds to be softer when using an auxiliary source, such as a Phonak Roger RM system. This perception is likely attributed to the 6 dB of attenuation that occurs at the sound processor microphone and the subsequent reduction in audibility for sounds arriving at the sound processor microphone rather than the Roger RM. To address this issue, Advanced Bionics has created "**Roger Ready**" mode, in which the processor is in "Mic Only" mode when no Roger input is present but automatically switches to the programmed mixing ratio when the Roger input is activated. In other words, the "Roger Ready" mode prevents the 6 dB attenuation at the Naída CI Q microphone when the Roger system is not in use, so the recipient's access to incidental and low-level sounds is uncompromised.

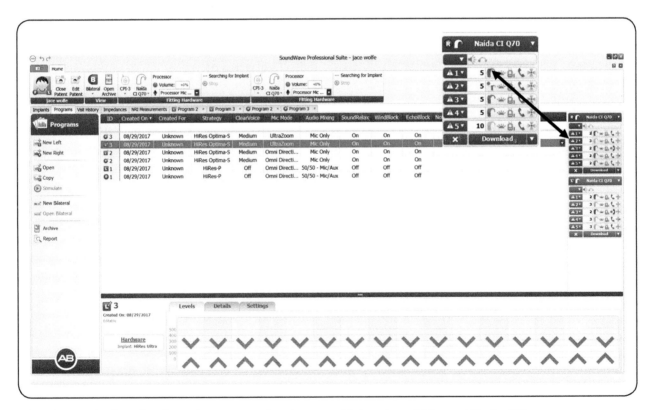

FIGURE 15–24. Configuration of sound processor settings. Image provided courtesy of Advanced Bionics, LLC.

Figure 15–25 provides an example of how the audiologist may enable/disable the Roger Ready mode when programming the sound processor at the end of the programming session.

For the Harmony, Auria, CII, and Platinum BTE (behind-the-ear) processors, microphone mixing (between the sound processor microphone and T-Mic) is controlled by adjusting the audio-mixing ratio. In other words, there is not an independent menu to adjust microphone mixing separate from mixing of the telecoil, FM, and so forth. When the T-Mic is connected to the direct audio input post of the Harmony, CII, or Platinum BTE, a 50/50 audio-mixing ratio results in equal emphasis being placed on the signals from the sound processor microphone and the T-Mic (but once again, the output of each microphone is attenuated by 6 dB to account for summation that occurs when microphones are active). The Aux Only program is commonly used with the T-Mic so that all of the sound input is captured by the T-Mic rather than the sound processor microphone. Gifford and Revit (2010) reported significantly better speech recognition in noise with a T-Mic only program relative to a program in which the sound processor microphone is enabled. This improvement is presumably due to placement of the T-Mic in the concha, allowing for preservation of the natural positive directivity of the auricle. For this reason, the authors recommend a default program of Aux Only along with the T-Mic for all Harmony, Auria, CII, and Platinum BTE users. The authors also recommend the T-Mic2 as the only input source for the default program for Naída CI Q users. To achieve this, the audiologist must select a "Mic Only" audio-mixing ratio and then select the T-Mic only option in the microphone source ("Mic Source") menu. The "Mic Only" is also used with the Naída and UltraZoom technology for a directional program for noisy situations.

Mic Mode

The "**Mic Mode**" parameter is an option for the Naída CI Q sound processor and determines whether the sound processor microphone will operate in omnidirectional or fully adaptive directional mode (shown on the right side of Figure 15–18). The three options in the drop-down "Mic Mode" menu are the "**Omni Directional**," "**UltraZoom**," and "**autoUltraZoom**" modes. The "Omni Directional" option is the default mode and results in the implementation of an omnidirectional polar plot pattern for the microphone of the Naída sound processor. The "UltraZoom" option enables the fully adaptive directional microphones (on board front and back microphones), which enable the directional microphone and adaptively adjust the microphone polar plot pattern so that the null of the polar plot pattern in the rear hemisphere is positioned toward the direction from which the

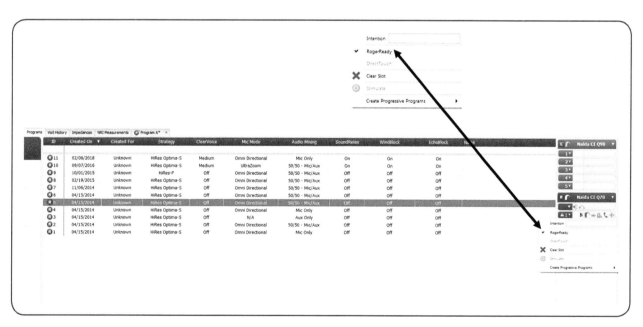

FIGURE 15–25. Activation of Roger Ready and creation of progressive programs. Image provided courtesy of Advanced Bionics, LLC.

most intense competing noise signal is arriving. As mentioned previously, the Naída CI Q possesses two omnidirectional microphones, and the electrical output from these two microphones may be analyzed to achieve the desired directional response. Research has shown that the UltraZoom pre-processing feature can provide very significant improvements in speech recognition in noise, particularly when paired with ClearVoice input processing (Hehrmann, Fredelake, Hammacher, Dyballa, & Büchner, 2012). The "autoUltraZoom" mode automatically switches from omnidirectional to directional mode when the recipient moves from a quiet to a noisy environment. The "autoUltraZoom" technology is only available in the Naída CI Q90 sound processor.

Internal Telecoil

The "**Internal Telecoil**" parameter simply enables the telecoil that is built into the Advanced Bionics ear-level sound processor (e.g., Naída and Harmony). The Neptune sound processor accesses the telecoil via the "T-Com" accessory. As mentioned earlier, for Naída CI Q and Harmony processors, the "Audio Mixing" parameter may be used to determine the relationship between the output from the sound processor microphone and the telecoil output. It should be noted that the T-Mic and the telecoil cannot be enabled at the same time because the Harmony considers each one as an auxiliary input.

Extended Filtering

Extended filtering will determine the lower cutoff frequency (i.e., high-pass cutoff) for the lowest frequency channel. In the default mode, Extended Low Filtering, the high-pass cutoff of channel 1, is set to 250 Hz with a center frequency of 333 Hz. In the Standard Filtering mode, the high-pass cutoff of channel 1 is increased to 350 Hz with a center frequency of 383 Hz. The vast majority of recipients will benefit from the extended low-frequency filtering. If an adult recipient persistently complains of annoyance of low-frequency weighted noise (e.g., traffic noise), the audiologist may choose to provide a program with Standard Filtering. Of note, because of the development and effectiveness of ClearVoice, the audiologist should rarely have to switch to Standard Filtering to address bothersome noise. However, if a recipient persistently complains of poor sound quality, including a prominent echo, intrusive ambient noise, or his or her own voice being too loud, then it may be beneficial to try Standard Filtering.

Lock

Advanced Bionics optimizes radio frequency (RF) power levels to establish efficient yet reliable bidirectional telemetry (i.e., "lock") between the sound processor and the cochlear implant internal device. The Naída CI Q sound processor manages requisite RF power settings using **AutoVoltage**. For the HiResolution strategies, the compliance voltage is 8 volts; therefore, AutoVoltage manages the pulse width and current so that the requested current amplitude voltage does not exceed voltage compliance limits available from an 8 volt power source. For the Optima strategy, the compliance voltage is reduced to 4 volts to increase power efficiency. In Optima, AutoVoltage manages the pulse width and maximum current so that the requisite current amplitude can be provided from a 4 volt power source.

The audiologist may also select manual RF power management for Naída CI Q users. This option should only be selected in rare cases, as the AutoVoltage mode is designed to optimize battery life for Naída CI Q users. For instance, in the rare occurrence that consistent lock could not be obtained with the AutoVoltage setting, the audiologist may select the manual mode and determine a manual power setting required to maintain lock. The manual RF power range spans from 1 to 15, and the audiologist may manually vary the number to determine the lowest setting required to maintain lock while an intense sound (e.g., loud clapping of hands) is delivered during "live speech mode." When manual power mode is used, the authors typically select a manual setting that is one step higher than the minimum setting required to maintain lock during the presence of an intense sound so as to reduce the likelihood of intermittencies during daily use.

For recipients who use the HiRes and HiRes with Fidelity 120 signal coding strategies, the HiRes 90K system possesses a unique feature called **PoEM** (Power Estimator), which is designed to optimize battery life as well as monitor and adjust the RF power needed to maintain a consistent signal across a variety of listening environments. The AutoVoltage and PoEM systems use high RF power levels only when absolutely necessary (i.e., high-level noise environments), and both systems automatically account for changes in skin-flap thickness that may occur over time (e.g., edema resides at the skin flap during the weeks after surgery, a haircut). These power management systems allow for a continuous estimation of power needs, and this is possible because the Advanced Bionics 90K and CII implants use two separate RF frequencies, one for forward telemetry (49 MHz) and another (10.7 MHz) for backward telemetry. This allows for a simultaneous exchange of information between the external and internal devices.

It should be noted that when programming within the conventional HiRes and HiRes with Fidelity 120 signal coding strategies, the audiologist may adjust the magnitude of the PoEM as well as the frequency in which the PoEM table is updated. The PoEM magnitude options are "low," "medium," and "high." The "high" PoEM setting is the default option and provides acceptable battery life in most instances. It is rare that the audiologist would ever want to stray from the "high" setting. Unlike HiRes Optima, the audiologist may also adjust the frequency in which the PoEM algorithm assesses the requisite power level needed to operate the cochlear implant. For conventional HiRes and HiRes with Fidelity 120 programs, the audiologist may select a "Check Interval" range from 10 to 50 msec in 10 msec intervals. The default setting is 20 msec, and once again, it is rare that the audiologist would need to deviate from the default setting. Experimentation with a different "Check Interval" setting may be attempted if a recipient reports that signal intermittencies and other troubleshooting options have been exhausted (i.e., replacement of transmitting cable/coil, processor, etc.).

Similar to the AutoVoltage feature, the PoEM mode may also be disabled, and the audiologist can manually adjust the RF level to a fixed setting. As before, the need for a manual RF adjustment is a rare occurrence and is necessary only when the recipient reports signal intermittencies across various environments. Manual adjustments are made in a similar manner as previously described for the HiRes Optima signal coding strategy.

For Harmony or Neptune sound processors, the audiologist may enable "**High Power Mode**." High Power Mode is a program-specific option that increases the power output of the processor for recipients with high power requirements. The "High Power Mode" setting will decrease battery life considerably, so the audiologist should only activate it as a last resort. It is disabled by default. The Naída sound processor manages power differently, and therefore, it does not utilize this parameter.

Ground (Return/Reference) Electrode

As previously noted, Advanced Bionics implants possess two ground (return) electrodes, one on the case and another "ring" electrode which resides on the electrode lead. The case electrode is the default ground electrode and is used as the ground electrode for the overwhelming majority of recipients. In rare cases, however, it may be necessary to switch to the ring ground electrode. Such instances include situations in which the case band ground electrode is determined to be faulty or when a non-auditory side effect (e.g., facial nerve stimulation) is present and cannot be resolved with other programming adjustments (i.e., increasing pulse width, channel clipping, or disabling one or more channels).

Channel Clipping

Channel clipping prevents stimulation from ever exceeding a predefined, fixed level. This is desirable when the user frequently adjusts the volume control, which results in adjustments to M levels. Clipping allows for an increase to stimulation on all channels except for the one in which clipping is implemented (clipping may be adjusted on a channel-by-channel basis). This is beneficial if stimulation at a certain level causes non-auditory side effects, such as facial nerve stimulation. In this case, clipping would be set at the highest stimulation level that does not provoke the undesired response. As previously discussed, intense, transient sounds exceeding 65 dB SPL are subjected to fast-acting AGC compression, which limits the amount by which stimulation will be provided above M level. If clipping is implemented at a certain level, then stimulation will never exceed that level, regardless of the nature or intensity of the input sound or of the nature of the input processing. Clipping may be accessed by right-clicking on an individual channel to expose a drop-down menu, from which "Clipping" may be selected (Figure 15–26). The programming audiologist may then use the up/down arrows to change the charge unit level at which clipping is applied, or a desired charge unit level may be entered into the field in the table residing below the programming level window.

DuoPhone. The **DuoPhone** feature utilizes the **Hearing instrument Body Area Network** (HiBAN) technology to stream a telephone signal from one Naída CI Q sound processor to the contralateral Naída CI Q

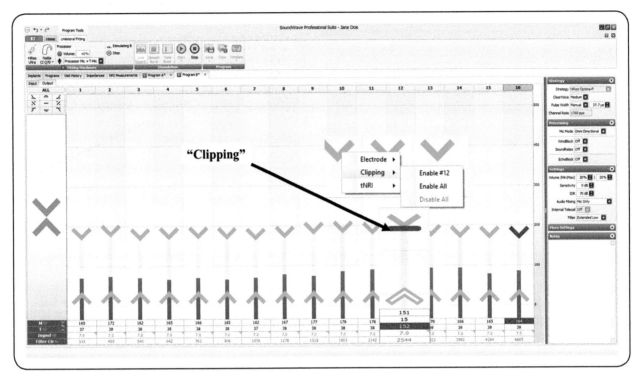

FIGURE 15–26. Clipping. Image provided courtesy of Advanced Bionics, LLC.

sound processor, allowing for bilateral telephone listening. Wolfe (2014) has shown that the DuoPhone improves speech recognition over the telephone for both cochlear implant and hearing aid users compared with the unilateral telephone condition. The DuoPhone feature is activated by the audiologist when the recipient's programs are loaded into the sound processor. The audiologist must select whether the telephone signal will be streamed from the left ear to the right ear or vice versa (Figure 15–27). Alternatively, the audiologist may activate "Direct Touch," which allows the recipient to choose the primary ear for telephone use. The telephone signal may be captured by the T-Mic 2, the sound processor microphone, or the telecoil and then streamed to the opposite sound processor. Of note, the microphone input at the opposite sound processor is attenuated by 10 dB to reduce the ambient noise captured at that ear. The DuoPhone technology is unavailable in the Naída CI Q30 sound processor. However, the DuoPhone technology may be used with the Naída Link hearing aid.

ZoomControl. **ZoomControl** must be set as a special feature in a program dedicated for special use cases in which the signal of interest arrives from the side of the listener. The audiologist must enable ZoomCon-

trol technology in one of the recipient's programs in order to allow for use of this feature. A microphone-enabled program is loaded into a program slot of the Naída CI Q70 or Q90 sound processor. Then, the audiologist must select the ZoomControl symbol (Figure 15–28), which resides adjacent to the program number loaded into each program slot. Once activated, the side of the ZoomControl icon that is highlighted (in red for the right ear and in blue for the left ear) indicates the side at which sound is captured to stream over to the opposite ear. Alternatively, the audiologist may activate "Direct Touch," which allows the recipient to choose the sound processor that will capture the signal of interest. When ZoomControl is in use, the microphone input at the opposite ear sound processor is attenuated by 12 dB to improve the signal-to-noise ratio of the desired signal.

The user may access ZoomControl in one of the five programs of the Naída CI Q70 or Q90 processors by using the program button on the processor or the AB myPilot to switch to a ZoomControl-enabled program. The myPilot allows the user to determine which ear is capturing the signal of interest and streaming it to the contralateral processor. ZoomControl may not be used in a program in which DuoPhone or UltraZoom has been enabled.

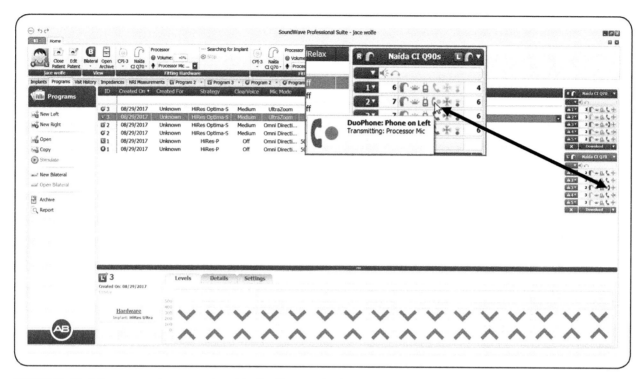

FIGURE 15–27. Adjustment and programming of the DuoPhone technology. Image provided courtesy of Advanced Bionics, LLC.

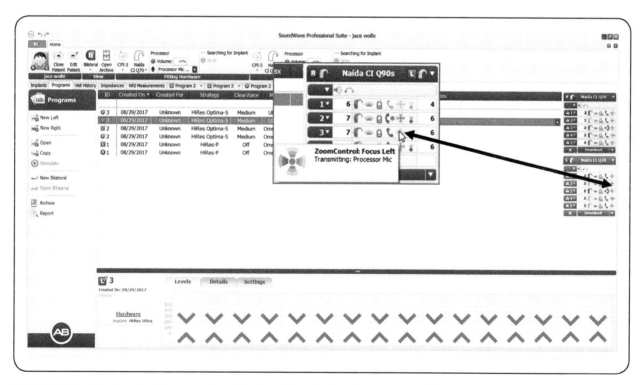

FIGURE 15–28. Adjustment and programming of the ZoomControl technology. Image provided courtesy of Advanced Bionics, LLC.

StereoZoom. StereoZoom is a noise-management technology that uses the HiBAN Binaural VoiceStream technology to exchange the audio information between bilateral Naída sound processors (or between the Naída sound processor and Naída Link hearing aid of a bimodal user) to create a binaural beam-former. When compared to directionality achieved via one sound processor or one hearing aid, a binaural beam-former can provide greater attenuation for sounds arriving from the rear hemisphere and more specific focus on sounds arriving from the front of the recipient. As a result, StereZoom may potentially provide better speech recognition in noise than what may be achieved with UltraZoom. The StereoZoom feature may be activated by the audiologist in a program created for noisy situations. The recipient must manually select the program in situations in which the speech signal of interest arrives from the front and the noise arrives from behind. StereoZoom is typically considered for adults and older children (e.g., teenagers) who experience difficulty with speech understanding in noise.

QuickSync. **QuickSync** is a feature that allows the user to change volume control or program settings for both ears simultaneously by pressing the control on just one processor. Although it is likely that QuickSync will not result in an improvement in speech understanding or hearing performance, it will facilitate a more convenient and simpler tactic to quickly adjust sound processor settings when needed. The audiologist may enable/disable the QuickSync feature when loading programs onto the recipient's sound processor.

Loading Programs into Advanced Bionics Sound Processors

To load programs into Advanced Bionics sound processors, the audiologist must select the "Programs" tab. On the far right-hand side of the screen, there will be a rectangular box (the Processor Pane) with a processor icon and a textual description of the type of sound processor that is connected to the programming computer (Figure 15–29). Because different programming options exist for the various Advanced Bionics sound processors, the following section will be divided into two categories, one for the Naída CI Q sound processor and another for all other Advanced Bionics sound processors.

When programming a unilateral Naída CI Q sound processor, the audiologist must first select whether the processor is to be loaded for the right

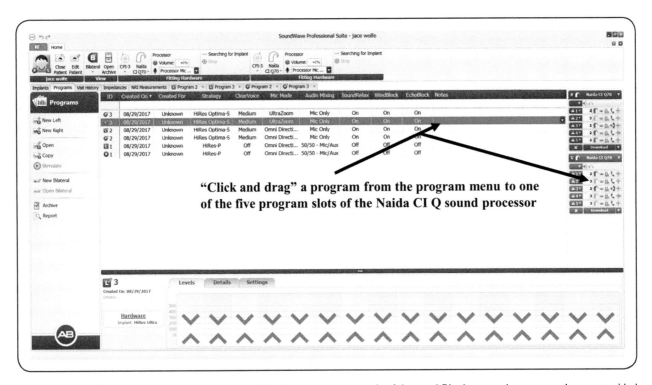

FIGURE 15–29. Visual example of the processing of loading programs onto the Advanced Bionics sound processor. Image provided courtesy of Advanced Bionics, LLC.

ear, the left ear, or as a bilateral processor. This may be achieved by "clicking" on the arrow in the upper right-hand corner of the processor box to open a drop-down menu which allows the audiologist to initialize the processor for the desired ear. For unilateral cochlear implant recipients, the Naída CI Q sound processor may also be initialized for use with the Naída Link hearing aid (for bimodal users) or the Naída Link CROS (Contralateral Routing of Signal; for recipients who have no usable hearing in the non-implanted ear). For the Naída CI Q sound processor, there will be five "slots" in which programs may be loaded. Programs are placed in each program slot by simply "clicking and dragging" the desired program from the menu of programs to the desired program slot (see Figure 15–29). When the desired number of programs is placed in the various program slots, the audiologist then "clicks" on the "Download" button to load the processor with the programs.

If the processor is initialized as a bilateral processor, up to 5 programs for each ear may be loaded into the same processor (for a total of 10 programs). When a recipient places the sound processor transmitting coil on his/her head (i.e., achieves lock), the IntelliLink feature automatically identifies the ear that is being stimulated, and the processor selects the programs that are loaded for that ear.

For each program that is dragged to a program slot, the audiologist may select multiple options that alter how the program functions for the recipient. As shown in Figure 15–30, the audiologist may enable/disable the LED light on the processor by simply highlighting/de-selecting the "light" icon. The audiologist may also enable/disable ComPilot streaming by activating/de-activating the ComPilot streaming icon. Furthermore, the audiologist may "click" on the arrow immediately to the right of each program slot number to access a drop-down menu, which provides access to numerous parameters.

For instance, the audiologist may determine the microphone source used for each program. ComPilot mixing (described later in this chapter) is also selected from this drop-down menu. Additionally, the audiologist may clear a program slot, enable/disable IntelliLink, and stimulate in live speech mode from a given program slot. Also, for bilateral recipients, the audiologist may confirm that the DuoPhone or Zoom-Control features are enabled for a given program by noting the presence of each feature's icon. Finally, the audiologist may "click" on the arrow to the left of the loudspeaker icon located immediately below the processor icon. This arrow opens another drop-down menu that allows the audiologist to adjust the settings of the internal alarm (e.g., whether internal

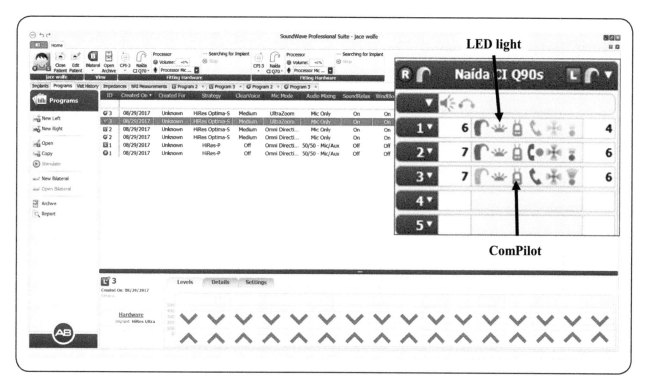

FIGURE 15–30. Adjustment of sound processor alerts, controls, and features. Image provided courtesy of Advanced Bionics, LLC.

alarm is enabled for various functions as well as the intensity and frequency of the alarm), and the audiologist may review a report of the estimated battery life (for a variety of different battery options) for each programming slot. The QuickSync feature (described earlier) may also be enabled in this menu for bilateral Naída users.

It should be noted that the audiologist may create progressive programs for the new recipient (i.e., a series of programs with progressively higher stimulation levels). Figure 15–31 provides an example of the progressive programs feature. When the "Create Progressive Programs" feature is used, four additional programs are automatically populated with progressively higher stimulation levels from the first program. The audiologist may select whether the M levels of each program globally increase by 5, 10, or 15 CU (current units).

Data Logging

The data logging feature provides the audiologist with valuable information about the recipient's usage patterns. As shown in Figure 15–32, the data logging report reveals the number of hours that the processor is used per day. It also breaks down the usage time into hours in which lock is obtained and hours in which lock is lost (e.g., the headpiece is not on the

head). It shows the hours per day that the processor is powered down. Furthermore, the data logging report indicates the programs the recipient uses, the types of environments in which the recipient resides, the frequency at which the recipient uses advanced features such as UltraZoom, DuoPhone, and so on, as well as usage patterns for the ComPilot, remote control, volume control, and program buttons. This data logging report is available for all Naída CI users. The audiologist should review this information at each programming session in an effort to ensure that the recipient (and his/her or family) is using the device appropriately (i.e., full-time use with children) and to assist in troubleshooting any recipient complaints.

Templates

A unique feature within the Advanced Bionics Sound-Wave programming software is the ability to create "**Templates**" that may be used to quickly retrieve a set of programming parameters that are likely to be appropriate for a given recipient. For instance, an "Adult" template could be created that would allow the audiologist to pull up a set of programming parameters that would be appropriate for the typical adult recipient (e.g., signal coding strategy, stimulation rate, pulse width, microphone mode, IDR, etc.; Figure 15–33). Templates may also be created to allow

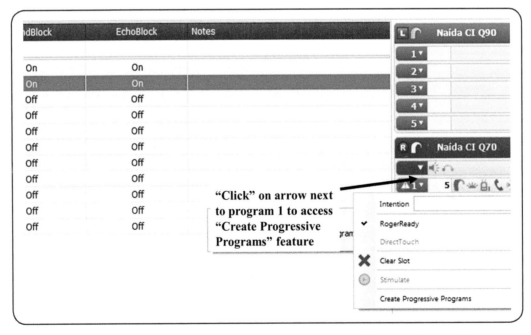

FIGURE 15–31. Creating progressive programs. Image provided courtesy of Advanced Bionics, LLC.

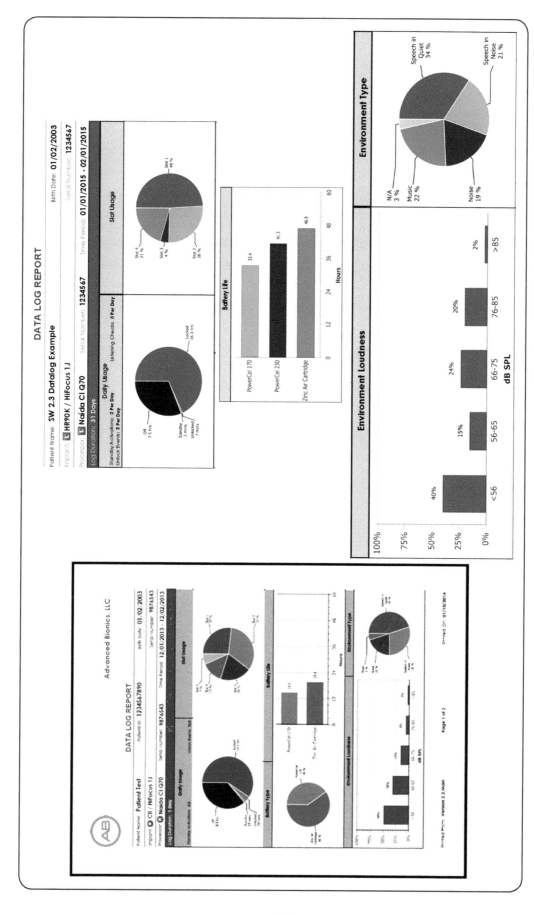

FIGURE 15–32. Data logging. Image provided courtesy of Advanced Bionics, LLC.

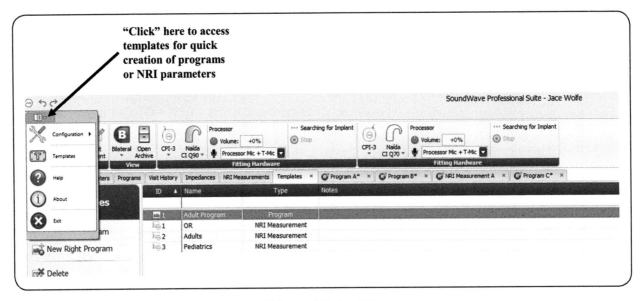

"Click" here to access templates for quick creation of programs or NRI parameters

FIGURE 15–33. Templates. Image provided courtesy of Advanced Bionics, LLC.

for quick access to the test parameters the audiologist prefers for Neural Response Imaging (NRI) assessment (e.g., electrodes that are evaluated, starting and ending levels).

Neural Response Imaging

NRI is the SoundWave platform used to measure the electrically evoked compound action potential. NRI is discussed further in Chapter 18.

Key Concepts

- Advanced Bionics cochlear implant systems may be programmed with use of SoundWave programming software.
- HiRes Optima S is the recommended signal coding strategy for new Advanced Bionics cochlear implant recipients, but a variety of signal coding strategies are available to meet the needs of individual recipients.
- The SoundWave programming software allows for control of a large number of parameters and signal processing technologies. The audiologist may adjust these parameters to optimize the listening needs of each individual recipient.

References

Advanced Bionics Corporation. (2003a). *New methodology for fitting cochlear implants.* Retrieved from https://www.advancedbionics.com/content/dam/advancedbionics/Documents/Regional/BR/New_Methodology_for_Fitting_Cochlear_Implants.pdf

Advanced Bionics Corporation. (2003b). *HiResolution sound processing.* Retrieved from https://www.advancedbionics.com/content/dam/advancedbionics/Documents/Global/en_ce/Professional/Technical-Reports/Sound-Processing/HiResolution_Sound_Processing_article.pdf

Advanced Bionics Corporation. (2009, March). *HiRes with Fidelity 120® clinical results.* Retrieved from http://www.advancedbionics.com/UserFiles/File/3-01009-A_HiRes120_Clinical%20Results%28Mar_05%29.pdf

Advanced Bionics. (2012). *HiRes Optima clinical results.* Valencia, CA: Author.

Advanced Bionics Corporation. (2003). *New methodology for fitting cochlear implants.* Retrieved from https://www.advancedbionics.com/content/dam/ab/Global/en_ce/documents/libraries/Professional%20Library/AB%20Technical%20Reports/Programming/New_Methodology_for_Fitting_Cochlear_Implants.pdf

Arora, K., Dawson. P., Dowell, R., & Vandali. A. (2009). Electrical stimulation rate effects on speech perception in cochlear implants. *International Journal of Audiology, 48*(8), 561–567.

Balkany, T., Hodges, A., Menapace, C., Hazard, L., Driscoll, C., Gantz, B., . . . Payne, S. (2007). Nucleus Freedom North American clinical trial. *Otolaryngology–Head and Neck Surgery, 136*(5), 757–762.

Baudhuin, J., Cadieux, J., Firszt, J. B., Reeder, R. M., & Maxson, J. L. (2012). Optimization of programming parameters in children with the advanced bionics cochlear implant. *Journal of the American Academy of Audiology, 23*(5), 302–312.

Buchner A., Frohne-Buchner, C., Battmer, R., & Lenarz, T. (2004) Two years of experience using stimulation rates between 800 and 5000 pps with the Clarion CI implant. *International Congress Series, 1273*, 48–51.

Büchner, A., Lenarz, T., Boermans, P. P., Frijns, J. H., Mancini, P., Filipo, R., ... Marco, J. (2012). Benefits of the HiRes 120 coding strategy combined with the Harmony processor in an adult European multicentre study. *Acta Otolaryngoloica, 132*(2), 179–187.

Buckler, L., & Overstreet, E. (2003). *Relationship between electrical stapedial reflex thresholds and Hi-Res program settings: Potential tool for pediatric cochlear-implant fitting.* Valencia, CA: Advanced Bionics.

Chang, Y. T., Yang, H. M., Lin, Y. H., Liu, S. H., & Wu, J. L. (2009). Tone discrimination and speech perception benefit in Mandarin-speaking children fit with HiRes fidelity 120 sound processing. *Otology and Neurotology, 30*(6), 750–757.

ClinicalTrials.gov. (2012). *ClinicalTrials.gov identifier: NCT010 66780.* Retrieved from https://clinicaltrials.gov/ct2/show/NCT01066780

Crukley, J., Scollie, S., & Parsa, V. (2011). An exploration of non-quiet listening at school. *Journal of Educational Audiology, 17*, 23–35.

Dunn , C., Tyler, R., Witt, S., & Gantz, B. (2006). Effects of converting bilateral cochlear implant subjects to a strategy with increased rate and number of channels. *Annals of Otology, Rhinology, and Laryngology, 115*(6), 425–432.

Gifford, R. H., & Revit, L. R. (2010). Speech perception for adult cochlear implant recipients a realistic background noise: Effectiveness of preprocessing strategies and external options for improving speech recognition in noise. *Journal of the American Academy of Audiology, 21*(7), 441–451.

Hehrmann, P., Fredelake, S., Hammacher, V., Dyballa, K. H., & Büchner, A. (2012). Improved speech intelligibility with cochlear implants using state-of-the-art noise reduction algorithms. *ITG-Fachbericht 236, Sprachkommunikation.* Braunschweig, Germany.

Holden, L. K., Reeder, R. M., Firszt, J. B., & Finley, C. C. (2011). Optimizing the perception of soft speech and speech in noise with the Advanced Bionics cochlear implant system. *International Journal of Audiology, 50*(4), 255–269.

Koch, D. B., Osberger, M. J., Segel, P., & Kessler, D. (2004). HiResolution and conventional sound processing in the HiResolution bionic ear: using appropriate outcome measures to assess speech recognition ability. *Audiology and Neurotology, 9*(4), 214–223.

Koch, D. B., Quick, A., Osberger M. J., Saoji, A., & Litvak, L. (2014). Enhanced hearing in noise for cochlear implant recipients: Clinical trial results for a commercially available speech-enhancement strategy. *Otology and Neurotology, 35*, 803–809.

Lee, E. R., Friedland, D. R., & Runge, C. L. (2012). Recovery from forward masking in elderly cochlear implant users. *Otology and Neurotology, 33*(3), 355–363.

Mancini, P., Bosco, E., D'Agosta, L., Traisci, G., Nicastri, M., Capelli, G., ... Filipo, R. (2009). Implementation of perceptual channels in children implanted with a HiRes 90K device. *Acta Otolaryngologica, 129*(12), 1442–1450.

Moore, B. C., & Glasberg, B. R. (1988). Gap detection with sinusoids and noise in normal, impaired, and electrically stimulated ears. *Journal of the Acoustical Society of America, 83*(3), 1093–1101.

Moore, B. C., Glasberg, B. R., & Stone, M. A. (1991). Optimization of a slow-acting automatic gain control system for use in hearing aids. *British Journal of Audiology, 25*(3), 171–182.

Pearsons, K. S. (1977). Effect of tone/noise combination on speech intelligibility. *Journal of the Acoustical Society of America, 61*(3), 884–886.

Pelosi, S., Rivas, A., Haynes, D. S., Bennett, M. L., Labadie, R. F., Hedley-Williams, A., & Wanna, G. B. (2012). Stimulation rate reduction and auditory development in poorly performing cochlear implant users with auditory neuropathy. *Otology and Neurotology, 33*(9), 1502–1506.

Spahr, A. J., Dorman, M. F., & Loiselle, L. H. (2007). Performance of patients using different cochlear implant systems: Effect of input dynamic range. *Ear and Hearing, 28*(2), 260–275.

Stone, M. A., Moore, B. C., Alcantara, J. I., & Glasberg, B. R. (1999). Comparison of different forms of compression using wearable digital hearing aids. *Journal of the Acoustical Society of America, 106*(6), 3603–3619.

Vandali, A., Whitford, L., Plant, K., & Clark, G. (2000). Speech perception as a function of electrical stimulation rate: Using the Nucleus 24 cochlear implant system. *Ear and Hearing, 21*, 608–624.

Verschuur, C. A. (2005). Effect of stimulation rate on speech perception in adult users of the Med-El CIS speech processing strategy. *International Journal of Audiology, 44*(1), 58–63.

Weber, B. P., Lai, W. K., Dillier, N., von Wallenberg, E. L., Killian, M. J., Pesch, J., ... Lenarz, T. (2007). Performance and preference for ACE stimulation rates obtained with Nucleus RP 8 and Freedom system. *Ear and Hearing, 28*(Suppl. 2), 46S–48S.

Wilson, B. (2006). Speech processing strategies. In H. R. Cooper & L. C. Craddock (Eds.), *Cochlear implants: A practical guide* (pp. 21–69). West Sussex, UK: Whurr.

Wolfe, J. (2014, December). *Benefit of bilateral hearing technology for understanding speech over the telephone.* Presented at the American Cochlear Implant Alliance Meeting, Nashville, Tennessee.

Wolfe, J., & Kasulis, H. (2008). Relationships among objective measures and speech perception in adult users of the HiResolution Bionic Ear. *Cochlear Implants International, 9*(2), 70–81.

Wolfe, J., Morais, M., Schafer, E., Agrawal, S., & Koch, D. (2015). Evaluation of speech recognition of cochlear implant recipients using adaptive, digital remote microphone technology and a speech enhancement sound processing algorithm. *Journal of the American Academy of Audiology, 26*(5), 502–508.

Wong, L. L., Vandali, A. E., Ciocca, V., Luk, B., Ip, V. W., Murray, B., ... Chung, I. (2008). New cochlear implant coding strategy for tonal language speakers. *International Journal of Audiology, 47*(6), 337–347.

Zhang, H., Runge-Samuelson, C., & Friedland, D. R. (2011). Effects of stimulation rate on speech perception in elderly cochlear implant users. *Laryngoscope, 121*(Suppl. 4), S199.

16

Programming Cochlear Nucleus Cochlear Implants

Jace Wolfe and Erin C. Schafer

Introduction to Programming Nucleus Cochlear Implants

This chapter will describe the principles, practices, and procedures pertaining to programming contemporary Nucleus cochlear implants.

Programming Nucleus Cochlear Implants

The primary programming platform for current Cochlear Nucleus sound processors is the **Custom Sound** software platform, which may be used to program all Nucleus sound processors, including the Nucleus 7, Nucleus 6, and Nucleus Kanso sound processors and all Nucleus cochlear implants described in Chapter 10. The following section describes programming of Cochlear Nucleus cochlear implants in the Custom Sound programming platform. The programming process will be described in the order in which the various steps are typically completed within the Custom Sound programming software.

Programming the Nucleus Sound Processors

The Nucleus 7, Nucleus 6, and Nucleus Kanso sound processors all possess several proprietary features that are potentially beneficial to the recipient. Fea-

tures of these processors include scene analysis with automatic adaptive directionality (SCAN), digital noise reduction (SNR-NR), wind noise reduction, data logging, and compatibility with a portfolio of proprietary wireless hearing assistance technologies (HATs). Additionally, the Nucleus 7 and 6 sound processors are equipped with an option to provide electroacoustic stimulation, the parameters of which are adjusted by the audiologist in the Custom Sound software. Moreover, the Nucleus 7 sound processor may be configured to work directly with Apple iPhones as well as in tandem with most contemporary GN ReSound hearing aids. Adjustments within Custom Sound, within the GN ReSound hearing aid fitting software, and within the recipient's iPhone are necessary to optimize performance of Nucleus 7 recipients who use iPhones and/or GN ReSound hearing aids on the non-implanted ear.

The hardware used to connect Nucleus processors to the computer (i.e., the programming pod and cable) is shown in Figure 16–1. Briefly, a programming interface, known as the **Cochlear Pod**, is connected to the sound processor with a specialized programming cable, and the pod is connected to the programming computer with a USB cable to a 2.0 or higher USB port. An array of programming cables are available to program the various Cochlear sound processors (Figure 16–2).

Cochlear also provides the **Cochlear Wireless Programming Pod**, which is an innovative and unique method to connect the programming computer to

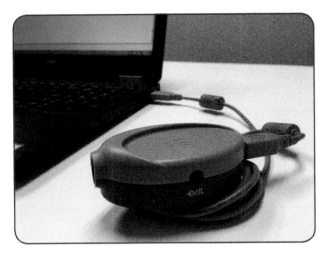

FIGURE 16–1. A visual example of the Cochlear Programming Pod. Image provided courtesy of Cochlear Americas, ©2018.

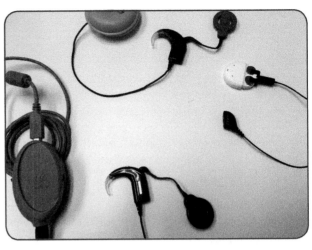

FIGURE 16–2. Cochlear programming cables. Image provided courtesy of Cochlear Americas, ©2018.

the sound processor via a wireless Bluetooth digital radio connection. As shown in Figure 16–3, the Cochlear Wireless Programming Pod is available in several configurations. For ear-level processors, the Wireless Programming Pod is connected to the base of the sound processor and to a Cochlear rechargeable battery. Because the connector of the Nucleus 7 sound processor is different from the Nucleus 5 and 6 sound processors, one Wireless Pod is available for the Nucleus 7 and a different Wireless Pod is available for the Nucleus 5 and 6 processors. Additionally, a short Kanso cable may be connected to the Nucleus 5/6 Wireless Pod along with a rechargeable battery connected to the base of the Pod to allow for quasi-wireless programming of the Kanso. The Wireless Pod contains an LED light to indicate connection to the computer and battery status. A Standard rechargeable battery will provide up to 4 hours of use of the Wireless Pod, whereas a Compact battery will provide up to 2.5 hours. The Wireless Programming Pod possesses a range of up to 9.8 feet (approximately 3 meters). Cochlear provides a Bluetooth transmitter that may be plugged into a 2.0 or higher USB port of the programming computer in order to wirelessly transmit data to and from the sound processor. Once the transmitter is connected, a Cochlear rechargeable battery must be connected to the Wireless Programming Pod to pair the Pod to the transmitter. If pairing does not occur, the audiologist may go into the settings menu of the computer and initiate the pairing process. Of note, it may be helpful to close Custom Sound software during the pairing process. Once the conventional Pod or Wireless Programming Pod is

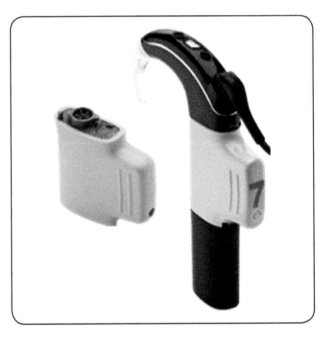

FIGURE 16–3. Cochlear wireless programming interface. Image provided courtesy of Cochlear Americas, ©2018.

connected to the computer, an icon of the particular programming Pod will appear in the ribbon bar at the bottom left side of the Custom Sound screen.

Creating a Recipient File

Prior to creating a program, the audiologist must create a file for the recipient and identify the implant(s) the recipient has received. In the Custom Sound software, this is accomplished by selecting the "Create" function on the right side of the "Recipient" "start-up" page (Figure 16–4). The recipient's first and last names, his/her date of birth, the type of implant the recipient has received, and the ear that has been implanted must be entered into the "Recipient Details" menu. Additional demographic information may also be entered as the audiologist desires. The audiologist must select the "Add" button in the "Recipient Details" menu to enter the implant the recipient has received. A pop-up menu is provided, and from this menu, the audiologist must enter the recipient implant model(s) and the ear(s) that was implanted (Figure 16–5).

Programming Process

In the Cochlear Custom Sound software, the basic programming process is essentially divided into four categories (Figure 16–6): (1) Measure Impedances, (2) Open or Create MAP, (3) Set Levels, and (4) Write to Processor. The audiologist may choose to incorporate other steps into the process as needed. Bilateral Balance should be used with bilateral cochlear implant recipients. Additional steps include: Per-

form Neural Response Telemetry (NRT) and Finalize Programming. The following description of programming Cochlear devices will be organized to correspond with the aforementioned categories. Of note, before programming can begin, the audiologist must indicate the connected processor(s) being programmed for a given ear. Designating the processor for programming with a particular ear is accomplished by clicking on the arrow in the right or left ear tab to access a drop-down menu which contains the processor(s) that are connected to the computer along with the serial number(s). The audiologist simply selects a processor to be programmed with the ear associated with the tab (Figure 16–7).

Measure Impedances

The first step involved in programming in Custom Sound is to measure electrode impedance in four different electrode coupling modes. Electrode impedances are measured by simply selecting the "Measure" button within the "Measure Impedance" platform (Figure 16–8). The results of the measurement are promptly displayed in the illustration of the electrode array and reference electrodes by depicting impedances falling within the normal range in a green color and any abnormal findings in a red color (Figure 16–9).

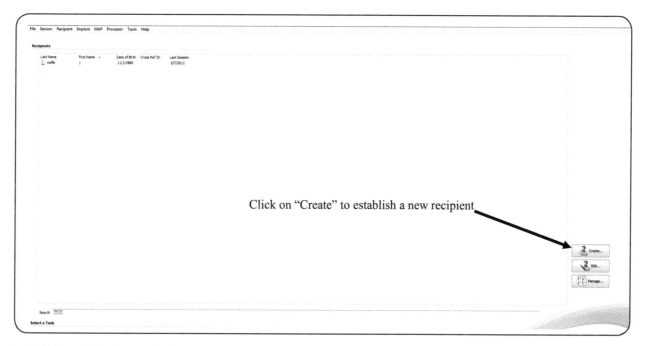

FIGURE 16–4. A visual example of the process of creating a new patient in Custom Sound. Image provided courtesy of Cochlear Americas, ©2018.

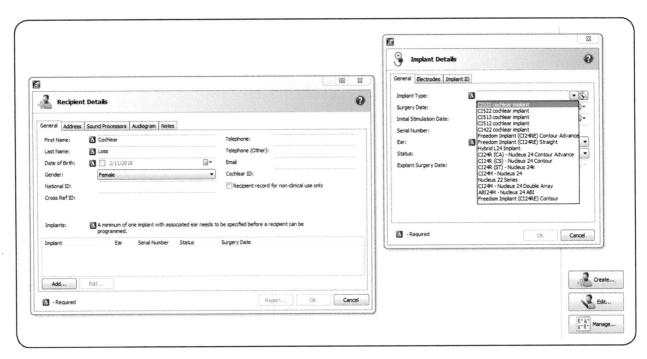

FIGURE 16–5. A visual example of the process of entering new patient information and cochlear implant information in Custom Sound. Image provided courtesy of Cochlear Americas, ©2018.

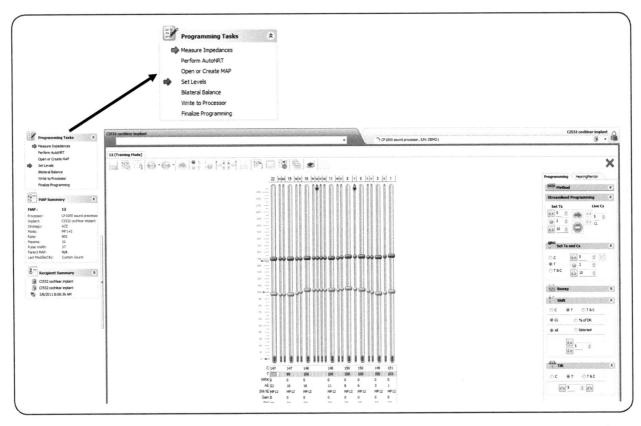

FIGURE 16–6. A visual example of the "Programming Tasks" menu in Custom Sound. Image provided courtesy of Cochlear Americas, ©2018.

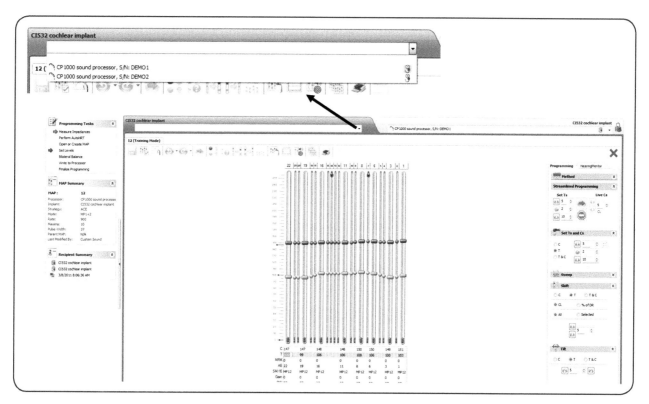

FIGURE 16–7. Selecting sound processor to program in Custom Sound. Image provided courtesy of Cochlear Americas, ©2018.

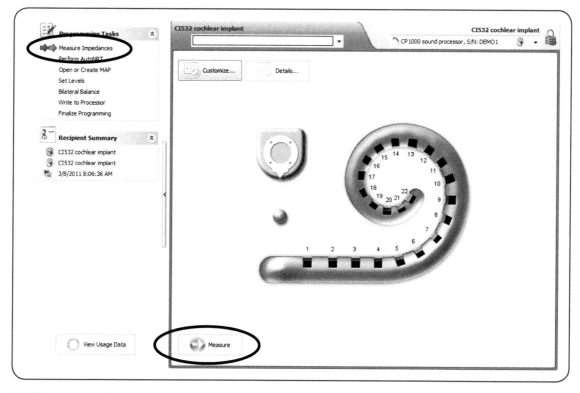

FIGURE 16–8. Impedance measurement in Custom Sound. Image provided courtesy of Cochlear Americas, ©2018.

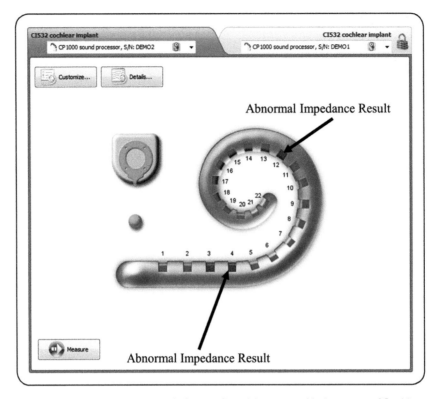

FIGURE 16–9. Impedance results in Custom Sound. Image provided courtesy of Cochlear Americas, ©2018.

The audiologist should select the "Details" button to review the electrode impedances in graphical and tabular form (Figure 16–10).

In each electrode coupling mode, a low-level electrical current (100 CL with a pulse width of 25 μsec), which is inaudible for many but not all recipients, is delivered sequentially to each intracochlear electrode contact. The impedance (in kOhms) is measured across the entire circuit as the current travels from the current source to the intracochlear electrode contact and finally to one or more reference electrodes.

Impedance is first measured in the common ground mode where the low-level current is delivered sequentially to each intracochlear electrode contact. Each of the remaining intracochlear contacts simultaneously serves as the return path. Because the common ground mode electrically couples each intracochlear electrode contact to the remaining intracochlear electrode contacts within the array, it is the most sensitive mode for detecting shorted electrode contacts. As a result, common ground is the preferred electrode coupling mode to detect anomalous intracochlear electrodes.

The Monopolar 1 and Monopolar 2 coupling modes measure electrode impedance by sequentially delivering the low-level current to each intracochlear electrode contact and by evaluating the impedance in the circuit from the current source to each intracochlear electrode and extracochlear reference electrode. Measuring electrode impedance in the Monopolar 1 and Monopolar 2 modes allows the audiologist to identify the status of the extracochlear reference electrodes (located on the end of the non-stimulating electrode lead and the implant case, respectively).

In the fourth mode, Monopolar 1+2, each intracochlear electrode is referenced to both the remote and case reference electrodes. In other words, the measure is completed by evaluating the impedance that exists in the circuit from the current source to each intracochlear electrode contact and finally to the reference, which comprises MP1 and MP2, which are electrically coupled to one another. The Monopolar 1+2 (MP1+2) mode is the default mode used for stimulation in the primary signal coding strategy used with Cochlear devices and the Advanced Combination Encoder (ACE) signal coding strategy (also in

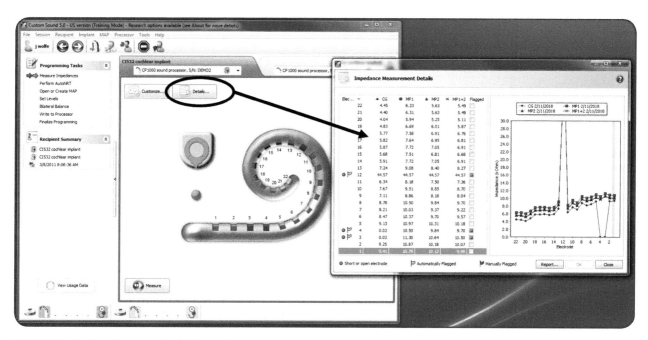

FIGURE 16–10. Impedance results in Custom Sound. Image provided courtesy of Cochlear Americas, ©2018.

the Continuous Interleaved Sampling [CIS] and Spectral-Peak [SPEAK] strategies). As a result, impedance measured in the MP1+2 mode closely reflects the typical impedance present during stimulation when the implant is used on a daily basis.

Cochlear considers electrode impedances below 565 ohms to be abnormally low and designates these electrode contacts as being part of "short" circuits, while electrode impedances greater than 30 kOhms for half-band electrode contacts are abnormally high and are referred to as "open" circuits. It should be noted that the open circuit limit for the electrode array with full-band electrode contacts (e.g., Nucleus Straight Array, Nucleus Double Array) is 20 kOhms. Electrodes with abnormal impedances are typically "flagged" and deactivated for programming and subsequent impedance assessments. In the "Measure Impedance" module, "flagged" electrodes are depicted in yellow for all subsequent impedance measurements. Flagged electrodes are also "grayed out" (disabled) in the programming/"Set Levels" module of Custom Sound (Figure 16–11).

At initial activation, impedance is frequently high but will generally decrease with routine implant use. Therefore, the audiologist should reassess the impedance of electrodes with abnormally high electrode impedance to determine whether impedance decreases to normal levels after stimulation of the electrodes. However, shorted electrodes will typi-

cally always remain as shorted electrodes and should be permanently disabled once they are identified. It should be reiterated that shorted electrodes are identified not only by their abnormally low impedance (i.e., less than 565 ohms) but also because the common ground mode allows for detection of two or more intracochlear electrodes that are electrically connected to one another.

For situations in which an electrode initially had abnormal impedance prior to stimulation and was subsequently flagged, the audiologist may re-activate the flagged electrode by accessing the "Recipient" tab at the top of the Custom Sound programming software and then selecting the "Edit" option within the "Recipient" tab. Then, the audiologist must highlight the implant of the affected ear, select the "Edit" option in the "Recipient Details" menu, and then select the "Electrodes" tab. From there, the audiologist may remove the "flag" from the electrode with an abnormal impedance value (Figure 16–12). Completing this series of steps will allow for reassessment and a subsequent determination of the integrity of a suspect electrode contact.

It should be noted that some researchers of Nucleus implants reported absolute impedance values that are within the aforementioned normal values but impedance results that nonetheless are atypical/abnormal and representative of a fault within the implant. Specifically, Zwolan et al. (2012) reported on

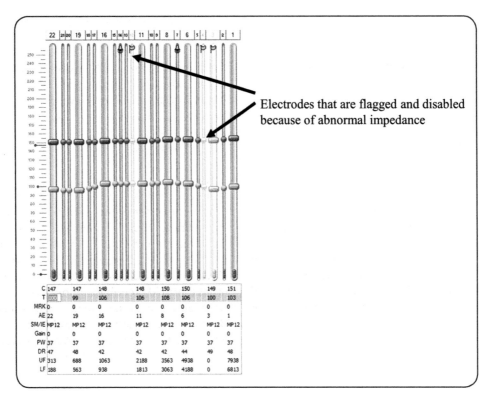

FIGURE 16–11. Flagged electrodes based on impedance results. Image provided courtesy of Cochlear Americas, ©2018.

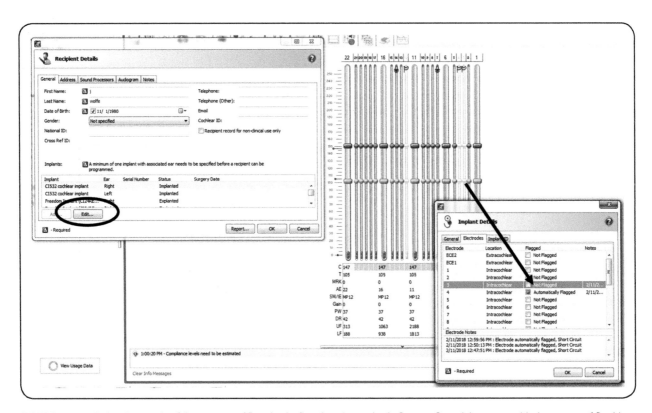

FIGURE 16–12. A visual example of the process of flagging/unflagging electrodes in Custom Sound. Image provided courtesy of Cochlear Americas, ©2018.

a retrospective review that they conducted with 635 recipients of Nucleus CI24R and CI24RE implants to inspect recipient performance and impedance data over the life of each recipient's implant use. They focused on electrode impedance results they defined as "atypical," which referred to results which were technically within normal limits but possessed findings that were uncharacteristic of a normal impedance assessment. The authors reported on the incidence of two types of atypical electrode impedance patterns found within Nucleus CI24R (Contour) and CI24RE (Freedom) implant recipients: (1) Zig-zag (sawtooth) defined as significantly decreased impedance on three or more all even or all odd numbered electrodes and (2) Low-flat defined as significantly decreased average impedance and impedance range on five or more successive electrodes.

More specifically, an atypical zig-zag pattern was defined as an impedance finding in which the graphed result possesses a sawtooth appearance, with a minimum of three "spikes" which are all found on either even-numbered or odd-numbered electrodes (Figure 16–13). Further, the electrode possessing the lower-value "spikes" must have impedance results that are at least 1.5 kOhms lower than both of their neighboring electrodes. The "spikes" must all fall on either even-numbered or odd-numbered electrodes. Zwolan et al. (2012) attributed the zig-zag pattern to a breach of the silicone insulation that covers the case

of the implant. All of the even-numbered electrode contacts are wired to one side of the implant case, while all of the odd-numbered electrode contacts are wired to the opposite side of the case. If a tear occurs on one side of the case, then body fluid ingress into that tear will potentially create a conduit for current to spread across either the even-numbered or odd-numbered electrode leads, depending on which side of the case the breach occurs. This type of fault is occasionally referred to as partial shorting.

A variety of management strategies exist for recipients who present with a zig-zag impedance finding. First, all of the electrodes with lower-numbered spike values may be disabled. When possible, the recipient may provide feedback about potential change or improvement in sound quality, and speech recognition may be evaluated to examine for improvement. Second, if the recipient notices degradation or no change in sound quality when suspect electrodes are disabled, and sound quality and speech recognition are both satisfactory, then all electrodes may remain enabled. In this case, the recipient's progress should be followed closely. Third, if the aforementioned strategies are unsuccessful, then the implant may be replaced.

According to Zwolan and colleagues (2012), a flat-low finding is defined by a number of specific characteristics. First, a flat-low finding must be determined by comparing the most recent impedance values and

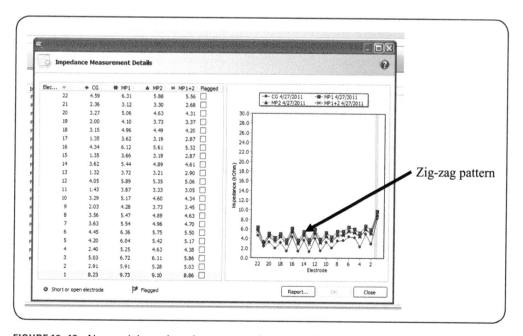

FIGURE 16–13. Abnormal zig-zag impedance pattern. Image provided courtesy of Cochlear Americas, ©2018.

a "baseline" measurement obtained at least 60 days after surgery. In order to meet the criteria to be classified as "flat-low" finding, at least five electrodes must be affected. The average impedance and impedance range of the group of low impedance electrodes must both decrease by at least 30% between the "baseline" and "current" values (see Figure 16–14 for an example).

For instance, in a "flat-low" impedance finding, impedances can decrease to approximately one-half of the value of the impedances measured a few months post-activation. A flat-low impedance finding may result from a tear in the insulation in the middle of the case, which would allow body fluid ingress to spread to even-numbered and odd-numbered electrode contacts. If sound quality and recipient performance are satisfactory in the presence of a low-flat finding, the recipient's progress should be followed closely over time. If performance is poorer than one would expect or if sound quality deteriorates over time, implant replacement should be considered.

Open or Create MAP

The next step involved in programming in Custom Sound is to select the signal coding strategy, stimulation rate, maxima, and other processing parameters. This is accomplished by selecting the "Open or Create MAP" module (Figure 16–15). The audiologist may select from a number of different parameters, including several signal coding strategies, electrode coupling modes, stimulation rates (pulses per second per channel), **maxima**, and pulse width. The ACE signal coding strategy is recommended initially because previous clinical trials show that it provides superior performance over CIS and SPEAK strategies (Beynon, Snik, & van den Broek, 2003; Manrique et al., 2005; Skinner et al., 2002). Moreover, previous research suggests that most subjects have optimal speech recognition performance when using a stimulation rate of 900 pps (see below for details pertaining to a study examining performance as a function of stimulation rate for Cochlear users) and at least 9 maxima (Balkany et al., 2007; Dorman, Loizou, Spahr, & Maloff, 2002). The author of this book recommends beginning with 10 maxima to provide sufficient detail for a speech signal embedded in competing noise and, with that number of maxima, a pulse width of 37 microseconds, which is the widest pulse width that still allows for a 900 pps stimulation rate. Of note, the default pulse width for ACE MAPs is 25 microseconds for cochlear implants with perimodiolar electrode

arrays and 37 microseconds for implants with lateral wall electrode arrays. The author recommends the 37 microsecond pulse width for all recipients over the software default pulse width of 25 microseconds, because a wider pulse width requires less current level for a given psychophysical percept, which reduces the likelihood that voltage compliance limits will be encountered. Additionally, the wider pulse width with lower current level may reduce the potential for deleterious channel interaction or non-auditory side effects (e.g., facial nerve stimulation). Along the same line of thinking, it may be useful to select a 50-microsecond pulse width for recipients who have lateral wall electrode arrays and who have stimulation levels that approach voltage compliance limits.

Additional Information on Stimulation Rate for Cochlear Recipients

The author of this book recommends the default stimulation of 900 pps for most Nucleus recipients. The overwhelming majority of nucleus recipients will perform very well with a 900 pps stimulation. However, some recipients may benefit from an adjustment to the stimulation rate. Balkany et al. (2007) reported on a study that was conducted to examine the preferred stimulation rate for 55 Nucleus Freedom recipients. Subjective preference and speech recognition were evaluated for six different stimulation rates (500, 900, 1200, 1800, 2400, and 3500 pps). Sixty-seven percent of the subjects preferred a stimulation rate of 1200 pps or lower, with most subjects preferring rates of 900 or 500 pps. Only 9 percent of subjects preferred stimulation rates higher than 1800 pps. Additionally, speech recognition did not improve with faster stimulation rates. The study authors concluded that most Nucleus Freedom recipients preferred slower stimulation rates (i.e., 900 pps or lower), and there was considerable variability in the ideal stimulation rate selected across subjects. In short, this study has several clinical implications. First, Nucleus recipients tend to perform better with moderate to low stimulation rates (e.g., 250 to 1200 pps). Second, the results of this study largely support the use of the default stimulation rate for Nucleus implants (e.g., 900 pps). Third, some recipients do perform better at alternative stimulation rates, and as a result, it may be worthwhile to consider stimulation rates other than 900 pps (i.e., default stimulation rate) for recipients who are struggling to adapt to the signal from their implant after several weeks of use. Of note, a slower stimulation rate may be particularly

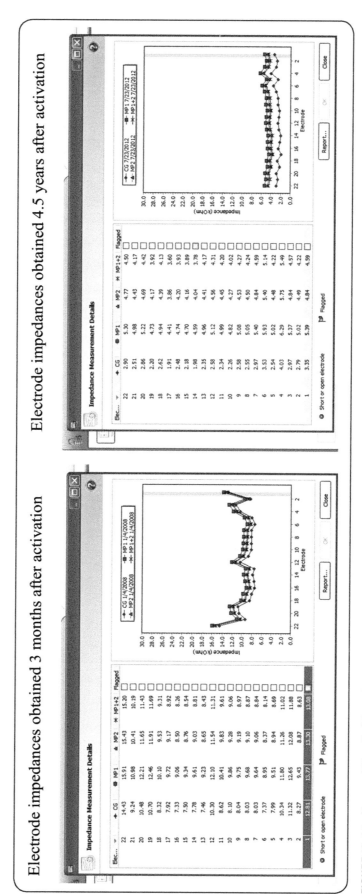

FIGURE 16–14. Abnormal "low flat" impedance pattern. Image provided courtesy of Cochlear Americas, ©2018.

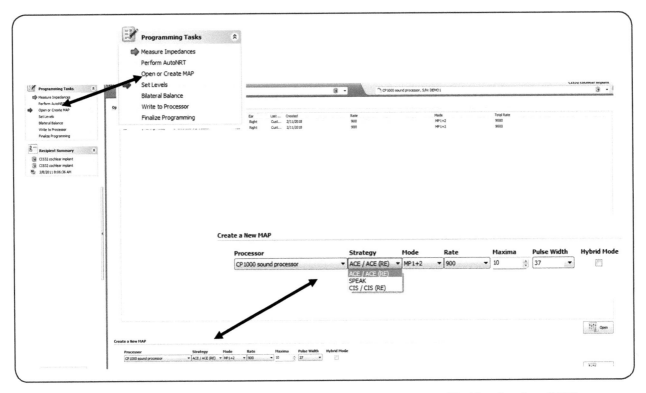

FIGURE 16–15. Selecting signal coding strategy in Custom Sound. Image provided courtesy of Cochlear Americas, ©2018.

useful for recipients who have evidence of neural dysfunction (e.g., auditory neuropathy spectrum disorder, cochlear nerve deficiency, multiple sclerosis, neural adaptation). Also, slower stimulation rates may be especially helpful for very elderly persons who are struggling with the default stimulation rate and for persons who have a lengthy duration of deafness (i.e., greater than 20 years).

Considerations for Additional Adjustments to Default Parameters

Once a MAP is created, the audiologist will have access to a substantial number of parameters in the "Set Levels" screen. The authors of this book often make adjustments to a couple of additional default parameters. Skinner, Holden, and Holden (1994, 1997) have shown that narrow frequency allocation in the mid-frequency channels results in better speech recognition. With that in mind, the authors also recommend setting the frequency allocation table's upper boundary out to approximately 8000 Hz for children but to approximately 7000 Hz for adults. The wider bandwidth is recommended for children because research has suggested that young children require an extended high-frequency response to adequately understand speech, especially when spoken by women and other children (Stelmachowicz, Pittman, Hoover, & Lewis, 2001).

Furthermore, for newly activated recipients, the authors recommend switching the volume control range from the default setting of 20% to 100%. The wider volume control range allows new recipients to select a minimal amount of stimulation, which the user may appreciate during the early acclimatization period of implant use, particularly when placing the coil on the head after a period of non-use (i.e., placing the coil on the head after awakening in the morning). A moderate volume control range (e.g., 30%–40%) is selected for most experienced implant users. A more detailed discussion on the effect of the volume control parameter is provided later in this chapter.

The authors recommend leaving all other processing parameters at the default settings for the initial program. If the recipient is not making satisfactory progress after approximately one month of implant use, then the audiologist may try alternative signal coding strategies or stimulation rates. It should, however, be noted that most recipients will experience satisfactory outcomes when the signal coding parameters are set to the default settings. Additional parameters for adjustment are discussed later in this chapter, but the reader should keep in mind that in many cases, adjustments to these parameters are not absolutely necessary. Again, the provision of appropriate T and C levels is the most important factor that influences recipient success.

Setting Stimulation Levels

The majority of the work (in terms of both time consumption and importance) involved in creating a program for a recipient is accomplished in the "Set Levels" module (Figure 16–16). This is where stimulation levels are set and where a number of programming parameters may be adjusted. When creating a new program in the Custom Sound fitting platform, five channels (22, 16, 11, 6, and 1) are highlighted for measurement. The streamlined approach to programming suggests that the audiologist measure stimulation levels on these five channels and interpolate the remaining values. As mentioned in Chapter 7, interpolation is only appropriate when using stimulation delivered via monopolar electrode coupling. This

procedure is supported by research, which shows equivalent performance for programs created with the streamlined and conventional approaches (Plant et al., 2005). However, to detect any potential variation across the array, the authors of this textbook also recommend measuring stimulation levels on at least one channel between each of these five highlighted channels as well as on channels 2, 3, and 4. Furthermore, if more than a 10 current level (CL) difference exists between the most closely spaced measured channels, then the authors recommend measuring a channel between the two channels in which the relatively large difference exists for T level.

It should be noted that the unit of stimulation in the Custom Sound software platform is referred to as a **current level (CL)** or clinical unit. The abbreviation "CL" will be used for the remainder of this chapter. The CL represents the product of the current amplitude and pulse width of the programming stimulus. The programming stimulus is a train of biphasic, rectangular pulses presented at a particular stimulation rate (e.g., default stimulation rate of 900 pulses per second). Stimulation level changes occur logarithmically and range from 0 CL (an amplitude of

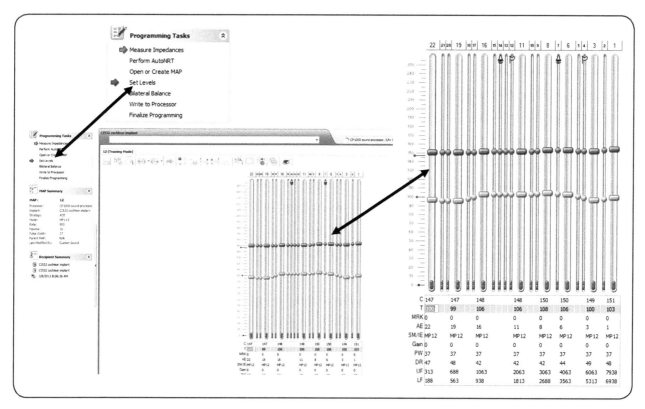

FIGURE 16–16. Selecting stimulation levels in Custom Sound. Image provided courtesy of Cochlear Americas, ©2018.

0 microamperes/phase) to 255 CL (an amplitude of 1.75 milliamperes/phase) at a given pulse width. The pulse width may vary from 9 to 400 microseconds/phase. Of note, the logarithmic growth of stimulus level in the Custom Sound programming platform results in relatively rapid loudness growth compared with the linear growth in stimulus levels present in the Advanced Bionics SoundWave software. As a result, the electrical dynamic range of Nucleus recipients is often narrower than that of Advanced Bionics recipients.

At appointments that follow the activation session, the audiologist should attempt to measure stimulation levels across a variety of channels so that, by one month of implant use, measurements are made on every channel at least one time. This action allows the audiologist to determine any channels that may possess particularly unusual levels. Alternatively, the audiologist may measure stimulation levels on the same subset of channels at each session and then balance loudness at C level across the electrode array and sweep at T level across the array to ensure comfort, a satisfactory auditory percept, and audibility across all channels. The latter approach may not be feasible with young children, but it achieves the objective of identifying anomalous channels for older children and adult users. It should be noted that measured channels should be highlighted, so the audiologist knows the channels on which T and C levels have been obtained. Highlighting measured channels is achieved by "clicking" (single click) on the channel or selecting "v" on the keyboard while the channel is being measured. A highlighted channel is represented by a yellow square (rather than white) encompassing the channel number (Figure 16–17).

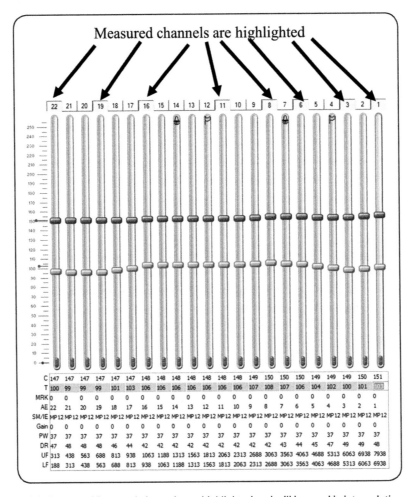

FIGURE 16–17. Measured channels are highlighted and will be used in interpolation if stimulation levels of all electrodes are not measured. Image provided courtesy of Cochlear Americas, ©2018.

As previously mentioned, the measurement of accurate T and C levels is crucial in providing a high-quality program. For the Nucleus cochlear implants, the T level is the lowest level of stimulation that the user can detect 100% of the time. At default settings, single-channel T- and C-level measurements are made with the presentation of a train of biphasic pulses with a stimulation rate of 900 pps and an on/off duty cycle of 500 msec. Recipients typically perceive these stimuli as similar to pure tones used during assessment of audiometric threshold. Typically, the authors present two trains of pulses each time the signal is presented (i.e., 500 msec on—500 msec off—500 msec on). However, for a recipient who is experiencing difficulty distinguishing the signal from his/her tinnitus, the authors may vary the number of pulse trains (usually between 1 and 5) that are presented and ask the recipient to count the number of "beeps" he/she hears. As previously mentioned, the "count-the-beeps" method allows the audiologist to determine whether the recipient is truly hearing the test signal, because he/she must report the correct number of pulse trains presented in order to indicate audibility.

Appropriate alternatives for measuring T levels are discussed in detail in Chapter 14 and 23, but typically the author of this book uses a "clinical-bracketing" (i.e., Hughson–Westlake [Carhart & Jerger, 1959]) approach with two stimulus presentations at each CL. At initial stimulation, a 5 CL ascending step-size and a 10 CL descending step-size is used. For experienced adults and attentive children, ascending and descending step-sizes may be set to 2 and 4 CL, respectively. Furthermore, small step-sizes should generally be used for all recipients who have narrow dynamic ranges (e.g., less than 15 CL).

Setting stimulation levels for Cochlear recipients differs from the default procedures used to determine stimulation levels for Advanced Bionics and MED-EL recipients. Measurement of T levels is an essential aspect of programming Nucleus implants, whereas default practice calls for the estimation of T level for Advanced Bionics and MED-EL recipients. When T levels are set too high, the user may complain of ongoing noise. This noise may arise from two sources. First, if T levels are set too high, the recipient may perceive a constant "buzzing" or "humming" sound secondary to suprathreshold low-level electrical stimulation. This is an unwanted percept, and the audiologist should attempt to eliminate it by decreasing T levels. Second, this noise may arise from the perception of ambient noise that normal-hearing persons hear every day but

that newly implanted persons may not have heard for quite some time (i.e., perception of ambient noise ranging from 25 to 50 dB SPL, such as the room's ventilation system or the fan on a computer). This percept is actually quite typical and intended, and the audiologist should encourage the recipient to attempt to acclimate to the low-level sound(s).

For many recipients, it is difficult to determine if the constant, low-level noise they are perceiving is attributed to excessive T-level stimulation or to audibility for low-level ambient sounds. One way to determine the culprit is to take the recipient inside a sound-treated audiometric test booth to see whether he/she is able to detect the sound. If the sound is eliminated, then it is likely the recipient was hearing low-level room noise, and he/she should be counseled to acclimate. It is worth mentioning that a constant noise secondary to excessively high T levels is possible with Nucleus recipients, but the use of the ACE (*n*-of-*m*) signal coding strategy does reduce the likelihood of this becoming a significant problem as might occur with CIS-based signal coding strategies.

Of course, it should be noted that the audiologist should evaluate warble tone thresholds once a stable program is established, with the goal of aided sound-field thresholds falling between 15 and 30 dB HL. Children should have warble tone soundfield thresholds no greater than 25 dB HL, whereas adults should have warble tone sound-field detection thresholds of no greater than 30 dB HL. If sound-field thresholds are substantially better than 15 dB HL, it may be prudent to consider slightly decreasing T-level stimulation. If soundfield detection thresholds are poorer than the aforementioned goals, then the audiologist should re-measure T levels with the goal of increasing T level on the same channels that correspond to the frequencies at which sound-field thresholds were elevated.

The upper stimulation levels, C levels, should be perceived by the user as "loud but comfortable." Approaches to measuring C levels are discussed in Chapters 14 and 23, but briefly, C levels may be set using a variety of techniques. When activating adult recipients, the authors of this text typically increase C levels globally from the T-level measurements in live speech mode (e.g., the processor microphone is activated so the recipient is able to hear speech and ambient environmental sounds) until the recipient reports that an optimal loudness and sound quality have been achieved. Then, loudness balancing is conducted two channels at a time across the array to ensure that loudness is equalized from channel to channel. The provision of equal loudness across channels typically optimizes sound quality and speech recognition.

After loudness balancing is completed, the C-level profile (e.g., shape across the array) is usually flatter than the T-level profile. In fact, as a general rule for Cochlear recipients, the C-level profile is usually flatter with less variation across the array than the T-level profile. After balancing is completed, the authors will once again adjust C levels globally (in 1–2 clinical-unit steps) in the live speech mode until the subject reports that loudness and sound quality are optimal. It is important to note that the authors typically will increase C levels to a point that just exceeds the recipient's most comfortable listening level in live speech mode or to a point that begins to degrade sound quality. Then, C levels are globally decreased back to an overall level that provides optimal listening comfort and sound quality. Increasing C levels to a level that just exceeds optimal comfort and sound quality allows the recipient to be certain that an optimal listening level and quality have been achieved.

For experienced recipients, the electrical dynamic range (range in CL between T level and C level) is typically from 20 to 60 CL, with most recipients possessing an electrical dynamic range around 40 to 50 CL (Botros, Banna, & Maruthurkkara, 2013). Some adult recipients who have a long duration of high-frequency hearing loss will have a narrower electrical dynamic range (15 to 30 CL) for high-frequency electrodes. The audiologist should be leery of electrodes for which the electrical dynamic range is significantly different from the typical range of 20 to 60 CL. Although the authors provide clinical services for recipients who have electrical dynamic ranges approaching 70 to 80 CL who achieve excellent performance with their cochlear implant, these cases are certainly the exception. The audiologist should be especially guarded against electrical dynamic ranges that are wider than normal in children, as studies have suggested that audiologists may be more apt to provide too much stimulation for children relative to adults (Zwolan & Overstreet, 2005).

Likewise, the audiologist should be concerned when the electrical dynamic range is very narrow (e.g., less than 20 CL), particularly when it is narrow across the array. In these cases, it may be prudent to attempt to gradually increase the electrical dynamic range over an extended period of time (i.e., increase the electrical dynamic range by 2 to 3 CL every four to six weeks over a six-month period). Of course, some recipients may not be able to tolerate this type of increase, even when the audiologist attempts to

provide it gradually across time. In these cases, the audiologist should avoid providing a signal that is uncomfortable. Regardless of the electrical dynamic range, the audiologist should gather outcome measurement data to ensure that a recipient's program is appropriate. Outcome measurements should include word recognition, sentence recognition in quiet and in noise, soundfield warble tone thresholds, and an assessment of subjective benefit/performance for recipients who can complete these measures. For younger children, outcome measures should include subjective questionnaires completed by caregivers (e.g., LittlEars, PEACH) as well as informal and formal assessment of speech, language, and auditory skill development by the child's Listening and Spoken Language Specialist or speech-language pathologist. Concern pertaining to deviant stimulation levels and/or an electrical dynamic range is heightened when outcome measurements suggest poor performance and progress.

Given the aforementioned discussion of stimulation levels and electrical dynamic range, it is helpful to administer a measure that serves as an objective guide to where C level should be set. The electrically evoked stapedial reflex threshold (ESRT) has been shown to correlate strongly to C level (Brickley et al.; Hodges et al., 1997; Lorens, Walkowiak, Piotrowska, Skarzynski, & Anderson, 2004). The use of ESRT as a guide to setting stimulation levels of Nucleus recipients will be discussed in Chapter 18. In short, the authors routinely use the ESRT to estimate and/or evaluate the appropriateness of C levels of Nucleus recipients.

Although the aforementioned techniques are the authors' preferred strategies to set C levels, other methods do exist. The audiologist may use psychophysical loudness scaling to set C levels to a "loud but comfortable" percept in several channels across the electrode array. The C levels for unmeasured channels are interpolated based on measured values. Then, C levels are decreased and the program is activated in live speech mode. Next, the audiologist globally increases C levels to the recipient's most comfortable listening level while in live speech mode.

The reader should remember that increases in stimulation in the Custom Sound software occur in a logarithmic fashion and may cause relatively large increases in loudness growth with small changes to C levels, particularly as stimulation levels approach the recipient's upper level of loudness comfort. While making global adjustments in live speech mode, small increases (e.g., 1–2 CL) may result in fairly large changes in loudness, clarity, and sound quality. As a result, it is important to make global adjustments in precise steps. Finally, the stimulation levels the recipient experiences while in live speech mode or while in everyday use are influenced by the volume control. The effect of the volume control parameter is discussed in detail in a later section of this chapter. The reader should pay special attention to the influence of the volume control on stimulation level.

Parameters That Influence How Acoustic Inputs Are MAPped into the Recipient's Electrical Dynamic Range

The previous section described how upper stimulation levels should be set for users of Cochlear Nucleus implants. In summary, T levels represent the lowest level of electrical stimulation the recipient can detect for each channel, and C levels represent the level of electrical stimulation at each channel that is loud but comfortable to the recipient. Collectively, the T and C levels define the user's electrical dynamic range (EDR). As previously discussed, a significant challenge facing engineers and designers of cochlear implants is the task of delivering a wide range of acoustic inputs (e.g., from whisper soft sounds of 20 dB SPL to very loud sounds of around 100 dB SPL and higher)

into the recipient's relatively narrow EDR (typically around 20 dB). The following section describes several parameters within the Cochlear Custom Sound programming platform that influence how a wide range of desirable acoustic inputs are delivered to an appropriate location within the narrow range of a recipient's electrical dynamic range. These parameters are all interrelated, so it is somewhat difficult to explain the effect that a given parameter has on the sound a recipient receives without having a thorough understanding of each of the other parameters. As a result, it may be necessary for the reader to review the following section more than once to acquire a full understanding of the influence of each parameter on the recipient's listening experience as well as how each parameter is interconnected in the sound processing of Cochlear sound processors. Of note, most of the following programming parameters may be adjusted in the "Parameters" tab, which is located in the "Set Levels" module (Figure 16–18).

IDR, IIDR, T-SPL, C-SPL, AGC, Sensitivity, and Autosensitivity Control

The input dynamic range (IDR) is not actually a programmable parameter found in the Custom Sound

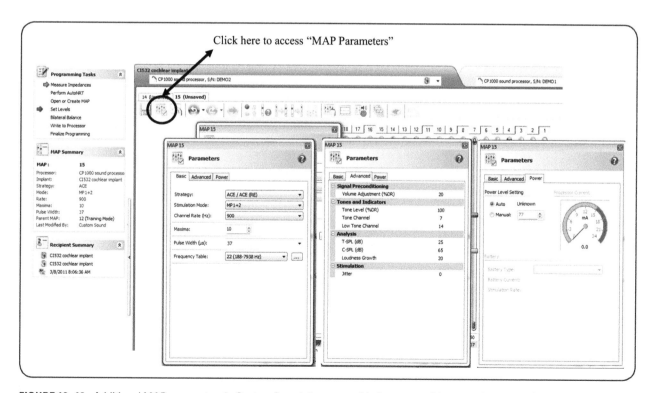

FIGURE 16–18. Additional MAP parameters in Custom Sound. Image provided courtesy of Cochlear Americas, ©2018.

programming software, but it is imperative to define it here and distinguish it from another parameter, the **instantaneous input dynamic range (IIDR)**, which is an important parameter within Custom Sound. Cochlear considers the IDR to refer to the maximum range of acoustic inputs that may be electronically captured by the sound processor without clipping or significant distortion. By this definition, the low end of the IDR for broadband sounds is determined by the noise floor of the microphone and is approximately 23 dB SPL. The upper end of the IDR may be determined by the limits of the A/D converter (i.e., the number of bits of the digital signal processor [DSP]). The upper range of the IDR of the Nucleus 7 sound processor is just over 100 dB SPL for broadband inputs, which results in an overall IDR of approximately 80 dB. It should be noted that the lower end of the IDR is actually lower for narrowband inputs (i.e., tones), especially in the mid-frequency range (1000 to 3000 Hz). This is due to the fact that the noise (i.e., microphone noise) present in any one channel is lower than the noise summed across all channels simultaneously for broadband inputs. As a result, the lower end of the IDR may reach as low as 9 dB SPL for narrowband inputs in the mid-frequency portion of the speech range.

As previously mentioned, the EDR of a typical recipient is usually around 10 to 25 dB, and as a result, some form of compression processing is needed to place this wide range of potential acoustic inputs (approximately 80 dB SPL for broadband inputs) at the front end of the processor into the narrow EDR. The signal processing engineers at Cochlear have developed a method to provide minimal fast-acting compression to a static speech signal while also allowing access to a wide range of dynamic signals (e.g., 20 to 100 dB SPL for broadband inputs) through the use of processing that is similar to a low-acting compressor (e.g., automatic volume control). In order to understand how this is accomplished, it is important to define some additional terminology. The IIDR is a parameter label that is specific to Cochlear Ltd. implants and is defined as the range of short-term, instantaneous fluctuations that are mapped without compression (or other types of attenuation, such as **Autosensitivity™ Control [ASC]**) into the recipient's electrical dynamic range at a given point in time. The default IIDR of contemporary Cochlear processors (Nucleus 7, Nucleus Kanso, Nucleus 6, Nucleus 5, and Nucleus Freedom) is 40 dB, which closely corresponds to the dynamic range of conversational level

speech. More specifically, when a talker speaks at an average conversational level, the peaks of the speech signal are near 65 dB SPL, whereas the minima of the speech signal fall near 25 dB SPL.

The default IIDR is defined by two parameters referred to as **T-SPL** and **C-SPL**. At default settings, the T-SPL is set at 25 dB SPL, which results in T-level stimulation for acoustic inputs of 25 dB SPL, whereas inputs below 25 dB SPL receive stimulation below level. If T levels are set appropriately (i.e., at a level that is just audible to the recipient), then inputs below 25 dB SPL should be inaudible to the user, while inputs at 25 dB SPL should be audible but very soft to the user.

At default settings, C-SPL is set to 65 dB SPL, which results in acoustic inputs at 65 dB SPL receiving C-level stimulation if the volume control of the sound processor is set to maximum position. All inputs that exceed 65 dB SPL are subjected to fast-acting infinite compression from a fast-acting **automatic gain control (AGC)** compressor with a high compression ratio. Acoustic inputs between 25 and 65 dB SPL receive electrical stimulation that falls between the T and C levels of the recipient.

It should be noted that the AGC of the Nucleus 6 and 7 sound processors are different from the AGC of the Nucleus 5 sound processor. In the Nucleus 5 sound processor, the AGC is a fast-acting mechanism that quickly attenuates high-level sounds with compression with a relatively high compression ratio. This may be undesirable if it distorts intensity/temporal cues that exist for high-level sounds. As a result, Cochlear developed a dual-action AGC for the Nucleus 6 and 7 sound processors. Moderate-level inputs are subjected to medium-speed (e.g., medium-acting time constant) compression with a modest compression ratio, whereas high-level sounds are subjected to fast-acting compression with relatively high compression ratios. The fast-acting component is more inclined to activate in response to high-level sounds with sudden onset. This dual-action AGC is designed to minimize distortion in response to the dynamic nature of everyday speech and environmental sounds. The dual-action AGC can be disabled in the Nucleus 6 sound processor and the AGC used in the Nucleus 5 processor may be restored by disabling the "Mid-loop Enabled" parameter, which is located in the "Program Settings" menu of the "Write to Processor" section of Custom Sound (Figure 16–19). The dual-action AGC cannot be disabled for the Nucleus 7 sound processor. The mid-loop component

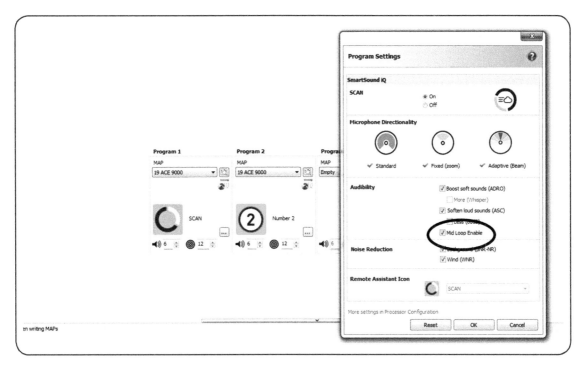

FIGURE 16–19. Enabling/disabling of mid-loop AGC for Nucleus 6 users. Image provided courtesy of Cochlear Americas, ©2018.

of the AGC is disabled when ASC is disabled in the Nucleus 7 sound processor. If the recipient is bothered by the dual-action AGC, then a separate program with ASC disabled may be created for use in situations in which the mid-loop feature is bothersome.

The audiologist may adjust the T-SPL (from 9 to 50 dB SPL) and C-SPL (from 65 to 84 dB SPL) parameters within the "Advanced" tab of the "Parameters" menu with the Set Levels section of Custom Sound (see Figure 16–18). However, as long as the audiologist counsels patients to allow for an adjustment period to new sounds, adjustments to T-SPL and C-SPL parameters are rarely needed. Indeed, a significant adjustment to these parameters alone may cause significant detriment to the listening experience of the recipient.

There are very few situations in which the audiologist may consider adjusting the T-SPL/C-SPL parameters. For example, when adults cannot acclimate to hearing low-level ambient noise (e.g., ventilation systems), the T-SPL parameter may be slightly increased to reduce the salience of low-level sounds. However, in most cases, adults do very well with a T-SPL of 25 dB, and newly implanted adults who complain of hearing low-level sounds will typically

acclimate to their newfound audibility with a short period of implant use. It should be stressed that it is unlikely that the T-SPL should ever be increased for young children.

Adjustments to C-SPL are generally not desired because decreases will result in compression of everyday inputs, and increases of the C-SPL without adjustment of other parameters (e.g., loudness growth, C Levels) will often make conversational speech too soft. However, if C-SPL is increased, then it is necessary for the audiologist to re-measure C levels to ensure that speech and environmental sounds are perceived with an appropriate loudness. It may also be beneficial to decrease the "Loudness Growth" from 20 to 15 after C-SPL is increased but before the C levels are re-measured. Again, it is worth reiterating that the C-SPL and "Loudness Growth" parameters rarely, if ever, need to be adjusted to optimize recipient performance.

The default IIDR of 40 dB with a T-SPL and C-SPL of 25 and 65 dB SPL, respectively, is very appropriate for use for listening to average conversational level speech in a quiet environment because the minima of the speech signal, which occur near 25 dB SPL, should be audible for the recipient. Likewise, little to no compression should be provided to the more intense components of speech, and as a result, the intensity cues of speech should be fairly well preserved. However, this IIDR would not be appropriate for all situations, as some components of soft-spoken speech would fall below 25 dB SPL and would not elicit stimulation. Also, loud speech and other high-level sounds would be subjected to fast-acting, high-level compression, which would likely compromise the identification and sound quality of these sounds.

In order to provide the recipient with access to a wide range of acoustic inputs without distortion and excessive compression, the IIDR window may be shifted in order to capture inputs below 25 dB SPL and to prevent excessive compression for all inputs exceeding 65 dB SPL. The sensitivity parameter controls the overall gain applied to the input signal from the microphone or direct auditory input (DAI). The sensitivity setting, which ranges from a minimum of "1" to a maximum of "20," may be adjusted by the recipient (if the audiologist provides the recipient with control over the sensitivity parameter), or it may be set to a fixed level by the audiologist. The default sensitivity setting is "12," which results in the IIDR being positioned from 25 dB SPL (T-SPL) to 65 dB SPL (C-SPL).

Figure 16–20 illustrates the effect of the sensitivity setting on the positioning of the IIDR. As shown, increasing the sensitivity setting moves the IIDR to a lower level, which provides the user with better access to low-level inputs but also results in a higher likelihood of high-level/excessive compression for moderate level inputs (e.g., average conversation-level speech). In contrast, decreasing the sensitivity

setting prevents moderate to high-level inputs from being overcompressed, but low-level inputs will be inaudible to the recipient.

ASC is a type of input processing that automatically adjusts the sensitivity setting when the ambient noise level at the processor input exceeds a default activation threshold of 57 dB SPL. In most moderate to high-level noise environments, talkers raise their voices so that their level exceeds the competing noise and the recipient is able to listen at a positive signal-to-noise ratio (SNR). ASC prevents excessive compression of the speech signal in noisy environments and enhances the likelihood of preserving a positive SNR in noisy listening conditions. Therefore, the total range of input levels the processor can encode without significant clipping or distortion is much wider than the IIDR.

Numerous studies have shown that use of ASC results in an improvement in the recipient's ability to understand speech in noise with no change in speech understanding in quiet (Gifford & Revit, 2010; Wolfe et al. 2009; Wolfe, Schafer, John, & Hudson, 2011; Wolfe et al., 2012). As a result, the audiologist should consider enabling ASC for the recipient's primary program to be used in most typical listening situations. It should be noted that ASC is enabled/disabled in the "Write to Processor" module, which will be discussed later in this chapter.

In most cases, Nucleus recipients do not have access to manual adjustment of the sensitivity control, and ASC (along with ADRO, which will be discussed later) is used with a fixed default sensitivity setting of "12" to provide access to a wide range of speech and environmental sounds. Audiologists may program the Cochlear Remote Assistants or Nucleus Smart App to allow the recipient to adjust the volume control and/or the sensitivity. However, in the typical case, remote controls are programmed to only allow for adjustment of the volume control. Figure 16–20 provides an indication of the effect of a manual sensitivity adjustment on the recipient's IIDR. It should be noted that a fixed sensitivity setting of "12" with ASC should always be used with young children and other recipients who are unable to appropriately adjust sensitivity settings manually. Because sensitivity is typically a fixed parameter, but the volume parameter is often recipient adjustable, the following section of this chapter will describe, in detail, the effect of the volume control.

The reader may ask when it would be appropriate to manually adjust the sensitivity control. Examples of situations in which recipients report that

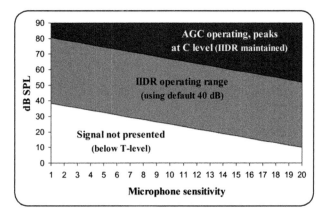

FIGURE 16–20. Adjustment of the sensitivity control setting on the instantaneous input dynamic range (IIDR). Image provided courtesy of Cochlear Americas, ©2018.

manual adjustment may be helpful include: (1) when speech and noise are too soft with ASC responding to background noise, it may be helpful to increase the sensitivity setting, (2) when better access to sounds originating from a distance (e.g., nature sounds when on a walk) is desired, it may be helpful to increase the sensitivity setting, and (3) when competing noise in a moderate-level noise environment continues to cause difficulty with speech recognition, it may be helpful to decrease the sensitivity setting even further. However, it should be stated again that the need for manual sensitivity adjustments are very infrequent, and as a result, the authors prefer to fix sensitivity setting at "12" and enable ASC for automatic adjustment of the sensitivity setting (Wolfe et al., 2009, 2011, 2012).

It should be noted that additional types of input processing also influence how acoustic inputs are delivered to a recipient's electrical dynamic range. For instance, ADRO is another adaptive form of input processing, which seeks to optimize the delivery of acoustic inputs to improve audibility for low-level inputs, while optimizing comfort for high-level inputs. Whisper is another type of input processing that aims to enhance the salience of low-level inputs. ASC, ADRO, Whisper, and other type of input processing are described in a later section of this chapter.

Volume Control. The **volume control** parameter has a large influence on the stimulation levels the recipient uses in his/her programs, and subsequently, it has the potential to substantially impact speech recognition and sound quality. As a result, it is imperative that the audiologist has a thorough understanding of the function of the volume control parameter as well as the impact of the volume control setting on the recipient's daily listening experience.

The volume control may be adjusted across 10 steps (from 1 to 10). The range over which the volume control adjusts C levels is programmable from 0 to 100% and is controlled by the "**Volume Adjustment (%DR)**" parameter, which is found in the "Advanced" tab of the "Parameters" menu (see Figure 16–18). It is important to remember that when a recipient is using his/her sound processor in a quiet environment at default settings (i.e., T-SPL, C-SPL, and sensitivity settings are all set to default), acoustic inputs at 25 dB SPL result in the provision of stimulation at T level, and acoustic inputs at 65 dB SPL and higher result in the provision of stimulation corresponding to the volume control setting (it should be noted that inputs exceeding 65 dB SPL are subjected to high-level com-

pression and result in stimulation corresponding to the volume control setting). The volume control parameter essentially has the effect of adjusting the upper level of stimulation (i.e., C levels) the recipient receives (i.e., the amount of stimulation for inputs >65 dB SPL). When the volume control is set to the maximum setting of "10," the recipient is provided with stimulation at the C level set for his/her MAP. Decreasing the volume control from the maximum position decreases the C-level stimulation the recipient receives for inputs of 65 dB SPL and higher.

The extent by which the volume control setting adjusts the stimulation level that the recipient receives for inputs equal to or exceeding 65 dB SPL is determined by the parameter referred to as "Volume Adjustment (%DR)" (hereafter referred to as "Volume Adjustment"). When the Volume Adjustment parameter is left at the default setting of 20%, decreasing the volume control from the maximum (i.e., 10) to the minimum (i.e., 1) results in a global reduction in C levels that corresponds to 20% of the recipient's electrical dynamic range. Therefore, a participant with an electrical dynamic range of 30 CL would experience a 6 CL decrease in stimulation when adjusting the volume control from 10 to 1 (30 CL * 20% = 6 CL). Table 16–1 provides examples of the effect of the volume control and the Volume Adjustment on the stimulation levels a recipient receives.

Several important considerations can be gleaned from Table 16–1. Specifically, wider Volume Adjustment ranges not only result in an overall wider effect of the volume control range, but each step adjustment of the volume control results in a relatively large change in the stimulation the recipient receives for moderate to high-level inputs. Note that for recipient #2 in Table 16–1, a Volume Adjustment range of 100% results in a change of 5 CL for each step adjustment of the volume control, whereas a Volume Adjustment range of 20% results in a change of 1 CL for each step adjustment of the volume control. In other words, small Volume Adjustment settings (i.e., 30% or less of DR) allow for more precise control over the stimulation the recipient receives for moderate to high-level inputs. Large changes to volume settings should not be necessary for experienced implant users as long as C levels are set appropriately, and as a result, the Volume Adjustment range should be relatively narrow (e.g., 30%–40%). A narrower Volume Adjustment range will allow experienced recipients to have more precise control over the stimulation they receive for moderate to high-level inputs. However, broader control over the C levels may be helpful to new implant

TABLE 16–1. Stimulation (in CL) Recipient Receives for Inputs Equaling or Exceeding 65 dB SPL

Recipient	T Level	C Level	DR	Volume Adjustment (% DR)	Volume Control (VC) Setting 1	2	4	6	8	10	Step Size/VC Setting
1	120	135	15	100%	120	121.7	125	128.3	131.7	135	1.67
1	120	135	15	50%	127.5	128.3	130	131.7	133.3	135	.83
1	120	135	15	20%	132	132.3	133	133.7	134.3	135	.33
1	120	135	15	0%	135	135	135	135	135	135	0
2	120	170	50	100%	120	125.6	136.7	147.8	158.9	170	5.56
2	120	170	50	50%	145	147.8	153.4	158.9	164.5	170	2.78
2	120	170	50	20%	160	161.1	163.3	165.6	167.8	170	1.11
2	120	170	50	0%	170	170	170	170	170	170	0
3	120	220	100	100%	120	131.1	153.3	175.6	197.8	220	11.11
3	120	220	100	50%	170	175.6	186.7	197.8	208.9	220	5.56
3	120	220	100	20%	200	202.2	206.7	211.1	215.6	220	2.22
3	120	220	100	0%	220	220	220	220	220	220	0

users, particularly when they first put the processor on in the morning or after a period of non-use.

Review of Table 16–1 also indicates that the effect of the volume control varies as a function of the size of the recipient's EDR. As shown, for recipients with narrow EDR, each step of the volume control (VC) adjustment results in a small change (in CL) in the stimulation provided to the recipient. In contrast, for recipients with wide EDR, each step of the VC results in a relatively large change (in CL) of stimulation. As a result, the audiologist should consider the recipient's EDR when selecting the Volume Adjustment parameter.

At initial activation, the authors typically provide a wide volume control range to allow the recipient or caregiver to adjust the volume down by 100% of their dynamic range. Parents are advised to start with the volume setting of "0" when the child first wakes up from sleep. The external transmitting coil should then be placed on the child's head and the volume of the processor should be increased to the desired setting (typically "10") over the next few seconds. If the child reacts negatively to the signal, the volume control should be adjusted to a comfortable setting, and the parent should attempt to increase the volume at a later point in the day. If the child shows no reaction, the next time the processor is placed on the child's head, the parent should begin at a volume setting of approximately "2" to "3" and gradually increase the starting volume setting over the next few days or weeks. Once the recipient is able to tolerate the program with the volume control at a stable position, the range of the Volume Adjustment parameter should be decreased or the control should be disabled (i.e., set to 0).

For most children who perform well and have stable stimulation levels, the authors of this text disable the volume control. If the family reports that the child occasionally reports that stimulation from the implant is too loud, then we will provide a narrow range for adjustment (e.g., 20%–30%) to allow the caregiver to provide a small decrease in stimulation in relatively precise steps. The family is encouraged to contact the clinic if the volume control must be substantially decreased to facilitate the child's comfort or if the child consistently complains of loudness discomfort. Parents are able to conveniently adjust the volume setting via the CR210 or CR230 wireless assistant; however, these changes must be warranted to justify alteration to the child's carefully programmed upper stimulation levels. As previously discussed, the audiologist should consider disabling the volume control for young children who have stable program levels. This may be accomplished by disabling the volume control in the Processor Configuration menu (to be discussed later) or by setting the Volume Adjustment range to 0 in the "Advanced Parameters" section of the "Set Levels" screen (Figure 16–21). The sensitivity control may be locked in the Processor Configuration menu (to be illustrated later) and should be routinely disabled for young children. There may be, however, some circumstances in which older children will desire to access the volume control.

For adults, the C levels are adjusted to provide a most comfortable loudness percept with the volume control set at a setting of 6 or 7, which allows the user to adjust the volume upward or downward from the recommended setting established during programming. The Volume Adjustment parameter is usually

set to 30% to 40%. For young children, comfortable upper stimulation levels are set with the volume control at the maximum setting (e.g., 10) to prevent increases in the volume control and a potentially uncomfortable loudness percept. As previously mentioned, for experienced pediatric recipients, the Volume Adjustment parameter is typically set between 0% and 20%.

It is the audiologist's responsibility to ensure that adults and older children understand the functions of the sensitivity and volume parameters to enable them to appropriately address difficulties they may experience across a variety of listening environments. It is often desirable to provide older children and adult recipients with the ability to adjust the volume control, but we tend to disable the manual sensitivity control and enable ASC. However, the manual sensitivity control is occasionally enabled for recipients who encounter a wide range of listening environments

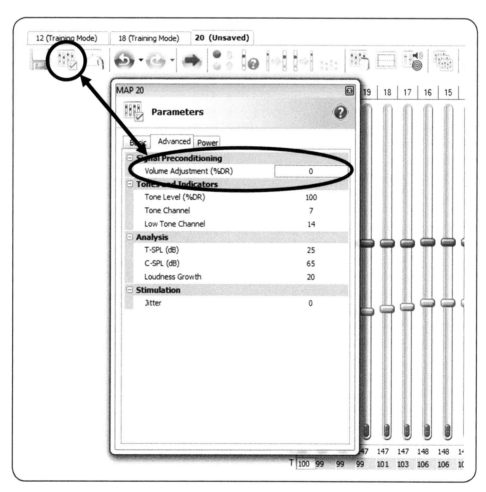

FIGURE 16–21. Volume control adjustment. Image provided courtesy of Cochlear Americas, ©2018.

and who request the freedom to exert more control over the manner in which their processor functions across these environments. It is critical that these recipients understand how to appropriately use the volume and sensitivity controls.

Once again, sensitivity influences the audibility of soft sounds and compression of loud sounds, whereas the volume control adjusts the stimulation the recipient receives for moderate to high-level inputs. Therefore, if patients feel that the overall loudness of a listening environment is too soft or loud, they should adjust the volume control up or down, respectively. However, if soft sounds from a distance are inaudible, especially in quiet situations, they can increase the sensitivity. In contrast, if background noise is preventing a user from understanding a talker located in close proximity, the recipient may choose to decrease the sensitivity setting. Understanding the function of these parameters will give experienced users the ability to address several common difficulties in quiet and noisy listening situations. It should be reiterated that when stimulation levels are set appropriately and

ASC is used, there is essentially no need to adjust the sensitivity setting manually. With ASC, most users are best served by adjusting the volume control instead.

It is also important to note that the sensitivity parameter affects the strength of the signal delivered from the sound processor microphone as well as the accessory or telecoil signal. For all earlier-generation processors (e.g., Freedom sound processor and earlier), the sensitivity adjustment affects only the strength of the signal from the microphone. Finally, it should be noted that the volume control and sensitivity settings may be adjusted in the "Set Levels" module to allow the recipient to experience the effect of these controls while listening to speech and environmental sounds during the programming process (Figure 16–22).

Frequency Allocation

As the name implies, the **frequency allocation** parameter determines how input acoustic frequencies are allocated or assigned across the active channels. At

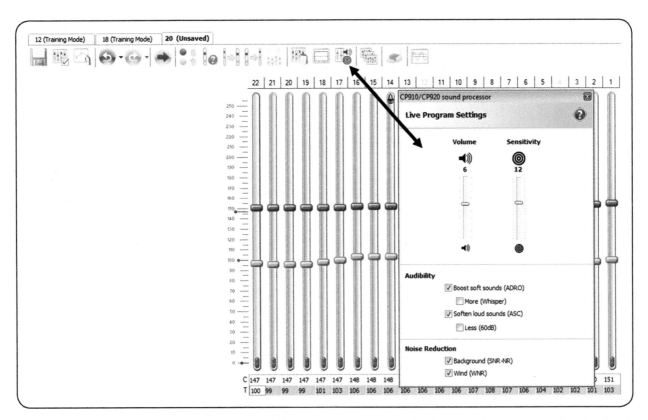

FIGURE 16–22. Accessing volume and sensitivity controls during live speech programming. Image provided courtesy of Cochlear Americas, ©2018.

default settings, the frequency range allocated across all 22 channels spans from 188 to 7938 Hz. The bandwidth of the low-frequency channels, 14 to 22, are narrow (125 Hz) relative to the mid-frequency channels, 10 to 13, which have a bandwidth of 250 Hz and high-frequency channels, 1 to 9, which have bandwidths ranging from 1000 to 375 Hz. The decision to provide narrower bandwidth channels in the low-frequency portion of the system is predicated upon the fact that the auditory filters of the peripheral auditory system are also narrower in the lower frequencies. Additionally, narrower channels are needed throughout the low- and mid-frequency range in order to distinguish formant frequencies of periodic vowels and consonants, which is essential for recognition of these phonemes. It is worth noting that the width of low-frequency channels is linearly spaced, while the width of high-frequency channels is logarithmically spaced. This spacing is based off psychoacoustic modeling of the normal auditory system (see Bark Scale in Zwicker, 1961).

The frequency allocation parameter may be adjusted within the "Frequency Table" drop-down menu (Figure 16–23). The default frequency allocation table is #22. As shown in Figure 16–23, the audiologist may reduce the upper bandwidth of the allocation range by selecting from one of five alternative frequency allocation tables; however, this adjustment is not imperative. The author of this book routinely leaves the frequency allocation table at the default setting for pediatric recipients in light of research that suggests children need a wider bandwidth for the recognition and production of speech (Stelmachowicz et al., 2001). However, the author of this book does frequently adjust the frequency allocation table to #22-B for adult recipients, who are not as reliant on an extended bandwidth are young children. Adjusting the frequency allocation table to #22-B does allow for a narrower bandwidth across several of the mid-frequency channels, which may improve the ability to distinguish speech sounds in that frequency range. Additional research of the frequency allocation parameter is needed to determine optimal settings for pediatric and adult recipients.

The audiologist may also manually control the assignment of input acoustic frequencies to each individual channel by selecting the rectangle icon to the right of the "Frequency Table" drop-down menu (see Figure 16–23). As shown in Figure 16–23, the "Frequency Bands" menu gives the audiologist access

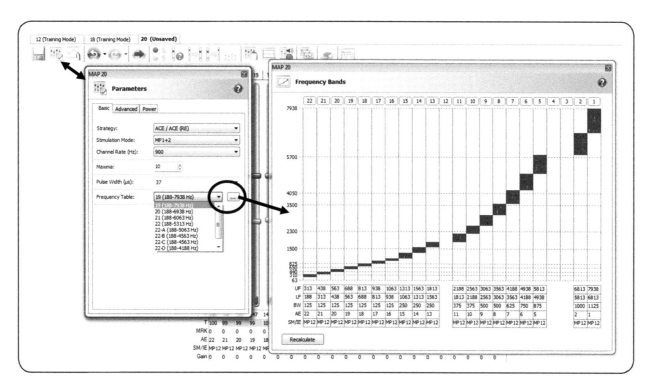

FIGURE 16–23. Frequency allocation adjustment. Image provided courtesy of Cochlear Americas, ©2018.

to a table in which the low- and high-frequency cut-offs of each channel may be determined by manually entering the desired value (in Hz) within each respective field.

The manufacturer suggests that the manual control of frequency allocation be used with caution. Indeed, the recipient's performance may be compromised if adjustments are made in a haphazard manner. With that said, there are two common uses for this module. First, audiologists may use this feature to control the cut-off between acoustic and electric stimulation for recipients who have usable residual hearing and utilize electro-acoustic stimulation (discussed in Chapter 10). Second, some legacy sound processors (e.g., ESPrit 3G, Spectra) used frequency allocation that was quite different from the defaults used in current sound processors. When these recipients upgrade to contemporary processors, they often reject the frequency allocation tables used with the current defaults. In such a case, the audiologist may manually re-create a frequency allocation that is similar to what the recipient used with his/her older sound processor. Again, additional research is needed to determine how audiologists may be able to adjust frequency allocation settings to optimize individual recipient performance.

Loudness Growth

The **loudness growth** parameter determines the steepness of the logarithmic function used to map input sounds into the recipient's electrical dynamic range. This parameter, which is also referred to as the **Q-value**, affects the slope of the amplitude growth function and determines the proportion of the user's EDR that is assigned to the upper 10 dB of the sound processor's input dynamic range. Lowering the loudness growth parameter (e.g., Q-value) results in a steeper loudness growth function slope, which should enhance the salience of low-level acoustic inputs (Figure 16–24). In other words, decreases and increases to loudness growth result in the mapping of inputs at higher or lower levels, respectively, in the user's electrical dynamic range. The loudness growth default setting is 20 but may be adjusted across a range from 10 to 50 within the "Advanced" tab of the "Parameters" menu (see Figure 16–18).

The author of this book rarely adjusts the loudness growth setting. However, a theoretical example of when an audiologist may choose to alter the loudness growth parameter would be if the recipient does not have adequate access to low-level sounds. In this case, the audiologist may decrease the loud-

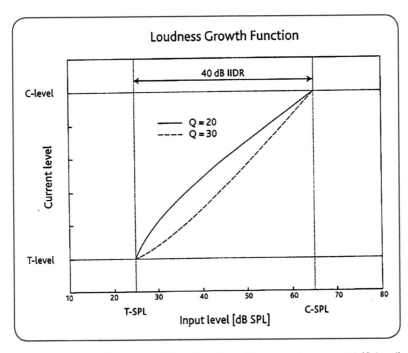

FIGURE 16–24. Loudness growth function at two different loudness growth (Q-level) settings. Image provided courtesy of Cochlear Americas, ©2018.

ness growth parameter from 20 to 10 to provide more salience for soft sounds. However, it is worth noting again that it is very unlikely that the audiologist will ever need to adjust this parameter. In general, access to low-level speech sounds and loudness normalization are satisfactory when stimulation levels are set appropriately.

Jitter

The **jitter** parameter is available only for the SPEAK signal coding strategy used by Nucleus 22 implant recipients. At low, fixed stimulation rates (e.g., 250 pps or lower), the recipient could perceive a continuous, low-pitched tonal sound that corresponds to the frequency of the stimulation rate. In essence, the auditory nerve is responding in a phase-locked manner to multiples of the stimulus rate, which is a normal auditory system function for pitch coding. Jitter causes the stimulation rate to vary randomly by a certain percentage (e.g., 10%) around the stimulation rate. This random variation around the dominant stimulation rate eliminates the user's perception of a continuous low-pitched sound. The need to adjust the jitter parameter is quite rare. When needed, the jitter parameter may be adjusted in the "Advanced" tab of the "Parameters" menu.

Channel Gains. **Channel gains** allow for frequency-specific adjustments of +10.5 dB/−12 dB to the input signal from the sound processor microphone. When using ACE, changes to channel gain will influence whether or not the channel will be selected as a maxima because the gain adjustment is implemented at the input before the signal is processed. High-frequency acoustic information contributes greatly to speech clarity, so it is not desirable to reduce the gain for high-frequency channels because doing so would reduce the likelihood that the high-frequency channels would be selected for stimulation. As a result, adjustment of channel gains in *n*-of-*m* strategies, such as ACE, should be avoided. Adjustments to stimulation levels to address sound quality issues would be preferred. The effect of adjusting channel gains within the CIS signal coding strategy is not as deleterious, but again, it is usually unnecessary when stimulation levels are set appropriately. When needed, channel gains may be adjusted by selecting the "Channel Gain" icon on the icon bar of the "Set Levels" module (Figure 16–25) or by accessing the

channel gain in the table below the stimulation levels in the "Set Levels" module (see Figure 16–25).

Voltage Compliance

Voltage compliance limits are measured in Custom Sound by clicking on the icon circled in Figure 16–26. Voltage compliance levels, indicated by red dashes on each channel (limit on channel 22 shown with arrow on Figure 16–26), show the maximum current amplitude available for stimulation. Voltage compliance levels are limited by the voltage capacity of the processor's power source (i.e., battery). Cochlear recommends that five or fewer channels are outside of voltage compliance limits by less than 10% on each channel. If these criteria are not met, the recipient will likely experience poor performance and sound quality because the loudness relationships across the channels will be compromised. Also, use of maximum current levels increases the likelihood of channel interaction and decreases battery life.

Voltage compliance issues are typically simple to address through programming adjustments. Specifically, the audiologist should increase the pulse width of the compromised channel and re-measure T and C levels. The increase in pulse width should decrease the current required to elicit a desired loudness percept. Again, the author of this book routinely increases the pulse width from the default of 25 μsec to 37 μsec, which reduces the likelihood that voltage compliance limits will be encountered while still allowing for a stimulation rate of 900 pps and 10 to 11 maxima. Once again, a 50-μsec pulse width may be necessary to avoid voltage compliance limits for recipients with lateral wall electrodes.

Prediction of Stimulation Levels from Other Programs

In Custom Sound, the question mark icon (Figure 16–27) can be used to estimate stimulation levels based on measured T and C levels in another program. Once a program is complete, the audiologist can begin a new program with the same signal coding strategy but a different stimulation rate or pulse width. Once the T and C levels are measured for one channel in the new program, the T and C levels of remaining channels can be predicted by clicking on the question mark icon. This feature allows for efficient creation of several programs with varying stimulation rates or a change in pulse width, which will aid the user in determining the optimal stimulus parameters for long-term use.

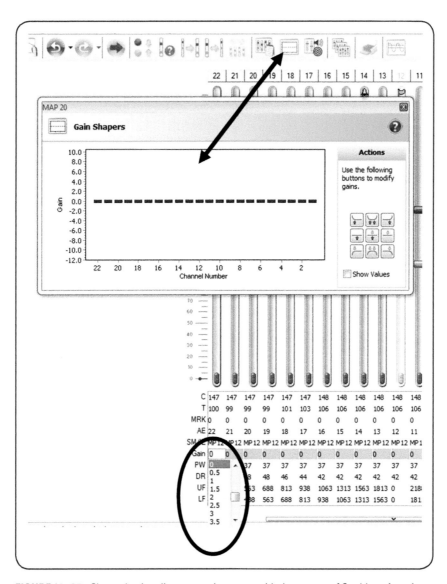

FIGURE 16–25. Channel gain adjustments. Image provided courtesy of Cochlear Americas, ©2018.

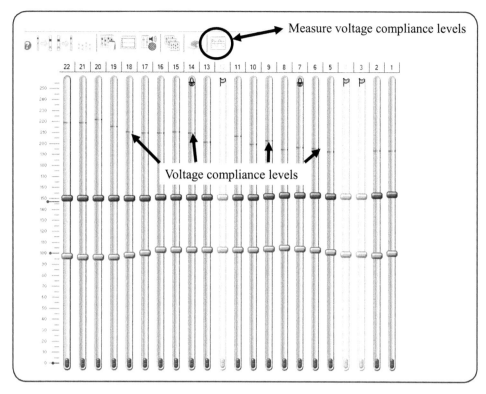

FIGURE 16–26. Voltage compliance measurement and results. Image provided courtesy of Cochlear Americas, ©2018.

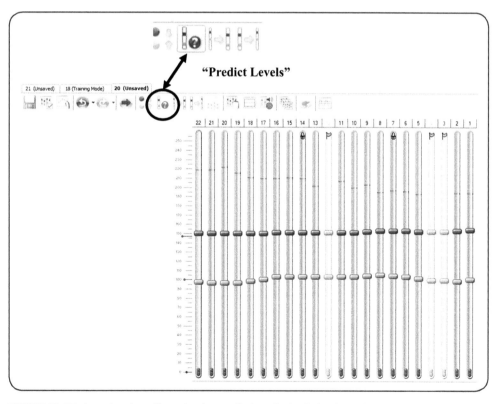

FIGURE 16–27. Location that allows for the prediction of stimulation levels based on limited measurements within a program and stimulation levels obtained with another program that used a different stimulation rate. Image provided courtesy of Cochlear Americas, ©2018.

Double Channel Mapping

The Custom Sound programming software also allows **double channel mapping**. This mapping involves directing the outputs of two channels into one intracochlear electrode contact, which may be desirable when the recipient has a restricted number of channels due to disabled electrodes. When patients have restricted channels, the range of input frequencies is limited (i.e., 5500 versus 7000 Hz). Double channel mapping results in an increased bandwidth assigned to each electrode contact and an increased overall bandwidth for the recipient. Double channel mapping is accomplished by right-clicking on the channel the audiologist wishes to link and selecting "Double Channel" from the list of options (Figure 16–28). Additionally, the audiologist may choose the channels that are linked by selecting in the table (located below the stimulation level grid within the "Set Levels" module) the "active electrode" that corresponds to the desired channel. It should be noted that the active electrode ("AE") and reference electrode/coupling mode (SM/IE) are not present by default in the table of the "Set Levels" module. However, the audiologist may enable these parameters to be included within the table by selecting "Tools" at the top of the Custom Sound software and then selecting the "My Preferences" tab. From there, the audiologist must access the "Display" tab and select the parameters that he/she desires to be displayed in the table (Figure 16–29).

Channel-to-Electrode Assignment

At default settings, the Cochlear system allocates 22 channels to the 22 active intracochlear electrode contacts. Electrode 1 (and channel 1) is assigned to the most basal contact, and the electrode contact/channel number becomes progressively higher toward the apical end of the cochlea. The audiologist can reassign a channel to a different electrode contact by clicking on the active electrode coordinate within the parameters/data table in the "Set Levels" and selecting the desired allocation. This procedure may be warranted on two rare occasions. First, it may be beneficial for recipients who do not have the expected tonotopic organization as determined by sweeping the programming stimulus across the electrode array. In this case, alterations are made to the channel-to-electrode

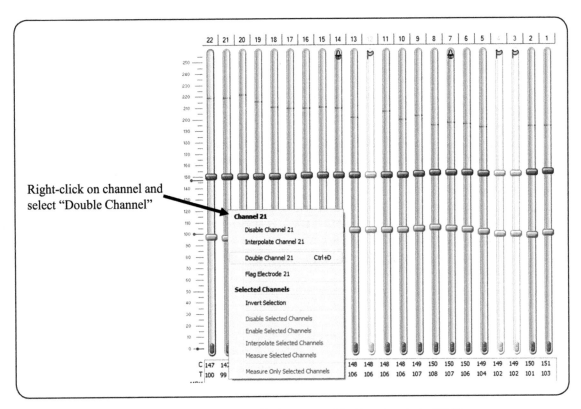

FIGURE 16–28. Double channel mapping. Image provided courtesy of Cochlear Americas, ©2018.

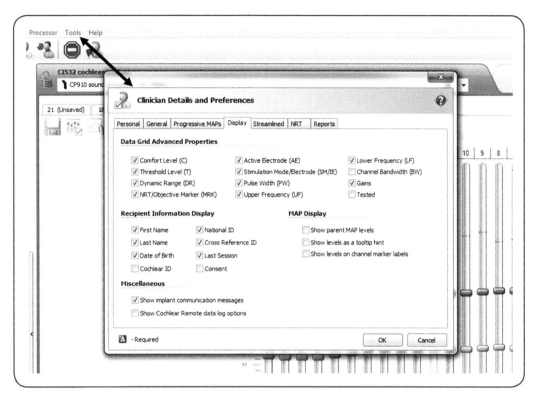

FIGURE 16–29. Preferences for parameters displayed within Custom Sound programming screen. Image provided courtesy of Cochlear Americas, ©2018.

assignment with the intention of restoring tonotopic organization. Second, if the recipient has a common cavity cochlea, the surgeon may choose to insert the electrode array through a cochleostomy made near the horizontal semicircular canal (i.e., opposite the typical direction). This procedure requires the audiologist to invert the channel-to-electrode assignment, which places the higher-numbered electrodes at the basal end of the cochlea and the lower-numbered electrodes at the apical end. It should be noted that the audiologist may also activate an icon button (circled in Figure 16–30) that automatically reverses the order in which channels are assigned as a function of frequency (i.e., high-frequency acoustic inputs are assigned to the most apical electrode contacts, while low-frequency acoustic inputs are assigned to the most basal electrode contacts). The "Reverse Electrode Order" option is only available for use with Nucleus Auditory Brainstem Implant recipients.

Additional Audiologist-Adjustable Parameters

The audiologist may also make several other adjustments by selecting icons within the "Set Levels" mod-

ule. Figure 16–31 identifies the icons that have not yet been discussed.

Write to Processor. Once a satisfactory MAP has been created in the programming platform, the audiologist must create programs for the recipient and load the programs onto the recipient's sound processor. This is accomplished in the "Write to Processor" section of the Custom Sound software (Figure 16–32). These programs may vary in stimulation levels or in preprocessing features. For example, new recipients may receive a different MAP in each program position so that they may have successively higher C levels to allow them to gradually acclimate to higher levels of stimulation. Once the audiologist believes that stimulation levels are appropriate and stable, the different programs will have identical stimulation levels (e.g., MAPs), but they may each possess different types of Smart Sound preprocessing (e.g., microphone mode, SNR-NR, WNR). Up to four programs may be loaded into a Nucleus 7, Nucleus Kanso, and Nucleus 6 sound processor. The Nucleus sound processor must be designated for use with either the right or left ear. In the default mode in the version of Custom

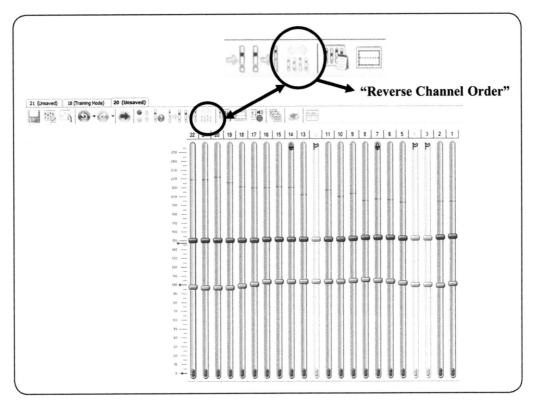

FIGURE 16–30. Reverse channel order option for auditory brainstem implant recipients. Image provided courtesy of Cochlear Americas, ©2018.

Sound that is used at the time of this writing, two user programs are populated from the MAP that was most recently created/selected, and these default programs differ for adult and pediatric recipients (i.e., under 6 years old). The two default programs for recipients 6 years old and older include the following: (1) "SCAN": which includes the SCAN acoustic scene analyzer with automatic implementation of Cochlear SmartSound iQ processing including Autosensitivity Control (ASC) + Adaptive Dynamic Range Optimization (ADRO) input processing, automatic selection of microphone mode, SNR-NR, and WNR; (2) "Number 2": SCAN is disabled but each of the following is enabled, ASC+ADRO, Standard microphone mode, SNR-NR, WNR. For pediatric recipients under 6 years of age, the two programs that are auto-populated are identical and include the following: (1) "Number 1": ASC+ADRO are enabled with the Standard microphone mode, but Scan, SNR-NR, and WNR are disabled; (2) "Number 2": the same preprocessing as program "Number 1." Of note, the author of this book routinely loads only one program for both children and adults, the SCAN program (with ASC+ADRO,

SNR-NR, and WNR) for adults and the "Number 1" program for children 3 years and younger. For children 4 years and older, the author typically loads only the SCAN program with ASC+ADRO, SNR-NR, and WNR.

These programs are shown in Figure 16–32. Also, as shown in this same figure, the default volume control setting is "6" and the sensitivity setting is fixed at "12." It should be noted that the volume control setting will change from a setting of "6" if the audiologist adjusted the volume setting in the "Set Levels" screen. The audiologist may also adjust the volume and sensitivity settings in the "Write to Processor" module.

The audiologist may review and adjust the type of input processing available within each program by selecting the small square icon toward the lower right-hand corner of each program box (Figure 16–33). These different types of input processing are described in detail below. The audiologist may also change the name of each program except for the SCAN program (which is fixed as "SCAN") by accessing the drop-down menu in the "Program Icon" section of the "Program Settings" menu (Figure 16–34).

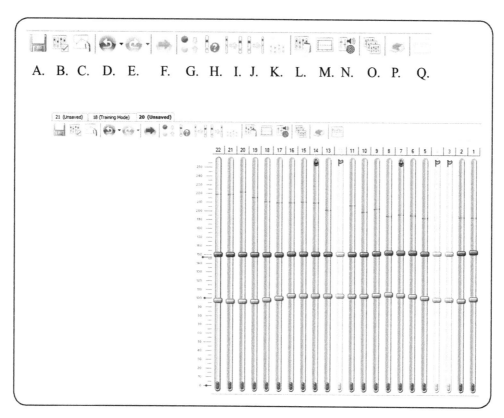

FIGURE 16–31. Adjustments and actions within the "Set Levels" screen: **A.** Saves the current program; **B.** Accesses a variety of additional MAP parameters; **C.** Accesses acoustic parameters for electric-acoustic users; **D.** Undo previous action; **E.** Redo previous step; **F.** Go Live: Activates sound processor so that recipient may hear in live speech mode; **G.** Hug T-profile—Superimposes C levels onto T levels; **H.** Predict levels—Predicts stimulation levels on the basis of a limited set of measurements; **I.** Makes all channels measureable; **J.** Makes only highlighted channels measurable; **K.** Reverses channel order; **L.** Notes—Allows audiologist to write notes for the program; **M.** Channel gain; **N.** Allows adjustment of volume control and sensitivity control; **O.** Creates progressive programs, each with C levels that are 5 CL higher than the preceding program; **P.** Prints program; **Q.** Measures voltage compliance levels. Image provided courtesy of Cochlear Americas, ©2018.

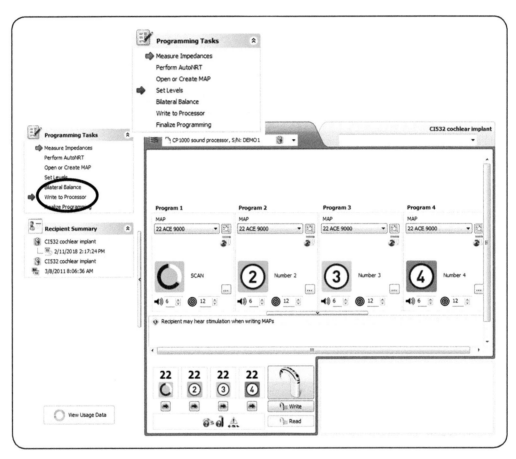

FIGURE 16–32. "Write to Processor" screen in which programs are loaded onto Nucleus sound processors. Image provided courtesy of Cochlear Americas, ©2018.

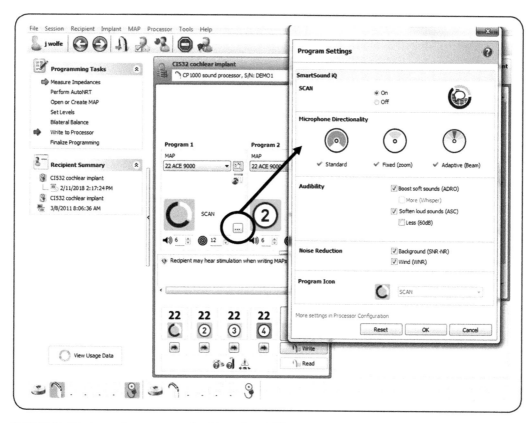

FIGURE 16–33. Accessing preprocessing (SmartSound iQ) settings within each program. Image provided courtesy of Cochlear Americas, ©2018.

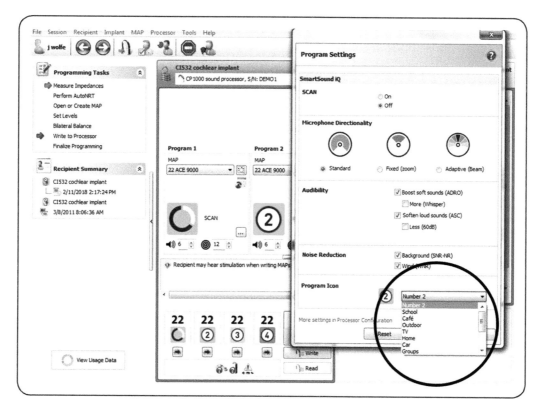

FIGURE 16–34. Labeling programs. Image provided courtesy of Cochlear Americas, ©2018.

This allows for the provision of different icons/labels for programs as they are displayed on the cochlear Remote Assistant. For instance, a program may be labeled numerically (e.g., Program 2) or descriptively (e.g., "Car," "Café," "Home"). The input processing schemes present in a program do not automatically change when an audiologist changes the program descriptor. In other words, if the audiologist changes the descriptor of the "Music" program, which at default includes the ADRO+Whisper input processing schemes, to be labeled as a "Car" program, the preprocessing will remain as ADRO+Whisper, which is unlikely to be ideal for the car. In such an example, the audiologist should adjust the input processing as well. Because cars are noisy places, it is probably most appropriate to disable Whisper (because Whisper can be detrimental to speech recognition in noise) and enable ASC and SNR-NR.

Input Processing

When selecting programs for the recipient in Custom Sound, the audiologist must consider the input preprocessing characteristics (i.e., **SmartSound iQ processing**), which include ASC, ADRO, Beam (multimicrophone directionality with adaptive positioning of the directional null), Zoom (fixed directionality), SNR-NR (channel-specific noise reduction), SCAN (fully automatic, adaptive directionality), and WNR (wind noise reduction), that will be provided to the recipient. The **SCAN** algorithm within SmartSound iQ is the cochlear implant industry's first input processing algorithm to perform acoustic scene analysis and automatically select the appropriate input signal processing with the goal of optimizing performance for the acoustic characteristics of a given listening situation. Based on previous research, optimal speech recognition for a variety of different speech sounds across a variety of listening environments can be achieved without the need for manual adjustment of processor controls by the combined use of ASC+ADRO in conjunction with SNR-NR, SCAN, and WNR (De Ceulaer et al., 2017; Plasmans et al., 2016; Wolfe et al., 2009, 2011. 2012, 2013, 2015). Access to low-level inputs is optimized by use of ADRO (James et al., 2002; Müller-Deile, Kiefer, Wyss, Nicolai, & Battmer, 2008), and performance in noisy environments is optimized by use of SCAN, ASC+ADRO, and SNR-NR (Wolfe et al., 2009, 2012, 2013). Therefore, the author of this book recommends simultaneous use of the following SmartSound iQ input processing schemes for adult recipients and children 4 years old

and up: ASC+ADRO, SNR-NR, SCAN, and WNR. The various input processing settings are selected in the "Write to Processor" screen, where new programs are loaded into the sound processor (to be discussed later in this chapter).

These different input processing schemes (e.g., Smart Sound iQ input processing) are described in detail below. All of the input processing schemes described below are available in the Nucleus 7, Nucleus Kanso, and Nucleus 6 sound processors.

SmartSound iQ Preprocessing

As mentioned earlier in this chapter, the Nucleus system offers several SmartSound preprocessing strategies that are designed to enhance listening abilities in a variety of situations. The effectiveness of these preprocessing strategies is well supported by research (De Ceulaer et al., 2017; Gifford & Revit, 2010; James et al., 2002; Müller-Deile, Kiefer, Wyss, Nicolai, & Battmer, 2008; Plasman et al., 2016; Wolfe et al., 2009, 2011, 2012, 2013, 2015). All of the different SmartSound iQ preprocessing options may be selected in the "Program Settings" menu, which may be accessed by clicking on the small square in the lower left-hand corner of each program box in the "Write to Processor" module (see Figure 16–33). As shown, two radio buttons exist to allow the audiologist to enable or disable SCAN. If SCAN is disabled, then the audiologist may choose from one of three microphone modes, including Standard, Fixed (Zoom), or Adaptive (Beam). ADRO and ASC may be selected in the "Audibility" window of the "Program Settings" menu. Finally, SNR-NR and WNR may be selected by enabling "Background" and "Wind," respectively, in the "Noise Reduction" window of the "Program Settings" menu. Each of the aforementioned preprocessing strategies is described in detail below.

Autosensitivity Control and Autosensitivity Control Breakpoint. As mentioned previously, **ASC** is a unique type of input preprocessing exclusive to the Cochlear Ltd. SmartSound programming platform. ASC essentially functions as a slow-acting AGC in noisy conditions. When the ambient noise level at the sound processor microphone exceeds 57 dB SPL, the ASC algorithm decreases the sensitivity of the sound processor microphone in an attempt to maximize the distance between the peaks of the speech signal and the ongoing competing noise.

As previously discussed, in quiet environments, ASC is not operational. However, ASC continuously analyzes the intensity of the competing noise during pauses in speech, and when the noise exceeds the default ASC breakpoint setting of 57 dB SPL, the digital ASC algorithm is engaged. The reduction in microphone sensitivity increases the input level that is subjected to high-level compression and prevents the peaks of speech from being compressed and embedded within the background noise. The reader is referred to Figure 16–20 for an illustration of how the sensitivity setting influences the positioning of the IIDR window. Previous research suggests that use of ASC significantly improves speech recognition in noise relative to performance with fixed sensitivity settings (Wolfe et al., 2009, 2012).

The **ASC breakpoint** may be increased from 3 dB to 60 dB SPL if the recipient complains that too much attenuation is provided in noisy environments. The ASC Breakpoint is adjusted in the "Program Settings" menu, which may be accessed by clicking on the small square (circled icon in Figure 16–33) in the lower left-hand corner of each program box in the Write to Processor module. The ASC Breakpoint may be adjusted to 60 dB by simply selecting the "Less (60dB)" option under the "Soften loud sounds (ASC)" option in the "Program Settings" menu. The ASC breakpoint rarely needs to be adjusted for new recipients. However, existing recipients who have not previously used ASC may report that ASC causes speech to be too soft in noisy environments. In this case, the Breakpoint should be increased to 60 dB SPL.

Adaptive Dynamic Range Optimization (ADRO). The objective of **ADRO** is to improve audibility for low-level sounds, maintain comfort for high-level inputs, and optimize the wide range of speech and other desirable acoustic inputs into the user's narrow electrical dynamic range. ADRO adaptively and constantly adjusts the gain in each of the channels of the sound processor based on an analysis conducted across three features of the input signal: the average input level, the level of the background noise, and the level of the loudest sounds. To maximize speech recognition, gains are increased in channels that possess a favorable SNR or include low-level speech. Conversely, to normalize loudness and prevent discomfort, gains are decreased in channels with high-intensity sounds.

Clinical studies evaluating speech recognition in noise with ADRO have found that it allows for an improvement in the recognition of low-level speech, but the benefits of ADRO for speech recognition in noise have been mixed. Dawson et al. (2004) studied speech recognition for a group of 15 children using ADRO with the Nucleus® SPrint™ body-worn sound processor. Speech recognition in quiet and in noise was significantly better with use of the ADRO program compared with the children's standard program, which did not include preprocessing. Additionally, everyday sounds were comfortable with ADRO (Dawson et al., 2004). In contrast, James and colleagues (2002) evaluated speech recognition in quiet and in noise for a group of 9 adults using ADRO with the SPrint sound processor and found that ADRO improved recognition of low-level speech in quiet relative to the standard program, but provided no significant improvement in speech recognition in noise. James et al. (2002) did report a significant improvement in perceptual sound quality with ADRO compared with the conventional program.

ADRO and ASC typically are used in conjunction with one another. ASC does not affect speech recognition in quiet as it automatically disengages in quiet settings, and it significantly improves speech recognition in noise (Wolfe et al., 2009). As a result, ASC should be used in conjunction with ADRO in order to optimize the recognition of speech in noise as well as the recognition of low-level speech in quiet.

Beam. **Beam** preprocessing, as used in the Focus program in the SmartSound iQ input processing scheme, utilizes the outputs of both processor microphones to create an adaptively varying directional microphone response. In noisy environments, the nulls of the Focus directional pattern are positioned to provide maximum attenuation for the locations in the rear hemisphere at which the most intense competing noise is arriving. However, this adaptive attenuation is disengaged when speech is the primary input present from the rear hemisphere (i.e., a positive SNR exists at the rear hemisphere). The focus mode significantly improves speech recognition in noise when speech is presented in front of the listener and the noise is from the side and back (Spriet et al., 2007). Focus should be used by adults in conjunction with ADRO and ASC, but it is most appropriate for use in noisy environments where the primary talker will be in close proximity (within 3–6 feet) in front of the user. In addition, the recipient must be counseled to face the talker and maintain a close proximity (i.e., 3–4 feet). Full-time use of Focus may limit access to speech and other important sounds that arrive from behind and from the sides of a recipient. It should be noted that the Beam algorithm is implemented across all channels in order to provide a frequency-specific directional response (i.e., theoretically, the polar plots of two different channels may vary depending on differences that exist in the signals present at those channels).

Zoom. **Zoom** preprocessing utilizes the two omnidirectional microphones to create a fixed, hypercardioid polar plot pattern with a maximum null at 120 degrees (in the horizontal plane) when worn on the right ear or 240 degrees (in the horizontal plane) when worn on the left ear (Figure 16–35) for an illustration of the polar plots associated with Beam, Zoom, and the Standard directional modes). Wolfe et al. (2012) reported that a large group of adult recipients received almost a 6 dB improvement in the SNR required for 50% sentence recognition with Zoom preprocessing relative to their performance with the conventional microphone mode. Cochlear reports that Zoom provides optimal attenuation of diffuse noise. It should be noted that Zoom does not function adaptively, but instead, it implements a fixed directional response. As a result, this setting is unlikely to be appropriate for full-time use, because it is likely that the recipient will at least occasionally need to hear sounds that arrive from the rear hemisphere.

The standard microphone mode of Nucleus sound processors is intended for use in quiet environments. It possesses a slightly positive directivity index (DI) as it seeks to mimic the directional response of the unaided ear. The manufacturer's objective was to avoid the use of an omnidirectional response for full-time use, because the classic omnidirectional response when worn on the head is most sensitive to sounds arriving from the side of the user. As a result, the conventional omnidirectional response has a negative DI, which may be detrimental for communication in face-to-face listening situations.

SCAN. **SCAN** preprocessing is the first signal processing algorithm available in a commercial cochlear implant sound processor to perform scene analysis and automatically switch from the conventional microphone response to an adaptive beam-forming mode. The SCAN scene analysis attempts to determine whether the acoustic environment primarily comprises speech in quiet, speech in noise, noise, quiet (low-level or no sound present), wind, or music. Based on the results of the scene analysis, SCAN automatically selects the most appropriate preprocessing schemes for the given environment. If speech in noise is the primary input, then the processor automati-

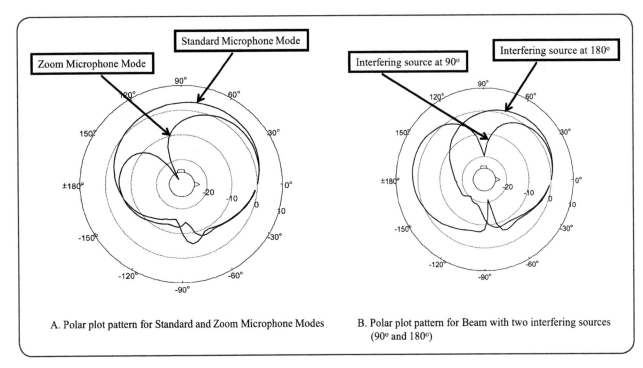

A. Polar plot pattern for Standard and Zoom Microphone Modes

B. Polar plot pattern for Beam with two interfering sources (90° and 180°)

FIGURE 16–35. Illustration of polar plot patterns associated with Beam, Zoom, and Standard microphone modes. These responses were measured on a B&K HATS mannequin. Image provided courtesy of Cochlear Americas, ©2018.

cally switches to the adaptive beam-forming mode. The activation threshold for activation to switch from the conventional microphone mode to a directional mode is 50 dB SPL. When noise is the only signal present, the sound processor will switch from the conventional microphone mode to the Zoom mode, which has a fixed, hypercardioid polar plot pattern. If speech and noise are both present, then SCAN will adaptively transition to beam-forming mode. At the time of this writing, there were no peer-reviewed publications reporting the potential benefits of SCAN. However, Wolfe et al. (2015) found an 18 percentage point improvement in speech recognition in noise with SCAN compared with performance without SCAN processing. Furthermore, word recognition in quiet was similar between the SCAN and conventional programs. Based on this study and others (De Ceulaer et al., 2017; Mauger et al., 2014; Plasmans et al., 2016), the author's preliminary recommendation is to select SCAN for adult recipients and school-age children.

However, the author of this book is not as clear on the use of SCAN for infants and young children. There are essentially no published studies examining the potential benefits and limitations of adaptive input processing schemes for young children. Similarly, there are a few published studies examining digital noise reduction and automatic, adaptive directionality for young children with hearing aids. In general, these studies have suggested that digital noise reduction in hearing aids does not degrade speech recognition in noise and may actually improve sound quality, comfort, and speech recognition, particularly when the competing noise is steady state in nature (Pittman, 2011; Pittman & Hiipakka, 2013; Stelmachowicz et al., 2010). In contrast, the evidence for the use of directional amplification with children is mixed. Some researchers have suggested that the benefits of an automatic, adaptive directional system outweigh any limitations (Ching et al., 2009; Dillon et al., 2012; King, 2010). Specifically, Dillon (2012) noted that directional amplification may improve speech understanding in noise and pointed out that young children frequently orient toward the signal of interest. Indeed, Ching and colleagues (2009) evaluated young children's tendency to orient toward the signal of interest and estimated simulated directional benefit based on the children's orientation toward speech present in their environment. Ching et al. (2009) concluded that the net detriment of directional use in real-world settings is likely to be negligible at worst.

Additionally, Dillon noted that directional amplification is not highly directional in real-world use because the automatic gain control present in most hearing aids partially nullifies the attenuation provided to sounds arriving from the rear hemisphere, and reverberation present in most realistic environments limits the directivity of a directional microphone. Finally, Dillon (2012) noted that modern automatic, adaptive hearing aids are unlikely to provide significant attenuation for rearward arriving sounds when the primary sound arriving from behind is speech. Consistent with the aforementioned information, the Australian Hearing's Protocol for Pediatric Amplification recommends providing automatic, adaptive directional hearing aids for infants and toddlers with hearing loss (King, 2010).

Although directional hearing aids can improve speech recognition in noise, there is an understandable reticence toward recommending directional technology with infants and young children. The primary concern stems from the potential for directional hearing aids to limit a child's access to important speech and environmental sounds arriving from behind or to the side of the child. Incidental listening refers to a listener's ability to attend to a message that is not directly intended for the listener. For instance, incidental listening occurs while a child is sitting in the corner of the room playing with a toy while also passively listening to a conversation his parents are having across the room. Estimates suggest that incidental listening accounts for 60% to 90% of what children learn about language (Ching et al., 2009; Cole & Flexer, 2007). If directional amplification limited access to incidental sounds arriving from behind a child, the child's model for language development may be compromised. Also, directional amplification may potentially hinder audibility for warning sounds arriving from behind (e.g., a car horn). Indeed, there are research studies that indicate that directional amplification can be detrimental to a child's speech understanding ability when the signal of interest arrives from behind the child (Ching et al., 2009; Ricketts, Galster, & Tharpe, 2007). Ricketts and colleagues (2007) evaluated the speech recognition in noise of 26 children who ranged in age from 10 to 17 years old and used hearing aids capable of switching between omnidirectional and directional mode. The evaluation was completed in a classroom environment, and the noise was presented from four loudspeakers located in the corners of the classroom. Speech recognition in noise was assessed while the signal of interest arrived from the front of as well as from behind the child. Compared with performance in the omnidirectional mode, children received a 2 dB improvement in the SNR with directional amplification when the signal of interest arrived from the front. However, when the signal of interest arrived from behind the children, the SNR required for 50% correct performance was 2 dB poorer in the directional mode. Ricketts et al. (2007) concluded that children should only use directional amplification when the signal of interest is located in the front hemisphere and that hearing aids should be equipped with the ability to switch between directional and omnidirectional modes. Consistent with the concern that directional amplification may hinder access to important speech and environmental sounds arriving from behind a child, the Ontario Infant Hearing Program's protocol for the provision of amplification in children indicates that audiologists refrain from fitting directional amplification on infants and toddlers (Bagatto, Scollie, Hyde, & Seewald, 2010).

The author of this book routinely provides automatic adaptive technology to school-aged children with hearing loss. These children are typically capable of describing their listening experience and are able to voice displeasure with limitations in the signal they receive. In contrast, infants and toddlers are typically unable to provide feedback pertaining to the signal they receive. As previously discussed, the language development of infants and toddlers is largely dependent on their ability to access sounds that arrive from all directions. Furthermore, infants and toddlers often fail to orient toward the speech signals present in their environment. As a result, a directional processor may hinder their full-time access to speech arriving from all directions in their environments. For now, the author of this text prefers to disable automatic adaptive directional programs (e.g., SCAN) for infants and toddlers (3 years and younger) and select the standard microphone mode for these recipients. Additional research is required to explore the benefits and limitations of real-world use of automatic adaptive directional systems for infants and toddlers with cochlear implants.

ForwardFocus. ForwardFocus is a feature that uses the two omnidirectional microphones of the Nucleus 7 sound processor to provide substantial attenuation to sounds arriving from the rear hemisphere. ForwardFocus is a clinician-enabled feature that may be loaded into a program that the recipient may enable in noisy situations in which the speech signal of interest arrives from the front and the noise is located behind

the recipient. ForwardFocus provides a greater reduction in sounds arriving from the rear hemisphere than Beam and Zoom, so recipients may consider switching to a program containing ForwardFocus when communication in noise is difficult with the use of Scan. Use of ForwardFocus may be undesirable in quiet situations, because it may reduce audibility of sounds the recipient may desire to hear. Recipients must be able to recognize situations in which ForwardFocus may improve speech recognition (i.e., in noisy environments when the speech is arriving from the front and the noise is arriving from behind), and the recipient must be able to position himself/herself so that the speech signal of interest does arrive from the front and the noise arrives from behind. ForwardFocus is generally considered appropriate for use with adults or older children (e.g., teenagers), because it is intended to be included in a program that is manually selectable for noisy situations. At the time of this writing, ForwardFocus is only available in the Nucleus 7 sound processor.

SNR-NR. **Signal-to-noise ratio noise reduction**, or **SNR-NR**, is a digital preprocessing algorithm that analyzes the SNR of each channel and automatically reduces the gain of channels comprising primarily noise. The primary goals of SNR-NR are to improve speech understanding and listening comfort in environments with steady-state noise, such as automobile or industrial noise. Dawson, Mauger, and Hersbach (2011) evaluated an early prototype of the SNR-NR algorithm with 13 experienced cochlear implant recipients and found about a 2 dB improvement in the SNR necessary for 50% sentence recognition compared with performance with conventional ACE signal coding. Mauger, Dawson, and Hersbach (2012) also evaluated a prototype of the SNR-NR algorithm and found that SNR-NR provided a 27 percentage point improvement in sentence recognition in the presence of steady-state competing noise and a 7 percentage point improvement in sentence recognition in the presence of babble noise relative to performance with conventional ACE signal coding. Likewise, Wolfe and colleagues (2015) evaluated SNR-NR and a group of 93 older children and adults and found a mean improvement of 8.5 percentage points on AzBio sentence recognition in noise with SNR-NR compared with performance without SNR-NR. The aforementioned improvements are quite impressive for a single-microphone noise reduction technology. The SNR-NR feature is only available in the Nucleus 6 sound processor.

Wind Noise Reduction. **Wind noise reduction (WNR)** automatically switches to a polar plot pattern more closely resembling an omnidirectional response because use of a directional microphone in wind enhances the level of the wind noise. Additionally, WNR reduces the gain for channels that are dominated by wind noise. Although no peer-reviewed publications examining the WNR existed at the time of this writing, Cochlear has reported on an in-house study with 13 experienced adult recipients and found a 22 percentage point improvement in sentence recognition in the presence of wind noise with the use of WNR relative to the WNR-disabled condition.

Whisper. The goal of **Whisper** is to enhance audibility for low-level signals or sounds that originate from a distance. At default settings, the Nucleus 6 sound processor provides audibility for inputs down to 25 dB SPL. In addition, ADRO enhances access to these low-level sounds. However, Whisper may also be used to further enhance the salience of low-level sounds. The primary function of Whisper is to place low-to-moderate level sounds (e.g., ≤52 dB SPL) into a higher position in the EDR relative to typical settings. This may be helpful for stimuli with a wide range of inputs, such as music or television, but it has been shown to potentially impair performance in noise (McDermott, Henshall, & McKay, 2002). Therefore, full-time use of Whisper is not recommended. Nevertheless, Whisper most likely should be enabled when listening to music, speech, or television in quiet environments. Whisper and ADRO are enabled in the "Music" program within the Custom Sound software.

Selecting SmartSound iQ Options for Various Programs. The aforementioned SmartSound iQ input processing schemes may be used simultaneously with one another. As stated previously, the audiologist selects which SmartSound iQ preprocessing schemes are available in each program slot in the "Write to Processor" section of Custom Sound. Within the "Program Settings" menu, the audiologist may access additional settings that affect how the sound processor is configured (Figure 16–36). The "Processor Configuration"

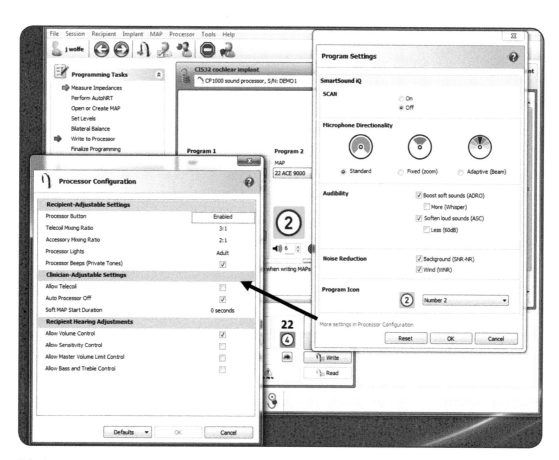

FIGURE 16–36. Processor configuration. Image provided courtesy of Cochlear Americas, ©2018.

menu may also be accessed by selecting the image of the processor in the lower middle section of the "Write to Processor" module (see Figure 16–36). The top one-third of the "Processor Configuration" menu allows the audiologist to set defaults for several parameters that are adjustable by the recipient using the Cochlear Remote Assistant. For instance, the audiologist may lock the buttons on the sound processor in order to prevent the recipient from inadvertently changing the program, telecoil, or volume settings. Also, the default telecoil and accessory-mixing ratios may be adjusted within this menu. The telecoil-mixing ratio determines the relative strength of signals from the telecoil and the sound processor microphone. The processor's built-in telecoil receives signals via electromagnetic induction and may be activated manually or in automatic mode for hearing on telecoil-compatible telephones or in conjunction with induction loop hearing-assistance technology (e.g., FM system with neckloop).

In Custom Sound, the default **Telecoil-Mixing** ratio is 3:1 for adults and 1:1 for children, but the user may adjust the ratio with the Cochlear Remote Assistants to allow for more or less emphasis from the sound processor microphone. A 3:1 mixing ratio provides 10 dB of attenuation to the signal from the processor microphone, whereas a 2:1 mixing ratio provides 6 dB of attenuation to the processor microphone. A 1:1 mixing ratio offers no attenuation to the signal from the sound processor microphone.

The **accessory-mixing ratio** functions exactly the same as the telecoil mixing ratio, but it influences the relative strength of signals from the sound processor microphone and the direct audio input source. The default accessory mixing ratio is 2:1 for adults and 1:1 for children (i.e., 6 dB reduction to processor microphone)

Furthermore, the audiologist may alter the operation of the sound processor's LED light, which indicates processor functionality or a fault condition. There are two choices: (1) Child: Indicator lights are displayed (flickers green) for microphone and DAI inputs exceeding 25 dB SPL, and the indicator light is displayed (flashes yellow) to indicate a fault condition and when Auto Processor Off has powered down the implant; (2) Adult: Indicator light flashes yellow to indicate a fault when the processor is off the head. The private tone indicator may also be enabled/disabled within the "Processor Configuration" menu.

Furthermore, the audiologist may alter several settings that cannot be altered by the recipient with the Cochlear Remote Assistant. For example, the audi-

ologist may determine whether the telecoil is enabled/disabled. The author of this book recommends disabling the telecoil for infants, young children, and all other recipients who do not possess the cognitive or motor abilities to manually activate the telecoil when appropriately needed. If the telecoil is enabled within this menu, the recipient may activate it by pressing the push button of the processor or by pressing the appropriate button on the Cochlear Remote Assistant. As a result, the telecoil may be inadvertently activated by recipients who do not understand its use or do not have good manual dexterity.

The **Auto Telecoil** may also be enabled/disabled within this section. As mentioned previously, the automatic telecoil engages when a fluctuating electromagnetic signal with desirable speech-like characteristics is present from a nearby telephone or induction loop system. When the Auto Telecoil is enabled in the Custom Sound software, the user may enable or disable the automatic telecoil feature with the Cochlear Remote Assistant; however, when this feature is disabled in the software, it is unavailable to the user even via the remote control. In this case, the user may manually engage and disengage the telecoil with the Cochlear Remote Assistant and with a button located on the upper spine of the processor.

The "**Auto Processor Off**" parameter controls a feature that powers down the processor if a link is not achieved between the sound processor and the recipient's implant over the course of two minutes. "Auto Processor Off" may be enabled/disabled within this menu. The author of this book recommends enabling the feature for adults but disabling it for children.

In the Processor Configuration screen, the audiologist may also enable and disable the **Master Volume Control and Bass and Treble Control** options. The Master Volume and Bass and Treble controls may be adjusted with use of their Nucleus Smart App for Nucleus 7 users or with the CR230 (in Advanced Mode) for Nucleus 6 users. The Master Volume Control gives the recipient the ability to adjust his/her C levels by ±10 CL (in 2 CL steps) from the C levels that the audiologist sets in the recipient's program. For instance, if the C levels are set to 150 CL, the recipient could use the Master Volume Control to adjust the C levels up to 160 CL or down to 140 CL. Of note, the C levels may not be adjusted above the voltage compliance limits. If the electrical dynamic range is less than 10 CL, then a reduction in the Master Volume Control will also decrease C and T levels in 2 CL steps (but when the Master Volume Control is increased again, then both

T and C levels will be increased). The purpose of the Master Volume Control is to provide the recipient with the ability to fine-tune his/her C levels based on listening experiences in daily environments. The conventional volume control setting adjusts stimulation levels within the electrical dynamic range that is established by the C levels the recipient has set with the Master Volume Control. The Master Volume Control may be used to independently set C levels at a preferred listening level for each program (i.e., C levels could be set to 156 CL for Program #1, 144 CL for Program #2, and 150 CL for Program #3. Of note, the Master Volume Control setting shown on the recipient's remote control corresponds to the average C level he/she is using (e.g., 156 CL in Program #1). The Master Volume Control cannot be enabled for programs with the following characteristics:

- Double electrode MAPping
- Electric-acoustic program
- CIS signal coding
- Programs with less than 12 active channels
- Programs in which the channel number and electrode number are not identical
- Programs in which voltage compliance limits have not been measured
- Programs with pulse width greater than 100 μsec or mixed pulse widths across channels

If the sound processor coil is off the recipient's head, then the Master Volume Control may not be increased. However, the Master Volume Control may be decreased while the sound processor coil is off of the recipient's head. When a recipient has adjusted the C levels with the Master Volume Control and his/her sound processor is connected to Custom Sound, a new program will be created in Custom Sound with the new preferred Master Volume Control C level. A red dot will appear next to the new program to indicate the fact that the program was created based on the recipient's adjustments.

The Bass and Treble Control allows the recipient to adjust the C levels for apical and basal channels by ±6 CL in 2 CL steps. The Bass and Treble Control is designed to provide the recipient with the opportunity to make fine-tuning adjustments to improve hearing performance and sound quality (e.g., too sharp, too tinny, too hollow). The recipient may adjust the Bass and Treble Control via the Nucleus Smart App for the Nucleus 7 sound processor and the CR230 Remote Assistant for the Nucleus 6 processor. As with the Master Volume Control, Bass and Treble Control

adjustments are included in a new program when the sound processor is connected to Custom Sound.

Once the desired programs are selected to be loaded onto the recipient's sound processor and the processor is configured as desired, the audiologist simply selects the "Write" button to program the processor with the selected programs and settings. It is necessary for the processor and transmitting coil to be in place on the recipient's head so that the radio frequency (RF) power level required to operate the processor may be measured and programmed into the processor. Once this measure is completed, the requisite RF power is saved in the recipient's file for that programming session and will be used when the same programs are loaded to processors at later dates (assuming the audiologist opens to file for the session date at which the desired programs were saved to the sound processor). RF power level is explained in detail below.

Power Level and Battery Life

The **power level** determines the strength of the RF signal necessary to deliver the requisite information from the external transmitting coil to the internal device without intermittencies or interruption. The power level is automatically estimated in Custom Sound when new programs are loaded onto the sound processor (Figure 16–37). Power level is determined by several factors, such as stimulation levels and impedance, but the primary determinant is the thickness of the recipient's skin flap. The power level should be measured at every programming session. An inaccurate power level will result in signal intermittencies or an unnecessary waste of power with reduced battery life. The Custom Sound software measurement of the automatic power level estimate is sufficient for the vast majority of recipients. However, if the recipient complains that the signal "cuts out" in noisy environments, the audiologist may want to set manually the RF power level to 10% higher than the estimated value.

A power level of 100% corresponds to the maximum voltage the processor can provide based on the power limits (i.e., voltage range) of the battery. Power level is determined by the amount of voltage necessary to deliver the RF signal across the skin flap and maintain a consistent, intermittent-free signal at the electrode with the highest power requirements (i.e., highest C levels and electrode impedance) while the recipient communicates in a high-level noise environment. Each sound processor and battery option

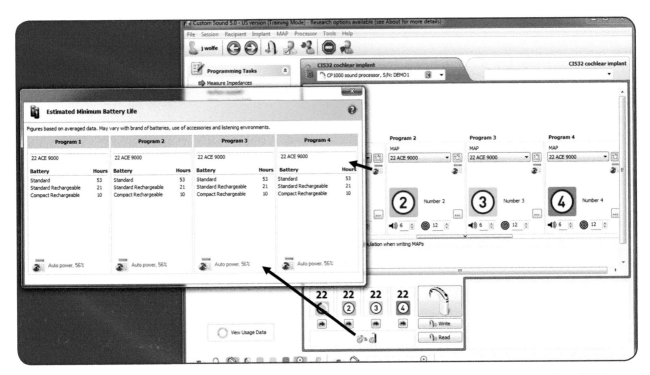

FIGURE 16–37. Power level for each program and estimated battery life. Image provided courtesy of Cochlear Americas, ©2018.

possesses a theoretical power level maximum limit. Because the maximum power level is determined on a processor-specific basis, it is not appropriate to compare power level required for one processor to the power level required for another model of processor.

The rechargeable batteries provide a 100% power level. As a result, recipient with thick skin flaps and high power needs (i.e., high stimulation levels) may be more inclined to experience a consistently intact signal without intermittencies and perform better with rechargeable batteries compared with the performance with two #675 zinc-air batteries. It should be noted that the rechargeable batteries can generally support higher power levels without signal intermittency, but excessively high power levels are generally associated with reduced battery life.

Given the power constraints of the different processors, explicit instructions are provided as to which battery options are suitable for use by a recipient. In most cases, all battery options are suitable, but in some rare cases, there may be some battery configurations that may not provide sufficient power, particularly toward the end of the battery life. Because children may not be able to report potential sound quality issues, they should use battery options that will guarantee suitable power.

It is important to note that it is occasionally difficult to accurately estimate power level for recipients with very thin skin flaps. In some cases, the telemetry may be interrupted when recipients with thin skin flaps operate their processors in daily use. In this event, the recipient may complain of signal intermittencies and/or the LED light, and data logging may indicate that a consistent lock is not obtained. If these issues occur, the audiologist may adhere a layer of mole skin to the underneath side of the coil or use a small plastic ring (spacer) provided by Cochlear to attach to the underneath side of the coil. Either solution artificially increases the width of the skin flap and allows for accurate provision of power level.

On the opposite end of the spectrum, it may be difficult to provide sufficient power to maintain a continuous lock and telemetry for recipients with unusually thick skin flaps. For recipients with thick skin flaps, it may be necessary to shave the hair over the skin flap to facilitate a connection. Typically, the pressure from the coil on the skin flap will result in "thinning" of the skin flap over time. Thick skin flaps are typically associated with high power levels, which will result in lower battery life. Also, it is more favorable to use rechargeable batteries, which possess a higher power level capacity than two zinc-air batteries. Finally, the RF power level may be changed to a manual mode in the "Parameters" menu ("Power" tab) of the "Set Levels" screen (see Figure 16–18). This adjustment is rarely needed. If a recipient complains of intermittencies, the audiologist can adjust the RF power level to an alternative setting in an attempt to eliminate the intermittency.

After power level is measured, the Custom Sound software also provides an estimate of the life (in hours) that a recipient should expect to receive from different battery configurations (see Figure 16–37). Battery life is influenced by skin flap thickness, stimulation levels, and electrode impedances. As one might expect, lower battery life is achieved for recipients with thicker skin flaps and higher stimulation levels and electrode impedances. It should be noted that the battery life measure is a general estimate of the life one should expect from a particular type of battery. Battery life will be shorter if the recipient uses a personal digital RF/FM receiver or wireless streaming (i.e., GN ReSound wireless accessories). Battery life will also be shorter if the recipient continually communicates in high-level noise environments.

Bilateral Mapping

The Custom Sound platform allows for simultaneous mapping of recipients with bilateral cochlear implants via two programming pod interfaces connected to the computer. The "**Bilateral Balancing**" tab allows for the activation of the bilateral sound processors in live speech mode (Figure 16–38). Global adjustments to T and C levels will ensure loudness balance between the two ears for speech and environmental sounds. Most users require a slight individualized reduction in C levels when listening in the bilateral mode compared with the unilateral conditions, which is likely related to binaural summation. The frequency allocation table for each processor may also be adjusted within the "Bilateral Balance" platform.

Neural Response Telemetry Measurement and AutoNRT

Neural Response Telemetry (NRT) is the feature within Custom Sound ("Perform AutoNRT") that allows the audiologist to measure the recipient's electrically evoked compound action potential (eCAP). The AutoNRT platform allows for the automatic

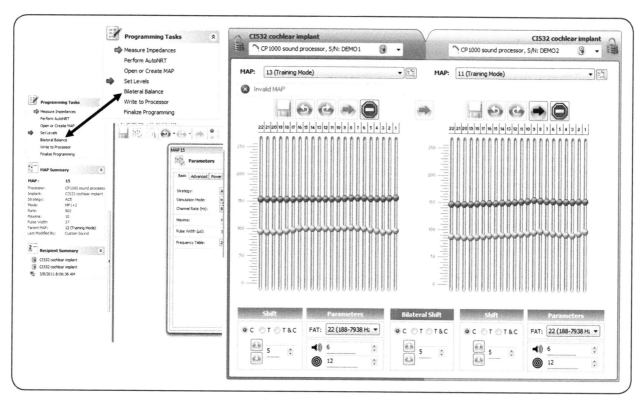

FIGURE 16–38. Bilateral cochlear implant programming. Image provided courtesy of Cochlear Americas, ©2018.

measurement and estimation of NRT thresholds. Measurement of the eCAP response in the autoNRT platform will be discussed further in Chapter 18.

View Usage Data

The View Usage Data platform allows the audiologist to review a data logging report that provides comprehensive information pertaining to the total use and usage patterns for the recipient since the previous programming session. The audiologist may review the number of hours the processor is used per day, the number of hours in which link is obtained/lost, the frequency in which programs are used, and acoustic characteristics of the environments the user encounters (Figure 16–39). This data logging feature was the first of its kind to be commercially introduced to the cochlear implant industry.

Finalize Programming

The "Finalize Programming" platform is simply a mechanism for the audiologist to record notes for a programming session and to generate both a clinic report (with MAP/Program parameters) as well as a report for the recipient to take home.

Programming Previous Generations of Nucleus Implants

Cochlear Ltd. has made a conscientious effort to offer the latest sound processor technology to its earliest recipients (Nucleus 22 users). However, due to limitations of the signal processor within the Nucleus 22 implant, as of now, it is only compatible for use with the Nucleus 6 sound processor.

In addition, the same programming software can be used across all generations of implants, which greatly simplifies programming for audiologists. The basic principles described in the previous section will enable an audiologist to program most Nucleus implants with a few exceptions.

Programming of the Nucleus 5 sound processor is essentially identical to the process of programming the Nucleus 6 sound processor described previously. The primary difference is that the Nucleus 5 sound processor is not capable of using SCAN, SNR-NR, and WNR input processing. As a result, the default "Everyday" program utilizes ASC+ADRO. The "Noise" program features Zoom+ASC+ADRO, whereas the "Focus"

program features Beam+ASC+ADRO. Finally, the "Music" program uses ADRO+Whisper. Additionally, the Nucleus 5 sound processor does not possess data logging, so that feature is obviously unavailable in Custom Sound. Finally, the wireless streaming accessories are unavailable with the Nucleus 5 sound processor.

The aforementioned programming differences between the Nucleus 5 and 6 sound processors also apply to the Freedom sound processor. Also, Zoom is unavailable in the Freedom sound processor, as is the Auto telecoil. Additionally, the Freedom sound processor does not have a remote assistant, so the telecoil- and accessory-mixing ratios must be made to individual programs that are loaded onto the Freedom sound processor.

There are also a handful of differences pertaining to the programming of Nucleus 22 implants as well. First, Nucleus 22 internal devices must use the SPEAK signal coding strategy, which typically uses bipolar (BP) electrode coupling (although it rarely occurs, the audiologist may also select common ground coupling). The current default electrode coupling mode is BP+3 where the reference electrode is four electrodes apical to the stimulating electrode. However, when the SPEAK was first introduced, the default mode was BP+1, and many users continue to use that today. As a result, the four most apical electrodes are disabled in the user's program. If adequate loudness growth cannot be achieved with this configuration, a wider bipolar coupling mode (e.g., BP+4) may be used. Finally, a "variable" electrode coupling mode in SPEAK allows the audiologist to vary the bipolar coupling mode (i.e., BP+1, BP+2, BP+3, etc.) from one electrode to the next. In the variable mode, the audiologist should ensure that the expected tonotopic organization exists by sweeping at C level from apex to base.

Second, the Nucleus 22 device is not capable of making telemetry measures. As a result, the RF power required to provide a signal with consistent integrity across a variety of environments will need to be measured. Also, the audiologist should perform a Skin Flap measure to estimate its thickness (i.e., density). This information is used to estimate and optimize the RF power used in the recipient's program. Of note, it is also not possible to record NRT measures with recipients of the Nucleus 24M cochlear implant.

Finally, stimulation levels in the Nucleus 22 device may be measured in Stimulus Level units or Current Level units, the same scale used for contemporary devices. When using Current Level units, the pulse width is set at a fixed value. However, with

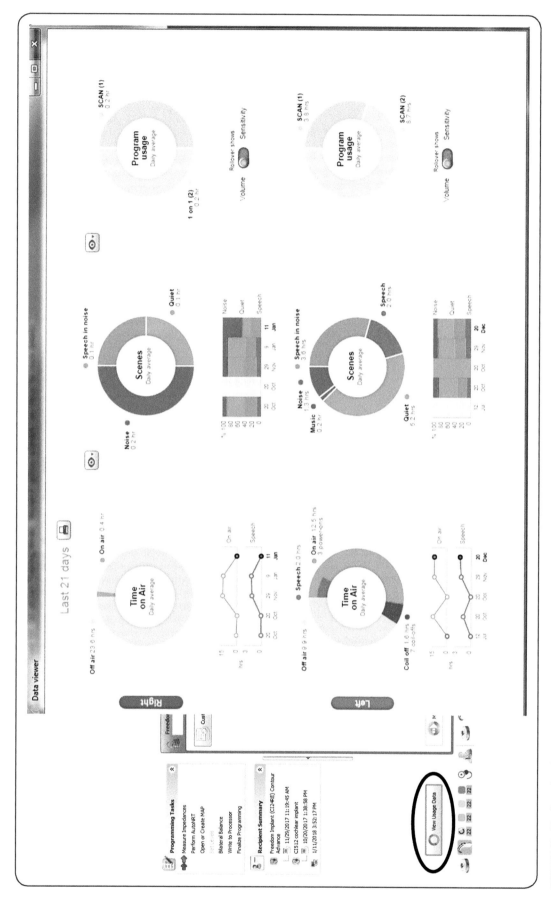

FIGURE 16–39. Data logging. Image provided courtesy of Cochlear Americas, ©2018.

Stimulus Level units, the pulse amplitude and the pulse width change in a complex manner in an attempt to minimize power as well as minimize time by providing the shortest possible pulse width. As a result, Stimulus Level units are preferred, but Current Level units may be used if manual determination of the pulse width is potentially advantageous.

Cochlear CR120 Remote Assistant

The Cochlear CR120 Remote Assistant may be used to measure electrode impedance and the electrically evoked compound action potential (i.e., NRT after the cochlear implant is inserted in the operating room or in an outpatient clinic (see Figure 16–40 for an example of the CR120 Remote Assistant). Cochlear has designed a fitting method to use the NRT thresholds to create a program that the recipient may use to have access to sound. The audiologist will then optimize the recipient's program using conventional programming methods.

Key Concepts

- Nucleus sound processors are programmed using the Custom Sound software.
- The primary and most important objective for programming Nucleus sound processors is to optimally set the recipient's T and C levels.
- Nucleus sound processors contain several types of adaptive signal processing, including ASC, ADRO, Scan, SNR-NR, WNR, and so forth. These

signal processing technologies have been shown to improve hearing performance in challenging listening situations and should be enabled for use by most recipients.
- ACE is the default signal coding strategy used by Nucleus recipients. Most Nucleus recipients perform quite well with ACE and the default stimulation rate of 900 pps. The programming audiologist may switch to alternate signal coding strategies and may adjust numerous other programming parameters to optimize the hearing performance of each individual recipient.

References

Bagatto, M., Scollie, S. D., Hyde, M., & Seewald, R. (2010). Protocol for the provision of amplification within the Ontario infant hearing program. *International Journal of Audiology, 49*(Suppl. 1), S70–S79.

Balkany, T., Hodges, A., Menapace, C., Hazard, L., Driscoll, C., Gantz, B., . . . Payne, S. (2007). Nucleus Freedom North American clinical trial. *Otolaryngology–Head and Neck Surgery, 136*(5), 757–762.

Beynon, A. J., Snik, A. F., & van den Broek, P. (2003). Comparison of different speech coding strategies using a disability-based inventory and speech perception tests in quiet and in noise. *Otology and Neurotology, 24*(3), 392–396.

Botros, A., Banna, R., & Maruthurkkara, S. (2013). The next generation of Nucleus® fitting: A multiplatform approach towards universal cochlear implant management. *International Journal of Audiology, 52*(7), 485–494. doi:10.3109/14992027.2013.781277

Brickley, G., Boyd, P., Wyllie, F., O'Driscoll, M., Webster, D., & Nopp, P. (2005). Investigations into electrically evoked stapedius reflex measures and subjective loudness percepts in

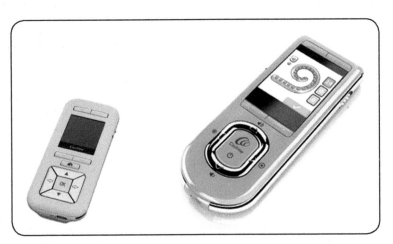

FIGURE 16–40. CR120 Remote Assistant. Image provided courtesy of Cochlear Americas, ©2018.

the MED-EL COMBI 40+ cochlear implant. *Cochlear Implants International*, *6*(1), 31–42.

Carhart, R., & Jerger, J. F. (1959). Preferred method for clinical determination of pure-tone thresholds. *Journal of Speech and Hearing Disorders*, *24*, 330–345.

Ching, T. Y. C., Dillon, H., Day, J., Crowe, K., Close, L., Chisholm, K., . . . Hopkins, T. (2009). Early language outcomes of children with cochlear implants: Interim findings of the NAL study on longitudinal outcomes of children with hearing impairment. *Cochlear Implants International*, *10*(Suppl. 1), 28–32.

Cole, E., & Flexer, C. (2007). *Children with hearing loss: Developing listening and talking, birth to six*. San Diego, CA: Plural.

Dawson, P. W., Decker, J. A., & Psarros, C. E. (2004). Optimizing dynamic range in children using the Nucleus cochlear implant. *Ear and Hearing*, *25*(3), 230–241.

Dawson, P. W., Mauger, S. J., & Hersbach, A. A. (2011). Clinical evaluation of signal-to-noise ratio based noise reduction in Nucleus cochlear-implant recipients, *Ear and Hearing*, *32*, 382–390.

De Ceulaer, G., Pascoal, D., Vanpoucke, F., & Govaerts, P. J. (2017). The use of cochlear's SCAN and wireless microphones to improve speech understanding in noise with the Nucleus 6® CP900 processor. *International Journal of Audiology*, *56*(11), 837–843.

Dillon, H. (2012). *Hearing aids* (2nd ed.). New York, NY: Thieme.

Dorman, M., Loizou, P., Spahr, A., & Maloff, E. (2002). A comparison of the speech understanding provided by acoustic models of fixed-channel and channel-picking signal processors for cochlear implants. *Journal of Speech, Language, and Hearing Research*, *45*(4), 783–788.

Gifford, R. H., & Revit, L. R. (2010). Speech perception for adult cochlear implant recipients a realistic background noise: Effectiveness of preprocessing strategies and external options for improving speech recognition in noise. *Journal of the American Academy of Audiology*, *21*(7), 441–451.

Hodges, A. V., Balkany, T. J., Ruth, R. A., Lambert, P. R., Dolan-Ash, S., & Schloffman, J. J. (1997). Electrical middle ear muscle reflex: Use in cochlear implant programming. *Otolaryngology–Head and Neck Surgery*, *117*(3 Pt. 1), 255–261.

James, C. J., Blamey, P. J., Martin, L., Swanson, B., Just, Y., & Macfarlane, D. (2002). Adaptive dynamic range optimization for cochlear implants: A preliminary study. *Ear and Hearing*, *23*(1 Suppl.), 49S–58S.

King A. (2010). The national protocol for paediatric amplification in Australia. *International Journal of Audiology*, *49*(Suppl. 1), S64–S69.

Lorens, A., Walkowiak, A., Piotrowska, A., Skarzynski, H., & Anderson, I. (2004). ESRT and MCL correlations in experienced paediatric cochlear implant users. *Cochlear Implants International*, *5*(1), 28–37.

Manrique, M., Huarte, A., Morera, C., Caballe, L., Ramos, A., Castillo, C., . . . Juan, E. (2005). Speech perception with the ACE and the SPEAK speech coding strategies for children implanted with the Nucleus cochlear implant. *International Journal of Pediatric Otorhinolaryngology*, *69*(12), 1667–1674.

Mauger, S. J., Dawson, P. W., & Hersbach, A. A. (2012). Perceptually optimized gain function for cochlear implant signal-to-noise ratio based noise reduction. *Journal of the Acoustical Society of America*, *131*(1), 327–336.

Mauger, S. J., Jones, M., Nel, E., & Del Dot, J. (2017). Clinical outcomes with the Kanso off-the-ear cochlear implant sound processor. *International Journal of Audiology*, *56*(4), 267–276.

Mauger, S. J., Warren, C. D., Knight, M. R., Goorevich, M., & Nel, E. (2014). Clinical evaluation of the Nucleus 6 cochlear implant

system: Performance improvements with SmartSound iQ. *International Journal of Audiology*, *53*(8), 564–576.

McDermott, H. J., Henshall, K. R., & McKay, C. M. (2002). Benefits of syllabic input compression for users of cochlear implants. *Journal of the American Academy of Audiology*, *13*, 14–24.

Muller-Deile, J., Kiefer, J., Wyss, J., Nicolai, J., & Battmer, R. (2008). Performance benefits for adults using a cochlear implant with adaptive dynamic range optimization (ADRO): A comparative study. *Cochlear Implants International*, *9*(1), 8–26.

Pittman A. (2011). Age-related benefits of digital noise reduction for short-term word learning in children with hearing loss. *Journal of Speech, Language, and Hearing Research*, *54*(5), 1448–1463. See more at: http://www.audiology.org/news/ Pages/20131017.aspx#sthash.o4AUO9iL.dpuf

Pittman, A. L., & Hiipakka, M. M. (2013). Hearing impaired children's preference for, and performance with, four combinations of directional microphone and digital noise reduction technology. *Journal of the American Academy of Audiology*, *24*, 832–844.

Plant, K., Law, M. A., Whitford, L., Knight, M., Tari, S., Leigh, J., . . . Nel, E. (2005). Evaluation of streamlined programming procedures for the Nucleus cochlear implant with the Contour electrode array. *Ear and Hearing*, *26*(6), 651–668.

Plasmans, A., Rushbrooke, E., Moran, M., Spence, C., Theuwis, L., Zarowski, A., Offeciers, E, . . . Mauger, S. J. (2016). A multicenter clinical evaluation of pediatric cochlear implant users upgrading to the Nucleus 6 system. *International Journal of Pediatric Otorhinolaryngology*, *83*, 193–199.

Ricketts, T., Galster, J., & Tharpe, A. M. (2007). Directional benefit in simulated classroom environments. *American Journal of Audiology*, *16*, 130–144.

Skinner, M., Holden, L., & Holden, T. (1994). Effect of frequency boundary assignment on speech recognition with the SPEAK speech-coding strategy. *Annals of Otology, Rhinology, and Laryngology*, *104*(Suppl. 166), 307–311.

Skinner, M. W., Holden, L. K., & Holden, T. A. (1997). Parameter selection to optimize speech recognition with the Nucleus implant. *Otolaryngology–Head and Neck Surgery*, *117*(3 Pt. 1), 188–195.

Skinner, M. W., Holden, L. K., Whitford, L. A., Plant, K. L., Psarros, C., & Holden, T. A. (2002). Speech recognition with the Nucleus 24 SPEAK, ACE, and CIS speech coding strategies in newly implanted adults. *Ear and Hearing*, *23*(3), 207–223.

Spriet, A., Van Deun, L., Eftaxiadis, K., Laneau, J., Moonen, M., van Dijk, B., . . . Wouters, J. (2007). Speech understanding in background noise with the two-microphone adaptive beamformer BEAM in the Nucleus Freedom cochlear implant system. *Ear and Hearing*, *28*(1), 62–72.

Stelmachowicz, P., Lewis, D., Hoover, B., Nishi, K., McCreery, R., & Woods, W. (2010) Effects of digital noise reduction on speech perception for children with hearing loss. *Ear and Hearing*, *31*(3), 345–355. See more at: http://www.audiology.org/news/ Pages/20100623.aspx#sthash.zMCu7V8y.dpuf

Stelmachowicz, P. G., Pittman, A. L., Hoover, B. M., & Lewis, D. E. (2001). Effect of stimulus bandwidth on the perception of /s/ in normal- and hearing impaired children and adults. *Journal of the Acoustical Society of America*, *110*(4), 2183–2190.

Wolfe, J., Neumann, S., Marsh, M., Schafer, E., Lianos, L., Gilden, J., . . . Jones, M. (2015). Benefits of adaptive signal processing in a commercially available cochlear implant sound processor. *Otology and Neurotology*, *36*(7), 1181–1190.

Wolfe, J., Parkinson, A., Schafer, E. C., Gilden, J., Rehwinkel, K., Mansanares, J., . . . Gannaway, S. (2012). Benefit of a commercially available cochlear implant processor with dual-microphone beamforming: A multi-center study. *Otology and Neurotology, 33*(4), 553–560.

Wolfe, J., Schafer, E. C., Heldner, B., Mulder, H., Ward, E., & Vincent, B. (2009). Evaluation of speech recognition in noise with cochlear implants and dynamic FM. *Journal of the American Academy of Audiology, 20*(7), 409–421.

Wolfe, J., Schafer, E. C., John, A., & Hudson, M. (2011). The effect of front-end processing on cochlear implant performance of children. *Otology and Neurotology, 32*(4), 533–538.

Wolfe, J., Schafer, E., Parkinson, A., John, A., Hudson, M., Wheeler, J., & Mucci, A. (2013). Effects of input processing and type of personal frequency modulation system on speech-recognition performance of adults with cochlear implants. *Ear and Hearing, 34*(1), 52–62.

Zwicker, E. (1961). Subdivision of the audible frequency range into critical bands. *Journal of the Acoustical Society of America, 33*(2), 248.

Zwolan, T., Heller, J., & McGreevy, C. (2012, May). *Atypical electrode impedance patterns and clinical outcomes.* Poster presentation at 12th International Conference on Cochlear Implants and Other Implantable Auditory Devices. Baltimore, MD.

Zwolan, T., & Overstreet, E. (2005). Setting upper program levels in children. In *Advanced Bionics auditory research bulletin* (pp. 54–56). Valencia, CA: Advanced Bionics Corporation.

17

Programming MED-EL Cochlear Implants

Jace Wolfe and Sara Neumann

Introduction to Programming MED-EL Cochlear Implants

This chapter will describe the principles, practices, and procedures pertaining to programming contemporary MED-EL cochlear implants.

Programming MED-EL Implants

The primary programming platform for current MED-EL sound processors is the **MAESTRO** software platform, which may be used to program essentially all existing sound processors, including the SONNET, RONDO, OPUS 2, OPUS 1, and the TEMPO+ sound processors. Recipients of any MED-EL cochlear implant (COMBI 40+, PULSAR CI100, SONATA TI100, CONCERT, and SYNCHRONY) may be programmed in the MAESTRO software. The following section describes programming of MED-EL cochlear implants in the MAESTRO programming platform. The programming process will be described in the order in which the various steps occur within the MED-EL programming software.

Patient Information Entry

Within the MAESTRO software, along the left side of the screen, there are multiple tabs. These tabs are referred to as the task column. The audiologist must select the first tab to enter or review patient information. If the patient is an established user who has transferred from another clinic, the audiologist must simply hook up the patient's sound processor to the MAX programming interface box. A pop-up box will automatically appear and auto-populate the patient's information into the programming software platform.

For a new patient, the audiologist must select the "New Patient" option, which is made available by selecting the "New" icon in the upper left corner of the MAESTRO homepage. The audiologist will then be prompted to enter the standard information, including name, date of birth, as well as sex/gender, and then she/he must select the tab with the implanted ear (Figure 17–1). The notifications pane in the lower third of the screen will prompt you to input requisite information, and those messages will disappear as the required information is entered. The audiologist should enter several pieces of information regarding the patient's internal (e.g., cochlear implant model and serial number, electrode array, surgery date) and external devices (e.g., sound processor model and external coil type) (Figures 17–2 and 17–3). Of note, if the audiologist does not have access to the serial number of the recipient's implant, then the audiologist may click on the "Read Serial" button on the right side of the screen. The MAESTRO software will interact with the implant's telemetry system to read the serial number as long as the audiologist has obtained a lock with the MED-EL Diagnostic MAX Coil S (for

487

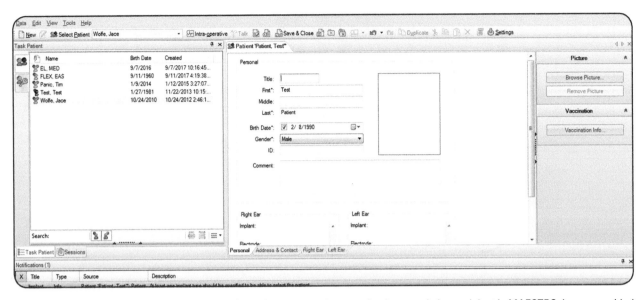

FIGURE 17–1. A visual example of the process of creating a new patient or selecting an existing recipient in MAESTRO. Image provided courtesy of MED-EL Corporation.

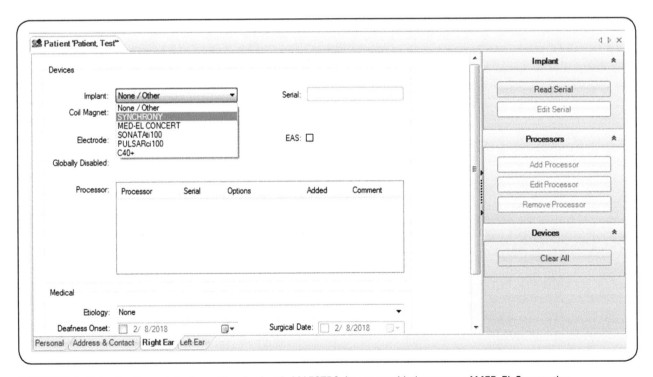

FIGURE 17–2. Selecting the recipient's cochlear implant in MAESTRO. Image provided courtesy of MED-EL Corporation.

use with SYNCHRONY implants) or MAX Coil (for use with all MED-EL implants developed prior to the SYNCHRONY) (Figure 17–4). Also of note, the audi-ologist must click on the "Add Processor" button on the right side of the screen to enter the processor and external coil information.

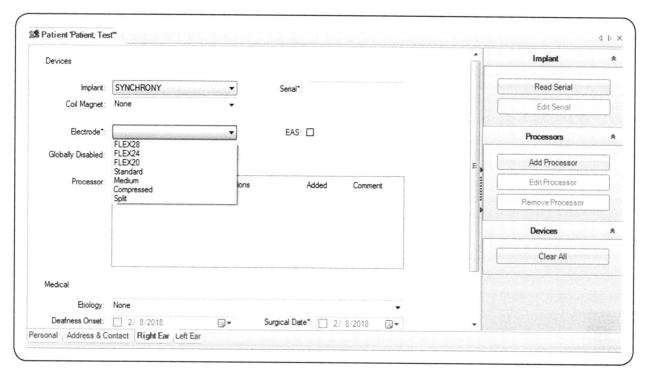

FIGURE 17–3. Selecting the recipient's electrode array in MAESTRO. Image provided courtesy of MED-EL Corporation.

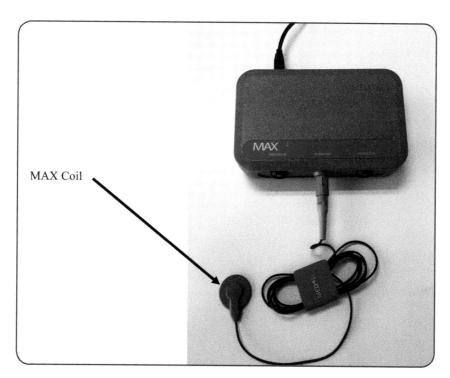

MAX Coil

FIGURE 17–4. The MED-EL MAX programming interface with MAX diagnostic coil. Image provided courtesy of MED-EL Corporation.

Connecting the Sound Processor and Conducting the Electrode Impedance Measurement

The **MED-EL MAX** programming interface is used to program MED-EL cochlear implants (Figure 17–5). The MAX connects to the programming computer by way of a USB cable to plugs into the standard USB 2.0 port of the computer and into the USB Type B socket on the back of the MAX. There are four additional ports on the Max: (1) two "Processor" sockets that allow for a connection to the recipient's sound processor via a proprietary programming cable, (2) one "Telemetry" socket to which the diagnostic telemetry coils (i.e., MAX Coil S or MAX Coil) may be connected, and (3) a "Trigger Connector" that allows for connection to an evoked potential system to signify the delivery of stimuli for electrically evoked brainstem response or cortical auditory evoked response assessment. LED lights reside above each socket to indicate that the respective device is connected and for which ear it is connected. A red light indicates that a right ear sound processor is connected, and a blue light indicates that a left ear sound processor is connected. A color-coded indicator is also present in a status bar at the bottom of the MAESTRO programming screen (Figure 17–6). The colors of the middle ring in the status bar are grayed out except for when the audiologist opens a menu that requires telemetry assessment (e.g., **impedance field telemetry**

[IFT] for electrode impedance assessment). When the diagnostic MAX coil is plugged into the "Telemetry" socket, the ring will turn red or blue depending upon whether the measure is being made on the right or left ear, respectively. Two working modes are available with the MAX interface: dynamic and fixed modes. The dynamic mode allows the audiologist to program a right or left sound processor with either "Processor" socket, whereas the fixed mode requires for the left socket to be used to program right ear sound processors and the right socket to be used for left ear sound processors. In dynamic mode, the rings in the status bar associated with the "Processor" socket are red and blue, whereas in the fixed mode, one ring in the status bar is blue and the other is red. When a processor is connected to the socket, a colored (red for right and blue for left) circle appears within the "Processor" ring (see Figure 17–6). If the incorrect processor is connected, an "X" will appear within the ring. Additionally, a dot will appear within the "Telemetry" ring if the MAX coil is correctly connected and a telemetry task is opened within the MAESTRO software. Furthermore, the status bar indicates the name of the connected processor and implant as well as the volume and sensitivity settings. Three different programming cables are available to allow for connection to the SONNET, RONDO, and other MED-EL behind-the-ear sound processors (Figure 17–7). The MAX is powered by the programming computer.

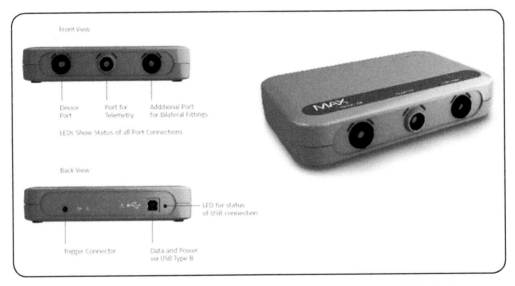

FIGURE 17–5. The MED-EL MAX programming interface. Image provided courtesy of MED-EL Corporation.

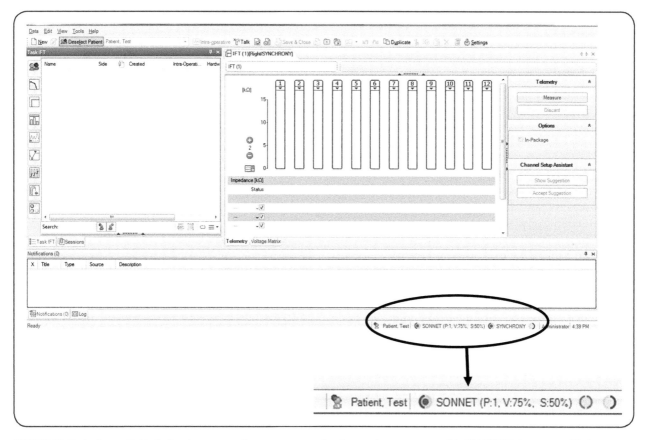

FIGURE 17–6. Indicator lights indicating connection to processor (and ear to be programmed) in MAESTRO. Image provided courtesy of MED-EL Corporation.

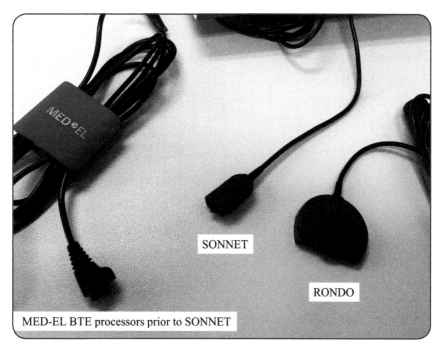

SONNET

RONDO

MED-EL BTE processors prior to SONNET

FIGURE 17–7. Programming cables used to program MED-EL sound processors. Image provided courtesy of MED-EL Corporation.

Electrode Impedance

The first step in programming MED-EL cochlear implants is to complete **IFT** measurements, which are used to provide an objective evaluation of the integrity of the implant electrode contacts and leads as well as the status of the electrode contact/tissue interface (see Figure 17–8 for an example of a normal setting). The audiologist must use a special diagnostic cable to complete telemetry measures in the MED-EL programming platform. Two diagnostic coils are available for MED-EL telemetry measures, the MAX Coil S and the MAX Coil. The audiologist must use the MAX Coil S when completing telemetry measures with recipients who have SYNCHRONY implants and the MAX Coil for recipients of CONCERT, SONATA TI100, PULSAR CI100, and the COMBI 40+ implants.

Once the correct MAX coil is selected for use, electrode impedances are measured at the 12 intracochlear electrode contacts relative to the reference electrode. The IFT task also allows for measurement of voltage distribution across all intracochlear electrodes when one active electrode is stimulated. These IFT measurements ensure the device is functioning properly and may guide or influence programming choices. Once the audiologist has selected a patient,

the IFT tab (the second tab in the task bar on the left side of the MAESTRO display) will automatically open.

Impedance results of the 12 intracochlear electrode contacts and one reference/ground electrode contact are displayed in kOhms in the IFT table. The impedance of the reference/ground electrode is affected by the surrounding tissue, the current conduction through the extracochlear medium, and the mechanical status of the electrode. The electrode impedance of the intracochlear electrode contacts is influenced by the status and integrity of the electrode leads and contacts as well as the characteristics of the surrounding cochlear fluids and tissues (i.e., fibrous tissue growth, perilymph, macrophages, proteins, etc.).

The impedance value of intracochlear electrode contacts will typically fall within 5 to 15 kOhms, while the typical ground path impedance is approximately 1 kOhm. The overall status of each electrode is provided under the impedance value and includes one of the following five categories. First, the "OK" status suggests that the voltage is within normal limits and suitable for stimulation (Figure 17–9). Second, the "Hi" status indicates that the voltage exceeds the normal limits of the system (open circuit) and cannot provide sufficient electrical current flow (see

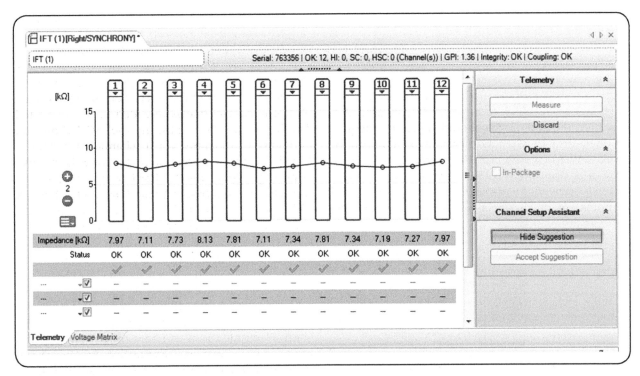

FIGURE 17–8. Impedance measurement with normal impedance results in MAESTRO. Image provided courtesy of MED-EL Corporation.

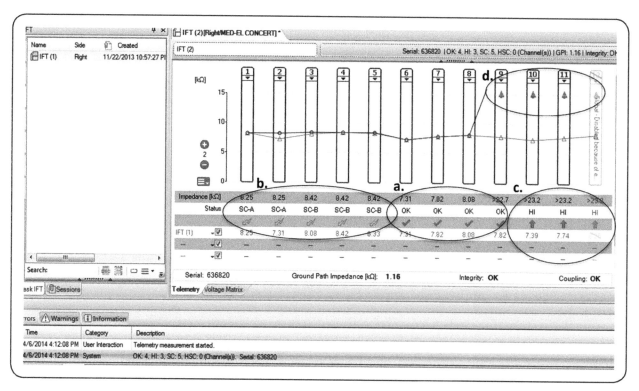

FIGURE 17–9. Impedance measurement with normal and abnormal impedance results in MAESTRO. Image provided courtesy of MED-EL Corporation.

Figure 17–9 c and d). Channels identified as open circuits (i.e., "Hi") should be deactivated. The software may also indicate an electrical impedance that is abnormal by noting a "greater than" (>) sign next to the impedance value. When the "greater than" (>) sign is seen next to a number, it indicates that the impedance is too high to be accurately measured. In that case, the audiologist should check for adequate loudness growth when measuring maximum comfort levels (MCLs) (see Figure 17–9 c and d). If loudness growth is considered to be okay, then the audiologist may leave that electrode active; however, if a full complement of channels is available for mapping, most audiologists elect to deactivate any "greater than" channels. If loudness growth is insufficient, then the audiologist should consider disabling the electrode contact. It should be noted that the impedance of the ground electrode of COMBI 40+ and PULSAR implants is typically higher (although it is still within normal limits) than the impedance of the ground electrode of SONATA, CONCERT, and SYN-CHRONY implants. The relatively higher (but normal) electrode impedance value measured on the ground electrode of the COMBI 40+ and PULSAR implants is

a relatively common finding that does not signify a problem with these implants but rather is due to the design of the ground electrode for those devices.

Third, the "SC-x" status refers to a short circuit and indicates that the signal also is traveling to another intracochlear electrode along with the electrode contact that is intended to be stimulated. The letter (e.g., "x") following the "SC-" allows the audiologist to identify which channels are shorted together in the event that more than one short circuit is present (Figure 17–9b). For instance, Figure 17–9 indicates that electrodes 1 and 2 are each labeled at "SC-a," whereas electrodes 3, 4, and 5 are labeled as "SC-b." These findings indicate that electrodes 1 and 2 are shorted together, and electrodes 3, 4, and 5 are shorted together. Fourth, the "SC?" or "HSC?" status indicates the rare situation where the software was unable to confirm the status of a possible shorted electrode and is intended to cue the audiologist to check the voltage table manually for a possible short. Electrode shorts can be manually identified by reviewing the **"Voltage Distribution Profile" (VDP)** table, which is described in the next section. If the voltage table confirms the presence of a short circuit, each (or all) of the electrode contacts that are determined to be shorted together should typically be disabled. However, if additional shorts are identified, the audiologist should consider contacting a MED-EL clinical representative to report that abnormality and to seek further direction.

Fifth, the "HSC-x" status suggests abnormally high electrode impedance in addition to electrical coupling to another electrode. The result of this test is generally intended to identify possible short circuits when the implant is tested in its sterile packaging, prior to implantation. It identifies possible short circuits even in the presence of very high impedance on the channels (as would be expected when the electrode and ground contacts are not contacting fluid or tissue). Finally, an "HSC?" status is shown when the reference electrode impedance is not measured correctly (although this is a rare finding when measured in vivo). Again, the VDP table will aid the audiologist with electrode management and review current spread on any given electrode.

In addition to the impedance value and status, the electrode impedance results table also displays the serial number of the internal SYNCHRONY, CONCERT, SONATA TI100, and PULSAR CI100 devices and the total number of functional, shorted, and open electrodes. Furthermore, the table describes the "integrity of the internal device electronics" and the quality of the coupling between the diagnostic MAX coil and the internal device. On the Integrity test, an "OK" status indicates normal functioning of the internal device electronics. If a "—" status is measured along with normal electrode impedance results, the audiologist should contact the MED-EL representative for further assessment of the internal device.

The quality of coupling may be described as either "OK," "Weak," "Faint," or "Poor." If the software indicates an "OK" status, it has determined that there is successful communication with the internal device. "Weak" or "Faint" classifications mean that only partial data can be obtained. If there is insufficient coupling between the diagnostic MAX coil and the implant, then the audiologist should reposition the MAX coil over the recipient's implant and/or attempt to improve the implant-to-coil distance to facilitate better adherence of the coil and the desired measurement. In the case of "poor" coupling, the audiologist should confirm that the MAX, cable, and diagnostic coils are adequately connected and functioning properly. If the coupling problem continues, the audiologist should contact the MED-EL representative.

The VDP table shows voltages measured across all electrodes when stimulating each electrode contact individually and provides a picture of how current fields spread in the cochlea. In the typical case, the voltage distributed to the stimulated electrode contact should be substantially greater than that at any of the other intracochlear electrodes. For example, if electrode 4 is the stimulated electrode contact and the voltage distributed to that electrode is 2.35 volts, then the voltage distributed across the other electrodes should be significantly lower than 2.35 volts (i.e., 0.3 volts may be measured across electrode 1). In practice, a small amount of voltage should be distributed across adjacent electrode contacts, but the values should be less than 50% of the voltage distributed across the stimulated contact. If voltages distributed across any other channel and the stimulated electrode are similar, it is likely that these two channels are shorted together. Figure 17–10 provides an example of the voltage distribution matrix/profile obtained for a normal IFT measurement). If the audiologist has concerns or questions pertaining to the recipient's IFT measures or interpretation of IFT results, then he/she should send the recipient's file to a MED-EL representative for further review.

Creating a Program in MAESTRO

Creating a program in Maestro is a fairly simple process requiring several steps that are discussed in the next few sections. To create a new program, the audiologist must right-click on the "Fitting" icon on the right side of the screen and select "New Fitting" (Figure 17–11).

Selecting a Signal Coding Strategy

The first step in creating a program in the MAESTRO programming platform is to select a signal coding strategy. The audiologist must access the "**Strategy**" tab to select the signal coding strategy that the recipient will use (Figure 17–12). As described in Chapter 8, there are four MED-EL signal coding strategies from which the audiologist may select: Fine Structure Processing (FSP), FS4, FS4-p, and one envelope coding strategy known as High Definition CIS (HDCIS). It should be noted that the FDA has not approved the use of the FS signal coding strategies with children in the prelingual age group in the USA. Most audiologists in the USA use these strategies with young children with success (i.e., off-label use).

Previous research suggests that the FSP strategies may yield better performance and sound quality relative to the older HDCIS strategy (see Chapter 8

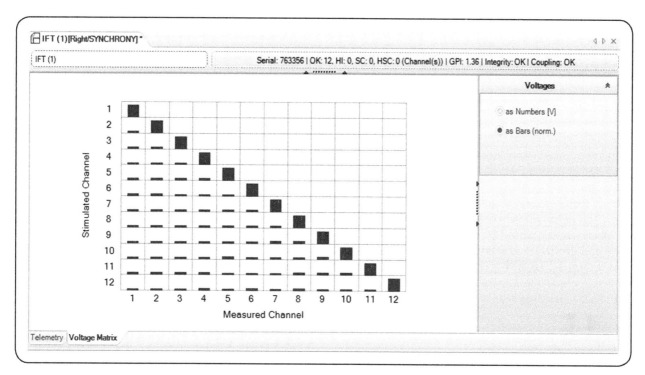

FIGURE 17–10. Voltage distribution table. Image provided courtesy of MED-EL Corporation.

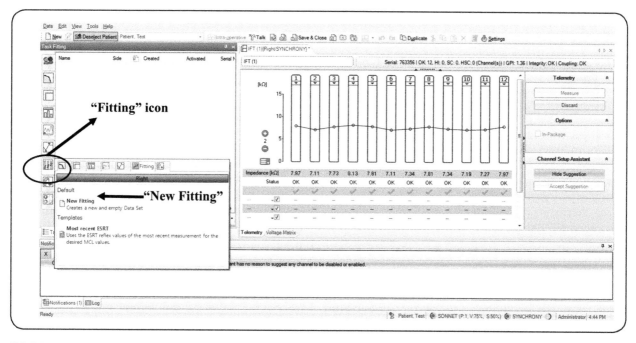

FIGURE 17–11. Creating a new program in MAESTRO. Image provided courtesy of MED-EL Corporation.

for a description of MED-EL signal coding strategies and a discussion of research exploring outcomes with MED-EL signal coding). FS4 and FS4-p provide fine structure processing over a larger number of apical channels (i.e., fine structure processing is provided to every channel which has a bandpass frequency

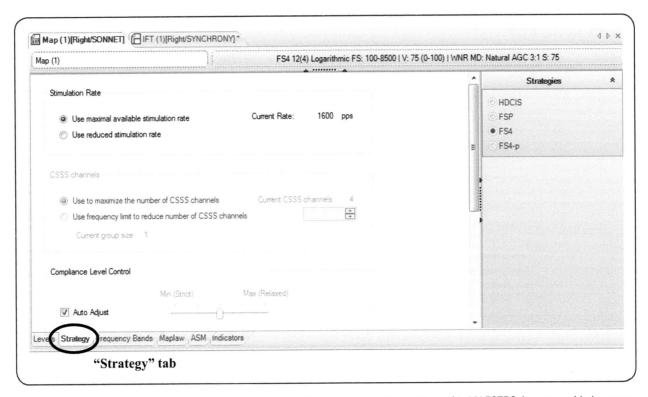

FIGURE 17–12. Selecting a signal coding strategy (along with stimulation rate, pulse width, etc.) in MAESTRO. Image provided courtesy of MED-EL Corporation.

that is entirely below 1000 Hz; for recipients with all 12 electrode contacts enabled, fine structure will be provided over the four most apical channels; if electrode contacts are disabled, then fine structure may be provided on three [or fewer] channels because the frequency up to 1000 Hz may be allocated across a smaller number of channels), which results in the provision of fine structure processing over a wider frequency range) compared with the traditional FSP strategy (i.e., typically just the first or second most apical channels). Therefore, the authors of this text recommend initial use of one of the newer generation of the FS strategies. Of note, FS4 is the default signal coding strategy in the Signal Coding Strategy tab of the MAESTRO software. If the recipient is not performing well with the FS strategies after several weeks of use, the HDCIS strategy may be used. It should be noted that the FS4-p strategy possesses a novel algorithm referred to as Channel Interaction Compensation (CIC), which seeks to minimize channel interaction. To maintain sufficient stimulation while minimizing channel interaction, CIC determines the current amplitudes for parallel stimulation so that the compound current amplitude is equal to the current

amplitude that would occur with sequential stimulation. FS4-p will stimulate two of the apical fine structure channels if and only if the zero-crossing detector recognizes that a zero crossing occurred within two fine structure channels during the last sample. The presence of multiple zero crossings within one sample happens only some small percentage of the time. However, when a zero crossing does occur within two fine structure channels within one sample, two fine structure channels will be stimulated simultaneously. CIC is needed in such a case in order to avoid unintentionally creating a virtual channel, so that both channels will be correctly represented without channel interaction.

Once the signal coding strategy is selected, the audiologist may also select from several other parameters related to stimulation within the coding strategy. For all MED-EL signal coding strategies, the audiologist may alter the stimulation rate. As with all signal coding strategies, the maximum stimulation rate is at least to an extent determined by the pulse width on individual channels. The primary unit of stimulation in the MAESTRO software is charge-based. As the charge delivered to a particular channel is increased, either the current amplitude or pulse width (duration) (or both) must increase. By default, the MAESTRO software attempts to provide the highest stimulation rate possible without exceeding voltage compliance limits. As a result, amplitude current initially increases when the audiologist increases the stimulation (in charge units). To avoid encountering voltage compliance limits, the MAESTRO software will eventually begin to increase pulse width as well. As pulse width is automatically increased, the maximum stimulation rate will decrease. If the level of stimulation necessary for a recipient requires the use of a wider pulse width than what is called for with the default settings, which is common for most recipients, the stimulation rate will automatically decrease. Of note, a higher stimulation rate is possible with deactivation of one or more of the 12 channels.

Because the MAESTRO platform attempts to provide the highest stimulation rate possible without exceeding voltage compliance limits, the default selection within the "Stimulation Rate" parameter menu is the "Use maximal available stimulation rate" (see Figure 17–12). As previously mentioned, the peer-reviewed literature indicates limited benefit for stimulation rates exceeding approximately 1500 pps (Arora, Dawson, Dowell, & Vandali, 2009; Balkany et al., 2007; Buchner, Frohne-Buchner, Battmer, & Lenarz 2004; Vandali, Whitford, Plant, & Clark, 2000; Verschuur, 2005; Weber et al., 2007). The audiologist should strive to maintain a stimulation rate of at least 800 pps. For the HDCIS and FSP signal coding strategies, the audiologist may select the "Use reduced stimulation rate" option and then adjust the stimulation rate in 10 unit steps down to 193 pps. For the FS4 and FS4-p signal coding strategies, when the "Use reduced stimulation rate" option is selected, the stimulation rate is fixed at a reduced rate (e.g., 750 pps) that is non-adjustable by the audiologist. The stimulation rate for FS4 strategies may not be reduced as low as it may for HDCIS and FSP, because the stimulation rate of FS4 strategies must be high enough to code zero crossings through the four most apical channels. Of note, MED-EL has not officially adopted the position that the audiologist should reduce the stimulation rate below the maximum available stimulation rate, and indeed, many MED-EL recipients will perform quite well with use of the maximum stimulation rate. Once again, however, research has generally failed to show that the typical recipient achieves higher levels of speech recognition with stimulation rates exceeding 1500 pps. For elderly recipients and individuals with a history of cochlear nerve dysfunc-

tion (e.g., auditory neuropathy spectrum disorder, cochlear nerve aplasia, abnormal neural adaptation), it may be beneficial to decrease the stimulation rate below the maximum rate available.

The **"CSSS channels"** parameter allows the audiologist to adjust the implementation of the fine structure stimulation (see Figure 17–12). The CSSS parameters are only adjustable for the FSP signal coding strategy. CSSS is unavailable in the HDCIS strategy and is automatically implemented across four channels in the FS4 strategies. For the FSP strategy, the audiologist may choose the frequency range for CSSS and the corner frequency above which CSSS will not be implemented. When the audiologist selects the "Use frequency limit to reduce number of CSSS channels" option, the default range of CSSS stimulation is set to 300 Hz, which allows for one channel of CSSS stimulation. Increasing the cutoff frequency will allow for implementation of CSSS over a larger number of apical channels. Because most audiologists will likely choose to provide FS4 or FS4-p for the recipients they serve, the CSSS parameter will be available for adjustment. Additionally, for FSP recipients, there is seldom a need to adjust the default CSSS parameters. Of note, the channels with FS/CSSS stimulation for all of the FS strategies are denoted by a music note icon next to the channel number in the programming screen.

The audiologist may also manage voltage compliance within the Signal Coding Strategy menu tab. The **Compliance Level Control** is an adjustable slider bar that determines how voltage compliance limits are measured. In short, the parameter determines how vigilant the system is at avoiding voltage compliance problems. These may be determined by: (1) measured values (i.e., electrode impedance), (2) strict voltage compliance estimation, or (3) theoretical maximum limits using relaxed voltage compliance estimation.

The Compliance Level Control default, which is typically used by most audiologists for most recipients, is Auto Adjust. The Auto Adjust setting seeks to strike a balance between avoiding voltage compliance issues, maximizing stimulation rate, and setting the pulse width to allow for FSP coding in as many apical channels as possible. If the user is not experiencing adequate loudness growth with default settings, manual adjustments to the "Compliance Level Control" may improve performance. Moving the slider bar of the Compliance Level Control toward the "Min (Strict)" direction will result in a wider pulse width to avoid voltage compliance limits. Conversely, moving the slider bar toward the "Max (Relaxed)" direction will result in the use of a narrower pulse width, which may allow for faster stimulation rates but will also increase the chance that the requested current amplitude will exceed voltage compliance limits.

The audiologist may also adjust the function of the volume control in the "Volume Mode" (Figure 17–13). The two volume options available within MAESTRO include the **IBK (Innsbruck)**, which is the default, and the **RTI (Research Triangle Institute)** modes. The RTI volume control mode is rarely used by audiologists who are fitting modern processors. For the RTI mode, when the volume control is set to the minimum position, no stimulation is provided. As the volume control is increased, the minimum and maximum stimulation levels are increased toward threshold (THR) and MCL, respectively. One disadvantage of the RTI mode is that some inputs may be inaudible when lower volume settings are used.

With the IBK mode (MAESTRO default), volume control settings correspond to stimulation at a percentage of the electrical dynamic range 0% to 100%. When IBK is selected, two parameters can be adjusted within the "Levels" tab of the MAESTRO software: the "minimum" and "maximum" volume control effects, which determine the overall range of the volume control. The minimum and maximum parameters denote the level that will be presented when the volume is turned all the way down or up, respectively. The upper range of the volume control determines the maximum stimulation that the recipient will receive (re. MCL setting of the program). The upper range should be set to 100%, which will be appropriate for the recipient if the audiologist has ensured during that programming session that MCL values are comfortable for the recipient.

Setting the lower end of the volume range to 0 will allow the recipient to decrease the stimulation level to THR. For most patients, the range should be set from a minimum of 80% to a maximum of 100%. This will allow the user to achieve a reasonable decrease in stimulation if needed, while also providing a manageable volume control range. When the lower end of the volume range is set to 80% (with an upper end of 100%), then the user must decrease the volume control of the FineTuner by 16 steps to go from the maximum to minimum of the volume range. Setting the lower end to 0 with an upper end of 100% (which is not a practice recommended by MED-EL) will require the recipient to decrease the FineTuner volume control by 64 steps (i.e., presses

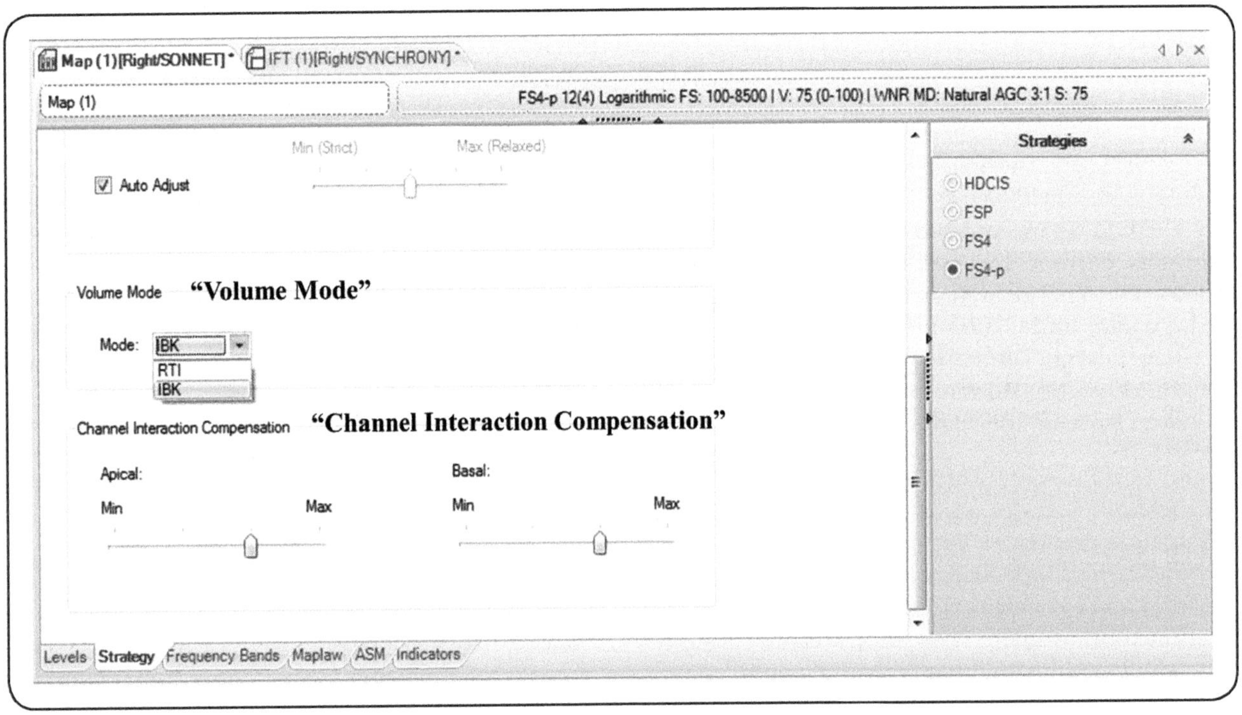

FIGURE 17–13. Adjustment of the volume control mode and channel interaction compliance. Image provided courtesy of MED-EL Corporation.

or clicks). A narrower range can be used to deactivate the volume control (e.g., Fine Tuner Volume Range minimum and maximum values both set to 100%), which may be helpful for children and adults who cannot reliably adjust their volume controls. In addition, the volume buttons on the FineTuner remote control can be deactivated.

If the FS4-p signal coding strategy is selected, MED-EL's **Channel Interaction Compensation (CIC)** algorithm is enabled (see Figure 17–13). CIC seeks to minimize the negative effects of channel interaction so that when neighboring channels are stimulated in parallel, the independent information on each channel is preserved (rather than aggregating to form a "virtual" channel). Of note, for the overwhelming majority of recipients, there is no need to adjust the CIC parameters. However, the audiologist may adjust two CIC parameters, "Apical" and "Basal," each of which alters the extent to which the stimulation on neighboring channels is adjusted to compensate for potential channel interaction.

Finally, it should be noted that even the oldest internal devices can be programmed using the newest strategies such as FS4, FS4-p, and FSP, with one notable exception. The FS4-p strategy is available only in MED-EL implants with the i100 signal processing chip (i.e., PULSAR, SONATA, CONCERT, SYNCHRONY, or later).

Setting Stimulation Levels

In the MAESTRO software platform, stimulation levels are adjusted in **charge units (qu)**. Charge units are defined as the product of the amplitude of the stimulus current and the pulse width divided by 1000—i.e., charge unit = (amplitude of current × pulse width/1000). This unit of stimulation represents constant charge. The system automatically adjusts the amplitude of the stimulus current and/or the pulse width to provide the requested magnitude of stimulation/loudness while avoiding voltage compliance limits and attempting to maximize stimulation rate. The range of stimulation levels are approximately 0 to 282.2 qu.

Stimulation levels are measured in the "**Levels**" tab of the MAESTRO Fitting menu. The primary stimulation level set in the MED-EL program is the MCL, the maximum comfort level, and is the upper level of stimulation for MED-EL implants. By definition, MCL refers to the maximum level of stimulation that is perceived as very loud but not uncomfortable or

painful with user volume control set to 100%. It is important to note that when the volume setting is adjusted to 100%, a 100 dB SPL input will receive MCL stimulation. Inputs between 25 and 100 dB SPL are mapped in between THR (electrical threshold) and MCL based on a logarithmic function referred to as Maplaw (to be discussed later). As a result, when conversation (at an average conversational level of 60–65 dB SPL) is occurring in live speech mode during the programming process, it is likely that the stimulation the recipient receives will be well below the MCL value and will occur at a comfortable level.

The MCL level can be manipulated using the handle on the right-hand side of each channel (Figure 17–14). When measured with a psychophysical approach, the recipient completes loudness scaling while 200-msec bursts of electrical biphasic pulses (during "Dynamic" stimulation) are delivered to a single electrode contact. Typically, the audiologist begins with MCL measurement on an electrode located in the middle of the array (electrodes 5 through 8), then measure on an electrode at the apical end of the array (electrodes 1 through 4), and then an electrode at the basal end (8 through 12). Then, MCLs may be measured on the intermediate channels. MED-EL also recommends that the audiologist re-measure the MCL on the first channel or two that were initially measured in order to ensure the reliability of those measurements (MED-EL Fitting Guide). **It should be noted that most recipients of MED-EL implants have MCL values between 5 and 25 charge units. MCL values exceeding 40 charge units are uncommon.**

Alternatively, MCLs may be set by globally increasing all MCL values in live speech mode (i.e., "flat MAP") to the recipient's MCL value. Then, channel-specific MCL values may be made based on the recipient's report or via loudness balancing. MED-EL recommends that loudness balancing be completed at 80% of the MCL value. Achieving loudness balance at 80% of the MCL should result in equal loudness across the array for input levels that approximate typical speech signals encountered in realistic listening situations. Of note, the percentage within the EDR at which stimulation is delivered is determined by the "Dynamics" parameter, which is located toward the top of the right side of the MAESTRO Levels screen. The percentage of the EDR at which stimulation is delivered is adjustable in 10 percentage point steps from 0 (THR) to 100% (MCL). To present speech in live speech mode, the audiologist selects the "Live" button on the right side of the MAESTRO "Levels" screen. When activating in live speech mode, the

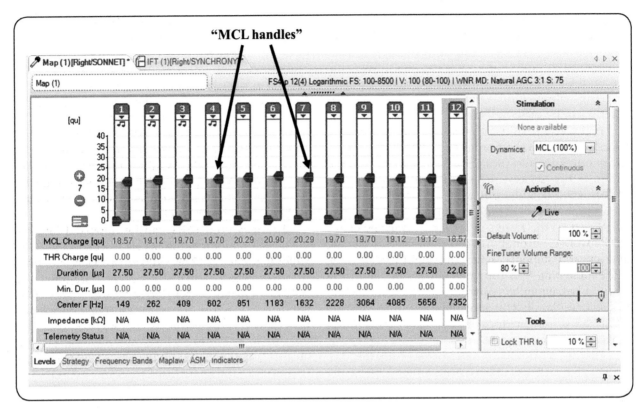

FIGURE 17–14. Adjustment of MCLs in MAESTRO. Image provided courtesy of MED-EL Corporation.

audiologist may choose the percentage of the electrical dynamic range where stimulation will be presented. When activating the device, the audiologist should select "Live," which turns the processor microphones on (selecting "Live" again, the sound processor microphones are off). MED-EL recommends activating in live speech mode with the volume control set to a reduced setting (e.g., 60% or lower) that is certain to avoid recipient discomfort. Then, the user test volume should be increased to 100%. If the recipient expresses signs of discomfort with the user test volume set to 100%, then the audiologist should globally decrease MCL values until optimal comfort and clarity for speech are achieved at a volume setting of 100%. Ideally, the "Default Volume" should be set to "100%" so that a 100 dB SPL sound results in MCL stimulation and average conversational level speech (60–65 dB SPL) is comfortable to the recipient.

Loudness balancing for two channels may be completed by using the computer mouse to highlight the MCL of two neighboring channels while pressing the shift key. Pressing the keyboard space bar will then present stimulation at the selected percentage of MCL.

Sweeping may be completed by holding down the shift key and highlighting all of the channels across the array. Pressing the space bar will sweep stimulation across all selected channels at the indicated percentage of the MCL. Pressing the control key will allow the audiologist to highlight channels that are not adjacent to one another. Pressing the space bar will then allow for stimulation of the selected channels. During sweeping/balancing, the MCL stimulus is delivered with a duration of 300 msec and an interstimulus gap of 500 msec. The reader is referred to Chapters 7, 14, and 23 for additional information on determination of upper stimulation levels.

Stimulation is delivered by clicking on the MCL slider of a channel and then pressing the "Dynamic" icon/radio button (with "Dynamic" set to 100% for MCL stimulation) in the upper right-hand corner of the "Levels" menu screen. Additionally, the space bar may be used to deliver stimulation. The audiologist may use the "Page up/down" keys to change stimulation levels by 15% of the MCL. Furthermore, the "arrow up/down" keys and the "+/−" keys may be used to change stimulation levels by 3% and 1%, respectively. Of note, during "Dynamic" stimulation, the audiologist may select the "Continuous" option so that the MCL signal is presented repeatedly with a 200-msec duration and a 500-msec interstimulus gap until the audiologist manually stops the signal presentation by hitting the keyboard space bar or by selecting the "Dynamic" button on the right side of the screen. The MAESTRO software provides an alert message (near the bottom of the MAESTRO screen) anytime the audiologist increases the stimulus level by more than 25% between stimulus presentations (Figure 17–15). The audiologist must dismiss this message prior to delivering stimulation.

Based on the results of research (Brickley et al., 2005), MED-EL strongly advocates the use of electrically evoked stapedial reflex threshold (ESRT) as a guide for setting MCL for patients who are unable to respond behaviorally to setting an MCL level (MED-EL ESRT Guide). ESRT can be obtained in the normal fitting screen, but a special platform in MAESTRO provides a method to track and better manage ESRT measurements. Figure 17–16 provides an overview of the ESRT platform features. In the ESRT platform,

the stimulus burst has a longer duration (i.e., 500 msec at default) than the stimulus used to determine MCL. The longer duration of the stimulus will result in a longer duration of the stapedial reflex, which will allow for easier observation of measurement of the ESRT with use of an acoustic immittance system. Within the ESRT platform, the audiologist can mark the response as a reflex using the following key strokes: mark as reflex (R), mark as no reflex (N), or mark as undefined (M). Additionally, the audiologist may use the "Mark as reflex" button located toward the bottom of the left side of the ESRT screen to mark the ESRT stimulation level.

The measured ESRT can be imported into the recipient's program in the Levels screen in the ESRT platform. Figure 17–17 provides an overview of options to transfer ESRTs into the recipient's program. The ESRT has a strong correlation to MCL (Brickley et al., 2005) and, therefore, the audiologist should attempt to measure it in all recipients without tympanostomy tubes or obvious middle ear dysfunction. In general, most recipients perform quite well when MCL values are set to the same levels that elicited to ESRT. The

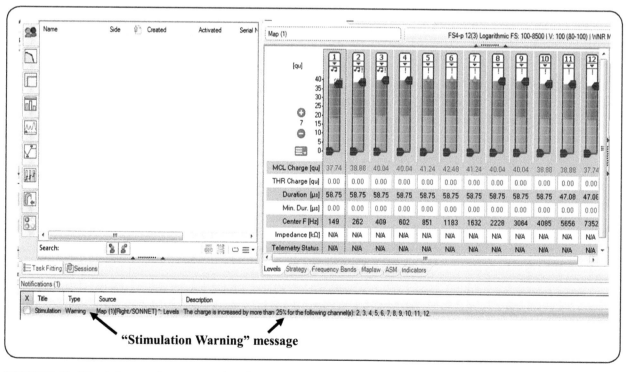

FIGURE 17–15. Stimulation warning message denoting an increase in stimulation level of more than 25% since last stimulation. The audiologist must dismiss this warning (i.e., "check" the box) before further programming may be completed. Image provided courtesy of MED-EL Corporation.

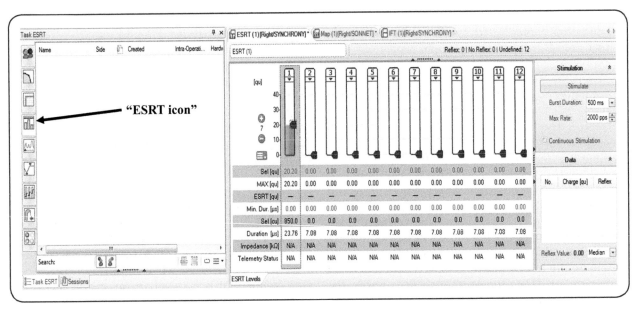

FIGURE 17–16. Electrically evoked stapedial reflex threshold (ESRT) measurement module. Image provided courtesy of MED-EL Corporation.

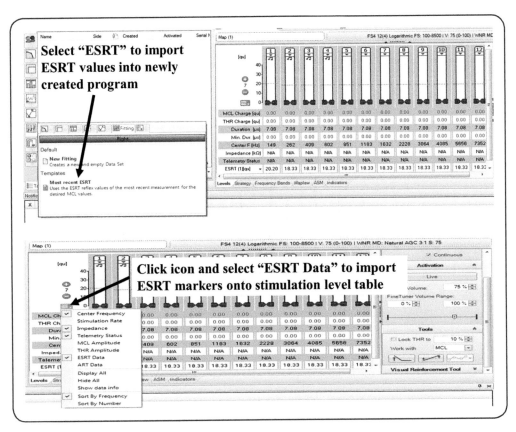

FIGURE 17–17. Importing ESRT measurements into a program. Image provided courtesy of MED-EL Corporation.

audiologist should be suspicious of MCL values that are 10% to 15% higher than the ESRT. This may indicate that the MCL values are excessive.

After the ESRT is measured, the authors of this book suggest that the audiologist conduct loudness balancing at 80% of the MCL across the electrode array (MED-EL Fitting Guide). Loudness balancing after ESRT measurement will ensure equal loudness across the frequency range. Furthermore, the audiologist should consider conducting sweeping (at 100% of MCL) at the end of the session to ensure that all MCLs do not exceed the user's discomfort threshold and do not elicit any other non-auditory side effects.

In the MAESTRO software, the electrical threshold is referred to as "THR" and is defined as the highest level at which a response is not obtained. The handle on the left-hand side of each channel is used to manipulate THR (Figure 17–18). As a result, the audiologist may obtain threshold via typical audiologic procedures, and if the recipient complains of a persistent humming/frying/static noise, then the programming audiologist would most likely need to provide a global decrease in the THR values until the recipient reports that the low-level sound is

eliminated. For young children who may not be able to reliably report on the presence of a continuous low-level noise, then the audiologist should consider globally decreasing THR values by at least 10% to 20% below the measured value. As mentioned earlier, the threat of a constant, audible low-level noise is a concern for recipients using Continuous Interleaved Sampling (CIS)–based signal coding strategies. The signal coding strategies used with the MED-EL system stimulate all activated channels with every frame of data (i.e., CIS based). If an analysis band (channel) does not contain information during a frame of stimulation, then that channel is stimulated at the THR level. As a result, when THR is set at a level that is consistently audible to the recipient, it is likely that a continuous sound (e.g., buzzing, humming, frying, static) will be detected when in quiet situations. Of note, when THR is manually measured in the MAESTRO fitting platform, the THR signal is delivered with a duration of 300 msec and an interstimulus interval of 500 msec.

It should be reiterated that MED-EL indicates that THR values should be estimated on the basis of the MCL settings (MED-EL Fitting Guide) for most

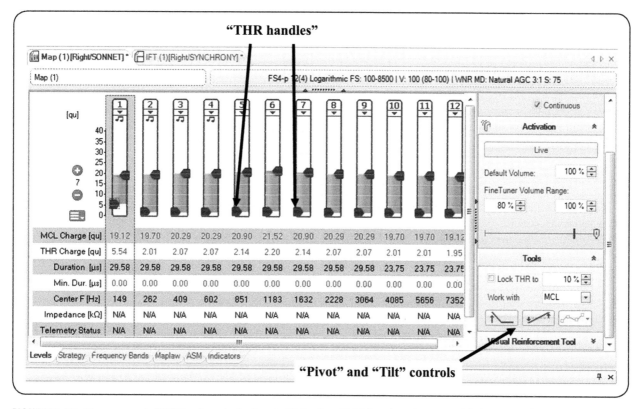

FIGURE 17–18. Measurement of THR levels and adjustment of "pivot" and "tilt" functions. Image provided courtesy of MED-EL Corporation.

patients. Specifically, THR may be set at 0 to 10% of MCL. Of note, it is suggested that THR be set at 0 for channels with FS/CSSS in order to reliably prevent audibility for low-level noise secondary to electrical stimulation. Previous research has shown similar performance is achieved when using a THR set to 10% of the upper stimulation level versus a measured THR (Spahr & Dorman, 2005). If a recipient is not performing well and the audiologist determines that Maplaw has been optimized, then the audiologist may consider measuring THR and setting the THR to just below the level of audibility. The "lock THR to" option is selected on the right-hand side of the "Levels" screen and will automatically set thresholds to a level determined by the audiologist (10% of MCL, 0, etc.) (see Figure 17–18). At default settings, THR is measured using 300 msec bursts of electrical pulses, but it is common practice to create programs with estimated THR levels. When estimated THR levels are used, the stimulation levels for low-level inputs are based on the measured upper stimulation levels.

As previously mentioned, adequate audibility for soft sounds may be determined by measuring soundfield detection thresholds in the audiometric test booth. If sound-field thresholds are elevated (>30 dB HL), the audiologist could consider increasing MCL values, selecting a steeper Maplaw function, or measuring THR levels. After these programming changes are made, sound-field measurements should be repeated to confirm adequate access to low-level sounds. Of note, if soundfield detection thresholds are elevated, the audiologist should refrain from increasing MCL to an inappropriate level. Obviously, MCL should not be increased to a level that is uncomfortable to the recipient. Additionally, the audiologist should exercise caution if an increase in MCL results in upper stimulation levels exceeding the ESRT by more than 10 to 15%. Furthermore, the audiologist should exercise caution if MCL is increased to a level that is atypical for MED-EL recipients (i.e., >25 charge units). Additional parameters to improve audibility of low-level sounds will be discussed in the following sections.

If the patient notes a humming sound, especially in quiet environments, it is an indication that at least one threshold value is set to an audible level. The audiologist needs to identify the channel that has an audible threshold and lower the THR level to a point where it is not audible to the patient. This can be achieved by sweeping through each channel at the THR level to determine what channel's THR is set to an audible level. Of course, the THR value of the offending channel would then be reduced. Alternative approaches involve globally decreasing the THR values until the low-level sound ceases or setting THR values to 0% to 10%.

Within the software, there are additional tools that can be used to streamline the process, including pivot, shift, and tilt (see Figure 17–18). These tools are generally used to quickly address the complaints of adult recipients (e.g., too tinny, too hollow, not sharp enough). It should be noted that these tools provide a coarse adjustment to the recipient's program, and the use of ESRT and loudness balancing tends to be more successful in addressing these types of complaints.

Additional Programming Parameters

Frequency Bands

The **Frequency Bands** screen allows the audiologist to control how input sound frequencies are allocated across the active channels (Figure 17–19). As stated in Chapter 11, MED-EL has the longest commercially available electrode array in the cochlear implant industry, which provides access to more apical sites of the cochlea. As a result, the MAESTRO software has a low cutoff of 70 Hz, which is quite lower than the low end of the frequency range of the implant systems of competing manufacturers. The overall frequency range spans from 70 to 8500 Hz. The lower end of the frequency range may be adjusted in 10 Hz steps from 70 to 350 Hz (default = 100 Hz for FS strategies), while the upper end of the range can be adjusted in 500 Hz steps from 3500 to 8500 Hz (default = 8500 Hz). Setting the upper end of the frequency range slightly lower (e.g., 7000 Hz) may be beneficial because it will create channels with narrower bandwidths in the speech frequencies. However, the upper range of 8500 Hz will serve most recipients well. The authors recommend setting the frequency range to span from 70 to 8500 Hz.

Frequencies within the defined input range are reallocated to existing channels using one of five approaches. The default and recommended allocation for the majority of participants is **Logarithmic FS**, in which the input frequencies are assigned to logarithmically spaced bands. The second option, **LinLog**, separates the lower frequencies into linear bands and the higher frequencies into logarithmic bands. This mode results in narrower low-frequency bands, which could theoretically provide better spectral resolution in the low frequencies. Improved

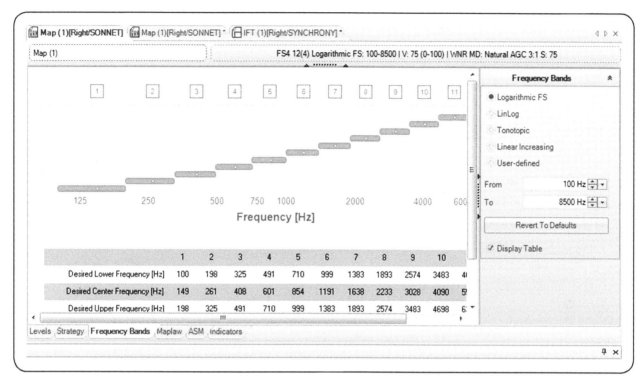

FIGURE 17–19. Frequency allocation menu. Image provided courtesy of MED-EL Corporation.

spectral resolution may be helpful for discriminating common speech and environmental sounds. The **Tonotopic** approach attempts to mimic the tonotopic organization observed in the normal cochlea. Theoretically, this mode will produce the most normal frequency percept. Furthermore, **Linear Increasing** divides the input frequencies into linear bands with increased bandwidth from the apical to basal direction. This strategy results in wider bandwidths for low-frequency channels relative to Logarithmic FS, but the highest-frequency channels are narrower. This mode may be helpful if the recipient exhibits confusion patterns with high-frequency sounds (e.g., /f/ vs. /s/ vs. /h/). Finally, the "**User-defined**" option allows the audiologist to manually select the cutoffs of each channel. In most cases, the audiologist should avoid the "User-defined" option, because the other frequency allocation options within MAESTRO are based on speech science and research. Arbitrarily adjusting the cutoff frequencies of the 12 analysis bands is unlikely to improve performance over the options provided by MED-EL. However, the "User-defined" option may be beneficial for allocating stimulation for recipients who have usable low-frequency hearing and who use electric-acoustic stimulation.

Also of note, the Frequency Band screen allows the audiologist to reorder how channels are allocated to electrode contacts, which is necessary (and should be performed first) when programming a split electrode. Figure 17–20 provides a view of the Frequency Bands tab in the map parameters.

It should also be noted that the audiologist may change the order in which the channels are allocated to the 12 stimulating electrode contact sites. This is accomplished by using the computer mouse to select a channel and then drag it to a desired location. It is very unlikely that the audiologist will have to re-order the channel to electrode assignment.

Maplaw

The **Maplaw** screen allows the audiologist to control the logarithmic function used to map acoustic inputs into the recipient's electrical dynamic range (Figure 17–21). The default choice in the Maplaw menu is "**Logarithmic Maplaw**," which maps lower-level inputs to a higher point in the electrical dynamic range. The other logarithmic function, "**S-shaped Maplaw**," provides less amplification for low-level sounds and a steep increase in amplification for moderate- and

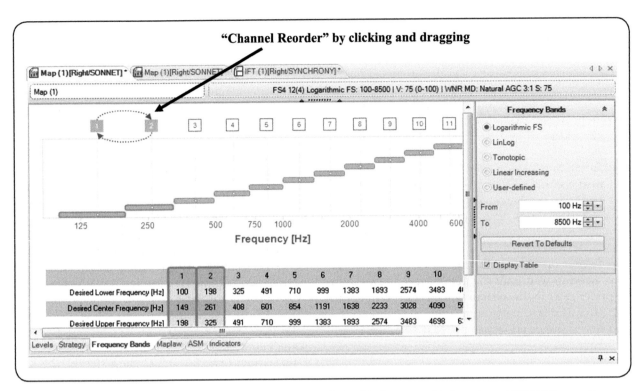

FIGURE 17–20. An illustration of re-ordering channel-to-electrode relationship. Image provided courtesy of MED-EL Corporation.

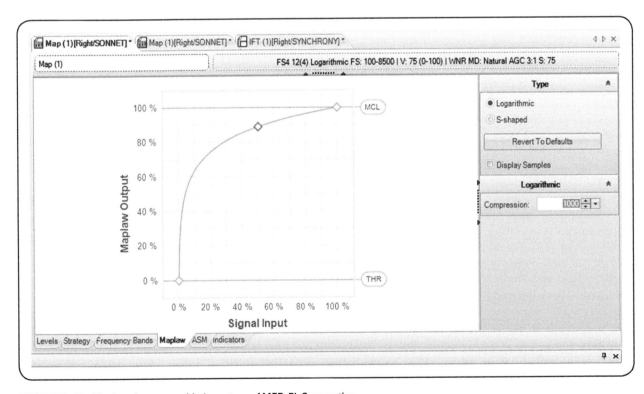

FIGURE 17–21. Maplaw. Image provided courtesy of MED-EL Corporation.

high-level inputs. The S-shaped Maplaw can be helpful in controlling constant background noise and can be used with patients who need to manage a specific noisy situation (i.e., sitting near a ventilation fan at work).

The audiologist also may adjust the default compression coefficient (i.e., 500) used to define the logarithmic function. Higher coefficients map softer inputs to a higher point in the electrical dynamic range. The **Maplaw compression coefficient** of 500 is suitable for most recipients. However, increasing the Maplaw compression coefficient to 1000 may improve audibility for recipients who have insufficient access to low-level sounds. At initial stimulation of adult recipients, a Maplaw of 750 to 1000 may be perceived as too "crisp" or "sharp." In this case, the audiologist may need to wait until the patient has a few days of experience with the system before attempting to use a higher Maplaw. Long-term, improved audibility of low-level sounds should improve performance.

Automatic Sound Management (ASM)

The **ASM** screen allows the audiologist to adjust input processing characteristics of the system, such as **automatic gain control (AGC).** Figure 17–22 provides a view of the ASM tab. The MED-EL system is designed to use dual-action front-end processing (ASM: adaptive compression with two compression thresholds, one with a relatively low kneepoint and slow response times and another with a higher kneepoint with faster response times) to provide a wide input dynamic range (IDR) of 75 dB by way of AGC, with an adaptive sound window of 55 dB that roves based on the input to the sound processor. This effectively maps inputs from as soft as 25 dB to as loud as 100 dB SPL. Within the ASM menu, the two parameters that may be adjusted include compression ratio and microphone sensitivity.

The **compression ratio** of the AGC system may be disabled (although it would typically be undesirable to do so) or set to one of four ratios (i.e., 2:1, 2.5:1, 3:1, or 3.5:1). The default ratio is 3:1. A lower ratio may be selected if the user reports that loud sounds are too soft (e.g., music). At lower compression ratio settings (e.g., 2:1, 2.5:1), the difference between loud and soft sounds is increased, which may be useful in high-level noise environments, because the background noise may be reduced. Higher compression ratios (e.g., 3.5:1) may address reports that loud

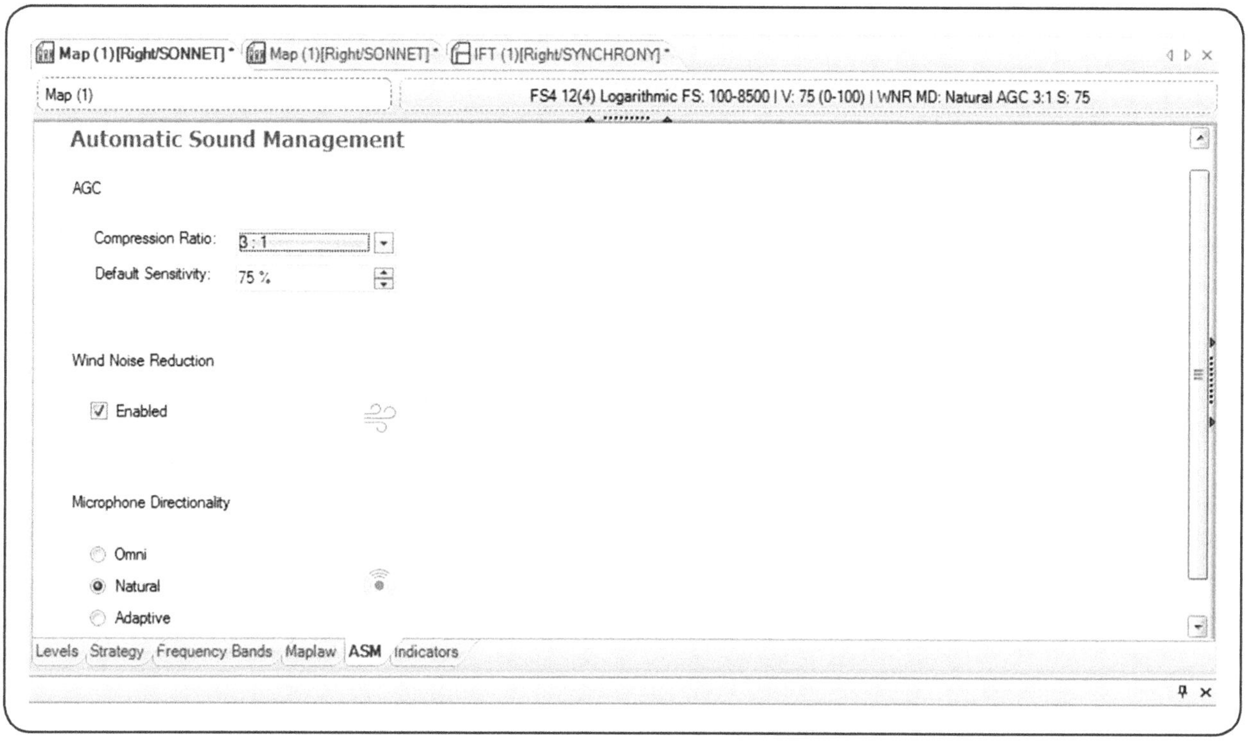

FIGURE 17–22. Automatic Sound Management menu. Image provided courtesy of MED-EL Corporation.

sounds are uncomfortable (although this complaint also should prompt the audiologist to re-evaluate and possibly decrease MCL levels). At a 3.5:1 compression ratio, the difference between low-level and high-level sounds will likely become less noticeable for the recipient. Background noise will be perceived as being louder.

The **microphone sensitivity** controls the gain of the microphone of the sound processor. The sensitivity parameter may be adjusted over a range from 0 to 100%. Higher sensitivity settings will provide better audibility of very soft sounds that are nearby; however, moderate-level sounds may be too loud, and performance in noise may deteriorate. In contrast, lower sensitivity settings may improve performance and comfort in noise, but soft sounds will not be audible. The default setting of 75% is appropriate for most recipients. The patient can control sensitivity with the MED-EL remote control.

Furthermore, the audiologist may enable/disable MED-EL's wind noise reduction and determine the **microphone mode** of the SONNET sound processor. Four microphone modes are available: (1) Omnidirectional, (2) Natural (slight directionality to mimic the directivity of the unaided auricle), (3) Adaptive

(directional mode with automatic activation), and (4) Auto-Adaptive (uses an omnidirectional setting in soft environments and then switches to Adaptive [directional] in louder environments). The audiologist can adjust the cut-off between omni and adaptive to be either 55 dB SPL or 60 dB SPL. MED-EL recommends starting at the default of 55.

Setting Sound Processor Indicators

The "**Indicators**" tab allows access to the sound processor indicators, including the LED light and private audible alarm. The LED light may be enabled/disabled to indicate the status of the processor (i.e., sound processor functioning correctly, a low battery, or communication with the remote control). The private alarm (a chime that is only audible to the recipient) can also alert the recipient to a problem (e.g., low battery) and can confirm a change in sound processor function (e.g., program change, volume control change). Additionally, the audiologist can adjust the loudness of enabled alerts according to user preferences. Figure 17–23 provides a view of options on the Indicators page.

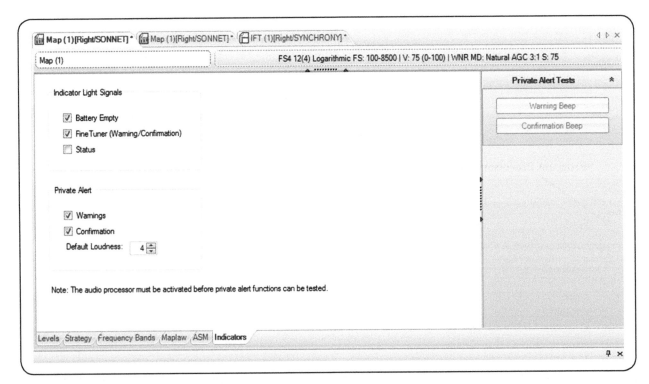

FIGURE 17–23. Adjustment of processor indicators. Image provided courtesy of MED-EL Corporation.

Loading Programs onto MED-EL Sound Processors

The final steps in saving the programs and configuring both the processor and FineTuner can be completed in the last tab: Configuration. The audiologist can load the desired programs into each individual slot by clicking on the drop-down arrow and selecting a program. Up to four programs may be loaded onto the sound processor (there are four program slots, but as few as one slot must be filled). Once the desired programs are selected, the audiologist simply clicks on "Program Processor," which is located on the right side of the "Configuration" screen (Figure 17–24).

In the "**Configuration**" screen, the audiologist may also access the "Data Logging" tab to review data logging statistics The audiologist may select "Options" to make several user-related adjustments. For example, the audiologist can also activate and deactivate the different buttons of the volume control by simply clicking on each button on the screen. The telecoil control may also be deactivated for children (Figure 17–25). Additionally, the audiologist may disable the "Automatic Coil Power Off," which automatically powers down the sound processor when the sound processor coil (DL Coil) is not in communication with the cochlear implant for 2 minutes. The audiologist may disable the LED light on the DL Coil. The LED light is particularly important for children, as it indicates that the implant and coil are in communication, and it may be used to ensure that the correct processor is on the correct ear for bilateral recipients.

Finally, the audiologist may adjust the strength of the MED-EL **Wind Noise Reduction (WNR)** (mild or strong) and alter the function of the adaptive directional microphone. Within the Adaptive Microphone Directionality mode, the audiologist can determine whether the sound processor always remains in the directional mode (if "Adaptive" directional mode was selected in the ASM tab) or if the microphone switches to directional mode at either 55 or 60 dBA. MED-EL strongly recommends that WNR be on whenever directionality features are enabled, as two microphones can increase the impact of wind turbulence over the microphones. WNR has no impact when turbulence is not present, so it is appropriate for it to be enabled at all times.

Electric-Acoustic Stimulation of MED-EL Recipients

For recipients who have usable hearing after cochlear implant surgery, the audiologist may program the

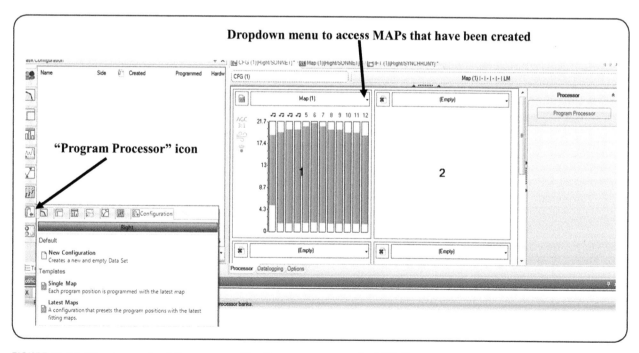

FIGURE 17–24. Visual example of the process of loading programs onto the MED-EL sound processor. Image provided courtesy of MED-EL Corporation.

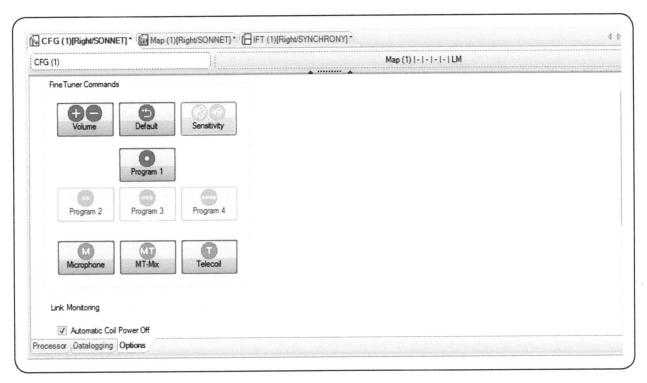

FIGURE 17–25. Adjustments to the Fine Tuner controls. Image provided courtesy of MED-EL Corporation.

SONNET sound processor to provide electric-acoustic stimulation. When the recipient information is entered in the "New Patient" menu, the audiologist must select the "**EAS**" option (Figure 17–26). Then, the audiologist must enter the recipient's most current postoperative audiogram into the "Audiogram" menu. Next, the audiologist measures stimulation levels in the "Fitting" screen. After stimulation levels are determined, the audiologist may adjust the frequency allocation in the "Frequency Bands" tab. The default crossover frequency up to which acoustical stimulation is delivered is the frequency at which the hearing loss crosses 65 dB on the audiogram. The audiologist may select the "Use Crossover As Minimum" button to adjust the electric stimulation to begin at the frequency at which the acoustic stimulation ends (850 Hz in the example shown in Figure 17–27). Of note, the audiologist may also manually adjust the frequency at which electrical stimulation begins in 10-Hz steps using the up/down arrows under the "Frequency Bands" menu on the right side of the screen. Finally, the audiologist may select the "Acoustic Fitting" mode on the ribbon task bar located at the left side of the screen (Figure 17–28). Within the "Acoustic Fitting" menu, the audiologist may adjust the overall gain of 48 dB SPL and a maximum power output as well as adjust gain and maximum power output (MPO) across six channels that range up to 2000 Hz.

MED-EL Specific Troubleshooting

In situations where a patient is reporting difficulty with the equipment, there are several options to complete troubleshooting to determine the problem source. The Speech Processor Test Device (SPTD) can be used to check for shorts in the cable or intermittencies in the coil. The audiologist should move the cable around while saying a long vowel (i.e., ahhh-hhh) to check for shorts. If there does not seem to be any obvious short, but the patient is still experiencing intermittencies, try simply replacing the cable first. Replacing the coil should be the second troubleshooting step. In the case of poor sound quality or decreased sound quality, the Microphone Test Device (MTD) can be used. The audiologist can use earbuds to listen to the microphone input to determine the integrity of the microphones.

The processors also have light indicators that may help with troubleshooting. The company provides

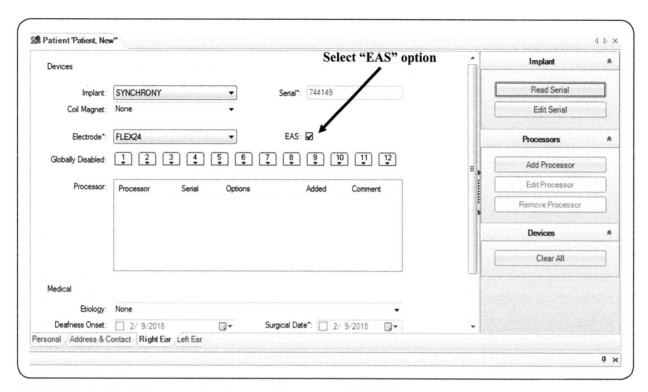

FIGURE 17–26. Enabling EAS programming. Image provided courtesy of MED-EL Corporation.

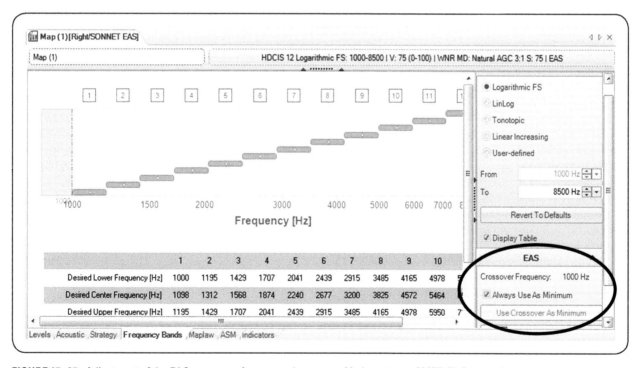

FIGURE 17–27. Adjustment of the EAS crossover frequency. Image provided courtesy of MED-EL Corporation.

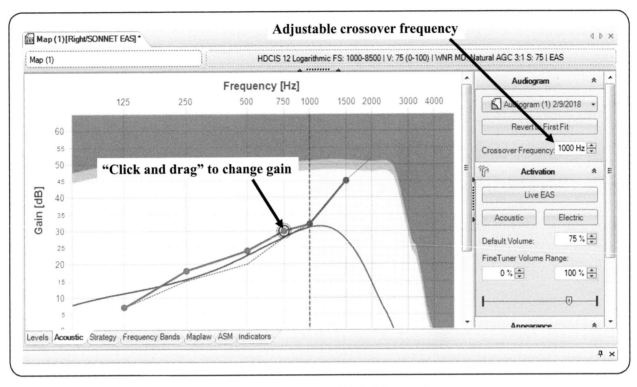

FIGURE 17–28. Adjustment of EAS settings. Image provided courtesy of MED-EL Corporation.

a troubleshooting guide that includes various error patterns that may be emitted by the indicator lights. If you get an indicator that you do not recognize, turn the processor off and back on. If the abnormal indicators persist, consult the troubleshooting guide or contact the company for assistance.

Additional Considerations

If the audiologist would like to share a recipient's MAPping information with another clinic or a MED-EL representative, or if programs need to be remotely loaded onto a recipient's replacement processor prior to being sent to the patient, then the audiologist may access the "Data" drop-down menu, select "export," and check the information that must be exported. The file should be saved as a packed data file (.mpd) so it can be opened in MAESTRO, and the audiologist must also send MAP numbers and configuration via email to expedite remote loading. If statistical analysis is the purpose of the export, then the file should be saved as an XML file.

Auditory Response Telemetry and Electrically Evoked Auditory Brainstem Response

The **Auditory Response Telemetry (ART)** platform is used to record the electrically evoked compound action potential (ECAP) of the cochlear nerve in response to electrical stimulation from the MED-EL cochlear implant system. The EABR platform allows the audiologist to interface with an auditory evoked response instrument to measure the electrically evoked auditory brainstem response (EABR). The reader is referred to Chapter 18 in this book for information pertaining to ART and EABR.

Key Concepts

- MED-EL cochlear implant systems may be programmed with use of MAESTRO programming software.
- FS4-p is the recommended signal coding strategy for new MED-EL cochlear implant recipients, but

a variety of signal coding strategies are available to meet the needs of individual recipients.

- The MAESTRO programming software allows for control of a large number of parameters and signal processing technologies. The audiologist may adjust these parameters to optimize the listening needs of each individual recipient.

References

Arora, K., Dawson. P., Dowell, R., & Vandali. A. (2009). Electrical stimulation rate effects on speech perception in cochlear implants. *International Journal of Audiology, 48*(8), 561–567.

Balkany, T., Hodges, A., Menapace, C., Hazard, L., Driscoll, C., Gantz, B., . . . Payne, S. (2007). Nucleus Freedom North American clinical trial. *Otolaryngology–Head and Neck Surgery, 136*(5), 757–762.

Brickley, G., Boyd, P., Wyllie, F., O'Driscoll, M., Webster, D., & Nopp, P. (2005). Investigations into electrically evoked stapedius reflex measures and subjective loudness percepts in the MED-EL COMBI 40+ cochlear implant. *Cochlear Implants International, 6*(1), 31–42.

Buchner A., Frohne-Buchner, C., Battmer, R., & Lenarz, T. (2004) Two years of experience using stimulation rates between 800 and 5000 pps with the Clarion CI implant. *International Congress Series, 1273,* 48–51.

Vandali, A., Whitford, L., Plant, K., & Clark, G. (2000). Speech perception as a function of electrical stimulation rate: Using the Nucleus 24 cochlear implant system. *Ear and Hearing, 21,* 608–624.

Verschuur, C. A. (2005). Effect of stimulation rate on speech perception in adult users of the Med-El CIS speech processing strategy. *International Journal of Audiology, 44*(1), 58–63.

Weber, B. P., Lai, W. K., Dillier, N., von Wallenberg, E. L., Killian, M. J., Pesch, J., . . . Lenarz, T. (2007). Performance and preference for ACE stimulation rates obtained with Nucleus RP 8 and Freedom system. *Ear and Hearing, 28*(2 Suppl.), 46S–48S.

18

Objective Measures of Cochlear Implant Function

Jace Wolfe

Introduction

Objective measures are those that evaluate the function of the auditory system or of hearing technology without a volitional behavioral response from the patient. Audiologists are typically familiar with objective measures, because they are used quite frequently to evaluate auditory function and the function of hearing aid technology. Examples of objective measures commonly used in the field of audiology include tympanometry, auditory brainstem response, auditory steady-state response, otoacoustic emissions, electroacoustic assessment of hearing aid function (i.e., 2-cc coupler measures), and real ear probe microphone measures. In contrast, behavioral measures are those that involve assessment of a patient's perception of sound or of the impact of the patient's hearing abilities on communication function. Examples of behavioral measures commonly used in audiology include visual reinforcement audiometry, conditioned play audiometry, conventional audiometry, speech recognition assessment, loudness scaling, and subjective questionnaires of auditory function and communication ability (e.g., Hearing Handicap Inventory for Adults, Parent Evaluation of Aural/Oral Performance of Children [PEACH], Abbreviated Profile of Hearing Aid Benefit). Of note, many objective measures do require an audiologist to subjectively evaluate the physiologic response of the patient. For example, for

auditory brainstem response assessment, an audiologist typically analyzes electroencephalographic (EEG) waveforms to determine whether a response is present, and if so, whether the response meets a certain set of criteria associated with that of a normal/typical response (although automated statistical analysis of auditory brainstem response [ABR] waveforms is also available). Because of the subjectivity involved in the audiologist's analysis of the patient's physiologic response, many have contended that it may be more appropriate to refer to objective measures as electrophysiologic measures of auditory function. However, some objective measures, such as electroacoustic assessment of hearing aid function or in the case of cochlear implants, electrode impedance, are not necessarily measures of physiologic function. Consequently, the term "objective measures" will be used for this book with the realization that it may not be the perfect term to describe each of the measures discussed in this chapter.

Several different types of objective measures play an important role in the management of the clinical care of cochlear implant recipients. Objective measures of cochlear implant function may be divided into two broad categories, (1) electrophysiologic measures and (2) electrical measures. **Electrophysiologic measures** are those that evaluate a physiologic response of the auditory system in response to electrical stimulation from the cochlear implant. Examples of electrophysiologic measures used in the management of cochlear implant recipients include:

- Electrically evoked compound action potential
- Electrically evoked stapedial reflex
- Electrically evoked auditory brainstem response
- Electrically evoked cortical auditory evoked responses
- Transtympanic promontory/round window electrical stimulation

Electrophysiologic measures of auditory function may be recorded with stimulation delivered outside the cochlea (i.e., extracochlear stimulation; on the promontory or round window) or inside the cochlea (i.e., intracochlear stimulation). Intracochlear stimulation is completed by delivering electrical stimuli to the intracochlear electrode contacts of the cochlear implant. Preoperative measurements are completed with extracochlear stimulation, whereas postoperative measurements are typically completed with intracochlear stimulation.

Electrical measures are those that evaluate the function of the cochlear implant system without the assessment of a physiologic response from the recipient. Examples of electrical measures used to evaluate cochlear implant function include:

- Electrode impedance assessment
- Radio frequency (RF) coupling/power assessment
- Voltage compliance assessment
- Electrical field imaging
- Average electrode voltages

The aforementioned electrophysiologic and electrical measures will be discussed in this chapter. The first section of this chapter will address electrophysiologic measures of auditory responsiveness to cochlear implant stimulation. The second section will discuss electrical measures of cochlear implant function. Of note, electrode impedance assessment, RF coupling, voltage compliance assessment, and electrical field imaging were discussed in Chapter 7, and as a result, coverage in this chapter of electrical measures will center on average electrode voltage measures.

Electrophysiologic Measures

The electrically evoked compound action potential and the electrically evoked stapedial reflex response are the two electrophysiologic measures that are primarily used in the clinical management of cochlear implant recipients. The electrically evoked auditory brainstem response and the cortical auditory evoked response can also be quite useful for the evaluation of auditory function of cochlear implant recipients, but these measures are used less frequently than the electrically evoked compound action potential and the electrically evoked stapedial reflex response. These measures will be discussed in isolation in the following paragraphs.

Electrically Evoked Compound Action Potential

The **electrically evoked compound action potential (ECAP)** is a synchronous response that is: (1) generated by a large number of cochlear nerve fibers, (2) stimulated by brief electrical pulses delivered to an intracochlear electrode contact of the cochlear implant, and (3) recorded on an intracochlear electrode contact that is typically located one to two electrode contacts away (in the apical direction) from the stimulated electrode. Figure 18–1 provides an example of an ECAP recorded from a cochlear implant recipient. The typical ECAP contains a negative "peak" that is referred to as "N1" and that occurs at a latency of approximately 0.2 to 0.4 msec (Abbas et al., 1999; Brown, Abbas, & Gantz, 1998; Cullington, 2000). The amplitude of N1 typically is around 25 to 30 microvolts at threshold but can be as large as 1500 microvolts, which is much larger than the peaks of ABR waveforms, which are rarely greater than 1 microvolt. In some but not all cases, there is a positive peak that follows N1. This positive peak is referred to as P2 and occurs between 0.6 and 0.8 msec. Additionally, a small trough, referred to as N2, may appear between N1 and P2. As shown in the amplitude growth function displayed in Figure 18–2, the amplitude of N1 is rather large for stimuli presented well above threshold, and P2 is typically only present at suprathreshold stimulus levels. Of note, the ECAP can be successfully measured in around 95% of cochlear implant recipients (Botros et al., 2007; Cafarelli Dees et al., 2005; van Dijk et al., 2007). Exceptions in which the ECAP cannot be recorded most often include recipients with cochlear nerve deficiency and those with auditory neural dysfunction (He et al., 2017).

The ECAP represents a synchronous response from the cochlear nerve, with the spiral ganglion cell bodies being the most likely generator of the ECAP. The amplitude of the ECAP response is much larger than the amplitude of typical auditory evoked responses measured with surface electrodes, because

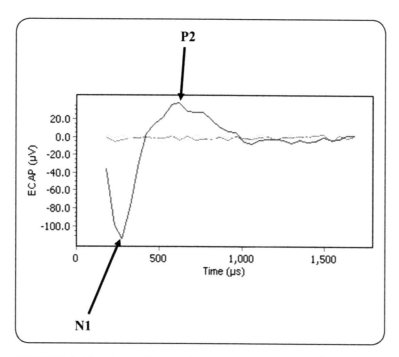

FIGURE 18–1. The electrically evoked compound action potential (ECAP). Image provided courtesy of Cochlear Americas, ©2018.

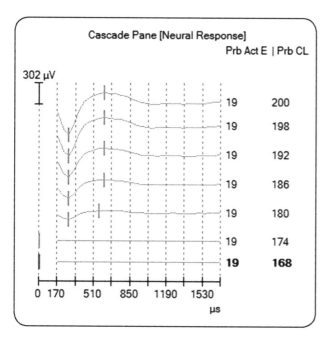

FIGURE 18–2. An electrically evoked compound action potential amplitude growth function. Image provided courtesy of Cochlear Americas, ©2018.

the recording electrodes used for the ECAP measure are located in close proximity to the neural generator (i.e., cochlear nerve; near-field generator). Addition-

ally, there is little to no interference from myogenic activity, because the stimulating and recording electrodes are located within and insulated by the temporal bone. Consequently, the ECAP may be recorded from children without the need of sedation or even for the child to be still and quiet during the measurement. Furthermore, because the ECAP is a peripheral auditory response, it is unaffected by sleep and anesthesia and may be successfully recorded during cochlear implant surgery or while a child takes a nap. However, successful recording of the ECAP is challenging nonetheless because the electrical artefact from the stimulus delivered from the cochlear implant is much larger than the auditory evoked response. As a result, artefact reduction techniques are required to extract the cochlear nerve response from the competing electrical artefact from the cochlear implant.

Measurement of the ECAP

A biphasic electrical pulse is the typical stimulus used to elicit the ECAP. The biphasic electrical pulses are typically delivered to one intracochlear electrode contact via monopolar electrode coupling (with an extracochlear ground electrode typically serving as the reference electrode) at a rate ranging from 30 to 80 pulses per second (pps) which is a much slower rate than that used for most cochlear implant signal coding strategies (e.g., 500 to 5000 pps). The ECAP stimulus is usually delivered at stimulus levels similar to those used for measuring stimulation levels during the implant MAPping process. In fact, most recipients are able to tolerate ECAP stimulus levels that are higher than the stimulation levels used for their MAPs, because the faster stimulus rates used for MAPing and in modern signal coding strategies elicit a louder auditory percept due to temporal summation. Of note, the ECAP stimulus typically possesses a relatively brief pulse width (e.g., 25–40 microseconds), because stimuli with longer pulse widths may saturate the recording amplifier.

The ECAP is typically recorded with use of an intracochlear electrode contact that is located one or two electrodes apical to the stimulated electrode and referenced to an extracochlear ground electrode. When the most apical electrode contact is stimulated for an ECAP measurement, the recording electrode contact is typically located one or two electrodes basal to the stimulated electrode contact. The electrical activity captured at the intracochlear and reference electrode contacts is delivered to a recording amplifier that is located in the electronics package housed inside the titanium case of the cochlear implant. The recording amplifier "switches on" shortly after the presentation of the ECAP stimulus so that it may capture and magnify the electrical activity from the recording and reference electrodes and deliver it to the DSP of the cochlear implant, where it is converted to a digital code. That digital code is then converted to an electromagnetic signal that is delivered from the coil of the cochlear implant to the coil of the external sound processor or measurement device located on the head. Then, the signal captured at the external coil is delivered to the programming computer, where it is processed, analyzed, and displayed on the monitor of the programming computer.

Of note, because the ECAP amplitude is a near-field response with a rather large amplitude, a relatively small number of averages are required to successfully measure the response. For instance, the ECAP can typically be recorded with 32 to 50 sweeps, whereas the acoustic ABR used to estimate hearing sensitivity in the audiology clinic usually requires several hundred to a couple of thousand sweeps. Likewise, the cochlear implant stimulus-related electrical artefact in the cochlea is very large and can overdrive (saturate) the recording amplifier. Additionally, the short latency of the ECAP increases the risk that stimulus-related artefact will still be present when the amplifier is "switched on" to record the

ECAP. Numerous artefact-reduction techniques have been developed to minimize or eliminate the stimulus-related artefact and allow for successful recording of the ECAP.

Forward-Masking Subtraction Artefact Reduction. The Cochlear Nucleus CI24M, which was commercially approved for commercial distribution by the FDA in 1998, was the first cochlear implant capable of completing the ECAP measurement. The Cochlear Nucleus CI24M, and all subsequently developed Nucleus cochlear implants, use an artefact reduction method developed by Paul Abbas and Carolyn Brown (Abbas et al., 1999; Brown et al., 1998). The **forward-masking subtraction technique** is unlike any artefact reduction method that is typically used for auditory evoked response measurement. The forward-masking subtraction technique uses four stimulus phases for each ECAP response acquired during the averaging process. Figure 18–3 provides a visual illustration of the forward-masking subtraction technique. Briefly, in the first phase, the stimulus, which is referred to as the "**probe**," is presented and the amplifier is switched on shortly thereafter to record the cochlear nerve's neural response as well as the stimulus-related electrical artefact. In the second phase, a **masker** and probe are both presented with a very short time interval separating the masker that precedes the probe. The time interval between the masker and probe is referred to as the **masker-probe interval (MPI)** and is generally within a range of 300 to 500 microseconds (Miller et al., 2000). For this second phase, the masker generates a neural response from the cochlear nerve as well as the electrical artefact. However, the probe that follows the masker only generates stimulus-related electrical artefact, because the cochlear nerve units were in their refractory state after responding to the masker that just preceded the probe. As a result, when the amplifier is switched on after the presentation of the pulse, a neural response is recorded to the masker, and a stimulus-related electrical artefact is recorded to both the masker and the probe. When the second interval is subtracted from the first interval, the stimulus-related electrical artefact related to the probe is subtracted, whereas the neural response elicited by the probe in the first interval is left intact. However, when subtraction is completed after the second interval, the recording amplifier has also captured a neural response and stimulus-related artefact associated with the masker presented during the second phase. A third phase is completed to eliminate the masker-related artefact and neural response.

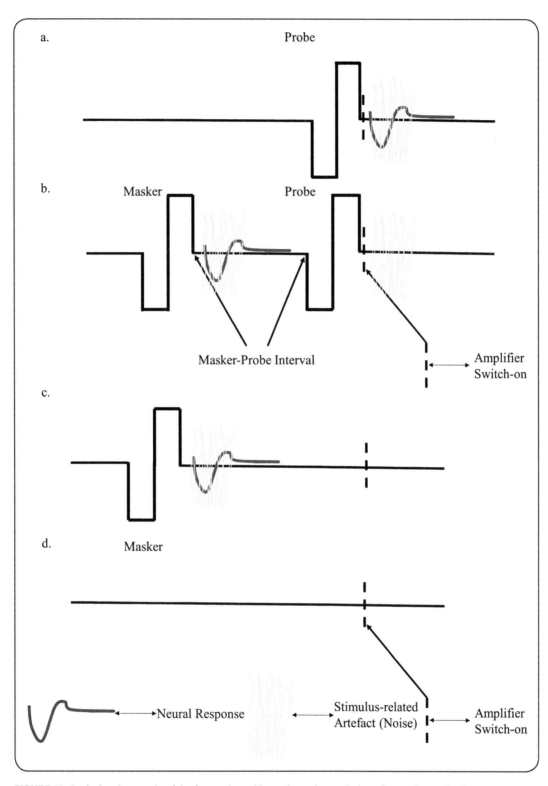

FIGURE 18–3. A visual example of the forward-masking subtraction technique for artefact reduction.

In the third phase, the masker is presented without the probe and the amplifier is switched on to capture the electrical activity related to the masker. When the electrical activity captured during the third phase is subtracted from the activity recorded during the second phase, the neural response and electrical artefact associated with the masker is cancelled out, leaving only the neural response elicited by the probe in the first phase. In the fourth and final phase, neither the masker nor the probe is presented, but the amplifier is switched on. During amplifier switch on, a small electrical artefact is created. Subtracting the artefact created in the fourth phase from the artefact created in the first phase removes this amplifier-elicited artefact and leaves only the neural response evoked by the probe. Research has suggested that the forward-masking subtraction technique is the most effective artefact reduction technique in that it provides the largest amplitude ECAP response with the lowest ECAP threshold and most robust morphology (Baudhuin, Hughes, & Goehring, 2016). The forward-masking subtraction technique is the default artefact reduction technique used with the Cochlear Nucleus cochlear implant system but is unavailable in the Advanced Bionics and MED-EL telemetry systems.

Numerous parameters may be adjusted to optimize ECAP recordings made with the forward masking subtraction technique. The three parameters that are most commonly adjusted are the amplifier gain, the amplifier delay, and the recording electrode contact. The **amplifier gain** is measured in dB and typically ranges from 40 to 70 dB. Setting the amplifier gain to a higher level (e.g., 60 to 70 dB) will improve the potential of recording low-level ECAP responses but will increase the risk of saturating the recording amplifier. Setting the amplifier gain at a lower value (e.g., 40 dB) reduces the risk of amplifier saturation but may not offer enough amplification to allow for successful recording of the ECAP.

The **amplifier delay** refers to the amount of time that elapses between the presentation of the signals and the "switch on" of the amplifier (Figure 18–4). The amplifier delay typically ranges from 50 to 125 microseconds. If the amplifier gain is set too short, then the stimulus-related electrical artefact may still be present at high levels and may saturate the amplifier. If the amplifier delay is set too long, then the neural response of the cochlear nerve may have already occurred and will be cut off or missed when the amplifier is switched on (Figure 18–5). Finally, the **recording electrode contact** may be adjusted in an attempt to avoid amplifier saturation while also allowing for the recording of a robust ECAP. The recording electrode contact is typically located two electrode contacts apical to the stimulating electrode contact but may be set to be as close as one electrode contact away or several electrode contacts away from the stimulating electrode contact. Also, the recording electrode contact may be located basally from the stimulating electrode contact. Of note, in the NRT platform, Cochlear offers a feature referred to as "Optimize recording parameters," which measures NRT at a suprathreshold stimulus level with a combination of different amplifier gains and delays as well as recording electrode contacts to identify the set of parameters to yield the optimal ECAP response.

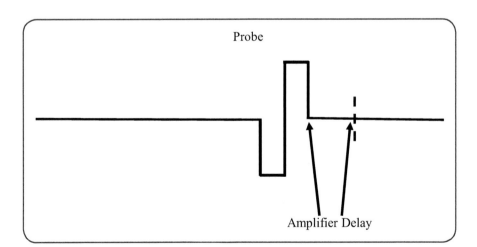

FIGURE 18–4. A visual example of the delay that exists between the offset of the stimulus and the "switch-on" of the recording amplifier (i.e., amplifier delay).

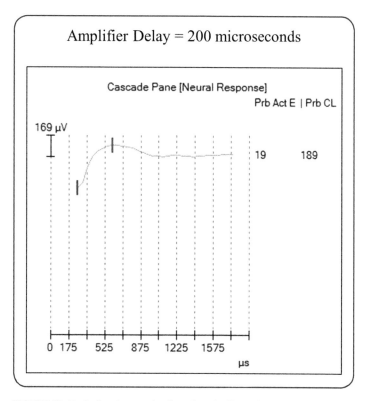

FIGURE 18–5. A visual example of an electrically evoked compound action potential response that is not fully captured because the amplifier delay was too long. Image provided courtesy of Cochlear Americas, ©2018.

Alternating Polarity Artefact Reduction. The **alternating polarity** artefact reduction scheme is commonly used in clinical auditory evoked response measurements to minimize or eliminate extraneous electrical signals or non-neural physiologic responses. Figure 18–6 provides a visual depiction of the alternating polarity technique. As shown, the biphasic electrical pulses alternately switch from cathodic-leading (i.e., negative polarity first) to anodic-leading (i.e., positive polarity first) throughout the duration of the measurement. As discussed in Chapter 3, neurons assume a positive polarity (i.e., positive charge) when stimulated (i.e., when an action potential is evoked). This stimulus-evoked change toward a positive potential occurs regardless of the leading polarity of the stimulus. In other words, whether the biphasic pulse begins with a cathodic or anodic phase, the cochlear neurons will always respond by producing an action potential with a sudden spike in positivity. Therefore, when the neural responses that are recorded to a cathodic- and then to an anodic-leading biphasic pulse are summed together at the recording amplifier, the neural responses to the two stimuli are similar and are amplified and preserved relatively intact. In contrast, the stimulus-related artefact changes in polarity with changes in stimulus polarity. Consequently, alternating the polarity of the stimulus results in a reduction or elimination of stimulus-related artefact when the responses to cathodic- and anodic-leading stimuli are summed together at the recording amplifier (see Figure 18–6).

At this point, the reader may be asking the question, "If the cochlear neurons always assume a positive charge when stimulated, then why is the peak of the ECAP plotted with a negative direction?" In short, the activity from the intracochlear electrode contact and the extracochlear reference electrode is delivered to two separate inputs of the differential amplifier, one with a positive polarity (i.e., non-inverting) and another with a negative polarity (i.e., inverting). The activity from the cochlear nerve that is captured by the intracochlear electrode contact is delivered to the amplifier input with the inverting polarity, which serves to invert the polarity of the cochlear nerve response.

A drawback of the alternating polarity artefact reduction method is the fact that there may be minor

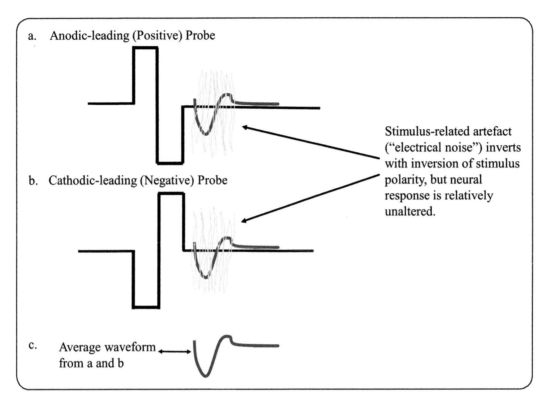

a. Anodic-leading (Positive) Probe

b. Cathodic-leading (Negative) Probe

Stimulus-related artefact ("electrical noise") inverts with inversion of stimulus polarity, but neural response is relatively unaltered.

c. Average waveform from a and b

FIGURE 18–6. A visual example of the alternating polarity technique for artefact reduction.

differences in amplitude and latency of the cochlear nerve's response to cathodic- and anodic-leading biphasic electrical pulses (Miller et al., 1998). Consequently, when summed together, the collective responses to cathodic- and anodic-leading biphasic pulses may have a slightly smaller amplitude, a slightly higher threshold, and a less prominent or robust morphology than the ECAP that is measured with the forward-masking subtraction technique (Frijns et al., 2002; Hughes et al., 2003). Of note, the alternating polarity scheme is the artefact reduction method used to measure the ECAP with Advanced Bionics cochlear implants (i.e., Neural Response Imaging [NRI]) and is also the default method used to measure the ECAP with MED-EL cochlear implants (Auditory Response Telemetry [ART]). Alternating polarity is not the default method but may also be used to measure the ECAP with Cochlear Nucleus cochlear implants (Neural Response Telemetry [NRT]).

Scaled Template Subtraction Artefact Reduction. The **scaled template subtraction technique** is another artefact reduction method that is available for use with Cochlear Nucleus NRT and MED-EL ART measurements. Figure 18–7 provides a visual example of

the scaled template subtraction technique. In short, the ECAP is measured with the use of two stimulus phases. In the first phase, the stimulus is presented at a level that is well below the ECAP threshold, and as a result, the amplifier captures stimulus-related artefact, but no neural response is present. In the second phase, a higher-level, suprathreshold stimulus is presented and electrical activity captured at the amplifier is analyzed. During analysis after the second phase, a template of the artefact is created by scaling up the artefact captured during the first phase by a factor equivalent to the ratio of the stimulus presented in phase two relative to phase one. This artefact template is subtracted from the electrical activity captured by the amplifier during phase two to essentially cancel out the stimulus-related artefact and leave the stimulus-evoked neural response largely intact.

Determining ECAP Threshold

Audiologists typically aim to determine an ECAP threshold for several different electrode contacts across the electrode array. ECAP thresholds are often obtained through the measurement of an ECAP **amplitude growth function (AGF)**. An AGF is obtained

a. Probe delivered at a level that is below neural response threshold (subthreshold)

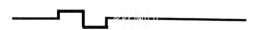

b. Artefact is "scaled up" by a multiple that is identical to the increase in probe level in "c" below

c. Probe delivered at a suprathreshold level

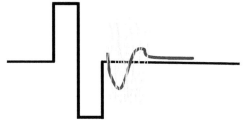

d. Neural waveform with artefact eliminated by template subtraction

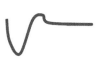

FIGURE 18–7. A visual example of the scaled template technique for artefact reduction.

by completing serial ECAP measurements on the same intracochlear electrode contact but at different stimulation levels. AGF typically includes measures completed at a stimulation level or stimulation levels that are below the ECAP threshold and several ECAP measures completed at suprathreshold stimulation levels. Figure 18–2 provides an example of an ECAP AGF. The change in stimulus level between measurements (i.e., step size) should be large enough to allow for an efficient determination of ECAP threshold (i.e., quickly proceed to a stimulus level that evokes

an ECAP threshold response) but small enough to allow for relatively precise resolution of the ECAP threshold.

As with most auditory evoked responses, the amplitude of the ECAP increases as the stimulus level is increased above the response threshold. Also, the morphology of the response becomes more robust with the P2 component becoming more prominent. In contrast to auditory evoked responses obtained to acoustic stimulation, the latency of the ECAP essentially remains unchanged with changes in stimulus level. The increase in response latency that typically occurs with a decrease in stimulus level for auditory evoked responses elicited by acoustic stimuli is primarily attributed to the cochlear traveling wave. Because the cochlea is bypassed during cochlear implant-elicited ECAP measurements, there is little to no change in the latency of the ECAP response with changes in stimulus level. Of note, the AGF can be measured with use of ascending (i.e., beginning at a higher, presumably suprathreshold stimulus level and progressively decreasing the stimulus level across serial measurements) or descending stimulus levels (i.e., from low to high stimulus levels). The advantage of a descending approach is that the audiologist may terminate the measurement once the ECAP response is observed and quickly proceed to a lower stimulus level. Another advantage is the fact that the audiologist may terminate the ECAP measure once threshold on a particular electrode is determined and proceed to measure the ECAP on another electrode contact. The disadvantages of the descending approach is that several suprathreshold ECAP measures may be completed before ECAP threshold is determined and the recipient may find the relatively high starting level to be uncomfortable. However, it should be noted that most recipients are able to comfortably tolerate ECAP stimulus levels that are equal to or moderately greater than the stimulation levels used in their daily program. The advantage of the ascending approach is that the starting stimulus level will likely be comfortable for the recipient. A disadvantage of the ascending approach is the possibility that several ECAP measures will be completed before an ECAP response is obtained.

The ECAP threshold may be calculated from the AGF by way of two different approaches, (1) visual analysis and (2) regression analysis. **Visual determination** of the ECAP threshold is completed in the same manner in which the auditory brainstem response is analyzed to estimate behavioral thresholds in infants and young children. In short, the audiologist tracks the ECAP AGF down to a stimulus level at which an identifiable ECAP can no longer be observed. In Figure 18–2, the ECAP threshold as determined by visual analysis is between 175 and 180 CL. As with a threshold search in conventional auditory brainstem response assessment, if the audiologist is uncertain of whether an ECAP response is present, then the ECAP measured at the next highest stimulation level should be analyzed and examined for the expected increase in response amplitude and enhancement in morphology. Of note, the ECAP threshold may be

obscured by the noise floor of the recording amplifier, which is typically around 5 to 25 microvolts for most cochlear implant systems. As a general rule of thumb, ECAP waveforms with amplitudes lower than 20 to 25 microvolts are generally considered to be within the noise floor of the measurement system.

The second method used to determine ECAP is to calculate a **linear regression** line that best fits the ECAP amplitude points obtained in the AGF (Figure 18–8). The **regression-derived ECAP threshold** is determined by identifying the stimulus level value at which the linear regression line crosses the x-axis (i.e., the stimulus level corresponding to an ECAP value of 0 microvolts as determined by extrapolation of the regression line; see Figure 18–8). The regression-derived ECAP threshold is oftentimes referred to as the T-ECAP (e.g., T-NRT for Cochlear Nucleus implants and t-NRI for Advanced Bionics implants). In order for the regression-derived NRI to provide an accurate estimation of the ECAP threshold, it is important that the ECAP AGF includes measures completed with at least four to five stimulus levels as well as an ECAP response that is obtained near or at the visual ECAP threshold. The regression-derived ECAP threshold may be misleading in some recipients, because the ECAP AGF does not always possess a linear shape. Also, the slope of the ECAP AGF can vary considerably across recipients, which will also affect where the regression line crosses the x-axis after extrapolation. Regression-derived ECAP thresholds are typically lower than visually determined ECAP thresholds. Potential advantages of the regression-derived ECAP threshold are: (1) a threshold can be quickly calculated based on a few suprathreshold responses and (2) the ECAP threshold may be better estimated for cochlear implant systems with higher noise floors. In contrast, disadvantages of the regression-derived ECAP approach are: (1) the ECAP threshold may be underestimated if the AGF function is non-linear, (2) the ECAP threshold may be underestimated if the slope of the AGF function is shallow and an ECAP response near threshold is not included in the AGF, and (3) for recipients with loudness tolerance issues, it may be difficult to obtain the four to five suprathreshold ECAP responses necessary to create an AGF that will provide a reasonable prediction of the ECAP threshold.

Of note, the slope of the linear regression line plotted through the AGF has also received interest as a variable that may be used to predict hearing performance and/or status of the auditory system. The slope of the AGF regression line indicates the rate of

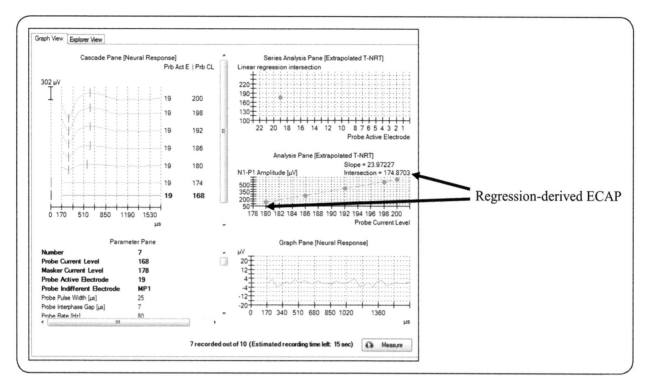

FIGURE 18–8. A visual example of an electrically evoked compound action potential (ECAP) amplitude growth function with regression analysis to predict the ECAP threshold. Image provided courtesy of Cochlear Americas, ©2018.

ECAP amplitude growth (in microvolts) as a function of stimulus level (in charge units or clinical units). The slope of the AGF regression line is typically steeper for persons with greater degrees of cochlear nerve neural survival (Charasse et al., 2004). Also, ECAP AGF slope is typically steeper for monopolar stimulation versus bipolar stimulation (Hoth, Spitzer, & Praetorius, 2018). AGF slope has not been shown to correlate with speech recognition or MAP stimulation levels (Hoth, Spitzer, & Praetorius, 2018).

Primary Clinical Applications of the ECAP

The ECAP may be clinically useful in a number of ways. For instance, the presence of a recordable ECAP indicates that the cochlear implant is providing stimulation and the cochlear nerve is responding to the stimulation. This information can be very reassuring to a recipient's family members. Additionally, the ECAP provides a baseline representation of physiologic function that may be helpful to recipient performance changes over time. Research has shown that the ECAP threshold remains fairly stable across time. Telmesani and Said (2016) evaluated ECAP thresholds across time for a group of 25 children with

Nucleus 24 implants and reported that ECAP thresholds were significant lower at activation compared with the ECAP measured intraoperatively. However, there was not a statistically significant difference in mean ECAP thresholds measured at initial activation and at 3, 6, and 12 months post-activation. Of note, Telmesani and Said did find a significant increase in T and C levels at activation compared with T and C levels at the 12-month post-activation point. Hughes et al. (2001) examined ECAP thresholds obtained intraoperatively and at different points in time throughout the 2-year post-activation period with 35 children and 33 adults using Nucleus CI24M implants. Hughes and colleagues (2001) reported that ECAP threshold decreased from the intraoperative measurement through one month post-activation but remained stable from the one-month to two-year post-activation period. Likewise, Spivak et al. (2011) recorded the ECAP in 71 children and adults and reported that ECAP thresholds measured at initial activation were lower than ECAP thresholds measured intraoperatively but there was no change in ECAP thresholds measured at the initial activation and 3-month post-activation appointments. The aforementioned studies show the ECAP threshold to be relatively stable across time after activation of the cochlear implant. Consequently, the ECAP serves as an indicator of physiologic and implant function over time. An absence of or significant change in ECAP over time may serve as an objective indicator of a problem with the cochlear implant or auditory function.

The Role of the ECAP in Cochlear Implant Programming. The ECAP has received a considerable amount of interest as a measure that may aid the audiologist in determining behavioral stimulation levels (i.e., electrical threshold and upper-stimulation levels). Research has shown that electrically evoked auditory response thresholds have a moderately strong correlation to behavioral electrical threshold (i.e., T level) when a similar stimulus is used to elicit each type of response (Abbas & Brown, 1991; Brown et al., 1994; McKay, Fewster, & Dawson, 2005; Shallop et al., 1991; Zimmerling & Hochmair, 2002). However, the stimulus that is typically used to elicit the ECAP is considerably different from the stimuli used to program cochlear implants as well as from the electrical signal used in most modern signal coding strategies. Specifically, the ECAP response is obtained to a single biphasic electrical pulse presented at a slow rate (30 to 80 pps), whereas implant stimulation occurs via a train of biphasic pulses that are delivered at a rate of 250 to 5000 pps for an extended period of time (e.g., continuously when the implant is used in realistic situations and for 300 to 500 milliseconds when stimuli are presented for T and upper-stimulation level measurements). Faster stimulation rates cannot be used to measure the ECAP because the response will deteriorate because the period of the stimulus will be less than the refractory period of the cochlear nerve and neural adaptation will occur. Furthermore, it is impractical to use the same slow rate of ECAP measurements (30–80 pps) for stimulation in a modern signal coding strategy, because research has shown a benefit for faster stimulation rates (e.g., several hundred to 1500 pps). Consequently, there is not a one-to-one relationship between the ECAP threshold and T level or upper-stimulation level.

Early work examining the ECAP as a tool to determine T and upper-stimulation levels suggested a weak relationship between the ECAP (80 pps stimulation rate) and behavioral stimulation levels measured at a 250 pps stimulation rate (Brown et al., 2000; Franck & Norton, 2001). Later research studies have generally shown an even poorer correlation between ECAP threshold and T and upper-stimulation level when the latter are measured at the faster stimula-

tion rates used in modern signal coding strategies (McKay, Fewster, & Dawson, 2005; Potts et al., 2007; Zimmerling & Hochmair, 2002).

In an effort to improve upon the potential of using the ECAP to estimate cochlear implant stimulation levels, several researchers have developed procedures in which the ECAP threshold is combined with a limited number of behavioral stimulation level measures to develop recipient-specific offset correction factors. For example, Hughes and colleagues (2000) proposed a method in which the ECAP threshold is measured on all active intracochlear electrode contacts. Next, behavioral T and upper-stimulation levels are measured for one electrode contact (typically in the middle of the array), and an offset (i.e., difference value: difference between T level and ECAP threshold and upper-stimulation level and ECAP threshold for the channel on which the behavioral measures are obtained) is determined between the ECAP and the measured T and upper-stimulation levels for that channel. Then, the offset measured at that electrode is used to estimate T levels (by subtracting the offset value from the ECAP threshold measured at each electrode contacts) and upper-stimulation levels (by adding the offset value to the ECAP threshold measured at each electrode) for the rest of the active channels. Figures 18–9, 18–10, and 18–11 provide a visual example of Hughes method. Although the addition of measured behavioral levels on one electrode contact may provide some improvement in the ability to use the ECAP threshold to estimate behavioral stimulation levels, research evaluating this method has suggested that the correlation between ECAP and behavioral stimulation levels was still weak to moderate at best (Hughes et al., 2000; Franck, 2002).

Smoorenburg, Willeboer, and van Dijk (2002) proposed another method in which behavioral measures were combined with the ECAP threshold in an attempt to estimate T and upper-stimulation levels across the electrode array. These researchers have also proposed that the audiologist measure the ECAP threshold for every intracochlear electrode contact within the array. Next, both T and upper-stimulation levels are set to the same level as the ECAP threshold across the electrode array (i.e., match the ECAP threshold profile). Then, the T and upper-stimulation levels are globally decreased to a level that was inaudible to the recipient. In many cases, the T and upper-stimulation levels are separated by a small amount (i.e., narrow EDR). After this is accomplished, the audiologist activates this program in live speech mode, and the T and upper-stimulation levels are

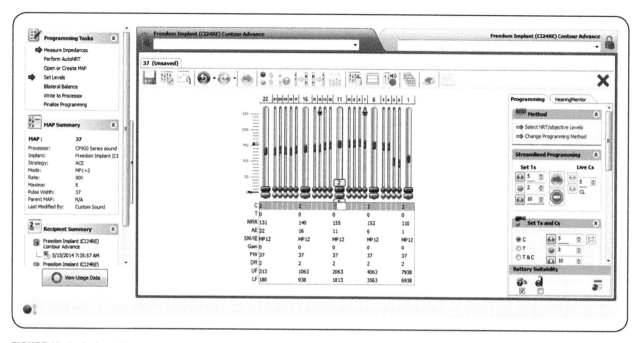

FIGURE 18–9. A visual illustration of the off-set method in which the electrically evoked compound action potential is combined with limited behavioral measures to predict stimulation levels across the entire electrode array (see text for detailed explanation). Image provided courtesy of Cochlear Americas, ©2018.

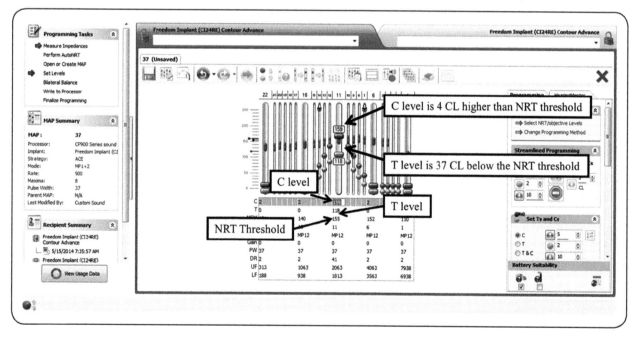

FIGURE 18–10. A visual illustration of the off-set method in which the electrically evoked compound action potential is combined with limited behavioral measures to predict stimulation levels across the entire electrode array (see text for detailed explanation). Image provided courtesy of Cochlear Americas, ©2018.

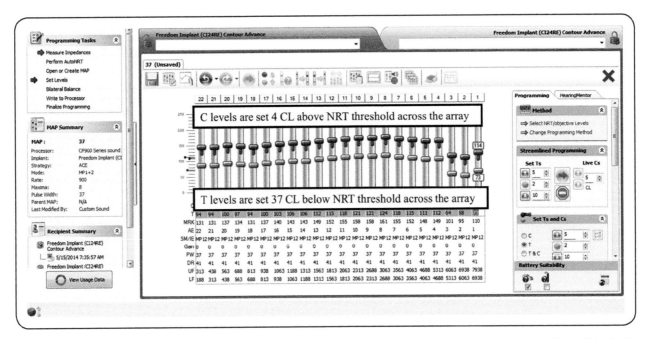

FIGURE 18–11. A visual illustration of the off-set method in which the electrically evoked compound action potential is combined with limited behavioral measures to predict stimulation levels across the entire electrode array (see text for detailed explanation). Image provided courtesy of Cochlear Americas, ©2018.

globally increased while the audiologist observes for a behavioral response to the stimulation. T levels were set to the point where a behavioral response to live speech is initially observed, and then upper-stimulation levels are globally increased to a level that should provide adequate stimulation without discomfort (i.e., ideally at a level that offers optimal clarity for speech and that is most comfortably loud to the recipient). Of course, even with this approach, identifying optimal upper-stimulation levels is very subjective and difficult when working with recipients who are unable to provide reliable verbal feedback about the loudness of the signals they receive. Again, these researchers reported weak to moderate correlations between the ECAP threshold and behavioral stimulation levels with the use of this method (Smoorenburg et al., 2002).

In summary, the majority of studies examining the ECAP as a tool to create cochlear implant program levels have suggested that it is quite limited in its ability to predict both T and upper-stimulation levels. It is difficult to pinpoint the exact cause of the weak relationship typically reported between ECAP and T/upper stimulation levels, but three possibilities exist. First, there are potentially substantial inter- and intrarecipient differences in the geometric orientation and physical distance between the stimulating electrode and recording contacts across the electrode array. The geometric orientation between the stimulating and recording electrodes as well as to the auditory neural elements has a substantial impact on the electrical potentials recorded via a near field approach (Moller, Colletti, & Fiorino, 1994), such as ECAP with cochlear implants. For instance, a recording electrode facing perpendicular to (i.e., directly toward) the auditory nerve will most likely capture a more robust ECAP response than a recording electrode facing at a 45-degree angle to the neural elements. Additionally, a recording electrode placed very close to the modiolus would likely capture a more robust ECAP response than an electrode that is located next to the lateral wall. Indeed, research has shown lower ECAP thresholds for recipients with perimodiolar electrode arrays compared with recipients with lateral wall electrode arrays (Telmesani & Said, 2015), a finding that may be attributed to both the greater amount of stimulation available from an electrode contact located proximal to the modiolus as well as to the fact that the recording electrode is located closer to the responding neural elements.

Second, as previously discussed, intersubject differences in neural refractory properties may affect the relationship of the ECAP response measured to a slow rate (e.g., 30–80 pps) compared with a behavioral response measured to a pulse train with a stimulation rate of several hundred to several thousand pps. Differences in intersubject neural refractoriness of auditory nerve fibers may contribute to the significant intersubject variability observed between ECAP threshold and behavioral stimulation levels. These differences may be especially prominent in CI programs/MAPs using faster stimulation rates (e.g., several thousand pps). Third, there may be differences among electrode arrays and the impact they may have on the stimulus and recording characteristics of the ECAP. For instance, the size and shape of the intracochlear electrode is likely to have an effect on the recording of auditory evoked potentials. Intracochlear electrode contacts with a larger surface area are likely to record a more robust ECAP response than electrode contacts with a smaller surface area. Given the manner in which these factors vary across recipients, a single ECAP-based correction factor is unlikely to provide an accurate estimation of T and upper-stimulation levels.

Botros and Psarros (2010a, 2010b) recently proposed another reason for the relatively poor relationship reported between ECAP threshold and behavioral stimulation levels. In a study examining NRT thresholds of Nucleus recipients, these researchers noted that a limitation of previous studies examining ECAP as predictor of behavioral stimulation level was the fact that each electrode within the electrode array was treated as a single, independent data point. Instead, Botros and Psarros proposed that the overall profile (i.e., shape) of the T and upper stimulation levels across the array should influence how these levels are set. Specifically, they noted that the profiles of the T and upper stimulation levels typically flattens as stimulation levels increase. At lower stimulation levels, Botros and Psarros noted that behavioral stimulation levels often take a similar shape or profile as the ECAP threshold profile. However, at higher stimulation levels, the profile of behavioral stimulation levels tends to flatten. Along this line of thinking, Botros and Psarros contended that the upper-stimulation level profile is typically flatter than the T level profile, particularly for recipients with wide EDRs. In short, Botros and Psarros concluded that the profile of T levels often takes the same shape as the ECAP-threshold profile, especially for recipients who have relatively low T levels, and whereas the upper-stimulation level profile may roughly mimic the ECAP-threshold profile, the upper-stimulation level profile tends to be flatter.

Botros and Psarros (2010a, 2010b) proposed that the flatter profiles at higher stimulation levels were due to a couple of factors. First, channel interaction is more prevalent at higher stimulation levels, which results in a greater similarity in the way the audi-

tory nerve responds from one channel (e.g., electrode contact) to the next. Hence, the psychophysical responses are more similar at higher levels where channel interaction is more substantial. Second, more neurons are recruited by the electrical stimulation at higher levels, and the loudness growth functions are steeper. As a result, each increment change in stimulus intensity results in a larger change in loudness, which leads to fewer level differences between adjacent electrodes. Again, this results in a flatter profile for higher stimulation levels (which especially affects the upper stimulation levels).

Botros and Psarros (2010a, 2010b) evaluated their hypothesis with a group of 15 Nucleus recipients who were able to provide feedback about loudness percept and sound quality. They developed a scaling factor to account for the flattening of the profile of stimulation levels associated with a given loudness percept that is particularly observed at higher stimulation levels. Then, they used this scaling factor to estimate the profile T and upper-stimulation levels for 29 Nucleus recipients on the basis of the ECAP threshold and compared this estimation to estimates that were based: (1) solely on the ECAP threshold, (2) on population mean estimates, and (3) on a flat profile. For each of the methods used to estimate T and upper-stimulation levels, the profiles developed from the respective approaches were globally increased so that T levels were set to a level that was just noticeable, and upper stimulation levels were set to a level that was loud but comfortable. They reported that the scaled ECAP estimates provided a significantly better estimate of the recipients measured T and C levels than any of the other methods used to estimate behavioral stimulation levels. Additionally, the majority of the subjects preferred programs created by the scaled ECAP approach relative to the other methods used to estimate behavioral stimulation levels. Botros, Banna, and Maruthurkkara (2013) further noted that the T and upper-stimulation levels may be further optimized by tilting the profile, that is, increasing/decreasing the emphasis of the low (bass) or high (treble) frequencies based on the recipient's feedback pertaining to the sound quality and clarity of speech and other environmental sounds. The interested reader is referred to the Botros and colleagues (2010a, 2010b, 2013) articles for more detailed information on conducting this procedure.

Although the Botros and Psarros (2010a, 2010b) approach of using scaled ECAP thresholds to estimate stimulation levels appears to hold promise, its clinical application is somewhat limited because of several factors. First, at the time of this writing, the scaling model that they used to shape the behavioral stimulation levels is not readily available in clinical software or by simple calculation by the audiologist. Second, even if the scaling model were readily available for clinical use, the audiologist must still be able to obtain a behavioral threshold to speech or environmental sounds to set the global T-level profile as well as determine the optimal level at which to set the global upper-stimulation level profile. Both of these tasks may prove to be difficult when creating cochlear implant programs for young and difficult-to-test recipients, who may not respond until the stimulus reaches suprathreshold levels, whose responses may be subtle

or difficult to interpret, and for whom objective measures are the most helpful. Third, the relationship between the ECAP and behavioral-stimulation levels is variable across recipients and may even be variable across the electrode array within an individual recipient. Subjects may have ECAP thresholds that fall near T levels, near upper-stimulation levels, or in the middle of their electrical dynamic range. Although the scaled ECAP approach may serve to account for some of this variability, it certainly does not capture it to the full extent for each individual.

For example, Figure 18–12 and Figure 18–13 show NRT thresholds superimposed over program

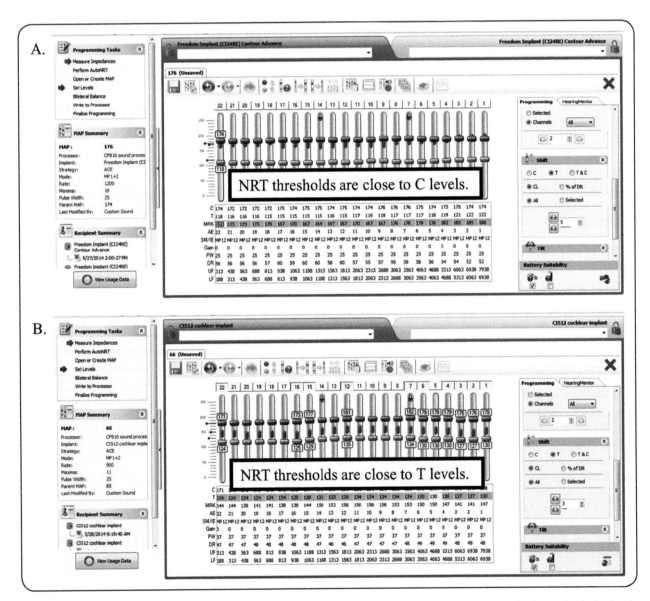

FIGURE 18–12. The relationship between electrically evoked compound action potential thresholds and behavioral stimulation levels (i.e., T and C levels) for an adult recipient who has achieved excellent outcomes. Image provided courtesy of Cochlear Americas, ©2018.

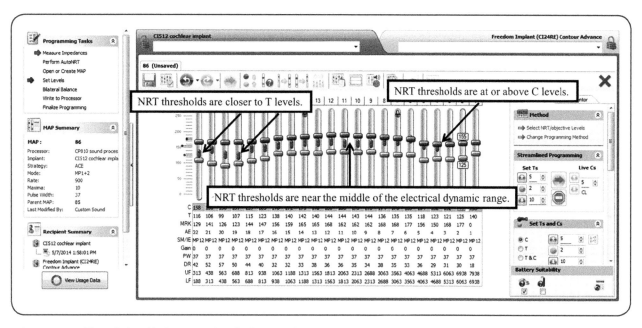

FIGURE 18–13. The relationship between electrically evoked compound action potential thresholds and behavioral stimulation levels (i.e., T and C levels) for an adult recipient who has achieved excellent outcomes. Image provided courtesy of Cochlear Americas, ©2018.

levels for reliable adults who have excellent open-set speech recognition abilities with their cochlear implants and for whom valid T and C levels were established from behavioral measures. As shown in the first two examples (see Figures 18–12A and 18-12B), the NRT threshold may approach the upper-stimulation level (i.e., C level) for some recipients and T levels for another. In contrast, for the recipient shown in Figure 18–13, the ECAP threshold falls near upper-stimulation level at some segments of the array, within the middle of the EDR at other segments of the array, and above upper-stimulation level for other channels. If the audiologist used any of the aforementioned ECAP-based approaches in isolation to set behavioral levels, then suboptimal stimulation levels would likely be provided for this recipient. Given the variable relationship of ECAP to measured stimulation needs, the audiologist should exercise caution when using the ECAP threshold to estimate T and upper-stimulation levels. Behavioral and/or ESRT measures serve as better indicators of ideal program levels, and it is simply inappropriate to create cochlear implant programs solely from ECAP thresholds when reliable behavioral (or ESRT in the case of upper-stimulation levels) measures can be obtained. In short, the audiologist should always strive to obtain valid behavioral levels (e.g., VRA, conditioned play audiometry, or conventional audiometry and loudness scaling) to determine T and

upper-stimulation levels as well as acquire the ESRT to corroborate upper-stimulation levels.

However, the audiologist will undoubtedly encounter recipients who are unable to cooperate for behavioral and ESRT measures to be measured, and as a result, the audiologist will have to rely on the ECAP threshold as a guide to estimate appropriate T and upper-stimulation levels. Examples of these recipients who are unable to cooperate for behavioral stimulation levels and/or ESRT to be completed include: (1) young children who exhibit inconsistent or subtle responses to auditory stimuli during the early stages of implant use, (2) recipients with multiple disabilities that complicate the measurement of behavioral stimulation levels, (3) recipients who have pressure equalization (PE) tubes that prevent the recording of the ESRT, (4) recipients who do not have measurable ESRT, and (5) recipients who will not tolerate the presence of the acoustic immittance probe for the completion of the ESRT. In these cases, the authors of this book have adopted a modified approach that is largely influenced by the protocols proposed by both Smoorenburg et al. (2002) and Botros and Psarros (2010a, 2010b). First, the audiologist should measure the ECAP threshold for all intracochlear electrode contacts across the array (see markers in Figure 18–14). Second, the T and upper-stimulation levels should be set to approximate the profile of the of the ECAP thresholds (Figure 18–15).

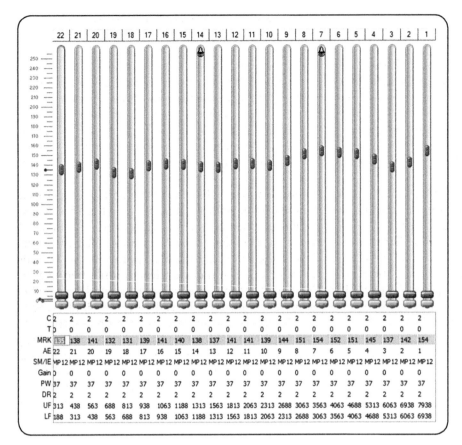

FIGURE 18–14. A visual illustration of the process of setting stimulation levels based on the electrically evoked compound action potential and observation of behavioral responses to sound in live speech mode (see text for a detailed explanation). Image provided courtesy of Cochlear Americas, ©2018.

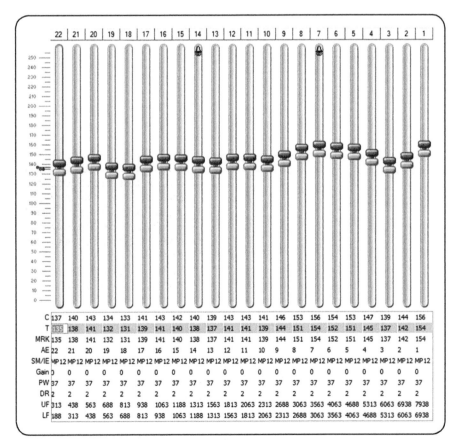

FIGURE 18–15. A visual illustration of the process of setting stimulation levels based on the electrically evoked compound action potential and observation of behavioral responses to sound in live speech mode (see text for a detailed explanation). Image provided courtesy of Cochlear Americas, ©2018.

It should be noted that when abrupt differences in ECAP thresholds exist across the array (i.e., ECAP thresholds that are markedly different at one or a small subset of electrodes relative to the remaining or neighboring electrodes), the audiologist should consider arbitrarily "smoothing" the T and upper-stimulation level profiles so that there are not significant fluctuations in the T and upper-stimulation levels across the array (Figure 18–16). Third, the T and upper -stimulation-level profiles are offset by a small amount (e.g., 10 CL/10% of ECAP threshold: if ECAP threshold is 150 CU, then offset by 15 charge units), and both are globally decreased to a level that the audiologist is certain will be inaudible to the recipient (Figure 18–17). Fourth, the implant is activated in live speech mode, and the T and upper-stimulation levels are gradually increased while the programming audiologist and assistant observe for a behavioral response from the recipient. T levels are set at the minimal level that elicits a response or just below the level that elicits a behavioral response (Figure 18–18). Fifth, upper-stimulation levels are increased slowly and set to a level that the audiologist believes will allow for adequate loudness normalization (i.e., loud sounds will be loud but comfortable to the recipient) and optimal speech recognition, while avoiding loudness discomfort. As upper-stimulation levels are increased, the audiologist should arbitrarily flatten the upper-stimulation level profile so that it continues to roughly approximate the ECAP threshold profile but is smoother or flatter in shape (Figure 18–19). This adjustment is based on the Botros and Psarros (2010a, 2010b) work, which suggests that the stimulation profile will flatten as stimulation levels are increased. Again, as stimulation levels approach higher current levels, then it is likely more appropriate to provide a flatter upper-stimulation level profile because the increased channel interaction associated with higher stimulation levels will lead to more similar requisite levels (i.e., flatter shape) from one electrode to the next. Of note, if stimulation levels are relatively high compared with what is typical for a particular implant system and electrode array, the audiologist may also consider flattening the T levels to a lesser extent than the flattening provided to the upper-stimulation level profile. Additionally, the audiologist

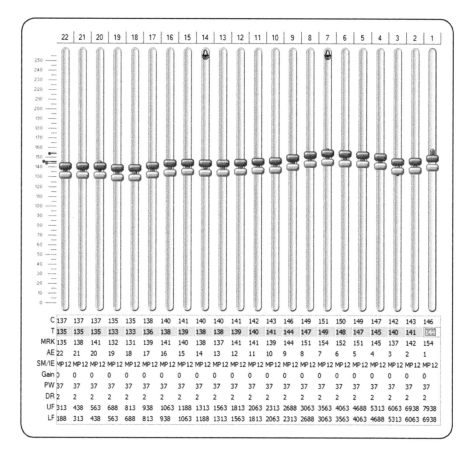

FIGURE 18–16. A visual illustration of the process of setting stimulation levels based on the electrically evoked compound action potential and observation of behavioral responses to sound in live speech mode (see text for a detailed explanation). Image provided courtesy of Cochlear Americas, ©2018.

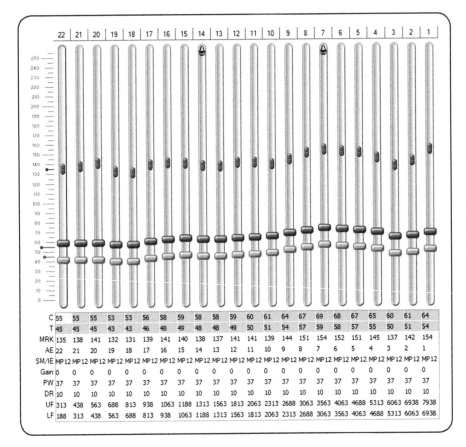

FIGURE 18–17. A visual illustration of the process of setting stimulation levels based on the electrically evoked compound action potential and observation of behavioral responses to sound in live speech mode (see text for a detailed explanation). Image provided courtesy of Cochlear Americas, ©2018.

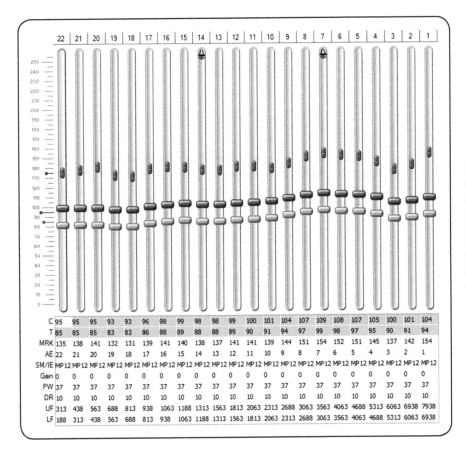

FIGURE 18–18. A visual illustration of the process of setting stimulation levels based on the electrically evoked compound action potential and observation of behavioral responses to sound in live speech mode (see text for a detailed explanation). Image provided courtesy of Cochlear Americas, ©2018.

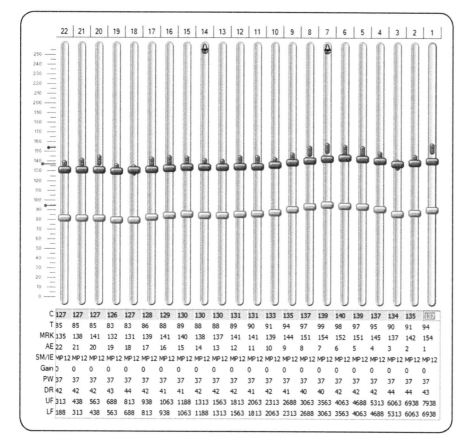

	22	21	20	19	18	17	16	15	14	13	12	11	10	9	8	7	6	5	4	3	2	1
C	127	127	127	126	127	128	129	130	130	130	131	131	133	135	137	139	140	139	137	134	135	167
T	85	85	85	83	83	86	88	89	88	88	89	90	91	94	97	99	98	97	95	90	91	94
MRK	135	138	141	132	131	139	141	140	138	137	141	141	139	144	151	154	152	151	145	137	142	154
AE	22	21	20	19	18	17	16	15	14	13	12	11	10	9	8	7	6	5	4	3	2	1
SM/IE	MP12	MP12	MP12	MP12	MP12	MP12	MP12	MP12	MP12	MP12	MP12	MP12	MP12	MP12	MP12	MP12	MP12	MP12	MP12	MP12	MP12	MP12
Gain	0	0	0	0	0	0	0	0	0	0	0	0	0	0	0	0	0	0	0	0	0	0
PW	37	37	37	37	37	37	37	37	37	37	37	37	37	37	37	37	37	37	37	37	37	37
DR	42	42	42	43	44	42	41	41	42	42	42	41	42	41	40	40	42	42	42	44	44	43
UF	313	438	563	688	813	938	1063	1188	1313	1563	1813	2063	2313	2688	3063	3563	4063	4688	5313	6063	6938	7938
LF	188	313	438	563	688	813	938	1063	1188	1313	1563	1813	2063	2313	2688	3063	3563	4063	4688	5313	6063	6938

FIGURE 18–19. A visual illustration of the process of setting stimulation levels based on the electrically evoked compound action potential and observation of behavioral responses to sound in live speech mode (see text for a detailed explanation). Image provided courtesy of Cochlear Americas, ©2018.

should use his/her knowledge about typical stimulation levels of a system to serve as a guide for estimating upper-stimulation levels. For example, most Nucleus recipients have an electrical dynamic range approaching 40 to 50 CL (typical range between 20 to 60 CL). As a result, an appropriate goal would be to set upper-stimulation levels so that the electrical dynamic range is approximately 40 to 50 CL. Additionally, most Advanced Bionics recipients have M levels in the 100 to 250 range (with some recipients possessing M levels up to 300 CU), whereas most MED-EL recipients have MCL in the 5 to 25 CU range with MCLs in excess of 40 CU being exceedingly rare. As a result, the audiologist should strive for upper-stimulation levels that approach typical levels and exercise caution when upper-stimulation levels fall well outside of a typical range for an implant make and model and for a particular electrode array.

The audiologist should be hesitant to adjusting upper-stimulation levels to a point that is markedly higher than what is necessary for the typical recipient with a given make and model of implant/electrode array, although there may be some exceptional cases

in which it is appropriate to do so. Of course, the audiologist should avoid setting upper-stimulation levels to a point that elicits aversive responses (e.g., eye blinking, anxiety, discomfort, tendency to remove the device). The reader is referred to Chapter 14 for more guidance on setting upper-stimulation levels for young children and adults. Admittedly, the protocol described here for estimating T and upper-stimulation levels from ECAP thresholds requires a certain degree of subjective judgment on the part of the audiologist, which is why the use of behavioral measures and the ESRT is recommended as the primary approach to determine cochlear implant program levels. However, in instances in which behavioral levels and the ESRT cannot be measured, the modified version of the Smoorenburg et al. (2002) and Botros/Psarros (2010a, 2010b) approaches described above is a reasonable substitute for estimating program levels.

Additional Uses for ECAP Measurement

Advanced variations of ECAP measurements may be completed to gather additional information about the auditory system's responsiveness to electrical stimulation. These advanced measures include rate of recovery measures and spread of excitation measures. Rate of recovery and spread of excitation measures have both received a good deal of interest in the research arena, but for the most part, these measures are rarely conducted as part of the clinical management of cochlear implant recipients. Nonetheless, a brief introduction of rate of recovery and spread of excitation measures will be provided in the next two sections.

Rate of Recovery ECAP Measurement. The **rate of recovery** ECAP measurement is a variation of the forward-masking subtraction technique. In short, multiple ECAP measurements are made with varying MPIs. Figure 18–20 provides a visual representation of the rate of recovery measure. As shown, no ECAP is measured with a very short MPI (500 microseconds and less) because the cochlear nerve units are still in a refractory state from the presentation of the masker preceding the probe. As the MPI lengthens (750 microseconds and longer), cochlear neural units begin to recover from the refractory state and produce an ECAP response to the probe. The amplitude of the ECAP reaches asymptotic levels when the MPI is approximately 520 milliseconds and greater.

Research examining the clinical applicability of rate of the recovery ECAP measurement has generally been less than promising. Shpak and colleagues (2004) initially reported that recipients with faster rate of recovery functions preferred faster stimulation rates, but in later reports, Shpak (2005) found no relationship between rate of recovery ECAP responses and preferred stimulation rate. Brown et al. (1990) and Kiefer et al. (2001) reported better speech recognition scores for recipients with faster rate of recovery ECAP functions. In contrast, however, a host of other research studies found no relationship between ECAP rate of recovery and speech recognition (Abbas & Brown, 1991; Battmer et al., 2005; Finley et al., 1997; Turner et al., 2002). Additionally, Muller-Deile and colleagues (2003) examined the ECAP rate of recovery function as a tool to predict the intersubject differences that exist between the relationship of ECAP threshold to behavioral electrical threshold (i.e., T level). Muller-Deile et al. concluded that the ECAP rate of recovery has limited potential to improve the potential of using NRT to individually predict behavioral electrical threshold.

In a paper describing the influence of cochlear nerve neural population on the ECAP rate of recov-

ery function, Botros and Psarros (2010b) sought to explain why the ECAP rate of recovery measurement has generally been limited in its ability to predict preferred stimulation rate, stimulation levels, and speech recognition. Botros and Psarros noted that there are several complexities that are associated with the outcome of a recipient's ECAP rate of recovery function and that these complexities complicate the task of using the rate of recovery measure for clinical management of implant recipients. Specifically, Botros and Psarros acknowledged that the ECAP is a "collective response of numerous neurons" and "when a given neuron exhibits a refractory period on firing, the capacity of the whole nerve to be excited might not be diminished if there are many other neurons in a non-refractory state." Furthermore, if a recipient has a larger number of surviving cochlear nerve units, there is a greater opportunity (relative to a recipient with a spare number of surviving cochlear neural elements) that a portion of these neurons may not be in refractory state for a given stimulus. Given these statements, it is possible that the whole (i.e., collective) nerve may recover more quickly during rate of recovery measures if the recipient has a larger number of surviving cochlear nerve units, because there is a theoretically higher likelihood that the recipient will have more functional neurons that are available to respond at a given point in time.

Additionally, Botros and Psarros recognized the fact that electrical threshold and loudness can be influenced not only by how often a neuron fires (which is influenced by its refractory properties) but also by how many neurons fire. Indeed, the ECAP response and the ECAP rate of recovery have been shown to change as a function of stimulus level (Battmer et al., Brown et al., 1990; Finley et al., 1997; Stypulkowski & van den Honert, 1984). Consequently, it is reasonable to assume that the ECAP rate of recovery is related not only to the refractoriness of the cochlear nerve fibers but also to the number of cochlear nerve units that are contributing to the production of the ECAP. Interestingly, Botros and Psarros found faster rate of recovery functions to be associated with a longer duration of deafness. They attributed this finding to a hypothesis that the rate of recovery function is influenced by the extent of surviving cochlear nerve units, and consequently, slower rate of recovery functions are associated with a larger population of cochlear nerve units. As a result, the participants with a shorter duration of deafness are likely to have more surviving cochlear nerve cells and thus slower rate of recovery functions.

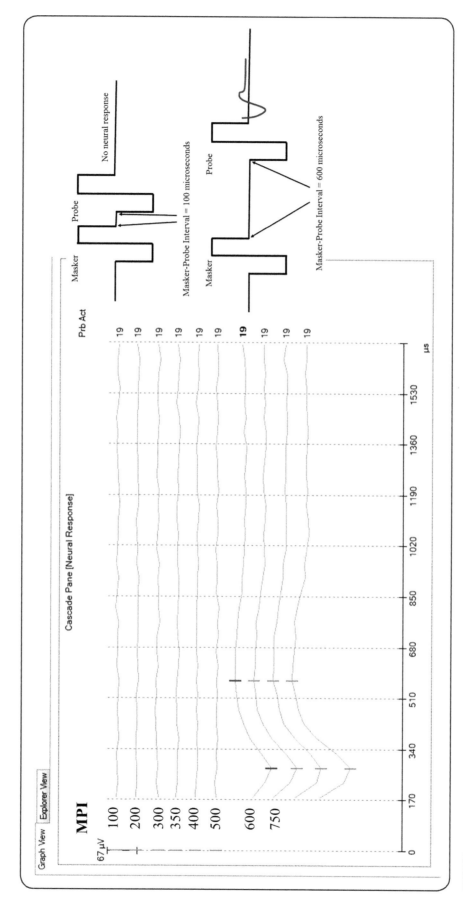

FIGURE 18–20. Rate of recovery electrically evoked compound action potential measurement.

As can be derived from this discussion of the complexities underlying an individual's ECAP rate of recovery function, the temporal response properties (i.e., refractoriness) of the cochlear nerve cannot easily be surmised from a rate of recovery function. For that reason, the rate of recovery function has seldom been applied in clinical settings. Additional research is required to unravel the complexities of the relationship between ECAP rate of recovery functions and cochlear nerve refractoriness in order for the former to be applied in a clinical setting to determine optimal stimulation rate and/or to predict recipient performance.

Spread of Excitation ECAP Measurement. The **spread of excitation** measurement is another advanced ECAP procedure that may be completed by manipulating the conventional ECAP measurement parameters. The spread of excitation may refer to the amount of electrical current spread from a stimulated electrode contact to surrounding electrode contacts. The spread of excitation may also refer to the spread of neural excitation in response to electrical stimulation on a particular electrode contact. The spread of neural excitation is obviously related to the spread of electrical current throughout the modiolus. The spread of excitation ECAP measurement may be completed via two different approaches. One approach simply involves the completion of multiple ECAP measurements with stimulation to the same intracochlear electrode contact but by changing the recording electrode from one measure to another (Cohen et al., 2004; Hughes & Stille, 2010). For instance, the first ECAP measure is made with the stimulus probe delivered to electrode 11 and with electrode 12 serving as the recording electrode. Then, subsequent measures may be completed with the recording occurring at electrodes 13, 14, 15, 16, and so forth. as well as 10, 9, 8, 7, and so forth. In most cases, the amplitude of the ECAP should diminish as the recording electrode is successively located farther from the electrode used to deliver the stimulus probe. This method, in which the recording electrode is successively adjusted from one measure to the next, measures spread of electrical current and neural excitation. Spread of excitation functions with steep slopes (i.e., decrease in ECAP amplitude as recording electrode is located farther away from stimulus probe electrode) implies less spread of excitation (i.e., channel interaction), which would theoretically be associated with better hearing performance.

The second method for measuring spread of excitation is a variant of the clinical forward-masking subtraction technique. In short, serial ECAP measurements are made with the stimulation delivered to the same electrode contact but with successive variation in the location of the masker electrode. As the location of the masker electrode is moved farther from the stimulated electrode, the masker becomes less effective at eliciting a state of refractoriness in the neurons that respond to the stimulating electrode. As a result, the neural response recorded on the second phase of the forward subtraction paradigm is intact and subtracted from the neural response recorded in the first phase (i.e., the unmasked, baseline condition). Therefore, as the masker is moved farther from the stimulated electrode, the amplitude of the recorded ECAP should reduce, and eventually, the ECAP should be eliminated.

Although the ECAP spread of excitation measurement may provide an indication of channel interaction, research has generally failed to establish the ECAP spread of excitation as a tool to effectively predict a recipient's performance or to determine whether certain electrode contacts should be disabled to avoid channel interaction. However, several researchers and audiologists have shown the spread of excitation ECAP to be useful for detecting electrode array tip foldover, as the shape of the spread of excitation function will change in an atypical manner when the electrode contacts involved with the foldover are used as a masker (Cohen, Saunders, & Richardson, 2004; Grolam et al., 2008; Zuniga et al., 2017).

ECAP Measurement in Modern Cochlear Implant Systems

All three cochlear implant manufacturers that have FDA approval to commercially distribute cochlear implants offer a platform to measure the ECAP with use of their clinical programming software. These manufacturer-specific programs will be described very briefly in the flowing sections.

Neural Response Imaging in the Advanced Bionics Cochlear Implant System. The ECAP may be recorded in the **Neural Response Imaging (NRI)** platform within the Advanced Bionics SoundWave software. NRI measurements may be set up on multiple channels, and once the audiologist initiates the measurement, the software will then automatically complete NRI measurements on each selected channel. The audiologist may alter measurement parameters at any time during the process of completing the NRI assessment on each of the channels. Additionally, the audiologist may create an NRI "template" that may be imported into the NRI platform to allow for quick initiation of NRI assessment across several channels.

The NRI platform may be accessed by selecting the "NRI Measurements" tab in the SoundWave software. The NRI measures are completed by delivering biphasic, rectangular electrical pulses at a rate of 30 pulses per second on the channel selected for stimulation and recording the ECAP captured at an electrode located two channels apical from the stimulated channel. When stimulating channels one and two, the recording electrode is located two channels basal to the stimulated channel. The audiologist selects the minimum and maximum stimulation levels that will be used for the NRI measurement (Figure 18–21). The audiologist may also select the number of measurements made between the measures made at the minimum and maximum values by entering the desired number of measures in the "Data Points" field in the table that resides underneath the NRI measurement window. The default number of measurement points is five, but the authors recommend that the distance

between successive measures be no more than 20 to 25 charge units.

NRI measures can be obtained with stimulation starting at the maximum value and progressing toward the minimum value or vice versa. The authors recommend beginning the NRI at a stimulation level that should be loud but not uncomfortable for the recipient and then decreasing in 15 to 25 charge unit steps. The descending stimulation approach allows for attainment of a clear NRI response at a relatively high stimulation level and termination of the NRI measure on a given channel as soon as the audiologist observes that the response is no longer present. Of note, as soon as the audiologist observes a clear NRI response, the "Skip to Next Data Point" button may be pressed to immediately proceed to the next stimulus level in the sequence. Also, as soon as the visual NRI is confidently identified, the audiologist may select the "Skip to Next Electrode" button to proceed to measurement on the next electrode contact in the sequence. The number of sweeps (e.g., stimulus presentations) on each channel is defined by the "Averages per Data Point" parameter. The default value is 32 sweeps, which is often sufficient to record

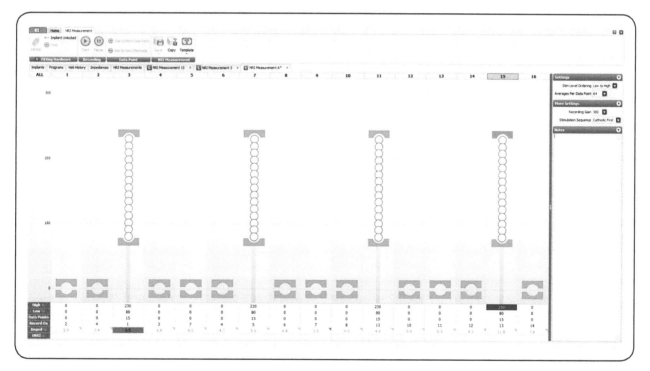

FIGURE 18–21. Setting starting and stopping stimulation levels in the Advanced Bionics Neural Response Imaging (NRI) platform. Image provided courtesy of Advanced Bionics, LLC.

a response. However, the authors typically select 128 sweeps and then choose to manually advance the measure to the next stimulus level once a clear response or no response has unequivocally been obtained. If the audiologist does not wish to manually advance to the next data point or electrode contact, then the use of 32 or 64 sweeps provides a good balance of efficiency and attainment of a reliable response. The recording gain of the amplifier is set to a default of 300 (i.e., amplified by a factor of 300). The amplifier gain can be set to 1000 times of amplification, but this adjustment is rarely needed. Finally, the NRI platform alternates the polarity of the biphasic stimulus to reduce stimulus-related artefact. The audiologist may select whether the stimulus leads with a cathodic (default) or anodic phase, but again, this adjustment is rarely needed.

It should be noted that NRI measurements may also be completed within the programming platform. The audiologist must simply "right click" on a channel to access a menu that includes "tNRI." Then, the software automatically attempts to measure a tNRI response, which is an estimated NRI threshold based on where a best-fit regression line (calculated from the amplitude of NRI responses made at the various stimulation levels) crosses 0 charge units on the *x*-axis

(Figure 18–22). The stimulation levels the software selects for tNRI assessment are based on the T levels and M levels determined for a given channel. The tNRI responses obtained from either the NRI measurement platform or the NRI measurement obtained within the programming screen are imported to a recipient's program.

Neural Response Telemetry in the Cochlear Nucleus Cochlear Implant System. **Neural Response Telemetry (NRT)** is the feature within Custom Sound ("Perform AutoNRT") that allows the audiologist to measure the recipient's electrically evoked compound action potential (ECAP). The **AutoNRT** platform allows for the automatic measurement and estimation of NRT thresholds. The default AutoNRT settings call for measurement of the NRT response on five electrodes (22, 16, 11, 6, and 1). The audiologist may choose to measure the NRT response on all electrodes by selecting the "All" option under the "Number of Electrodes" that are tested (Figure 18–23). The audiologist may also choose the starting level and the step size (both in Current Level [CL]) used for assessment. AutoNRT uses an artificial intelligence algorithm developed by Botros and colleagues (2007) to automatically identify ECAP responses and to automatically determine

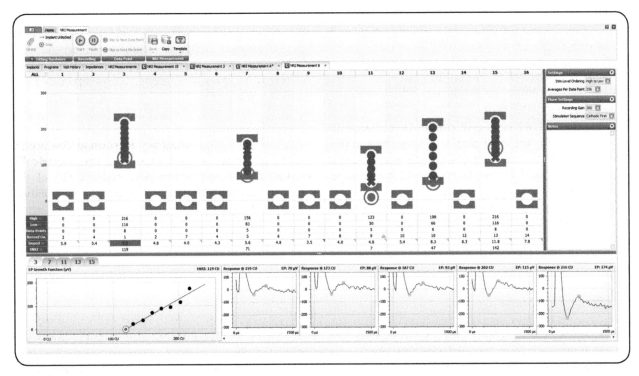

FIGURE 18–22. Advanced Bionics Neural Response Imaging (NRI) measurements. Image provided courtesy of Advanced Bionics, LLC.

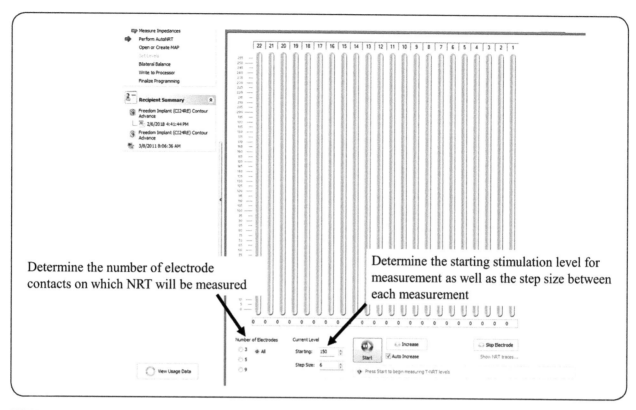

Determine the number of electrode contacts on which NRT will be measured

Determine the starting stimulation level for measurement as well as the step size between each measurement

FIGURE 18–23. Setting measurement parameters for Neural Response Telemetry (NRT) measurement in the Cochlear Custom Sound AutoNRT platform. Image provided courtesy of Cochlear Americas, ©2018.

the ECAP threshold. Research has shown that ECAP thresholds obtained with AutoNRT agree closely with the ECAP thresholds audiologists determine with use of the manual NRT platform (Spivak et al., 2011). Figure 18–24 provides an example of the ECAP obtained in the AutoNRT platform.

When the NRT response cannot be successfully measured in the AutoNRT platform, then the audiologist can attempt to adjust measurement parameters in the Custom Sound EP application, which is a separate program that provides comprehensive control of stimulation parameters pertaining to the ECAP as well as to other electrically evoked auditory evoked responses such as the electrically evoked auditory brainstem response and the cortical auditory evoked response. Within the Custom Sound EP software, the audiologist may adjust amplifier delay and gain as well as adjust the recording electrode and electrode coupling modes used to measure the NRT. Additionally, the audiologist may select from a variety of artefact rejection methods (e.g., forward masking subtraction, scaled template subtraction, alternating polarity) and can complete advanced ECAP measurements such as

the spread of excitation and rate of recovery measures discussed earlier. It should be noted that it is definitely the rare exception when the ECAP cannot be recorded from an experienced recipient in the AutoNRT platform.

Auditory Response Telemetry in the MED-EL Cochlear Implant System. The **Auditory Response Telemetry (ART)** platform is used to record the electrically evoked compound action potential (ECAP) of the auditory nerve in response to electrical stimulation from the MED-EL cochlear implant system. First, to conduct ART measurements, the audiologist must access the "ART" icon in the MED-EL MAESTRO software. Also, the diagnostic MAX coil must be used to administer the ART assessment. Then, the audiologist must define the maximum and minimum stimulation levels that encompass an amplitude growth series that may be used to determine the ECAP threshold (Figure 18–25). Of note, the stimulus levels are defined in clinical units (i.e., current amplitude), but the maximum value is also shown in charge units as well. The audiologist may adjust several other ECAP

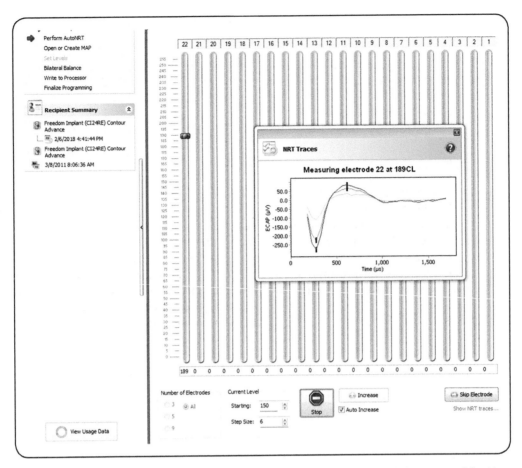

FIGURE 18–24. Measurement of Neural Response Telemetry (NRT). Image provided courtesy of Cochlear Americas, ©2018.

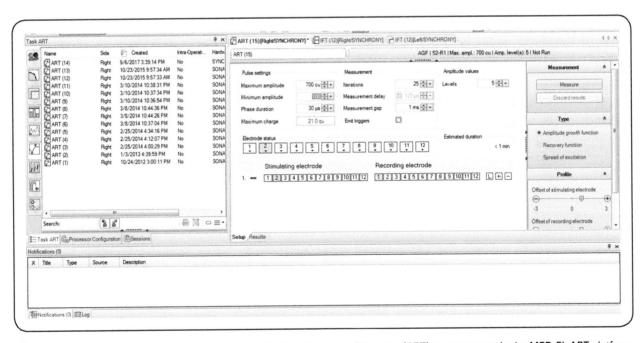

FIGURE 18–25. Setting measurement parameters for Auditory Response Telemetry (ART) measurement in the MED-EL ART platform. Image provided courtesy of MED-EL Corporation.

parameters, including the pulse width, amplifier delay, recording electrode contact, and number of ECAP measurements completed within the maximum and minimum stimulus levels. The ECAP threshold obtained in ART may be determined via visual analysis (similar the ABR assessment) or may estimate the ECAP threshold via the zero-crossing of the *x*-axis from the linear regression line calculated from the measures obtained in the amplitude growth series (Figure 18–26). Additionally, the ART platform allows the audiologist to complete the spread of excitation and rate of recovery measures. It is important to note that MED-EL advocates for the use of ART to measure auditory responsiveness to the cochlear implant but does not endorse the use of ART for estimating THR and MCL values.

Electrically Evoked Stapedial Reflex Response

The **electrically evoked stapedial reflex threshold (ESRT)** is the only objective, electrophysiologic measure that has been shown to be a good predictor of cochlear implant stimulation levels. Specifically, the ESRT has been shown to be an excellent predictor of upper-stimulation level (Gordon et al., 2004; Hodges et al., 1997; Lorens, Walkowiak, Piotrowska, Skarzynski, & Anderson, 2004). The electrically evoked

stapedial reflex response is a contraction of the stapedius muscle in the middle ear that is a time-locked response to an electrical stimulus which is generally considered to be loud but not uncomfortable to the recipient. Like the acoustic reflex measured in the diagnostic audiology clinic, the ESRT requires a synchronous response of cochlear nerve neurons to the eliciting stimulus. The afferent response from the stimulated cochlear nerve is delivered to the cochlear nucleus in the brainstem and then to: (1) the ipsilateral motor nucleus of the facial nerve as well as (2) across the trapezoid body to the superior olivary complex and then to the motor nucleus of the facial nerve on the side contralateral to the ear of stimulation. Next, the efferent stapedial branch of the facial nerve elicits a reflexive contraction of the stapedius muscle in both middle ears. As such, the ESRT is a bilateral response (i.e., the stapedial muscle contracts in both ears in response to stimulation in only one ear).

Given all the auditory structures involved in the production of the electrically evoked stapedial reflex response, adequate function is required at several levels of the auditory system in order for the ESRT to be measurable. Of great importance, middle ear function must be completely normal for the ESRT to be measurable, because even clinically insignificant changes in middle ear conduction (i.e., an increase in middle ear stiffness) will prevent the measurement

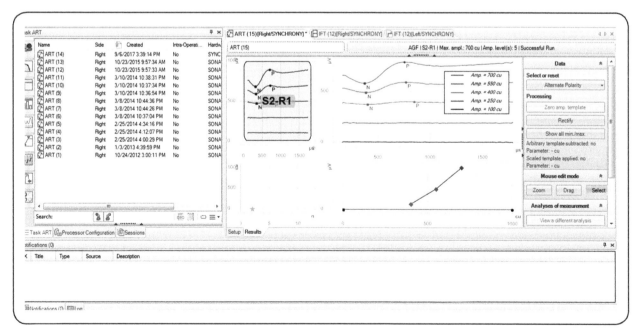

FIGURE 18–26. MED-EL Auditory Response Telemetry (ART) amplitude growth function. Image provided courtesy of MED-EL Corporation.

of further changes in middle ear stiffness that occur secondary to the contraction of the stapedius muscle and that are identified by a time-locked decrease in acoustic admittance. In other words, when the middle ear is stiffened, the stapedius muscle may contract, but the stiffness present in the middle ear does not allow for acoustic admittance measurements to recognize a further change in stiffness resulting from that contraction of the stapedius muscle. As a result, it is unlikely that the ESRT will be recordable when the acoustic admittance probe is placed in an ear with a pressure equalization (PE) tube, in an ear with significant middle ear dysfunction, or even in an ear with a subtle decrease in middle ear admittance. Of note, Wolfe, Gilbert, and colleagues (2017) suggested that the ESRT may be less likely to be recorded when the admittance probe is placed in an ear that has undergone cochlear implantation. It is possible that the cochlear implant surgery may have resulted in a negligible and clinically insignificant decrease in middle ear admittance resulting in a decrease in the likelihood to record the ESRT with the measurement probe in the implanted ear. Of importance, Wolfe, Gilbert, and colleagues (2017) also showed that the ESRT may be recorded with a higher level of success with use of a 678 or 1000 Hz probe tone relative to the use of a 226 Hz probe tone. The greater success associated with use of a higher frequency probe tone may be attributed to the fact that many middle ear disorders increase the stiffness of the middle ear system. Because stiffness affects the transmission of low-frequency sounds, an increase in stiffness may result in a decrease in the likelihood to measure a change in admittance of a 226 Hz probe tone but not of higher-frequency probe tones (i.e., 678 and 1000 Hz). It is also prudent to note at this point that for unilateral cochlear implant recipients, the acoustic admittance probe is typically placed in the non-implanted ear to avoid encountering any possible changes in middle ear function that may be associated with cochlear implant surgery.

Along with the middle ear, several other components of the auditory system must be functional in order for the ESRT to be measurable. The cochlear nerve must be intact and capable of producing s synchronous response to a high-level stimulus. Also, the auditory neurons of the cochlear nucleus and superior olivary complex must be capable of producing synchronous responses to high-level stimuli. Finally, the stapedial branch of the facial nerve must be intact, and the stapedius muscle must be functional.

Measurement of the ESRT

Measurement of the ESRT is straightforward and is relatively simple to complete with a conventional middle ear analyzer. First, the audiologist places an acoustic immittance probe into the external ear canal. If only one ear is implanted, the measurement probe is placed in the non-implanted ear (Figure 18–27). If both ears are implanted, the audiologist should consider initially placing the probe in the ear that appears to have the most normal middle ear compliance as indicated by tympanometry (i.e., ear that has peak compensated static acoustic admittance values within normal limits; if both ears are within normal limits, then begin with the ear with the highest peak compensated static acoustic admittance value). Once the probe ear is determined, acoustic admittance is continuously recorded, and the programming stimulus (for obtaining upper-stimulation level) is delivered to the cochlear implant in an ascending manner. Typically, the programming stimulus is a train of electrical pulses occurring at the same stimulation rate used in the signal coding strategy and with a duration of 300 to 500 msec. Also, the audiologist should typically present three to four pulse trains (i.e., "beeps") at each stimulus level. Of practical importance, it is often helpful to leave on the audible indicator of the programming computer so the audiologist may associate the time-locked relationship of the audible cue of the stimulus presentation to the change in admittance observed on the display of the middle ear analyzer. Most audiologists measure the ESRT with a 226 probe tone delivered to the probe ear. However, it may be useful to measure with a 678 or 1000 Hz probe tone for recipients who have bilateral cochlear implants or for whom no ESRT is measured to a 226 Hz probe tone. When the level of the stimulus from the implant is sufficiently intense to elicit the stapedial reflex, the audiologist will observe a decrease in admittance, which is time-locked with stimulus presentations (Figure 18–28). Because the stapedial reflex is a bilateral response, the time-locked, stimulus-induced decrease in admittance may be observed in the ear ipsilateral and contralateral to the cochlear implant. If the audiologist is uncertain of whether movement on the admittance meter is attributed to the stapedial response or to movement-related artefact, the stimulus level should be increased. If an ESRT is present, the time-locked changes in admittance should increase in amplitude (see Figure 18–28). Once the audiologist is confident the electrically evoked stapedial response is present, the stimulus level should

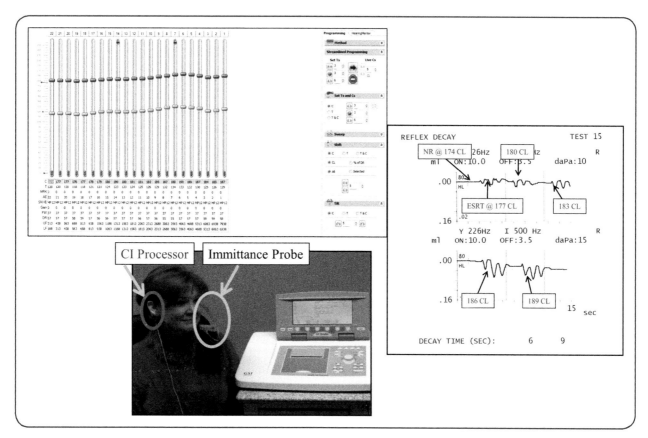

FIGURE 18–27. Measurement of the electrically evoked stapedial reflex threshold.

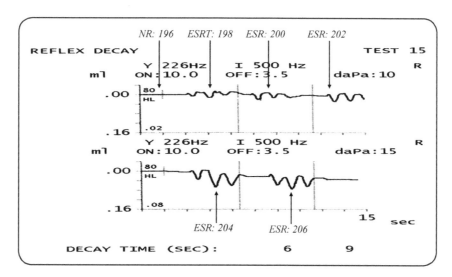

FIGURE 18–28. Visual illustration of the electrically evoked stapedial reflex threshold obtained from a cochlear implant recipient.

be decreased until the response is no longer present. Then, the stimulus level is increased again until the response is once again observed. The ESRT is the lowest stimulus level that elicits a time-locked change in admittance on two ascending trials.

Clinical Utility of ESRT to Cochlear Implant Stimulation Levels

A number of researchers have reported a strong correlation between the ESRT and upper-stimulation level (i.e., C level, M level, and MCL) (Allum et al., 2002; Brickley et al., 2005; Gordon et al., 2004; Hodges et al., 1997; Lorens et al., 2004; Shallop & Ash, 1995; Spivak & Chute, 1994; Stephan & Welzl-Muller, 2000; Walkowiak et al., 2011). In fact, correlation coefficients between ESRT and upper-stimulation levels are strong and range from 0.79 to 0.92 (Brickley et al., 2005; Hodges et al., 1997; Lorens et al., 2004; Stephan & Welzl-Muller, 2000). The strong relationship between ESRT and upper-stimulation level has been shown to exist for recipients of multiple makes and models of cochlear implants. For example, Hodges et al. (1999) measured the ESRT in pediatric recipients of Advanced Bionics Clarion C1 cochlear implants and concluded that M levels should be set at 90% of the ESRT. In another study, Hodges et al. (1997) measured the ESRT in 17 out of 25 adult Advanced Bionics implant users and reported that the ESRT was obtained just below the behavioral loudness discomfort threshold for all of these participants (ESRT is typically within about 10% of M level). Research examining the relationship between ESRT and C level of Nucleus recipients has generally found the ESRT to be obtained within 10 to 20 clinical units of the ESRT (i.e., ESRT is typically at or 10 to 20 clinical units higher than C level) (Battmer et al., 1990; Bresnihan et al., 2001; Opie et al., 1997). Furthermore, research with MED-EL recipients has found the ESRT to occur at or just below (i.e., typically within 10%) MCL (Lorens et al., 2004; Stephan & Welz-Muller, 2000). In short, the ESRT is a valid predictor of upper-stimulation level for the majority of cochlear implant recipients for whom the measure may be obtained.

Also of note, researchers have suggested that use of the ESRT to set implant stimulation levels results in upper-stimulation levels that are equally loud across the electrode array, which is a desirable goal of the cochlear implant fitting process (Hodges, Butts, & King, 2003). As previously discussed, balancing of loudness across the electrode array should result

in optimal sound quality and speech recognition. Indeed, a number of research studies have shown comparable or even better speech recognition with programs based on the ESRT compared with programs based on conventional behavioral stimulation levels. For instance, Spivak and colleagues (1994) found comparable speech recognition outcomes obtained with ESRT- and behaviorally based C levels. Wolfe and Kasulis (2008) reported a slight but statistically significant improvement in word recognition with ESRT-based upper-stimulation levels relative to performance with behaviorally based upper-stimulation levels for a group of Advanced Bionics cochlear implant recipients. Likewise, Hodges et al. (1997) found better speech recognition with ESRT-based programs for a group of adults using Nucleus cochlear implants. Furthermore, Lorens et al. (2004) found that parents reported that ESRT-based programs provided at least as good if not better performance for a group of children with MED-EL cochlear implants.

Of note, the ESRT may not be successfully obtained in all cochlear implant recipients. For instance, Hodges and colleagues (1997) successfully measured the ESRT in 17 out of 25 (68%) adult participants and 31 out of 40 (78%) pediatric participants. A review of peer-reviewed literature discussing ESRT indicates the percentage of recipients for whom an ESRT may be successfully measured ranges from 63% to 80% (Caner et al., 2007; Gordon et al., 2004; Hodges et al., 1997, 1999; Opie et al., 1997; Spivak & Chute, 1994). Although many studies typically do not report the frequency of the probe tone used to measure the ESRT, it is likely that default probe frequency of 226 Hz was selected for most studies. In contrast, Wolfe et al. (2017) measured the ESRT using 226, 678, and 1000 Hz probe tones with a group of adult Advanced Bionics cochlear implant recipients and reported that the ESRT was measured in 82% of subjects with use of the 226 Hz probe tone and 100% of the subjects with use of the 678 or 1000 Hz probe tones.

Using ESRT to Estimate Upper-Stimulation Levels

The ESRT should be measured on as many channels as possible and remaining channels should be estimated via interpolation. Accordingly, measurement of the ESRT across the electrode array will result in the upper-stimulation level profile being set according to the ESRT profile. Typically, ESRT is measured on every second or third electrode contact. For children who may become intolerant to the measurement after a short time, it is recommended that the audiologist begin the ESRT measurement on an apical channel. Then, the audiologist should proceed to a basal channel, then a channel located in the middle of array, and from that point, the audiologist may skip to different segments of the electrode array until a satisfactory number of channels are evaluated. Once the ESRT is measured for a sufficient number of electrode contacts, the audiologist should globally decrease upper-stimulation levels to a level that the audiologist is certain will be comfortable for the recipient (i.e., near threshold). Next, while the recipient listens to speech and environmental sounds in live speech mode, the upper-stimulation levels are gradually increased globally (in small increments) to a level that provides optimal speech recognition, sound quality, and comfort. For Advanced Bionics recipients, M levels are typically set approximately 10% lower than the ESRT. C levels of Nucleus recipients are typically set 10 to 15 clinical units below the ESRT. MCL of MED-EL recipients are typically set at ESRT or just below.

It should be noted that the upper-stimulation levels may be set close to ESRT for all cochlear implant systems but should not typically be set higher than the ESRT. Setting upper-stimulation levels higher than the ESRT would likely result in continuous elicitation of the stapedial reflex threshold to moderately intense sounds, such as average conversational speech. This is not typical for persons with normal hearing and should not be a reality for cochlear implant users. Of note, while slowly increasing the stimulation levels toward the ESRT, the audiologist should carefully observe the recipient while moderate to loud sounds are present in the environment (e.g., hand clapping, musical instruments, such as a xylophone, noise makers). If the recipient shows any signs of aversiveness or distress to the increase in stimulation levels, the audiologist should not provide further increases in stimulation, even if the upper-stimulation levels are far removed from the ESRT. It is possible that the recipient may require more time to acclimate to stimulation from the cochlear implant and to an increase in stimulation.

Alternatively, an individual recipient may simply perform well with and prefer upper-stimulation levels that are considerably lower than ESRT. Furthermore, the audiologist should refrain from providing further increases in upper-stimulation level if the recipient begins to produce eye-blinks (i.e., aural-palpebral reflex) in response to moderate to high-level stimulation from the implant. Adults who used high-power

hearing aids for many years frequently will desire upper-stimulation levels that are excessively high, but setting the upper-stimulation levels at erroneously high levels may hamper performance. In these cases, the ESRT can serve as a good guide to determine an appropriate limit for upper-stimulation levels.

Once assessment of upper-stimulation level is completed, the audiologist may consider sweeping the programming stimulus at upper-stimulation level across the electrode array. Sweeping simply involves the sequential presentation of the programming stimulus across the electrode array. Sweeping is conducted to ensure that upper level stimulation is comfortable to the user at every intracochlear electrode contact and to ensure that the recipient does not experience problems with sound quality or non-auditory side effects (e.g., facial nerve stimulation).

Other Electrophysiologic Auditory Evoked Responses

The audiologist may measure a number of additional electrically evoked auditory evoked responses. Some measures, such as the electrically evoked middle latency response (EMLR), acoustic change complex (EACC) (Brown et al., 2008; He et al., 2015), mismatch negativity (EMMN) (Kraus et al., 1993), and the P300 (EP300) (Friedman et al., 1975), have received interest in the research arena but have not generally been used in the clinic. The remainder of the discussion of electrically evoked auditory responses will center on the electrically evoked auditory brainstem response, the electrically evoked cortical auditory evoked response, and transtympanic promontory/round window electrically evoked auditory responses.

Electrically Evoked Auditory Brainstem Response

The **electrically evoked auditory brainstem response (EABR)** is a series of peaks present in electroencephalograph that is recorded from electrodes located on the head and that are produced by the synchronous firing of auditory-responsive neurons in the auditory brainstem in response to electrical stimulation from the cochlear implant. The EABR is similar to its acoustic counterpart but also contains some differences as well. Like the acoustic ABR, the EABR contains a robust wave V and possibly a wave III (Figure 18–29) (Shallop et al., 1990). The amplitude of waves III and V increases with increases in stimulus level (Brown

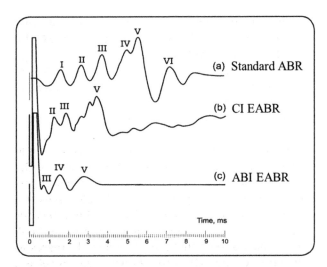

FIGURE 18–29. Visual illustration of the electrically evoked auditory brainstem response obtained from a cochlear implant recipient. Image provided courtesy of Cochlear Americas, ©2018.

et al., 1994; Shallop et al., 1991). Additionally, waves III and V are likely generated by multiple groups of neurons within the pons and midbrain of the brainstem (Hall, 2007). However, unlike the acoustic ABR, changes in stimulus level result in little to no change in the latencies of waves III and V (see Figure 18–29) (Firszt et al., 2002; Kileny et al., 1997). The change in latency that occurs with changes in stimulus level is primarily attributable to changes in the traveling wave in the cochlea. Because the EABR is produced by direct stimulation of the cochlear nerve, there is little to no change in latency with changes in stimulus level. Additionally, the latency of waves III and V of the EABR typically occur about 1 to 1.5 msec earlier than waves III and V of the acoustic ABR (Shallop et al., 1990). Once again, the waves of the EABR occur at earlier latencies, because the cochlear nerve is stimulated directly, and as a result, the signal does not have to travel through the ear canal and middle ear and then along the traveling wave within the cochlea. Furthermore, waves I and II of the EABR are often not visible in the recording, because they are obscured by the implant-generated electrical artefact.

The EABR is typically recorded by interfacing the cochlear implant programming system with a clinical auditory evoked response system. The electrical stimulus is delivered from the programming software to an external sound processor or to a diagnostic transmitting coil and then to the cochlear implant. The interface that couples the sound processor or diagnostic transmitting coil to the sound processor

must send a trigger pulse to the clinical auditory evoked response system to signify the presentation of the stimulus and the need to record the auditory evoked response. Once triggered, the auditory evoked response system records the EEG captured by electrodes located on the surface of the head. The box below contains stimulus and recording parameters typically used to acquire the EABR.

The primary purpose of the EABR is to confirm implant function and/or auditory responsiveness to implant stimulation for recipients whose implants do not contain telemetry systems. With the advent of telemetry systems and the capability to measure the ECAP, the clinical utility of the EABR was greatly diminished. The ECAP is generally easier to record than the EABR, may be recorded without sedation because it is largely immune to movement-related artefact, and does not require the use of a separate auditory evoked response system. Of note, the EABR may be useful in cases in which the ECAP cannot be recorded because of cochlear abnormalities (e.g., cochlear ossification). Also, the ECAP does evaluate auditory responsiveness through the auditory brainstem rather than just of the cochlear nerve as with ECAP. As with ECAP, the presence of an EABR response indicates that the signal should be audible to the recipient at the stimulus level used to elicit the

---

Stimulus and recording parameters typically used to acquire the electrically evoked auditory brainstem response.

EABR Measurement Parameters

Stimulus Parameters

- Biphasic electrical pulse
- Alternating polarity
- Stimulation rate: 10–80 Hz
- Pulse width: 25–400 microseconds
- Number of stimuli: 500 to 2000

Acquisition Parameters

- Non-inverting electrode: Cz or high forehead
- Inverting electrode: contralateral mastoid or earlobe
- Reference electrode: low forehead
- Analysis window: 10 msec
- "Block" first 1.0 msec of analysis window
- Filter settings: 100 Hz to 3000 Hz
- Artifact rejection: +/– 15 microvolts

response. However, the EABR is not a good predictor of T or upper-stimulation level.

Electrically Evoked Cortical Auditory Evoked Response

The **electrically evoked cortical auditory evoked response (ECAER)** is a series of peaks present in electroencephalograph that is recorded from electrodes located on the head and that are produced by the synchronous firing of auditory-responsive neurons in the auditory thalamus and cortex in response to electrical stimulation from the cochlear implant (refer to Figure 18–30 for an example of the ECAER). The typical ECAER comprises three peaks, a P1, N1, and P2. The amplitude of the peaks increases with stimulus level. Also, the amplitude, morphology, and latency of the ECAER changes as a function of age. In particular, N1 and P2 are often absent in infants and newly implanted children and develop throughout childhood. Also, the latency of P1 is quite late for normal-hearing infants (i.e., 300 msec) and decreases to approximately 100 to 150 msec in the pre-school years at approximately 60 msec by young adulthood (Dorman et al., 2007; Hall, 1992). N1 and P2 occur at approximately 75 to 150 msec and 150 to 210 msec, respectively.

The ECAER may be measured with two different approaches. The electrical stimulus may be delivered from the implant programming software directly to the cochlear implant as previously described with the EABR. With direct stimulation, a trigger pulse is needed to signify to the auditory evoked response system that the signal has been delivered and that averaging/analysis should commence. The ECAER may also be measured by delivering test signals (e.g., speech signals, tone bursts) from a loudspeaker in the soundfield and recording the response collected by the auditory evoked response system.

The CAER may be used to indicate that stimulation from the cochlear implant is resulting in a response from neurons in the auditory cortex. Additionally, the presence of the CAER indicates that the response is audible to the recipient. Furthermore, the latency of the P1 component of the CAER serves as a biomarker of the maturation of the auditory nervous system. As shown in Figure 18–31, Sharma and colleagues have shown that the P1 latency decreases as a function of age. Of note, children who receive a cochlear implant at an early age (i.e., 3 years old and younger) typically have P1 latencies that fall within the typical range for children with normal hearing, a finding that suggests typical maturation of the auditory nervous system. In contrast, the latency of the CAER almost invariably falls outside of the normal range for children who are born with severe to profound hearing loss and who do not receive a cochlear implant until 7 years of age and older, a finding that suggests arrested development of the auditory system. Variable results are seen for children implanted between 3 and 7 years of age, with some children possessing CAER P1 latencies that approximate that of children with normal hearing aids and others possessing CAER P1 latencies that fall outside of the normal range.

Researchers affiliated with Australian Hearing Services (AHS) have also used the CAER to determine whether children with auditory neuropathy spectrum disorder (ANSD) should be considered for cochlear implantation (Gardner-Berry, Hou, & Ching, in press). Briefly, the CAER is administered while the child uses hearing aids. A present aided CAER suggests that use of the hearing aid allows for a synchronous response from the auditory nervous system. In contrast, an absent CAER suggests that the auditory nervous system is unable to produce a synchronous response to acoustic signals delivered from the hearing aid. As a result, the child should be considered for cochlear implantation.

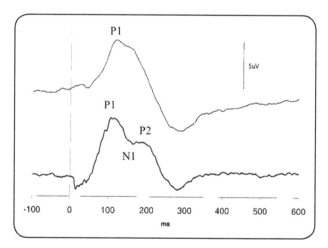

FIGURE 18–30. Visual illustration of the electrically evoked cortical auditory evoked response obtained from a cochlear implant recipient.

Transtympanic Promontory/Round Window Electrical Stimulation

Transtympanic electrical stimulation differs from the other measurements discussed in this chapter,

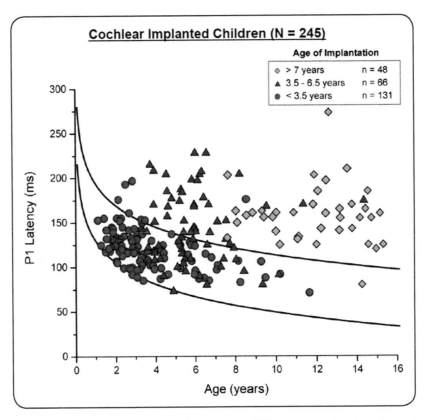

FIGURE 18–31. Cortical auditory evoked response P1 latency as a function of age at implantation. Modified from Sharma, Dorman, and Spahr, 2002; image provided courtesy of Anu Sharma

because the stimulation is extracochlear in nature rather than intracochlear. In other words, the electrical stimulation is delivered to the outer wall of the cochlea (i.e., the promontory) and/or to the round window. Typically, a cochlear implant surgeon places long needle electrodes through the tympanic membrane and onto the promontory (just anterior and inferior to the round window) or round window. An audiologist delivers electrical pulses to the stimulating needle, and the response of the auditory system is captured by disc/cup electrodes placed on the patient's head. The activity captured by the surface electrodes is delivered to a clinical auditory evoked response system for averaging and analysis. The electrically evoked ABR is the auditory response that has been most commonly measured in response to transtympanic stimulation. However, it is possible to also record other types of auditory responses to transtympanic stimulation (e.g., ECAP, ECAER). The ECAP is not typically recorded to transtympanic stimulation, because due to the short latency of the CAP, it is

difficult to separate the response from the stimulus artefact. The ECAER is not typically recorded to transtympanic stimulation, because the measures are often made under sedation/anesthesia, which diminishes the amplitude of the CAER. The recording parameters of the **transtympanic EABR (T-EABR)** are similar to those used for the recording of the conventional acoustic ABR. The characteristics of the T-EABR are similar to the EABR described previously. In short, waves III and V are usually attainable, but wave I is often obscured by the electrical artefact. Additionally, the latency of T-EABR components is typically 1 to 1.5 msec earlier than the latency of the same components of the acoustic ABR counterpart. The amplitude of the T-EABR typically increases with increases in stimulus level, but there is often a minimal change in latency with changes in stimulus level.

Various examiners have used differing techniques to deliver stimulation. For example, Brown and Abbas (2006) have used bipolar stimulation to deliver electrical current to the promontory. Abbas and Brown

(2006) have reported that the use of bipolar stimulation minimizes the electrical artefact captured at the recording electrodes placed on the patient's head. In contrast, Kileny et al. (1994) have reported great success with the recording of the EABR with use of monopolar needle electrodes located on the promontory. Of note, the presence/absence and amplitude of the T-EABR can vary considerably depending upon the placement of the needle electrode (Gardi, 1985). For example, the T-EABR may be absent on the initial measurement, but after the surgeon moves the stimulating needle electrode by less than a few millimeters, a robust T-EABR may be recorded, a finding that is likely related to more robust stimulation being delivered during the latter attempt. In an effort to provide more consistent, robust stimulation to the cochlear nerve via extracochlear stimulation, Gibson and colleagues (2017) have developed a "golf-club" electrode which has a large surface area at its tip to allow for stimulation to be delivered to a broader location. Gibson et al. have reported good success with eliciting the EABR with the golf-club electrode placed on the round window or in the niche of the round window.

Clinical Utility of the Transtympanic Electrically Evoked Auditory Brainstem Response

When cochlear implants were first introduced, several researchers explored the use of T-EABR to predict outcomes following cochlear implantation and to determine the ear to be implanted. In general, these studies included adults and children who were profoundly deafened and who had received little to no benefit from hearing aids prior to cochlear implant surgery. However, research initially indicated that the T-EABR was of limited value in predicting success. For instance, Nikolopoulos and colleagues (2000) measured the T-EABR in 47 children and obtained robust responses in 35 children and absent response in 12 children. In spite of these differences in T-EABR outcomes, postoperative speech recognition of the children with absent T-EABR was similar to that of children with present T-EABR. In sum, T-EABR is no longer routinely used to determine ear of implantation or prognosis of success with a cochlear implant.

The T-EABR may be helpful to determine whether cochlear implantation is suitable for children with certain types of etiologies and/or hearing disorders. For example, Kim et al. (2008) completed preoperative T-EABR in 39 children with inner ear malforma-

tions, including some children who had a narrow internal auditory canal, which is often associated with an absent or deficient cochlear nerve. Kim and colleagues reported that poorer postoperative outcomes were associated with higher T-EABR thresholds, absent T-EABR, and/or smaller T-EABR wave V amplitude. Additionally, Walton and colleagues (2008) recorded with T-EABR with use of their golf-club electrode placed on the promontory of children with cochlear hearing loss and children with auditory neuropathy spectrum disorder (ANSD). Walton et al. reported that the children with cochlear hearing loss had present and typically robust T-EABRs. They also found that some of the children with ANSD had robust T-EABRs, whereas other children with ANSD had absent or abnormal T-EABRs. Of note, the children who had absent or abnormal T-EABRs had poorer postoperative speech recognition abilities compared with the children who had normal T-EABRs. To summarize, the T-EABR is not routinely used to select ear of implantation or to predict cochlear implant outcome. However, the T-EABR may help to identify whether a child is likely to benefit from cochlear implantation if the child has been diagnosed with ANSD or severely abnormal cochlear anatomy.

Electrical Measures

Electrical measures are diagnostic tests that evaluate the electrical function of the cochlear implant system without requiring a physiologic response from the recipient. Electrode impedance and average electrode voltage measurements are examples of electrical measures. Electrical impedance measures were covered in detail in Chapter 7. Average electrode voltage measurements will be discussed in the following section.

Average Electrode Voltage Measurements

Average electrode voltage measurements (AEVs) are tests that are completed with disc/cup electrodes that are placed on the head to capture the electrical signal generated by the cochlear implant and that are conducted throughout the head. AEVs are completed by generating biphasic electrical pulses from the cochlear implant system, capturing the resultant electrical signal that is volume-conducted throughout the head by electrodes located on the head, and delivering the captured signal to an auditory evoked response system for averaging and analysis. Three surface electrodes are typically used to measure AEVs with the following montage:

- Non-inverting electrode (+): Located at ipsilateral mastoid/earlobe
- Inverting electrode (–): Located at contralateral mastoid/earlobe
- Ground: May be located essentially anywhere on the body (e.g., forehead, wrist, shoulder)

Of note, some examiners have completed AEVs with the inverting electrode located at the forehead and the ground located elsewhere. Often, a low-pass filter (cutoff at 10,000 Hz) is often used to reduce contamination from the RF signal delivered by the implant.

AEVs are typically measured with the biphasic electrical pulses delivered via a monopolar stimulation mode, but for Nucleus recipients, common ground stimulation mode is also used. Use of multiple stimulation modes is beneficial, because each stimulation mode can provide novel information regarding the function of the implant. For example, use of monopolar coupling results in large amplitude pulses that are captured at the recording electrodes. The absence of a large amplitude pulse following stimulation of a given electrode would be suggestive of an open circuit. Furthermore, because the common ground stimulation mode uses a return path that includes all intracochlear electrode contacts, short circuits are best identified by common ground stimulation.

For AEV assessment, stimulation is usually delivered at a level that is at or below the recipient's behavioral threshold for electrical hearing. However, the electrical current delivered throughout the head is typically much larger than the recipient's myogenic activity, so sedation is usually not required to complete AEV measures. The response collected and displayed by the evoked potential system should resemble a series of biphasic electrical pulses. The AEV stimulus is typically delivered at a rate of 50 to 250 pps. In most cases, the AEV stimulus is delivered at multiple levels to evaluate whether the signal that is recorded also grows in amplitude in an expected manner. Although audiologists may record AEVs with a clinical evoked potential system, in many cases, a representative from the cochlear implant manufacturer is present to conduct the AEV test with the use of a special recording system and software designed for AEV analysis of cochlear implant function.

Outcomes of AEV Measurements

AEV outcomes are primarily assessed by evaluating the amplitude, polarity, and shape of the AEV waveforms. The following findings may indicate a problem with the cochlear implant:

- The AEV amplitude is smaller than expected, does not increase with stimulus level increase as expected, or is different with stimulation of one (or additional) intracochlear electrode contact compared with the other electrode contacts in the array. The amplitude of the AEV response recorded from basal channels is typically larger than the AEV amplitude recorded from apical channels, because the basal intracochlear electrode contacts are located more closely to the recording electrodes.
- The polarity of the AEV waveform is opposite of what is expected. Of note, in the common ground mode, AEV polarity will invert at a middle point in the electrode array. However, any other change in response polarity is atypical. With the standard electrode recording montage, the biphasic pulses recorded from basal electrodes possess a negative-leading polarity, and the pulses recorded from apical electrodes possess a positive-leading polarity.
- Because the AEV stimulus is biphasic, an AEV with a monophasic shape is abnormal. Also, the shape of the AEV waveform should be similar across the electrode array.
- An absent or intermittent AEV response may be suggestive of a faulty receiver/stimulator or broken electrode leads, particularly when the AEV is absent to stimulation on all channels. An absent AEV on one channel is indicative of an open circuit for that channel.

Clinical Application of AEV Measurement

The role of AEV in the clinical management of cochlear implant recipients has diminished with the introduction of telemetry systems within the cochlear implant. Open- and short-circuited electrodes are some of the most common electrical faults in modern cochlear implant systems, and both types of faults are identifiable with electrode impedance assessment and/or electrical field imaging available in contemporary cochlear implant systems. Furthermore, a faulty cochlear implant receiver or DSP would reveal itself in an inability to establish telemetry (e.g., lock/link) with use of the programming computer. Likewise, a faulty stimulator would reveal itself as an inability to provide stimulation from the programming computer despite attainment of lock/link with the implant. If lock/link to the implant is obtained but no stimulation can be delivered, the audiologist should attempt to change the return electrode (e.g., reference/ground) and/or increase the RF power used to deliver the signal from the sound processor to the cochlear implant.

For cochlear implants with telemetry systems, AEV measures often simply serve to corroborate the diagnostic findings obtained via telemetry measures. In short, the primary utility of AEVs is to evaluate the electrical function of older cochlear implant systems that do not possess functioning telemetry systems.

Key Concepts

- Objective measures provide valuable information about the status of the cochlear implant and the responsiveness of the auditory system to stimulation from the cochlear implant. Objective measures should be routinely included in the cochlear implant programming process.
- The electrically evoked compound action potential (ECAP) provides an indication of the cochlear nerve's neural response to electrical stimulation from the cochlear implant. The ECAP threshold cannot be reliably used to estimate stimulation levels. However, the ECAP is a valuable clinical tool that provides useful information to the audiologist.
- The electrically evoked stapedial reflex threshold is an excellent predictor of upper-stimulation level.

References

Abbas, P. J., & Brown, C. J. (1991a). Electrically evoked auditory brainstem response: Growth of response with current level. *Hearing Research, 51*(1), 123–137.

Abbas, P. J., & Brown, C. J. (1991b). Electrically evoked auditory brainstem response: Refractory properties and strength-duration functions. *Hearing Research, 51*(1), 139–147.

Abbas, P., Brown, C., & Etler, C. (2006). Electrophysiology and device telemetry In S. Waltzman & N. Cohen (Eds.), *Cochlear implants* (2nd ed.). New York, NY: Thieme.

Abbas, P. J., Brown, C. J., Shallop, J. K., Firszt, J. B., Hughes, M. L., Hong, S. H., & Staller, S. J. (1999). Summary of results using the Nucleus CI24M implant to record the electrically evoked compound action potential. *Ear and Hearing, 20*(1), 45–59.

Allum, J. H., Greisiger, R., & Probst, R. (2002). Relationship of intraoperative electrically evoked stapedius reflex thresholds to maximum comfortable loudness levels of children with cochlear implants. *International Journal of Audiology, 41*(2), 93–99.

Battmer, R. D., Lai, W. K., Dillier, N., Pesch, J., Killian, M. J., & Lenarz, T. (2005). *Correlation of NRT recovery function parameters and speech perception results for different stimulation rates.* Presented at Fourth International Symposium and Workshops: Objective Measures in Cochlear Implants, Hannover, Germany.

Battmer, R. D., Laszig, R., & Lehnhardt, E. (1990). Electrically elicited stapedius reflex in cochlear implant patients. *Ear and Hearing, 11*(5), 370–374.

Baudhuin, J. L., Hughes, M. L., & Goehring, J. L. (2016). A comparison of alternating polarity and forward masking artifact-reduction methods to resolve the electrically evoked compound action potential. *Ear and Hearing, 37*(4), e247–e255.

Botros, A., Banna, R., & Maruthurkkara, S. (2013). The next generation of Nucleus((R)) fitting: A multiplatform approach towards universal cochlear implant management. *International Journal of Audiology, 52*(7), 485–494.

Botros, A., & Psarros, C. (2010a). Neural response telemetry reconsidered: I. The relevance of ECAP threshold profiles and scaled profiles to cochlear implant fitting. *Ear and Hearing, 31*(3), 367–379.

Botros, A., & Psarros, C. (2010b). Neural response telemetry reconsidered: II. The influence of neural population on the ECAP recovery function and refractoriness. *Ear and Hearing, 31*(3), 380–391.

Botros, A., van Dijk, B., & Killian, M. (2007). AutoNR: An automated system that measures ECAP thresholds with the Nucleus Freedom cochlear implant via machine intelligence. *Artificial Intelligence in Medicine, 40*(1), 15–28.

Bresnihan, M., Norman, G., Scott, F., & Viani, L. (2001). Measurement of comfort levels by means of electrical stapedial reflex in children. *Archives of Otolaryngology–Head and Neck Surgery, 127*(8), 963–966.

Brickley, G., Boyd, P., Wyllie, F., O'Driscoll, M., Webster, D., & Nopp, P. (2005). Investigations into electrically evoked stapedius reflex measures and subjective loudness percepts in the MED-EL COMBI 40+ cochlear implant. *Cochlear Implants International, 6*(1), 31–42.

Brown, C. J., Abbas, P. J., Fryauf-Bertschy, H., Kelsay, D., & Gantz, B. J. (1994). Intraoperative and postoperative electrically evoked auditory brainstem responses in Nucleus cochlear implant users: Implications for the fitting process. *Ear and Hearing, 15*(2), 168–176.

Brown C. J., Abbas P. J., & Gantz, B. (1990). Electrically evoked whole-nerve action potentials: Data from human cochlear implant users. *Journal of the Acoustical Society of America, 88*, 1385–1391.

Brown, C. J., Abbas, P. J., & Gantz, B. J. (1998). Preliminary experience with neural response telemetry in the Nucleus CI24M cochlear implant. *American Journal of Otology, 19*(3), 320–327.

Brown, C. J., Etler, C., He, S., O'Brien, S., Erenberg, S., Kim, J. R., . . . Abbas, P. J. (2008). The electrically evoked auditory change complex: Preliminary results from Nucleus cochlear implant users. *Ear and Hearing, 29*(5), 704–717.

Brown, C. J., Hughes, M. L., Luk, B., Abbas, P. J., Wolaver, A., & Gervais, J. (2000). The relationship between EAP and EABR thresholds and levels used to program the Nucleus 24 speech processor: Data from adults. *Ear and Hearing, 21*(2), 151–163.

Cafarelli Dees, D., Dillier, N., Lai, W. K., von Wallenberg, E., van Dijk, B., Akdas, F., . . . Smoorenburg, G. F. (2005). Normative findings of electrically evoked compound action potential measurements using the neural response telemetry of the Nucleus CI24M cochlear implant system. *Audiology and Neurootology, 10*(2), 105–116.

Caner, G., Olgun, L., Gultekin, G., & Balaban, M. (2007). Optimizing fitting in children using objective measures such as neural response imaging and electrically evoked stapedius reflex threshold. *Otology and Neurotology, 28*(5), 637–640.

Charasse, B., Thai-Van, H., Chanal, J. M., Berger-Vachon, C., & Collet, L. (2004). Automatic analysis of auditory nerve electrically evoked compound action potential with an artificial neural network. *Artificial Intelligence in Medicine, 31*(3), 221–229.

Cohen, L. T., Saunders, E., & Richardson, L. M. (2004). Spatial spread of neural excitation: comparison of compound action potential and forward-masking data in cochlear implant recipients. *International Journal of Audiology, 43*(6), 346–355.

Cullington, H. (2000). Preliminary neural response telemetry results. *British Journal of Audiology, 34*(3), 131–140.

Dorman, M. F., Sharma, A., Gilley, P., Martin, K., & Roland, P. (2007). Central auditory development: Evidence from CAEP measurements in children fit with cochlear implants. *Journal of Communication Disorders, 40*(4), 284–294.

Finley, C. C., Wilson, B., van den Honert, C., Lawson, D. (1997). *Speech processors for auditory prostheses. Sixth quarterly progress report,* NIH Project N01-DC-5-2103.

Firszt, J. B., Chambers, R. D., Kraus, & Reeder, R. M. (2002). Neurophysiology of cochlear implant users I: Effects of stimulus current level and electrode site on the electrical ABR, MLR, and N1-P2 response. *Ear and Hearing, 23*(6), 502–515.

Franck, K. H. (2002). A model of a nucleus 24 cochlear implant fitting protocol based on the electrically evoked whole nerve action potential. *Ear and Hearing, 23*(1 Suppl), 67S–71S.

Franck, K. H., & Norton, S. J. (2001). Estimation of psychophysical levels using the electrically evoked compound action potential measured with the neural response telemetry capabilities of Cochlear Corporation's CI24M device. *Ear and Hearing, 22*(4), 289–299.

Friedman, D., Simson, R., Ritter, W., & Rapin, I. (1975) Cortical evoked potentials elicited by real speech words and human sounds. *Electroencephalography and Clinical Neurophysiology, 38,* 13–19.

Frijns, J. H., Briaire, J. J., de Laat, J. A., & Grote, J. J. (2002). Initial evaluation of the Clarion CII cochlear implant: Speech perception and neural response imaging. *Ear and Hearing, 23*(3), 184–197.

Gardi, J. N. (1985). Human brain stem and middle latency responses to electrical stimulation: Preliminary observations. In R. A. Schindler & M. M. Merzenich (Eds.), *Cochlear implants* (pp. 351–363). New York, NY: Raven.

Gardner-Berry, K., Hou, S. Y. L., & Ching, T. Y. C. (in press). Managing infants and children with auditory neuropathy spectrum disorder (ANSD). In J. Madell, C. Flexer, J. Wolfe, & E. Schafer (Eds.), *Pediatric audiology: Diagnosis, technology, and management* (3rd ed.). New York, NY: Thieme.

Gibson, W. P. (2017). The clinical uses of electrocochleography. *Frontiers in Neuroscience, 11,* 274.

Gordon, K., Papsin, B. C., & Harrison, R. V. (2004). Programming cochlear implant stimulation levels in infants and children with a combination of objective measures. *International Journal of Audiology, 43*(Suppl. 1), S28–S32.

Grolman, W., Maat, A., Verdam, F., Simis, Y., Carelsen, B., Freling, N., & Tange, R. A. (2008). Spread of excitation measurements for the detection of electrode array foldovers: A prospective study comparing 3-dimensional rotational x-ray and intraoperative spread of excitation measurements. *Otology and Neurotology, 30,* 27–33.

Hall, J. W. III. (1992). *Handbook of auditory evoked responses.* Needham Heights, MA: Allyn & Bacon.

Hall, J. W. (2007). *New handbook of auditory evoked responses.* Upper Saddle River, NJ: Pearson.

He, S., Grose, J. H., Teagle, H. F., Woodard, J., Park, L. R., Hatch, D. R., . . . Buchman, C. A. (2015). Acoustically evoked auditory change complex in children with auditory neuropathy spectrum disorder: A potential objective tool for identifying cochlear implant candidates. *Ear and Hearing, 36*(3), 289–301.

He, S., Shahsavarani, B. S., McFayden, T. C., Wang, H., Gill, K. E., Xu, L., . . . He, N. (2017). Responsiveness of the electrically stimulated cochlear nerve in children with cochlear nerve deficiency. *Ear and Hearing, 39*(2), 238–250.

Hodges, A. V., Balkany, T. J., Ruth, R. A., Lambert, P. R., Dolan-Ash, S., & Schloffman, J. J. (1997). Electrical middle ear muscle reflex: use in cochlear implant programming. *Otolaryngology-Head and Neck Surgery, 117*(3 Pt 1), 255–261.

Hodges, A. V., Butts, S., Dolan-Ash, S., & Balkany, T. J. (1999). Using electrically evoked auditory reflex thresholds to fit the CLARION cochlear implant. *Annals of Otology, Rhinology, and Laryngology, Supplement, 177,* 64–68.

Hodges A. V., Butts S, King J. (2003) Electrically evoked stapedial reflexes: Utility in cochlear implant patients. In H. Cullington (Ed.), *Cochlear implants objective measures* (pp. 81–93). Philadelphia, PA: Whurr.

Hoth, S., Spitzer, P., & Praetorius, M. (2018). A new approach for the determination of ECAP thresholds. *Cochlear Implants International, 19*(2), 104–114.

Hughes, M. L., Brown, C. J., Abbas, P. J., Wolaver, A. A., & Gervais, J. P. (2000). Comparison of EAP thresholds with MAP levels in the Nucleus 24 cochlear implant: Data from children. *Ear and Hearing, 21*(2), 164–174.

Hughes, M. L., Goehring, J. L., & Baudhuin, J. L. (2017). Effects of stimulus polarity and artifact reduction method on the electrically evoked compound action potential. *Ear and Hearing, 38*(3), 332–343.

Hughes, M. L., & Stille, L. J. (2010). Effect of stimulus and recording parameters on spatial spread of excitation and masking patterns obtained with the electrically evoked compound action potential in cochlear implants. *Ear and Hearing, 31*(5), 679–692.

Hughes, M. L., Vander Werff, K. R., Brown, C. J., Abbas, P. J., Kelsay, D. M., Teagle, H. F., & Lowder, M. W. (2001). A longitudinal study of electrode impedance, the electrically evoked compound action potential, and behavioral measures in Nucleus 24 cochlear implant users. *Ear and Hearing, 22*(6), 471–486.

Kiefer, J., Hohl, S., Sturzebecher, E., Pfennigdorff, T., & Gstoettner, W. (2001). Comparison of speech recognition with different speech coding strategies (SPEAK, CIS, and ACE) and their relationship to telemetric measures of compound action potentials in the Nucleus CI 24M cochlear implant system. *Audiology, 40*(1), 32–42.

Kileny, P. R., Zwolan, T. A., Boerst, A., & Telian, S. A. (1997). Electrically evoked auditory potentials: Current clinical applications in children with cochlear implants. *American Journal of Otology, 18*(6 Suppl.), S90–S92.

Kileny, P. R., Zwolan, T. A., Zimmerman-Phillips, S., & Telian, S. A. (1994). Electrically evoked auditory brainstem response in pediatric patients with cochlear implants. *Archives of Otolaryngology–Head and Neck Surgery, 120*(10), 1083–1090.

Kim, A. H., Kileny, P. R., Arts, H. A., El-Kashlan, H. K., Telian, S. A., & Zwolan, T. A. (2008). Role of electrically evoked auditory brainstem response in cochlear implantation of children with inner ear malformations. *Otology and Neurotology, 29*(5), 626–634.

Kraus, N., Micco, A. G., Koch, D. B., McGee, T., Carrell, T., Sharma, A., . . . Weingarten, C. Z. (1993). The mismatch negativity cortical evoked potential elicited by speech in cochlear-implant users. *Hearing Research, 65*(1–2), 118–124.

Lorens, A., Walkowiak, A., Piotrowska, A., Skarzynski, H., & Anderson, I. (2004). ESRT and MCL correlations in experienced paediatric cochlear implant users. *Cochlear Implants International, 5*(1), 28–37.

McKay, C. M., Fewster, L., & Dawson, P. (2005). A different approach to using neural response telemetry for automated cochlear implant processor programming. *Ear and Hearing, 26*(4 Suppl), 38S–44S.

Miller, C. A., Abbas, P. J., & Brown, C. J. (2000). An improved method of reducing stimulus artifact in the electrically evoked whole-nerve potential. *Ear and Hearing, 21*(4), 280–290.

Miller, C. A., Abbas, P. J., Rubinstein, J. T., Robinson, B. K., Matsuoka, A. J., & Woodworth, G. (1998). Electrically evoked compound action potentials of guinea pig and cat: responses to monopolar, monophasic stimulation. *Hearing Research, 119*(1–2), 142–154.

Moller, A. R., Colletti, V., & Fiorino, F. G. (1994). Neural conduction velocity of the human auditory nerve: Bipolar recordings from the exposed intracranial portion of the eighth nerve during vestibular nerve section. *Electroencephalography and Clinical Neurophysiology, 92*, 316–320.

Müller-Deile, J. (2004). Versorgung mit cochlear implantaten [Care with cochlear implants]. *Sprache Stimme Gehör, 28*, 1–14.

Nikolopoulos, T. P., Mason, S. M., Gibbin, K. P., & O'Donoghue, G. M. (2000). The prognostic value of promontory electric auditory brainstem response in pediatric cochlear implantation. *Ear and Hearing, 21*(3), 236–241.

Opie, J. M., Allum, J. H., & Probst, R. (1997). Evaluation of electrically elicited stapedius reflex threshold measured through three different cochlear implant systems. *American Journal of Otology, 18*(6 Suppl.), S107–S108.

Potts, L. G., Skinner, M. W., Gotter, B. D., Strube, M. J., & Brenner, C. A. (2007). Relation between neural response telemetry thresholds, T- and C-levels, and loudness judgments in 12 adult Nucleus 24 cochlear implant recipients. *Ear and Hearing, 28*(4), 495–511.

Shallop, J. K., & Ash, K. R. (1995). Relationships among comfort levels determined by cochlear implant patient's self-programming, audiologist's programming, and electrical stapedius reflex thresholds. *Annals of Otology, Rhinology, and Laryngology, Supplement, 166*, 175–176.

Shallop, J. K., Beiter, A. L., Goin, D. W., & Mischke, R. E. (1990). Electrically evoked auditory brainstem responses (EABR) and middle latency responses (EMLR) obtained from patients with the Nucleus multichannel cochlear implant. *Ear and Hearing, 11*(1), 5–15.

Shallop, J. K., VanDyke, L., Goin, D. W., & Mischke, R. E. (1991). Prediction of behavioral threshold and comfort values for Nucleus 22-channel implant patients from electrical auditory brainstem response test results. *Annals of Otology, Rhinology, and Laryngology, 100*(11), 896–898.

Sharma, A., Dorman, M., & Spahr, A. (2002). A sensitive period for the development of the central auditory system in children with cochlear implants: Implications for age of implantation. *Ear and Hearing, 23*(6), 532–539.

Sharma, A., Martin, K., Roland, P., Bauer, P., Sweeney, M. H., Gilley, P., & Dorman, M. (2005). P1 latency as a biomarker for central auditory development in children with hearing impairment. *Journal of the American Academy of Audiology, 16*(8), 564–573.

Shpak T. (2005, June). *Correlations between rate preference and NRT.* Presented at 12th NRT Research Workshop, Hannover, Germany.

Shpak, T., Berlin, M., & Luntz, M. (2004). Objective measurements of auditory nerve recovery function in Nucleus CI 24 implantees in relation to subjective preference of stimulation rate. *Acta Otolaryngologica, 124*(6), 679–683.

Smoorenburg, G. F., Willeboer, C., & van Dijk, J. E. (2002). Speech perception in Nucleus CI24M cochlear implant users with processor settings based on electrically evoked compound action potential thresholds. *Audiology and Neurootology, 7*(6), 335–347.

Spivak, L., Auerbach, C., Vambutas, A., Geshkovich, S., Wexler, L., & Popecki, B. (2011). Electrical compound action potentials recorded with automated neural response telemetry: Threshold changes as a function of time and electrode position. *Ear and Hearing, 32*(1), 104–113.

Spivak, L. G., & Chute, P. M. (1994). The relationship between electrical acoustic reflex thresholds and behavioral comfort levels in children and adult cochlear implant patients. *Ear and Hearing, 15*(2), 184–192.

Stephan, K., & Welzl-Muller, K. (2000). Post-operative stapedius reflex tests with simultaneous loudness scaling in patients supplied with cochlear implants. *Audiology, 39*(1), 13–18.

Stypulkowski, P. H., & van den Honert, C. (1984). Physiological properties of the electrically stimulated auditory nerve. I. Compound action potential recordings. *Hearing Research, 14*(3), 205–223.

Telmesani, L. M., & Said, N. M. (2015). Effect of cochlear implant electrode array design on auditory nerve and behavioral response in children. *International Journal of Pediatric Otorhinolaryngology, 79*(5), 660–665.

Telmesani, L. M., & Said, N. M. (2016). Electrically evoked compound action potential (ECAP) in cochlear implant children: Changes in auditory nerve response in first year of cochlear implant use. *International Journal of Pediatric Otorhinolaryngology, 82*, 28–33.

Turner, C., Mehr, M., Hughes, M., Brown, C., & Abbas P. (2002). Within-subject predictors of speech recognition in cochlear implants: A null result. *Acoustic Research Letters Online, 3*, 95–100.

van Dijk, B., Botros, A. M., Battmer, R. D., Begall, K., Dillier, N., Hey, M., . . . Offeciers, E. (2007). Clinical results of AutoNRT, a completely automatic ECAP recording system for cochlear implants. *Ear and Hearing, 28*(4), 558–570.

Walkowiak, A., Lorens, A., Polak, M., Kostek, B., Skarzynski, H., Szkielkowska, A., & Skarzynski, P. H. (2011). Evoked stapedius reflex and compound action potential thresholds versus most comfortable loudness level: assessment of their relation for charge-based fitting strategies in implant users. *ORL—Journal of Otorhinolaryngology and Related Specialties, 73*(4), 189–195.

Walton, J., Gibson, W. P., Sanli, H., & Prelog, K. (2008). Predicting cochlear implant outcomes in children with auditory neuropathy. *Otology and Neurotology, 29*(3), 302–309.

Wolfe, J., Gilbert, M., Schafer, E., Litvak, L. M., Spahr, A. J., Saoji, A., & Finley, C. (2017). Optimizations for the electrically-evoked stapedial reflex threshold measurement in cochlear implant recipients. *Ear and Hearing, 38*(2), 255–261.

Wolfe, J., & Kasulis, H. (2008). Relationships among objective measures and speech perception in adult users of the HiResolution Bionic Ear. *Cochlear Implants International, 9*(2), 70–81.

Zimmerling, M. J., & Hochmair, E. S. (2002). EAP recordings in ineraid patients—correlations with psychophysical measures and possible implications for patient fitting. *Ear and Hearing, 23*(2), 81–91.

Zuniga, M. G., Rivas, A., Hedley-Williams, A., Gifford, R. H., Dwyer, R., Dawant, B. M., . . . Labadie, R. F. (2017). Tip fold-over in cochlear implantation: Case series. *Otology and Neurotology, 38*(2), 199–206.

19

Considerations for Vestibular Assessment and Management of Cochlear Implant Candidates and Recipients

Jamie M. Bogle

Introduction

The numerous and substantial advantages of cochlear implantation are discussed throughout this book. Most recipients receive considerable benefit from their cochlear implant; however, with all interventions, there are risks. One common risk following cochlear implantation is dizziness and/or imbalance due to damage to the vestibular end organs. Understanding who may be most at risk, as well as developing appropriate management for those who do experience dizziness following cochlear implantation, is key to providing comprehensive management to patients undergoing this procedure.

Vestibular Anatomy and Physiology

Many patients with hearing loss experience dizziness and/or imbalance. Various underlying pathologies can lead to these symptoms, which may or may not be related to the inner ear. The balance system requires appropriate sensory signal detection and integration from the vestibular, visual, and proprioceptive systems; however, it is the vestibular system that may be most at risk for altered function during cochlear implantation (Handzel, Burgess, & Nadol, 2005; Tien & Linthicum, 2002). The inner ear is located within the temporal bone, housing both the cochlear and vestibular systems. The auditory and vestibular systems are closely related phylogenetically and anatomically. The vestibular system is ancient, developing over 450 million years ago to monitor rotational and linear head movement (Gray, 1955). Interestingly, the vestibular system took on another role—hearing, leading to the development of the cochlea in mammals. Vestibular end organs have maintained some level of sound detection (Cazals, Aran, Erre, Guilhaume, & Aurosseau, 1983; McCue & Guinan, 1995; Moffat & Caprianica, 1976; Wit, Bleeker, & Mulder, 1983; Young, Fernández, & Goldberg, 1977). The primitive ear arises from the same tissues during embryological development and divides into two sections. The dorsal portion develops into the semicircular canals, utricle, and endolymphatic duct, whereas the ventral area develops into the saccule and cochlea (Sadler, 2004; Zemlin, 1998).

There are five vestibular end organs in each inner ear to detect both angular and linear movements (Figure 19–1). Three semicircular canals act as an internal gyroscope and are responsible for detecting and encoding information regarding angular accelerations or determining when an individual is turning the head. These organs lie orthogonally

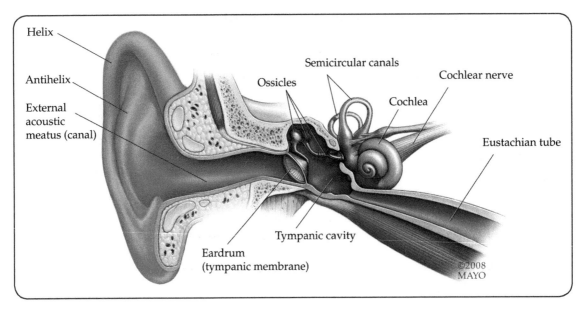

FIGURE 19–1. The inner ear is housed within the temporal bone and includes the cochlea, semicircular canals, and otolith organs. Image provided courtesy of Mayo Clinic.

from one another and detect head movement in yaw, pitch, and roll planes (Breuer, 1874; Camis & Creed, 1930; Hillman & McLaren, 1979; Lysakoswki & Goldberg, 2004; McLaren & Hillman, 1979). Information detected from these vestibular end organs triggers the vestibulo-ocular reflex pathway, leading to maintenance of stable vision during movement.

The two remaining vestibular end organs are the saccule and utricle, collectively described as the otolith organs. The otolith organs detect and encode information regarding linear translations, including those induced by gravity and head tilts (Fernández & Goldberg, 1976; Goldberg, Desmadryl, Baird, & Fernández, 1990; Lysakowski & Goldberg, 2004; Uchino et al., 1997). These sensory inputs are important for maintaining postural stability through the vestibulo-collic and vestibulo-spinal reflexes. The otolith organs are heavily involved in gross motor skill development, including learning to sit, stand, and walk (Kaga, Shinjo, Jin, & Takegoshi, 2008).

Vestibular Function and Hearing Loss

Hearing and vestibular loss often co-occur, likely related to common underlying inner ear pathology (Table 19–1). Vestibular function in patients with significant hearing loss can range from normal to bilateral areflexia, or absent vestibular responses. Up to 72% of children and adults with significant sensorineural hearing loss have some level of vestibular dysfunction (Buchman, Joy, Hodges, Telischi, & Balkany, 2004; Chiong, Nedzelski, McIlmoyl, & Shipp, 1994; Huygen, Van Den Broek, Spies, Mens, & Admiraal, 1994; Ito, 1998; Krause, Wechtenbruch, Rader, & Gürkov, 2009; Szirmai, Ribári, & Répássy, 2001); however, this is likely to depend on the underlying inner ear pathology (see Table 19–1). For instance, patients with hearing loss following meningitis generally all demonstrate abnormal semicircular canal function, but variable otolith responses. On the other hand, patients with hearing loss related to Connexin 26 are more likely to demonstrate otolith dysfunction than semicircular canal impairment (Cushing, Gordon, Rutka, James, & Papsin, 2013).

Although there are five vestibular end organs, common clinical protocols have evaluated only the horizontal semicircular canal, leading to limited understanding of vestibular function in patients with hearing loss. Common vestibular diagnostic and functional measures are provided in Table 19–2. Vestibular clinical presentation for patients under evaluation for cochlear implantation varies significantly, but in general, semicircular canal abnormalities are noted in up to half of cases (Buchman et al., 2004; Krause et al., 2009), with

TABLE 19–1. Common Disorders Associated with Both Hearing and Vestibular Dysfunction

Genetic		Acquired	
Usher syndrome (Type I)	Connexin 26	Prematurity	Aging
Pendred syndrome	Inner ear malformations	Anoxia	Ménière disease
Waardenburg syndrome	Enlarged vestibular aqueduct	Fetal alcohol syndrome	Labyrinthitis
Cogan syndrome	Otosclerosis	Meningitis	Autoimmune inner ear disease
Brachio-oto-renal syndrome	Charcot-Marie-Tooth disease	Cytomegalovirus	
CHARGE		Ototoxicity	Trauma

TABLE 19–2. Common Vestibular Diagnostic and Functional Measures

Measure	Targeted End Organ	Reflex Pathway
Caloric Test[a]	Horizontal SCC	Vestibulo-ocular reflex
Video Head Impulse Test[a]	Horizontal, superior, posterior SCC	Vestibulo-ocular reflex
Rotational Chair Test[a]	Horizontal SCC	Vestibulo-ocular reflex
Cervical Vestibular Evoked Myogenic Potential (cVEMP)[a]	Saccule	Vestibulo-collic reflex
Ocular Vestibular Evoked Myogenic Potential (oVEMP)[a]	Utricle	Vestibulo-ocular reflex
Sensory Organization Test (SOT)[b]		Vestibulo-spinal reflex
Dynamic Visual Acuity Test[b]	Horizontal SCC	Vestibulo-ocular reflex

SCC: Semicircular canal; [a]diagnostic measures of vestibular function; [b]functional measures of vestibular/balance function.

abnormal otolith function described in up to 44% (Ibrahim, da Silva, Segal, & Zeitouni, 2017; Melvin, Della Santina, Carey, & Migliaccio, 2009).

Pediatric Considerations

Children with severe to profound sensorineural hearing loss are likely to demonstrate additional vestibular impairment (Brookhouser, Cyr, & Beauchaine, 1982). The prevalence of vestibular dysfunction is highly associated with underlying inner ear pathology. Children with congenital sensorineural hearing loss demonstrate both semicircular canal (41%) and otolith (42%) dysfunction (Inoue et al., 2013) with approximately equal proportions of bilateral and uni-

lateral vestibular loss (Inoue et al., 20130; Kaga et al., 2008). Acquired hearing loss may demonstrate variable risk for vestibular dysfunction. For example, Cushing et al. (2009) described abnormal horizontal semicircular canal function in all eight children evaluated following meningitis infection. Unfortunately, as most children present with unknown hearing loss etiology, subsequent vestibular dysfunction may not be evaluated.

The importance of vestibular function in children is commonly overlooked as it relates to general development, educational outcomes, and safety. The vestibular system in children matures and integrates into the balance system throughout the first few years of life (Shumway-Cook & Woollacott, 1985). Although children demonstrate a remarkable ability to compensate for reduced vestibular function, congenital or early-onset vestibular dysfunction may lead to significant delays in motor skill development (Martin, Jelsma, & Rogers, 2012; Suarez et al., 2007). These deficits may not be apparent until the child fails to meet gross motor development milestones as gross motor skills require appropriate vestibular system information (Shall, 2009). Children with significant sensorineural hearing loss are known to have delays in gross motor skill development likely related to concurrent vestibular loss. These delays can be identified early through intervention or diagnostic services (Inoue et al., 2013; Rine et al., 2000). Understanding vestibular system limitations (i.e., severity of vestibular system dysfunction) can aid in the development of appropriate early intervention services.

Educational outcomes are monitored for children with hearing loss due to their reduced access to auditory information; however, the impact of vestibular dysfunction on the skills needed for educational achievement is not well described. Bilateral vestibular dysfunction leads to oscillopsia (i.e., lack of visual stability during head movement), which generally creates difficulty with reading and classroom tasks such as taking notes and working on a computer. Braswell and Rine (2006) reported on 14 children with sensorineural hearing loss and noted that those with vestibular hypofunction demonstrated significantly poorer reading ability than those children with appropriate vestibular function and typically developing children. This work highlights the likely impact of vestibular system dysfunction in the educational achievement of children with significant sensorineural hearing loss. Further work is needed to understand the likely relationship between these outcomes and the vestibular system as well as to develop appropriate rehabilitation measures for young children learning to read.

Safety is a significant consideration for children at risk for vestibular dysfunction, especially in situations with reduced visual input. Children with poor vestibular function may have difficulty participating in typical activities, such as learning to ride a bicycle or catching a ball, especially when running. This may limit their abilities to participate in typical childhood activities or increase their risk for injury due to reduced balance or visual stability (Martin et al., 2012). Importantly, children with vestibular dysfunction should take considerable care when around water. Children, and adults, should never swim alone and should ensure appropriate use of life vests and goggles. Swimming creates a significant dependence on the vestibular system, especially the otolith organs, in determining the location of the water's surface. In cases of poor visibility, such as in murky water or with the eyes closed, this becomes especially challenging and should be viewed with caution.

Impact of Cochlear Implantation on the Vestibular System

Cochlear implantation requires insertion of an electrode array into the inner ear, which may lead to altered function throughout the vestibular system. The changes in vestibular system function may lead to dizziness and/or imbalance in some patients, but it is important to remember that long-term concerns regarding the vestibular system occur in less than 10% of cases (Hansel et al., 2018). There may be numerous mechanisms for significant inner ear damage following cochlear implantation which may or may not lead to significant functional challenges related to dizziness and/or imbalance. Electrode array insertion is associated with end organ structural changes, including otolith membrane distortion and collapse, reactive neuromas, and vestibulofibrosis (Gstoettner et al., 1997; Handzel et al., 2005; Katsiari et al., 2013; Tien & Linthicum, 2002). During cochlear implantation, an electrode array is gently advanced creating contact pressure as it moves along the tissues within the cochlea (Chen, Clark, & Jones, 2003; Rebscher et al., 1999). The area of highest pressure has been modeled at approximately 175° or 10 mm from the round window (Verbist et al., 2009). This corresponds with the basal turn of the cochlea, or the area of first resistance encountered during electrode array insertion. The saccule is the closest vestibular end organ to the first point of resistance, which may put this end organ at specific risk for damage. Two studies have evaluated the vestibular end organs of donor temporal bones. Tien and Linthicum (2002) evaluated 11 pairs of temporal bones, each with a cochlear implant placed during the donor's lifetime, and found notable vestibular end organ damage in 72%. Damage was noted mostly within the saccule, with less damage observed in the utricle and semicircular canals. Additionally, 75% of those with damage to the basal turn of the cochlea also demonstrated damage to the saccule, possibly associated with electrode placement. Handzel et al. (2005) further explored the anatomical changes that can occur following cochlear implantation, noting that most of their temporal bones ($n =$ 19) exhibited evidence of cochlear hydrops (83%), saccular collapse (56%), and saccular hydrops (22%). These findings suggest that patients may be at risk for atypical accumulation of endolymph following surgery, possibly leading to endolymphatic hydrops or Ménière disease symptoms. These studies, although limited, suggest that structural changes to the vestibular system are common. The high prevalence of structural changes noted in histopathological studies provides information regarding the possibility of altered inner ear function. It is important to remember that as cochlear implantation electrode arrays and surgical techniques evolve to preserve inner ear structures, the vestibular system may demonstrate fewer alterations as well.

Dizziness Post-Cochlear Implantation

Dizziness is a common complication after cochlear implantation. Although up to 74% of adults report some level of dizziness and/or imbalance after surgery (Enticott, Tari, Koh, Dowell, & O'Leary, 2006; Fina et al., 2003; Kubo, Yamamoto, Iwaki, Doi, & Tamura, 2001; Steenerson, Cronin, & Gary, 2001), these symptoms generally resolve within 30 days (Parmar et al., 2012). Dizziness is often described as a feeling of lightheadedness or imbalance, whereas others describe rotational vertigo (Fina et al., 2003; Steenerson et al., 2001). The time course of dizziness presentation varies. Of those with dizziness, about half report symptoms within a week after cochlear implantation, suggesting changes to the inner ear likely due to surgical interventions (Ito, 1998; Krause et al., 2009; Parmar et al., 2012). Children are not immune to post-surgical dizziness. Jacot et al. (2009) reported on a series of 89 children ranging in age from 7 months to 16 years, finding that 27% demonstrated vestibular systems such as dizziness and vomiting during the first 48 hours following surgery. Furthermore, children may demonstrate additional imbalance during at least the first week following implantation (Birman, Gibson, & Elliott, 2015).

Interestingly, dizziness symptoms may not occur immediately, suggesting a change in inner ear status over time. González-Navarro et al. (2015) described 25 patients with dizziness symptoms that began over one month post-cochlear implantation. They found that most patients described a sense of imbalance

(48%). Others (20%) described recurrent vertigo episodes with aural fullness and tinnitus that were consistent with possible endolymphatic hydrops. Positional vertigo (i.e., benign paroxysmal positional vertigo or BPPV) was noted in another 20%, which was resolved with repositioning maneuvers. Although this work only evaluated patients with late-onset dizziness symptoms, the authors estimated that delayed dizziness occurred in approximately 4% of their patient population. Other work has found similar delays in dizziness. Kubo et al. (2001) described dizziness in 94 patients, noting that 34% had acute onset of vertigo symptoms, aural fullness, and tinnitus between one and three months postoperatively, again similar to symptoms associated with endolymphatic hydrops. This delayed onset was further described by Fina and colleagues (2003), who found a median onset of dizziness symptoms of 74 days (interquartile range: 26–377 days). Although it is assumed that dizziness/imbalance related to cochlear implantation should occur immediately due to the surgical intervention, there may be a later onset for some patients.

Pediatric Considerations

Children provide an interesting cohort for balance evaluation, as they do not have established vestibular reflexes at the time of implantation. Some etiologies of hearing loss are also related to concurrent vestibular dysfunction. This area of research is emerging, but studies are finding not only reduced balance function in children with significant sensorineural hearing loss, but also possible effects of cochlear implantation in this population. In some studies, significant differences in balance function have been reported in children with and without cochlear implants (De Kegel, Maes, Van Waelvelde, & Dhooge, 2015; Ebrahimi, Movallali, Jamshidi, Haghgoo, & Rahgozar, 2016; Oyewumi et al., 2016). Ebrahimi et al. (2016) evaluated 85 children (7–12 years old) with profound sensorineural hearing loss and compared their balance with control children. They found significant differences in balance function between children with hearing loss and controls, suggesting that children with significant hearing loss may also have challenges with the vestibular system. Furthermore, they noted that balance was reduced for children with cochlear implants compared with children who had hearing loss but did not have a cochlear implant, suggesting a possible reduction in balance ability for children following cochlear implantation. This is not completely established, and cochlear implantation has not always been associated with reduced balance. Eustaquio and colleagues (Eustaquio, Berryhill, Wolfe, & Saunders, 2011) noted no differences in balance function between those children with and without cochlear implants. The mean balance for these children was significantly reduced compared with normative values, indicating that the cause of deafness may have also impaired vestibular function. These data indicate that not all children with cochlear implants demonstrate a larger reduction in balance function compared with other children with significant hearing loss. Longitudinal balance development data have also been reported to describe the possible effect of cochlear implantation. De Kegel et al. (2015) monitored a group of children ($n = 48$) through two years of age using various developmental scales and clinical diagnostic testing. Although all children were cochlear implant candidates, only 23 received an implant during the evaluation period. The children who received a cochlear implant demonstrated a significant drop in gross motor performance between 6 and 18 months, with recovery at the 24-month evaluation. Additionally, some children ($n = 7$) demonstrated absent otolith function, suggesting reduced vestibular end organ function. None of these children were walking by 18 months of age, demonstrating a significant delay in gross motor development. The authors concluded that cochlear implantation can lead to a change in gross motor development trajectory that may require intervention services. They hypothesized that this could be due to significant surgically induced vestibular dysfunction, but also conceded that the dominant focus on auditory skill development likely after a cochlear implant could contribute to delayed gross motor skill performance. Understanding that these children may be at increased risk for gross motor delay could reduce the delay in initiating habilitation or rehabilitation services (De Kegel et al., 2015; Rine et al., 2004).

Importantly, children with dizziness and imbalance may be at increased risk for cochlear implant device failure. Wolter et al. (2015) noted that children with reduced vestibular function were 7.6 times more likely to experience cochlear implant device failure than those with intact vestibular system. The authors hypothesized that the higher risk for falls in these children may lead to additional head trauma and subsequent failure. Identification of children who may be at a higher risk of falling may lead to reduced device failure and less need for reimplantation.

Vestibular Function Post-Cochlear Implantation

Cochlear implantation has been shown to cause structural changes in histopathological studies (Handzel et al., 2005; Tien & Linthicum, 2002) and functional changes are also described, although quite variable. In general, cochlear implantation has been shown to disrupt semicircular canal function in up to half of cases (Brey et al., 1995; Enticott et al., 2006; Huygen et al., 1995; Krause et al., 2009; Vibert, Hausler, Kompis, & Vischer, 2001).

Semicircular canal function, typically evaluated using caloric testing, has long been used to describe vestibular function in patients experiencing dizziness and imbalance. Caloric testing relies on a reflex pathway describing the function of the horizontal semicircular canal, superior vestibular nerve, and subsequent vestibulo-ocular reflex pathway (Jacobson & Shepard, 2016). Although up to half of patients demonstrate a significant change in this response following surgery (Batuecas-Caletrio et al., 2015; Krause, Louza, Wechtenbruch, & Gürkov, 2010; Schwab, Durisin, & Kontorinis, 2010), not all patients report significant dizziness in association with this change, highlighting the variability in clinical diagnostic evaluation and self-perceived symptoms (Krause et al., 2010).

Temporal bone studies have suggested that the saccule may be the vestibular end organ most at risk for injury following cochlear implantation (Handzel et al., 2005; Tien & Linthicum, 2002) and evaluation of this end organ should provide improved insight into changes in vestibular function postoperatively. Saccular reflex testing has evolved over the last two decades, providing a method of describing otolith function (Colebatch, Halmagyi, & Skuse, 1994). Cervical vestibular evoked myogenic potentials (cVEMPs) are used clinically to describe function of the saccule, inferior vestibular nerve, and subsequent descending vestibulo-collic reflex pathway—an important postural stability reflex pathway. Numerous studies have demonstrated a significant change in this response following implantation (Chen, Chen, Zhang, & Qin, 2016; Katsiari et al., 2013; Krause et al., 2010; Robard, Hitier, Lebas, & Moreau, 2015; Todt, Basta, & Ernst, 2008). Abnormalities in this reflex pathway have been noted in up to 44% of patients (Ibrahim et al., 2017).

The unpredictability in reported changes described in patients following cochlear implantation likely is due to multiple variables. First, the underlying variability in study samples should be considered, as this will lead to various vestibular outcomes. This is difficult to quantify due to the large proportion of individuals with unknown hearing loss etiology and subsequent vestibular pathology. Second, the protocols utilized over time to describe vestibular system function have evolved, providing information on additional end organ function.

Pediatric Considerations

Previous literature regarding vestibular function in patients with cochlear implants was focused mostly on adults and older children; however, age limitations are no longer a considerable concern due to new technology. In general, children are tolerant of various vestibular protocols (Cushing, Gordon, Rutka, James, & Papsin, 2013). Current protocols allow for evaluation of semicircular canal function in children as young as 3 months of age (Wiener-Vacher & Wiener, 2017) and saccule function soon after birth (Erbek et al., 2007) (Table 19–3).

Vestibular presentation is variable in children postimplantation as well, with up to half demonstrating reduced vestibular function (Ajalloueyan, Saeedi,

TABLE 19–3. Example Vestibular Protocol by Age for Cochlear Implant Candidates

Age	Semicircular Canal	Otolith	Balance/Gross Motor Skills
>1 year	vHIT	cVEMP	PDMS-2
			AIMS
1–3 years	vHIT	cVEMP	AIMS
			GDBT
3–7 years	vHIT	cVEMP, oVEMP	GDBT
			Single leg stance
			Romberg test
			SOT
>7 years	vHIT, caloric	cVEMP, oVEMP	Single leg stance
			Romberg test
			SOT

vHIT = video head impulse test; cVEMP = cervical vestibular evoked myogenic potential; oVEMP = ocular vestibular evoked myogenic potential; PDMS-2 = Peabody Developmental Motor Scales (Darrah, Magill-Evans, Volden, Hodge, & Kembhavi, 2007); AIMS = Alberta Infant Motor Scale (Darrah, Piper, & Watt, 1998); GDBT = Ghent Developmental Balance Test (De Kegel et al., 2012); SOT = sensory organization test.

Sadeghi, & Zamiri Abdollahi, 2017; Cushing et al., 2013; Devroede, Pauwels, Le Bon, Monstrey, & Mansbach, 2016; Jacot, Van Den, Abbeele, Debre, & Wiener-Vacher, 2009; Thierry et al., 2015). Cushing et al. (2013) provided a large sample ($N = 153$) of pediatric subjects, describing some amount of postoperative semicircular canal dysfunction in half. Presentation was varied, however, with 35% demonstrating bilateral areflexia and 21% demonstrating mild to moderate loss. Unfortunately, no preimplantation vestibular data were available for comparison, leaving interpretation regarding the impact of surgical intervention on vestibular function unclear. Jacot et al. (2009) evaluated 224 children (7 months–16 years old) to provide a comparison of pre- versus post-cochlear implantation vestibular responses. Prior to implantation, half demonstrated significant vestibular dysfunction. For the remaining children after surgery, 17% demonstrated reduced function, 10% had absent responses, and 7% had hyperactive responses, suggesting irritation within the vestibular system. The remaining 60% demonstrated no significant changes, which is consistent with adult findings (Enticott et al., 2006). A group of these children was re-evaluated within seven years postimplantation. Although the majority (63%) demonstrated stable responses, 11% demonstrated a decrease in responses. Interestingly, 19% presented with significant improvement in responses. These findings indicate that it is possible to experience long-term variations in vestibular function associated with cochlear implantation.

Most noted changes to the semicircular canals have been described using caloric testing, a low-frequency response (Jacobson & Shepard, 2016). Higher frequency evaluation using the video head impulse test (vHIT) allows for testing of younger patients due to increased tolerance of the procedure (Wiener-Vacher & Wiener, 2017), but may not be as sensitive to postsurgical changes. Ajalloueyan et al. (2017) noted that there were no changes in vHIT responses in children between 12 and 56 months of age. Nassif et al. (2016) evaluated this response in children over 5 years of age, again finding no significant differences in vHIT responses between children with cochlear implants and controls. Furthermore, they did not find any significant differences when comparing implanted and nonimplanted sides. This is not altogether surprising, as caloric testing and vHIT are often in disagreement, especially for mild dysfunction (McCaslin, Jacobson, Bennett, Gruenwald, & Green, 2014). Additional work is needed to better understand the usefulness of vHIT, especially in young children, as this metric is more commonly used clinically, due to its increased tolerance and reduced expense.

Otolith function is especially important for pediatric patients due to its relationship to gross motor skill development. Xu et al. (2015) noted a significant reduction in cVEMPs after implantation in children (*n* = 31) between 3 and 12 years of age. Preimplantation, 69% demonstrated appropriate responses, while only 31% demonstrated repeatable responses postoperatively. Furthermore, those with present postoperative responses were described as having significantly reduced amplitude, suggesting reduced saccular responses. Devroede et al. (2016) noted fewer changes in their study of 16 children. Although a similar percentage demonstrated appropriate preimplantation responses (79%), this study found fewer changes postoperatively (62%). In sum, however, otolith dysfunction is noted in over half of patients postoperatively (Ajalloueyan et al., 2017; Cushing et al., 2013; Devroede et al., 2016; Jacot et al., 2009; Janky & Givens, 2015; Xu et al., 2015).

Improved Postoperative Vestibular Function

It is expected that cochlear implantation may lead to reduced vestibular function; however, some studies have demonstrated an increase in vestibular response hypothesized to be due to electrical current spread (Ribári, Küstel, Szirmai, & Répássy, 1999). In fact, initial concern regarding the impact of cochlear implantation on the vestibular system was focused on the possible complication of electrical current spread to the vestibular system. Black (1977) first reported on the possible vestibular system effects of cochlear implantation by noting alterations in postural stability when the sound processor was turned on. He hypothesized that the electrical current was spreading from the cochlea to nearby vestibular nerve fibers. Further work emphasized this possibility, especially for patients with high amplitude stimulation strategies (Black, Lilly, Peterka, Fowler, & Simmons, 1987). More recent work has demonstrated differences in diagnostic function with the sound processor on versus off. For example, Nassif et al. (2016) compared vHIT responses in children with the sound processor on and off, finding increased VOR gain with the sound processor turned on, but only in patients with unilateral cochlear implants. No differences were noted in bilaterally implanted patients, suggesting that asymmetric electrical current spread could lead to changes in underlying vestibular function. It is

unclear whether this represents a significant functional finding, and further work should investigate the possibility of increased vestibular input obtained due to electrical current spread.

Risk Factors for Reduced Vestibular Function

Several risk factors may predict postoperative dizziness. These factors include both individual patient as well as technological considerations. Improved understanding of these risks should allow for improved patient counseling and management.

Preimplantation Dizziness Status

Patients with and without preimplantation vestibular dysfunction may be at risk for postoperative dizziness for different reasons. First, those patients with appropriate preoperative vestibular function may be more at risk for dizziness postimplantation, as those patients have substantial function that could be lost. On the other hand, those patients with preoperative dizziness may be at risk due to an underlying vestibular pathology (Fina et al., 2003). Those patients may have less stable vestibular structures, which may be more likely to succumb to damage.

Age Effect

Although there are likely numerous patient-specific factors that increase risk for dizziness following cochlear implantation, age appears to be a common consideration. Brey et al. (1995) noted that patients over 60 years of age were more likely to demonstrate significant reduction in vestibular function. Fina et al. (2003) later supported this finding, noting that there was a statistically significant age effect for patients with postimplantation dizziness, with those over 59 years more likely to demonstrate significant issues. More recent work has found that while age is still a significant factor in postoperative dizziness, the age for concern may be somewhat older. Rohloff et al. (2017) noted significantly more dizziness reported in patients over 70 years of age, with no influence of bilateral versus unilateral implantation. Of note, not all older patients will experience postoperative dizziness. Mosnier and colleagues (2014) found no age effect for postoperative dizziness, even though 25% of all subjects over 65 years of age demonstrated a decrease in caloric response. Increased risk of dizziness due to age is a significant consideration due to increased risk of falls and significant injury in this population. Falls are common in patients with hearing loss. Criter and Honaker (2013) reported that half of patients seen in a university audiology clinic experienced a fall within the previous 12 months. As this reported prevalence of falls is well above that reported in the general population (25%) (Sarmiento & Lee, 2017), this may emphasize the relationship between hearing loss and vestibular dysfunction (Zuniga et al., 2012). Additionally, as noted in the pediatric population (Wolter et al., 2015), falls may increase the likelihood of device failure. This has not yet been evaluated in the adult population, but should be considered.

Electrode Considerations

Surgical variations also contribute to postoperative dizziness. Electrode location within the inner ear greatly influences dizziness outcomes. Clearly, an electrode misplaced within the vestibule is likely to cause significant dizziness as well as provide less than adequate cochlear stimulation (Tange, Grolman, & Maat, 2006). Furthermore, research suggests that electrode array position within the scala vestibuli may also contribute to postoperative dizziness symptoms (Nordfalk, Rasmussen, Hopp, Greisiger, & Jablonski, 2014). Even in cases of appropriate electrode location, dizziness outcomes vary between those implanted using a round window approach versus an antero-posterior approach. Todt et al. (2008) noted that subjective dizziness was reduced when using a round window approach for electrode placement.

The electrode itself should also be considered. Although manufacturer differences have not been noted (Enticott et al., 2006; Frodlund, Harder, Mäki-Torkko, & Ledin, 2016; Louza et al., 2015), other factors such as electrode stiffness and insertion depth have been considered. Frodlund et al. (2016) found a significant reduction in caloric response and increased dizziness when using a stiff electrode array, but no differences between precurved or flexible straight electrode options provided by Cochlear Corporation (New South Wales, Australia) and Med-El Corporation (Innsbruck, Austria). This likely relates to the increased pressure along the cochlear lateral wall as previously described. Interestingly, recent work evaluating insertion depth has found no significant differences in dizziness outcomes (Louza et al., 2015; Nordfalk et al., 2016).

Current surgical techniques that utilize a slow insertion speed (Rajan, Kontorinis, & Kuthubutheen,

2013), steroid use (Enticott, Eastwood, Briggs, Dowell, & O'Leary, 2011; Rajan, Kuthubutheen, Hedne, & Krishnaswamy, 2012), and atraumatic electrode arrays (Mirsalehi et al., 2017) aim to reduce trauma in order to preserve cochlear structures and therefore acoustic hearing. These techniques also demonstrate promise in reducing the possible damage to vestibular end organ structures, as well as subsequent inner ear systemic changes associated with cochlear implantation.

Bilateral Cochlear Implantation

The impact of simultaneous or sequential cochlear implantation on the vestibular system should be considered, especially when reflecting on the vestibular influence on gross motor development in young children or when determining fall risk in the adult population. Both groups provide an interesting discussion regarding the effects of acute bilateral vestibular dysfunction. The impact of acute unilateral or bilateral otolith dysfunction has not been well described in children or adults, but could pose a safety concern for imbalance, especially in situations with reduced visual or proprioceptive information (case example provided in Figure 19–2).

Pre-cochlear implantation vestibular evaluation can provide guidance regarding the effects of bilateral cochlear implantation. Knowledge of these structures can guide the clinician in counseling patients and their families regarding the risk of dizziness and imbalance following surgery. Consider the possible guideline for considering a second implant. If asymmetric vestibular function is found pre-cochlear implantation, consider initial implantation of the ear with poorer vestibular function. Retest vestibular function postoperatively to determine if vestibular function was preserved before deciding to pursue a second cochlear implant. For those with decreased postoperative vestibular responses, consider not pursuing the second implant. However, if the second implant is desired, the patient and his or her family should be counseled on the risk of bilateral vestibular hypofunction. See case example provided in Figure 19–2. In cases of preimplantation bilateral vestibular dysfunction, such as described in meningitis, consider simultaneous bilateral cochlear implantation due to the already reduced/absent vestibular responses (Wiener-Vacher, Obeid, & Abou-Elew, 2012), likelihood of cochlear ossification (Nichani et al., 2011), and reduced number of surgical interventions.

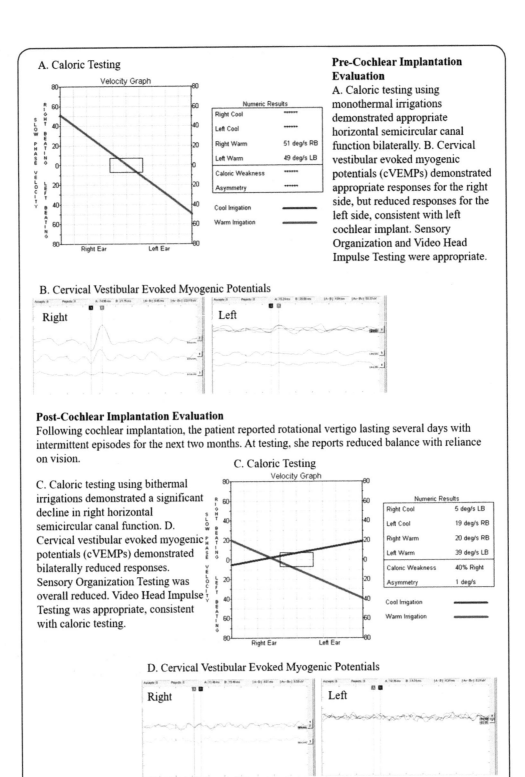

A. Caloric Testing

Velocity Graph

Numeric Results

Right Cool	******
Left Cool	******
Right Warm	51 deg/s RB
Left Warm	49 deg/s LB
Caloric Weakness	******
Asymmetry	******

Cool Irrigation —————
Warm Irrigation —————

Pre-Cochlear Implantation Evaluation
A. Caloric testing using monothermal irrigations demonstrated appropriate horizontal semicircular canal function bilaterally. B. Cervical vestibular evoked myogenic potentials (cVEMPs) demonstrated appropriate responses for the right side, but reduced responses for the left side, consistent with left cochlear implant. Sensory Organization and Video Head Impulse Testing were appropriate.

B. Cervical Vestibular Evoked Myogenic Potentials

Right

Left

Post-Cochlear Implantation Evaluation
Following cochlear implantation, the patient reported rotational vertigo lasting several days with intermittent episodes for the next two months. At testing, she reports reduced balance with reliance on vision.

C. Caloric testing using bithermal irrigations demonstrated a significant decline in right horizontal semicircular canal function. D. Cervical vestibular evoked myogenic potentials (cVEMPs) demonstrated bilaterally reduced responses. Sensory Organization Testing was overall reduced. Video Head Impulse Testing was appropriate, consistent with caloric testing.

C. Caloric Testing

Velocity Graph

Numeric Results

Right Cool	5 deg/s LB
Left Cool	19 deg/s RB
Right Warm	20 deg/s RB
Left Warm	39 deg/s LB
Caloric Weakness	40% Right
Asymmetry	1 deg/s

Cool Irrigation —————
Warm Irrigation —————

D. Cervical Vestibular Evoked Myogenic Potentials

Right

Left

Follow Up Recommendations: Patient initialized vestibular rehabilitation to improve balance function and further facilitate vestibular compensation. She was counselled regarding taking increased care in situations with reduced proprioception, especially as her vision continues to deteriorate.

FIGURE 19–2. Case example of vestibular effects post-cochlear implantation. Patient is a 45-year-old female under evaluation for a second cochlear implant. Her left cochlear implant was placed 10 years prior with no associated dizziness or imbalance reported. She has history of Usher syndrome (Type II). No baseline vestibular evaluation results were available.

Dizziness Management and Rehabilitation

A substantial number of individuals will experience some level of dizziness and/or imbalance following cochlear implantation. Fortunately, this is generally short lived. In some cases, however, cochlear implantation may lead to vestibular dysfunction and subsequent symptoms including significant imbalance and vertigo. This generally resolves over time due to underlying mechanisms of vestibular compensation, meaning that the central vestibular system will adapt to the altered vestibular input and rebalancing its expectation for incoming signals (Lacour, Helmchen, & Vidal, 2016). Some patients who experience continued dizziness symptoms following implantation may need to be referred to vestibular rehabilitation. Physical therapists can provide exercises to improve postural stability as well as help the vestibulo-ocular reflex to adapt to its new sensory input (Whitney, Alghwiri, & Alghadir, 2015).

Transient Vestibular Pathology

Evaluation for positional vertigo, or BPPV, should occur in those patients with postimplantation dizziness, especially if the patient reports dizziness with position changes such as rolling over in bed or tipping the head back. Up to 66% of patients may demonstrate positive BPPV findings that require management with canalith repositioning maneuvers (i.e., Epley maneuvers) (Zanetti, Campovecchi, Balzanelli, & Pasini, 2007). This has not been reported in children.

Conclusions

Cochlear implantation is an integral option for children and adults with significant sensorineural hearing loss, providing access to the auditory environment. Although improving access to sound leads to improved speech development and understanding, the effects of cochlear implantation on other inner ear structures should be considered. Research demonstrates that cochlear implantation may lead to anatomical changes, especially to the saccule, and may be associated with cochlear trauma especially at the basal turn (Handzel et al., 2005; Tien & Linthicum, 2002). The results of pre-cochlear implantation vestibular testing may provide valuable information regarding the status of the inner ear, assisting in determining the most appropriate ear to implant. Vestibular testing is a reasonable addition to the cochlear implant candidacy evaluation and can assist the clinician in providing appropriate counseling of candidates and their families regarding the possible effects of cochlear implantation on the vestibular system.

Key Concepts

* Most recipients receive considerable benefit from their cochlear implant; however, with all interventions, there are risks. One common risk following cochlear implantation is dizziness and/or imbalance due to damage to the vestibular end organs.
* Understanding who may be most at risk, as well as developing appropriate management for those who do experience dizziness following cochlear implantation, is key to providing comprehensive management to patients undergoing this procedure.
* Audiologists should adhere to evidence-based protocols to evaluate vestibular function as needed prior to and after cochlear implantation. Current assessment protocols allow for assessment of vestibular function in infants, children, and adults.
* Audiologists should be aware of risk factors for reduced vestibular function.
* If chronic vestibular symptoms persist after cochlear implantation, vestibular rehabilitation and management can be quite helpful in reducing the symptoms that the recipient experiences.

References

Ajalloueyan, M., Saeedi, M., Sadeghi, M., & Zamiri Abdollahi, F. (2017). The effects of cochlear implantation on vestibular function in 1 to 4-year-old children. *International Journal of Pediatric Otorhinolaryngology, 94*, 100–103.

Batuecas-Caletrio, A., Klumpp, M., Santacruz-Ruiz, S., González, F. B., Sánchez, E. G., & Arriaga, M. (2015). Vestibular function in cochlear implantation: Correlating objectiveness and subjectiveness. *Laryngoscope, 125*(10), 2371–2375.

Birman, C. S., Gibson, W. P. R., & Elliott, E. J. (2015). Pediatric cochlear implantation: Associated with minimal postoperative pain and dizziness. *Otology and Neurotology, 36*(2), 220–222.

Black, F. O. (1977). Present vestibular status of subjects implanted with auditory prostheses. *Annals of Otology, Rhinology, and Laryngology, Supplement, 38,* 49–56.

Black, F. O., Lilly, D. J., Peterka, R. J., Fowler, L. P., & Simmons, F. B. (1987). Vestibulo- ocular and vestibulospinal function before and after cochlear implant surgery. *Annals of Otology, Rhinology, and Laryngology, 96*(1 Pt. 2), 106–108.

Braswell, J., & Rine, R. M. (2006). Evidence that vestibular hypofunction affects reading acuity in children. *International Journal of Pediatric Otorhinolaryngology, 70*(11), 1957–1965.

Breuer, J. (1874). Über die function der Bogengänges des Ohrlabrinthes. *Wiener Medizinisches Jahrbuch, 4,* 72–124.

Brey, R. H., Facer, G. W., Trine, M. B., Lynn, S. G., Peterson, A. M., & Suman, V. J. (1995). Vestibular effects associated with implantation of a multiple channel cochlear prosthesis. *American Journal of Otology, 16*(4), 424–430.

Brookhouser, P. E., Cyr, D. G., & Beauchaine, K. A. (1982). Vestibular findings in the deaf and hard of hearing. *Otolaryngology–Head and Neck Surgery, 90*(6),773–777.

Buchman, C., Joy, J., Hodges, A., Telischi, F. F., & Balkany, T. J. (2004). Vestibular effects of cochlear implantation. *Laryngoscope, 114*(10 Pt. 2, Suppl. 103), 1–22.

Camis, M., & Creed, R. S. (1930). *The physiology of the vestibular apparatus.* Oxford, UK: Clarendon Press.

Cazals, Y., Aran, J. M., Erre, J. P., Guilhaume, A, & Aurosseau, C. (1983). Vestibular acoustic reception in the guinea pig: A saccular function. *Acta Oto-Laryngologica, 95*(1–4), 211– 217.

Chen, B. K., Clark, G. M., & Jones, R. (2003). Evaluation of trajectories and contact pressures for the straight nucleus cochlear implant electrode array—a two-dimensional application of finite element analysis. *Medical Engineering and Physics, 25*(2), 141–147.

Chen, X., Chen, X., Zhang, F., & Qin, Z. (2016). Influence of cochlear implant on vestibular function. *Acta Oto-Laryngologica, 136*(7), 655–659.

Chiong, C. M., Nedzelski, J. M., McIlmoyl, L. D., & Shipp, D. B. (1994). Electro-oculographic findings pre- and post-cochlear implantation. *Journal of Otolaryngology, 23*(6), 447–449.

Colebatch, J. G., Halmagyi, G. M., & Skuse, N. F. (1994). Myogenic potentials generated by a click-evoked vestibulocollic reflex. *Journal of Neurology, Neurosurgery, and Psychiatry, 57*(2), 190–197.

Criter, R. E., & Honaker, J. A. (2013). Falls in the audiology clinic: A pilot study. *Journal of the American Academy of Audiology, 24*(10), 1001–1005.

Cushing, S. L., Gordon, K. A., Rutka, J. A., James, A. L., & Papsin, B. S. (2013). Vestibular end-organ dysfunction in children with sensorineural hearing loss and cochlear implants: An expanded cohort and etiologic assessment. *Otology and Neurotology, 34*(3), 422–428.

Cushing, S. L., Papsin, B. C., Rutka, J. A., James, A. L., Blaser, S. L., & Gordon, K. A. (2009). Vestibular end-organ and balance deficits after meningitis and cochlear implantation in children correlate poorly with functional outcome. *Otology and Neurotology, 30,* 488–495.

Darrah, J., Magill-Evans, J., Volden, J., Hodge, M., & Kembhavi, G. (2007). Scores of typically developing children on the Peabody Ddevelopmental Motor Scales: Infancy to preschool. *Physical and Occupational Therapy in Pediatrics, 27*(3), 5–19.

Darrah, J., Piper, M., & Watt, M. J. (1998). Assessment of gross motor skills of high-risk infants: Predictive validity of the alberta infant motor scale. *Developmental Medicine and Child Neurology, 40*(7), 485–491.

De Kegel, A., Baetens, T., Peersman, W., Maes, L., Dhooge, I., & Van Waelvelde, H. (2012). Ghent developmental balance test: A new tool to evaluate balance performance in toddlers and preschool children. *Physical Therapy, 92*(6), 841–852.

De Kegel, A., Maes, L., Van Waelvelde, H., & Dhooge, I. (2015). Examining the impact of cochlear implantation on the early gross motor development of children with a hearing loss. *Ear and Hearing, 36*(3), e113–e121.

Devroede, B., Pauwels, I., Le Bon, S. D., Monstrey, J., & Mansbach, A. L. (2016). Interest of vestibular evaluation in sequentially implanted children: Preliminary results. *European Annals of Otorhinolaryngology, Head and Neck Diseases, 133,* S7–S11.

Ebrahimi, A., Movallali, G., Jamshidi, A., Haghgoo, H. A., & Rahgozar, M. (2016). Balance performance of deaf children with and without cochlear implants. *Acta Medica Iranica, 54*(11), 738–742.

Enticott, J. C., Eastwood, H. T., Briggs, R. J., Dowell, R. C., & O'Leary, S. J. (2011). Methylprednisolone applied directly to the round window reduces dizziness after cochlear implantation: A randomized clinical trial. *Audiology and Neurotology, 16*(5), 289–303.

Enticott, J. C., Tari, S., Koh, S. M., Dowell, R. C., & O'Leary, S. J. (2006). Cochlear implant and vestibular function. *Otology and Neurotology, 27*(6), 824–830.

Erbek, S., Erbek, S. S., Gokman, Z., Ozkiraz, S., Tarcan, A., & Ozluoglu, L. N. (2007). Clinical application of vestibular evoked myogenic potentials in healthy newborns. *International Journal of Pediatric Otorhinolaryngology, 71*(8), 1181–1185.

Eustaquio, M. E., Berryhill, W., Wolfe, J. A., & Saunders, J. E. (2011). Balance in children with bilateral cochlear implants. *Otology and Neurotology, 32*(3), 424–427.

Fernández, C., & Goldberg, J. M. (1976). Physiology of peripheral neurons innervating otolith organs of the squirrel monkey. III. Response dynamics. *Journal of Neurophysiology, 39,* 996–1008.

Fina, M., Skinner, M., Goebel, J., Piccirillo, J. F., Neely, J. G., & Black, O. (2003). Vestibular dysfunction after cochlear implantation. *Otology and Neurotology, 24*(2), 234–242.

Frodlund, J., Harder, H., Mäki-Torkko, E., & Ledin, T. (2016). Vestibular function after cochlear implantation. *Otology and Neurotology, 37*(10), 1535–1540.

Goldberg, J. M., Desmadryl, G., Baird, R. A., & Fernández, C. (1990). The vestibular nerve of the chinchilla. V. Relation between afferent discharge properties and peripheral innervation patterns in the utricular macula. *Journal of Neurophysiology, 63,* 791–804.

González-Navarro, M., Manrique-Huarte, R., Manrique-Rodríguez, M., Huarte-Irujo, A., & Pérez-Fernández, N. (2015). Long-term follow-up of late onset vestibular complaints in patients with cochlear implant. *Acta Oto-Laryngologica, 135*(12), 1245–1252.

Gray, O. (1955). A brief survey of the phylogenesis of the labyrinth. *Journal of Laryngology and Otology, 69*(3), 151–159.

Gstoettner, W., Plenk, H. J., Franz, P., Hamzavi, J., Baumgartner, W., Czemy, C., & Ehrenberger, K. (1997). Cochlear implant deep electrode insertion: Extent of insertional trauma. *Acta Oto-Laryngologica, 117*(2), 274–277.

Handzel, O., Burgess, B. J., & Nadol, J. B. (2005). Histopathology of the peripheral vestibular system after cochlear implantation in the human. *Otology and Neurotology, 27*(1), 57–64.

Hänsel, T., Gauger, U., Bernhard, N., Behzadi, N., Ventura, M. E. R., Hofmann, V., . . . Coordes, A. (2018). Meta-analysis of subjective complaints of vertigo and vestibular tests after cochlear implantation. *Laryngoscope*. Advance online publication.

Hillman, D. E. & McLaren, J. W. (1979). Displacement configuration of semicircular canal cupulae. *Neuroscience, 4*(12), 1989–2000.

Huygen, P. L. M., Hinderink, J. B., Van Den Broek, P., Van Den Borne, S., Brokx, J. P. L., Mens, L. H. M., & Admiraal, R. J. C. (1995). The risk of vestibular function loss after intracochlear implantation. *Acta Oto-Laryngologica, 115*(Suppl. 520), 270–272.

Huygen, P. L. M., Van Den Broek, P., Spies, T. H., Mens, L. H. M., & Admiraal, R. J. C. (1994). Does intracochlear implantation jeopardize vestibular function? *Annals of Otology, Rhinology, and Laryngology, 103*, 609–614.

Ibrahim, I, da Silva, S. D, Segal, B., & Zeitouni, A. (2017). Effect of cochlear implant surgery on vestibular function: Meta-analysis study. *Journal of Otolaryngology–Head and Neck Surgery, 46*(1), 44.

Inoue, A, Iwasaki, S., Ushino, M., Chihara, Y., Fujimotor, C., Egami, N., & Yamasoba, T. (2013). Effect of vestibular dysfunction on the development of gross motor function in children with profound hearing loss. *Audiology and Neurotology, 18*(3), 143–151.

Itayem, D. A., Sladen, D., Driscoll, C. L., Neff, B. A., Beatty, C. W., & Carlson, M. L. (2017). Cochlear implant associated labyrinthitis: A previously unrecognized phenomenon with a distinct clinical and electrophysiological impedance pattern. *Otology and Neurotology.* Advance online publication.

Ito, J. (1998). Influence of the multichannel cochlear implant on vestibular function. *Otolaryngology–Head and Neck Surgery, 118*(6), 900–902.

Jacobson, G., & Shepard, N. (2016). *Balance function assessment and management* (2nd ed.). San Diego, CA: Plural.

Jacot, E., Van Den Abbeele, T., Debre, H. R., & Wiener-Vacher, S. R. (2009). Vestibular impairments pre- and post-cochlear implant in children. *International Journal of Pediatric Otorhinolaryngology, 73*(2), 209–217.

Janky, K., & Givens, D. (2015). Vestibular, visual acuity and balance outcomes in children with cochlear implants: A preliminary report. *Ear and Hearing, 36*(6), e364–e372.

Kaga, K., Shinjo, Y., Jin, Y., & Takegoshi, H. (2008). Vestibular failure in children with congenital deafness. *International Journal of Audiology, 47*(9), 590–599.

Katsiari, E., Balatsouras, D. G., Sengas, J., Riga, M., Korres, G. S., & Xenelis, J. (2013). Influence of cochlear implantation on the vestibular function. *European Archives of Oto-Rhino-Laryngology, 270*(2), 489–495.

Krause, E., Louza, J. P. R., Wechtenbruch, J., & Gürkov, R. (2010). Influence of cochlear implantation on peripheral vestibular receptor function. *Otolaryngology–Head and Neck Surgery, 142*(6), 809–813.

Krause, E., Wechtenbruch, J., Rader, T., & Gürkov, R. (2009). Influence of cochlear implantation on sacculus function. *Otolaryngology–Head and Neck Surgery, 140*(1), 108–113.

Kubo, T., Yamamoto, K., Iwaki, T., Doi, K., & Tamura, M. (2001). Different forms of dizziness occurring after cochlear implant. *European Archives of Oto-Rhino-Laryngology, 258*(1), 9–12.

Lacour, M., Helmchen, C., & Vidal, P. P. (2016). Vestibular compensation: the neuro-otologist's best friend. *Journal of Neurology, 263*(Suppl. 1), S54–S64.

Louza, J., Mertes, L., Braun, T., Gürkov, R., & Krause, E. (2015). Influence of insertion depth in cochlear implantation on vertigo symptoms and vestibular function. *American Journal of Otolaryngology–Head and Neck Medicine and Surgery, 36*(2), 254–258.

Lysakowski, A., & Goldberg, J. M. (2004). Morphophysiology of the vestibular sensory periphery. In S. M. Highstein, R. R. Fay, & A. N. Popper (Eds.), *The vestibular system*. Berlin, Germany: Springer-Verlag.

Martin, W., Jelsma, J., & Rogers, C. (2012). Motor proficiency and dynamic visual acuity in children with bilateral sensorineural hearing loss. *International Journal of Pediatric Otorhinolaryngology, 76*(10), 1520–1525.

McCaslin, D. L., Jacobson, G. P., Bennett, M. L., Gruenwald, J. M., & Green, A. P. (2014). Predictive properties of the vestibular head impulse test: Measures of caloric symmetry and self-report dizziness handicap. *Ear and Hearing, 35*(5), e185–e191.

McCue, M. P., & Guinan, J. J. (1995). Spontaneous activity and frequency selectivity of acoustically responsive vestibular afferents in the cat. *Journal of Neurophysiology, 74*(4), 1563–1572.

McLaren, J. W., & Hillman, D. E. (1979). Displacement of the semicircular canal cupula during sinusoidal rotation. *Neuroscience, 4*(12), 2001–2008

Melvin, T. -A., N., Della Santina, C. C., Carey, J. P., & Migliaccio, A. A. (2009). The effects of cochlear implantation on vestibular function. *Otology and Neurotology, 30*(1), 87–94.

Mirsalehi, M., Rau, T. S., Harbch, L., Hugl, S., Mohebbi, S., Lenarz, T., & Majdani, O. (2017). Insertion force and intracochlear trauma in temporal bone specimens implanted with a straight atraumatic electrode array. *European Archives of Otorhinolaryngology, 274*(5), 2131–2140.

Moffat, A. J. M., & Capranica, R. R. (1976). Auditory sensitivity of the saccule in the American toad (Bufo americanus). *Journal of Comparative Physiology, 105*(1), 1–8.

Mosnier, I., Bebear, J. -P., Marx, M., Fraysse, B., True, E., Lina-Granade, G., . . . Sterkers, O. (2014). Predictive factors of cochlear implant outcomes in the elderly. *Audiology and Neurotology, 19*(1), 15–20.

Nassif, N., Balzanelli, C., & Redaelli de Zinis, L. O. (2016). Preliminary results of video head impulse testing (vHIT) in children with cochlear implants. *International Journal of Pediatric Otorhinolaryngology, 88*, 30–33.

Nichani, J., Green, K., Hans, P., Bruce, I., Henderson, L., & Ramsden, R. (2011). Cochlear implantation after bacterial meningitis in children: Outcomes in ossified and nonossified cochleas. *Otology and Neurotology 32*(5), 784–789.

Nordfalk, K. F., Rasmussen, K., Hopp, E., Bunne, M., Silvola, J. T., & Jablonski, G. E. (2016). Insertion depth in cochlear implantation and outcome in residual hearing and vestibular function. *Ear and Hearing, 37*(2), 129–137.

Nordfalk, K. F., Rasmussen, K., Hopp, E., Greisiger, R., & Jablonski, G. E. (2014). Scalar position in cochlear implant surgery and outcome in residual hearing and the vestibular system. *International Journal of Audiology, 53*(2), 121–127.

Oyewumi, M., Wolter, N. E., Heon, E., Gordon, K. A., Papsin, B. C., & Cushing, S. L. (2016). Using balance function to screen for vestibular impairment in children with sensorineural hearing loss and cochlear implants. *Otology and Neurotology, 37*(7), 926–932.

Parmar, A., Savage, J., Wilkinson, A., Hajioff, D., Nunez, D. A., & Robinson, P. (2012). The role of vestibular caloric tests in cochlear implantation. *Otolaryngology–Head and Neck Surgery, 147*(1), 127–131.

Rajan, G. P., Kontorinis, G., & Kuthubutheen, J. (2013). The effects of insertion speed on inner ear function during cochlear implantation: A comparison study. *Audiology and Neurotology, 18*(1), 17–22.

Rajan, G. P., Kuthubutheen, J., Hedne, N., & Krishnaswamy, J. (2012). The role of preoperative, intratympanic glucocorticoids for hearing preservation in cochlear implantation: A prospective clinical study. *Laryngoscope, 122*(1), 190–195.

Rebscher, S. J., Hellmann, M., Bruszewski, W., Talbot, N. H., Snyder, R. L., & Merzenich, M. M. (1999). Strategies to improve electrode positioning and safety in cochlear implants. *IEEE Transactions on Biomedical Engineering, 46*(3), 340–352.

Ribári, O., Küstel, M., Szirmai, A., & Répássy, G. (1999). Cochlear implantation influences contralateral hearing and vestibular responsiveness. *Acta Oto-Laryngologica, 119*(2), 225–228.

Rine, R. M., Braswell, J., Fisher, D., Joyce, K., Kalar, K., & Shaffer, M. (2004). Improvement of motor development and postural control following intervention in children with sensorineural hearing loss and vestibular impairment. *International Journal of Pediatric Otorhinolaryngology, 68*(9), 1141–1148.

Rine, R M., Cornwall, G., Gan, K., LoCascio, C., O'Hare, T., Robinson, E., & Rice, M. (2000). Evidence of progressive delay of motor development in children with sensorineural hearing loss and concurrent vestibular dysfunction. *Perceptual and Motor Skills, 90*(3 Pt. 2), 1101–1112.

Robard, L., Hitier, M., Lebas, C., & Moreau, S. (2015). Vestibular function and cochlear implant. *European Archives of Oto-Rhino-Laryngology, 272*(3), 523–530.

Rohloff, K., Koopmann, M., Wei, D., Rudack, C., & Savvas, E. (2017). Cochlear implantation in the elderly: Does age matter? *Otology and Neurotology, 38*(1), 54–59.

Sadler, T. W. (2004). *Langman's medical embryology* (9th ed.). Baltimore, MD: Lippincott, Williams & Wilkins.

Sarmiento, K., & Lee, R. (2017). STEADI: CDC's approach to make older adult fall prevention part of every primary care practice. *Journal of Safety Research.* Advance online publication.

Schwab, B., Durisin, M., & Kontorinis, G. (2010). Investigation of balance function using dynamic posturography under electrical-acoustic stimulation in cochlear implant recipients. *International Journal of Otolaryngology, 2010,* 978594.

Shall, M. S. (2009). The importance of saccular function to motor development in children with hearing impairments. *International Journal of Otolaryngology, 2009,* 972565.

Shumway-Cook, A., & Woollacott, M. H. (1985). The growth of stability: Postural control from a development perspective. *Journal of Motor Behavior, 17*(2), 131–147.

Steenerson, R. L., Cronin, G. W., & Gary, L. B. (2001). Vertigo after cochlear implantation. *Otology and Neurotology, 22*(6), 842–843.

Suarez, H., Angeli, S., Suarez, A., Rosales, B., Carrera, X., & Alonso, R. (2007). Balance sensory organization in children with profound hearing loss and cochlear implants. *International Journal of Pediatric Otorhinolaryngology, 71*(4), 629–637.

Szirmai, Á, Ribári, O., & Répássy, G. (2001). Air caloric computer system application in monitoring vestibular function changes after cochlear implantation. *Otolaryngology–Head and Neck Surgery, 125*(6), 631–634.

Tange, R. A., Grolman, W., & Maat, A. (2006). Intracochlear misdirected implantation of a cochlear implant. *Acta Oto-Laryngologica, 126*(6), 650–652.

Thierry, B., Blanchard, M., Leboulanger, N., Parodi, M., Wiener-Vacher, S. R., Garabedian, E. N., & Loundon, N (2015). Cochlear implantation and vestibular function in children. *International Journal of Pediatric Otorhinolaryngology, 79*(2), 101–104.

Tien, H. C., & Linthicum, F. H. (2002). Histopathologic changes in the vestibular after cochlear implantation. *Otolaryngology–Head and Neck Surgery, 127*(4), 260–264.

Todt, I., Basta, D., & Ernst, A. (2008). Does the surgical approach in cochlear implantation influence the occurrence of postoperative vertigo? *Otolaryngology–Head and Neck Surgery, 138*(1), 8–12.

Uchino, Y., Sato, H., Sasaki, M., Imagawa, M., Ikegami, H., Isu, N., & Graf, W. (1997). Sacculocollic reflex arcs in cats. *Journal of Neurophysiology, 77,* 3003–3012.

Verbist, B. M., Ferrarini, L., Briaire, J. J., Zarowski, A., Admiraal-Behloul, F., Olofsen, H., . . . Frijns, J. H. M. (2009). Anatomic considerations of cochlear morphology and its implications for insertion trauma in cochlear implant surgery. *Otology and Neurotology, 30*(4), 471–477.

Vibert, D., Hausler, R., Kompis, M., & Vischer, M. (2001). Vestibular function in patients with cochlear implantation. *Acta Oto-Laryngologica Supplement, 545,* 29–34.

Whitney, S. L., Alghwiri, A., & Alghadir, A. (2015). Physical therapy for persons with vestibular disorders. *Current Opinion of Neurology, 28*(1), 61–68.

Wiener-Vacher, S. R., Obeid, R., & Abou-Elew, M. (2012). Vestibular impairment after bacterial meningitis delays infant posturomotor development. *Journal of Pediatrics, 161*(2), 246–251.

Wiener-Vacher, S. R., & Wiener, S. I. (2017). Video head impulse tests with a remote camera system: normative values of semicircular canal vestibulo-ocular reflex gain in infants and children. *Frontiers in Neurology.* Advance online publication.

Wit, H. P., Bleeker, J. D., & Mulder, H. H. (1983). Responses of pigeon vestibular nerve fibers to sound and vibration with audio frequencies. *Journal of the Acoustical Society of America, 75*(1), 202–208.

Wolter, N. E., Gordon, K. A., Papsin, B. C., & Cushing, S. L. (2015). Vestibular and balance impairment contributes to cochlear implant failure in children. *Otology and Neurotology, 36*(6), 1029–1034.

Xu, X., Zhang, X. T., Zhang, Q., Hu, J., Chen, Y. F., & Xu, M. (2015). Ocular and cervical vestibular-evoked myogenic potentials in children with cochlear implant. *Clinical Neurophysiology, 126*(8), 1624–1631.

Young, E. D., Fernández, C., & Goldberg, J. M. (1977). Responses of squirrel monkey vestibular neurons to audio-frequency sound and head vibration. *Acta Oto-Laryngologica, 84*(1–6), 352–360.

Zanetti, D., Campovecchi, C. B., Balzanelli, C., & Pasini, S. (2007). Paroxysmal positional vertigo after cochlear implantation. *Acta Oto-Laryngologica, 127*(5), 452–458.

Zemlin, W. R. (1998). *Speech and hearing science: Anatomy and physiology* (4th ed.). Needham Heights, MA: Allyn & Bacon.

Zuniga, M. G., Dinkes, R. E., Davalos–Bichara, M., Carey, J. P., Schubert, M. C., King, W. M., . . . Agrawal, Y. (2012). Association between hearing loss and saccular dysfunction in older individuals. *Otology and Neurotology, 33*(9), 1586–1592.

Additional Consideration in the Management of Cochlear Implants for Children and Adults

Jace Wolfe

Introduction

This chapter addresses a variety of topics that are relevant to the clinical management of persons with cochlear implants. Specific items of discussion include bimodal technology, bilateral cochlear implantation, single-sided deafness, hearing assistive technology for cochlear implant users, cochlear implant reliability, and music aptitude following cochlear implantation.

The Benefits of Binaural Hearing

The benefits of **binaural hearing** are discussed in Chapter 3. In short, the binaural auditory system utilizes interaural time and intensity differences to allow for better detection and identification of acoustic signals in noise (van Hoesel, 2004). Binaural auditory squelch, head shadow effect, and summation all contribute to better hearing in noisy and reverberant environments. The binaural auditory system also allows for spatial hearing, which supports sound localization and speech recognition in noise (Churchill et al., 2014). Also, binaural auditory function allows for ready access to sound arriving from both sides of a listener. Because of the importance of binaural auditory function, audiologists should strive to optimize auditory function of each ear with hearing loss. Audiologic intervention for persons with bilateral hearing loss may come in the form of a binaural

hearing aid fitting, bilateral cochlear implantation, or bimodal use (i.e., use of a cochlear implant and a hearing aid in the nonimplanted ear). Additionally, cochlear implantation may be considered for persons with single-sided deafness. The following sections provide relevant information pertaining to bimodal hearing technology, bilateral cochlear implantation, and cochlear implantation for persons with single-sided deafness.

Bimodal

During the early years in which cochlear implantation was provided as a clinical service, most cochlear implant recipients only used one cochlear implant and did not use a hearing aid on the nonimplanted ear. Many audiologists were concerned that the signals provided by a cochlear implant and hearing aid would be "incompatible" and would be difficult for the implant user to discern (Ching et al., 2001; Dooley et al., 1993). Specifically, some audiologists feared that the differences that existed in electric and acoustic signals and the response elicited within the auditory system by each would lead to poorer quality in the bimodal condition compared with the monaural cochlear implant condition. However, in the 1990s and early 2000s many researchers began to demonstrate an improvement in speech recognition in noise in the bimodal condition relative to the monaural cochlear implant condition (Armstrong et al., 1997; Ching et al., 2001; Dooley et al., 1993; Shallop et al., 1992). In the current context, **bimodal** technology refers to the use of a cochlear implant along with a hearing aid for the nonimplanted ear. It should be noted that the term "bimodal" has also been used to refer to the use of two modes of language, particularly sign language and listening and spoken language.

Ching and colleagues (2001) were among the first group of researchers who demonstrated the merits of bimodal hearing technology for children. Ching et al. (2001) evaluated speech recognition in quiet and in noise and the localization abilities of 16 children who used a cochlear implant along with a hearing aid in the nonimplanted ear. Of note, the children typically had profound hearing loss in the nonimplanted ear. The children achieved statistically significant improvements in speech recognition in quiet and in noise as well as in localization in the bimodal condition relative to the monaural cochlear implant condition. Of note, Ching et al. pointed out that the hearing aids of the children in this study were fitted to the NAL-RP prescriptive targets with an overall gain adjustment made to the hearing aid to achieve loudness balance between the implanted and aided ears. Subsequently, a number of other researchers have shown improvements in hearing performance with the use of bimodal hearing technology relative to the monaural cochlear implant condition (Morera et al., 2005).

Likewise, a number of researchers have also demonstrated bimodal benefit for adult recipients (Blamey et al., 1997; Ching, Incerti, & Hill, 2004; Gifford et al., 2007; Shallop et al., 1992). For instance, Ching, Incerti, and Hill (2004) evaluated bimodal benefit in 21 adults who used a cochlear implant along with a hearing aid for the nonimplanted ear. Ching and colleagues reported a mean improvement in speech recognition in noise of greater than 10 percentage points in the bimodal condition relative to the monaural cochlear implant condition. Also, a small but significant improvement in localization was achieved in the bimodal condition relative to the monaural cochlear implant condition. Ching et al. noted that the hearing aids of the participants in their study were fitted to the NAL-NL1 prescriptive targets. They concluded that the NAL-NL1 prescribed frequency response was well received by most participants and resulted in binaural loudness balance. Additionally, Gifford et al. (2007) evaluated the word recognition in quiet, sentence recognition in quiet, and sentence recognition in noise of 11 adult cochlear implant recipients and found that bimodal use resulted in a

mean improvement of 15 to 20 percentage points in all conditions relative to the use of a cochlear implant alone. Also of note, Sheffield and Gifford (2014) have shown that bimodal benefit is available even to recipients who have functional hearing only within a limited frequency range. Specifically, Sheffield and Gifford studied the effect that acoustic bandwidth had on 12 adult bimodal users. They reported that the provision of acoustic amplification from 0 to 250 Hz in the nonimplanted ear improved CNC word recognition and sentence recognition in noise for stimuli spoken by a female talker compared with use of the cochlear implant alone. Furthermore, the provision of acoustic amplification from 0 to 125 Hz in the nonimplanted ear improved sentence recognition in noise for stimuli spoken by a male talker compared with use of the cochlear implant alone. Of note, for both word recognition and sentence recognition in noise, expanding the bandwidth from 250 Hz to the full acoustic bandwidth condition (which typically provided acoustic audibility beyond 750 Hz or higher) resulted in further improvements in performance compared with the condition in which only the cochlear implant was used.

Sheffield, Jahn, and Gifford (2015) have attributed the improvement in speech recognition that comes with the availability of low-frequency acoustic information to one of two different hypotheses. First, they note that Li and Loizou's (2008) "**glimpsing theory**" could explain the improvement in speech recognition in noise that occurs with the availability of an acoustic signal. The glimpsing theory suggests that the temporal peaks of the low-frequency portion of the speech signal can be accessed during the troughs of the noise. If the glimpsing theory does explain the improvement in speech recognition in noise that occurs with the provision of a low-frequency acoustic signal, then improvement in speech recognition in noise can be achieved whether the acoustic signal is provided in the nonimplanted ear (for bimodal users) or in the implanted ear as well (for recipients who have preservation of low-frequency hearing after cochlear implant surgery). Another hypothesis that may explain the improvement observed in speech recognition in noise with the provision of an acoustic signal is related to Qin and Oxenham's (2006) "**source segregation theory**," which suggests that the auditory system extracts the various types of acoustic information present in the electric and acoustic signals and integrates the information to allow for better performance than would be possible with the use of either signal (acoustic or electric) alone. Presumably, integration of the cues available in the acoustic and electric signals would be more effective when both cues are available in the same ear as would be the case for a recipient who uses electric-acoustic stimulation (but not necessarily the case for a bimodal user who would have to extract the acoustic signal from one ear and the electric signal from the other ear and then integrate the information). Indeed, Fu, Galvin, and Wang (2017) demonstrated that a low-frequency acoustic signal and a mid- to high-frequency electric signal may be more effectively integrated in the same ear compared with across ears.

It should be noted that studies of the localization abilities of bimodal users have shown mixed results, with some studies showing that bimodal use results in improvement in spatial hearing abilities over the monaural implant condition (Ching, Incerti, & Hill, 2004; Ching et al., 2006; Dunn et al., 2010; Potts et al., 2009; Seeber, Baumann, & Fastl, 2004; Tyler et al., 2002) and other studies showing limited to no bimodal benefit (Litovsky et al., 2006). In general, bimodal recipients typically perform above chance levels on spatial hearing tasks (Ching, Incerti, & Hill, 2004; Ching et al., 2006; Dunn et al., 2010; Potts et al., 2009; Seeber, Baumann, & Fastl, 2004; Tyler et al., 2002). However, the spatial hearing abilities of bimodal recipients are typically much poorer than those of persons with normal hearing. Specifically, persons with normal hearing can typically localize a sound to 1° to 2° for low-frequency signals that are presented from 0 degrees azimuth (Mills, 1958). In contrast, the localization error of bimodal users typically ranges from 10° to 60° (Ching, Incerti, & Hill, 2004; Ching et al., 2006; Dunn et al., 2010; Litovsky et al., 2006; Potts et al., 2009; Seeber, Baumann, & Fastl, 2004; Tyler et al., 2002). Of note, studies have shown that bimodal use can provide some improvement in spatial hearing abilities even when unaided hearing sensitivity is in the severe to profound hearing loss range (Ching et al., 2004; Dunn et al., 2005).

It is important to remember the fundamental factors that likely limit bimodal recipients from achieving excellent spatial hearing abilities. Many bimodal users have severe to profound high-frequency hearing loss, and as a result, the ear with the hearing aid does not have good access to high-frequency sounds. Consequently, high-frequency (greater than 1500 Hz) interaural level differences are not available to support localization. Additionally, most cochlear implant

recipients are unable to process temporal cues beyond several hundred hertz (Clark et al., 1978; Eddington et al., 1978; Simmons, 1966; Tong & Clark, 1985; Tong et al., 1979), and the processing of low-frequency temporal information (i.e., fine temporal structure occurring between 50 to several hundred Hz) via electrical stimulation is likely to be poorer than processing of low-frequency temporal information via acoustic stimulation (Dorman et al., 2016; Loiselle et al., 2016). As a result, the bimodal user does not have ready access to low-frequency interaural (below 1500 Hz) cues that also support localization. It should be noted that Loiselle et al. (2015) studied sound localization in a group of adult bimodal users. Some of the participants had symmetrical low-frequency hearing after cochlear implant surgery, whereas others experienced some low-frequency hearing loss in the implanted ear and had asymmetrical low-frequency hearing thresholds between the implanted and nonimplanted ears. Loiselle and colleagues found that the individuals with symmetric low-frequency hearing developed relatively good localization abilities (albeit not as good as normal-hearing listeners), whereas the individuals with asymmetric low-frequency hearing sensitivity after implant surgery performed near chance levels on localization tasks. Additionally, use of a hearing aid for the nonimplanted ear resulted in a degradation in the localization of a wideband signal for some of the participants (both with and without asymmetric low-frequency hearing). Loiselle et al. hypothesized that the poorer localization performance in the wideband condition may have been due to amplification being provided in a cochlear dead region. As such, Loiselle and colleagues recommended that the audiologist evaluate for the presence of cochlear dead regions in bimodal recipients and exercise caution to avoid over-amplification in regions with severe to profound hearing loss.

Although there is a paucity of peer-reviewed publications examining the topic, bimodal hearing most likely will provide improvements in music perception and appreciation, pitch perception, and sound quality compared with use of only a cochlear implant (Dorman et al., 2008; Gfeller et al., 2007; Gifford, Dorman, & Brown, 2010). The interested reader is referred to the studies cited in the previous sentence for more information regarding the potential benefits of bimodal hearing on music perception, pitch perception, and sound quality.

In order to optimize the benefit bimodal users receive from hearing aid use for the nonimplanted ear, the audiologists must ensure that the hearing aid is properly fitted. At a minimum, a hearing aid fitting for a bimodal user should involve several requisite steps:

- Determine air and bone conduction pure-tone hearing thresholds at octave and inter-octave audiometric frequencies from 125 to 8000 Hz.
- Measure the user's real-ear-to-coupler difference (RECD) and plot the user's hearing thresholds in dB SPL on the display of the hearing aid analyzer.
- Conduct real-ear probe microphone measures to match the hearing aid output to an evidence-based prescriptive target. Many cochlear implant audiologists match the output of a bimodal user's hearing aid to the NAL-NL2 target, because the researchers at the National Acoustic Laboratory have conducted extensive research showing satisfactory results when amplification is fitted to NAL targets (Ching et al., 2001; 2004). Ideally, hearing aid output should be matched to prescriptive targets for test signals presented at 55, 65, and 75 dB SPL inputs. For young children who cannot remain still in order for probe microphone measurements to be completed, simulated probe microphone measurements should be conducted in a hearing aid coupler.
- The maximum output of the hearing aid (i.e., Real-Ear Aided Response–90—REAR-90) should be evaluated and deemed to be appropriate and comfortable. For children and adults, the REAR-90 should be set to prescriptive target and determined not to exceed safe limits. For listeners who can provide verbal feedback about their perception of loud sounds, the audiologist should ensure that a swept pure tone presented at 85 to 90 dB SPL does not produce an aided output that is uncomfortable to the listener. It may also be useful to measure loudness discomfort thresholds, especially for those who have limited dynamic ranges (Mueller & Bentler, 2005).
- The audiologist should ensure that interaural loudness is achieved while the bimodal user wears the hearing and cochlear implant. Changes should be made to the hearing aid overall gain as necessary to achieve interaural loudness balance.
- Ching et al. (2004) also suggest that it may be useful to provide bimodal users with alternative frequency responses. In particular, Ching and colleagues suggest the provision of a frequency response that has a 6 dB/octave "cut" from 2000

to 250 Hz relative to the NAL-NL2 target and a 6 dB/octave "boost" from 250 to 2000 Hz relative to the NAL-NL2 target. These alternative frequency responses will accommodate users who may prefer a little more or a little less low-frequency gain than is prescribed by the NAL-NL2 prescriptive target.
- Zhang and colleagues (2014) used the Threshold Equalization Noise (TEN) test (Moore et al., 2000, 2004) to identify cochlear dead regions in the nonimplanted ear of 11 bimodal users. Cochlear dead regions are areas in the cochlea at which there is substantial inner hair cell loss. Zhang et al. then measured word recognition in quiet and sentence recognition in noise in several conditions: (1) hearing aid alone, (2) cochlear implant alone, (3) bimodal condition with the hearing aid set to provide wideband, high-frequency amplification, and (4) bimodal condition with the hearing aid set to provide a reduction in gain in frequency regions in which cochlear dead regions exist. Zhang et al. reported that word recognition in quiet and sentence recognition in noise were significantly better in the bimodal conditions compared with the hearing aid alone and cochlear implant alone conditions. Furthermore, word recognition in quiet and sentence recognition in noise were better in the bimodal condition with the limited gain at frequencies with cochlear dead regions compared with performance in the bimodal condition with the wideband frequency response. Likewise, Davidson et al. (2015) reported that pediatric bimodal users achieved better hearing performance with bimodal use relative to either unilateral listening condition and preferred a restricted bandwidth and nonlinear frequency compression over a wideband frequency response. Considering the findings of the Zhang et al. and Davidson studies, audiologists should consider measuring for the presence of cochlear dead regions and reducing hearing aid gain in frequency regions in which a dead region exists.
- Finally, it is worthwhile to note that Gifford et al. (2017) have shown that bimodal users may achieve better speech recognition when the low-frequency cutoff for electrical stimulation is increased from the full cochlear implant bandwidth condition. In most cases, cochlear implants provide electrical stimulation from 100 to 200 Hz up to approximately 8000 Hz. Gifford

et al. evaluated the AzBio sentence recognition in noise of 11 experienced adult bimodal users and found that many individuals (but not all) achieved their best speech recognition in noise when the low-frequency electrical cutoff was raised from the default (e.g., 100–200 Hz) to higher cutoff (e.g., 313–563 Hz). Gifford and colleagues hypothesized that the improvement in bimodal recipients' speech recognition in noise observed with an increased electrical cutoff frequency may be attributed to "less perceptual distraction from overlap of the physical transmission of the electric and acoustic stimulus" (i.e., a reduced risk of masking between the two signals). Also, they noted that increasing the low-frequency cutoff may have the effect of coding sound at the place in the cochlea at which it was intended to be coded. Specifically, the Cochlear Nucleus Contour Advance and Slim Straight electrode arrays are generally inserted to a depth of approximately 360 to 440 degrees (Boyer et al., 2015; Franke-Trieger & Murbe, 2015; Landsberger et al., 2015; Mukherjee et al., 2012), which is roughly to the place in the cochlea at which sounds in the range of 700 to 900 Hz are coded. Increasing the low-frequency electrical cut-off to 313 to 563 Hz may have provided a better match to frequency being processed through the cochlear implant analysis band (e.g., channel) and the characteristic frequency at the location of the electrode contact corresponding to the given analysis band. Fowler and colleagues (2016) have also reported improvements in speech recognition with increases in the low-frequency electrical cutoff for bimodal users.

Bilateral Cochlear Implantation

Throughout the 1990s and into the early 2000s, unilateral cochlear implantation was the standard of care for persons with severe to profound hearing loss. However, beginning in the early- to mid-2000s, peer-reviewed reports of the benefits of **bilateral cochlear implantation** began to emerge as an opportunity to improve the hearing abilities and quality of life of individuals with bilateral severe to profound hearing loss (Buss et al., 2008; Gantz et al., 2002; Litovsky et al., 2004, 2006; Nopp, Schleich, & D'Haese, 2004; Schleich, Nopp, & D'Haese, 2004; Tyler et al., 2002; van Hoesel & Tyler, 2003).

Bilateral Cochlear Implantation and Speech Recognition in Noise

The overwhelming majority of published research studies have shown significant improvement in speech recognition in noise with use of two cochlear implants compared with one for both children and adults, particularly when the speech and noise sources were spatially separated (Buss et al., 2008; Ramsden & O'Driscoll, 2002; Reeder et al., 2017; Schafer et al., 2007, 2011; Smulders et al., 2016). Of note, several studies have shown that bilateral cochlear implantation provides limited to at best modest improvement in speech recognition in noise when the speech and noise are delivered from the same loudspeaker located in front of the recipient (Buss et al., 2008; Schafer et al., 2007, 2011; van Hoesel, Ramsden, & O'Driscoll, 2002; Wackym et al., 2017). The fact that bilateral cochlear implantation provides better speech recognition noise improvement when the speech and noise are spatially separated rather than coincident is likely attributed to the fact that cochlear implant users are better able to capitalize on interaural intensity differences compared with interaural timing differences (see Chapter 3 for a review). Interaural timing/phase cues are likely to play a role in the auditory system's ability to extract a signal of interest that is spatially embedded in competing noise, and consequently, bilateral benefit may be limited when the speech and noise are spatially coincident.

Ching, van Wanrooy, and Dillon (2007) conducted a literature review of a large number of studies that evaluated speech recognition in noise in bimodal and bilateral users. In general, these studies showed improvement in speech recognition in noise in both the bimodal and bilateral conditions relative to the monaural cochlear implant conditions. Ching et al. (2007) reported that the magnitude of binaural benefit was similar between the bilateral and bimodal conditions. They also noted that there was considerable variability in the binaural benefit experienced by participants in both the bimodal and bilateral groups.

Furthermore, research has shown that recipient's feedback given in self-report questionnaires indicates that bilateral cochlear implantation provides an improvement in speech recognition in noise over unilateral cochlear implant use (Kraaijenga et al., 2017; Smulders et al., 2016; Vincent et al., 2012; Wackym et al., 2007). Of note, some studies do suggest that the improvement in speech recognition noise is less for recipients who have long periods of deafness in the second implanted ear (Mosnier et al., 2009; Reeder et al., 2017; Schafer & Thibodeau, 2006). In contrast, other studies have shown considerable improvement in speech recognition in noise in spite of a lengthy duration of deafness for the second implanted ear (Peters et al., 2007; Wolfe et al., 2007).

Spatial Hearing and Bilateral Cochlear Implantation

Research has almost unequivocally found that bilateral cochlear implantation improves localization in noise compared with the unilateral cochlear implant condition (Grieco-Calub & Litovsky, 2012). For instance, Nopp, Schleich, and D'Haese (2004) measured localization in 18 adult bilateral cochlear implant recipients and found almost a 30° improvement in the minimum audible angle obtained in the bilateral condition (less than 20°) compared with the unilateral condition (>30°). Likewise, Kerber and Seeber (2012) reported median root-mean-squared error minimum audible angles ranging from 2.8° to 7.3°, 14.8° to 44.8°, and 28.8° to 65.5° in the normal-hearing, bilateral cochlear implant, and unilateral cochlear implant conditions, respectively. Three important conclusions may be taken from the Kerber and Seeber study. First, bilateral cochlear implantation typically allows for significant improvement in spatial hearing relative to unilateral cochlear implant use. Second, a significant amount of variability exists in the spatial hearing abilities of bilateral cochlear implant recipients. Third, bilateral cochlear implant recipients typically achieve poorer spatial hearing performance compared with persons with normal hearing.

Given the limitations that exist in the processing of interaural temporal information with electrical stimulation of the cochlear nerve, the improvement in localization provided by bilateral cochlear implantation is most likely attributed primarily to interaural intensity cues. It should be noted that persons with bilateral cochlear implants are often able to localize sound more effectively than bimodal users (Ching, van Wanrooy, & Dillon, 2007). For instance, Ching and colleagues (2007) conducted an extensive literature review of 10 peer-reviewed publications and found that about half of the adult subjects and 62% of pediatric subjects in these studies showed significant bimodal benefit for localization. In contrast, 89% of adult subjects and 65% of pediatric subjects achieved better localization in the bilateral condition compared with the best monaural condition. Ching et al. (2007) noted that many of the subjects in the bimodal studies had poor hearing in the nonimplanted ear, and

consequently, they may have been unable to derive benefit from hearing aid use. However, they also reported that there was no systematic relationship between pure-tone average in the aided ear and bimodal benefit.

The better localization skills observed in bilateral cochlear implant recipients relative to many bimodal recipients is likely attributed to the limited availability of usable interaural cues to bimodal users. Although interaural timing cues are often difficult to process via bilateral electrical stimulation of the cochlear nerve, high-frequency interaural intensity cues should be readily available and may be used to localize high-frequency and broadband sounds. In contrast, many bimodal users have poor high-frequency hearing sensitivity, so high-frequency interaural level differences are unavailable because of insufficient high-frequency audibility in the aided ear. Moreover, the fact that fast temporal cues are not readily processed when the cochlear nerve is stimulated electrically limits access to low-frequency interaural temporal cues.

Audiologists should inform recipients that an extended period of bilateral cochlear implant use may be necessary to allow for localization skills to develop. Research has suggested that 3 to 12 months of bilateral cochlear implant use is needed to develop spatial hearing abilities. For instance, Litovsky, Parkinson, and Arcaroli (2009) evaluated spatial hearing in 17 adult cochlear implant recipients. Litovsky et al. (2009) reported that 82% of the participants demonstrated bilateral benefit on lateralization tasks (i.e., right/left discrimination) after just 3 months of bilateral use. However, only 47% of the participants had demonstrated bilateral benefit on localization tasks after 3 months of bilateral implant use. Overall, the group did show a mean improvement in localization abilities after only 3 months of bilateral implant use. Litovsky and colleagues (2009) concluded that bilateral cochlear implantation improves spatial hearing for adult recipients, but precise localization seems to "require more refined mechanisms," which may be supported by the development of spatial maps in the auditory cortex. Of note, research suggests that adults with longer durations of deafness prior to implantation may develop poorer localization skills and may require a longer period of bilateral cochlear implant use prior to the development of spatial hearing abilities (Reeder et al., 2014).

Litovsky et al. (2006) evaluated spatial hearing abilities in 13 children with bilateral cochlear implants (obtained in sequential surgical procedures with varying delays in implantation of the second ear) and

6 children who used bimodal technology. Litovsky and colleagues found that most children with bilateral cochlear implant localized sound better in the bilateral condition compared with the unilateral condition. They did, however, report a large variability in the spatial hearing abilities of children with bilateral cochlear implants. Importantly, they noted that progress in localization abilities was observed across at least two years of bilateral cochlear implant use in some participants. Furthermore, they noted that many children with a lengthy duration of deafness in the second implanted ear (e.g., 10 to 12 years old at the time when the second ear was implanted) received considerable improvement in their localization abilities with the use of bilateral cochlear implantation compared with the unilateral condition. Moreover, Litovsky et al. (2006) reported that the children with bilateral cochlear implants generally had better spatial hearing abilities compared with the children who used bimodal technology. In another study, Grieco-Calub and Litovsky (2012) evaluated spatial hearing in children with bilateral cochlear implants and showed significantly better localization for children who had more than 12 months of bilateral use compared with children with less than 12 month of bilateral use. Also of note, Litovsky noted that spatial hearing abilities did not emerge in children with unilateral cochlear implants, a fact that underscores the vital importance of adequate auditory stimulation of both ears of children with bilateral hearing loss.

Bimodal Versus. Bilateral Cochlear Implant Use

Research has shown that bimodal and bilateral cochlear implant use typically allows for better speech recognition in noise compared with the monaural cochlear implant condition. Research has also shown that some bimodal and most bilateral cochlear implant users achieve better localization in the binaural condition relative to the monaural cochlear implant condition. However, bilateral cochlear implant use typically allows for better localization than bimodal use. The use of a hearing aid in the nonimplanted ear may provide fine temporal structure and access to pitch and music melody (Gfeller et al., 2006), whereas these features are more difficult to access with electrical stimulation of the cochlear nerve. Of course, the benefit obtained from hearing aid use in the nonimplanted ear is likely to be greater if the nonimplanted ear has better functional hearing.

Determination of bimodal versus bilateral cochlear implant candidacy for children was discussed in

Chapter 6. For adults, the audiologist should evaluate the overall needs of the unilateral cochlear implant recipient to determine whether the recipient is more likely to benefit from bimodal or bilateral cochlear implant use. If the bimodal recipient reports difficulty in noise and clinical assessment of speech recognition in noise shows no improvement in the bimodal condition compared with the monaural cochlear implant condition, then bilateral cochlear implantation should be considered. Because clinical audiology is largely devoid of tests that allow for assessment of localization and music appreciation, the audiologist should ask the bimodal recipient to compare localization and music appreciation in real-world settings with and without a hearing aid in the nonimplanted ear. The recipient will be able to determine whether hearing aid use improves spatial hearing abilities and sound quality compared with monaural cochlear implant use and will be able to determine with the audiologist's counsel whether bilateral cochlear implant use may offer improvement.

Simultaneous Versus. Sequential Bilateral Cochlear Implantation

Simultaneous bilateral cochlear implantation refers to the provision of two cochlear implants during the same surgical procedure. **Sequential** cochlear implantation refers to the provision of two cochlear implants during two separate surgical procedures occurring at different points in time. Several investigators have explored the merits and limitations of simultaneous versus sequential cochlear implantation for children and adults. The safety of simultaneous versus sequential is an important consideration. Ramsden and colleagues (2009) reported on the medical outcomes of 50 children who received bilateral cochlear implants in the same procedure and reported that the complication rates were similar for simultaneous bilateral cochlear implantation versus unilateral cochlear implantation. Santa Maria and Oghalai (2013) point out that sequential implantation exposes the recipient to two anesthesia induction and intubation cycles rather than the one that is required with simultaneous cochlear implantation. The induction (i.e., the beginning) and emergence (i.e., the end) of anesthesia are generally considered to be stages of anesthesia in which complications are most likely to arise. Two surgical procedures require two separate inductions and emergences. As a result, the patient is exposed to both stages twice as often as would be the case with simultaneous procedures. It should, however, be noted that the rate of anesthesia complications is minimal for cochlear implant cases. Some researchers do acknowledge the associated risk (although weak) of developmental delay and dementia associated with anesthesia. (Barton et al., 2018; Jiang et al., 2017). Further research is needed to determine if the deleterious effects of anesthesia are potentially greater with one longer procedure versus two shorter procedures.

Age is another important factor in the decision to pursue simultaneous versus sequential cochlear implantation. Infants between the ages of 6 to 12 months have a relatively small blood volume (i.e., total volume of blood in the circulatory system). For instance, the average adult has a blood volume of 4.7 to 5.5 liters (i.e., 1.2 to 1.5 gallons), whereas the blood volume of a 6-month-old infant is about one-tenth of an average adult (i.e., similar to a can of soda pop) (Darrow, Soule, & Buckman, 1928). As a result, blood loss is an important consideration in cochlear implant surgery for infants. Obviously, blood loss will be greater when two implants are provided in the same procedure. With that said, infants between the ages of 6 to 12 months have routinely undergone simultaneous bilateral cochlear implantation without complication (O'Connell et al., 2016). Of important note, simultaneous cochlear implantation is likely to be a more suitable consideration when performed by experienced cochlear implant surgeons. To avoid exposure to a very long period of anesthesia, sequential cochlear implantation may be preferred for surgeons who require longer operating times.

Audiologists must also take into account the development of the binaural auditory system when determining whether to recommend simultaneous versus sequential bilateral cochlear implantation. Gordon and colleagues compared interaural auditory brainstem response (ABR) wave V latency differences for 15 children who received bilateral cochlear implants in the same procedure, 15 children who received bilateral cochlear implants with a short delay (less than one year) between procedures, and 16 children who received bilateral cochlear implants with a long delay (greater than 2 years) between procedures. There was no difference between ears in ABR latencies and morphology for the children who received bilateral cochlear implants in the same procedure. The ABR recorded at activation had longer latencies on the later implanted ear for children who received their cochlear implants in sequential procedures. The delayed latencies persisted at 3 and 9 months postactivation in the later implanted ear for the children who had greater than two years between

implant surgeries. However, the interaural ABR latencies were similar for the children who underwent bilateral cochlear implantation with two surgical procedures spaced closely in time. Gordon et al. (2008) concluded that children who had bilateral cochlear implants with a long delay between procedures had significantly longer differences in the latency of neural conduction between the two sides of the auditory nervous system. In contrast, Sparreboom et al. (2010) evaluated ABR latencies for 30 children who received bilateral cochlear implants in sequential procedures with a delay between surgeries ranging from 18 to 86 months. Sparreboom found no differences in interaural ABR latencies when measured at 12 months postactivation of the second-implanted ear. Further research is required to elucidate the physiologic and functional outcomes associated with simultaneous versus sequential cochlear implantation. However, Gordon et al. (2008) and conventional wisdom suggest that simultaneous bilateral cochlear implantation or a short delay between sequential procedures is likely to promote optimal development of the binaural auditory system.

It is important to mention that sequential bilateral cochlear implantation can still be beneficial for persons who receive their implants in sequential procedures with long delays between surgeries. Wolfe et al. (2007) evaluated word recognition in quiet in the first and second implanted ears in monaural conditions and speech recognition in noise in the bilateral and monaural conditions for a group of 12 children who all received their first cochlear implant during the first two years of life and their second cochlear implant at various ages ranging from 1 year, 8 months to 9 years, 6 months. There was not a statistically significant difference in word recognition in quiet for the first and second implanted ears for children who received their second cochlear implant prior to 4 years of age. In contrast, word recognition in quiet was significantly poorer for the second implanted ear of children who received their second cochlear implant after 4 years of age. However, use of bilateral cochlear implants provided significantly better speech recognition in noise relative to use of the first implanted ear alone for all children, regardless of the age at which the second ear was implanted. In short, although speech recognition was poorer in the second implanted ear of children who received their implant at a later age, bilateral cochlear implant benefit was still present in spite of the late age at implantation of the second implanted ear. Similarly, Peters et al. (2007) evaluated speech recognition in quiet and in noise for a group of 30 children and found better speech recognition for each ear when bilateral cochlear implantation was provided at an earlier age. Again, however, even the children who received a second cochlear implant at a later age (e.g., 8 to 13 years old) generally obtained better speech recognition in noise in the bilateral condition compared with the unilateral condition. As previously mentioned, Litovsky et al. (2006) also reported that bilateral cochlear implantation provided significant improvement in spatial hearing abilities for children who received their second cochlear implant in their preteen or teenage years.

Moreover, Reeder et al. (2014) evaluated speech recognition in quiet and in noise and localization in 21 adults who received bilateral cochlear implants in sequential procedures and who had varying durations of deafness in the second implanted ear. Reeder and colleagues reported that participants with longer durations of deafness (i.e., greater than 30 years) achieved poorer outcomes in the second implanted ear. Once again, though, all participants received benefit from bilateral cochlear implantation relative to the best unilateral condition. In short, the hearing performance of each ear of bilateral cochlear implant recipients will be optimized with a shorter duration of deafness for each ear and a shorter delay between cochlear implant surgeries for each ear. However, children and adults who have a lengthy duration of deafness and/or a lengthy delay between procedures for each ear are still generally able to achieve better overall hearing outcomes with bilateral cochlear implantation compared with monaural cochlear implant use. For recipients who perform well with their first cochlear implant but have a lengthy duration of deafness in the nonimplanted ear, the audiologist should provide counsel that the outcomes of the second-implanted ear will likely never be as good as the first-implanted ear and may even be quite poor depending on the length of auditory deprivation for the second-implanted ear. Nonetheless, performance in the bilateral condition is likely to be better than performance in the second-implanted ear alone (Peters et al., 2007; Reeder et al., 2014, 2017; Wolfe et al., 2007). The audiologist should also inform the recipient that several months or even a year or longer may be required to realize bilateral benefit (Litovsky et al., 2006). Finally, because the performance of the second-implanted ear may be limited if that ear has a lengthy duration of deafness, it is imperative that the recipient may very well be motivated to pursue bilateral cochlear implantation. Otherwise, the recipient

may become discouraged if outcomes are not satisfactory in the early stages of use of the second implant and then become a nonuser of the second implant.

Cochlear Implantation for Persons with Single-Sided Deafness

Single-sided deafness (SSD) refers to a diagnosis of severe to profound hearing loss in the poorer ear with normal or near-normal hearing sensitivity in the opposite ear. Over 18 million persons in the United States have SSD (Lin, Niparko, & Ferrucci, 2011). Because it prevents bilateral auditory input to the auditory nervous system, SSD typically impairs speech recognition in noise and spatial hearing abilities. Single-sided deafness may also impair speech recognition in quiet when the signal of interest arises from the side of the poorer ear. Additionally, single-sided deafness can lead to a degradation in the quality of life of adults and academic difficulties for children (Bess & Tharpe, 1986; Oyler, Oyler, & Markin, 1988). For instance, Bess and Tharpe (1986) reported that children with unilateral hearing loss are 10 times more likely to fail a grade in school than their peers with normal hearing. Furthermore, Bess and Tharpe noted that in addition to the 35% of children who had unilateral hearing loss and failed a grade in school, another 13% required specialized academic support. Moreover, many persons with single-sided deafness experience tinnitus in the poorer hearing ear (Fetterman, Saunders, & Luxford, 1996; Friedmann et al., 2016; Sladen et al., 2017).

A number of different intervention options are available for persons with single-sided deafness. First, audiologists should counsel persons with single-sided deafness and their families to proactively manage their environments in an attempt to mitigate the deleterious effects of single-sided deafness. For example, children with hearing loss may attempt to sit in a position in the classroom that provides good proximity to the signal of interest. Also, whenever possible, the listener should be positioned so that the signal of interest arises from the side of the better hearing ear. Furthermore, if possible, the noise level of the room should be minimized (e.g., turn off television if nobody is watching), and reverberation levels should be minimized (e.g., place rugs over hard floors, hang curtains or drapes over windows). The families of infants and young children with unilateral hearing loss should seek to expose the child to as much intelligible speech as possible. Carol Flexer,

Ph.D., pediatric audiologist, recommends reading at least 10 books a day and speaking in melodic tones to better engage both hemispheres of the brain of children with single-sided deafness (Flexer, 2015). Of course, the audiologist should also recommend that the person with single-sided deafness should attempt to prevent noise-induced hearing loss in the better hearing ear by avoiding high-level noise or by using hearing protection when in the presence of high-level noise.

Secondly, audiologists may recommend a number of different hearing technologies for persons with single-sided deafness. A contralateral-routing-of-signal (CROS) hearing aid contains a microphone that is worn on the poorer ear to capture sounds on the ear with hearing loss and wirelessly transfer the signal to a low-gain hearing aid that is worn on the better hearing ear. Similarly, an osseointegrated bone conduction hearing device may be used on the poorer ear to capture sounds on the ear with hearing loss and transfer the signal to the better hearing ear via bone conduction. CROS aids and osseointegrated bone conduction hearing devices both are successful in overcoming the head shadow effect and improving speech recognition in quiet and in noise when the signal of interest arises from the side of the poorer ear (Finbow et al., 2015). However, CROS aids and osseointegrated bone conduction hearing devices do not restore auditory function to the poorer ear, and as a result, improvement is limited or nonexistent for speech recognition in noise when the signal arrives from in front of the listener or to the side of the better ear. Additionally, CROS aids and osseointegrated bone conduction hearing devices do not alleviate tinnitus that may be present at the poorer hearing ear. The audiologist may also recommend a remote microphone system, which contains a microphone that is worn near the mouth of the talker of interest to capture the talker's speech and wirelessly deliver the signal of interest to a receiver that is worn at the listener's better hearing ear. Remote microphone technology can provide significant improvement in speech recognition in noise for the talker who wears the microphone, but remote microphone systems do not improve the listener's ability to hear others in the environment, nor do they improve spatial hearing abilities or tinnitus in the poorer hearing ear.

Over the past several years, several peer-reviewed publications have described the potential benefits and limitations of cochlear implantation for persons with single-sided deafness (Arndt et al., 2015; Blasco & Redleaf, 2014; Firszt et al., 2012; Friedmann et al.,

2016; Sladen et al., 2016, 2017; Vermiere & Van de Heyning, 2009; Vincent et al., 2015). In general, research studies examining cochlear implantation for persons with single-sided deafness suggest that cochlear implantation improves speech recognition in quiet and in noise as well as spatial hearing abilities (Arndt et al., 2015; Blasco & Redleaf, 2014; Firszt et al., 2012; Friedmann et al., 2016; Sladen et al., 2016, 2017; Vermiere & Van de Heyning, 2009; Vincent et al., 2015). Additionally, persons who have single-sided deafness and receive a cochlear implant generally report that the cochlear implant improves their hearing abilities. Of note, research unequivocally shows improvement in speech recognition in noise when the signal arrives from the side of the poorer ear, whereas when the signal of interest and noise both arrive from in front of the listener, some studies show significant improvement in speech recognition in noise whereas others do not (Blasco & Redleaf, 2014; Friedmann et al., 2016; Sladen et al., 2016, 2017). Cochlear implantation represents the only opportunity to restore binaural auditory input for persons with single-sided deafness. Additionally, most persons with single-sided deafness have reported that cochlear implantation eliminated or reduced the severity of their tinnitus (Blasco & Redleaf, 2014; Friedmann et al., 2016; Sladen et al., 2016, 2017). Additional research is required to determine the effect of cochlear implantation on speech, language, and academic development of children with single-sided deafness.

Although there is a paucity of peer-reviewed publications describing research examining cochlear implantation for infants and young children with single-sided deafness, preliminary reports suggest that cochlear implantation does improve speech recognition in noise, functional hearing abilities, and spatial hearing abilities in infants and young children with congenital hearing loss and hearing loss acquired during the perilingual period (Arndt et al., 2015; Thomas et al., 2017). This research does suggest that better outcomes are likely for children who receive their cochlear implant at an early age so that the period of auditory deprivation for the poorer ear is limited (Arndt et al., 2015; Tavora-Vieirea & Rajan, 2015). In a paper describing the results of a study on cochlear implant outcomes of children with single-sided deafness, Arndt and colleagues (2015) stated that cochlear implantation for children with congenital single-sided deafness "should take place before the age of 4 years." However, it should be noted that children who had progressive hearing loss or who had sufficient audibility at an early age from hearing aid use in the ear with hearing loss may benefit from cochlear implantation at later ages. Arndt et al. (2015) theorized that the poor outcomes observed in later-implanted children who have congenital single-sided deafness are likely attributed to reorganization of the secondary auditory cortex (Kral et al., 2013) and to an inability to facilitate development of the binaural auditory system during its critical sensitive period (Gordon et al., 2013).

The etiology of the hearing loss of persons with single-sided deafness also affects outcomes after cochlear implantation. Persons who have single-sided deafness due to cochlear nerve deficiency are likely to achieve poor outcomes from cochlear implantation, particularly those who have absent (aplastic) cochlear nerves (Arndt et al., 2015). Children and adults with unilateral cochlear nerve deficiency are likely to reject a cochlear implant because the auditory signal it provides is substantially inferior to the better hearing ear. Additionally, the implanted ear with cochlear nerve deficiency is unlikely to preserve enough auditory information to allow for robust interaural auditory cues necessary for improvements in speech recognition in noise and spatial hearing abilities. Of note, as many as 50% of children with congenital single-sided deafness have cochlear nerve deficiency (Clemmens et al., 2013; Levi et al., 2013; Nakano, Arimoto, & Matsunaga, 2013). In fact, Clemmens and colleagues evaluated 128 children who had unilateral hearing loss and who underwent high-resolution MRI and indicated that 100% of infants with profound sensorineural hearing loss had cochlear nerve deficiency. In short, it is imperative that a high-resolution MRI of the temporal bone is completed prior to implantation of children with congenital single-sided deafness to ensure the presence of an intact cochlear nerve. Cochlear implantation is not recommended for infants and children who have cochlear nerve deficiency.

Cytomegalovirus (CMV) is another potential etiology of congenital single-sided deafness. There is actually a paucity of peer-reviewed publications that determine the incidence of CMV in patients with single-sided deafness, but CMV is recognized as the most common environmental cause of congenital hearing loss, with estimates suggesting that as many as one-third of nongenetic congenital hearing loss can be attributed to CMV (Nassetta, Kimberlin, & Whitley, 2009). As mentioned in Chapter 22, CMV may lead to a loss in spiral ganglion survival and to significant neurocognitive deficits (Carraro, Park, & Harrison,

2016). As a result, research has shown that some children who have CMV and bilateral hearing loss make limited progress with spoken language development after cochlear implantation, a fact that has been attributed to the cognitive/neurological deficits associated with CMV (Hoey et al., 2017; Yoshida et al., 2017). Consequently, audiologists should counsel families of children with single-sided deafness regarding the potential effect of CMV on the central nervous system and the possibility that benefit from cochlear implantation may be limited. Similarly, bacterial meningitis may be the cause of single-sided deafness in children and adults. If cochlear ossification has occurred after bacterial meningitis, the likelihood is remote that cochlear implantation will be successful for the person with single-sided deafness.

Enlarged vestibular aqueduct has also been shown to be a relatively common cause of single-sided deafness in children (Arndt et al., 2015). As long as the duration of deafness prior to implantation is short, most children with single-sided deafness from enlarged aqueduct syndrome will do quite well with a cochlear implant. Again, if a child is born with severe to profound single-sided hearing loss due to enlarged vestibular aqueduct, cochlear implantation should ideally be provided by 1 year of age. The most common causes of single-sided deafness in adults are sudden hearing loss (likely due to viral or autoimmune disorders) and labyrinthitis (Arndt et al., 2011). Adults with single-sided deafness due to sudden hearing loss and labyrinthitis should perform well after cochlear implantation, particularly if they have a short duration of deafness prior to receiving a cochlear implant.

Audiologists should take into account several variables when determining cochlear implant candidacy for persons with single-sided deafness. Adults should be highly motivated to pursue cochlear implantation. Friedmann et al. (2016) have suggested that adults who have single-sided deafness and bothersome tinnitus in the affected ear are more motivated to use their cochlear implant during all waking hours to eliminate the perception of their tinnitus. Adults and children with single-sided deafness are likely to perform better if cochlear implantation is provided after a short period of deafness. In particular, children who are born with single-sided deafness should undergo cochlear implantation by 1 year of age if MRI has confirmed the presence of an intact cochlear nerve. Friedmann et al. (2015) also recommend cochlear implantation with a simultaneous labyrinthectomy for persons who have single-sided deafness and vertigo with an etiology of Meniere's disease. Likewise, Hansen et al. (2013) reported that cochlear implantation resulted in a significant improvement in the word and sentence recognition of a group of adults with single-sided deafness attributed to Meniere's disease. Cochlear implantation should definitely be promptly considered for children who have single-sided deafness with an etiology associated progressive hearing loss (e.g., enlarged vestibular aqueduct syndrome, ototoxicity) because of the threat of a decline in hearing in the better hearing ear as well.

Cochlear Implants and Hearing Assistive Technology (HAT)

Most cochlear implant recipients are able to understand speech relatively well in quiet listening environments (Gifford et al, 2008; Helms et al, 2004; Wolfe et al., 2013). However, many cochlear implant recipients so experience substantial difficulty with understanding speech in noise. For example, relative to performance in quiet, a cochlear implant recipient's speech recognition in noise is typically 30 to 60 percentage points poorer when evaluated at a signal-to-noise ratio (SNR) that is common in real-world listening situations (e.g., +5 dB SNR) (Schafer & Thibodeau, 2003, 2004; Spahr et al., 2007; Wolfe et al., 2013). Furthermore, many cochlear implant recipients experience difficulty with understanding speech in other challenging listening situations such as understanding speech over the telephone (Ito, Nakatake, & Fuijita, 1999) and the television (Duke et al., 2016).

Use of **hearing assistive technology (HAT)** can provide significant improvement in speech recognition in the challenging listening situations mentioned above (Duke et al., 2016; Fitzpatrick et al., 2009; Wolfe et al., 2013, 2016). A variety of HAT devices are available for use with modern cochlear implant systems. Indeed, cochlear implant manufacturers provide HATs that are designed to improve speech recognition in noise, speech perception over the telephone, and hearing performance when using consumer electronics (e.g., television, computers, tablets, MP3 players). Figure 20–1 provides examples of wireless remote-microphone systems that are intended to improve speech recognition in noise (Wolfe et al., 2009, 2012, 2013). A personal, wireless, remote microphone system typically includes a microphone that is worn in close proximity to the talker's mouth (i.e., within 6 to 8 inches) in order to capture the speech signal of interest near the source and to consequently improve the SNR. In most of these systems, a directional microphone is used to further enhance the SNR of the speech signal captured at the remote microphone. In conventional use, the audio signal captured at the microphone is delivered to a radio transmitter that delivers the signal of interest via a wireless radio signal to a miniature radio receiver that is integrated within or coupled to the cochlear implant recipient's sound processor.

Remote microphone systems come in several configurations. Remote microphone accessory systems feature a remote microphone that delivers audio signals directly to a small digital receiver that is housed within the sound processor or hearing aid (i.e., integrated receiver). In general, **remote microphone**

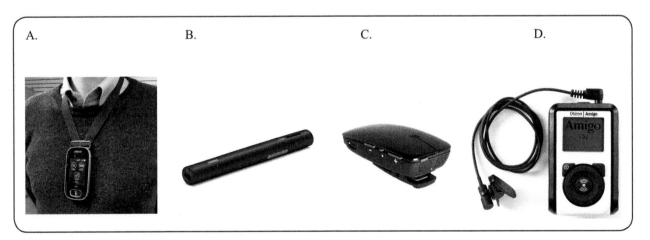

A.   B.   C.   D.

FIGURE 20–1. Examples of remote microphone transmitters. Images provided courtesy of Phonak, Cochlear, and Oticon.

accessory systems may only be used with the hearing aids or cochlear implant sound processors that are developed by the manufacturer who created the remote microphone accessory system. For example, Cochlear partnered with GN ReSound to include the GN ReSound wireless technology in Nucleus sound processors. As a result, GN ReSound wireless remote microphone accessory technology (i.e., Mini Mic 2+) may only be used with GN ReSound hearing aids and Nucleus sound processors.

Personal remote microphone systems are typically able to be used with hearing aids and cochlear implant sound processors made by all major hearing technology manufacturers. For example, the Phonak Roger remote microphone system may be used with Phonak hearing aids but may also be used with other makes of hearing aids and with all makes of cochlear implant sound processors. Typically, a special adaptor is needed to connect the radio receiver of a personal remote microphone system to the hearing aid or sound processor of another manufacturer.

Some remote microphone systems use Bluetooth radio frequency transmission to deliver the audio signal to a Bluetooth receiver worn on the recipient's body. Then, the Bluetooth receiver delivers the audio signal to the recipient's sound processor via digital near-field magnetic induction (e.g., the Phonak/Advanced Bionics ComPilot streamer) or via electromagnetic induction to the sound processor's telecoil.

Figure 20–2 provides an example of several HAT devices that are intended to improve communication over the telephone. These HATs typically operate by delivering the signal to and from a mobile telephone via Bluetooth transmission and then delivering the

audio signal from the HAT device to the cochlear implant sound processor via a proprietary digital radio signal or via near-field magnetic induction (NFMI). However, Cochlear's Nucleus 7 sound processor can directly stream audio to and from an Apple iPhone via a proprietary "Made for iPhone" (MFi) digital radio signal (i.e., no HAT interface is required). Wolfe and colleagues (2016a, 2016b) have shown that wireless HAT devices improve word recognition over the telephone by an average 15 to 25 percentage points in quiet and 25 to 40 percentage points in noise. These wireless telephone HAT devices also allow for hands-free mobile telephone use.

Additionally, many of these HATs are able to wirelessly stream audio signals to both ears of bilateral and bimodal users (depending on the make and model of the recipient's hearing aid). Research has shown that bilateral/bimodal telephone use allows for significantly better speech recognition compared with the best monaural condition (Wolfe et al., 2016a). Bimodal telephone use allows the recipient access to the fine temporal structure of the acoustic signal in the aided ear and the amplitude envelope across the speech frequency range in the implanted ear. Furthermore, wireless streaming of music to a hearing aid and cochlear implant sound processor provides a significant improvement in music appreciation and lyric recognition for bimodal users compared with listening to either device alone (Wolfe et al., 2016a). Once again, the finding that bimodal listening improves the enjoyment of music is not surprising given the fact that the low-frequency acoustic signal at the hearing aid ear is necessary to convey fine temporal structure, whereas the high-frequency signal from the cochlear

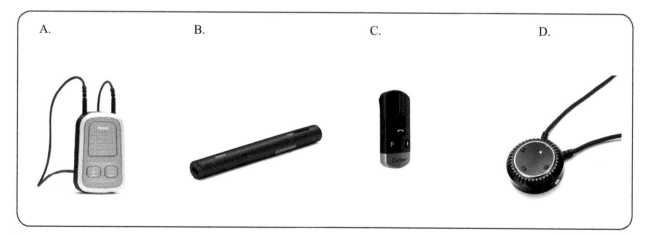

A. B. C. D.

FIGURE 20–2. Examples of hearing assistive technologies that may receive Bluetooth signals and then transmit an audio signal to the cochlear implant sound processor. Images provided courtesy of Phonak, Cochlear, and ClearSounds.

implant is likely to improve lyric recognition and to provide access to sounds that may be inaudible with a hearing aid alone.

The Advanced Bionics Naída cochlear implant sound processor possesses a unique technology that allows the recipient to hear the telephone signal in both ears at the same time. The Naída's Binaural Voice-Stream Technology uses NFMI to wirelessly deliver the the telephone audio signal captured at one ear to the Naída sound processor or Phonak Naída Link hearing aid worn at the opposite ear (Figure 20–3). Wolfe (2014) has shown that use of the DuoPhone improves word recognition over the telephone by approximately 20 percentage points relative to the monaural condition.

Wireless HAT may also be used to deliver the audio signal from the television directly to the recipient's sound processor(s) and/or hearing aid. Figure 20–4 provides examples of HATs that are used to wirelessly deliver audio signals from the television to a recipient's cochlear implant sound processor(s) and/or hearing aid via digital radio transmission. Duke, Wolfe, and Schafer (2016) have shown that these types of television HAT devices can improve the recognition of speech delivered from a television by an average of 23 percentage points.

Adjustable Parameters That Influence Performance Obtained with HAT

Audiologists may adjust a variety of parameters to meet the needs of the cochlear implant user. Programming adjustments may typically be made to three different components within the HAT: (1) the transmitter of the HAT (e.g., remote microphone system), (2) the receiver of the sound processor and/or hearing aid, and/or (3) the sound processor.

Adjustable Transmitter Settings. The **transmitter** of modern remote microphone RF systems typically possess several programmable/adjustable parameters. For example, many transmitters possess a volume control that increases the strength of the signal delivered from the wireless transmitter to the receiver of the recipient's sound processor and/or hearing aid. In theory, increasing the volume control setting will increase the level of the audio signal from the HAT, resulting in an improvement in the SNR of the audio signal delivered by the HAT. However, Musgrave et al. (2015) evaluated the effect of the volume control setting on speech recognition in noise of recipients using the Cochlear Nucleus Mini Mic and found no change in performance with changes in the volume control setting. Musgrave and colleagues proposed that the Autosensitivity Control (ASC) processing of the Nucleus 6 sound processor had already reduced the competing noise captured at the sound processor microphone, and as a result further increases in the gain of the signal from the remote microphone did not improve the SNR. Also, Musgrave and colleagues proposed that the AGC processing within the Nucleus 6 may have compressed the gain increases that occurred with volume control adjustments.

Additional parameters that may be adjusted in modern transmitters include the use of data logging, the use of multiple microphone/transmitter networks

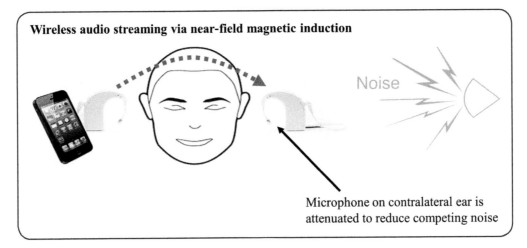

FIGURE 20–3. A visual example of the Advanced Bionics DuoPhone technology. Image provided courtesy of Advanced Bionics, LLC.

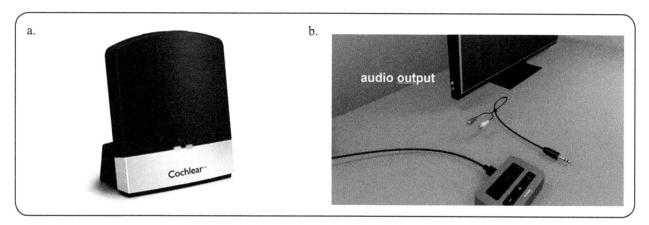

FIGURE 20–4. A visual example of hearing assistive technologies that can stream audio signals from a television to a cochlear implant sound processor. Images provided courtesy of Cochlear and Phonak.

that allow for team teaching or group activities, adjustment of the frequency used to transmit a radio signal, adjustment between use of a microphone or telecoil to capture the signal of interest, adjustment of the microphone mode used by the transmitter to capture the signal (e.g., omnidirectional, directional with fixed polar plot, adaptive directional), the monitoring of ambient noise levels and signal integrity, and so forth.

Adjustable Radio Receiver Settings. The **receiver** may also be adjusted to optimize a recipient's listening performance and experience. For instance, the **receiver gain** is an important programmable parameter that may influence recipient performance. The receiver gain refers to the strength of the signal delivered from the receiver to the sound processor. In general, a higher receiver gain setting provides a greater emphasis on the signal from the receiver relative to the signal from the sound processor microphone, resulting in an improvement in the SNR.

Schafer and colleagues (2009) evaluated the influence of receiver gain on speech recognition in noise for a group of recipients of Advanced Bionics Auria sound processors ($N = 14$) and Cochlear Freedom sound processors ($N = 8$). They found that higher receiver gain settings resulted in better speech recognition in noise for Advanced Bionics users. In contrast, increases in receiver gain settings did not improve speech recognition in noise for recipients using the Cochlear Nucleus Freedom sound processor. Another study by Wolfe et al. (2009) indicated that the lack of an improvement in speech recognition with receiver gain increases for Cochlear Freedom

users was likely associated with the input processing that was selected for the Freedom sound processor. In particular, ASC signal processing must be enabled in Cochlear Nucleus processors in order to allow for improvements in speech recognition with receiver gain increases.

Although the aforementioned studies were all conducted with receivers with a **fixed gain** (i.e., the gain of the radio receiver was fixed at one level regardless of the competing noise level in the listening environment). It has long been recognized that a fixed-gain FM receiver often fails to deliver the optimal gain for a specific situation (Wolfe et al., 2009). For example, in a quiet environment, a moderate fixed-gain setting may be greater than what is preferred by the recipient (i.e., too loud), but in a high-level noise environment, the moderate fixed-gain setting may be insufficient. **Adaptive remote microphone systems** were developed with this dilemma in mind. Adaptive remote microphone systems automatically increase the receiver gain when the ambient noise level increases. For example, in a quiet environment, the gain of an adaptive receiver is set to a low to moderate level when speech is presented to the microphone of the transmitter. If no speech is present, then the transmitter is muted. When the ambient noise level exceeds 57 dB SPL, the gain of the receiver automatically increases (Figure 20–5).

Wolfe et al. (2009) evaluated speech recognition in quiet and in classroom noise presented at multiple levels for 13 Advanced Bionics recipients and 11 Cochlear recipients. Performance was measured with use of fixed-gain remote microphone receivers as well as with adaptive, frequency-modulated (FM) receivers.

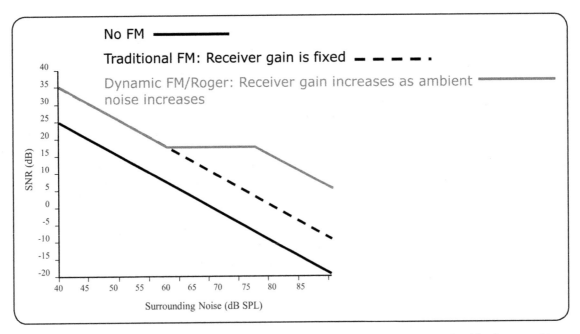

FIGURE 20–5. An example of the signal-to-noise ratio (SNR) as a function of the ambient noise level for three conditions, (1) no remote microphone (No FM), (2) a fixed-gain remote microphone system, and (3) an adaptive gain remote microphone system. Image provided courtesy of Phonak.

Wolfe and colleagues reported that there was no difference in speech recognition in quiet between use of the fixed-gain and adaptive FM systems, but the adaptive FM receiver provided substantially better speech recognition in moderate- to high-level noise (e.g., noise levels ranging from 65 to 75 dBA). When the competing noise level was 70 dBA (which is commonly encountered in realistic environments), use of adaptive FM improved speech recognition by about 50 percentage points relative to performance with the fixed-gain system. Thibodeau (2010) reported that adaptive FM provided similar improvement in speech recognition in noise for hearing aid users relative to their performance with fixed-gain FM.

Wolfe et al. (2013) also evaluated speech recognition in quiet and in noise for a group of cochlear implant recipients using fixed-gain (analog) FM, adaptive (analog) FM, and adaptive digital radio remote microphone systems. Significantly better speech recognition in noise was obtained with adaptive FM systems over fixed-gain FM systems. Moreover, speech recognition in noise obtained with the adaptive digital radio system was significantly better than that obtained with the adaptive FM system. Wolfe and colleagues (2013) attributed the improvement obtained with the digital system to the fact that digital signal processing allowed for greater control in the adap-

tive increases in receiver gain that occurred with increases in competing noise level. To summarize, adaptive digital remote microphone technology is likely to provide the best speech recognition in environments with moderate- to high-level noise.

Cochlear Implant Sound Processor Settings. The cochlear implant sound processor also contains several programmable parameters that affect recipient performance with HAT. For example, the **mixing ratio** is an adjustable parameter that controls the relative strength of the signals from the sound processor microphone and the receiver of the remote microphone RF system. In Advanced Bionics sound processors, the audio mixing ratio controls the strength of the signals from both the telecoil and the direct auditory input. For Cochlear processors, the telecoil mixing ratio controls the strength of the signals from the sound processor microphone and telecoil, whereas the accessory mixing ratio controls the relative strength of the signals from the sound processor microphone and direct auditory input and wireless audio signals (e.g., MFi, Mini Mic 2+, Phone Clip, TV Streamer). MED-EL cochlear implants do not contain the mixing ratio parameter, and by default, equal emphasis is provided on signals delivered from the sound processor microphone and direct audio input and telecoil.

In Advanced Bionics implants, a 50/50 mixing ratio results in an equal emphasis being placed on the signals from the sound processor microphone and telecoil, whereas a 30/70 mixing ratio results in 10 dB of attenuation to the sound processor microphone. However, it is important to note that even with use of a 50/50 mixing ratio, Advanced Bionics sound processors provide 6 dB of attenuation to the signals from the sound processor microphone and the HAT. As a result, when the 50/50 mixing ratio is in use, the recipient will experience a slight attenuation for sounds arriving at the sound processor microphone. However, the audiologist may enable "Roger Ready" mode, which only provides the simultaneous attenuation when an audio signal is present at the remote microphone receiver of the Naída sound processor. Of note, the "Aux Only" mixing ratio deactivates the sound processor microphone, allowing the recipient to attend to only the input from the HAT.

In Cochlear implants, use of a 1:1 mixing ratio results in equal emphasis being placed on the signals from the sound processor microphone and the input from either the telecoil or direct auditory input. A 2:1 mixing ratio offers 6 dB attenuation to the signal from the sound processor microphone, and a 3:1 mixing ratio results in 10 dB attenuation to the signal from the sound processor microphone. Finally, use of "Accessory Only" mixing ratio results disables the sound processor microphone, allowing the recipient to hear only the signal from the HAT.

Wolfe and Schafer (2008) evaluated the effect of the audio mixing ratio on the speech recognition in quiet and in noise of 12 Advanced Bionics Auria users. There was a trend toward better sentence recognition in noise with use of the 30/70 mixing ratio, but word recognition in quiet at the 50 dBA presentation level was significantly poorer (a reduction of 66 percentage points) with use of the 30/70 mixing ratio when the signal of interest was delivered to the sound processor microphone rather than the FM microphone. Wolfe and Schafer (2008) attributed the poorer word recognition associated with the 30/70 mixing ratio to the 10 dB attenuation at the sound processor microphone and concluded that a 30/70 mixing ratio is not appropriate for school-aged children. The 10 dB attenuation to the signal from the sound processor microphone will potentially hinder access to signals of interest that are not directed to the remote microphone (i.e., other students in the class asking or answering questions). Wolfe and Schafer (2008) recommended the 50/50 mixing ratio for use with children.

In contrast, Musgrave et al. (2015) evaluated speech recognition in quiet and in noise whereas Nucleus recipients used the Mini Mic 2+ and ASC signal processing with various mixing ratios. Musgrave and colleagues reported no significant change in speech recognition of the Nucleus users when the mixing ratio was altered. In short, the accessory mixing ratio is likely to have little impact on speech recognition in noise during remote microphone use for Nucleus recipients. However, the accessory mixing ratio will likely improve speech perception in noise when the recipient uses the TV Streamer and Phone Clip because the audio signal is delivered directly from the television or telephone and possesses a favorable SNR. In short, a 1:1 mixing ratio is recommended for infants and children, and a default 2:1 mixing ratio is recommended for adults.

As previously discussed, Wolfe et al. (2009) reported that ASC must be enabled to allow for satisfactory benefit from remote microphone use for Nucleus users (e.g., Nucleus 5, Nucleus 6, Nucleus 7, Kanso) (see Chapter 16 for a description of ASC). Wolfe et al. (2009) found that the speech recognition in noise of Nucleus recipients was very poor when ASC was disabled (i.e., 0% correct at competing noise levels of 65 dB SPL and higher). Furthermore, increases in receiver gain FM did not result in improvement in speech recognition in noise for Nucleus recipients when ASC was disabled. The lack of remote microphone benefit that was observed when ASC was disabled was attributed to the fact that the speech and noise signal were both being compressed substantially, resulting in an unfavorable SNR. At the default instantaneous IDR (IIDR) and sensitivity settings of 40 dB and 12, respectively, the Nucleus sound processor maps acoustic inputs from approximately 25 to 65 dB SPL into the recipients EDR. Acoustic inputs greater than 65 dB SPL are infinitely compressed. The signal from the remote microphone transmitter is typically delivered to the sound processor at 72 dB SPL, and as a result, the signal from the receiver is subjected to high-level compression when the sensitivity control is fixed at a level of 12. Consequently, the signal from the remote microphone is embedded in the noise when the noise level is 65 dB SPL and higher. Additionally, the significant compression for inputs of 65 dB SPL and higher results in compression of the receiver gain increases provided from an adaptive system. Therefore, ASC is needed to automatically adjust the IIDR and prevent compression of the signal from the remote microphone system. Of note, ASC was disabled in the Schafer et al. (2009) study, a fact that likely explains the poor performance obtained by the Nucleus Freedom users in that study as well as the finding that manual increases in receiver gain did not improve performance.

The second influential parameter, sensitivity, also affects how Cochlear sound processors map acoustic inputs into the EDR. The sensitivity control shifts the IIDR window up or down depending on the setting of the control (Figure 20–6). An increase in the sensitivity setting shifts the IIDR window downward so that lower-level inputs (i.e., <25 dB SPL) are mapped into the EDR, but infinite compression occurs for signals with input levels above 65 dB SPL. This would most likely improve audibility for low-level (e.g., soft) sounds, but it would degrade speech recognition in noise. In contrast, decreases in the microphone sensitivity setting shifts the IIDR upward so low-level sounds are presented below electrical threshold, but high-level speech sounds are less likely to be subjected to high-level compression. As a result, audibility for low-level sounds would be reduced, but speech recognition in noise would likely improve.

Control of the sensitivity setting can be automated with the ASC input processing option. ASC adaptively adjusts the sensitivity control in order to prevent infinite compression of high-level speech signals in noisy environments (i.e., sensitivity is decreased when ambient noise exceeds 57 dB SPL), with a primary objective of improving listening comfort and speech recognition in noise. Research has indicated that use of ASC significantly improves speech recognition in noise and comfort for adults and children with cochlear implants relative to a fixed sensitivity setting (Wolfe et al., 2009, 2011).

When ASC is enabled and remote microphone technology is used in moderate to high level noise environments, the automatic decrease in sensitivity reduces the compression that is provided to the signal from the remote microphone RF system. As a result, speech recognition in noise with use of a personal remote microphone RF system is significantly better with ASC enabled. Specifically, Wolfe et al. (2009) found that use of ASC with remote microphone RF technology improved speech recognition in noise by up to 70 percentage points relative to performance with remote microphone technology when ASC is disabled. In summary, ASC should be enabled when Nucleus recipients use HAT (in particular, when remote microphone technology is used).

Counseling Cochlear Implant Recipients Regarding the Appropriate Use of HAT

The preceding sections clearly demonstrate that the use of HAT can improve the hearing performance of cochlear implant recipients in challenging listening situations, particularly when modern HAT is adjusted and programmed appropriately by the audiologist. In order for a cochlear implant recipient to benefit from the use of HAT, however, the audiologist must convince the recipient and/or his or her family of the importance of using HAT, and the audiologist must inform the recipient (and his/her caregivers) of the appropriate care, use, and maintenance of HAT. Many cochlear implant recipients and caregivers may be reluctant to use HAT. Some may be intimidated by the task of learning to effectively use new technology, some may not want to be burdened with the task of operating and maintaining additional hearing technology, some may feel that there is a cosmetic stigma attached to the use of HAT, some may believe that hearing performance is satisfactory without the use of HAT, and still others may not believe that they can afford HAT. The caregivers of young children should be informed of the importance of access to intelligible speech the during critical sensitive period of auditory brain development (see Chapter 3). The use of remote microphone technology will optimize a child's access to speech originating from a distance or speech that is present in noisy and reverberant environments.

Audiologists should counsel caregivers about the importance of using remote microphone technology with infants and young children in situations in which the child will not have satisfactory access to intelligible speech without the use of remote micro-

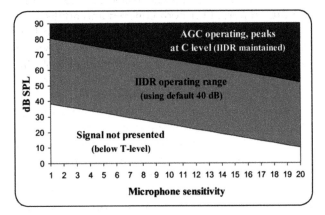

FIGURE 20–6. A visual example of the effect of the sensitivity control on the instantaneous input dynamic range (IIDR) of Nucleus sound processors. Image provided courtesy of Cochlear, Ltd.

phone technology (e.g., traveling in the backseat of a car, traveling on loud public transportation, riding in a stroller in a noisy department store). Additionally, school-age children who have cochlear implants should routinely use remote microphone technology in classroom situations. Moreover, older children and adults should use remote microphone technology and other HATs in situations in which they cannot hear well with the use of their cochlear implant(s) alone.

One strategy to encourage older children and adults to use HAT is to complete a Client Oriented Scale of Improvement (COSI) (Dillon, James, & Ginis, 1997) form to identify the recipient's greatest hearing needs (Figure 20–7). The COSI requires the recipient to work with the audiologist to identify four or five specific situations in which the recipient would like to hear better. For example, the recipient may indicate that he/she wants to understand his/her spouse better while eating at their favorite restaurant, understand his/her grandchildren better over the telephone, and understand the television newscaster better. These COSI responses would provide the audiologist with the opportunity to suggest a remote microphone, a wireless telephone HAT device, and a wireless television HAT device as strategies to improve hearing performance in the situations that are most difficult for the recipient. Additionally, the recipient should consider demonstrating the function of HAT in the clinic. Many recipients are initially reluctant to use HAT but become convinced of the potential benefit of HAT after experiencing the improvement that can be obtained.

Although it may seem trivial, the audiologist must properly inform the recipient of how to operate HAT. The audiologist should verbally explain how HAT is operated. Then, the audiologist should show the recipient how to operate HAT. Next, the audiologist should give the recipient the opportunity to operate the HAT and provide support and answer questions as necessary. Finally, the audiologist should provide the recipient with multiple resources that may be accessed if questions or problems arise related to future use of the HAT. For example, the audiologist should provide the recipient with written materials describing the proper use and care of HAT as well as inform the recipient of where to access video descriptions if available (e.g., YouTube, manufacturer's website). Also, the audiologist should provide the recipient with a plan for whom the recipient should contact if problems or questions arise. Of note, it is imperative that the audiologist provide ample instruction and support to school professionals who are supporting children who use HAT in school settings.

Cochlear Implant Reliability

Cochlear implants are manufactured to last a lifetime and generally have impressive track records for durability. However, cochlear implants contain electronic components that are housed in fairly small packages and that reside in an environment that is rather hostile to electronics (i.e., the moist and warm environment of the temporal bone). **Reliability** is a term that is frequently used to describe the durability of the cochlear implant (i.e., the probability that a cochlear implant performs to the manufacturer's specifications under typical operating conditions for an intended period of time) (International Standards Organization [ISO] 5842-2:2014; Maurer, Marangos, & Ziegler, 2005). The ISO standard 5841-2:2014 is the current standard that addresses reliability of pulse generators or leads for cardiac pacemakers and has been adopted by cochlear implant manufacturers as the standard that will be used to determine cumulative survival rates of cochlear implant makes and models and for reporting cochlear implant failures to the appropriate regulatory body (e.g., FDA). A **cochlear implant failure** is the term used to describe a cochlear implant that is unable to perform its intended function according to the manufacturer's specifications (Maurer, Marangos, & Ziegler, 2005). A **hard failure** describes a cochlear implant that has totally lost function (i.e., no stimulation may be delivered to elicit an auditory sensation). A **soft failure** describes a cochlear implant that deviates from the manufacturer's specifications but has not totally lost function. The **cumulative survival rate (CSR)** describes the percentage of a particular make and model of cochlear implant that are still functional at a given point in time. The CSR is typically reported on an annual basis. The CSR is also typically reported for both children and adults.

Cochlear implants that are deemed to be hard failures are typically removed and replaced with a new cochlear implant. Often, the process of replacing a faulty cochlear implant with a new cochlear implant is referred to as a cochlear implant revision. Anecdotal experiences and published reports have generally shown that cochlear implant revisions result in a successful outcome when the decision to replace a cochlear implant is based on sound clinical judgment (Zeitler, Budenz, & Roland, 2009). Soft cochlear implant failures present a more pressing dilemma to the cochlear implant team. Some soft failures may present with objective indicators that suggest that the function of the implant is compromised. For instance, average electrode voltage (AEV) assessment may

National Acoustic Laboratories
A division of Australian Hearing

NAL
CLIENT ORIENTED SCALE OF IMPROVEMENT

Name : _____

Audiologist : _____   Category. _____

Date : _____ 1. Needs Established _____

       2. Outcome Assessed _____

New Return

SPECIFIC NEEDS

Indicate Order of Significance

Degree of Change

	Worse	No Difference	Slightly Better	Better	Much Better

CATEGORY

Final Ability (with hearing aid)

Person can hear

10% 25% 50% 75% 95%

	Hardly Ever	Occasionally	Half the Time	Most of Time	Almost Always

Categories

1. Conversation with 1 or 2 in quiet
2. Conversation with 1 or 2 in noise
3. Conversation with group in quiet
4. Conversation with group in noise
5. Television/Radio @ normal volume
6. Familiar speaker on phone
7. Unfamiliar speaker on phone
8. Hearing phone ring from another room
9. Hear front door bell or knock
10. Hear traffic
11. Increased social contact
12. Feel embarrassed or stupid
13. Feeling left out
14. Feeling upset or angry
15. Church or meeting
16. Other

FIGURE 20–7. Client Oriented Scale of Improvement (COSI). Copyright © National Acoustics Laboratories.

indicate that electrical pulses generated by the implant do not behave in an expected manner (e.g., pulse amplitude does not increase as expected with increases in stimulation). In other cases, there may be no obvious signs of implant malfunction, but the recipient's progress is poorer than expected or performance diminishes over time. The audiologists involved in the care of the recipient should rule out all other potential factors that may compromise outcomes before considering revision surgery. Factors to explore include patient-specific factors (e.g., neuro-cognitive deficits, age at implantation, duration of deafness, etiology), device wear time, adequate exposure to intelligible speech to allow for development of the auditory system of children, adequate function of the external sound processor, optimal cochlear implant program/map, and so forth. If exhaustive trouble-shooting has ruled out other factors as the primary cause of the recipient's unsatisfactory outcome, the cochlear implant team should consider cochlear implant revision.

An International Consensus Group for Cochlear Implant Reliability Reporting was formed to develop a system for defining cochlear implant failures and for reporting failures to cochlear implant clinics and to the FDA (Battmer et al., 2010). When a device is explanted, the cochlear implant team should return it to the cochlear implant manufacturer for analysis. If the manufacturer's analysis indicates that the cochlear implant is operating outside of the specifications of the device, then the failure should be included in the CSR of the implant make and model. Furthermore, if a manufacturer's assessment indicates that a device is faulty in vivo, but the implant is not surgically removed, then the device should be deemed a failure and included in the CSR. The manufacturer should notify the cochlear implant team within 60 days of receipt of the implant regarding whether the implant was functioning within specifications. The cochlear implant team and the manufacturer should continue to monitor the progress of all recipients who undergo revision surgery and whose implant is deemed to be operating within the specification of the device. If an explanted device is deemed to be within specification, but the patient performs better with the replacement cochlear implant, the manufacturer should consider the device a failure and include it in the CSR. If a device is removed and found to be within specification and the recipient does not experience better performance after six months of use of the replacement implant, then the revision does not count as a failure and is not included in the calculation of the CSR.

The CSR of each of the cochlear implant manufacturers is rather impressive. Many cochlear implant recipients are still using cochlear implants that they received 20 to 30 years ago. With that said, all cochlear implant manufacturers have produced at least one make and model of a cochlear implant that has been plagued with a critical fault. However, over time, implant manufacturing practices have been refined and improved, and implant reliability has also improved. Nonetheless, cochlear implants are still susceptible to failure. For instance a blow to the implant can result in a tear in the silicone insulation and a subsequent ingress of body fluid into the implant. The prudent audiologist should counsel the implant candidate that it is possible (and even likely in the case of infants and young children) that the cochlear implant will need to be replaced in the recipient's lifetime. Again, cochlear implant revision procedures typically result in a favorable outcome.

Cochlear implant reliability is often primarily focused on the cochlear implant (i.e., the internal components). However, the reliability of the external sound processor is also very important. As with the cochlear implant, improvements have been made in the design and durability of cochlear implant sound processors, transmitting cables, and transmitting coils. Audiologists should also consider the reliability of the cochlear implant external equipment when counseling a cochlear implant candidate about the cochlear implant system that best meets his/her needs. For example, a recipient who is routinely exposed to moisture (albeit swimming, perspiration, humidity, etc.) or debris (e.g., dirt, dust) should consider a sound processor that has a robust ingress protection (IP) rating (i.e., 57 or better).

Cochlear Implants and Music

Many recipients of cochlear implants are able to understand speech presented without visual cues (Balkany et al., 2007, 2013; Gifford et al., 2010; Gifford, Shallop, & Peterson, 2008; Plant et al., 2015) and are able to successfully communicate via listening and spoken language (Dettman et al., 2016; Geers et al., 2011, 2017). However, music perception of cochlear implant users continues to be quite limited, particularly with severe deficits observed in pitch and timbre perception. Numerous research studies have shown that most cochlear implant users experience significant difficulty with **pitch**-based tasks such as **melody** recognition (e.g., recognizing simple melodies, especially when rhythmic cues are removed), pitch ranking (determining if the pitch of a test signal is higher or lower than a reference signal) and discrimination (determining if two signals have the same or a different pitch), and pitch production (e.g., "singing in tune/on pitch") (Donnelly, Guo, & limb, 2009; Galvin, Fu, & Nogaki, 2007; Gfeller et al., 2002, 2007, 2008; Hsiao, 2008; Kang et al., 2009; Kong et al., 2004; Limb & Rubinstein, 2012; Stordahl, 2002; Sucher & McDermott, 2007; Vongpaisal et al., 2006). It should be noted that although performance on pitch-based tasks is generally poor for most implant users, there is variability across recipients, with a small minority achieving relatively good performance. For instance, Gfeller and colleagues (2007) showed that many pediatric cochlear implant recipients were unable to detect interval changes smaller than 3 to 8 semitones, whereas a small number of children in the study could detect changes as small as one semitone. A semitone is the smallest interval used in classical Western music and is equal to 1/12 of an octave.

The difficulty of cochlear implant users to accurately perceive pitch and melody can be attributed to at least two factors. First, modern cochlear implant systems possess 12 to 22 physical electrode contacts, whereas the normal cochlea possesses 3,500 inner

hair cells to code spectral information. Speech recognition in quiet typically requires a relatively broad analysis of spectral information. For example, Figure 20–8 shows vowel formant ellipses, which are spread across a fairly broad frequency range requiring rather gross spectral analysis. In contrast, musical notes are separated by 1/12 of an octave, and consequently, much greater spectral resolution is required to discriminate between the individual notes in music. The smaller number of perceptual channels available to cochlear implant users results in difficulty in tasks requiring fine spectral resolution (e.g., melody recognition, recognition of different musical instruments, speech recognition in noise, recognition of pitch of a talker's voice). As mentioned in Chapters 7 and 8, cochlear implant manufacturers have attempted to use current steering/virtual channels in attempts to increase the number of spectral channels available to process pitch, signals in noise, etc. However, research has shown little to at best modest improvement in music perception with the use of signal coding strategies incorporating current steering/virtual channels (Berenstein et al., 2008).

Second, as previously mentioned in Chapter 3, the spectral content of a sound is processed by two cues in the auditory system, place cues and temporal

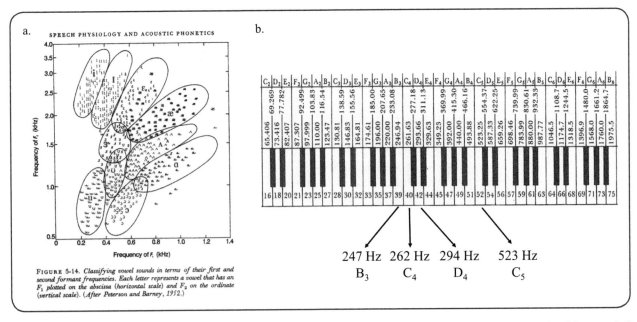

FIGURE 5-14. *Classifying vowel sounds in terms of their first and second formant frequencies. Each letter represents a vowel that has an F₁ plotted on the abscissa (horizontal scale) and F₂ on the ordinate (vertical scale). (After Peterson and Barney, 1952.)*

FIGURE 20–8. A. Vowel formant ellipses. Reproduced from Peterson and Barney, "Control methods used in a study of the vowels," *The Journal of the Acoustical Society of America*, (1952), 24(175), with permission of the Acoustical Society of America. **B.** Frequencies associated with musical notes on a piano keyboard. Image provided courtesy of Advanced Bionics, LLC.

cues. Place cues originate in the cochlea and are generally associated with the exact place in the cochlea that is maximally stimulated by the stimulating sound (i.e., low-frequency sounds are coded at the apical end of the cochlea, whereas high-frequency sounds are coded at the basal end). The tonotopic organization that begins in the cochlea persists throughout the auditory nervous system. Temporal cues refer to the fact that phase-locking within the cochlear nerve causes cochlear nerve units to fire at integer multiples of the frequency of the stimulating sound. In the normal auditory system, the cochlear nerve fires at integer multiples of the stimulating frequency up to at least 5000 Hz (Moeller, 2001, 2013). Several studies have suggested that a phase-locked response only occurs up to 200 to 400 Hz in response to electrical stimulation of the cochlear nerve (Clark, 1969, 1970; Moxon, 1971). As a result, cochlear implant recipients are limited in their ability to use temporal cues to process spectral information for pitch-based tasks such as melody recognition as well as pitch production and discrimination. Some modern signal coding strategies vary the electrical stimulation rate so that it coincides with the frequency of the incoming sound (e.g., FSP, FS4, FS4-p). However, research has generally shown limited to at best modest improvement in music perception with the use of these signal coding strategies (McDermott, 2004).

Research has also shown that many cochlear implant users experience considerable difficulty with **timbre** recognition (Gfeller et al., 1997, 1998; Looi et al., 2008a, 2008b). Timbre refers to quality or character of a sound made by a voice or musical instrument. Timbre recognition is often evaluated by asking cochlear implant recipients to identify/discriminate different musical instruments, a task with which most cochlear implant recipients experience significant difficulty (Gfeller, 1997, 1998; Nimmons et al., 2008). Timbre perception may also be evaluated by asking a listener to rate the pleasantness or to characterize the quality of a tone (e.g., rich vs. dull; full vs. sparse). Research has typically shown that cochlear implant recipients generally rate music to be less pleasant with poorer sound quality compared with the ratings offered by persons with normal hearing.

In contrast to the findings of studies evaluating pitch and timbre perception, numerous research studies have shown that cochlear implant users are able to perceive **rhythm** with accuracy similar to that of persons with normal hearing (Gfeller & Lansing, 1991; Gfeller et al., 1997; Looi et al., 2008a, 2008b;

McDermott, 2004; Vongpaisal, Trehub, & Schellenberg, 2006). Rhythmic cues typically vary relatively slowly across time and are effectively coded with electrical stimulation of the cochlear nerve (similar to the fact that amplitude envelope cues are coded more accurately than fine temporal structure in response to electrical stimulation from a cochlear implant). Because of their relatively good ability to follow rhythmic cues, many cochlear implant users are able to enjoy "the beat" of music as well as many percussive instruments. Of note, the perception of rhythmic cues allows many cochlear implant users to recognize rhythmic melodies, such as "Mary Had a Little Lamb" and "Happy Birthday," which would be difficult to perceive based on melodic cues alone.

Research has shown that a cochlear implant recipient's perception and enjoyment of music may improve with musical training (Looi, Gfeller, & Driscoll, 2012). Additionally, it should be noted that many pediatric cochlear implant recipients are more likely to enjoy music than postlingually deafened adults, because children have only known music available via electrical stimulation of the auditory system, whereas adults have more stringent expectations due to their previous experiences with music when their hearing was normal. For adult recipients, it may be easier to recognize and eventually enjoy music with which they were familiar prior to receiving a cochlear implant. Extensive exposure to and practice with music is likely to improve music perception and appreciation over time. Many children with cochlear implants are able to learn to play musical instruments, dance to music, and enjoy a variety of different genres of music. Considering the wide variability in musical aptitudes across cochlear implant users, it may be valuable for a musical instructor to evaluate the musical aptitude of an individual child and develop goals and instruction that are customized to suit the child's abilities. Hsaio and Gfeller (2012) also recommend that the cochlear implant recipient be provided with opportunities to visually observe an instrument as it is being played or a singer who is singing a song in order to receive visual cues that support the music that is being heard. Also, visual cues may be provided through the use of written lyrics and/or musical scores. Finally, Hsaio and Gfeller recommend providing contextual cues (such as a description of what is producing the music or the emotions and meaning underlying a song) to aid in music perception and to provide the listener with ample exposure to music of interest.

Future Considerations in Cochlear Implants

As can be gathered from the descriptions in this book describing cochlear implant hardware and signal processing as well as the outcomes obtained with cochlear implants, countless improvements in technology and hearing performance have been achieved over the past 40-plus years. Audiologists who work with cochlear implant candidates and recipients have a responsibility to continue to pursue innovative changes that will advance the state-of-the-art of cochlear implantation as well as to stay abreast of the rapid changes that will inevitably occur with cochlear implant technology and practices. This section provides a general summary of several factors that are likely to impact the future of cochlear implant technology and practices.

Future Advances in Cochlear Implant Surgery

Cochlear implant outcomes are certainly dependent on the success of cochlear implant surgery. Ideally, the cochlear implant electrode array should be inserted entirely within the scala tympani and should avoid causing trauma to the delicate sensory and supporting structures of the organ of Corti. Numerous studies have shown better outcomes for recipients whose electrode arrays are housed entirely within the scala tympani compared with those whose electrode arrays leave the scala tympani and dislocate to the scala media and/or scala vestibuli (Aschendorff, 2007; Holden et al., 2013). Trans-scalar dislocation undoubtedly results in damage to the organ of Corti and other cochlear structures (e.g., vascular structures of the cochlea) (De Seta et al., 2017) as well as results in the electrode contacts being positioned in a suboptimal orientation and location relative to the modiolus and underlying sensory neurons (Finley et al., 2008). Avoidance of cochlear trauma during electrode array insertion is necessary to preserve acoustic hearing for individuals who have functional low-frequency hearing and are likely to benefit from electric-acoustic stimulation (Wanna et al., 2014, 2015). Furthermore, minimizing cochlear trauma also is likely to improve outcomes of conventional cochlear implant recipients for whom preservation of acoustic hearing is not an objective. Damage to cochlear sensory and structural cells likely results in retrograde degeneration of cochlear nerve fibers, which is likely to impair hearing performance with the implant (Spoendlin, 1975). Additionally, cochlear trauma secondary to electrode array insertion is likely to result in the formation of scar tissue in the cochlea (Ishiyama et al., 2016), a fact that is likely to adversely affect how electrical current travels from the electrode array to the cochlear nerve. Moreover, research has shown that cochlear implant outcomes are better when the electrode array is inserted to the appropriate angular insertion depth (O'Connell et al., 2016).

Given the importance of electrode array placement on hearing preservation and the outcomes of all cochlear implant recipients, the future will undoubtedly bring advances that will improve the surgeon's ability to achieve a complete scala tympani insertion and to minimize cochlear trauma. Clearly, the evolution of cochlear implant electrode array and technology and surgical procedures have increased the likelihood of hearing preservation (Aschendorff, 2007; Aschendorff et al., 2017), and cochlear manufacturers will most certainly continue to improve electrode array design and surgical procedures in efforts to achieve even better outcomes. For instance, investigators have already begun to explore the possibility of using robotics to drill through the mastoid bone and to enter into the cochlea via the round window or a cochleostomy as well as to assist with insertion of the electrode array (Caversaccio et al., 2017; Weber et al., 2017; Zhang et al., 2006). Robotic systems have the benefit of allowing for precise measurement and control in insertion forces applied during drilling and during electrode array insertion. Also, robotic systems can precisely control the speed at which drilling progresses and the speed of electrode array insertion. Imaging may be used to assist the robot in determining the ideal path for drilling through the mastoid bone in an effort to avoid the facial nerve and other delicate structures. Imaging may also be used to allow for better control of electrode array insertion. Imaging is likely to be used in other ways to enhance cochlear implant surgery. For instance, it is likely that audiologists will make a common practice of using preoperative imaging to estimate cochlear duct length to determine ideal electrode array choice and angular depth of insertion. Additionally, fluoroscopic imaging will likely be used routinely to allow for real-time visualization of the cochlea during electrode array insertion so that the surgeon can determine whether an optimal electrode array insertion is being achieved (Coelho, Waltzman, & Roland, 2008; Fishman et al., 2003). In particular, fluoroscopic imaging may be of importance in complicated cases such as those with cochlear malformations.

At the time of this writing, MED-EL announced the release of OTOPLAN, a tablet-based ontologic software program that translates radiologic images into three-dimensional images of the temporal bone. The cochlear implant surgeon may use the OTOPLAN-derived three-dimensional reconstructed images (i.e., models) to plan surgery, preoperatively identify important anatomical landmarks and potential complications, select the ideal electrode array to best suit an individual's unique anatomy, preoperatively determine a desired insertion depth (e.g., determine the insertion depth necessary to reach a certain frequency place in the cochlea), conduct postoperative analysis to perform a quality check and verify insertion status from postoperative images. Almost assuredly in the future, surgeons and audiologists will routinely use programs like OTOPLAN to optimize cochlear implant surgery outcomes and programming approaches.

In the future, it is also likely that surgeons will administer pharmacologic agents to improve the outcomes of cochlear implant recipients. Research has shown that the steroids administered systemically or directly to the cochlea may improve hearing preservation after cochlear implant surgery (Santa Maria et al., 2014), but no consensus exists regarding the dosage, schedule (i.e., when and how often steroids should be administered), and the manner (e.g., orally, intravenously, direct to the cochlea) the steroids should be administered. Most likely, a consensus will develop in the future so that steroid treatment can be provided to reduce cochlear inflammation and improve the likelihood of hearing preservation after cochlear implant surgery. Additionally, in the future, it is possible that drug-eluting cochlear implant electrode arrays will be developed to administer steroids or possibly even brain-derived neurotrophins (Dabdoub & Nishimura, 2017). Neurotrophins are proteins that facilitate the survival and potentially the growth and development of neurons (Huang & Reichardt, 2001). Preliminary research conducted with guinea pigs has shown that a drug-eluting electrode array that administered neurotrophins into the cochlea allowed for preservation and development of cochlear nerve dendrites as well as lower current levels required to elicit and auditory response (Browne et al., 2016; Pinyon et al., 2014; Ramekers et al., 2015).

Future Advances in Cochlear Implant Technology

Manufacturers and researchers will also make continual improvements in cochlear implant hardware and technology. Within the next decade or two, it is likely that at least one of the manufacturers will obtain commercial approval to distribute a totally implantable cochlear implant. As discussed in the chapter on middle ear implantable hearing devices, totally implantable hearing technology already exists and is approved for commercial use. Totally implantable hearing devices typically use piezoelectric transducers located on a middle ear structure or a subcutaneous microphone (located underneath the skin) to capture the audio signal of interest. Briggs et al. (2008) reported on the results of three recipients who were implanted with a totally implantable cochlear implant (referred to as the TIKI) developed by Cochlear Ltd. Briggs and colleagues reported surgical or major postoperative complications related to the totally implantable cochlear implant. The TIKI implant could be used in the "invisible hearing" mode in which sound was captured by the subcutaneous microphone or in conventional mode in which the recipient used an Esprit 3G behind-the-ear sound processor to capture sound and deliver a signal to the cochlear implant via near-field electromagnetic induction (i.e., short-range radio frequency transmission from the coil of the sound processor). Sound-field warbled tone thresholds and speech recognition were significantly poorer in the invisible hearing mode relative to the conventional mode, a finding the authors attributed to attenuation of the audio signal as it passed across skin to the subcutaneous microphone in the invisible mode. Additionally, Briggs and colleagues reported that some recipients were annoyed by the salience of body noise interference when using the subcutaneous microphone. Because of the limitations observed in this research trial, the TIKI was not developed for commercial use. However, Cochlear Ltd. has purchased the implantable hearing technologies developed by Otologics Carina and Implex, two totally implantable middle ear hearing devices, an acquisition that would seem to indicate that Cochlear Ltd. is still actively pursuing the development of totally implantable hearing technology. Given the competitive nature that exists in the development of technology across the major cochlear implant manufacturers, each of the cochlear implant manufacturers is undoubtedly exploring the development of a totally implantable cochlear implant. Along those same lines, there will be a continued effort to miniaturize the cochlear implant and to increase the power efficiency of the cochlear implant, as both of these characteristics will enhance cosmetics and improve the likelihood that a totally implantable cochlear implant will provide hearing through an entire day on one battery charge.

Researchers have also explored the possibility of stimulating the cochlear nerve with optical stimulation instead of electrical current. It is well known that the broad current spread that occurs with electrical stimulation results in channel interaction that leads to suboptimal frequency resolution and speech recognition (Fishman, Shannon, & Slattery, 1997; Friesen et al., 2001; Noble et al., 2014). Several researchers have explored the possibility of improving spectral resolution through the use of laser stimulation of the cochlear nerve (Hernandez et al., 2014; Izzo et al., 2006, 2008). Other researchers have explored the possibility of using genetic therapy (delivered via a viral vehicle) to develop light-sensitive ion channels in the cochlear nerve (Hernandez et al., 2014). The development of the light-sensitive ion channels in the cochlear nerve facilitated an auditory response to optical stimulation (i.e., micro-LED-based stimulators). Although several obstacles (e.g., ensuring safety of the cochlear nerve, providing adequate loudness growth) exist to the development of a cochlear implant that can provide optical stimulation, use of optical stimulation does possess the potential to improve hearing performance, and researchers will continue to explore the feasibility of optical stimulation of the cochlear nerve (Kallweit et al., 2016).

Changes and improvements will also undoubtedly occur with external cochlear implant hardware and technology. As discussed in Chapter 8, signal coding strategies and signal processing have evolved considerably over the past 30 years, and recipient outcomes have improved because of these advances. Most certainly, cochlear implant manufacturers will continue to develop new signal coding strategies (e.g., new forms of current steering, signal coding based on cochlear modeling and psychoacoustics, etc.), new variations in signal processing (e.g., beam-forming, noise reduction, de-reverberation, speech enhancement), new stimuli (e.g., monophasic, multi-phasic), and new electrode coupling options (e.g., tripolar). Cochlear implant manufacturers will also continue to miniaturize the external sound processors, improve the durability of the sound processor (e.g., waterproof, shatterproof), and offer improvements in power options (e.g., improved efficiency, rechargeable battery integrated into sound processor). Moreover, manufacturers will continue to expand the ability of cochlear implant hardware to interface with personal electronic devices (e.g., mobile telephone, tablet, computer, television, etc.), wireless technologies (e.g., Bluetooth, Wi-Fi), and hearing assistive technologies. Additionally, manufacturers are likely to develop cochlear implant sound processors that integrate the signal between the two ears of the user in an attempt to optimize binaural auditory processing for bilateral and bimodal cochlear implant users. Furthermore, manufacturers are likely to continue to develop new wearing options (e.g., off-the-ear) that will provide flexibility to meet the diverse needs of cochlear implant recipients across the age and lifestyle spectrum.

Future Advances in Cochlear Implant Programming

The future will also bring changes to the way in which cochlear implants are programmed. More than likely, patient-driven programming will become prevalent in the future. Dwyer et al. (2016) compared the hearing performance obtained with use of an audiologist-generated program versus a patient-generated program for 18 experienced adult recipients and found no statistically significant difference in speech recognition in quiet and in noise, sound quality, and spectral modulation detection obtained with the two programs. Dwyer and colleagues advocated for the use of patient-generated programming, because the growth of individuals receiving cochlear implants is expected to increase at a rate of at least 11% per year (Laaman & Rutledge, 2012), and as a result, audiologists will be unable to meet the demand of recipients who need cochlear implant programming.

Govaerts and colleagues at the Eargroup at the University of Antwerp in Belgium have developed a software-based program called Fitting to Outcomes eXpert (FOX) that also attempts to automate the cochlear implant programming process (Govaerts et al., 2010). The FOX program incorporates the results of four psychoacoustic measures and generates a cochlear implant program (i.e., MAP) based on the recipient's outcomes on each of the four measures, which include: (1) detection thresholds obtained with use of the cochlear implant (250 to 8000 Hz), (2) psychophysical loudness scaling to a tonal-like stimulus at 250, 1000, and 4000 Hz, (3) Auditory Speech Sounds Evaluation, which is a phoneme discrimination test containing 20 pairs of isolated vowels and consonants; the individual phonemes that make up a given pair of phonemes contain different spectral compositions, and the recipient's task is to discriminate between the two phonemes in the pair; the objective of the Auditory Speech Sounds Evaluation is to gain a clinical indication of the frequency discriminating power of the auditory system (Vaerenberg et al., 2011) (Figure 20–9 shows an illustration

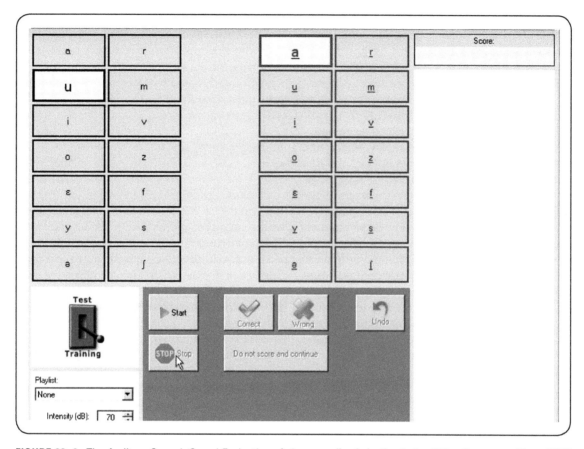

FIGURE 20–9. The Auditory Speech Sound Evaluation of phoneme discrimination in the Fitting Outcomes eXpert (FOX) programming suite. Image provided courtesy of Paul Govaerts.

of the Auditory Speech Sound Evaluation of phoneme discrimination), and (4) word recognition testing conducted at multiple presentation levels (e.g., 40, 55, 70, and 85 dB SPL).

The data obtained for the measures within the FOX program may be manually entered (after completing the measurements in an audiometric test booth), or ideally, the measurements are automatically administered by the FOX software from the cochlear implant programming computer, which is directly coupled to the recipient's sound processor (an approach which is referred to as "direct connect"). Administering the measurements included within the FOX program from the computer directly to the recipient's sound processor requires the completion of a calibration process so that the input level of test stimuli are accurate. An obvious advantage of directly administering the stimuli from the programming computer to the recipient's sound processor is the fact that it removes the need for an audiometric test booth.

The FOX software incorporates the recipient's outcome for each of the four measures with the software's knowledge of the cochlear implant system's signal coding and MAPping parameters to generate a cochlear implant program designed to optimize the recipient's hearing performance. Additionally, the FOX software takes into account all of the previous changes that the software has made to recipients' MAPs over the life of the FOX software program and analyzes how those changes have affected hearing performance in the four measurements made within the FOX software program. Associating changes in recipient performance with changes that FOX makes to MAPs allows for the FOX software program to use artificial intelligence to determine which MAPping changes are most likely to improve an individual recipient's performance. Currently, the FOX software program considers the impact that tens of millions of previous MAPping adjustments have had on recipients' performance when determining the programming adjustments to recommend for an individual recipient. Theoretically, the use of **artificial intelligence** will allow for continued improvement in the programming recommendations that FOX software makes based on the results of the measurement data it receives. Almost assuredly, this concept of artificial intelligence will be commonly applied to the process of determining cochlear implant candidacy as well as to the practice of programming cochlear implants

FOX may also be used to activate new recipients. For new activations, FOX initially generates a series of programs with stimulation levels that are typical of the cochlear implant system (e.g., make, model, electrode array) used by the recipient. The recipient initially uses the program that has the highest stimulation levels that are deemed to be comfortable to the recipient. The recipient is provided with multiple programs, each with successively higher stimulation levels, and is instructed to progress through the programs over the next several days as long as the program is not uncomfortable. Eventually, the outcome data from the four different psychoacoustical measures will also be incorporated to generate programs that are designed to optimize the recipient's hearing performance.

The initial peer-reviewed publications describing research studies that have evaluated FOX are encouraging. Battmer et al. (2015) compared the time required to create audiologist-generated versus FOX-generated programs for 27 adult implant recipients seen at several cochlear implant centers in Europe. They reported that the use of FOX reduced programming time during the first two weeks of cochlear implant use but that there was no difference in programming time between FOX- and audiologist-generated programs when compared over a 6-month period. Buechner and colleagues (2015) compared hearing performance obtained with FOX- versus audiologist-generated programs for 10 experienced adult cochlear implant recipients. They reported that soundfield detection thresholds were significantly better with the FOX-based program but that there were no difference in speech recognition obtained with the two programs. Meeuws et al. (2017) also compared speech recognition obtained with audiologist-generated versus FOX-generated programs. The 25 participants were experienced adult cochlear implant users. Use of the FOX programs provided a small but statistically significant improvement in speech recognition.

Cochlear Ltd. purchased a license to be the exclusive provider of the FOX software system. Clinical trials are currently underway with the likely objective being to incorporate FOX into Cochlear's Custom Sound programming software. It is not difficult to envision a possibility of the FOX software-based program being administered remotely from the recipient's smartphone. The stimuli for the four different measurements could be delivered via Cochlear's wireless audio streaming, and programming adjustments could also be made wirelessly from the smartphone to the recipient's sound processor. As of now, it is unknown how automated programming systems, such as FOX, will affect the audiologist's role in the cochlear implant programming process.

Remote programming of cochlear implants is a practice that is likely to become commonplace in the future. Many recipients find it difficult to travel to a clinic for programming (e.g., elderly, young children, recipients who are ill or who live in rural locations), particularly for the several programming sessions that are necessary during the first few months of implant use. Several researchers have demonstrated the feasibility of remote cochlear implant programming and have demonstrated satisfactory recipient outcomes obtained with programs that are created remotely (Eikelboom et al., 2014; Goehring & Hughes, 2017; Kuzokov et al., 2014; Ramos et al., 2009; Vroegop et al., 2017). With the proliferation of smartphone technology and online communication that has occurred around the world as well as the trend toward telehealth in all sectors of health care (Foster et al., 2014), remote cochlear implant programming will likely be a routine practice in the future.

In the future, it is also likely that audiologists will adopt new and innovative measures that will enhance cochlear implant programming and improve recipient outcomes. For example, Noble and colleagues (2014) have explored the use of modeling and high-resolution CT imaging to evaluate the position of the electrode array in the cochlea and predict electrode contacts that may cause excessive overlap in stimulation (i.e., channel interaction). The researchers disabled electrode contacts that were predicted to cause channel interaction. Preliminary results have shown that this image-guided programming technique has the potential to improve the hearing performance of some recipients (Labadie et al., 2016; Noble et al., 2016), with up to 90% of adult recipients showing equivocal or better performance with a program with disabled electrodes based on the findings of the CT imaging. Given these positive findings, it is possible that image-guided programming will be used to improve recipient outcomes in the future.

It is likely that additional measures will be developed to improve the cochlear implant programming process. Several investigators have explored the potential of using complex measures, such as spread-of-excitation, rate-of-recovery, temporal processing, spectral resolution, and so forth, to determine the ideal programming parameters (e.g., stimulation rate, potential to benefit from current steering or the provision of fine temporal structure, electrodes that should be disabled) for a recipient (Cohen et al., 2003; He, Teagle, & Buchman, 2017; Hughes, 2008; Hughes & Abbas, 2006; van der Beek et al., 2012). Unfortunately, however, research exploring a link between advanced psychophysical measures and cochlear implant outcomes has failed to identify a measure that can assist in the determination of the ideal programming parameters for a recipient (Caner et al., 2007). Of note, Gifford, Hedley-Williams, and Spahr (2014) have shown that performance on a spectral modulation task correlated with monosyllabic word recognition obtained with a cochlear implant, which suggests that there is a potential relationship between performance on advanced measures and the outcomes achieved after cochlear implantation. Researchers will continue to seek measurements that audiologists can complete to improve the ability to determine ideal cochlear implant programming parameters, and it is possible that these measures will be available for clinical use in the future. Additionally, it is possible that the telemetry system of the cochlear implant will be used to complete measures of cochlear nerve function and adjust the settings of the cochlear implant to optimize the cochlear nerve's response. Moreover, data from telemetry measures of cochlear nerve function could conceivably be remotely transmitted to the audiologist via the recipient's audiologist, who could monitor the data and determine whether audiologic intervention could improve the recipient's outcome. Indeed, the telemetry system of cardiac pacemakers is already used to monitor the device, and the data compiled are delivered to the managing physician for management (Burri & Senouf, 2009).

Future Advances in Cochlear Implant Assessment

The future will also likely bring changes in the assessment practices of audiologists who serve cochlear implant recipients. At the time of this writing, the FDA-approved indications of use for the Nucleus CI532 cochlear implant with adults indicate that the device should be considered for individuals who have sentence recognition scores in the best aided condition of no better than 50% correct in the ear to be implanted and no more than 60% correct in the

nonimplanted ear. These indications for use, which have been unchanged since the year 2000, represent the most lax speech recognition criteria approved by the FDA for cochlear implantation in the United States. However, researchers have shown that many individuals who have aided speech recognition scores that are better than the current indications for use are often able to receive considerable benefit from and improvement in hearing performance with a cochlear implant (Gifford et al., 2010). In the future, the indications for use of cochlear implants will likely become more lax to allow for more individuals with moderate to profound hearing loss to benefit from cochlear implant technology. For example, Cochlear Americas is currently conducting a multiple-center clinical trial that explores the use of CNC monosyllabic words in the best aided condition with a criterion of no better than 40% correct for the ear to be implanted and no better than 50% correct in the nonimplanted ear. Assuming favorable results are obtained in this trial along with the efforts of other cochlear implant manufacturers, it is likely that the speech materials used for cochlear implant candidacy assessment with both adults and children as well as the indications of use will change in the future.

Interestingly, Govaerts (2016) has argued that formal indications of use for cochlear implantation should be abolished. Govaerts contended that the decision to proceed with cochlear implantation should be made on a case-by-case basis in order to best meet the unique needs of each individual. He suggested that experienced hearing health care professionals are best suited to determine cochlear implant candidacy on an individual basis, and he noted that liberalizing the indications for use is unlikely to have a big impact on current practices or the budgets of the entities that pay for cochlear implant services.

We hope, the future will also bring advances in measurements that may be used to determine appropriate candidates for cochlear implantation. For instance, it may be possible that preimplant aided performance on an acoustic version of the spectral modulation detection task described in Gifford, Hedley-Williams, and Spahr (2014) may predict individuals who are more likely to perform well with a cochlear implant. Further research is needed to determine whether preimplant performance on a task of spectral modulation detection (or on other advanced psychoacoustic measures) could assist in predicting outcomes with cochlear implantation.

Additionally, researchers have shown a relationship between findings on brain imaging studies and cochlear implant outcomes. For instance, Lee and colleagues (2001) used PET scan imaging to show that the auditory cortex of poorly performing cochlear implant recipients was active in the absence of sound, a finding they attributed to colonization of the auditory system by other sensory modalities such as vision. Also, Mortensen et al. (2006) used PET scan imaging to show greater levels of activity in the left inferior prefrontal cortex of recipients who had higher levels of open-set speech recognition. In the future, brain imaging will likely be used in clinical settings to predict cochlear implant outcomes prior to implant surgery as well as postoperatively to identify whether stimulation from the cochlear implant is facilitating auditory-related responses in the brain that are expected in recipients who achieve satisfactory outcomes after implantation.

Key Concepts

- Cochlear implant recipients generally achieve better hearing performance with the use of bilateral cochlear implants or the use of a hearing aid and a cochlear implant (i.e., bimodal use) compared with the use of a single cochlear implant alone. The audiologist should strive to optimize the programming of the hearing technology used for each ear in order to maximize the recipient's hearing performance. Bilateral cochlear implant outcomes are generally better when the duration of deafness is short.
- Cochlear implantation is a viable option for individuals with single-sided deafness, particularly when the duration of deafness is short. Children born with single-sided deafness should ideally receive a cochlear implant within the first two years of life. Cochlear nerve aplasia should be ruled out as a cause of single-sided deafness prior to pursuing cochlear implantation.
- Hearing assistive technology can provide substantial improvement in speech recognition in challenging listening situations and should routinely be used in difficult listening environments.
- Cochlear implant recipients generally have poorer music perception than speech recognition. In particular, perception of melody and timbre is frequently poor.
- Future advances in cochlear implantation will undoubtedly lead to improvements in the outcomes of recipients.

References

Armstrong, M., Pegg, P., James, C., & Blamey, P. (1997). Speech perception in noise with implant and hearing aid. *American Journal of Otology, 18*(6 Suppl.), S140–S141.

Arndt, S., Laszig, R., Aschendorff, A., Beck, R., Schild, C., Hassepass, F., . . . Wesarg, T. (2011). [Unilateral deafness and cochlear implantation: Audiological diagnostic evaluation and outcomes]. *HNO, 59*(5), 437–446.

Arndt, S., Prosse, S., Laszig, R., Wesarg, T., Aschendorff, A., & Hassepass, F. (2015). Cochlear implantation in children with single-sided deafness: Does aetiology and duration of deafness matter? *Audiology and Neurotology, 20*(Suppl. 1), 21–30.

Aschendorff, A., Briggs, R., Brademann, G., Helbig, S., Hornung, J., Lenarz, T., . . . James, C. J. (2017). Clinical investigation of the Nucleus Slim Modiolar Electrode. *Audiology and Neurotology, 22*(3), 169–179.

Aschendorff, A., Kromeier, J., Klenzner, T., & Laszig, R. (2007). Quality control after insertion of the Nucleus Contour and Contour Advance electrode in adults. *Ear and Hearing, 28*(2 Suppl.), 75S–79S.

Balkany, T., Hodges, A., Menapace, C., Hazard, L., Driscoll, C., Gantz, B., . . . Payne, S. (2007). Nucleus Freedom North American clinical trial. *Otolaryngology–Head and Neck Surgery, 136*(5), 757–762.

Barton, K., Nickerson, J. P., Higgins, T., & Williams, R. K. (2018). Pediatric anesthesia and neurotoxicity: What the radiologist needs to know. *Pediatric Radiology, 48*(1), 31–36.

Battmer, R. D., Backous, D. D., Balkany, T. J., Briggs, R. J., Gantz, B. J., van Hasselt, A., . . . International Consensus Group for Cochlear Implant Reliability, R. (2010). International classification of reliability for implanted cochlear implant receiver stimulators. *Otology and Neurotology, 31*(8), 1190–1193.

Battmer, R. D., Borel, S., Brendel, M., Buchner, A., Cooper, H., Fielden, C., . . . Vanat, Z. (2015). Assessment of "Fitting to Outcomes Expert" FOX with new cochlear implant users in a multi-centre study. *Cochlear Implants International, 16*(2), 100–109.

Berenstein, C. K., Mens, L. H., Mulder, J. J., & Vanpoucke, F. J. (2008). Current steering and current focusing in cochlear implants: Comparison of monopolar, tripolar, and virtual channel electrode configurations. *Ear and Hearing, 29*(2), 250–260.

Bess, F. H., & Tharpe, A. M. (1986). Case history data on unilaterally hearing-impaired children. *Ear and Hearing, 7*(1), 14–19.

Blamey, P., Artieres, F., Baskent, D., Bergeron, F., Beynon, A., Burke, E., . . . Lazard, D. S. (2013). Factors affecting auditory performance of postlinguistically deaf adults using cochlear implants: An update with 2251 patients. *Audiology and Neurotology, 18*(1), 36–47.

Blasco, M. A., & Redleaf, M. I. (2014). Cochlear implantation in unilateral sudden deafness improves tinnitus and speech comprehension: Meta-analysis and systematic review. *Otology and Neurotology, 35*(8), 1426–1432.

Boyer, E., Karkas, A., Attye, A., Lefournier, V., Escude, B., & Schmerber, S. (2015). Scalar localization by cone-beam computed tomography of cochlear implant carriers: A comparative study between straight and periomodiolar precurved electrode arrays. *Otology and Neurotology, 36*(3), 422–429.

Briggs, R. J., Eder, H. C., Seligman, P. M., Cowan, R. S., Plant, K. L., Dalton, J., . . . Patrick, J. F. (2008). Initial clinical experience with a totally implantable cochlear implant research device. *Otology and Neurotology, 29*(2), 114–119.

Browne, C. J., Pinyon, J. L., Housley, D. M., Crawford, E. N., Lovell, N. H., Klugmann, M., & Housley, G. D. (2016). Mapping of Bionic array electric field focusing in plasmid DNA-based gene electrotransfer. *Gene Therapy, 23*(4), 369–379.

Buechner, A., Vaerenberg, B., Gazibegovic, D., Brendel, M., De Ceulaer, G., Govaerts, P., & Lenarz, T. (2015). Evaluation of the 'Fitting to Outcomes eXpert' (FOX®) with established cochlear implant users. *Cochlear Implants International, 16*(1), 39–46.

Burri, H., & Senouf, D. (2009). Remote monitoring and follow-up of pacemakers and implantable cardioverter defibrillators. *Europace, 11*(6), 701–709.

Buss, E., Pillsbury, H. C., Buchman, C. A., Pillsbury, C. H., Clark, M. S., Haynes, D. S., . . . Barco, A. L. (2008). Multicenter U.S. bilateral MED-EL cochlear implantation study: Speech perception over the first year of use. *Ear and Hearing, 29*(1), 20–32.

Caner, G., Olgun, L., Gultekin, G., & Balaban, M. (2007). Optimizing fitting in children using objective measures such as neural response imaging and electrically evoked stapedius reflex threshold. *Otology and Neurotology, 28*(5), 637–640.

Carraro, M., Park, A. H., & Harrison, R. V. (2016). Partial corrosion casting to assess cochlear vasculature in mouse models of presbycusis and CMV infection. *Hearing Research, 332*, 95–103.

Caversaccio, M., Gavaghan, K., Wimmer, W., Williamson, T., Anso, J., Mantokoudis, G., . . . Weber, S. (2017). Robotic cochlear implantation: surgical procedure and first clinical experience. *Acta Otolaryngologica, 137*(4), 447–454.

Ching, T. Y., Incerti, P., & Hill, M. (2004). Binaural benefits for adults who use hearing aids and cochlear implants in opposite ears. *Ear and Hearing, 25*(1), 9–21.

Ching, T. Y., Incerti, P., Hill, M., Brew, J., Priolo, S., & Rushbrook, E. (2004). Would children who did not wear a hearing aid after implantation benefit from using a hearing aid with a cochlear implant in opposite ears? *Cochlear Implants International, 5*(Suppl. 1), 92–94.

Ching, T. Y., Incerti, P., Hill, M., & van Wanrooy, E. (2006). An overview of binaural advantages for children and adults who use binaural/bimodal hearing devices. *Audiology and Neurotology, 11*(Suppl. 1), 6–11.

Ching, T. Y., Psarros, C., Hill, M., Dillon, H., & Incerti, P. (2001). Should children who use cochlear implants wear hearing aids in the opposite ear? *Ear and Hearing, 22*(5), 365–380.

Ching, T. Y., van Wanrooy, E., & Dillon, H. (2007). Binaural-bimodal fitting or bilateral implantation for managing severe to profound deafness: A review. *Trends in Amplification, 11*(3), 161–192.

Churchill, T. H., Kan, A., Goupell, M. J., & Litovsky, R. Y. (2014). Spatial hearing benefits demonstrated with presentation of acoustic temporal fine structure cues in bilateral cochlear implant listeners. *Journal of the Acoustical Society of America, 136*(3), 1246.

Clark, G. M. (1969). Responses of cells in the superior olivary complex of the cat to electrical stimulation of the auditory nerve. *Experimental Neurology, 24*(1), 124–136.

Clark, G. M. (1970). Study of the vesicle content and distribution of nerve endings in the medial superior olive of the cat. *Journal of Anatomy, 106*(Pt. 1), 200.

Clark, G. M., Tong, Y. C., Bailey, Q. R., Black, R. C., & Martin, L. F. (1978). A multiple-electrode cochlear implant. *Journal of the Otolaryngology Society of Australia, 4*, 208–212.

Clemmens, C. S., Guidi, J., Caroff, A., Cohn, S. J., Brant, J. A., Laury, A. M., . . . Germiller, J. A. (2013). Unilateral cochlear nerve deficiency in children. *Otolaryngology–Head and Neck Surgery, 149*(2), 318–325.

Coelho, D. H., Waltzman, S. B., & Roland, J. T., Jr. (2008). Implanting common cavity malformations using intraoperative fluoroscopy. *Otology and Neurotology, 29*(7), 914–919.

Cohen, L. T., Richardson, L. M., Saunders, E., & Cowan, R. S. (2003). Spatial spread of neural excitation in cochlear implant recipients: Comparison of improved ECAP method and psychophysical forward masking. *Hearing Research, 179*(1–2), 72–87.

Dabdoub, A., & Nishimura, K. (2017). Cochlear implants meet regenerative biology: State of the science and future research directions. *Otology and Neurotology, 38*(8), e232–e236.

Darrow, D. C., Soule, H. C., & Buckman, T. E. (1928). Blood volume in normal infants and children. *Journal of Clinical Investigation, 5*(2), 243–258.

Davidson, L. S., Firszt, J. B., Brenner, C., & Cadieux, J. H. (2015). Evaluation of hearing aid frequency response fittings in pediatric and young adult bimodal recipients. *Journal of the American Academy of Audiology, 26*(4), 393–407.

De Seta, D., Torres, R., Russo, F. Y., Ferrary, E., Kazmitcheff, G., Heymann, D., . . . Nguyen, Y. (2017). Damage to inner ear structure during cochlear implantation: Correlation between insertion force and radio-histological findings in temporal bone specimens. *Hearing Research, 344*, 90–97.

Dettman, S. J., Dowell, R. C., Choo, D., Arnott, W., Abrahams, Y., Davis, A., . . . Briggs, R. J. (2016). Long-term communication outcomes for children receiving cochlear implants younger than 12 months: A multicenter study. *Otology and Neurotology, 37*(2), e82–e95.

Dillon, H., James, A., & Ginis, J. (1997). Client Oriented Scale of Improvement (COSI) and its relationship to several other measures of benefit and satisfaction provided by hearing aids. *Journal of the American Academy of Audiology, 8*(1), 27–43.

Donnelly, P. J., Guo, B. Z., & Limb, C. J. (2009). Perceptual fusion of polyphonic pitch in cochlear implant users. *Journal of the Acoustical Society of America, 126*(5), EL128–133.

Dooley, G. J., Blamey, P. J., Seligman, P. M., Alcantara, J. I., Clark, G. M., Shallop, J. K., . . . Menapace, C. M. (1993). Combined electrical and acoustical stimulation using a bimodal prosthesis. *Archives of Otolaryngology–Head and Neck Surgery, 119*(1), 55–60.

Dorman, M. F., Gifford, R. H., Spahr, A. J., & McKarns, S. A. (2008). The benefits of combining acoustic and electric stimulation for the recognition of speech, voice and melodies. *Audiology and Neurotology, 13*(2), 105–112.

Dorman, M. F., Liss, J., Wang, S., Berisha, V., Ludwig, C., & Natale, S. C. (2016). Experiments on auditory-visual perception of sentences by users of unilateral, bimodal, and bilateral cochlear implants. *Journal of Speech, Language, and Hearing Research, 59*(6), 1505–1519.

Duke, M. M., Wolfe, J., & Schafer, E. (2016). Recognition of speech from the television with use of a wireless technology designed for cochlear implants. *Journal of the American Academy of Audiology, 27*(5), 388–394.

Dunn, C. C., Perreau, A., Gantz, B., & Tyler, R. S. (2010). Benefits of localization and speech perception with multiple noise sources in listeners with a short-electrode cochlear implant. *Journal of the American Academy of Audiology, 21*(1), 44–51.

Dunn, C. C., Tyler, R. S., & Witt, S. A. (2005). Benefit of wearing a hearing aid on the unimplanted ear in adult users of a cochlear implant. *Journal of Speech, Language, and Hearing Research, 48*(3), 668–680.

Dwyer, R. T., Spahr, T., Agrawal, S., Hetlinger, C., Holder, J. T., & Gifford, R. H. (2016). Participant-generated cochlear implant programs: Speech recognition, sound quality, and satisfaction. *Otology and Neurotology, 37*(7), e209–e216.

Eddington, D., Dobelle, W., Brackmann, D., Mladejovsky, M., & Parkin, J. (1978). Place and periodicity pitch elicited by stimulation of multiple scala tympani electrodes in deaf volunteers. *Transacations of the American Society for Artificial Internal Organs, 24*, 1–5.

Eikelboom, R. H., Jayakody, D. M., Swanepoel, D. W., Chang, S., & Atlas, M. D. (2014). Validation of remote mapping of cochlear implants. *Journal of Telemedicine and Telecare, 20*(4), 171–177.

Fetterman, B. L., Saunders, J. E., & Luxford, W. M. (1996). Prognosis and treatment of sudden sensorineural hearing loss. *American Journal of Otology, 17*(4), 529–536.

Finbow, J., Bance, M., Aiken, S., Gulliver, M., Verge, J., & Caissie, R. (2015). A comparison between wireless CROS and bone-anchored hearing devices for single-sided deafness: A pilot study. *Otology and Neurotology, 36*(5), 819–825.

Finley, C. C., Holden, T. A., Holden, L. K., Whiting, B. R., Chole, R. A., Neely, G. J., . . . Skinner, M. W. (2008). Role of electrode placement as a contributor to variability in cochlear implant outcomes. *Otology and Neurotology, 29*(7), 920–928.

Firszt, J. B., Holden, L. K., Reeder, R. M., Waltzman, S. B., & Arndt, S. (2012). Auditory abilities after cochlear implantation in adults with unilateral deafness: A pilot study. *Otology and Neurotology, 33*(8), 1339–1346.

Fishman, A. J., Roland, J. T., Jr., Alexiades, G., Mierzwinski, J., & Cohen, N. L. (2003). Fluoroscopically assisted cochlear implantation. *Otology and Neurotology, 24*(6), 882–886.

Fishman, K. E., Shannon, R. V., & Slattery, W. H. (1997). Speech recognition as a function of the number of electrodes used in the SPEAK cochlear implant speech processor. *Journal of Speech Language and Hearing Research, 40*(5):1201–1215.

Fitzpatrick, E. M., Seguin, C., Schramm, D. R., Armstrong, S., & Chenier, J. (2009). The benefits of remote microphone technology for adults with cochlear implants. *Ear and Hearing, 30*(5), 590–599.

Flexer, C. (2015). *Listening brain as the foundation for language and literacy.* Oral presentation at the Mississippi Speech and Hearing Association, March 31, 2015, Jackson, Mississippi. Retrieved October 31, 2017, from https://www.z2systems.com/neon/resource/msha/files/Handouts/2015/Listening%20Brain%20as%20the%20Foumdation%20for%20Language%20%26%20Literacy.pdf

Fowler, J. R., Eggleston, J. L., Reavis, K. M., McMillan, G. P., & Reiss, L. A. (2016). Effects of removing low-frequency electric information on speech perception with bimodal hearing. *Journal of Speech Language and Hearing Research, 59*(1), 99–109.

Franke-Trieger, A., & Murbe, D. (2015). Estimation of insertion depth angle based on cochlea diameter and linear insertion depth: A prediction tool for the CI422. *European Archives of Otorhinolaryngology, 272*(11), 3193–3199.

Friedmann, D. R., Ahmed, O. H., McMenomey, S. O., Shapiro, W. H., Waltzman, S. B., & Roland, J. T., Jr. (2016). Single-sided deafness cochlear implantation: Candidacy, evaluation, and outcomes in children and adults. *Otology and Neurotology, 37*(2), e154–e160.

Friesen, L. M., Shannon, R. V., Baskent, D., & Wang, X. (2001). Speech recognition in noise as a function of the number of spectral channels: Comparison of acoustic hearing and cochlear implants. *Journal of the Acoustical Society of America, 110*(2):1150–1163.

Fu, Q. J., Galvin, J. J., 3rd, & Wang, X. (2017). Integration of acoustic and electric hearing is better in the same ear than across ears. *Scientific Reports, 7*(1), 12500.

Galvin, J. J., 3rd, Fu, Q. J., & Nogaki, G. (2007). Melodic contour identification by cochlear implant listeners. *Ear and Hearing, 28*(3), 302–319.

Gantz, B. J., Tyler, R. S., Rubinstein, J. T., Wolaver, A., Lowder, M., Abbas, P., . . . Preece, J. P. (2002). Binaural cochlear implants placed during the same operation. *Otology and Neurotology, 23*(2), 169–180.

Geers, A. E., Brenner, C. A., & Tobey, E. A. (2011). Long-term outcomes of cochlear implantation in early childhood: Sample characteristics and data collection methods. *Ear and Hearing, 32*(1 Suppl.), 2S–12S.

Geers, A. E., Mitchell, C. M., Warner-Czyz, A., Wang, N. Y., Eisenberg, L. S., & Team, C. D. I. (2017). Early sign language exposure and cochlear implantation benefits. *Pediatrics, 140*(1), e20163489.

Gfeller, K., Knutson, J. F., Woodworth, G., Witt, S., & DeBus, B. (1998). Timbral recognition and appraisal by adult cochlear implant users and normal-hearing adults. *Journal of the American Academy of Audiology, 9*(1), 1–19.

Gfeller, K., & Lansing, C. R. (1991). Melodic, rhythmic, and timbral perception of adult cochlear implant users. *Journal of Speech and Hearing Research, 34*(4), 916–920.

Gfeller, K., Oleson, J., Knutson, J. F., Breheny, P., Driscoll, V., & Olszewski, C. (2008). Multivariate predictors of music perception and appraisal by adult cochlear implant users. *Journal of the American Academy of Audiology, 19*(2), 120–134.

Gfeller, K. E., Olszewski, C., Turner, C., Gantz, B., & Oleson, J. (2006). Music perception with cochlear implants and residual hearing. *Audiology and Neurootology, 11*(Suppl. 1), 12–15.

Gfeller, K., Turner, C., Mehr, M., Woodworth, G., Fearn, R., Knutson, J. F., . . . Stordahl, J. (2002). Recognition of familiar melodies by adult cochlear implant recipients and normal-hearing adults. *Cochlear Implants International, 3*(1), 29–53.

Gfeller, K., Turner, C., Oleson, J., Zhang, X., Gantz, B., Froman, R., & Olszewski, C. (2007). Accuracy of cochlear implant recipients on pitch perception, melody recognition, and speech reception in noise. *Ear and Hearing, 28*(3), 412–423.

Gfeller, K., Woodworth, G., Robin, D. A., Witt, S., & Knutson, J. F. (1997). Perception of rhythmic and sequential pitch patterns by normally hearing adults and adult cochlear implant users. *Ear and Hearing, 18*(3), 252–260.

Gifford, R. H., Davis, T. J., Sunderhaus, L. W., Menapace, C., Buck, B., Crosson, J., . . . Segel, P. (2017). Combined electric and acoustic stimulation with hearing preservation: Effect of cochlear implant low-frequency cutoff on speech understanding and perceived listening difficulty. *Ear and Hearing, 38*(5), 539–553.

Gifford, R. H., Dorman, M. F., & Brown, C. A. (2010). Psychophysical properties of low-frequency hearing: Implications for perceiving speech and music via electric and acoustic stimulation. *Advances in Otorhinolaryngology, 67*, 51–60.

Gifford, R. H., Dorman, M. F., McKarns, S. A., & Spahr, A. J. (2007). Combined electric and contralateral acoustic hearing: Word and sentence recognition with bimodal hearing. *J Speech Lang Hearing Research, 50*(4), 835–843.

Gifford, R. H., Dorman, M. F., Shallop, J. K., & Sydlowski, S. A. (2010). Evidence for the expansion of adult cochlear implant candidacy. *Ear and Hearing, 31*(2), 186–194.

Gifford, R. H., Hedley-Williams, A., & Spahr, A. J. (2014). Clinical assessment of spectral modulation detection for adult cochlear implant recipients: A non-language based measure of performance outcomes. *International Journal of Audiology, 53*(3), 159–164.

Gifford, R. H., Shallop, J. K., & Peterson, A. M. (2008). Speech recognition materials and ceiling effects: Considerations for cochlear implant programs. *Audiology and Neurootology, 13*(3), 193–205.

Goehring, J. L., & Hughes, M. L. (2017). Measuring sound-processor threshold levels for pediatric cochlear implant recipients using conditioned play audiometry via telepractice. *Journal of Speech and Language Hearing Research, 60*(3), 732–740.

Gordon, K. A., Valero, J., van Hoesel, R., & Papsin, B. C. (2008). Abnormal timing delays in auditory brainstem responses evoked by bilateral cochlear implant use in children. *Otology and Neurotology, 29*(2), 193–198.

Gordon, K. A., Wong, D. D., & Papsin, B. C. (2013). Bilateral input protects the cortex from unilaterally-driven reorganization in children who are deaf. *Brain, 136*(Pt. 5), 1609–1625.

Govaerts, P. J. (2016). Expert opinion: Time to ban formal CI selection criteria? *Cochlear Implants International, 17*(Suppl. 1), 74–77.

Govaerts, P. J., Vaerenberg, B., De Ceulaer, G., Daemers, K., De Beukelaer, C., & Schauwers, K. (2010). Development of a software tool using deterministic logic for the optimization of cochlear implant processor programming. *Otology and Neurotology, 31*(6), 908–918.

Grieco-Calub, T. M., & Litovsky, R. Y. (2012). Spatial acuity in 2- to 3-year-old children with normal acoustic hearing, unilateral cochlear implants, and bilateral cochlear implants. *Ear and Hearing, 33*(5), 561–572.

Hansen, M. R., Gantz, B. J., & Dunn, C. (2013). Outcomes after cochlear implantation for patients with single-sided deafness, including those with recalcitrant Meniere's disease. *Otology and Neurotology, 34*(9), 1681–1687.

He, S., Teagle, H. F. B., & Buchman, C. A. (2017). The electrically evoked compound action potential: From laboratory to clinic. *Frontiers in Neuroscience, 11*, 339.

Helms, J., Weichbold, V., Baumann, U., von Specht, H., Schon, F., Muller, J., . . . D'Haese, P. (2004). Analysis of ceiling effects occurring with speech recognition tests in adult cochlear-implanted patients. *ORL Journal of Otorhinolaryngology and Related Specialties, 66*(3), 130–135.

Hernandez, V. H., Gehrt, A., Reuter, K., Jing, Z., Jeschke, M., Mendoza Schulz, A., . . . Moser, T. (2014). Optogenetic stimulation of the auditory pathway. *Journal of Clinical Investigation, 124*(3), 1114–1129.

Hoey, A. W., Pai, I., Driver, S., Connor, S., Wraige, E., & Jiang, D. (2017). Management and outcomes of cochlear implantation in patients with congenital cytomegalovirus (cCMV)-related deafness. *Cochlear Implants International, 18*(4), 216–225.

Holden, L. K., Finley, C. C., Firszt, J. B., Holden, T. A., Brenner, C., Potts, L. G., . . . Skinner, M. W. (2013). Factors affecting open-set word recognition in adults with cochlear implants. *Ear and Hearing, 34*(3), 342–360.

Hsiao, F. (2008). Mandarin melody recognition by pediatric cochlear implant recipients. *Journal of Music Therapy, 45*(4), 390–404.

Hsiao, F., & Gfeller, K. (2012). Music perception of cochlear implant recipients with implications for music instruction: A review of literature. *Update University South Carolina Department of Music, 30*(2), 5–10.

Huang, E. J., & Reichardt, L. F. (2001). Neurotrophins: roles in neuronal development and function. *Annual Review of Neuroscience, 24*, 677–736.

Hughes, M. L. (2008). A re-evaluation of the relation between physiological channel interaction and electrode pitch ranking in cochlear implants. *Journal of the Acoustical Society of America, 124*(5), 2711–2714.

Hughes, M. L., Abbas, P. J. (2006). The relation between electrophysiologic channel interaction and electrode pitch ranking in cochlear implant recipients. *Journal of the Acoustical Society of America, 119*, 1527–1537.

International Organization for Standardization (ISO) 5841-2:2014. (2014, August). *Implants for surgery—cardiac pacemakers—Part 2: Reporting of clinical performance of populations of pulse generators or leads.* Retrieved February 6, 2018, from https://www.iso.org/standard/60541.html

Ishiyama, A., Doherty, J., Ishiyama, G., Quesnel, A. M., Lopez, I., & Linthicum, F. H. (2016). Post hybrid cochlear implant hearing loss and endolymphatic hydrops. *Otology and Neurotology, 37*(10), 1516–1521.

Ito, J., Nakatake, M., & Fujita, S. (1999). Hearing ability by telephone of patients with cochlear implants. *Otolaryngology-Head and Neck Surgery, 121*(6), 802–804.

Izzo, A. D., Richter, C. P., Jansen, E. D., & Walsh, J. T., Jr. (2006). Laser stimulation of the auditory nerve. *Lasers in Surgery and Medicine, 38*(8), 745–753.

Izzo, A. D., Walsh, J. T., Jr., Ralph, H., Webb, J., Bendett, M., Wells, J., & Richter, C. P. (2008). Laser stimulation of auditory neurons: Effect of shorter pulse duration and penetration depth. *Biophysical Journal, 94*(8), 3159–3166.

Jiang, J., Dong, Y., Huang, W., & Bao, M. (2017). General anesthesia exposure and risk of dementia: A meta-analysis of epidemiological studies. *Oncotarget, 8*(35), 59628–59637.

Kallweit, N., Baumhoff, P., Krueger, A., Tinne, N., Kral, A., Ripken, T., & Maier, H. (2016). Optoacoustic effect is responsible for laser-induced cochlear responses. *Scientific Report, 6*, 28141.

Kang, R., Nimmons, G. L., Drennan, W., Longnion, J., Ruffin, C., Nie, K., . . . Rubinstein, J. (2009). Development and validation of the University of Washington Clinical Assessment of Music Perception test. *Ear and Hearing, 30*(4), 411–418.

Kerber, S., & Seeber, B. U. (2012). Sound localization in noise by normal-hearing listeners and cochlear implant users. *Ear and Hearing, 33*(4), 445–457.

Kong, Y. Y., Cruz, R., Jones, J. A., & Zeng, F. G. (2004). Music perception with temporal cues in acoustic and electric hearing. *Ear and Hearing, 25*(2), 173–185.

Kraaijenga, V. J. C., Ramakers, G. G. J., Smulders, Y. E., van Zon, A., Stegeman, I., Smit, A. L., . . . Grolman, W. (2017). Objective and subjective measures of simultaneous vs sequential bilateral cochlear implants in adults: A randomized clinical trial. *JAMA Otolaryngology-Head and Neck Surgery, 143*(9), 881–890.

Kral, A., Heid, S., Hubka, P., & Tillein, J. (2013). Unilateral hearing during development: Hemispheric specificity in plastic reorganizations. *Frontiers in Systems Neuroscience, 7*, 93.

Kuzovkov, V., Yanov, Y., Levin, S., Bovo, R., Rosignoli, M., Eskilsson, G., & Willbas, S. (2014). Remote programming of MED-EL cochlear implants: users' and professionals' evaluation of the remote programming experience. *Acta Otolaryngologica, 134*(7), 709–716.

Laaman, S., & Rutledge, J. (2012). *Cochlear*. Morgan Stanley Research, November 28.

Labadie, R. F., Noble, J. H., Hedley-Williams, A. J., Sunderhaus, L. W., Dawant, B. M., & Gifford, R. H. (2016). Results of postoperative, CT-based, electrode deactivation on hearing in prelingually deafened adult cochlear implant recipients. *Otology and Neurotology, 37*(2), 137–145.

Landsberger, D. M., Svrakic, M., Roland, J. T., Jr., & Svirsky, M. (2015). The relationship between insertion angles, default frequency allocations, and spiral ganglion place pitch in cochlear implants. *Ear and Hearing, 36*(5), e207–e213.

Lee, D. S., Lee, J. S., Oh, S. H., Kim, S., Kim, J., Chung, J., Lee, M. C., & Kim, C. S. (2001). Deafness: Cross-modal plasticity and cochlear implants. *Nature, 409*, 149–150.

Levi, J., Ames, J., Bacik, K., Drake, C., Morlet, T., & O'Reilly, R. C. (2013). Clinical characteristics of children with cochlear nerve dysplasias. *Laryngoscope, 123*(3), 752–756.

Li, N., & Loizou, P. C. (2008). Effect of spectral resolution on the intelligibility of ideal binary masked speech. *Journal of the Acoustical Society of America, 123*(4), EL59–64.

Limb, C. J., & Rubinstein, J. T. (2012). Current research on music perception in cochlear implant users. *Otolaryngology Clinics of North America, 45*(1), 129–140.

Lin, F. R., Niparko, J. K., & Ferrucci, L. (2011). Hearing loss prevalence in the United States. *Archives in Internal Medicine, 171*(20), 1851–1852.

Litovsky, R. Y., Johnstone, P. M., Godar, S., Agrawal, S., Parkinson, A., Peters, R., & Lake, J. (2006). Bilateral cochlear implants in children: Localization acuity measured with minimum audible angle. *Ear and Hearing, 27*(1), 43–59.

Litovsky, R. Y., Parkinson, A., & Arcaroli, J. (2009). Spatial hearing and speech intelligibility in bilateral cochlear implant users. *Ear and Hearing, 30*(4), 419–431.

Litovsky, R. Y., Johnstone, P. M., & Godar, S. P. (2006). Benefits of bilateral cochlear implants and/or hearing aids in children. *International Journal of Audiology, 45*(Suppl. 1), S78–91.

Litovsky, R. Y., Parkinson, A., Arcaroli, J., Peters, R., Lake, J., Johnstone, P., & Yu, G. (2004). Bilateral cochlear implants in adults and children. *Archives of Otolaryngology-Head and Neck Surgery, 130*(5), 648–655.

Litovsky, R., Parkinson, A., Arcaroli, J., & Sammeth, C. (2006). Simultaneous bilateral cochlear implantation in adults: A multicenter clinical study. *Ear and Hearing, 27*(6), 714–731.

Loiselle, L. H., Dorman, M. F., Yost, W. A., Cook, S. J., & Gifford, R. H. (2016). Using ILD or ITD cues for sound source localization and speech understanding in a complex listening environment by listeners with bilateral and with hearing-preservation cochlear implants. *Journal of Speech Language and Hearing Research, 59*(4), 810–818.

Loiselle, L. H., Dorman, M. F., Yost, W. A., & Gifford, R. H. (2015). Sound source localization by hearing preservation patients with and without symmetrical low-frequency acoustic hearing. *Audiology and Neurootology, 20*(3), 166–171.

Looi, V., Gfeller, K., & Driscoll, V. (2012). Music appreciation and training for cochlear implant recipients: A review. *Seminars in Hearing, 33*(4), 307–334.

Looi, V., McDermott, H., McKay, C., & Hickson, L. (2008a). Music perception of cochlear implant users compared with that of hearing aid users. *Ear and Hearing, 29*(3), 421–434.

Looi, V., McDermott, H., McKay, C., & Hickson, L. (2008b). The effect of cochlear implantation on music perception by adults with usable pre-operative acoustic hearing. *International Journal of Audiology, 47*(5), 257–268.

Maurer, J., Marangos, N., & Ziegler, E. (2005). Reliability of cochlear implants. *Otolaryngology-Head and Neck Surgery, 132*(5), 746–750.

McDermott, H. J. (2004). Music perception with cochlear implants: A review. *Trends in Amplification, 8*(2), 49–82.

Meeuws, M., Pascoal, D., Bermejo, I., Artaso, M., De Ceulaer, G., & Govaerts, P. J. (2017). Computer-assisted CI fitting: Is the learning capacity of the intelligent agent FOX beneficial for speech understanding? *Cochlear Implants International, 18*(4), 198–206.

Mills, A. W. (1958). On the minimum audible angle. *Journal of the Acoustical Society of America, 30*(4), 237.

Moller, A. R. (2001). Neurophysiologic basis for cochlear and auditory brainstem implants. *American Journal of Audiology, 10*(2), 68–77.

Moller, A. R. (2013). *Hearing: Anatomy, physiology, and disorders of the auditory system* (3rd ed.). San Diego: Plural Publishing, Inc.

Moore, B. C., Glasberg, B. R., & Stone, M. A. (2004). New version of the TEN test with calibrations in dB HL. *Ear and Hearing, 25*(5), 478–487.

Moore, B. C., Huss, M., Vickers, D. A., Glasberg, B. R., & Alcantara, J. I. (2000). A test for the diagnosis of dead regions in the cochlea. *British Journal of Audiology, 34*(4), 205–224.

Morera, C., Manrique, M., Ramos, A., Garcia-Ibanez, L., Cavalle, L., Huarte, A., . . . Estrada, E. (2005). Advantages of binaural hearing provided through bimodal stimulation via a cochlear implant and a conventional hearing aid: A 6-month comparative study. *Acta Otolaryngologica, 125*(6), 596–606.

Mortensen, M. V., Mirz, F., & Gjedde, A. (2006). Restored speech comprehension linked to activity in left inferior prefrontal and right temporal cortices in postlingual deafness. *Neuroimage, 31*(2), 842–852.

Mosnier, I., Sterkers, O., Bebear, J. P., Godey, B., Robier, A., Deguine, O., . . . Ferrary, E. (2009). Speech performance and sound localization in a complex noisy environment in bilaterally implanted adult patients. *Audiology and Neurootology, 14*(2), 106–114.

Moxon, E. C. (1971). *Neural and mechanical responses to electrical stimulation of the cat's inner ear.* Ph.D. thesis, MIT, Cambridge, MA.

Mueller, H. G., & Bentler, R. A. (2005). Fitting hearing aids using clinical measures of loudness discomfort levels: An evidence-based review of effectiveness. *Journal of the American Academy of Audiology, 16*(7), 461–472.

Mukherjee, P., Uzun-Coruhlu, H., Wong, C. C., Curthoys, I. S., Jones, A. S., & Gibson, W. P. (2012). Assessment of intracochlear trauma caused by the insertion of a new straight research array. *Cochlear Implants International, 13*(3), 156–162.

Musgrave, E., Wolfe, J., Duke, M., & Neumann, Z. (2015). Presented at American Cochlear Implant Alliance meeting on October 17, 2015 in Washington, D.C.

Nakano, A., Arimoto, Y., & Matsunaga, T. (2013). Cochlear nerve deficiency and associated clinical features in patients with bilateral and unilateral hearing loss. *Otology and Neurotology, 34*(3), 554–558.

Nassetta, L., Kimberlin, D., & Whitley, R. (2009). Treatment of congenital cytomegalovirus infection: Implications for future therapeutic strategies. *Journal of Antimicrobial Chemotherapy, 63*(5), 862–867.

Nimmons, G. L., Kang, R. S., Drennan, W. R., Longnion, J., Ruffin, C., Worman, T., . . . Rubenstein, J. T. (2008). Clinical assessment of music perception in cochlear implant listeners. *Otology and Neurotology, 29*(2), 149–155.

Noble, J. H., Gifford, R. H., Hedley-Williams, A. J., Dawant, B. M., & Labadie, R. F. (2014). Clinical evaluation of an image-guided cochlear implant programming strategy. *Audiology and Neurootology, 19*(6), 400–411.

Noble, J. H., Hedley-Williams, A. J., Sunderhaus, L., Dawant, B. M., Labadie, R. F., Camarata, S. M., & Gifford, R. H. (2016). Initial results with image-guided cochlear implant programming in children. *Otology and Neurotology, 37*(2), e63–e69.

Nopp, P., Schleich, P., & D'Haese, P. (2004). Sound localization in bilateral users of MED-EL COMBI 40/40+ cochlear implants. *Ear and Hearing, 25*(3), 205–214.

O'Connell, B. P., Cakir, A., Hunter, J. B., Francis, D. O., Noble, J. H., Labadie, R. F., . . . Wanna, G. B. (2016). Electrode location and angular insertion depth are predictors of audiologic outcomes in cochlear implantation. *Otology and Neurotology, 37*(8), 1016–1023.

O'Connell, B. P., Holcomb, M. A., Morrison, D., Meyer, T. A., & White, D. R. (2016). Safety of cochlear implantation before 12 months of age: Medical University of South Carolina and Pediatric American College of Surgeons-National Surgical Quality improvement program outcomes. *Laryngoscope, 126*(3), 707–712.

Oyler, F., Oyler, A. L., & Matkin, N. D. (1988). Unilateral hearing loss: Demographics and educational impact. *Language, Speech, and Hearing Services in Schools, 19*, 201–210.

Peters, B. R., Litovsky, R., Parkinson, A., & Lake, J. (2007). Importance of age and postimplantation experience on speech perception measures in children with sequential bilateral cochlear implants. *Otology and Neurotology, 28*(5), 649–657.

Pinyon, J. L., Tadros, S. F., Froud, K. E., Wong, A. C. Y., W., Thompson, I. T., Crawford, E. N., . . . Housley, G. D. (2014). Close-field electroporation gene delivery using the Cochlear implant electrode array enhances the bionic ear. *Science Translational Medicine, 6*(233), 233ra254.

Plant, K. L., van Hoesel, R. J., McDermott, H. J., Dawson, P. W., & Cowan, R. S. (2015). Clinical outcomes for adult cochlear implant recipients experiencing loss of usable acoustic hearing in the implanted ear. *Ear and Hearing, 36*(3), 338–356.

Potts, L. G., Skinner, M. W., Litovsky, R. A., Strube, M. J., & Kuk, F. (2009). Recognition and localization of speech by adult cochlear implant recipients wearing a digital hearing aid in the nonimplanted ear (bimodal hearing). *Journal of the American Academy of Audiology, 20*(6), 353–373.

Qin, M. K., & Oxenham, A. J. (2006). Effects of introducing unprocessed low-frequency information on the reception of envelope-vocoder processed speech. *Journal of the Acoustical Society of America, 119*(4), 2417–2426.

Ramekers, D., Versnel, H., Strahl, S. B., Klis, S. F., & Grolman, W. (2015). Temporary neurotrophin treatment prevents deafness-induced auditory nerve degeneration and preserves function. *Journal of Neuroscience, 35*(36), 12331–12345.

Ramos, A., Rodriguez, C., Martinez-Beneyto, P., Perez, D., Gault, A., Falcon, J. C., & Boyle, P. (2009). Use of telemedicine in the remote programming of cochlear implants. *Acta Otolaryngologica, 129*(5), 533–540.

Ramsden, J. D., Papsin, B. C., Leung, R., James, A., & Gordon, K. A. (2009). Bilateral simultaneous cochlear implantation in children: Our first 50 cases. *Laryngoscope, 119*(12), 2444–2448.

Reeder, R. M., Firszt, J. B., Cadieux, J. H., & Strube, M. J. (2017). A longitudinal study in children with sequential bilateral cochlear implants: Time course for the second implanted ear and bilateral performance. *Journal of Speech Language and Hearing Research, 60*(1), 276–287.

Reeder, R. M., Firszt, J. B., Holden, L. K., & Strube, M. J. (2014). A longitudinal study in adults with sequential bilateral cochlear implants: Time course for individual ear and bilateral performance. *Journal of Speech Language and Hearing Research, 57*(3), 1108–1126.

Santa Maria, P. L., Gluth, M. B., Yuan, Y., Atlas, M. D., & Blevins, N. H. (2014). Hearing preservation surgery for cochlear implantation: A meta-analysis. *Otology and Neurotology, 35*(10), e256–e269.

Santa Maria, P. L., & Oghalai, J. S. (2014). When is the best timing for the second implant in pediatric bilateral cochlear implantation? *Laryngoscope, 124*(7), 1511–1512.

Schafer, E. C., Amlani, A. M., Paiva, D., Nozari, L., & Verret, S. (2011). A meta-analysis to compare speech recognition in noise with bilateral cochlear implants and bimodal stimulation. *International Journal of Audiology, 50*(12), 871–880.

Schafer, E. C., Amlani, A. M., Seibold, A., & Shattuck, P. L. (2007). A meta-analytic comparison of binaural benefits between bilateral cochlear implants and bimodal stimulation. *Journal of the American Academy of Audiology, 18*(9), 760–776.

Schafer, E. C., & Thibodeau, L. M. (2003). Speech recognition performance of children using cochlear implants and FM systems. *Journal of Educational Audiology, 11*, 15–26.

Schafer, E. C., & Thibodeau, L. M. (2004). Speech recognition abilities of adults using cochlear implants interfaced with FM systems. *Journal of the American Academy of Audiology, 15*(10), 678–691.

Schafer, E. C., & Thibodeau, L. M. (2006). Speech recognition in noise in children with cochlear implants while listening in bilateral, bimodal, and FM-system arrangements. *American Journal of Audiology, 15*(2), 114–126.

Schafer, E. C., Wolfe, J., Lawless, T., & Stout, B. (2009). Effects of FM-receiver gain on speech-recognition performance of adults with cochlear implants. *International Journal of Audiology, 48*(4), 196–203.

Schleich, P., Nopp, P., & D'Haese, P. (2004). Head shadow, squelch, and summation effects in bilateral users of the MED-EL COMBI 40/40+ cochlear implant. *Ear and Hearing, 25*(3), 197–204.

Seeber, B. U., Baumann, U., & Fastl, H. (2004). Localization ability with bimodal hearing aids and bilateral cochlear implants. *Journal of the Acoustical Society of America, 116*(3), 1698–1709.

Shallop, J., Arndt, P., & Turnacliff, K. (1992). Expanded indications for cochlear implantation: Perceptual results in seven adults with residual hearing. *Journal of Speech-Language Pathology and Applied Behavior Analysis, 16*, 141–148.

Sheffield, S. W., & Gifford, R. H. (2014). The benefits of bimodal hearing: Effect of frequency region and acoustic bandwidth. *Audiology and Neurootology, 19*(3), 151–163.

Sheffield, S. W., Jahn, K., & Gifford, R. H. (2015). Preserved acoustic hearing in cochlear implantation improves speech perception. *Journal of the American Academy of Audiology, 26*(2), 145–154.

Simmons, F. B. (1966). Electrical stimulation of the auditory nerve in man. *Archives of Otolaryngology, 84*(1), 2e54.

Sladen, D. P., Carlson, M. L., Dowling, B. P., Olund, A. P., Teece, K., DeJong, M. D., . . . Driscoll, C. L. (2017). Early outcomes after cochlear implantation for adults and children with unilateral hearing loss. *Laryngoscope, 127*(7), 1683–1688.

Sladen, D. P., Frisch, C. D., Carlson, M. L., Driscoll, C. L., Torres, J. H., & Zeitler, D. M. (2017). Cochlear implantation for single-sided deafness: A multicenter study. *Laryngoscope, 127*(1), 223–228.

Smulders, Y. E., van Zon, A., Stegeman, I., Rinia, A. B., Van Zanten, G. A., Stokroos, R. J., . . . Grolman, W. (2016). Comparison of bilateral and unilateral cochlear implantation in adults: A randomized clinical trial. *JAMA Otolaryngology-Head and Neck Surgery, 142*(3), 249–256.

Smulders, Y. E., van Zon, A., Stegeman, I., van Zanten, G. A., Rinia, A. B., Stokroos, R. J., . . . Grolman, W. (2016). Cost-utility of bilateral versus unilateral cochlear implantation in adults: A randomized controlled trial. *Otology and Neurotology, 37*(1), 38–45.

Spahr, A. J., Dorman, M. F., & Loiselle, L. H. (2007). Performance of patients using different cochlear implant systems: Effects of input dynamic range. *Ear and Hearing, 28*(2), 260–275.

Sparreboom, M., Beynon, A. J., Snik, A. F., & Mylanus, E. A. (2010). Electrically evoked auditory brainstem responses in children with sequential bilateral cochlear implants. *Otology and Neurotology, 31*(7), 1055–1061.

Spoendlin, H. (1975). Retrograde degeneration of the cochlear nerve. *Acta Otolaryngologica, 79*(3–4), 266–275.

Stordahl, J. (2002). Song recognition and appraisal: a comparison of children who use cochlear implants and normally hearing children. *Journal of Music Therapy, 39*(1), 2–19.

Sucher, C. M., & McDermott, H. J. (2007). Pitch ranking of complex tones by normally hearing subjects and cochlear implant users. *Hearing Research, 230*(1–2), 80–87.

Tavora-Vieira, D., & Rajan, G. P. (2015). Cochlear implantation in children with congenital and noncongenital unilateral deafness. *Otology and Neurotology, 36*(8), 1457–1458.

Thibodeau, L. (2010). Benefits of adaptive FM systems on speech recognition in noise for listeners who use hearing aids. *American Journal of Audiology, 19*(1), 36–45.

Thomas, J. P., Neumann, K., Dazert, S., & Voelter, C. (2017). Cochlear implantation in children with congenital single-sided deafness. *Otology and Neurotology, 38*(4), 496–503.

Tong, Y. C., Black, R. C., Clark, G. M., Forster, I. C., Millar, J. B., O'Loughlin, B. J., & Patrick, J. F. (1979). A preliminary report on a multiple-channel cochlear implant operation. *Journal of Laryngology and Otology, 93*, 679e695.

Tong, Y. C., & Clark, G. M. (1985). Absolute identification of electric pulse rates and electrode positions by cochlear implant patients. *Journal of the Acoustical Society of America, 77*, e1881–e1888.

Tyler, R. S., Gantz, B. J., Rubinstein, J. T., Wilson, B. S., Parkinson, A. J., Wolaver, A., . . . Lowder, M. W. (2002). Three-month results with bilateral cochlear implants. *Ear and Hearing, 23*(1 Suppl.), 80S–89S.

Tyler, R. S., Parkinson, A. J., Wilson, B. S., Witt, S., Preece, J. P., & Noble, W. (2002). Patients utilizing a hearing aid and a cochlear implant: speech perception and localization. *Ear and Hearing, 23*(2), 98–105.

Vaerenberg, B., Govaerts, P. J., de Ceulaer, G., Daemers, K., & Schauwers, K. (2011). Experiences of the use of FOX, an intelligent agent, for programming cochlear implant sound processors in new users. *International Journal of Audiology, 50*(1), 50–58.

van der Beek, F. B., Briaire, J. J., & Frijns, J. H. (2012). Effects of parameter manipulations on spread of excitation measured with electrically-evoked compound action potentials. *International Journal of Audiology, 51*(6), 465–474.

van Hoesel, R. J. (2004). Exploring the benefits of bilateral cochlear implants. *Audiology and Neurootology, 9*(4), 234–246.

van Hoesel, R. J., & Tyler, R. S. (2003). Speech perception, localization, and lateralization with bilateral cochlear implants. *Journal of the Acoustical Society of America, 113*(3), 1617–1630.

van Hoesel, R., Ramsden, R., & Odriscoll, M. (2002). Sound-direction identification, interaural time delay discrimination, and speech intelligibility advantages in noise for a bilateral cochlear implant user. *Ear and Hearing, 23*(2), 137–149.

Vermeire, K., & Van de Heyning, P. (2009). Binaural hearing after cochlear implantation in subjects with unilateral sensorineural deafness and tinnitus. *Audiology and Neurootology, 14*(3), 163–171.

Vincent, C., Arndt, S., Firszt, J. B., Fraysse, B., Kitterick, P. T., Papsin, B. C., . . . Marx, M. (2015). Identification and evaluation of cochlear implant candidates with asymmetrical hearing loss. *Audiology and Neurootology, 20*(Suppl. 1), 87–89.

Vincent, C., Bebear, J. P., Radafy, E., Vaneecloo, F. M., Ruzza, I., Lautissier, S., & Bordure, P. (2012). Bilateral cochlear implantation in children: Localization and hearing in noise benefits. *International Journal of Pediatric Otorhinolaryngology, 76*(6), 858–864.

Vongpaisal, T., Trehub, S. E., & Schellenberg, E. G. (2006). Song recognition by children and adolescents with cochlear implants. *Journal of Speech and Language Hearing Research, 49*(5), 1091–1103.

Vroegop, J. L., Dingemanse, J. G., van der Schroeff, M. P., Metselaar, R. M., & Goedegebure, A. (2017). Self-adjustment of upper electrical stimulation levels in CI programming and the effect on auditory functioning. *Ear and Hearing, 38*(4), e232–e240.

Wackym, P. A., Runge-Samuelson, C. L., Firszt, J. B., Alkaf, F. M., & Burg, L. S. (2007). More challenging speech-perception tasks demonstrate binaural benefit in bilateral cochlear implant users. *Ear and Hearing, 28*(2 Suppl.), 80S–85S.

Wanna, G. B., Noble, J. H., Carlson, M. L., Gifford, R. H., Dietrich, M. S., Haynes, D. S., . . . Labadie, R. F. (2014). Impact of electrode design and surgical approach on scalar location and cochlear implant outcomes. *Laryngoscope, 124*(Suppl. 6), S1–S7.

Wanna, G. B., Noble, J. H., Gifford, R. H., Dietrich, M. S., Sweeney, A. D., Zhang, D., . . . Labadie, R. F. (2015). Impact of intrascalar electrode location, electrode type, and angular insertion depth on residual hearing in cochlear implant patients: Preliminary results. *Otology and Neurotology, 36*(8), 1343–1348.

Weber, S., Gavaghan, K., Wimmer, W., Williamson, T., Gerber, N., Anso, J., Bell, B., . . .Caversaccio, M. (2017, March). Instrument flight to the inner ear. *Science Robotics, 2*(4).

Wolfe, J. (2014). *Benefit of bilateral hearing technology for understanding speech over the telephone.* Presented at the American Cochlear Implant Alliance Meeting, December 11, 2014, Nashville, Tennessee.

Wolfe, J., Baker, S., Caraway, T., Kasulis, H., Mears, A., Smith, J., . . . Wood, M. (2007). 1-year postactivation results for sequentially implanted bilateral cochlear implant users. *Otology and Neurotology, 28*(5), 589–596.

Wolfe, J., Morais, M., & Schafer, E. (2015). Improving hearing performance for cochlear implant recipients with use of a digital, wireless, remote-microphone, audio-streaming accessory. *Journal of the American Academy of Audiology, 26*(6), 532–539.

Wolfe, J., Morais, M., & Schafer, E. (2016a). Speech recognition of bimodal cochlear implant recipients using a wireless audio streaming accessory for the telephone. *Otology and Neurotology, 37*(2), e20–25.

Wolfe, J., Morais Duke, M., Schafer, E., Cire, G., Menapace, C., & O'Neill, L. (2016b). Evaluation of a wireless audio streaming accessory to improve mobile telephone performance of cochlear implant users. *International Journal of Audiology, 55*(2), 75–82.

Wolfe, J., Morais, M., Schafer, E., Mills, E., Mulder, H. E., Goldbeck, F., . . . Lianos, L. (2013). Evaluation of speech recognition of cochlear implant recipients using a personal digital adaptive radio frequency system. *Journal of the American Academy of Audiology, 24*(8), 714–724.

Wolfe, J., Parkinson, A., Schafer, E. C., Gilden, J., Rehwinkel, K., Mansanares, J., . . . Gannaway, S. (2012). Benefit of a commercially available cochlear implant processor with dual-microphone beamforming: A multi-center study. *Otology and Neurotology, 33*(4), 553–560.

Wolfe, J., & Schafer, E. C. (2008). Optimizing the benefit of sound processors coupled to personal FM systems. *Journal of the American Academy of Audiology, 19*(8), 585–594.

Wolfe, J., Schafer, E. C., Heldner, B., Mulder, H., Ward, E., & Vincent, B. (2009). Evaluation of speech recognition in noise with cochlear implants and dynamic FM. *Journal of the American Academy of Audiology, 20*(7), 409–421.

Wolfe, J., Schafer, E. C., John, A., & Hudson, M. (2011). The effect of front-end processing on cochlear implant performance of children. *Otology and Neurotology, 32*(4), 533–538.

Yoshida, H., Takahashi, H., Kanda, Y., Kitaoka, K., & Hara, M. (2017). Long-term outcomes of cochlear implantation in children with congenital cytomegalovirus infection. *Otology and Neurotology, 38*(7), e190–e194.

Zeitler, D. M., Budenz, C. L., & Roland, J. T., Jr. (2009). Revision cochlear implantation. *Current Opinion in Otolaryngology-Head and Neck Surgery, 17*(5), 334–338.

Zhang, J., Xu, K., Simaan, N., & Manolidis, S. (2006). A pilot study of robot-assisted cochlear implant surgery using steerable electrode arrays. *Medical Image Computing and Computer-Assisted Intervention, 9*(Pt 1), 33–40.

Zhang, T., Dorman, M. F., Gifford, R., & Moore, B. C. (2014). Cochlear dead regions constrain the benefit of combining acoustic stimulation with electric stimulation. *Ear and Hearing, 35*(4), 410–417.

Factors Affecting the Outcomes of Adults with Cochlear Implants

Jace Wolfe

Introduction

Research has identified several factors that may influence the outcomes adults achieve after cochlear implantation. Example of factors that have been shown to affect cochlear implant outcomes include but are not limited to duration of severe to profound hearing loss, location of the electrode array within the cochlea, age at implantation, etiology of the hearing loss, and preoperative aided speech recognition (Blamey et al., 2103; Holden et al., 2013; Holden et al., 2016; Lazard et al., 2012; Plant et al., 2015; Roditi et al., 2009; Rubenstein et al., 1999; Zwolan et al., 2014). Although several factors have been shown to impact cochlear implant outcomes in adults, it should also be noted that research studies have found a great amount of intersubject variability in cochlear implant outcomes and that the variability cannot be fully explained or predicted by preimplant factors (Blamey et al., 1996; Blamey et al., 2013; Dowell et al., 2004; Gifford et al., 2008; Heydebrand et al., 2007; Lazard et al., 2012; Roditi et al., 2009; Shea et al., 1990; Summerfield & Marshall, 1995; Waltzman et al., 1995). For example, for a group of 143 experienced adult unilateral cochlear implant recipients, Gifford et al. (2008) reported mean speech recognition scores of 84.8%, 55.7%, and 72.1% correct on the HINT sentence test in quiet, CNC monosyllabic word test, and AzBio sentence test in quiet, respectively. However,

the range of speech recognition scores for these 143 recipients ranged from approximately 15% to 100% correct, 15% to 95% correct, and 10% to 98% correct for the HINT, CNC, and AzBio tests, respectively. Additionally, research studies examining the factors that affect cochlear implant outcomes have reported that anywhere from 10% to 80% of the intersubject variance in postoperative speech recognition scores can be explained by preimplant factors (Blamey et al., 2013; Lazard et al., 2012; Roditi et al., 2009; Waltzman et al., 1995). This chapter will provide a review of numerous factors that may influence outcomes adults achieve with cochlear implant technology. The first section of this chapter will provide a summary of several landmark studies that have explored the factors that affect the outcomes of a relatively large number of adult cochlear implant recipients. The second section of this chapter will highlight specific factors that have been shown to influence the outcomes of adult cochlear implant recipients and provide detailed information regarding the effect of these factors on cochlear implant outcomes.

A Review of Studies Examining Factors That Influence Cochlear Implant Outcomes of Adults

The following section will summarize several recent studies that have explored the factors that influence the outcomes of adult cochlear implant recipients.

Residual Speech Recognition and Cochlear Implant Performance: Effects of Implantation Criteria—Rubinstein et al., 1999

Rubinstein and colleagues (1999) conducted a landmark study examining factors that predict postimplant speech recognition. Specifically, Rubinstein et al. explored the relationship between postimplant CNC word recognition (in the unilateral condition) and preimplant aided Central Institute of the Deaf (CID) sentence recognition in quiet and duration of deafness. Rubinstein reported that better preimplant aided CID sentence scores were associated with better postimplant CNC word recognition scores. Also, participants with a shorter duration of deafness typically obtained better postimplant CNC word recognition scores. However, it should be noted that the extremes of the data sets were responsible for these correlations. For instance, when preimplant aided CID sentence recognition scores of 0% were removed from the analysis, there was not a significant relationship between preimplant CID sentence recognition and postimplant CNC word recognition. Likewise, when participants with a duration of deafness of greater than 20 years were removed from the analysis, there was not a significant relationship between duration of deafness and postimplant CNC word recognition. In summary, Rubinstein and colleagues concluded that a lengthy duration of deafness (i.e., exceeding 20 years) was predictive of limited word recognition capacity after cochlear implantation. They also concluded that better preimplant speech recognition was suggestive of a prognosis of good postimplant speech recognition. Rubinstein et al. hypothesized that cochlear implant candidates with a shorter duration of deafness and better aided preimplant speech recognition were more likely to have a larger contingent of functioning spiral ganglion cells.

Predictors of Audiological Outcome Following Cochlear Implantation in Adults—Green et al., 2007

Green and colleagues (2007) evaluated the potential relationship between several different pre- and postimplant factors and postimplant sentence recognition for 117 postlingually deafened adult cochlear implant recipients. There was no relevant relationship between postimplant sentence recognition and gender, age at implantation, etiology of hearing loss, preoperative hearing sensitivity, implant brand, signal coding strategy, and the number of intracochlear electrodes inserted into the cochlea. The only factor that was shown to influence postimplant sentence recognition was the duration of deafness. Specifically, recipients with a longer duration of profound deafness generally had poorer speech recognition with their cochlear implant. Of note, however, there was a wide spread of results for participants who had a duration of deafness of less than 20 years, whereas the recipients who had a duration of deafness exceeding 20 years typically achieved poor sentence recognition with their cochlear implant. Additionally, there appeared to be no relationship between duration of deafness and postimplant speech recognition for the participants whose duration of deafness was less than 20 years. Of note, the duration of deafness only accounted for 9% of the variability in sentence recognition observed for the group. Green and colleagues concluded that other factors (e.g., auditory processing, auditory nervous system changes) likely contributed to the large amount of variability observed across participants.

Factors Affecting Auditory Performance of Postlinguistically Deaf Adults Using Cochlear Implants: An Update with 2251 Patients—Blamey et al., 2013

Blamey et al. (2013) reported on the largest study examining pre- and postimplant factors that affect performance of adult cochlear implant recipients. This study explored the outcomes of 2251 postlingually deafened adult cochlear implant recipients who were served across multiple cochlear implant centers located in multiple countries. Of note, this study served as an update to an earlier study that was published in 1996 and that also examined factors that influence postimplant word recognition performance (Blamey et al., 1996). The earlier Blamey (1996) study found that the largest factor affecting postimplant speech recognition outcomes was the duration of deafness. Poorer postimplant scores were also generally found for recipients who were older at implantation and for recipients with hearing loss caused by bacterial meningitis.

In the Blamey et al. (2013) study, better postimplant speech recognition was associated with a shorter duration of deafness, a younger age at implantation, longer experience with the cochlear implant, and a younger age at the onset of severe to profound hearing loss. Specifically, Blamey and colleagues found that a duration of deafness longer than 20 years was typically associated with poorer outcomes but that the negative effect of duration of deafness was not as detrimental as it was in the earlier (1996) study, a finding they attributed to improvements in cochlear implant technology and surgical practices as well as to improvements in hearing aid technology for persons with significant hearing loss. Blamey et al. also noted that poorer implant outcomes were observed for persons over 65 years of age, but they also pointed out that most of the older participants did receive considerable improvement in their speech recognition relative to the preimplant aided condition.

Blamey and colleagues also found that etiology affected postimplant outcomes. Better performance was generally found in recipients whose hearing loss was sudden/idiopathic, had a genetic cause, or was attributed to Meniere's disease, whereas poorer performance was found in recipients with hearing loss cause by temporal bone fracture, acoustic neuroma, and auditory neuropathy. The negative effect of bacterial meningitis was not as great as what was observed in the 1996 study, a fact that Blamey et al. attributed to the clinical practice of earlier provision of a cochlear implant for those whose deafness is caused by meningitis.

Finally, Blamey and colleagues noted that performance improved throughout the first 3.5 years of implant use with the majority of this improvement occurring within the first 12 months of use. Of note, Blamey and colleagues reported that the factors included in their predictive model only accounted for 10% of the variability observed in the performance of this large group of adult implant recipients. They hypothesized that the unexplained variability may have been partially attributed to differences that are likely to exist in auditory processing, in the auditory nervous system, and in cognitive abilities of the participants. Blamey et al. theorized that central effects were probably more likely to explain variability in implant outcomes than were differences in peripheral auditory status (e.g., spiral ganglion survival). Blamey and colleagues also acknowledged that additional factors that were unaccounted for in their study, such as hearing aid use, implant brand, duration of moderate hearing loss, and so forth, may have also impacted implant outcomes.

In an analysis of the same group of 2251 implant recipients, Lazard et al. (2012) explored the effect of a host of additional pre-, per-, and postimplant factors on speech recognition obtained with a unilateral cochlear implant. Lazard found the following to have a negative effect on postimplant speech recognition outcomes:

- Longer duration of severe to profound hearing loss
- Longer duration of moderate hearing loss
- Lack of or sporadic hearing aid use

- Poorer pure-tone average in the better ear
- Poorer pure-tone average in the implanted ear
- Older age at implantation
- Poorer preimplant speech recognition
- Larger number of disabled intracochlear electrode contacts
- Inappropriate insertion depth of electrode array

Of note, gender and level of education did not influence speech recognition achieved after cochlear implantation.

Again, Lazard and colleagues attributed poorer postimplant outcomes to deleterious changes in the auditory nervous system and in auditory processing abilities. They noted that the negative effects of auditory deprivation were at least partially offset by the consistent use of hearing aids, and they stressed the critical importance of prompt provision of well-fitted hearing aids with the onset of mild to moderate hearing loss. Additionally, Lazard et al. acknowledged the importance of cochlear implant function on postoperative outcome. The study results illustrated the importance of the surgical placement of the implant, because participants whose electrode arrays were inserted to an inappropriate depth performed more poorly. Also, recipients who had nonfunctioning electrodes tended to perform more poorly. Furthermore, Lazard and colleagues found that a significant difference in performance was a function of the manufacturer of the implant used by the participants. The brand type was anonymized, so no specific statements were made about the potential superiority of one type of cochlear implant system over its competitors, but the fact that different results were obtained as a function of implant brand does underscore the importance of cochlear implant technology. Of note, Lazard et al. acknowledged the fact that most of the participants have upgraded to newer external sound processors and were no longer using the sound processor that was used during study testing. As a result, the differences in performance across cochlear implant manufacturers may no longer exist with changes in sound processor technology.

Factors Affecting Open-Set Word Recognition in Adults with Cochlear Implants—Holden et al., 2013

Holden and colleagues sought to determine the sources of variability in cochlear implant outcomes by measuring CNC word recognition in 114 postlingually deafened adult unilateral cochlear implant recipients. Specifically, CNC word recognition was assessed at 2 weeks postimplantation and then at frequent intervals through the first two years of implant use. Holden et al. examined several recipient-specific factors such as age of implantation, cognitive status, educational level, duration of hearing loss, duration of deafness, hearing aid use, preimplant audiometric thresholds and speech recognition, and the like. Additionally, they explored the influence of audibility on cochlear implant speech recognition outcomes by measuring sound-field warbled tone detection thresholds obtained with use of the cochlear implant. Furthermore, a three-dimensional CT scan was completed with each participant to evaluate the scalar location of the electrode array as well as the distance of the electrode array from the modiolus.

The mean CNC word recognition score of the participants in the Holden et al. study was 61.5% correct, with one subject scoring above 90% correct and the lowest-performing subjects scoring near 10% correct. The CNC word recognition test was not routinely administered in the preoperative condition, but the mean score for the preoperatively administered HINT sentence test in quiet, which is generally considered to be far simpler than the CNC word test, was 16.4% correct. Of note, the CNC word score for the majority of the participants reached an asymptotic level at approximately 6 months postimplantation.

Holden and colleagues identified several recipient-specific factors that were associated with better postoperative CNC word recognition performance, including younger age at implantation (e.g., 65 years old and younger), shorter duration of hearing loss and of severe to profound hearing loss, better preoperative aided sentence recognition score, and consistent use of hearing aids prior to implantation. Moreover, higher cognitive abilities were associated with better word recognition with a cochlear implant, but it should be noted that a larger number of the older participants obtained lower scores on the cognitive measures. After controlling for the factor of age, cognitive ability was no longer a factor that influenced cochlear implant outcomes.

Clinician-related parameters also affected word recognition outcomes. Better CNC word recognition scores were typically obtained by the participants who had lower sound-field warbled tone detection thresholds with their cochlear implant. Of note, Holden et al. reported that throughout the study, the programming audiologists followed the cochlear implant program's typical policy of adjusting T levels, IDR, gain, and so forth for all participants in an attempt to obtain sound-field warbled tone detection thresholds of 30 dB HL or less.

Additionally, Holden and colleagues found that the position of the electrode array had a significant effect on word recognition scores. For instance, participants who had electrode arrays that were located more closely to the modiolus (i.e., perimodiolar placement) generally achieved better word recognition scores. Also, poorer word recognition scores were obtained for recipients who had intracochlear electrode contacts that were not located in the scala tympani (i.e., intracochlear electrode contact located in the scala vestibuli). Furthermore, poorer word recognition scores were generally obtained by recipients for whom the electrode array was inserted to a deeper depth than intended by the implant manufacturer.

Factors Affecting Outcomes in Cochlear Implant Recipients Implanted with a Perimodiolar Electrode Array Located in the Scala Tympani—Holden et al., 2016

In acknowledgment of the importance and impact of the proper placement of the electrode array within the scala tympani, Holden and colleagues (2016) conducted a follow-up study to identify the effect of audiologic and biographic factors on postimplant speech recognition for a group of 39 adult recipients (40 ears) for whom radiographic assessment confirmed that their perimodiolar electrode array was located entirely within the scala tympani. Holden et al. found no correlation between postimplant speech recognition in duration of severe to profound hearing loss, duration of hearing loss, preoperative aided speech recognition, preoperative pure-tone hearing loss, or duration of hearing aid use. The only factor that was found to be negatively correlated to postimplant speech recognition was the age at implantation. Holden and colleagues hypothesized that changes in auditory processing and cognitive decline associated with the aging process may be responsible for the poorer speech recognition observed for older participants. However, they also noted that the study participants who were older than 65 years of age had a mean preimplant CNC word score of 8.4% correct and a mean postimplant CNC word score of 72% correct. Although speech recognition may have been poorer for the older participants, it is obvious that the older participants did receive considerable benefit from cochlear implantation.

Holden et al. acknowledged the fact that their finding of no relationship between duration of deafness and postimplant speech recognition differed from most other studies, which have shown a robust negative relationship of duration of deafness and postimplant speech recognition. Holden and colleagues noted that 37 of the 39 participants were consistent users of hearing aids prior to implantation, a fact that may have staved off the negative effects of auditory deprivation. Furthermore, Holden found greater variability in postimplant speech recognition in noise relative to performance in quiet. Holden et al. theorized that the greater variability observed in speech recognition in noise was likely due to differences in auditory processing abilities across participants. Finally, it should be noted that the mean performance of the participants in the Holden et al. (2016) study was 76%, 87%, and 52% correct for the CNC word, AzBio sentences in quiet, and AzBio sentences in noise tests, respectively. These mean scores are considerably better than the typical performance of previous studies (Mahmoud & Ruckenstein, 2014). Holden and colleagues attributed the overall high level of speech recognition observed in this study to the proper placement of the electrode array in the scala tympani.

Factors Predicting Postoperative Unilateral and Bilateral Speech Recognition in Adult Cochlear Implant Recipients with Acoustic Hearing—Plant et al., 2016

Plant and colleagues (2016) examined factors that affect speech recognition obtained with a cochlear implant, but their study differed from previous studies in several important ways. First, Plant et al. evaluated 65 postlingually deafened recipients who scored at least 46% correct on preimplant monosyllabic word recognition testing, which is considerably better preimplant hearing performance relative to other studies that have examined factors that influence implant outcomes. The inclusion of participants with better preimplant auditory function is relevant because of the recent trend for audiologists to recommend cochlear implantation for patients who struggle to hear with hearing aids but who may not meet indications for use. Secondly, Plant and colleagues evaluated postimplant speech recognition for the implanted ear as well as in the bimodal condition (i.e., cochlear implant along with hearing aid in nonimplanted ear or use of natural hearing in the nonimplanted ear). Evaluation of performance in the bimodal condition is important, because performance in the bimodal condition is often better than the unilateral condition. Also, the bimodal condition is likely to more closely represent the recipients' hearing performance in realistic situations because recipients listen with two ears in the real world. Third, speech recognition was compared

between the preoperative condition and the postoperative condition at 12 months postimplantation by evaluating both monosyllabic word recognition and sentence recognition in noise.

Word recognition in the unilateral implant condition was generally poorer for recipients who had a longer duration of severe to profound hearing loss and for those who had a better pure-tone average on the nonimplanted ear. The finding of poorer word recognition in the unilateral implant condition for persons with better hearing in the nonimplanted ear is most likely attributed to the likelihood that those recipients were at least partially dependent on the information received from the nonimplanted ear to understand speech. As a result, word recognition was poorer in the unilateral implant condition, because the valuable input from the nonimplanted ear was removed. It should be noted that most participants achieved poor word recognition in the unilateral cochlear implant condition when the pure-tone average in the nonimplanted ear was 40 dB HL or better. Also of importance, there was a wide spread of word recognition scores in the unilateral cochlear implant condition for recipients with a duration of deafness that was less than 20 years. In contrast, all subjects achieved poor word recognition in the unilateral condition when the duration of deafness exceeded 20 years. Of note, age at implantation and degree of hearing loss in the implanted ear were not factors that affected implant outcomes. Also of note, the predictive factors accounted for 34% of the variability observed in word recognition in the unilateral across the participants.

In the bimodal listening condition, word recognition in quiet and sentence recognition in noise were poorer for persons with a longer duration of deafness, older age at implantation, and a poorer pure-tone average in the nonimplanted ear. The finding of better speech recognition in the bimodal condition for persons with better hearing sensitivity in the nonimplanted ear underscores the potential importance of hearing aid use in the nonimplanted ear. Of note, there was a wide spread of word recognition scores in the bimodal condition for recipients who had a pure-tone average of 50 dB HL or poorer in the nonimplanted ear. In contrast, most every recipient achieved excellent word recognition in the bimodal when the pure-tone average was better than 50 dB HL. As with the unilateral condition, there was a wide spread of bimodal word recognition scores for recipients with a duration of deafness of less than 20 years. In contrast, most every recipient (with the exception of one) achieved poor bimodal word recognition scores when the duration of deafness exceeded 20 years. Also of importance, the recipients generally achieved excellent bimodal word recognition performance when their age at implantation was less than 50 years, whereas a wide spread of performance existed for recipients who had an age at implantation of greater than 50 years. Additionally, although sentence recognition in noise tended to be better for recipients with a shorter duration of deafness, younger age at implantation, and better hearing in the nonimplanted ear, a fairly wide spread of speech recognition in noise performance existed even for the youngest recipients who had shorter durations of deafness and better hearing in the nonimplanted ear. The greater variability observed in sentence recognition in noise is consistent with numerous studies showing a wide spread in speech recognition in noise as a function of pure-tone hearing thresholds, age, and so forth. (Roberts et al., 2013). The predictive variables explained 36% of the variability observed in bimodal word recognition in quiet and 30% of the bimodal sentence recognition in noise.

Individual Factors That Affect Postoperative Outcomes with Cochlear Implants

The audiologist should have a thorough understanding of the factors that influence postoperative outcomes that adults achieve with cochlear implants. A working knowledge of the factors that affect implant outcomes allows the audiologist to effectively identify appropriate candidates for cochlear implantation and to appropriately counsel the candidate and his/her family regarding realistic expectation of cochlear implantation. The following sections provide a brief review of the individual factors that affect postoperative outcomes of adults with cochlear implants.

Duration of Hearing Loss and Deafness

As may be seen in the review of the studies previously reviewed in this chapter, most studies have shown that a longer duration of deafness negatively impacts cochlear implant outcomes (Blamey et al., 1996; 2013; Gantz et al., 1993; Green et al., 2007; Holden et al., 2013; Lazard et al., 2012; Leung et al., 2005; Plant et al., 2016; Rubinstein et al., 1999). The poorer performance observed for recipients with a longer duration of deafness is most likely attributable to changes in the auditory nervous system (e.g.,

cross-modal plasticity and colonization of the auditory cortices) and auditory processing. Indeed, several researchers have shown the deleterious effect of auditory deprivation on the auditory nervous system (Champoux et al., 2009; Doucet et al., 2006; Giraud & Lee, 2007; Glick & Sharma, 2017; Lee et al., 2007; Lin et al., 2014; Moore & Shannon, 2009; Rouger et al., 2007; Strelnikov et al., 2010). Of note, it is logical to also hypothesize that a longer duration of deafness would lead to a decrease in spiral ganglion cell bodies because of the loss of trophic factors delivered from the cochlea. Further, it is also logical to assume that a loss of spiral ganglion cell bodies would result in a reduction in speech recognition obtained with a cochlear implant. However, most studies have failed to show a relationship between spiral ganglion cell body survival and cochlear implant outcomes (Blamey, 1997; Fayad & Linthicum, 2006; Fayad et al., 1991; Gassner, Shallop, & Driscoll, 2005; Linthicum et al., 1991; Nadol et al., 2001)). For instance, substantial open-set speech recognition has been observed in cochlear implant recipients for whom postmortem studies have shown less than 10% of the normal complement of auditory neural elements (Fayad et al., 1991; Linthicum et al., 1991). Blamey (1997) stated that the lack of a relationship between spiral ganglion survival and cochlear implant outcome may be attributed to the fact "that the minimum number of cells required for good speech perception is quite low, and the majority of implant users exceed this minimum requirement." In contrast, it should also be noted that some researchers have reported a positive relationship between spiral ganglion cell count and word recognition scores (Seyyedi, Viana, & Nadol, 2014). In short and as one may expect, the function of the auditory nervous system is probably the most important factor influencing the relationship between duration of deafness and cochlear implant outcomes; however, although a relatively sparse number of spiral ganglion cell bodies can allow for good open set speech recognition, the best outcomes are obtained by recipients who have more intact and better functioning peripheral and central auditory structures.

It is important to note that research examining the effect of the duration of deafness on cochlear implant outcomes has typically found no relationship so long as the duration of deafness does not exceed 20 years (Mosnier et al., 2014). In other words, many recipients who have a duration of deafness between 0 and 20 years will perform quite well with their cochlear implants. In contrast, many recipients who have a duration of deafness exceeding 20 years will struggle to achieve excellent speech recognition with their cochlear implants (Migirov et al., 2010). However, exceptions to this rule do exist. Indeed, peer-reviewed research and anecdotal clinical experience do suggest that long-term deafened adults often achieve better speech recognition with a cochlear implant than they do with hearing aids. Additionally, the duration of deafness is likely to be less detrimental for a recipient who has consistently worn well-fitted hearing aids to provide satisfactory audibility for the speech-frequency range, thus staving off some of the deleterious effects of auditory deprivation (Holden et al., 2016). The lack of full-time hearing aid use may also be detrimental for persons with moderate hearing loss. Indeed, Lazard et al. (2012) showed that the duration of moderate hearing loss also negatively influenced cochlear implant outcomes. It is important to note that cochlear implantation may be beneficial for persons who have a duration of deafness exceeding 20 years along with less than ideal hearing aid use. For instance, the cochlear implant may improve sound awareness and access to speech and environmental sounds. In such a case, the audiologist must carefully inform the candidate in order to establish realistic expectations.

Finally, it is important to mention that it may be difficult to determine the duration of deafness for some cochlear implant candidates. Many candidates do not bring serial audiograms to their appointments so that audiologists can obtain a clear indication of the length and progression of hearing loss. A common practice is to estimate the duration of deafness based on how long it has been since the candidate has been able to converse over the telephone. For persons with flat audiometric configurations, estimating duration of deafness based on telephone use is probably a valid practice. However, many candidates have a severe to profound high-frequency hearing loss which causes substantial difficulty with communication in many listening situations, but their functional low-frequency hearing allows for reasonable use of the telephone. Anecdotally, the author has served several patients who have functional low-frequency hearing with a lengthy (greater than 20 years) duration of profound high-frequency hearing loss. Many of these recipients struggled to acclimate to the high-frequency stimulation received from the cochlear implant. Again, this difficulty was likely due to changes that occurred in the auditory nervous system (e.g., cross-modal plasticity in the auditory cortex). In short, these patients generally performed better with their cochlear implant and a hearing aid

in the nonimplanted ear than they did in the pre-implant, binaurally aided condition, and as such, implantation was beneficial. However, the prudent audiologist should be aware not only of the duration of deafness, but also of the duration of severe to profound high-frequency hearing loss and carefully counsel such candidates about the potential for limited benefit after implantation.

Age at Implantation

Numerous studies have shown poorer outcomes for recipients implanted at later ages (Hiel et al., 2016; Holden et al., 2013; Strelnikov et al., 2013, 2015). Once again, the reduced outcomes for older recipients are most likely attributable to changes in auditory processing and to the auditory nervous system. However, it should be noted that several studies have found no effect of advanced age on cochlear implant outcomes, particularly when the analysis accounts for duration of deafness, which is naturally likely to be greater for older persons (Carlson et al., 2010; Green et al., 2007; Holden et al., 2013). Also, some studies have found little to no difference in the outcomes observed between elderly and younger recipients. For instance, Carlson et al. (2010) measured word recognition and sentence recognition in quiet and in noise for two groups, 208 recipients between 18 and 79 years old and 50 recipients who were at least 80 years old. Postoperative speech recognition was essentially identical for the two groups. The effect of age on cochlear implant outcomes is best summarized with the following statements:

- Some studies have shown a slight to modest trend of poorer performance in elderly recipients compared with younger recipients (Ghiselli et al., 2016; Strelnikov et al., 2013, 2015), whereas other studies have shown comparable performance (Carlson et al., 2009; Green et al., 2007).
- Poorer outcomes in elderly recipients could be due to changes in auditory processing. If so, the audiologist should be prepared to provide aural rehabilitation to assist the recipient in overcoming the negative effects of auditory processing difficulties. Also, the audiologist should counsel the recipient that additional time may be required to acclimate to the cochlear implant.
- The overwhelming majority of elderly cochlear implant recipients receive substantial benefit from cochlear implantation. In fact, studies have

shown cochlear implantation to be beneficial for recipients who are 90 years old and older (Carlson et al., 2010).

- It is imperative that elderly candidates undergo medical evaluation to ensure suitable fitness for cochlear implant surgery.
- A minority of elderly persons live a relatively isolated lifestyle. The audiologist should identify a means for these recipients to be exposed to intelligible speech to allow for acclimatization to the cochlear implant.
- Some elderly recipients may have difficulties with fine motor control and/or dexterity. The audiologist should identify these issues and assist the recipient in identifying approaches to successfully use his/her cochlear implant technology. Additionally, the audiologist should plan to allow for additional time for counseling regarding the appropriate use of cochlear implant technology.

Preoperative Hearing Status

Numerous studies have examined preoperative auditory function as a factor that affects postoperative speech recognition. Specifically, research has primarily focused on the effect of preoperative pure-tone average and of aided speech recognition on cochlear implant outcomes. In general, most studies have failed to show a correlation between preoperative pure tone hearing thresholds and postoperative speech recognition with a cochlear implant (Battmer et al., 1995; Blamey et al., 1992; Ching, Incerti, & Hill, 2004; Ching et al., 2001; Gantz et al., 1988, 1993; Potts et al., 2009; Waltzman et al., 1995). Likewise, as previously mentioned, one may assume that poorer hearing thresholds would be associated with poorer spiral ganglion survival, but even if that is the case, multiple studies have failed to show a correlation between spiral ganglion survival and postoperative speech recognition (Fayad & Linthicum, 2006; Fayad et al., 1991; Gassner, Shallop, & Driscoll, 2005; Linthicum et al., 1991; Nadol et al., 2001). Additionally, adults who have profound hearing loss are likely to be a rather heterogeneous group in regard to the cause of the hearing loss. For example, the etiology underlying profound hearing loss may include sudden, idiopathic loss, autoimmune conditions, and ototoxicity, and each of these etiologies is typically associated with a good outcome following cochlear implantation.

It should be acknowledged that many of the studies that are cited here and that did not find a relationship between preoperative audiometric thresholds and postoperative speech recognition were conducted at a time (1980s and 1990s) when most recipients had profound hearing loss prior to implantation. Currently, many cochlear implant clinics are recommending cochlear implants for persons who may have hearing thresholds in the severe hearing loss range or that have substantial amounts of hearing in the low-frequency range with severe to profound high-frequency hearing loss. Many recipients who do not meet the current FDA indications for cochlear implantation perform very well with cochlear implants (Gifford et al., 2010; Mudery et al., 2017; Sladen et al., 2017). With the movement toward a more lax set of audiometric criteria for cochlear implantation, it is quite possible and maybe even probable that recipients who have substantial amounts of preoperative hearing will be expected to achieve excellent outcomes after cochlear implantation. Indeed, Lazard et al. (2012) did find better unilateral cochlear implant speech recognition for persons with better preoperative hearing thresholds. Of note, Lazard and colleagues reported that participants who had better preoperative hearing thresholds in either the implanted or nonimplanted ear achieved better speech recognition after cochlear implantation. Lazard et al. hypothesized that "speech performance with a cochlear implant does not rely more on the peripheral structures of the implanted ear, but more on the integrity of central processing. This possibility is consistent with the strong relationship between PTA (pure-tone average) in the better ear and preoperative speech recognition scores. Whichever ear is implanted, what seems to matter is that the brain was not deprived of auditory inputs preoperatively."

Additionally, Lazard and colleagues suggested that hearing aid use is likely an important factor associated with preoperative hearing status. Specifically, in order to take advantage of any functional preoperative hearing, recipients must use hearing aids that provide adequate audibility prior to implantation in order to prevent the negative effects of auditory deprivation on the auditory nervous system. Accordingly, Lazard et al. stated that "auditory processing and central preservation probably depend more on aided thresholds than unaided PTA, thus hearing aid use may tend to reduce the observed effect of PTA." Indeed, many recipients who have better preoperative hearing status and consistent use of well-fitted hearing aids are more likely to also have greater survival of spiral ganglion cells and better auditory nervous function.

Research examining the relationship between pre- and postoperative speech recognition scores has generally found that persons with better preoperative aided speech recognition achieve better speech recognition after cochlear implantation (Lazard et al., 2012; Roditi et al., 2009; Rubinstein et al., 1999). Once again, higher aided preoperative speech recognition scores may suggest better spiral ganglion survival (Ylikoski & Savolainen, 1984) and better preservation of auditory nervous system function. Several statements are pertinent in regard to the relationship of preoperative aided speech recognition to postoperative speech recognition obtained with a cochlear implant:

- A poor aided preoperative speech recognition score does not confine a recipient to a poor outcome following cochlear implantation. The classic paper by Rubinstein et al. (1999) showed monosyllabic word recognition scores after obtained implantation ranging from 0 to 70% correct for a participants who obtained a score of 0% correct in the preoperative aided condition. As with a profound pure-tone hearing loss, an aided preoperative speech recognition score may be obtained with persons who have an etiology of hearing loss (e.g., sudden idiopathic, autoimmune, ototoxicity) that is typically associated with a favorable cochlear implant outcome.
- Persons who have higher preoperative aided speech recognition scores often achieve satisfactory speech recognition after cochlear implantation. A number of research studies have shown that recipients with preoperative speech recognition scores exceeding FDA indications for use often achieve postoperative speech recognition scores that are above average for what is expected of the typical cochlear implant recipient (Gifford et al., 2010; Mudery et al., 2017; Plant et al., 2015; Sladen et al., 2017).
- Postoperative speech recognition obtained after cochlear implantation is likely to be better for recipients who consistently used well-fitted hearing aids prior to cochlear implantation. It is logical to assume that the consistent use of well-fitted hearing aids will promote better aided preoperative speech recognition. The consistent use of well-fitted hearing aids likely limits

the deleterious effects of auditory deprivation (e.g., spiral ganglion degeneration, cross-modal colonization of the auditory cortex).
- Aided preoperative speech recognition is not a fail-proof indicator of postoperative speech recognition. Some recipients with poor aided preoperative speech recognition will obtain excellent postoperative speech recognition, whereas some recipients who have modest amounts of aided preoperative speech recognition may not achieve excellent postoperative speech recognition.

Etiology

Historically, most studies have failed to show a strong relationship between hearing loss etiology and cochlear implant outcomes except for a finding of poorer performance for recipients whose hearing loss was caused by bacterial meningitis and better than average performance for recipients whose hearing loss was attributed to Meniere's disease (Blamey et al., 1996; Clark, 2003). However, in a more recent study of 2251 implant recipients, Blamey and colleagues (2013) did find that the etiology of the participants' hearing loss did have a significant influence on cochlear implant outcomes. As previously discussed, participants with sudden idiopathic hearing loss performed better than the average recipient, as did recipients with Meniere's disease and a genetic cause of hearing loss. In contrast, participants with temporal bone fracture, acoustic neuroma, and auditory neuropathy spectrum disorder (ANSD) performed more poorly than the typical recipient. Of note, participants whose hearing loss was caused by bacterial meningitis performed close to the group average. Recipients who have suffered a sudden idiopathic loss of hearing are expected to do well after cochlear implantation, because their duration of deafness is short and degeneration of peripheral auditory nerve fibers and of the auditory cortex is most likely to be minimal. Recipients with Meniere's disease are likely to perform well after cochlear implantation, because their site of lesion is at the cochlea, and the cochlear implant bypasses the pathologic peripheral organ and stimulates the relatively healthy cochlear nerve. Likewise, many genetic causes of hearing loss also affect the cochlea, which leads to a satisfactory result with cochlear implantation. In contrast, transverse temporal bone fractures often cause trauma (severance) to the cochlear nerve, rendering cochlear implantation unsuccessful. Similarly, acoustic neuromas often cause severe degeneration of the cochlear nerve, and in many cases, the cochlear nerve is sectioned during tumor removal. Finally, the site of lesion for adult-onset ANSD may exist at the cochlear nerve and/or auditory nervous system pathways. In such cases, a cochlear implant will most likely only be marginally successful in mitigating the dyssynchronous neural responsiveness of the auditory system.

Bacterial Meningitis. Several studies have indicated that recipients whose hearing loss is due to bacterial meningitis perform more poorly than the average cochlear implant recipient (Battmer et al., 1995; Blamey et al., 1996; de Brito et al., 2013; Philippon et al., 2010; Waltzman et al., 1995). Bacterial meningitis causes inflammation in the cochlear labyrinth, which leads to hair cell loss and possibly to ossification in the cochlear scalae, and it also has been shown to result in a substantial loss of spiral ganglion cell bodies and auditory neurons in the brainstem (El-Kashlan et al., 2003; Lu & Schuknecht, 1994; Nadol & Hsu, 1991). The potential damage to the neurons of the cochlear nerve and brainstem are likely to limit auditory responsiveness to electrical stimulation from the cochlear implant. Furthermore, the bony growth in the cochlea adversely affects the spread of electrical current from the electrode array to the cochlear nerve. Additionally, the cochlear ossification may prevent an adequate insertion of the electrode array into the cochlea. Indeed, prompt provision of cochlear implantation is imperative for persons who have suffered a severe to profound hearing loss secondary to bacterial meningitis in order to improve the likelihood of insertion of the electrode array into the cochlea prior to the onset of ossification. Blamey and colleagues (2013) attributed the prompt provision of cochlear implantation to the better outcomes observed for adults with bacterial meningitis relative to what was observed in their previous study (Blamey et al., 1996). Of note, Axon et al. (1998) found that when cochlear ossification does occur, it is likely complete within a few months following the onset of the infection. Also of note, Caye-Thomasen et al. (2012) performed a radiologic study on the cochlear anatomy of 47 ears (34 recipients) affected by bacterial meningitis. They concluded that cochlear ossification was present in 26% of the ears (35% of the participants) under study, a finding that is comparable to previous studies which have found ossification in 34% to 73% of persons who are deafened because of bacterial meningitis (Axon et al., 1998; Beijen et

al., 2009; Nikolopoulos et al., 1997; Yune, Miyamoto, & Yune, 1991). Caye-Thomasen and colleagues also reported that *Streptococcus pneumoniae* caused ossification more frequently than Neisseria meningitis. It should be mentioned that bacterial meningitis may also lead to significant neurological insults, which may also limit communication abilities following cochlear implantation. Finally, the programming audiologist should consult with the cochlear implant surgeon to determine an estimate for how many electrodes are in the cochlea and for whether cochlear ossification is likely to complicate cochlear implant programming and recipient progress. Recipients who have significant cochlear ossification are likely to need wider electrical pulse widths and may also require different electrode coupling modes (e.g., bipolar, pseudomonopolar) to avoid facial nerve stimulation.

Otosclerosis. Some persons with advanced otosclerosis may develop significant cochlear hearing loss resulting in little to no benefit from conventional hearing aids and/or osseointegrated bone conduction devices. Several reports have shown cochlear implantation to provide significant benefit and excellent outcomes for persons with advanced otosclerosis (Castillo et al., 2014; Profant, Kabatova, & Varga, 2016; Psillas et al., 2007; Sainz et al., 2007). Of note, advanced otosclerosis often leads to a progression of bony growth/otospongiotic material into the basal end of the cochlear labyrinth. As a result, electrical stimulation of the most basal intracochlear electrode contacts may lead to facial stimulation and/or to inadequate loudness growth (Psillas et al., 2007; Sainz et al., 2009). The programming audiologist may need to be prepared to disable basal electrode contacts, widen the electrical pulse width, and/or change the electrode coupling mode to manage these issues.

Auditory Neuropathy Spectrum Disorder. Adult-onset of ANSD is often associated with a peripheral neuropathy disorder that may also affect vision, motor functions, and tactile sensations. Examples of late-onset ANSD include Friedrich's ataxia, Leber's hereditary optic neuropathy, Charcot-Marie Tooth disease, Riboflavin transporter deficiency, Mohr Tranebjaeg syndrome, and OPA1. The pathologic progression of many of these disorders results in gradual dysfunction of peripheral dendrites, ganglion cells, axons, and/or the myelin sheath. When persons with these conditions perform poorly with hearing aids, a number of research studies have shown that benefit may be obtained from cochlear implantation (Goswamy et al.,

2012; Huang, Santarelli, & Starr, 2009; Santarelli et al., 2015). However, as found in the Blamey et al. (2013) study, many adults with late-onset ANSD will achieve poorer outcomes following cochlear implantation compared with the typical implant recipient. The site of lesion of the ANSD is the most likely factor influencing the recipient's outcome. If an ANSD profile is associated with a cochlear or synaptic site of lesion, cochlear implant outcomes will likely be excellent. If the myelin sheath is affected, neural synchrony will be compromised for acoustic stimulation, but it is possible that the robust synchronization facilitated by electrical stimulation will allow for better hearing performance. However, performance is unlikely to be as good as it would be for a recipient with a fully myelinated cochlear nerve. If ANSD results in degeneration of cochlear nerve elements and/or neurons of the auditory brainstem, the benefit of cochlear implantation is likely to be limited. However, as previously mentioned, research has shown relatively favorable cochlear implant outcomes for recipients with sparse spiral ganglion survival (Blamey, 1997). As such, cochlear implantation may prove to be beneficial for persons who have some neural degeneration due to ANSD. The audiologist should carefully counsel the candidate with late-onset ANSD in order to establish realistic expectations. The presence of a robust cochlear-implant-elicited ECAP response (e.g., NRT) is a prognostic indicator of possible success with a cochlear implant. The programming audiologist may choose to use slower stimulation rates and/or wider electrical pulse widths if signs of neural pathology exist.

Stimulation Levels and Electrophysiologic Responses

Several examiners have observed changes that occur with cochlear implant stimulation levels and electrophysiologic responses over time. Most researchers have reported that the electrical thresholds (i.e., T levels) of adult recipients remain relatively stable from implant activation onward (Brown et al., 1995; Dorman et al,. 1992; Hughes et al., 2001, Waltzman et al., 1991). In contrast, upper-stimulation levels tend to increase throughout the first year of implant use, a fact that is most likely attributed to the adult recipient's acclimation to electrical stimulation of the auditory system and to an increased tolerance for louder sounds. In particular, adults with a long duration of high-frequency severe to profound hearing

loss often require several weeks or months to tolerate adequate stimulation to the basal portion of the electrode array. Electrode impedances typically decrease throughout the first few days of implant use and stabilize thereafter. The electrically evoked compound action potential (ECAP) threshold measured in the operating room is typically much higher than the ECAP threshold measured at activation. The ECAP threshold tends to remain relatively stable from activation onward (Hughes et al., 2001). Likewise, the ESRT tends to remain relatively stable or increases slightly throughout the first year of implant use (Greisiger et al., 2007).

Assessment of Postoperative Cochlear Implant Outcomes

The prudent audiologist will conduct a thorough periodic assessment of cochlear implant outcomes. The cochlear implant outcome assessment battery should include:

- Informal interview to inquire about recipient's progress/difficulties
- Otoscopic evaluation and inspection of cochlear implant site
- An evaluation of the recipient's hearing technology (e.g., microphone check, inspection of the integrity of cables, connectors, batteries, assessment of sound processor acoustic component, assessment of hearing aid)
- Evaluation of sound-field warbled tone thresholds
- Assessment of word recognition in quiet and sentence recognition in noise and possibly in quiet for each ear separately and in the bilateral/bimodal condition
- Administration of a questionnaire to evaluate subjective performance and/or benefit

"Aided" Warbled Tone Threshold Assessment

The audiologist should measure sound-field warbled tone detection thresholds to ensure that the recipient has good access to low-level sounds. A reasonable goal is to obtain sound-field warbled tone thresholds of 20 to 25 dB HL from 250 to 6000 Hz in the unilateral cochlear implant condition (each unilateral cochlear implant condition for bilateral recipients) (Holden et al., 2013; Skinner et al., 1997). Attainment of sound-field warbled tone detection thresholds near 20 dB HL from 250 to 6000 Hz should ensure access to the low-level components of soft speech. It is not desirable to obtain sound-field detection thresholds below 15 dB HL, because in realistic environments, there is unlikely to be an abundance of speech information below 15 to 20 dB HL. Also, low-level noise is primarily present below 20 dB HL and will likely mask any important sounds that may exist below that level. Furthermore, the microphone noise floor of modern cochlear implant sound processors likely prevents detection of sounds below 15 to 20 dB HL.

It should be noted that sound-field detection thresholds should be measured to warbled tones rather than to narrowband noise. The latter is not typically designed for assessment of hearing sensitivity and may be higher in level and will be wider in bandwidth than warbled tones. Additionally, the audiologist should ensure that the recipient is located in the spot in the sound booth in which calibration was completed. Ideally, the loudspeaker should be calibrated for presentation of test signals from 0 degrees. If not, the audiologist should account for correction factors associated with the calibration of the loudspeaker at 45 or 90 degrees.

Assessment of Speech Recognition

Speech recognition should be evaluated with the use of recorded speech materials. As mentioned in the chapters discussing cochlear implant candidacy assessment, the use of recorded materials eliminates the variability inherent in monitored live voice speech testing. Also, several studies have shown that live voice speech recognition assessment overestimates the speech recognition capacity of both adults and children (Roeser & Clark, 2008; Uhler, Biever, & Gifford, 2016). The audiologist should administer the same measures that were administered in the Minimal Speech Test Battery (MTSB) used to evaluate cochlear implant candidacy. Ideally, monosyllabic word recognition assessment (e.g., CNC words) should be conducted in quiet at a presentation level of 60 dBA. Additionally, sentence recognition in noise should be completed at a +10 dB SNR. If the recipient scores less than 20% to 25% correct, then assessment should be conducted at a more favorable SNR (e.g., +15 dB SNR). If the recipient scores near ceiling, then assessment should be conducted at a +5 dB SNR. The prudent audiologist should also evaluate sentence recognition in quiet at a presentation level of 60 dBA. If the recipient scores below 20% to 25% correct on

sentence recognition in quiet assessment, then the audiologist should complete evaluation with a simpler measure of speech recognition. Examples of easier speech recognition measures include HINT sentences in quiet, Overlearned sentences, CID sentences, Four-choice Spondee test, and so forth. Recorded speech recognition should be conducted in each unilateral condition as well as in the bilateral/bimodal condition. Speech recognition assessment should be attempted at the one-month postactivation appointment and at every appointment thereafter.

A minimum recommended postoperative follow-up schedule is:

- One-day postactivation checkup
- One-week postactivation checkup with sound-field warbled tone detection thresholds
- One-month postactivation checkup with sound-field warbled tone detection thresholds and aided speech recognition
- Three-month postactivation checkup with sound-field warbled tone detection thresholds and aided speech recognition
- Six-month postactivation checkup with sound-field warbled tone detection thresholds and aided speech recognition
- One-year postactivation checkup with sound-field warbled tone detection thresholds and aided speech recognition
- Biannual to annual checkups with sound-field warbled tone detection thresholds and aided speech recognition

Key Concepts

- Research has shown a high level of variability in the speech, language, auditory, academic, and social outcomes adults achieve after cochlear implants.
- In general, better outcomes are associated with a shorter duration of deafness, younger age at implantation, a closer proximity of the electrode array to the modiolus, and a complete insertion of the electrode array in the scala tympani (i.e., no translocation of the electrode array into the scala media and/or scala vestibuli).
- Adults with hearing loss should use well-fitted hearing aids prior to cochlear implantation in an attempt to stave off the deleterious effects of auditory deprivation.

- In general, poorer outcomes after implantation are associated with bacterial meningitis, injury to the cochlear nerve, and lengthy duration of severe to profound hearing loss.
- Audiologists should administer a battery of measures to evaluate the outcomes of each adult recipient.

References

Axon, P. R., Temple, R. H., Saeed, S. R., & Ramsden, R. T. (1998). Cochlear ossification after meningitis. *American Journal of Otology, 19*(6), 724–729.

Battmer, R. D., Gupta, S. P., Allum-Mecklenburg, D. J., & Lenarz, T. (1995). Factors influencing cochlear implant perceptual performance in 132 adults. *Annals of Otology, Rhinology, and Laryngology Supplement, 166*, 185–187.

Beijen, J., Casselman, J., Joosten, F., Stover, T., Aschendorff, A., Zarowski, A., . . . Mylanus, E. (2009). Magnetic resonance imaging in patients with meningitis-induced hearing loss. *European Archives of Otorhinolaryngology, 266*(8), 1229–1236.

Blamey, P. (1997). Are spiral ganglion cell numbers important with a cochlear implant? *American Journal of Otology, 18*(6), S11–S12.

Blamey, P., Arndt, P., Bergeron, F., Bredberg, G., Brimacombe, J., Facer, G., . . . Whitford, L. (1996). Factors affecting auditory performance of postlinguistically deaf adults using cochlear implants. *Audiology and Neurotology, 1*(5), 293–306.

Blamey, P., Artieres, F., Baskent, D., Bergeron, F., Beynon, A., Burke, E., . . . Lazard, D. S. (2013). Factors affecting auditory performance of postlinguistically deaf adults using cochlear implants: An update with 2251 patients. *Audiology and Neurotology, 18*(1), 36–47.

Blamey, P. J., Pyman, B. C., Gordon, M., Clark, G. M., Brown, A. M., Dowell, R. C., & Hollow, R. D. (1992). Factors predicting postoperative sentence scores in postlinguistically deaf adult cochlear implant patients. *Annals of Otology, Rhinology, and Laryngology, 101*(4), 342–348.

Brown, C. J., Abbas, P. J., Bertschy, M., Tyler, R. S., Lowder, M., Takahashi, G., . . . Gantz, B. J. (1995). Longitudinal assessment of physiological and psychophysical measures in cochlear implant users. *Ear and Hearing, 16*(5), 439–449.

Carlson, M. L., Breen, J. T., Gifford, R. H., Driscoll, C. L., Neff, B. A., Beatty, C. W., . . . Olund, A. P. (2010). Cochlear implantation in the octogenarian and nonagenarian. *Otology and Neurotology, 31*(8), 1343–1349.

Castillo, F., Polo, R., Gutierrez, A., Reyes, P., Royuela, A., & Alonso, A. (2014). Cochlear implantation outcomes in advanced otosclerosis. *American Journal of Otolaryngology, 35*(5), 558–564.

Caye-Thomasen, P., Dam, M. S., Omland, S. H., & Mantoni, M. (2012). Cochlear ossification in patients with profound hearing loss following bacterial meningitis. *Acta Otolaryngologica, 132*(7), 720–725.

Champoux, F., Lepore, F., Gagne, J. P., & Theoret, H. (2009). Visual stimuli can impair auditory processing in cochlear implant users. *Neuropsychologia, 47*(1), 17–22.

Ching, T. Y., Dillon, H., & Byrne, D. (2001). Children's amplification needs—same or different from adults? *Scandinavian Audiology Supplement*, (53), 54–60.

Ching, T. Y., Incerti, P., & Hill, M. (2004). Binaural benefits for adults who use hearing aids and cochlear implants in opposite ears. *Ear and Hearing, 25*(1), 9–21.

Clark, G. (2003). Cochlear implants in children: Safety as well as speech and language. *International Journal of Pediatric Otorhinolaryngology, 67*(Suppl. 1), S7–20.

de Brito, R., Bittencourt, A. G., Goffi-Gomez, M. V., Magalhaes, A. T., Samuel, P., Tsuji, R. K., & Bento, R. F. (2013). Cochlear implants and bacterial meningitis: A speech recognition study in paired samples. *International Archives of Otorhinolaryngology, 17*(1), 57–61.

Dorman, M. F., Smith, L. M., Dankowski, K., McCandless, G., & Parkin, J. L. (1992). Long-term measures of electrode impedance and auditory thresholds for the Ineraid cochlear implant. *Journal of Speech and Hearing Research, 35*(5), 1126–1130.

Doucet, M. E., Bergeron, F., Lassonde, M., Ferron, P., & Lepore, F. (2006). Cross-modal reorganization and speech perception in cochlear implant users. *Brain, 129*(Pt. 12), 3376–3383.

Dowell, R. C., Hollow, R., & Winton, E. (2004). Outcomes for cochlear implant users with significant residual hearing: Implications for selection criteria in children. *Archives of Otolaryngology–Head and Neck Surgery, 130*(5), 575–581.

El-Kashlan, H. K., Ashbaugh, C., Zwolan, T., & Telian, S. A. (2003). Cochlear implantation in prelingually deaf children with ossified cochleae. *Otology and Neurotology, 24*(4), 596–600.

Fayad, J. N., & Linthicum, F. H., Jr. (2006). Multichannel cochlear implants: Relation of histopathology to performance. *Laryngoscope, 116*(8), 1310–1320.

Fayad, J., Linthicum, F. H., Jr., Otto, S. R., Galey, F. R., & House, W. F. (1991). Cochlear implants: Histopathologic findings related to performance in 16 human temporal bones. *Annals of Otology, Rhinology, and Laryngology, 100*(10), 807–811.

Gantz, B. J., Tyler, R. S., Knutson, J. F., Woodworth, G., Abbas, P., McCabe, B. F., . . . et al. (1988). Evaluation of five different cochlear implant designs: Audiologic assessment and predictors of performance. *Laryngoscope, 98*(10), 1100–1106.

Gantz, B. J., Woodworth, G. G., Knutson, J. F., Abbas, P. J., & Tyler, R. S. (1993). Multivariate predictors of audiological success with multichannel cochlear implants. *Annals of Otology, Rhinology, and Laryngology, 102*(12), 909–916.

Gassner, H. G., Shallop, J. K., & Driscoll, C. L. (2005). Long-term clinical course and temporal bone histology after cochlear implantation. *Cochlear Implants International, 6*(2), 67–76.

Ghiselli, S., Nedic, S., Montino, S., Astolfi, L., & Bovo, R. (2016). Cochlear implantation in postlingually deafened adults and elderly patients: Analysis of audiometric and speech perception outcomes during the first year of use. *Acta Otorhinolaryngologica Italica, 36*(6), 513–519.

Gifford, R. H., Dorman, M. F., Shallop, J. K., & Sydlowski, S. A. (2010). Evidence for the expansion of adult cochlear implant candidacy. *Ear and Hearing, 31*(2), 186–194.

Gifford, R. H., Shallop, J. K., & Peterson, A. M. (2008). Speech recognition materials and ceiling effects: Considerations for cochlear implant programs. *Audiology and Neurotology, 13*(3), 193–205.

Giraud, A. L., & Lee, H. J. (2007). Predicting cochlear implant outcome from brain organisation in the deaf. *Restorative Neurology and Neuroscience, 25*(3–4), 381–390.

Glick, H., & Sharma, A. (2017). Cross-modal plasticity in developmental and age-related hearing loss: Clinical implications. *Hearing Research, 343*, 191–201.

Goswamy, J., Bruce, I. A., Green, K. M., & O'Driscoll, M. P. (2012). Cochlear implantation in a patient with sensorineural deafness secondary to Charcot-Marie-Tooth disease. *Cochlear Implants International, 13*(3), 184–187.

Green, K. M., Bhatt, Y., Mawman, D. J., O'Driscoll, M. P., Saeed, S. R., Ramsden, R. T., & Green, M. W. (2007). Predictors of audiological outcome following cochlear implantation in adults. *Cochlear Implants International, 8*(1), 1–11.

Greisiger, R., Shallop, J. K., Hol, P. K., Elle, O. J., & Jablonski, G. E. (2015). Cochlear implantees: Analysis of behavioral and objective measures for a clinical population of various age groups. *Cochlear Implants International, 16*(Suppl. 4), 1–19.

Heydebrand, G., Hale, S., Potts, L., Gotter, B., & Skinner, M. (2007). Cognitive predictors of improvements in adults' spoken word recognition six months after cochlear implant activation. *Audiology and Neurotology, 12*(4), 254–264.

Hiel, A. L., Gerard, J. M., Decat, M., & Deggouj, N. (2016). Is age a limiting factor for adaptation to cochlear implant? *European Archives of Otorhinolaryngology, 273*(9), 2495–2502.

Holden, L. K., Finley, C. C., Firszt, J. B., Holden, T. A., Brenner, C., Potts, L. G., . . . Skinner, M. W. (2013). Factors affecting open-set word recognition in adults with cochlear implants. *Ear and Hearing, 34*(3), 342–360.

Holden, L. K., Firszt, J. B., Reeder, R. M., Uchanski, R. M., Dwyer, N. Y., & Holden, T. A. (2016). Factors affecting outcomes in cochlear implant recipients implanted with a perimodiolar electrode array located in scala tympani. *Otology and Neurotology, 37*(10), 1662–1668.

Hughes, M. L., Vander Werff, K. R., Brown, C. J., Abbas, P. J., Kelsay, D. M., Teagle, H. F., & Lowder, M. W. (2001). A longitudinal study of electrode impedance, the electrically evoked compound action potential, and behavioral measures in nucleus 24 cochlear implant users. *Ear and Hearing, 22*(6), 471–486.

Lazard, D. S., Giraud, A. L., Gnansia, D., Meyer, B., & Sterkers, O. (2012). Understanding the deafened brain: Implications for cochlear implant rehabilitation. *European Annals of Otorhinolaryngology, Head, and Neck Disorders, 129*(2), 98–103.

Lazard, D. S., Vincent, C., Venail, F., Van de Heyning, P., Truy, E., Sterkers, O., . . . Blamey, P. J. (2012). Pre-, per- and postoperative factors affecting performance of postlinguistically deaf adults using cochlear implants: A new conceptual model over time. *PLoS One, 7*(11), e48739.

Lee, H. J., Truy, E., Mamou, G., Sappey-Marinier, D., & Giraud, A. L. (2007). Visual speech circuits in profound acquired deafness: A possible role for latent multimodal connectivity. *Brain, 130*(Pt. 11), 2929–2941.

Leung, J., Wang, N. Y., Yeagle, J. D., Chinnici, J., Bowditch, S., Francis, H. W., & Niparko, J. K. (2005). Predictive models for cochlear implantation in elderly candidates. *Archives of Otolaryngology–Head and Neck Surgery, 131*(12), 1049–1054.

Lin, F. R., Ferrucci, L., An, Y., Goh, J. O., Doshi, J., Metter, E. J., . . . Resnick, S. M. (2014). Association of hearing impairment with brain volume changes in older adults. *Neuroimage, 90*, 84–92.

Linthicum, F. H., Jr., Fayad, J., Otto, S. R., Galey, F. R., & House, W. F. (1991a). Cochlear implant histopathology. *American Journal of Otology, 12*(4), 245–311.

Linthicum, F. H., Jr., Fayad, J., Otto, S., Galey, F. R., & House, W. F. (1991b). Inner ear morphologic changes resulting from cochlear implantation. *American Journal of Otology, 12*(Suppl.), 8–10; discussion 18–21.

Lu, C. B., & Schuknecht, H. F. (1994). Pathology of prelingual profound deafness: Magnitude of labyrinthitis fibro-ossificans. *American Journal of Otology, 15*(1), 74–85.

Mahmoud, A. F., & Ruckenstein, M. J. (2014). Speech perception performance as a function of age at implantation among post-

lingually deaf adult cochlear implant recipients. *Otology and Neurotology, 35*(10), e286–e291.

Migirov, L., Taitelbaum-Swead, R., Drendel, M., Hildesheimer, M., & Kronenberg, J. (2010). Cochlear implantation in elderly patients: Surgical and audiological outcome. *Gerontology, 56*(2), 123–128.

Moore, D. R., & Shannon, R. V. (2009). Beyond cochlear implants: Awakening the deafened brain. *Nature Neuroscience, 12*(6), 686–691.

Mosnier, I., Bebear, J. P., Marx, M., Fraysse, B., Truy, E., Lina-Granade, G., . . . Sterkers, O. (2014). Predictive factors of cochlear implant outcomes in the elderly. *Audiology and Neurotology, 19*(Suppl. 1), 15–20.

Mudery, J. A., Francis, R., McCrary, H., & Jacob, A. (2017). Older individuals meeting Medicare cochlear implant candidacy criteria in noise but not in quiet: Are these patients improved by surgery? *Otology and Neurotology, 38*(2), 187–191.

Nadol, J. B., Jr., & Hsu, W. C. (1991). Histopathologic correlation of spiral ganglion cell count and new bone formation in the cochlea following meningogenic labyrinthitis and deafness. *Annals of Otology, Rhinology, and Laryngology, 100*(9 Pt. 1), 712–716.

Nadol, J. B., Jr., Shiao, J. Y., Burgess, B. J., Ketten, D. R., Eddington, D. K., Gantz, B. J., . . . Shallop, J. K. (2001). Histopathology of cochlear implants in humans. *Annals of Otology, Rhinology, and Laryngology, 110*(9), 883–891.

Nikolopoulos, T. P., O'Donoghue, G. M., Robinson, K. L., Holland, I. M., Ludman, C., & Gibbin, K. P. (1997). Preoperative radiologic evaluation in cochlear implantation. *American Journal of Otology, 18*(6 Suppl.), S73–S74.

Pasanisi, E., Bacciu, A., Vincenti, V., Guida, M., Barbot, A., Berghenti, M. T., & Bacciu, S. (2003). Speech recognition in elderly cochlear implant recipients. *Clinical Otolaryngology and Allied Sciences, 28*(2), 154–157.

Philippon, D., Bergeron, F., Ferron, P., & Bussieres, R. (2010). Cochlear implantation in postmeningitic deafness. *Otology and Neurotology, 31*(1), 83–87.

Plant, K., McDermott, H., van Hoesel, R., Dawson, P., & Cowan, R. (2016). Factors predicting postoperative unilateral and bilateral speech recognition in adult cochlear implant recipients with acoustic hearing. *Ear and Hearing, 37*(2), 153–163.

Plant, K. L., van Hoesel, R. J., McDermott, H. J., Dawson, P. W., & Cowan, R. S. (2015). Clinical outcomes for adult cochlear implant recipients experiencing loss of usable acoustic hearing in the implanted ear. *Ear and Hearing, 36*(3), 338–356.

Potts, L. G., Skinner, M. W., Litovsky, R. A., Strube, M. J., & Kuk, F. (2009). Recognition and localization of speech by adult cochlear implant recipients wearing a digital hearing aid in the nonimplanted ear (bimodal hearing). *Journal of the American Academy of Audiology, 20*(6), 353–373.

Profant, M., Kabatova, Z., & Varga, L. (2016). Otosclerosis and cochlear implantation. *Surgery of Stapes Fixations*, 105–112.

Psillas, G., Kyriafinis, G., Constantinidis, J., & Vital, V. (2007). Far-advanced otosclerosis and cochlear implantation. *B-ENT, 3*(2), 67–71.

Roberts, D. S., Lin, H. W., Herrmann, B. S., & Lee, D. J. (2013). Differential cochlear implant outcomes in older adults. *Laryngoscope, 123*(8), 1952–1956.

Roditi, R. E., Poissant, S. F., Bero, E. M., & Lee, D. J. (2009). A predictive model of cochlear implant performance in postlingually deafened adults. *Otology and Neurotology, 30*(4), 449–454.

Roeser, R., Clark, J. (2008). Live voice speech recognition audiometry: Stop the madness. *Audiology Today, 20*, 32–33.

Rouger, J., Lagleyre, S., Fraysse, B., Deneve, S., Deguine, O., & Barone, P. (2007). Evidence that cochlear-implanted deaf patients are better multisensory integrators. *Proceedings of the National Academy of Sciences United States of Aemrica, 104*(17), 7295–7300.

Rubenstein, J., Parkinson, W., Tyler, R., & Gantz, B. (1999). Residual speech recognition and cochlear implant performance: Effects of implantation criteria. *American Journal of Otology, 20*(4), 445–452.

Sainz, M., Garcia-Valdecasas, J., Garofano, M., & Ballesteros, J. M. (2007). Otosclerosis: Mid-term results of cochlear implantation. *Audiology and Neurotology, 12*(6), 401–406.

Santarelli, R., Rossi, R., Scimemi, P., Cama, E., Valentino, M. L., La Morgia, C., . . . Carelli, V. (2015). OPA1-related auditory neuropathy: Site of lesion and outcome of cochlear implantation. *Brain, 138*(Pt. 3), 563–576.

Seyyedi, M., Viana, L. M., & Nadol, J. B., Jr. (2014). Within-subject comparison of word recognition and spiral ganglion cell count in bilateral cochlear implant recipients. *Otology and Neurotology, 35*(8), 1446–1450.

Shea, J. J., 3rd, Domico, E. H., & Orchik, D. J. (1990). Speech recognition ability as a function of duration of deafness in multichannel cochlear implant patients. *Laryngoscope, 100*(3), 223–226.

Skinner, M. W., Holden, L. K., & Holden, T. A. (1997). Parameter selection to optimize speech recognition with the Nucleus implant. *Otolaryngology–Head and Neck Surgery, 117*(3 Pt. 1), 188–195.

Sladen, D. P., Gifford, R. H., Haynes, D., Kelsall, D., Benson, A., Lewis, K., . . . Driscoll, C. L. (2017). Evaluation of a revised indication for determining adult cochlear implant candidacy. *Laryngoscope, 127*(10), 2368–2374.

Strelnikov, K., Marx, M., Lagleyre, S., Fraysse, B., Deguine, O., & Barone, P. (2015). PET-imaging of brain plasticity after cochlear implantation. *Hearing Research, 322*, 180–187.

Strelnikov, K., Rouger, J., Demonet, J. F., Lagleyre, S., Fraysse, B., Deguine, O., & Barone, P. (2010). Does brain activity at rest reflect adaptive strategies? Evidence from speech processing after cochlear implantation. *Cerebral Cortex, 20*(5), 1217–1222.

Strelnikov, K., Rouger, J., Demonet, J. F., Lagleyre, S., Fraysse, B., Deguine, O., & Barone, P. (2013). Visual activity predicts auditory recovery from deafness after adult cochlear implantation. *Brain, 136*(Pt. 12), 3682–3695.

Summerfield, A. Q., & Marshall, D. H. (1995). Preoperative predictors of outcomes from cochlear implantation in adults: Performance and quality of life. *Annals of Otology, Rhinology, and Laryngology Supplement, 166*, 105–108.

Uhler, K., Biever, A., & Gifford, R. H. (2016). Method of speech stimulus presentation impacts pediatric speech recognition: Monitored live voice versus recorded speech. *Otology and Neurotology, 37*(2), e70–e74.

Waltzman, S. B., Cohen, N. L., & Shapiro, W. H. (1991). Effects of chronic electrical stimulation on patients using a cochlear prosthesis. *Otolaryngology–Head and Neck Surgery, 105*(6), 797–801.

Waltzman, S. B., Fisher, S. G., Niparko, J. K., & Cohen, N. L. (1995). Predictors of postoperative performance with cochlear implants. *Annals of Otology, Rhinology, and Laryngology Supplement, 165*, 15–18.

Ylikoski, J., & Savolainen, S. (1984). The cochlear nerve in various forms of deafness. *Acta Otolaryngologica, 98*(5–6), 418–427.

Yune, H. Y., Miyamoto, R. T., & Yune, M. E. (1991). Medical imaging in cochlear implant candidates. *American Journal of Otology, 12*(Suppl.), 11–17; discussion 18–21.

Zwolan, T. A., Henion, K., Segel, P., & Runge, C. (2014). The role of age on cochlear implant performance, use, and health utility: A multicenter clinical trial. *Otology and Neurotology, 35*(9), 1560–1568.

22

Factors Affecting the Outcomes of Children with Cochlear Implants

Jace Wolfe

Introduction

Over the past 25 years, a number of research studies have examined the outcomes of children with cochlear implants and the factors that influence the progress that children make after cochlear implantation (Blamey et al., 2001; Ching & Dillon, 2013; Ching et al., 2018; Chiossi & Hyppolito, 2017; Cupples et al., 2016; Geers et al,. 2003, 2011; Kim et al., 2010; Moog & Geers, 2003; Nittrouer et al., 2012; Percy-Smith et al., 2010; Quittner et al., 2013; Tobey et al., 2003). As with adults, there is a significant amount of variability observed in the outcomes achieved by children with cochlear implants, and that variability cannot be entirely explained by any number of factors (Blamey et al., 2001; Ching & Dillon, 2013; Ching et al., 2018; Chiossi & Hyppolito, 2017; Cupples et al., 2016; Geers et al,. 2003, 2011; Janeschik et al., 2013; Kim et al., 2010; Moog & Geers, 2003; Nittrouer et al., 2012; Percy-Smith et al., 2010; Quittner et al., 2013; Tobey et al., 2003). However, research has also identified a host of factors that do generally tend to influence the outcome a child achieves after cochlear implantation. The following sections will review research that explores outcomes of children with cochlear implants and will highlight a number of factors that have been shown to affect cochlear implant outcomes in children. Additionally, a protocol for postoperative assessment will be discussed. Although several factors have been shown to influence pediatric cochlear implant outcomes, the reader should understand that there are very few factors that confine a child to a particular outcome. Indeed, in spite of the existence of factors that are often negatively associated with cochlear implant outcomes, the provision of excellent otologic, audiologic, and audition-based speech and language intervention along with a complete commitment from the family to meet a child's need will often result in a favorable outcome for the child and family.

Age at Identification, Intervention, and Implantation

Age of implantation is one of the most robust factors that influences the outcomes achieved by children with hearing loss. Specifically, and as one may expect after reading the discussion of auditory nervous system development in Chapter 3, better outcomes are typically obtained by children who receive a cochlear implant(s) at earlier ages (Ching & Dillon, 2013; Dettman et al., 2016; Houston et al., 2012; Houston & Miyamoto, 2010). Some of the most impressive findings demonstrating the importance of early implantation have come from a landmark Longitudinal Outcomes of Children with Hearing Impairment (LOCHI) study conducted by Teresa Ching and colleagues with the National Acoustic Laboratories (Ching & Dillon, 2013). The LOCHI study is an ongoing longitudinal study following the outcomes of 451 Australian children with hearing loss (born 2002–2007) from birth to early adulthood. The LOCHI study will examine the long-term speech, language, auditory, psychosocial, and educational outcomes of children who have hearing loss, many of whom use hearing aids and/or cochlear implants. The LOCHI study is unique and of great importance for several reasons. First, it includes a large number of children who were recruited from the entire country of Australia, and as such, the study should provide a representation of the typical population of children with hearing loss (rather than "cherry-picking" a certain type of subject that may yield a particular result but may not be representative of the broader population of children with hearing loss). Second, the study is longitudinal, which allows for the examination of outcomes over a long course of time and avoids biases that may occur when developing study questions during a retrospective review of a cohort of patients. Third, Australia contains a national health care system that offers hearing health care for all children. As a result, children should have access to newborn hearing screening and the services and technologies necessary to mitigate the potential effects of hearing loss. Additionally, Australian Hearing has published clinical protocols that specify the provision of evidence-based, modern hearing health care, so the children should have ready access to excellent services.

Ching and Dillon (2013) initially reported on the outcomes of 134 children who had cochlear implants and who were evaluated at 3 years of age. Forty-six of the children received their first cochlear implant before 12 months of age. Ching and Dillon examined the impact of the age of implantation on the global outcomes of the children. The global outcome represented a collective measure of the children's performance on measures of expressive and receptive language, speech production, social development, and auditory function. Ching and Dillon hypothesized that each of the individual outcome measures were all affected by the child's ability to understand speech and language. They reported that age at implantation was one of the strongest predictors of global language outcome measured at 3 years of age. The outcomes of children implanted at 12 months of age were significantly poorer than the outcomes of children implanted at 6 months of age. Of note, beginning at 6 months of age, a global outcome delay of 1/2 standard deviation occurs for every 6-month delay in cochlear implantation. As a result, the speech, language, and auditory development of a child whose cochlear implant is activated at 18 months of age will be on average one standard deviation poorer than a child whose cochlear

implant is activated at 6 months of age. Ching (2014) reported similar findings for 114 children whose outcomes were measured at 5 years of age. The global language scores of children implanted at 6 months of age were 0.7 standard deviation higher than those of children implanted at 12 months of age and were almost 1.5 standard deviations higher than children implanted at 24 months of age.

Dettman and colleagues (2016) reported on the outcomes of 403 school-aged children who underwent cochlear implantation between 6 months and 6 years of age. One-hundred and fifty-one of the children were implanted prior to 12 months of age. Dettman et al. (2016) found that 81% of children who received their cochlear implant prior to 12 months of age had a receptive vocabulary that was within the normal range for children with normal hearing when measured at school-entry age. In contrast, only 52% of the children implanted between 13 and 18 months of age achieved normal receptive vocabulary development, and less than 25% of children achieved normal receptive language development when implanted later than 18 months of age. Similarly, children implanted prior to 12 months of age achieved better speech recognition, expressive and receptive language, and speech production compared with children implanted after 12 months of age.

Houston and colleagues (2012) explored the ability of preschool children with normal hearing and preschool children with cochlear implants to learn new words through audition by examining the length of time at which the children gazed at target words in a closed set. Children with cochlear implants were evaluated 12 to 18 months after cochlear implant activation. Additionally, the children with cochlear implants were divided into two groups, (1) those activated between 7 to 13 months of age and (2) those implanted between 16 to 23 months of age. The children implanted prior to one year of age demonstrated similar word learning abilities as the children with normal hearing. In contrast, the later-implanted children struggled substantially to learn the new target words. Of note, the performance on the word-learning task correlated with later measures of vocabulary size.

Considering the impressive improvement in outcomes associated with cochlear implantation prior to one year of age, the prudent audiologist should consider the safety of cochlear implantation for infants. Colletti et al. (2005) reported on implantation in 10 children under 12 months of age and found no major complications. Likewise, James and Papsin (2004) reported no complications in 25 children who were implanted between 7 and 12 months of age. Additionally, Kalejaiye et al. (2017) evaluated the safety of cochlear implantation in 73 infants who underwent cochlear implantation prior to one year of age. Kalejaiye and colleagues also found no serious complication in their relatively large cohort of young infants. Furthermore, Kalejaiye et al. reported that the most commonly reported problem was soft tissue complication, which occurred in 1.33% of their cases. They noted that the incidence of soft tissue complication was similar to that of the general population.

Given the emerging body of research showing significantly better outcomes for children who undergo cochlear implantation prior to 12 months of age as well as the evidence of the safety of cochlear implantation for young infants, audiologists should strive to pursue cochlear implantation between 6 and 9 months for children born with profound hearing loss. However, several factors should be contemplated when the audiologist is considering cochlear implantation prior to a child's first birthday. First, a thorough medical evaluation must be conducted to ensure that the child is mature and healthy enough for cochlear implant surgery. Similarly, a pediatric anesthesiologist should be present to administer general anesthesia and monitor the child's vital signs throughout the surgical process. Second, it is imperative that the infant's hearing sensitivity and auditory status are evaluated by a pediatric audiologist who is experienced in electrophysiologic and behavioral assessment of auditory function. Because valid behavioral thresholds are often not obtained in infants until 8 to 10 months of age, it is probable that the infant's hearing thresholds will be estimated from auditory brainstem response (ABR) assessment. The audiologist should be experienced in the administration and analysis of electrophysiologic measures of auditory function. Additionally, the audiologist should administer subjective questionnaires to evaluate the family's impression of the child's auditory responsiveness. Third, as many as 40% of children with hearing loss have additional disabilities. It may be difficult to identify the presence of some cognitive/neurological disabilities during the first few months of a child's life, and as a result, the impact of such a disability on cochlear implant outcome will be unknown. As a result, the audiologist may not be able to adequately prepare/counsel the family regarding the impact of the disability on the child's progress with his/her cochlear implant. Nonetheless, earlier implantation is likely to optimize the child's outcome with his/her cochlear implant. Finally, some families may not be prepared to proceed with cochlear implantation when their child is 6 to 9 months of age. The wishes of the family should certainly be respected. With that said, the audiologist has an ethical responsibility to inform the families that the outcomes of their children may be irreparably harmed by waiting until after 12 months of age to pursue cochlear implantation.

Mode of Communication

Several research studies have also shown that the outcomes achieved by children with cochlear implants are also significantly influenced by the mode of communication used by the child and family (Ching & Dillon, 2013; Chu et al., 2016; Dettman et al., 2016; Geers et al., 2011, 2017; Moog & Geers, 2013). The mode of communication refers to the approach or method that the child and family use to exchange information in the expressive and receptive domains. Multiple modes of communication exist and can include approaches that are primarily based on auditory communication, approaches that are primarily based on visual communication, and approaches that are a combination of the two. Prior to a discussion on the research examining the impact of communication mode on cochlear implant outcomes, a brief description will be provided of the communication modes available to children with hearing loss and their families.

Auditory-Verbal

The auditory-verbal approach involves the use of hearing technology paired with specific audition-based techniques and strategies aimed to teach children to maximize their auditory abilities so that they may communicate through Listening and Spoken Language. No manual communication (i.e., sign language) is used, and the use of visual cues is discouraged. The auditory-verbal approach is underscored by the establishment of early identification of the hearing loss and the prompt provision of hearing aids and or cochlear implants so that the child has consistent access to intelligible speech at as early an age as possible. Auditory-verbal therapy seeks to empower and equip the child's caregivers to use their child's hearing as "the primary sensory modality in developing Listening and Spoken Language" and to "create environments that support Listening and Spoken Language throughout the child's daily activities" (AG Bell, 2017). A primary goal of the auditory-verbal approach is for children with hearing loss to be fully mainstreamed into educational settings with their peers with normal hearing.

Auditory-Oral

The auditory-oral approach also seeks to develop spoken language as the child's primary method of communication. As with the auditory-verbal approach, the auditory-oral method encourages active Listening and Spoken Language through the use of hearing aids and/or cochlear implants. However, the use of speech reading and other natural gestures are also encouraged with the auditory-oral method. Sign language is not used. The parents do participate in weekly therapy sessions that are intended to guide the parents in facilitating Listening and Spoken Language development throughout the child and family's daily routine. The ultimate goal of the auditory-oral approach is for the child to be fully mainstreamed in educational settings with his/her normal hearing peers, children may attend auditory-oral preschools designed to promote the spoken language of children with hearing loss.

Listening and Spoken Language

As hearing technology and audiology services have improved over the years, the necessity to rely on visual information has diminished. As a result, the auditory-oral and auditory-verbal approaches have become quite similar. In recognition of the unity between these two approaches, the term "Listening and Spoken Language" is now often used to refer to either approach, because the ultimate goal of each is to maximize the child's ability to listen and to communicate through spoken language. Of note, research suggests that 90% to 95% of children with hearing loss have parents with normal hearing (Mitchell & Karchmer, 2004). Consequently, the Listening and Spoken Language approach is the natural language of the family and does not require the family to become fluent in another language.

American Sign Language

According to a definition/description provided by the Alexander Graham Bell (2017), American Sign Language (ASL) is "a manual language taught as a child's primary language, with English taught as a second language. ASL is recognized as a true language in

its own right and does not follow the grammatical structure of English. This method is used extensively within the Deaf community, a group that views itself as having a separate culture and identity from mainstream hearing society." Most people who use ASL use it exclusively for communication (i.e., they do not speak English). Because the grammatical structure and rules of English and ASL are different, it is impossible to simultaneously speak English and ASL in entirety. Additionally, because the structure and grammatical rules of ASL do not coincide with English, written communication will differ from ASL, a fact that has likely served to limit the literacy outcomes of persons who use ASL. As a result, after language is developed through the use of ASL, many users will also attempt to learn English as a second language in order to enable literacy development. The terms bilingual and bicultural are sometimes used to refer to persons who have become fluent in both ASL and English. The term bilingual acknowledges the fact that ASL and English are two distinct languages. The term bicultural acknowledges the reality that ASL is often associated with its own unique culture (i.e., Deaf culture), and the use of both languages allows the user to transition between the Deaf and mainstream cultures. Of note, during the first few years of life, children who are born with severe to profound hearing loss and whose families choose ASL as their child's primary mode of communication must be exposed to adults who are fluent in sign language. Consequently, the family must become fluent in sign language or provide consistent exposure to adults who sign fluently. Many children who use ASL attend schools for the Deaf with other children who communicate exclusively through sign language. However, children who primarily communicate via ASL may also participate in mainstream settings with the assistance of a full-time sign language interpreter.

Manually Coded English

Manually coded English combines the signs from ASL with additional signs developed by educators as well as with finger spelling in an attempt to communicate in the same word order and with the same grammatical markers as used in English. Manually coded English was developed by educators so that the sign language would be entirely consistent with English, which will facilitate the development of literacy and writing skills. Every word (e.g., "an," "but," "A") and all morphemes within the spoken message are included within the signed message. For example, finger spelling and other novel signs are used to convey plurality, possessiveness, and verb status such as "ed" and "ing." Sign Exact English (SEE) is an example of manually coded English. Use of a manually coded English mode requires the child's caregivers to become fluent in sign language during the child's first few years of life. Additionally, the child's educators must also use manually coded English sign language, or an interpreter must be available in the classroom. Of note, simultaneous communication is a term used to describe the simultaneous use of manually coded English and spoken English.

Total Communication

According to a definition provided by the BEGINNINGS program, Total Communication (TC) is a "philosophy of using every and all means to communicate with deaf children. The child is exposed to a formal sign-language system (based on English), finger spelling (manual sign alphabet), natural gestures, speech reading, body language, oral speech, and the use of amplification" (e.g., hearing aids, cochlear implants) (Total Commuications, 2017). The child's caregivers should become fluent in sign language and should consistently use sign language from the child's birth and throughout his/her formative years, and the child's educators should use sign language in the classroom.

Cued Speech

Cued speech provides a manual supplement to spoken English. Eight different hand cues are produced by the mouth to represent different speech sounds that may not be differentiated by speech reading (i.e., the speech sounds are produced in the same manner on the lips). Cued speech was particularly helpful before the advent of cochlear implants because many children with severe to profound high-frequency hearing loss did not have access to high-frequency phonemes. The use of cued speech is intended to allow for the development of communication through spoken language. The child's caregivers must master the use of the cued speech system and teach the child how to use cued speech. Additionally, cued speech must be used in educational settings. The development of sophisticated hearing aid and cochlear implant technology allows most children with hearing loss to have access to every phoneme in his/her native language. As a result, cued speech is no longer used prevalently.

Research Examining the Effect of Mode of Communication on Outcomes of Children with Cochlear Implants

A number of studies have examined the relationship between the communication mode used by the child and family and the outcomes of children with cochlear implants (Ching & Dillon, 2013; Chu et al., 2016; Dettman et al., 2016; Geers et al., 2011, 2017; Moog & Geers, 2013; Percy-Smith et al., 2010; Phan et al., 2016). In general, these studies have found better auditory, speech, and language outcomes for children who communicate via a Listening and Spoken Language approach. Some of these studies will be briefly reviewed in the next few sections.

The LOCHI has explored the impact of communication mode on auditory, speech, and language outcomes. Ching, Zhang, and Hou (in press) reported better global language outcomes for children who used Listening and Spoken Language at home and in educational settings. According to Ching, Zhang, and Hou (in press),

> The advantage associated with the use of speech should not be interpreted as a causal effect, as the study did not randomly assign children to "speech" versus "speech plus sign" groups. Parental decisions on communication mode appeared to be influenced by information from professionals, family and friends; considerations of practicalities of communication within the family; children's individual characteristics; and parents' own aspirations about their children's future opportunities.

Geers and colleagues (2011) examined the outcomes of 112 teenagers from across North America. All subjects had been diagnosed with hearing loss prior to 3 years of age, had received at least one cochlear implant prior to 5 years of age, and had at least 10 years of cochlear implant experience prior to assessment. Sixty-one of the children used Listening and Spoken Language as their mode of communication, whereas 51 of the children used sign language or Total Communication. Geers, Brenner, and Tobey concluded that high school age children who communicated via Listening and Spoken Language obtained higher levels of speech perception, speech intelligibility, language, and literacy than the high school age children who communicated via sign language. Additionally, Geers and colleagues examined the relationship between verbal rehearsal speed and other outcomes and characteristics of the study participants. Verbal rehearsal speed, which is essentially an indication of speaking rate, was measured by estimating the average duration of each participant's production of 12 unique seven-syllable sentences. Pisoni and Geers (2000) have suggested that verbal rehearsal skills provide a representation of a child's underlying language processing skills, and previous research has indicated that verbal rehearsal speed may explain some of the variability inherent in the language outcomes of children with cochlear implants (Pisoni & Cleary, 2003). Indeed, Geers et al. (2011) reported that the variability in outcomes observed across the participants with cochlear implants was largely explained by their verbal reasoning skills. Furthermore, Geers and colleagues (2011) noted that their study "supports the hypothesis that verbal rehearsal speed and information processing capacity are basic/core mediators of verbal development in children with hearing loss. Continued reliance on sign to supplement spoken communication influences the underlying core information processing speed and verbal rehearsal of items in working memory. The more CI [cochlear implant] students' spoken language is augmented by sign, the slower their verbal rehearsal speed." In sum, the use of sign language seemed to have delayed the basic processing skills that are fundamental to speech, language, and literacy development. Of note, the language, reading, and social adjustment scores of the participants in the Geers et al. (2011) study were generally within one standard deviation of normative results obtained from a group of age-matched children with normal hearing. Also of note, the performance of these children measured during their high school years was highly correlated with their performance measured in elementary school, a fact that suggested relatively stable outcomes across time and that emphasized the importance of early intervention.

In another study, Geers et al. (2017) examined the impact of sign language on the outcomes of 97 children who were selected from the Childhood Development after Cochlear Implantation (CDaCI) study database. The CDaCI is a prospective multicenter, NIH-funded study examining the outcomes of 188 children who received cochlear implants from six large cochlear implant centers between November 2002 and December 2004. The 97 children selected for the Geers et al. (2017) study met the following criteria: (1) received cochlear implant by 38 months of age, (2) parents consistently reported communi-

cation mode, (3) testing completed near early and late elementary grades, and (4) the children received specialized intervention during first three years of implant use. The researchers classified the children into three groups: (1) Listening and Spoken Language with no use of sign language, (2) short-term sign use: use of sign language through no more than 12 months after cochlear implant activation, and (3) long-term sign use: use of sign language for at least three years. Geers and colleagues (2017) reported that children who had no history of sign language use achieved better speech recognition through the first three years of implant use, and at the end of their elementary school years, they also obtained significantly better spoken language and literacy skills compared with children who were short- or long-term sign users. Furthermore, 70% of the children who did not use sign language developed age-appropriate spoken language abilities, whereas only 39% of the children who used sign language developed age-appropriate spoken language. Additionally, the speech production of children who did not use sign language was significantly better than those who did. Geers and colleagues stated that "this study provides the most compelling support yet available in CI literature for the benefits of spoken language input for promoting verbal development in children implanted by three years of age" (Geers et al., 2017).

As with the Geers et al. (2011, 2013) studies, research has generally found that children who communicate via Listening and Spoken Language achieve better literacy skills than children who use sign language (Harris, Terlektsi, & Kyle, 2017). Historically, children who were deaf and used sign language to communicate read at approximately a third-grade level upon graduation from high school (Vermeulen et al., 2007). The relatively low literacy levels in deaf children who used sign language are likely attributed to the lack of phonemic awareness and to the fact that the structure and grammatical rules of ASL differ from those of English. Indeed, Harris, Terletski, and Kyle studied literacy development in 41 children with pre-longitudinal severe to profound hearing loss and found better literacy skills in children who communicated via Listening and Spoken Language relative to those who used sign language. Similarly, in a study of 27 children with cochlear implants, Nittrouer et al. (2012) found better literacy development in children with better Listening and Spoken Language abilities. Likewise, Desj-Jardin, Ambrose, and Eisenberg (2009) studied literacy development in 16 children with cochlear implants and reported that the children with better expressive oral language skills achieved better reading skills.

The physiological underpinning of the association between higher literacy skills and more proficiency Listening and Spoken Language abilities can be found in brain imaging studies that have shown that the areas of the brain that are active when we comprehend spoken language are also the same areas that are active when we read (Bisconti et al., 2016; Mortensen et al., 2006). Specifically, the left inferior prefrontal cortex has been shown to be active during the comprehension of spoken language and during activities requiring phonemic processing, which is the association of a particular phoneme with its respective sound (e.g., think "hooked on phonics"). To underscore the importance of phonemic awareness on literacy development, imagine if you are only fluent in the English language but are asked to read words that are written in Chinese characters. In the same way, deaf children (or children who do not have access to intelligible speech during the first few years of life) are being asked to recognize letters on a page, combine them for words, and understand the meanings of those words without ever having heard the sounds associated with the letters. For example, the word "dog" is simple to read for those who are fluent in English. You know the "duh" sound of D, the "ah" sound of A, and the "g" sound of G. And you immediately equate the combination of those sounds to a furry animal that says "woof." But what if you'd never heard the sounds of the letters, D, O, and G, either individually or strung together? What would those symbols mean to you? Even though you live in a country where the word "dog" is universally known and you can sign for the animal "dog," seeing D-O-G means nothing. That is the uphill battle that a deaf child has to traverse to learn to read. Sign language consists of motions that indicate meaning but are not English in its written form. Furthermore, ASL contains a structure and set of grammatical rules that are different than what are used in written English. Accordingly, Geers et al. (2011) found a close relationship between spoken language and literacy abilities and noted that the children with cochlear implants "who demonstrate the best spoken vocabulary and syntax in elementary grades achieve the highest literacy performance in high school." Finally, it is worth reiterating that in contrast to the historically low levels of literacy abilities of children with severe to profound hearing loss, in a group of teenagers who used cochlear implants and Listening and Spoken Language, Geers and colleagues found literacy skills that were typically within one standard deviation of age-matched normal hearing peers.

A Comment on Research Examining the Relationship Between Communication Mode and Outcomes After Cochlear Implantation. The overwhelming consensus finding of research studies examining the relationship between cochlear implant outcomes and the communication mode of the child and family is that children who communicate via Listening and Spoken Language achieve higher auditory, speech, spoken language, and literacy skills. However, these studies do possess limitations that are important to discuss. For instance, many of the children in the Geers et al. (2003, 2011) studies came from families who had high levels of education and family income. Additionally, many of these children were educated in preschools that provided intensive intervention and education designed to optimize auditory and spoken language development in children with hearing loss. As a result, these children may have had several advantages that contributed to their impressive outcomes but that are not available to all children with hearing loss. Furthermore, the children in the Geers (2003, 2011) studies did not have additional disabilities. Of course, children who have hearing loss and other disabilities, such as a neurocognitive disorder, may achieve poorer outcomes than the children in the Geers (2003, 2011) studies.

Moreover, the aforementioned studies do not firmly establish a causal relationship between mode of communication and outcomes following cochlear implantation. Instead, these studies simply establish a causative relationship between mode of communication and outcomes. To elaborate, it is quite possible that many children in these studies began with the use of sign language but transitioned to full-time use of Listening and Spoken Language after satisfactory progress in spoken language was achieved. In contrast, the children who continued to struggle with spoken language development also continued to use sign language. Consequently, a comparison made between the two groups at a later point in time may ultimately be a comparison between children who made progress after implantation and those who did not. Furthermore, because of ethical considerations, it is impossible to design a prospective study in which children are randomly assigned to different mode of communication groups. Families possess the right to choose their children's communication methodology. As such, it is possible that families who have several factors that predispose their children to a better postoperative outcome are also the families who choose to communicate with their child via Listening and Spoken Language. If this was indeed the case, the finding of better outcomes for children who use Listening and Spoken Language would be associative but not necessarily causal. An analogy would be the hypothesis that frequent exercise triggers a physiologic urge to eat healthier. Indeed, a study that explored exercise and eating habits would likely find that people who exercise more frequently tend to eat healthier. However, one cannot conclude that exercise triggers a physiologic urge to eat healthier. Instead, it may be more likely to assume that people who desire to live a healthy lifestyle choose to exercise frequently and to eat healthy. Once again, the relationship is one of association rather than causality. With that said, it is important to conclude that research examining the relationship between outcomes and communication mode typically find that an emphasis on Listening and Spoken Language results in better outcomes after cochlear implantation. Whether this relationship is associative or causal, families should be aware of these research findings, particularly when they desire for their children to maximize their Listening and Spoken Language abilities.

Etiology of Hearing Loss

For the most part, the etiology of a child's hearing loss does not impact outcomes achieved after a cochlear implantation. There are, however, some exceptions to this rule. The following sections will examine the hearing disorders that do influence outcomes after cochlear implantation.

Genetic Hearing Loss

About 50% of childhood hearing loss can be attributed to a genetic etiology (Gorlin, Toriello, & Cohen, 1995; Morton, 1991). Genetic hearing loss may be classified as nonsyndromic or syndromic with about 1/3 of genetic hearing loss being associated with a syndrome (Morton, 1991). Genetic hearing losses can be further categorized into the mode of inheritance, with approximately 77% being attributed to recessive inheritance, 22% to dominant inheritance, and 1% to X-linked inheritance. In general, children with a genetic etiology of hearing loss achieve satisfactory results after cochlear implantation (Abdurehim, Lehmann, & Zeitouni, 2017; Park et al., 2017; Stahr et al., 2017; Varga et al., 2014; Vesseur et al., 2016; Wu et al., 2015).

Approximately 50% of nonsyndromic recessive hearing loss is caused by a mutation in the GJB2

gene (DFNB1), which is responsible for encoding the connexin 26 protein (McGuirt & Smith, 1999). The connexin 26 protein is responsible for creating gap junction bonds in the stria vascularis and in supporting cells of the organ of Corti. Specifically, the connexin 26 gap junctions allow for the circulation of K+ ions from the stria vascularis to the scala media and then to the scala tympani and back to the stria vascularis. This circulation of K+ ions allows for the maintenance of the positive endocochlear resting potential necessary for cochlear transduction (i.e., hair cell depolarization). Connexin 26 mutations result in a reduction or elimination of the endocochlear testing potential, which will eventually result in a loss of inner hair cell function. However, the cochlear macroanatomy and the cochlear nerve are both intact. As a result, children with GJB2-type genetic deafness typically achieve excellent outcomes with cochlear implants (Park et al., 2017; Wu et al., 2015).

A mutation of the SLC26A4 gene is another common cause of autosomal recessive hearing loss. The SLC26A4 mutation is known to result in Pendred's syndrome, which is an autosomal recessive syndromic cause of hearing loss, as well as in DFNB4 hearing loss. Pendred's syndrome is characterized by enlarged vestibular aqueduct, cochlear dysplasia (e.g., Mondini's malformation, common cavity), and a thyroid disorder. DFNB4 is characterized by the same features except for the thyroid disorder (Usami et al., 1999). Of note, enlarged vestibular aqueduct is often associated with severe to profound high-frequency hearing loss and has also been associated with progressive hearing loss. Additionally, the progression of hearing loss can be exacerbated by minor head trauma (e.g., bumping head during sports or play). Because the site of lesion for enlarged vestibular aqueduct is outside the cochlea, most people achieve excellent benefit from and outcomes with cochlear implants (Park et al., 2017). Of course, if an SLC26A4 gene mutation also results in cochlear dysplasia, cochlear implant outcomes may be limited to some extent. A perilymphatic gusher/leak is a common complication during surgery for persons with enlarged vestibular aqueduct (Isaiah et al., 2017; Papsin, 2005).

Excellent outcomes from cochlear implantation occur from patients with a variety of different syndromes that cause hearing loss. Cochlear implantation is very beneficial for persons with Usher syndrome. The pathological mechanism underlying Usher syndrome results in dysfunction of the cochlear hair cells (Yan & Liu, 2010). As a result, cochlear implantation is quite successful at bypassing the disordered part of the inner ear and stimulating the functional cochlear nerve. Additionally, because Usher syndrome results in macular degeneration and blindness, hearing is particularly important to support localization and spatial awareness. Prompt provision of bilateral cochlear implants for persons who have Usher syndrome with severe to profound hearing loss and some residual vision is essential to allow for the development of localization skills through audition.

Research has shown that cochlear implantation results in improvement in auditory function for many children with CHARGE syndrome (Young et al., 2017). Young and colleagues found that children diagnosed with CHARGE syndrome obtained poorer outcomes than the typical child with a cochlear implant, but they did achieve better auditory outcomes compared with their performance with hearing aids. Of note, CHARGE is often associated with cochlear nerve deficiency and cognitive/neurological disorders, both of which are known to adversely affect cochlear implant outcomes.

Furthermore, cochlear implantation has been shown to provide satisfactory outcomes and benefits for children diagnosed with Waardenburg syndrome, which frequently results in cochlear dysfunction (the prevalence of hearing loss in children with Waardenburg syndromes varies by study with a range spanning from 35 to 75% (Bayrak et al., 2017; Broomfield et al., 2013; Koyama et al., 2016). There four different types of Waardenburg syndrome (Type I, Type II, Type III, and Type IV, and the prevalence of hearing loss varies across type. Bayrak and colleagues did report a perilymphatic gusher during surgery for all 11 subjects with Waardenburg in their study. Also, cochlear dysplasia is a common finding in patients who have severe to profound hearing loss from Waardenburg syndrome. Of note, Waardenburg syndrome is the most common cause of autosomal dominant sensorineural hearing loss.

Alport syndrome, Branchio-oto-renal syndrome, and Jervell and Lange-Nielsen syndrome can all cause sensorineural hearing loss with a cochlear site of lesion. As a result, cochlear implantation is expected to provide considerable benefit and result in satisfactory outcomes for persons who have severe to profound hearing loss because of these syndromes.

To summarize, many children with genetic causes of hearing loss will receive substantial benefit from and will achieve excellent outcomes with cochlear implant technology. Children who have genetic etiologies that result in a cochlear site of lesion but that leave the cochlear macro-anatomy intact are expected to achieve better outcomes than children who have sites of lesion that result in anatomical abnormalities of the cochlea (e.g., cochlear dysplasia) or cochlear nerve. Furthermore, genetic mutations that also result in cognitive/neurological disorders will most likely result in poorer outcomes after cochlear implantation. As a result, the audiologist should evaluate each child on an individual basis when determining a prognosis for cochlear implant outcome.

Aplasia/Deficiency of the Cochlear Nerve

The term **cochlear nerve deficiency** refers to the case in which the cochlear nerve is smaller than normal or absent as observed via magnetic resonance imaging (MRI) (Glastonbury et al., 2002). Cochlear aplasia refers to a complete lack of development of the cochlear nerve (i.e., absent cochlear nerve), whereas cochlear nerve hypoplasia refers to partial development of the cochlear nerve so that the caliber of the cochlear nerve is smaller than the other nerves in the internal auditory canal (i.e., small/thin cochlear nerve). In general, research has shown markedly reduced outcomes for children with cochlear nerve deficiency. For instance, Papsin studied 195 children who were identified with abnormal cochleovestibular anatomy as determined via CT scan assessment. Eleven of these children had an abnormally narrow internal auditory canal, which is typically associated with cochlear nerve deficiency. The majority of children with abnormal cochlear anatomy achieved good outcomes with and benefit from their cochlear implants, whereas the children with abnormally small internal auditory canals achieved significantly poorer outcomes and little to no improvement in speech recognition following cochlear implantation.

Several recent studies examining children with cochlear nerve deficiency have sought to predict cochlear implant benefit by evaluating the anatomy of the cochlear nerve via MRI. Birman et al. (2016) reported on outcomes for 50 children (100 ears) who had cochlear nerve deficiency for at least one ear as indicated by MRI. Cochlear aplasia (as defined by the presence of no cochlear nerve on MRI) was present in 64 ears, hypoplasia (abnormally small cochlear nerve on MRI) was present in 25 ears, and a normal cochlear nerve was present for 11 ears. Birman and colleagues collected information pertaining to several important factors, including cochlear nerve anatomy from the MRI, transtympanic EABR, cochlear implant–elicited ABR, intraoperative NRT, communication mode, and categories of auditory perception.

Birman et al. (2016) reported at least some ability to understand spoken language for about 47% of the ears with cochlear nerve aplasia and 89% of the ears with cochlear nerve hypoplasia. Furthermore, 51% of the children in the study used spoken language (with some supplementing spoken language with sign language), whereas 49% of the children communicated primarily by sign language. Children who had cochlear nerve aplasia were more likely to communicate via sign language. Of note, children who also had an additional disability were less likely to develop the ability to understand speech and to communicate via spoken language.

Peng and colleagues (2017) conducted a literature review of 18 studies with a total of 97 subjects with cochlear nerve deficiency. Several interesting findings were reported from this literature review. The auditory outcome following cochlear implantation was characterized into four different categories: (1) nonstimulation/minimal detection, (2) improved sound detection, (3) closed-set speech recognition, and (4) open-set speech recognition. Peng et al. (2017) reported that most studies showed at least some subjects who had developed some level of speech recognition following cochlear implantation. However, approximately 54% of the subjects did not develop any speech discrimination ability. As with the Birman study, subjects in the Peng et al. literature review who were diagnosed by MRI with cochlear nerve hypoplasia achieved better speech recognition than subjects with cochlear nerve aplasia. Specifically, 65% of children with hypoplastic cochlear nerves developed closed- or open-set speech recognition compared with only 30% of children with aplastic cochlear nerves. Also, subjects who were diagnosed with a syndrome were less likely to achieve a favorable auditory response than those with nonsyndromic cochlear nerve deficiency. Of note, almost 43% of children with a syndromic condition and cochlear nerve deficiency failed to demonstrate an auditory response to electrical stimulation. Peng and colleagues (2017) concluded that "while initial reports cast doubt that ears with absent cochlear nerve aplasia could benefit from cochlear implantation secondary to the lack of an afferent neural pathway, later studies have revealed that patients with cochlear nerve aplasia can derive meaningful CI use. This is likely secondary to cochlear nerve fibers traveling with other nerves within the internal auditory canal."

The following statements briefly summarize the effect of cochlear nerve deficiency on cochlear implant outcomes:

- Research has generally shown poorer outcomes for children diagnosed with cochlear nerve deficiency on MRI assessment.
- However, many children with cochlear nerve deficiency do achieve sound awareness with cochlear implant use, and some children develop some speech recognition capacity.
- As many as 50% of children with cochlear nerve deficiency are able to communicate via spoken language.
- Children who are diagnosed with cochlear nerve hypoplasia are more likely to achieve a favorable auditory and spoken language outcome than children with cochlear nerve aplasia.
- Children with additional disabilities and/or a syndromic diagnosis generally achieve poorer outcomes following cochlear implantation.
- Children with severe to profound hearing loss should undergo MRI assessment with temporal bone protocol to evaluate the status of the cochlear nerve. CT scan does not allow for adequate identification of cochlear nerve deficiency (Adunka, Jewells, & Buchman, 2007; Parry, Booth, & Roland, 2005). Of note, Buchman et al. (2006) reported that cochlear nerve deficiency affected only one ear in about half of the subjects in their study, which underscores the importance of MRI to identify ear of implantation.
- Children who have present EABR and ECAP (i.e., NRT) generally achieve better outcomes following cochlear implantation.

Abnormal Cochlear Anatomy

Numerous researchers have also looked at the effect of abnormal cochlear anatomy on outcomes following cochlear implantation. In general, most children with inner malformation receive substantial benefit from cochlear implantation, and the outcomes of children with cochlear abnormalities are better than the outcomes of children with cochlear nerve deficiency. Buchman et al. (2004) examined the outcomes of 28 children who had been diagnosed by CT scan with inner ear anatomical abnormalities. Buchman and colleagues found that the type of inner ear abnormality had a large impact on the outcome achieved after implantation. Specifically, children with enlarged vestibular aqueduct, Mondini's malformation, and partial semicircular canal aplasia perform very well, with 86% of children with these findings achieving open-set speech recognition. In contrast, poorer outcomes were observed in children who had been diagnosed with an isolated incomplete cochlear partition, cochlear hypoplasia, common cavity cochleae, or total semicircular canal aplasia. Of note, almost 60% of children diagnosed with more severe inner ear abnormalities also had been diagnosed with an additional disability which likely contributed to the their reduced outcome following cochlear implantation. Additionally, Buchman and colleagues noted that children diagnosed with CHARGE generally achieved poorer outcomes with their cochlear implants. CHARGE syndrome is often associated with cochlear nerve deficiency and significant cognitive/neurological delay, both of which may have hindered the children's progress. Overall, Buchman et al. concluded that cochlear implantation was beneficial for most of the children with inner ear abnormalities in their study, with 96% of the subjects using their implant on a daily basis and almost 2/3 developing either open- or closed-set speech recognition. However, speech recognition is often reduced for children with more extensive cochlear anomalies and for children with additional disabilities.

Papsin (2005) also evaluated the effect of cochleo-vestibular abnormalities on the outcomes of 298 children with cochlear implants. The outcomes of 140 children with inner ear abnormalities were compared with those of 158 children with normal inner ear anatomy. Papsin reported that the cochlear implant surgery was more challenging in 24% of the children with inner ear abnormalities, with 17.5% presenting with complications related to abnormal middle ear anatomy and 6.7% presenting with perilymphatic leakage. Of particular note, there was not a statistically significant difference in speech recognition between the children with inner ear abnormalities and the children with normal cochleovestibular anatomy. Additionally, both groups typically received significant benefit from cochlear implantation. In contrast, children diagnosed with an abnormally small internal auditory canal did tend to achieve poorer outcomes than the rest of the children. Most likely, the children with small internal auditory canals also had deficient cochlear nerves. Of importance, the children with hypoplastic cochleae and common cavity cochleae did require higher stimulation levels (typically with use of a wider pulse width) and were more likely to require more extensive implant programming to avoid facial nerve stimulation.

Isaiah et al. (2017) conducted a chart review of 381 children who underwent CT scan and/or MRI as part of a cochlear implant candidacy assessment. They reported that 102 (27%) of these children were determined to have an inner ear anatomical abnormality. As with Buchman et al. (2004) and Papsin (2005), Isaiah and colleagues reported that children with an enlarged vestibular aqueduct typically achieved excellent outcomes after cochlear implantation. In contrast, Isaiah et al. found poor outcomes for children with other types of inner ear abnormalities. Only 24% of children with cochlear dysplasia (e.g., Mondini's malformation, common cavity) developed speech recognition after cochlear implantation, whereas only 33% of children with vestibular dysplasia developed speech recognition after implantation. None of the children with a diagnosis of cochlear nerve deficiency developed speech recognition after cochlear implantation.

Collectively, the research examining the effects of inner abnormalities may be summarized as follows:

- Inner ear abnormalities are a risk factor for poorer outcomes with reduced benefit from a cochlear implant.
- Children with enlarged aqueducts are excellent candidates for cochlear implantation and typically achieve good outcomes.
- Many children with cochlear anatomical abnormalities can derive significant benefit from cochlear implantation, but it is likely that advanced programming techniques will be necessary to optimize performance. Frequent cochlear implant programming may be necessary to account for changes that may occur in requisite stimulus levels. Intensive habilitative therapy may also be necessary to maximize auditory performance.
- Surgical complications are likely with many cases of inner ear abnormalities.
- An abnormally small internal auditory canal is often associated with poor outcomes after cochlear implantation.
- Audiologists should carefully inform families of the potential impact of inner ear abnormalities on the outcomes and otologic/audiology/habilitative management of their children.

Auditory Neuropathy Spectrum Disorder

One may expect that children with auditory neuropathy spectrum disorder (ANSD) would perform poorly with cochlear implants, because the word "neuropathy" would seem to imply that the site of lesion is at the nerve or within the auditory nervous system. However, ANSD is a broad term that is used to describe a constellation of hearing disorders with a variety of different sites of lesion. ANSD manifests clinically as an absent or abnormal auditory brainstem response (ABR) with a present otoacoustic emission (OAE) and/or cochlear microphonic response (Declau et al., 2013; Starr & Rance, 2015). The actual site of lesion that results in an absent ABR in the presence of normal or near-normal outer hair cell function may reside within the cochlea (inner hair cells), at the cochlear synapse, at the cochlear nerve, or in the auditory brainstem (Rance, 2005). Children who have ANSD with a site of lesion in the cochlea or at the cochlear synapse will likely do very well with a cochlear implant (Berlin et al., 2003, 2010; Jeong et al., 2007; Peterson et al., 2003; Teagle et al., 2010; Walton et al., 2008). Additionally, many patients with a site of lesion at the cochlear nerve or auditory brainstem (e.g., hyperbilirubinemia) may achieve better hearing performance with a cochlear implant than with hearing aids (Berlin et al., 2003, 2010; Rance et al., 2005). For example, demyelinating disorders (e.g., demyelination that may occur following hyperbilirubinemia) will result in reduced capability of the auditory system to generate a compound synchronous response to acoustic stimulation. Because stimulation with electrical pulses results in an over-synchronization of the response of the cochlear nerve fibers, cochlear implantation may allow for a more favorable response to speech and environmental sounds.

Numerous research studies have explored the outcomes of children who have ANSD and receive cochlear implants. For example, Ching and colleagues (2013, 2018; Gardner-Berry et al., in press) have explored outcomes of children with ANSD and have found no difference in spoken language achievement and aided speech perception compared with children with cochlear hearing loss. Of note, Gardner-Berry, Hou, and Ching (in press) noted that the cortical auditory evoked response (CAER) was used to aid in the provision of early hearing aid fitting and in the determination of cochlear implant candidacy. In short, hearing aid gain and output was set at a level that resulted in the production of a present aided CAER. If no CAER was present with the hearing aids set for a severe to profound hearing loss, then cochlear implantation was pursued between 6 and 12 months of age. As a result, the children with ANSD received prompt provision of hearing aids or cochlear implants as needed. According to Gardner-Berry et al. (in press), "the use of CAEPs together with functional auditory assessments, such as the PEACH, enable us to reach decisions about the need

to provide amplification and to proceed with the early fitting of hearing aids in infants with ANSD. Current evidence shows that the provision of early amplification and/or cochlear implants is associated with better speech language outcomes in infants with hearing loss." Of note, Ching et al. (2013) reported that 30% of children with ANSD have at least one additional disability other than hearing loss. Audiologists and families of children with hearing loss should be aware of the potential of additional disabilities to limit outcomes after cochlear implantation. Also of note, Gardner-Berry et al. (in press) noted that ANSD diagnosed in the newborn period has a genetic cause in 40% of cases.

Teagle and colleagues (2010) reported on the outcomes of 52 children who had ANSD and received a cochlear implant for at least one ear. Forty-two percent of these children were born prematurely, and over half of the children in the study had additional disabilities. Also, an MRI indicated brain and/or inner abnormalities in 38% of the children. Teagle et al. reported that 50% of the children were able to develop open-set speech recognition following cochlear implantation. Of the children who were unable to participate in open-set speech recognition assessment, 30% had additional disabilities and/or were too young to complete open-set testing. Of the 26 children who did achieve open-set speech recognition, only 7 achieved a score of greater than 70% correct on the PBK-50 word recognition test. It is important to mention that only 4 of the 52 children in the Teagle et al. study received their cochlear implants prior to 18 months of age. As such, it is possible that speech recognition after cochlear implantation may have been better for these children if they would have received their cochlear implants at an earlier age. It should also be noted that none of the children who were diagnosed with cochlear nerve deficiency were able to develop open-set speech recognition after cochlear implantation. Teagle and colleagues noted the concern that CND may negatively influence cochlear implant benefit for children with CHARGE syndrome. Also of importance, children who had present ECAP responses (e.g., NRT) after cochlear implantation achieved good open-set speech recognition, whereas the children who had absent/abnormal ECAP responses did not achieve open-set speech recognition.

Berlin et al. (2010) reported on 260 patients diagnosed with ANSD across multiple clinical sites. Eighty-five of these patients had used hearing aids, and 49 received cochlear implants. Berlin and colleagues noted that 15% received at least "some benefit" (improvement in speech recognition) from hearing aids, whereas 85% received at least "some benefit" from cochlear implant use. Of note, Berlin et al. reported that none of the participants with ANSD caused by an otoferlin mutation achieved spontaneous spoken language development or open-set speech recognition with hearing aid use, whereas they were able to achieve good outcomes with cochlear implants.

Humphriss and colleagues (2013) reviewed 27 studies examining the outcomes persons with ANSD achieve following cochlear implantation. Humphriss et al. concluded that outcomes are generally favorable for children who receive cochlear implants but did note that many of the studies included a small number of children or were not formally designed with sound methodological characteristics. Similarly, Fernandes and colleagues (2015) reviewed 22 studies describing outcomes of children who were diagnosed with ANSD and received a cochlear implant and concluded that cochlear implantation "improved their performance of hearing skills." Fernandes et al. also reported that the children with ANSD had similar performance compared with children who had cochlear hearing loss and had received a cochlear implant.

As mentioned in Chapter 18 (Objective Measures of Cochlear Implant Function), Gibson and Sanli (2007) used transtympanic electrical stimulation at the round window to measure the electrically evoked electrocochleography (ECochG) and auditory brainstem responses (EABR) for 39 children (78 ears) with ANSD. The researchers reported that children who had ANSD and a robust transtympanic EABR achieved postimplant speech recognition that was at least as good as children who had received a cochlear implant after a diagnosis of severe to profound hearing loss with a cochlear site of lesion (i.e., sensory hearing loss). In contrast, the children with abnormal or absent transtympanic EABR achieved limited to poor open-set speech recognition following cochlear implantation. Gibson and Sanli concluded that the presence of a preimplant EABR may "indicate a significantly better outcome after cochlear implant surgery" compared with absent preimplant ABR in children.

The outcomes that children with ANSD achieve after cochlear implantation may be summarized as follows:

- Most studies indicate that most children with ANSD achieve significant benefit from and open-set speech recognition with cochlear implant use.

Research typically has found that most children with ANSD achieve postimplant outcomes that are similar to those in children with cochlear hearing loss.

- Ching et al. (2013) and Gardner-Berry, Hou, and Ching (in press) have suggested that children with ANSD will achieve better outcomes if a cochlear implant is provided at an early age (e.g., prior to 12 months of age). They also advocate for the use of cortical auditory evoked response assessment along with behavioral audiologic assessment, standardized questionnaires (e.g., PEACH, LittlEARS), and parent/therapist report to determine whether cochlear implantation should be provided at an early age for children with ANSD.
- The site of lesion of the ANSD likely influences outcomes after cochlear implantation. Children with a site of lesion at the cochlea or cochlear synapse are likely to receive excellent benefit from cochlear implantation, whereas children with cochlear nerve deficiency and/ or dysfunction along the afferent auditory pathway are likely to achieve relatively poor outcomes with cochlear implantation. Children with minor demyelinating conditions (e.g., hyperbilirubinemia) are likely to achieve benefit from cochlear implantation if progress with hearing aids is unsatisfactory.
- Cortical auditory evoked response assessment and electrocochleography (eCochG) may assist in the determination of site of lesion prior to cochlear implantation. Additionally, transtympanic electrically evoked eCochG and ABR assessment may assist in site of lesion identification and determination of prognosis for cochlear implantation.
- MRI with temporal bone protocol should be conducted to evaluate the status of the cochlear nerve.
- The presence of an ECAP (e.g., NRT, NRI, ART) following cochlear implantation suggests that a favorable outcome is likely after cochlear implantation.
- Many children with ANSD can develop age-appropriate spoken language communication abilities after cochlear implantation. For children with cochlear nerve deficiency or a site of lesion at the afferent auditory pathway, communication development may need to be supported by manual communication (sign language/cued speech along with auditory/spoken language).

Ototoxicity

Ototoxicity is believed to produce free radicals that alter the molecular composition of the inner ear and that result in damage to the cochlear hair cells through metabolic dysfunction and/or apoptosis (Selimoglu, 2007). Importantly, ototoxicity typically results in damage to the cochlear hair cells with little to no dysfunction at the cochlear nerve and afferent auditory pathways (Nakaizumi et al., 2004). As a result, persons who suffer severe to profound hearing loss after exposure to ototoxic agents will typically achieve excellent outcomes after cochlear implantation (Nichani et al., 2013).

Cytomegalovirus

Cytomegalovirus (CMV) is the leading cause of non-genetic hearing loss in infants, accounting for as much as 1/3 of hearing losses present at birth (Nassetta, Kimberlin, & Whitley, 2009). CMV causes hearing loss when the mother contracts the virus during pregnancy. Of note, 3% to 50% of women of child-bearing age have not been infected with CMV. Of the 1 to 4% of women who contract CMV during pregnancy, approximately 30% pass it to the infant. CMV may be transmitted to the infant through the placenta, during delivery, or from breast milk. Eighty percent of infants infected with CMV will not develop symptoms. Congenital CMV must be diagnosed within the first two to three weeks of life. Hearing loss from CMV is often progressive. It may be unilateral or bilateral, and the degree of hearing loss may be variable. The exact mechanism through which CMV causes hearing loss is not well understood. However, Carraro et al. (2017) have suggested that CMV may result in vascular changes that damage the stria vascularis. Importantly, CMV often causes neurological/cognitive deficits and may also result in damage to spiral ganglion cell bodies (Carraro, Park, & Harrison, 2016). Children who are deafened from CMV will typically receive benefit from cochlear implantation (Hoey et al., 2017; Yoshida et al., 2017). The fact that cochlear implantation is beneficial for children with CMV should not be surprising considering a probable cochlear site of lesion. However, research has also shown that some children with CMV make limited progress with spoken language development after cochlear implantation, a fact that has been attributed to the cognitive/neurological deficits often associated with CMV (Hoey et al., 2017; Yoshida et al., 2017). As a result, audiologists should consider cochlear implantation for children with CMV but should also counsel families regarding the potential effect of CMV on the central nervous system and the consequential effect on cochlear implant outcomes.

Child and Family Variables

A number of different research studies have shown that several child and family variables have a substantial impact on the outcomes a child achieves after cochlear implantation. For instance, several studies have found that maternal education level (e.g., high school, college, graduate school, doctoral degree) is positively associated with cochlear implant outcomes (Barnard et al., 2015; Ching et al., 2013; Fitzpatrick et al., 2007). The exact mechanisms responsible for the better outcomes observed for children whose mothers have higher educational levels are uncertain. It may be that families with higher educational levels have greater financial resources to obtain services and technology for their children. Likewise, families with higher educational levels may have greater access to transportation to allow for attendance at audiology and auditory verbal therapy appointments. Choo and Dettman (2017) reported on the influence that attendance at audiology appointments has on outcomes of 400 children with cochlear implants. They noted that the children who did not regularly attend audiology appointments had poorer receptive language abilities and open-set word recognition compared with the children who regularly attended audiology appointments. Of note, Choo and Dettman did note that the children who did not regularly attend appointments were also more likely to have additional disabilities. Additionally, it is possible that families with higher educational levels may have additional time to allow for the provision of therapy for their children in the home. Indeed, several studies have found better outcomes for children whose parents have greater sensitivity to their needs (Ching & Dillon, 2013; Quittner et al., 2013).

Several research studies have also shown better outcomes for children whose families have a higher socioeconomic status (SES) (Barnard et al., 2015; Ching & Dillon, 2013; Niparko et al., 2010; Tobey et al., 2003). Once again, the families with greater financial means are likely to have better access to the technology, services, and transportation children with hearing loss need to achieve optimal outcomes. Of note, Ching et al. (2014) did not find a statistically significant relationship between SES and outcomes that children with cochlear implants obtained at 5 years of age. It is important to acknowledge that Australia has a national health care system that provides access to care for all Australian citizens. As a result, SES may not have possessed as large of an effect, because the children had ready access to the technology and services needed to develop spoken language, regardless of the child's degree of hearing loss or the family's financial means.

Although it may seem obvious, children with cochlear implants will not achieve satisfactory progress if they do not use their cochlear implants. Risley and Hart (1995) have estimated that the typical child from an affluent family is exposed to 46 million words during the first four years of life. Throughout the preschool years, a child is awake approximately 10 to 13 hours per day. In a study examining the number of hours that children used hearing aids per day (as indicated by data logging collected by the children's hearing aids), Jones and Launer (2010) reported that children between birth and 4 years old used their hearing aids for an average of almost 6 hours per day. Let's say the typical child listens for 12 hours per day during the first four years of life to allow for exposure to 46 million words. If the child with hearing loss is only listening with hearing technology for half the time that a child with normal hearing listens each day, then the child with hearing loss will only be exposed to 23 million words through the first four years of life. Undoubtedly, the reduced exposure to intelligible speech will have deleterious consequences on auditory brain development and on the development of spoken language abilities. There is a paucity of research examining data logging in infants and children with cochlear implants. Guerzoni and Cuda (2017) reported better language outcomes for children for whom data logging had indicated longer cochlear implant use in the presence of speech in a quiet environment. Busch, Vanpoucke, and van Wieringen (2017) examined cochlear implant data logging records to determine daily use in hours and found that children from birth to 6 years old had an average of 6.5 hours of use per day, which compared unfavorably to 10.5 or more hours of use per day for older children and adults. In a large multi-center study of children who used hearing aids, Walker et al. (2015) found that children who used their hearing aids for more than 10 hours per day obtained better language outcomes than children who used their hearing aids for less than 10 hours per day. In short, in order to optimize individual potential and outcomes, children with cochlear implants must use their cochlear implants during all waking hours. It is

imperative for the audiologist to counsel families of the critical importance of full-time cochlear use (i.e., during all waking hours; "eyes open, ears on") from the day of activation onward.

Research has also explored the cochlear implant outcomes of children who speak English as a second language. In general, research has suggested that children who are bilingual achieve excellent outcomes in both languages following cochlear implantation (Bunta & Douglas, 2013; Bunta et al., 2016). Of note, to optimize outcomes in both languages, children with cochlear implants should receive intensive spoken-language-based intervention/therapy in early education settings, and the family should receive Listening and Spoken Language–based intervention in their native language with the goal of creating an auditory language-rich environment in the home. Once again, early implantation and full-time cochlear implant used during all waking hours will provide the child with the best opportunity to develop optimal receptive and expressive abilities in two or more spoken languages.

Several research studies have also explored the effect that additional disabilities/comorbidities have on outcomes after cochlear implantation. In short, the presence of an additional disability has a negative impact on the outcomes children achieve after cochlear implantation (Ching et al., 2013, 2014, 2018, in press). As previously noted, about 30% to 40% of children with hearing loss have an additional disability (Ching et al., 2013; Cupples et al., 2016; Gallaudet Research Institute, 2011; Picard, 2004). In particular, neurocognitive disabilities are most likely to have a negative effect on outcomes after cochlear implantation. However, it should be noted that numerous research studies and substantial anecdotal experience have indicated that most children who have severe to profound hearing loss with additional disabilities receive substantial benefit from cochlear implantation (Beer et al., 2012; Cupples et al., 2016; Hoey et al., 2017; Holt & Kirk, 2005; Palmieri et al., 2014; Waltzman et al., 2000; Yoshida et al., 2017). In general, studies have shown that children with hearing loss and additional disabilities benefit from cochlear implantation but generally perform more poorly than children without additional disabilities (Beer et al., 2012; Ching & Dillon, 2013; Cupples et al., 2016; Donaldson et al., 2004; Eshraghi et al., 2015; Hoey et al., 2017; Holt & Kirk, 2005; Palmieri et al., 2014; Wakil et al., 2014; Waltzman et al., 2000; Yoshida et al., 2017). Of note, many studies have shown that the parents of children with disabilities often report considerable benefit from cochlear implantation, even when negligible benefit is shown on objective measures of hearing and language abilities (Donaldson, Heavner, & Zwolan, 2004; Eshraghi et al., 2015). Also, several studies have suggested that children with additional disabilities may require more time to reach a given level of performance compared with children without disabilities (Cupples et al., 2016; Pyman et al., 2000; Waltzman et al., 2000).

Cupples et al. (2016) specifically examined the outcomes of 180 children with hearing loss and additional disabilities. These 180 children were part of a larger population study of 462 children who were diagnosed in Australia and included in the Longitudinal Outcomes of Children with Hearing Impairment (LOCHI) study. Expressive and receptive language, speech production, and nonverbal IQ were all evaluated. The children who used cochlear implants achieved similar outcomes across all domains compared with the children who used hearing aids. As a whole, the children's mean scores for receptive language assessment were 65.0, 77.1, and 83.2 for the Childhood Development Inventory (CDI), Pre-School Language Scale–4th Edition (PLS-4), and the Peabody Picture Vocabulary Test–4th Edition (PPVT-4), respectively. Mean scores for expressive language assessment were 62.8 and 74.4 for the CDI and PLS-4, respectively. The mean score for speech production assessment, as measured with the Diagnostic Evaluation of Articulation and Phonology (DEAP) was 96. In short, the average speech and language scores for the children with additional disabilities in the Cupples et al. study were significantly lower than the mean performance of their typically developing age-matched peers. Of note, children who communicated via spoken language achieved better outcomes on all language and speech measures compared with children who communicated via speech and sign language. Also, children with higher nonverbal IQ achieved better outcomes on all speech and language measures. Additionally, children whose mothers had higher levels of education scored higher on the PLS-4.

The outcomes that children with additional disabilities obtain after cochlear implantation may be summarized as follows:

- Children with severe to profound hearing loss and additional disabilities often receive considerable benefit from cochlear implantation. Most studies show significant improvement in speech, language, auditory, and social abilities following cochlear implantation. Also, parent report usually indicates substantial benefit from cochlear implantation, even when improvement may not be evident of formal measures of auditory and language abilities.

- The postimplant speech, language, and auditory outcomes of children with additional disabilities are often not as good as those of children with normal hearing and children who have hearing loss without additional disabilities. In many cases, the limited benefit of children with additional disabilities may be attributed to lower nonverbal IQ and neurocognitive disabilities. A reasonable postimplant goal for children with additional disabilities is that speech, language, and auditory outcomes as measured via norm-referenced, standardized assessments should be at least as good as the child's nonverbal IQ.

- Children with additional disabilities may require a longer time to develop auditory skills and spoken language after cochlear implantation compared with children who have hearing loss and no other disabilities.

- Children who have severe to profound hearing loss and additional disabilities should be considered for cochlear implantation as soon as the cochlear implant team determines that hearing aids will not adequately support speech and language development. Early implantation (e.g., 12 months old or less) will likely result in better outcomes.

- Children with additional disabilities will likely achieve better auditory, speech, and language outcomes when they communicate via spoken language. Cupples et al. (2016) showed poorer outcomes for children who used sign language. Intensive auditory-verbal therapy and focused auditory-oral education may be necessary to optimize outcomes of children with additional disabilities.

- The expressive language of a subset of some children with additional disabilities may be quite limited. For instance, many children with autism spectrum disorder (ASD) have delays in expressive communication (Eshraghi et al., 2015). Emphasis on audition and full-time cochlear implant will likely optimize receptive language and speech recognition. If expressive communication does not develop satisfactorily after implantation, a manual method of expressive communication (e.g., Picture Exchange Communication System [PECS]) should be considered. Of note, Eshraghi et al. (2015)

have shown that many children with ASD receive significant benefit from and make considerable progress after cochlear implantation.

Preoperative Hearing Status

A number of different studies have examined the effect of preoperative hearing status on postimplant outcomes (An, Kim, & Chung, 2012; Blamey et al., 2001; Eisenberg et al., 2004; Geers & Nicholas, 2006; Geers & Nicholas, 2007, Geers, Nicholas, & Moog. 2007; Gerard et al., 2010; Gordon et al., 2001; Gratacap et al., 2015; Kuo & Gibson, 2000; Leigh et al., 2011; Niparko et al., 2010). For the most part, these studies have found that children who have some residual hearing prior to implantation achieve better outcomes after cochlear implantation (An, Kim, & Chung, 2012; Geers & Nicholas, 2006, 2007; Geers, Nicholas, & Moog. 2007; Gordon et al., 2001; Gratacap et al., 2015; Niparko et al., 2010), but some studies have found no differences in the postimplant outcomes of children with and without preimplant residual acoustic hearing (Eisenberg et al., 2004; El-Hakim et al., 2002; Gerard et al., 2010; Leigh et al., 2011). For instance, Niparko et al. (2010) examined postimplant outcomes in 188 children who underwent cochlear implantation prior to 5 years of age and found that children with better preoperative hearing (i.e., better four-frequency pure tone average on the better ear) obtained better speech recognition following cochlear implantation. Similarly, Nicholas and Geers (2006) reported that children with better unaided and aided preoperative pure tone averages obtained better receptive language after cochlear implantation. The finding that better preoperative aided thresholds were associated with better postoperative implant outcomes underscores the importance of the provision of an audible aided signal with appropriately fitted hearing aids prior to implantation. In contrast, Leigh et al. (2011) examined postoperative speech recognition in 80 children who received a cochlear implant during their first three years of life and found no relationship between preoperative audiometric hearing thresholds and postoperative speech recognition obtained with a cochlear implant. It should be noted that many of the children in the Leigh et al. study underwent cochlear implantation during the first 12 to 18 months of life. As a result, the negative consequences of auditory deprivation that are likely to be greater for children with poorer preoperative hearing sensitivity are likely limited by the prompt provision of an audible signal via cochlear implantation. Also of note, Leigh and colleagues did note that children with cochlear implants achieved speech recognition that was as good as that of children who had a 65 dB HL pure-tone average and used hearing aids.

Chiossi and Hyppolito (2017) conducted an extensive literature review to summarize the results of studies that examined the outcomes of children who had at least some acoustic hearing prior to receiving a cochlear implant. They identified 22 different peer-reviewed articles exploring the topic and concluded that cochlear implantation will likely improve the hearing performance of children when their hearing impairment is "worse than 75 to 78 dB HL on pure-tone audiometry." Chiossi and Hyppolito noted that substantial variability exists in the findings of the 22 studies, with many concluding that children who had some residual hearing prior to cochlear implantation achieved better postimplant speech recognition and speech production (An, Kim, & Chung, 2012; Geers & Nicholas, 2006, 2007; Geers, Nicholas, & Moog. 2007; Gordon et al., 2001; Gratacap et al., 2015; Gupta, 2012; Niparko et al., 2010; Phan et al., 2016), whereas a smaller number of studies found no difference in speech recognition between children with and without residual hearing prior to cochlear implantation (Eisenberg et al., 2004; Gerard et al., 2010; Leigh et al., 2011). They did note that children with residual hearing prior to implantation tended to make faster progress after receiving a cochlear implant than children who had no hearing prior to implantation. Additionally, Chiossi and Hyppolito acknowledged that "there is not a determination of the amount of residual hearing considered necessary for granting better auditory performance for the cochlear user or the difference between children with different preoperative hearing thresholds." Furthermore, they stated that there is insufficient evidence to fully understand the impact of residual hearing prior to implantation on language outcomes obtained after implantation, because "language is a complex process affected by a multitude of variables not controlled in most studies." Finally, Chiossi and Hyppolito stressed the fact that several of the studies they reviewed concluded that the best postoperative speech recognition was obtained by children with residual hearing prior to implantation occurred in the bimodal condition (i.e., the children were using their cochlear implant along with a hearing aid in the nonimplanted ear).

Kuo and Gibson (2000) examined outcomes in 33 children who received a cochlear implant under

10 years of age and 12 children who received a cochlear implant between 10 and 15 years of age. As expected, Kuo and Gibson reported that speech recognition and language outcomes were better for the younger children. They did find better speech recognition and language outcomes for children with better preoperative residual hearing but only for the group of children who received an implant between 10 and 15 years of age. Once again, the finding that older children with better preoperative residual hearing achieved better postoperative outcomes likely underscores the importance of access to intelligible speech prior to implantation. Presumably, the older children who had better preoperative residual hearing were more likely to receive benefit from well-fitted hearing aids, and as a result, the auditory areas of the brain were stimulated through the provision of an audible aided signal. In contrast, the older children without preoperative residual hearing likely had a lengthy period of auditory deprivation resulting in colonization of the secondary auditory cortex by other sensory modalities and a subsequent reduction in performance with a cochlear implant (Kral & Eggermont, 2007; Kral et al., 2016; Sharma, Dorman, & Spahr, 2002; Wolfe et al., 2007).

To summarize:

* Many (but not all) studies have shown that children with better preoperative hearing sensitivity obtain better postoperative outcomes.
* The finding of better postoperative outcomes for children with better preoperative hearing may be due to multiple factors, including more favorable integrity of the peripheral and central auditory nervous system (e.g., normal cochlear anatomy, larger number of spiral ganglion cell bodies), smaller effect of auditory deprivation, greater potential to benefit from amplification prior to implantation, and so forth.
* The potential negative effects of poorer preoperative hearing sensitivity may be mitigated by early implantation.
* Appropriate fitting of hearing aids (i.e., real ear probe microphone assessment to ensure optimization of hearing aid output relative to the child's hearing thresholds) and full-time hearing aid use prior to implantation are necessary to capitalize on residual hearing that may exist prior to implantation, particularly for children who do not undergo cochlear implantation during early childhood.
* To optimize outcomes, children with functional acoustic hearing should continue to use a hearing

aid in the nonimplanted ear after cochlear implantation.

Cochlear Implantation in Older Children with Prelingual Deafness

As repeatedly discussed in this chapter, outcomes following cochlear implantation are significantly better when children receive a cochlear implant at an early age (Ching & Dillon, 2013; Dettman et al., 2016; Houston et al., 2012; Houston & Miyamoto, 2010; Mahmoud & Ruckenstein, 2014). To optimize outcomes, children who are born with severe to profound hearing loss should ideally undergo cochlear implantation before 12 months of age (Ching et al., 2013; Dettman et al., 2016). However, because of a variety of different circumstances, some children who are born with severe to profound hearing loss may not receive a cochlear implant until they are much older (e.g., elementary school, teenagers). As previously discussed, Sharma et al. (2002) have found deleterious changes in auditory brain function when cochlear implantation is provided after the first two to three years of life. Specifically, Sharma and colleagues found a delayed cortical auditory evoked response in most every child who received a cochlear implant after 7 years of age. The changes that occur in auditory brain development and function secondary to early-onset auditory deprivation result in a substantial reduction in the outcomes a child will receive from a cochlear implant (Arisi et al., 2010; Bosco et al., 2013; Galvin, Hughes, & Mok, 2010; Peters et al., 2007; Shpak et al., 2009; Wolfe et al., 2007; Zeitler et al., 2012). However, it should also be understood that many children who are born with severe to profound hearing loss are able to derive considerable benefit from cochlear implantation (Arisi et al., 2010; Shpak et al., 2009; Zeitler et al., 2012).

For instance, Shpak and colleagues (2009) examined speech recognition after implantation for 20 children who were born with severe to profound hearing loss and who underwent implantation between 8 and 18.5 years of age. Shpak et al. reported a mean improvement of almost 25 and 45 percentage points for word and sentence recognition, respectively, between preoperative aided performance and performance at the two-year postimplant point. Of note, Shpak and colleagues reported that their participants tended to require a longer period of time postoperatively to develop open-set speech recognition compared with postlinguistically deafened adult recipients. Interestingly, Shpak et al. also characterized each participant with the use of a preimplant assessment profile that explored eight items that are known to influence postoperative outcomes: (1) age at CI, (2) aided open-set preimplant speech recognition, (3) communication mode, (4) consistent participation in aural rehabilitation prior to implantation, (5) candidate's attitude to cochlear implantation, (6) educational placement, (7) family support and expectations, and (8) additional disabilities. In general, children who were prelingually deafened and received a cochlear implant during their teenage years were more likely to develop open-set speech recognition with younger age of implantation (8 to 13 years of age), some open-set speech recognition with hearing aids prior to implantation, use of an oral communication mode prior to implantation, and no additional disabilities. The children who received little to no benefit from cochlear implantation were those who had the lowest scores on the preimplant assessment profile.

Arisi and colleagues (2010) also examined postoperative speech recognition in 45 participants who received cochlear implants during their adolescent years. They also found that the group as a whole obtained significant improvement in their open-set speech recognition following cochlear implantation. However, there were 15 children who continued to have poor speech recognition following cochlear implantation. The children with a poor outcome tended to be those with a later age of diagnosis and poorer preoperative audiometric thresholds. These 15 children tended to use their cochlear implant less than the better performers. Similarly, Zeitler et al. (2012) examined postoperative speech recognition of 67 children who received cochlear implants during their adolescent years. Sentence and word recognition improved by 51.1 and 32.23 percentage points, respectively, between the pre- and 1-year postimplant conditions. The participants who had better hearing prior to implantation and who used oral communication prior to implantation were more likely to develop open-set speech recognition following cochlear implantation.

To summarize:

- Many adolescents who were born with severe to profound hearing loss are able to obtain substantial benefit from cochlear implantation.
- Children who had severe to profound hearing loss and who received a cochlear implant during their adolescent years tend to obtain better outcomes when they have better preoperative hearing, consistent use of well-fitted hearing aids prior to implantation, no additional disabilities

other than hearing loss, use of Listening and Spoken Language prior to implantation, an earlier age of identification of hearing loss and intervention, and a positive attitude about cochlear implant technology, listening, and spoken language.
- The audiologist should provide significant counseling prior to implantation so that adolescents with severe to profound hearing loss have realistic expectations regarding the benefit they will obtain from cochlear implantation. The counseling should take into account the preimplant otologic, speech and language, and developmental history of the child.
- Children with unfavorable preimplant profiles are less likely to perform well with their cochlear implants and are more likely to become nonusers of their cochlear implants.
- Consistent use of an appropriately fitted hearing aid prior to implantation is likely to facilitate success. Consistent hearing aid users should continue hearing aid use in the nonimplanted ear after implantation.

Stimulation Levels and Electrophysiologic Responses

In order to effectively manage the care of children with cochlear implants, the audiologist should have a good understanding of how stimulation levels and electrophysiologic levels are expected to change over time. Hughes et al. (2001) examined behavioral stimulation and electrophysiologic levels obtained for the first two years after activation for 21 children (age at implantation ranging from 16.5 months to 17.9 years old) and 29 adults with cochlear implants. Hughes and colleagues reported that the electrical thresholds (i.e., T levels) increased throughout the first few months for some children and decreased for others, but as a group, the children's T levels increased slightly from activation to the 3-month postactivation appointment but stabilized thereafter. In contrast, the T levels of adult recipients remained stable from activation throughout the first two years of implant use. Hughes et al. attributed the increase in the children's T levels during the first few months of CI use to "possible changes within the cochlea or changes in behavioral criterion level." Henkin et al. (2003) also reported an increase in T levels during the first three months of CI use for 25 children of severe to profound hearing loss of prelingual onset. The upper stimulation levels increased throughout the first year of use for both children and adults and stabilized thereafter. Of note, the T levels of pediatric and adult participants were pretty similar across the study sessions, whereas the children's upper stimulation levels were lower than the adults' upper stimulation levels at activation but increased at a much greater rate than adults. As a result, the children's upper stimulation levels were substantially higher than the adults' upper stimulation levels from 6 to 24 months postactivation. Additionally, the electrically evoked compound action potential (ECAP) increased through the first month of use and stabilized thereafter. Electrode impedances for both groups decreased from the activation appointment through the first days of implant use and stabilized from that point forward.

Gordon, Papsin, and Harrison (2004) examined behavioral and electrophysiologic levels across the first year of implant use for 88 pediatric cochlear implant recipients (age at implantation ranging from 7 months to 17 years). Almost one-half of the participants in the Gordon et al. study were under three years of age at activation. Gordon and colleagues also found that T levels increased throughout the first few weeks of implant use for some children and decreased for others, but for the group, mean T levels decreased slightly through the first year of implant use. Gordon and colleagues hypothesized that the decrease in T levels throughout the first year of implant use may be attributed to an enhancement in the children's attention to sound, an improvement in their ability to respond close to their true hearing threshold, and/or to the fact that behavioral observation audiometry may have been used with younger children and overestimated the child's threshold response. Similarly, Shapiro and Waltzman (1995) theorized that the significant changes they observed in children's T levels through the first three months of implant use (T levels increased for some and decreased for others) were due to an increase in the consistency and reliability of the children's responses over time. Gordon et al. reported that mean upper stimulation levels increased throughout the first 6 months of use and stabilized thereafter. Of note, whenever possible, the electrically evoked stapedial reflex threshold (ESRT) was used as a guide to estimate upper stimulation levels in the study participants. The ECAP thresholds decreased from the levels obtained in the operative room to the levels measured at activation and remained stable from activation throughout the first year of implant use. The ESRT was measured in the operative room and then at 3, 6, and 12 months postactivation. The ESRT measured at 3 months post-

activation was significantly lower (better) than the ESRT measured in the operating room, and a slight increase occurred in the ESRT obtained throughout the 3-month to 12-month postactivation period.

To summarize,

- The ESRT and ECAP thresholds measured in the operating room tend to be substantially higher than the ESRT and ECAP measures obtained at activation and subsequent appointments. The ECAP threshold tends to remain stable from activation throughout the first two years of implant use. The ESRT may increase slightly throughout the first year of implant use.
- Electrode impedances decrease throughout the first few days of implant use and stabilize thereafter.
- T levels are variable across children, but the true electrical threshold is most likely to remain relatively stable throughout implant use.
- Upper stimulation levels increase throughout the first few months of implant use as the recipient acclimates to the new auditory stimulus. However, audiologists should be careful to avoid unnecessary increases in upper stimulation levels at each appointment throughout the first one to two years of implant use. Adult upper stimulation levels tend to stabilize after 3 to 6 months of use, whereas studies show that children's upper stimulation levels tend to increase over a longer period of time. Audiologists should be reticent about increasing upper stimulation levels solely for the sake of increasing stimulation. The ESRT serves as an excellent guide to estimating upper stimulation levels. Chapters 14, 15, 16, 17, and 23, provide valuable information regarding typical upper stimulation levels and electrical dynamic ranges for modern cochlear implant systems.

Assessment of Postoperative Cochlear Implant Outcomes of Children

The prudent audiologist will conduct a thorough periodic assessment of cochlear implant outcomes. The cochlear implant outcome assessment battery should include:

- Informal interview of the parent and the child, if possible, to inquire about child's progress/difficulties

- Otoscopic evaluation and inspection of cochlear implant site(s)
- An evaluation of the child's hearing technology (e.g., microphone check, inspection of the integrity of cables, connectors, batteries, assessment of sound processor acoustic component, assessment of hearing aid). Inspection of the external equipment is especially important for children, because they are less likely than adults to be able to take care of their equipment, and young children may be unable to provide verbal feedback about the signal they are receiving from their cochlear implant.
- Evaluation of sound-field warbled tone thresholds
- Whenever possible, assessment of word recognition in quiet and sentence recognition in noise and possibly in quiet for each ear separately and in the bilateral/bimodal condition
- Administer questionnaire to evaluate subjective performance and/or benefit (e.g., LittlEARS, PEACH).

"Aided" Warbled Tone Threshold Assessment

The audiologist should measure sound-field warbled tone detection thresholds to ensure that the recipient has good access to low-level sounds. A reasonable goal is to obtain sound-field warbled tone thresholds of 20 to 25 dB HL from 250 to 6000 Hz in the unilateral cochlear implant condition (each unilateral cochlear implant condition for bilateral recipients) (Holden et al., 2013; Skinner et al., 1997). Attainment of sound-field warbled tone detection thresholds near 20 dB HL from 250 to 6000 Hz should ensure access to the low-level components of soft speech. It is not desirable to obtain sound-field detection thresholds below 15 dB HL, because in realistic environments, there is unlikely to be an abundance of speech information below 15 to 20 dB HL. Also, low-level noise is primarily present below 20 dB HL and will likely mask any important sounds that may exist below that level. Furthermore, the microphone noise floor of modern cochlear implant sound processors likely prevents detection of sounds below 15 to 20 dB HL.

It should be noted that sound-field detection thresholds should be measured to warbled tones rather than to narrowband noise. The latter is not typically designed for assessment of hearing sensitivity and may be higher in level and will be wider in bandwidth than warbled tones. Additionally, the audiologist should ensure that the recipient is located

in the spot in the sound booth in which calibration was completed. Ideally, the loudspeaker should be calibrated for presentation of test signals from 0 degrees. If not, the audiologist should account for correction factors associated with the calibration of the loudspeaker at 45 or 90 degrees. Finally, a test assistant should be able to facilitate a reliable and valid conditioned response for visual reinforcement and conditioned play audiometry. Also, multiple toys/activities should be available when conducting conditioned play audiometry with young children.

Assessment of Speech Recognition

Whenever possible, speech recognition should be evaluated with the use of recorded speech materials. As mentioned in the chapters discussing cochlear implant candidacy assessment, the use of recorded materials eliminates the variability inherent in monitored live voice speech testing. Also, several studies have shown that live voice speech recognition assessment overestimates the speech recognition capacity of both adults and children (Roeser & Clark, 2008; Uhler, Biever, & Gifford, 2016). The audiologist should administer the same measures that were administered in the Pediatric Minimal Speech Test Battery (PMSTB) used to evaluate cochlear implant candidacy. Ideally, monosyllabic word recognition assessment (e.g., LNT words) should be conducted in quiet at a presentation level of 60 dBA. Additionally, sentence recognition in noise should be completed at a +10 dB SNR. If the recipient scores less than 20% to 25% correct, then assessment should be conducted at a more favorable SNR (e.g., +15 dB SNR). If the recipient scores near ceiling, then assessment should be conducted at a +5 dB SNR. The prudent audiologist should also evaluate sentence recognition in quiet at a presentation level of 60 dBA. If the recipient scores below 20% to 25% correct on sentence recognition in quiet assessment, then the audiologist should complete evaluation with a simpler measure of speech recognition within the PMSTB. Aided speech recognition should be conducted in each unilateral condition as well as in the bilateral/bimodal condition.

A minimum recommended postoperative follow-up schedule is:

- One-day postactivation checkup
- One-week postactivation checkup with sound-field warbled tone detection threshold assessment if possible

- One-month postactivation checkup with sound-field warbled tone detection threshold assessment if possible
- Three-month postactivation checkup with sound-field warbled tone detection threshold assessment if possible
- Six-month postactivation checkup with sound-field warbled tone detection threshold and aided speech recognition assessment if possible
- One-year postactivation checkup with sound-field warbled tone detection threshold and aided speech recognition assessment if possible
- Quarterly checkups with sound-field warbled tone detection threshold and aided speech recognition assessment if possible until the child reaches 7 years of age and has at least two years of implant use. Children who are 7 years old and older and have at least two years of implant experience should be seen for biannual checkups.

Key Concepts

- Research has shown a high level of variability in the speech, language, auditory, academic, and social outcomes children achieve after cochlear implantation.
- In general, better outcomes are associated with an earlier age of implantation, a communication mode centered on Listening and Spoken Language, exposure to a robust listening-rich model of language (i.e., complex intelligible speech), higher levels of maternal support and maternal education, higher family levels of income, and higher nonverbal IQ.
- In general, poorer outcomes after implantation are associated with the presence of additional disabilities, cochlear nerve aplasia, bacterial meningitis, and severe cochlear aplasia.
- Of note, most children with severe to profound hearing loss and auditory neuropathy spectrum disorder can achieve impressive outcomes after cochlear implantation if they are equipped with appropriate technology that is programmed ideally by the audiologist to meet the needs of the child, and the child uses the cochlear implant during all waking hours and is exposed to a robust model of spoken language.
- Audiologists should administer a battery of measures to evaluate the outcomes of each child. Audiologists should also work closely with the child's speech-language pathologist to ensure that the child is making satisfactory progress in speech, language, and functional auditory skill development (e.g., at least one year of progress in speech and language development in one calendar year) pursuing language abilities that are commensurate with normal-hearing peers.

References

Abdurehim, Y., Lehmann, A., & Zeitouni, A. G. (2017). Predictive value of GJB2 mutation status for hearing outcomes of pediatric cochlear implantation. *Otolaryngoloy–Head and Neck Surgery, 157*(1), 16–24.

Adunka, O. F., Jewells, V., & Buchman, C. A. (2007). Value of computed tomography in the evaluation of children with cochlear nerve deficiency. *Otology and Neurotology, 28*(5), 597–604.

AG Bell > Home. (2017). Retrieved from https://www.agbell.org/

An, Y. S., Kim, S. T., & Chung, J. W. (2012). Preoperative voice parameters affect the postoperative speech intelligibility in patients with cochlear implantation. *Clinical and Experimental Otorhinolaryngology, 5*(Suppl. 1), S69–S72.

Arisi, E., Forti, S., Pagani, D., Todini, L., Torretta, S., Ambrosetti, U., & Pignataro, L. (2010). Cochlear implantation in adolescents with prelinguistic deafness. *Otolaryngology–Head and Neck Surgery, 142*(6), 804–808.

Barnard, J. M., Fisher, L. M., Johnson, K. C., Eisenberg, L. S., Wang, N. Y., Quittner, A. L., . . . Team, C. D. I. (2015). A Prospective longitudinal study of U.S. children unable to achieve open-set speech recognition 5 years after cochlear implantation. *Otology and Neurotology, 36*(6), 985–992.

Barnard, J., Grant, S. W., Hickey, G. L., & Bridgewater, B. (2015). Is social deprivation an independent predictor of outcomes following cardiac surgery? An analysis of 240,221 patients from a national registry. *BMJ Open, 5*(6), e008287.

Bas, E., Gupta, C., & Van De Water, T. R. (2012). A novel organ of Corti explant model for the study of cochlear implantation trauma. *Anatomical Record (Hoboken), 295*(11), 1944–1956.

Bayrak, F., Catli, T., Atsal, G., Tokat, T., & Olgun, L. (2017). Waardenburg syndrome: An unusual indication of cochlear implantation experienced in 11 patients. *Journal of International Advanced Otology, 13*(2), 230–232.

Beer, J., Harris, M. S., Kronenberger, W. G., Holt, R. F., & Pisoni, D. B. (2012). Auditory skills, language development, and adaptive behavior of children with cochlear implants and additional disabilities. *International Journal of Audiology, 51*(6), 491–498.

Berlin, C. I., Hood, L. J., Morlet, T., Wilensky, D., Li, L., Mattingly, K. R., . . . Frisch, S. A. (2010). Multi-site diagnosis and management of 260 patients with auditory neuropathy/dyssynchrony (auditory neuropathy spectrum disorder). *International Journal of Audiology, 49*(1), 30–43.

Berlin, C. I., Morlet, T., & Hood, L. J. (2003). Auditory neuropathy/dyssynchrony: Its diagnosis and management. *Pediatric Clinics of North America, 50*(2), 331–340, vii–viii.

Birman, C. S., Powell, H. R., Gibson, W. P., & Elliott, E. J. (2016). Cochlear implant outcomes in cochlea nerve aplasia and hypoplasia. *Otology and Neurotology, 37*(5), 438–445.

Bisconti, S., Shulkin, M., Hu, X., Basura, G. J., Kileny, P. R., & Kovelman, I. (2016). Functional near-infrared spectroscopy brain imaging investigation of phonological awareness and passage comprehension abilities in adult recipients of cochlear implants. *Journal of Speech, Language, and Hearing Research*, *59*(2), 239–253.

Blamey, P. J., Sarant, J. Z., Paatsch, L. E., Barry, J. G., Bow, C. P., Wales, R. J., . . . Tooher, R. (2001). Relationships among speech perception, production, language, hearing loss, and age in children with impaired hearing. *Journal of Speech, Language, and Hearing Research*, *44*(2), 264–285.

Bosco, E., Nicastri, M., Ballantyne, D., Viccaro, M., Ruoppolo, G., Ionescu Maddalena, A., & Mancini, P. (2013). Long term results in late implanted adolescent and adult CI recipients. *European Archives of Otorhinolaryngology*, *270*(10), 2611–2620.

Broomfield, S. J., Bruce, I. A., Henderson, L., Ramsden, R. T., & Green, K. M. (2013). Cochlear implantation in children with syndromic deafness. *International Journal of Pediatric Otorhinolaryngology*, *77*(8), 1312–1316.

Buchman, C. A., Copeland, B. J., Yu, K. K., Brown, C. J., Carrasco, V. N., & Pillsbury, H. C., 3rd (2004). Cochlear implantation in children with congenital inner ear malformations. *Laryngoscope*, *114*(2), 309–316.

Buchman, C. A., Roush, P. A., Teagle, H. F., Brown, C. J., Zdanski, C. J., & Grose, J. H. (2006). Auditory neuropathy characteristics in children with cochlear nerve deficiency. *Ear and Hearing*, *27*(4), 399–408.

Bunta, F., & Douglas, M. (2013). The effects of dual-language support on the language skills of bilingual children with hearing loss who use listening devices relative to their monolingual peers. *Language, Speech, and Hearing Services in the Schools*, *44*(3), 281–290.

Bunta, F., Douglas, M., Dickson, H., Cantu, A., Wickesberg, J., & Gifford, R. H. (2016). Dual language versus English-only support for bilingual children with hearing loss who use cochlear implants and hearing aids. *International Journal of Language and Communication Disorders*, *51*(4), 460–472.

Busch, T., Vanpoucke, F., & van Wieringen, A. (2017). Auditory environment across the life span of cochlear implant users: Insights from data logging. *Journal of Speech, Language, and Hearing Research*, *60*(5), 1362–1377.

Carraro, M., Almishaal, A., Hillas, E., Firpo, M., Park, A., & Harrison, R. V. (2017). Cytomegalovirus (CMV) infection causes degeneration of cochlear vasculature and hearing loss in a mouse model. *Journal of Associated Research in Otolaryngology*, *18*(2), 263–273.

Carraro, M., Park, A. H., & Harrison, R. V. (2016). Partial corrosion casting to assess cochlear vasculature in mouse models of presbycusis and CMV infection. *Hearing Research*, *332*, 95–103.

Ching, T. Y., Day, J., & Cupples, L. (2014). Phonological awareness and early reading skills in children with cochlear implants. *Cochlear Implants International*, *15*(Suppl. 1), S27–S29.

Ching, T. Y., Day, J., Van Buynder, P., Hou, S., Zhang, V., Seeto, M., . . . Flynn, C. (2014). Language and speech perception of young children with bimodal fitting or bilateral cochlear implants. *Cochlear Implants International*, *15*(Suppl. 1), S43–S46.

Ching, T. Y., Day, J., Seeto, M., Dillon, H., Marnane, V., & Street, L. (2013). Predicting 3-year outcomes of early-identified children with hearing impairment. *B-ENT, Suppl. 21*, 99–106.

Ching, T. Y., & Dillon, H. (2013). Major findings of the LOCHI study on children at 3 years of age and implications for audiological management. *International Journal of Audiology*, *52*(Suppl. 2), S65–S68.

Ching, T. Y. C., Dillon, H., Leigh, G., Cupples, L. (in press). Learning from the longitudinal outcomes of children with hearing impairment (LOCHI) study: Summary of 5-year findings and implications. *International Journal of Audiology*. Advance online publication. https://doi.org/10.1080/14992027.1385865

Ching, T. Y., Dillon, H., Marnane, V., Hou, S., Day, J., Seeto, M., . . . Yeh, A. (2013). Outcomes of early- and late-identified children at 3 years of age: Findings from a prospective population-based study. *Ear and Hearing*, *34*(5), 535–552.

Ching, T. Y. C., Zhang, V. W., & Hou, S. (in press). The importance of early intervention for infants and children with hearing loss. In J. R. Madell, C. Flexer, J. Wolfe, & E. C. Schafer (Eds.), *Pediatric audiology: Diagnosis, technology, and management* (3rd ed.). New York, NY: Thieme Medical.

Chiossi, J. S. C., & Hyppolito, M. A. (2017). Effects of residual hearing on cochlear implant outcomes in children: A systematic-review. *International Journal of Pediatric Otorhinolaryngology*, *100*, 119–127.

Choo, D., & Dettman, S. J. (2017). What can long-term attendance at programming appointments tell us about pediatric cochlear implant recipients? *Otology and Neurotology*, *38*(3), 325–333.

Chu, C., Choo, D., Dettman, S., Leigh, J., Traeger, G., Lettieri, G., . . . Dowell, R. (2016, May). *Early intervention and communication development in children using cochlear implants: The impact of service delivery practices and family factors.* Presented at Audiology Australia National Conference 2016, Melbourne, Australia.

Colletti, V., Carner, M., Miorelli, V., Guida, M., Colletti, L., & Fiorino, F. G. (2005). Cochlear implantation at under 12 months: Report on 10 patients. *Laryngoscope*, *115*(3), 445–449.

Cupples, L., Ching, T. Y. C., Button, L., Leigh, G., Marnane, V., Whitfield, J., . . . Martin, L. (2016). Language and speech outcomes of children with hearing loss and additional disabilities: Identifying the variables that influence performance at five years of age. *International Journal of Audiology*, 1–12.

Declau, F., Boudewyns, A., Van den Ende, J., & van de Heyning, P. (2013). Auditory neuropathy: A challenge for diagnosis and treatment. *B–ENT, Supplement 21*, 65–79.

DesJardin, J. L., Ambrose, S. E., & Eisenberg, L. S. (2009). Literacy skills in children with cochlear implants: The importance of early oral language and joint storybook reading. *Journal of Deaf Studies and Deaf Education*, *14*(1), 22–43.

Dettman, S., Choo, D., & Dowell, R. (2016). Barriers to early cochlear implantation. *International Journal of Audiology*, *55*(Suppl. 2), S64–S76.

Dettman, S. J., Dowell, R. C., Choo, D., Arnott, W., Abrahams, Y., Davis, A., . . . Briggs, R. J. (2016). Long-term communication outcomes for children receiving cochlear implants younger than 12 months: A multicenter study. *Otology and Neurotology*, *37*(2), e82–e95.

Donaldson, A. I., Heavner, K. S., & Zwolan, T. A. (2004). Measuring progress in children with autism spectrum disorder who have cochlear implants. *Archives of Otolaryngology–Head and Neck Surgery*, *130*(5), 666–671.

Eisenberg, L. S., Kirk, K. I., Martinez, A. S., Ying, E. A., & Miyamoto, R. T. (2004). Communication abilities of children with aided residual hearing: Comparison with cochlear implant users. *Archives of Otolaryngology–Head and Neck Surgery*, *130*(5), 563–569.

El-Hakim, H., Abdolell, M., Mount, R. J., Papsin, B. C., & Harrison, R. V. (2002). Influence of age at implantation and of residual hearing on speech outcome measures after cochlear implantation: Binary partitioning analysis. *Annals of Otology, Rhinology, and Laryngology Supplement, 189*, 102–108.

Eshraghi, A. A., Nazarian, R., Telischi, F. F., Martinez, D., Hodges, A., Velandia, S., . . . Lang, D. (2015). Cochlear implantation in children with autism spectrum disorder. *Otology and Neurotology, 36*(8), e121–e128.

Fernandes, N. F., Morettin, M., Yamaguti, E. H., Costa, O. A., & Bevilacqua, M. C. (2015). Performance of hearing skills in children with auditory neuropathy spectrum disorder using cochlear implant: A systematic review. *Brazilian Journal of Otorhinolaryngology, 81*(1), 85–96.

Fitzpatrick, E., Coyle, D. E., Durieux-Smith, A., Graham, I. D., Angus, D. E., & Gaboury, I. (2007). Parents' preferences for services for children with hearing loss: A conjoint analysis study. *Ear and Hearing, 28*(6), 842–849.

Gallaudet Research Institute. (2011). *Regional and national summary report of data from the 2009-2010 annual survey of deaf and hard of hearing children and youth.* Retrieved from http://research.gallaudet.edu/Demographics/ 2010_National_ Summary.pdf

Galvin, K. L., Hughes, K. C., & Mok, M. (2010). Can adolescents and young adults with prelingual hearing loss benefit from a second, sequential cochlear implant? *International Journal of Audiology, 49*(5), 368–377.

Gardner-Berry, K., Hou, S. Y. L., & Ching, T. Y. C. (in press). Managing infants and children with auditory neuropathy spectrum disorder. In J. R. Madell, C. Flexer, J. Wolfe, & E. C. Schafer (Eds.), *Pediatric audiology: Diagnosis, technology, and management* (3rd ed.). New York, NY: Thieme Medical.

Geers, A. E., Brenner, C. A., & Tobey, E. A. (2011). Long-term outcomes of cochlear implantation in early childhood: Sample characteristics and data collection methods. *Ear and Hearing, 32*(1 Suppl.), 2S–12S.

Geers, A. E., Davidson, L. S., Uchanski, R. M., & Nicholas, J. G. (2013). Interdependence of linguistic and indexical speech perception skills in school-age children with early cochlear implantation. *Ear and Hearing, 34*(5), 562–574.

Geers, A. E., Mitchell, C. M., Warner-Czyz, A., Wang, N. Y., Eisenberg, L. S., & Team, C. D. I. (2017). Early sign language exposure and cochlear implantation benefits. *Pediatrics, 140*(1), e20163489.

Geers, A. E., Nicholas, J. G., & Moog, J. S. (2007). Estimating the influence of cochlear implantation on language development in children. *Audiological Medicine, 5*(4), 262–273.

Geers, A. E., Nicholas, J. G., & Sedey, A. L. (2003). Language skills of children with early cochlear implantation. *Ear and Hearing, 24*(1 Suppl.), 46S–58S.

Geers, A. E., & Sedey, A. L. (2011). Language and verbal reasoning skills in adolescents with 10 or more years of cochlear implant experience. *Ear and Hearing, 32*(1 Suppl.), 39S–48S.

Geers, A. E., Strube, M. J., Tobey, E. A., Pisoni, D. B., & Moog, J. S. (2011). Epilogue: factors contributing to long-term outcomes of cochlear implantation in early childhood. *Ear and Hearing, 32*(1, Suppl.), 84S–92S.

Gerard, J. M., Deggouj, N., Hupin, C., Buisson, A. L., Monteyne, V., Lavis, C., . . . Gersdorff, M. (2010). Evolution of communication abilities after cochlear implantation in prelingually deaf children. *International Journal of Pediatric Otorhinolaryngology, 74*(6), 642–648.

Gibson, W. P., & Sanli, H. (2007). Auditory neuropathy: An update. *Ear and Hearing, 28*(2 Suppl.), 102S–106S.

Glastonbury, C. M., Davidson, H. C., Harnsberger, H. R., Butler, J., Kertesz, T. R., & Shelton, C. (2002). Imaging findings of cochlear nerve deficiency. *AJNR American Journal of Neuroradiology, 23*(4), 635–643.

Gordon, K. A., Papsin, B. C., & Harrison, R. V. (2004). Toward a battery of behavioral and objective measures to achieve optimal cochlear implant stimulation levels in children. *Ear and Hearing, 25*(5), 447–463.

Gordon, K. A., Twitchell, K. A., Papsin, B. C., & Harrison, R. V. (2001). Effect of residual hearing prior to cochlear implantation on speech perception in children. *Journal of Otolaryngology, 30*(4), 216–223.

Gorlin, R. J., Toriello, H. V., & Cohen, M. J. (1995). Hereditary hearing loss and its syndromes. *American Journal of Medical Genetics, 61*(1), 101.

Gratacap, M., Thierry, B., Rouillon, I., Marlin, S., Garabedian, N., & Loundon, N. (2015). Pediatric cochlear implantation in residual hearing candidates. *Annals of Otology, Rhinology, and Laryngology, 124*(6), 443–451.

Guerzoni, L., & Cuda, D. (2017). Speech processor data logging helps in predicting early linguistic outcomes in implanted children. *International Journal of Pediatric Otorhinolaryngology, 101*, 81–86.

Hart, B., & Risley, T. R. (1995). *Meaningful differences in the everyday experience of young American children.* Baltimore, MD: Paul H. Brookes.

Harris, M., Terlektsi, E., & Kyle, F. E. (2017). Concurrent and longitudinal predictors of reading for deaf and hearing children in primary school. *Journal of Deaf Studies and Deaf Education, 22*(2), 233–242.

Henkin, Y., Kaplan-Neeman, R., Muchnik, C., Kronenberg, J., & Hildesheimer, M. (2003). Changes over time in electrical stimulation levels and electrode impedance values in children using the Nucleus 24M cochlear implant. *International Journal of Pediatric Otorhinolaryngology, 67*(8), 873–880.

Hoey, A. W., Pai, I., Driver, S., Connor, S., Wraige, E., & Jiang, D. (2017). Management and outcomes of cochlear implantation in patients with congenital cytomegalovirus (cCMV)-related deafness. *Cochlear Implants International, 18*(4), 216–225.

Holden, L. K., Finley, C. C., Firszt, J. B., Holden, T. A., Brenner, C., Potts, L. G., . . . Skinner, M. W. (2013). Factors affecting open-set word recognition in adults with cochlear implants. *Ear and Hearing, 34*(3), 342–360.

Holt, R. F., & Kirk, K. I. (2005). Speech and language development in cognitively delayed children with cochlear implants. *Ear and Hearing, 26*(2), 132–148.

Houston, D. M., & Miyamoto, R. T. (2010). Effects of early auditory experience on word learning and speech perception in deaf children with cochlear implants: Implications for sensitive periods of language development. *Otology and Neurotology, 31*(8), 1248–1253.

Houston, D. M., Stewart, J., Moberly, A., Hollich, G., & Miyamoto, R. T. (2012). Word learning in deaf children with cochlear implants: Effects of early auditory experience. *Developmental Science, 15*(3), 448–461.

Hughes, M. L., Vander Werff, K. R., Brown, C. J., Abbas, P. J., Kelsay, D. M., Teagle, H. F., & Lowder, M. W. (2001). A longitudinal study of electrode impedance, the electrically evoked compound action potential, and behavioral measures in Nucleus 24 cochlear implant users. *Ear and Hearing, 22*(6), 471–486.

Humphriss, R., Hall, A., Maddocks, J., Macleod, J., Sawaya, K., & Midgley, E. (2013). Does cochlear implantation improve speech recognition in children with auditory neuropathy spectrum disorder? A systematic review. *International Journal of Audiology, 52*(7), 442–454.

Isaiah, A., Lee, D., Lenes-Voit, F., Sweeney, M., Kutz, W., Isaacson, B., . . . Lee, K. H. (2017). Clinical outcomes following cochlear implantation in children with inner ear anomalies. *International Journal of Pediatric Otorhinolaryngology, 93*, 1–6.

James, A. L., & Papsin, B. C. (2004). Cochlear implant surgery at 12 months of age or younger. *Laryngoscope, 114*(12), 2191–2195.

Janeschik, S., Teschendorf, M., Bagus, H., & Arweiler-Harbeck, D. (2013). Influence of etiologic factors on speech perception of cochlear-implanted children. *Cochlear Implants International, 14*(4), 190–199.

Jeong, S. W., Kim, L. S., Kim, B. Y., Bae, W. Y., & Kim, J. R. (2007). Cochlear implantation in children with auditory neuropathy: Outcomes and rationale. *Acta Otolaryngologica Supplementum*, (558), 36–43.

Jones C., & Launer S. (2010). Pediatric fittings in 2010: The Sound Foundations Cuper Project. In R. Seewald & J. Bamford (Eds.), A *Sound Foundation Through Early Amplification: Proceedings of the 2010 International Conference* (pp. 187–192). Chicago, IL: Phonak AG.

Kalejaiye, A., Ansari, G., Ortega, G., Davidson, M., & Kim, H. J. (2017). Low surgical complication rates in cochlear implantation for young children less than 1 year of age. *Laryngoscope, 127*(3), 720–724.

Kim, L. S., Jeong, S. W., Lee, Y. M., & Kim, J. S. (2010). Cochlear implantation in children. *Auris Nasus Larynx, 37*(1), 6–17.

Koyama, H., Kashio, A., Sakata, A., Tsutsumiuchi, K., Matsumoto, Y., Karino, S., . . . Yamasoba, T. (2016). The hearing outcomes of cochlear implantation in Waardenburg syndrome. *BioMed Research International, 2016*.

Kral, A., Eggermont, J. (2007). What's to lose and what's to learn: Development under auditory deprivation, cochlear implants and limits of cortical plasticity. *Brain Research Review, 56*(1), 259–269.

Kral, A., Kronenberger, W. G., Pisoni, D. B., O'Donoghue, G.M. (2016). Neurocognitive factors in sensory restoration of early deafness: A connectome model. *Lancet Neurology, 15*(6): 610–621.

Kuo, S. C., & Gibson, W. P. (2000). The influence of residual high-frequency hearing on the outcome in congenitally deaf cochlear implant recipients. *American Journal of Otology, 21*(5), 657–662.

Leigh, J., Dettman, S., Dowell, R., & Sarant, J. (2011). Evidence-based approach for making cochlear implant recommendations for infants with residual hearing. *Ear and Hearing, 32*(3), 313–322.

Mahmoud, A. F., & Ruckenstein, M. J. (2014). Speech perception performance as a function of age at implantation among postlingually deaf adult cochlear implant recipients. *Otology and Neurotology, 35*(10), e286–e291.

McGuirt, W. T., & Smith, R. J. (1999). Connexin 26 as a cause of hereditary hearing loss. *American Journal of Audiology, 8*(2), 93–100.

Mitchell, R. E., & Karchmer, M. A. (2004). When parents are deaf versus hard of hearing: patterns of sign use and school placement of deaf and hard-of-hearing children. *Journal of Deaf Studies and Deaf Education, 9*(2), 133–152.

Moog, J. S., & Geers, A. E. (2003). Epilogue: Major findings, conclusions and implications for deaf education. *Ear and Hearing, 24*(1 Suppl.), 121S–125S.

Mortensen, M. V., Mirz, F., & Gjedde, A. (2006). Restored speech comprehension linked to activity in left inferior prefrontal and right temporal cortices in postlingual deafness. *Neuroimage, 31*(2), 842–852.

Morton, N. E. (1991). Genetic epidemiology of hearing impairment. *Annals of the New York Academy of Science, 630*, 16–31.

Nakaizumi, T., Kawamoto, K., Minoda, R., & Raphael, Y. (2004). Adenovirus-mediated expression of brain-derived neurotrophic factor protects spiral ganglion neurons from ototoxic damage. *Audiology and Neurootology, 9*(3), 135–143.

Nassetta, L., Kimberlin, D., & Whitley, R. (2009). Treatment of congenital cytomegalovirus infection: Implications for future therapeutic strategies. *Journal of Antimicrobial Chemotherapy, 63*(5), 862–867.

Nichani, J., Bruce, I. A., Mawman, D., Khwaja, S., Ramsden, R., & Green, K. (2013). Cochlear implantation in patients deafened by ototoxic drugs. *Cochlear Implants International, 14*(4), 207–212.

Nicholas, J. G., & Geers, A. E. (2006). Effects of early auditory experience on the spoken language of deaf children at 3 years of age. *Ear and Hearing, 27*(3), 286–298.

Nicholas, J. G., & Geers, A. E. (2013). Spoken language benefits of extending cochlear implant candidacy below 12 months of age. *Otology and Neurotology, 34*(3), 532–538.

Nicholas, J. G., & Geers, A. E. (2007). Will they catch up? The role of age at cochlear implantation in the spoken language development of children with severe to profound hearing loss. *Journal of Speech, Language, and Hearing Research, 50*(4), 1048–1062.

Niparko, J. K., Tobey, E. A., Thal, D. J., Eisenberg, L. S., Wang, N. Y., Quittner, A. L., . . . Team, C. D. I. (2010). Spoken language development in children following cochlear implantation. *Journal of the American Medical Association (JAMA), 303*(15), 1498–1506.

Nittrouer, S., Caldwell, A., Lowenstein, J. H., Tarr, E., & Holloman, C. (2012). Emergent literacy in kindergartners with cochlear implants. *Ear and Hearing, 33*(6), 683–697.

Palmieri M, Berrettini S, Forli F, et al. (2012). Evaluating benefits of cochlear implantation in deaf children with additional disabilities. *Ear and Hearing, 33*(6):721–730.

Papsin, B. C. (2005). Cochlear implantation in children with anomalous cochleovestibular anatomy. *Laryngoscope, 115*(1 Pt. 2 Suppl. 106), 1–26.

Park, J. H., Kim, A. R., Han, J. H., Kim, S. D., Kim, S. H., Koo, J. W., . . . Choi, B. Y. (2017). Outcome of cochlear implantation in prelingually deafened children according to molecular genetic etiology. *Ear and Hearing, 38*(5), e316–e324.

Parkes, W. J., Gnanasegaram, J. J., Cushing, S. L., James, A. L., Gordon, K. A., & Papsin, B. C. (2017). Preliminary experience using a cochlear implant with a novel linear pedestal design. *International Journal of Pediatric Otorhinolaryngology, 93*, 42–46.

Parry, D. A., Booth, T., & Roland, P. S. (2005). Advantages of magnetic resonance imaging over computed tomography in preoperative evaluation of pediatric cochlear implant candidates. *Otology and Neurotology, 26*(5), 976–982.

Peng, K. A., Kuan, E. C., Hagan, S., Wilkinson, E. P., & Miller, M. E. (2017). Cochlear nerve aplasia and hypoplasia: Predictors of cochlear implant success. *Otolaryngology–Head and Neck Surgery, 157*(3), 392–400.

Percy–Smith, L., Caye–Thomasen, P., Breinegaard, N., & Jensen, J. H. (2010). Parental mode of communication is essential for speech and language outcomes in cochlear implanted children. *Acta Otolaryngologica, 130*(6), 708–715.

Peters, B. R., Litovsky, R., Parkinson, A., & Lake, J. (2007). Importance of age and postimplantation experience on speech perception measures in children with sequential bilateral cochlear implants. *Otology and Neurotology, 28*(5), 649–657.

Peterson, A., Shallop, J., Driscoll, C., Breneman, A., Babb, J., Stoeckel, R., & Fabry, L. (2003). Outcomes of cochlear implantation in children with auditory neuropathy. *Journal of the American Academy of Audiology, 14*(4), 188–201.

Phan, J., Houston, D. M., Ruffin, C., Ting, J., & Holt, R. F. (2016). Factors affecting speech discrimination in children with cochlear implants: Evidence from early-implanted infants. *Journal of the American Academy of Audiology, 27*(6), 480–488.

Picard M. (2004). Children with permanent hearing loss and associated disabilities: Revisiting current epidemiological data and causes of deafness. *Volta Review, 104*, 221–236.

Pisoni, D. B., & Cleary, M. (2003). Measures of working memory span and verbal rehearsal speed in deaf children after cochlear implantation. *Ear and Hearing, 24*(1 Suppl.), 106S–120S.

Pisoni, D. B., & Geers, A. E. (2000). Working memory in deaf children with cochlear implants: Correlations between digit span and measures of spoken language processing. *Annals of Otology, Rhinology, and Laryngology Supplement, 185*, 92–93.

Pyman, B., Blamey, P., Lacy, P., Clark, G., & Dowell, R. (2000). The development of speech perception in children using cochlear implants: Effects of etiologic factors and delayed milestones. *American Journal of Otology, 21*(1), 57–61.

Quittner, A. L., Cruz, I., Barker, D. H., Tobey, E., Eisenberg, L. S., Niparko, J. K., & Childhood Development after Cochlear Implantation Investigative, T. (2013). Effects of maternal sensitivity and cognitive and linguistic stimulation on cochlear implant users' language development over four years. *Journal of Pediatrics, 162*(2), 343–348 e343.

Rance, G. (2005). Auditory neuropathy/dys-synchrony and its perceptual consequences. *Trends in Amplification, 9*(1), 1–43.

Rance, G., Roper, R., Symons, L., Moody, L. J., Poulis, C., Dourlay, M., & Kelly, T. (2005). Hearing threshold estimation in infants using auditory steady-state responses. *Journal of the American Academy of Audiology, 16*(5), 291–300.

Roeser, R., & Clark, J. (2008). Live voice speech recognition audiometry: Stop the madness. *Audiology Today, 20*, 32–33.

Selimoglu, E. (2007). Aminoglycoside-induced ototoxicity. *Current Pharmaceutical Design, 13*(1), 119–126.

Shapiro, W., & Waltzman, S. (1995). Changes in electrical thresholds over time in young children implanted with the Nucleus cochlear prosthesis. *Annals of Otology, Rhinology, and Laryngology Supplement, 166*, 177–178.

Sharma, A., Dorman, M. F., & Spahr, A. J. (2002). A sensitive period for the development of the central auditory system in children with cochlear implants: Implications for age of implantation. *Ear and Hearing, 23*(6), 532–539.

Shpak, T., Koren, L., Tzach, N., Most, T., & Luntz, M. (2009). Perception of speech by prelingual preadolescent and adolescent cochlear implant users. *International Journal of Audiology, 48*(11), 775–783.

Skinner, M., Holden, L., & Holden, T. (1997). Parameter selection to optimize speech recognition with the Nucleus implant. *Otolaryngology–Head and Neck Surgery, 117*(3), 188–195.

Stahr, K., Kuechler, A., Gencik, M., Arnolds, J., Dendy, M., Lang, S., & Arweiler-Harbeck, D. (2017). Cochlear implantation in siblings with Refsum's disease. *Annals of Otology, Rhinology, and Laryngology, 126*(8), 611–614.

Starr, A., & Rance, G. (2015). Auditory neuropathy. *Handbook of Clinical Neurology, 129*, 495–508.

Teagle, H. F., Roush, P. A., Woodard, J. S., Hatch, D. R., Zdanski, C. J., Buss, E., & Buchman, C. A. (2010). Cochlear implantation in children with auditory neuropathy spectrum disorder. *Ear and Hearing, 31*(3), 325–335.

Tobey, E. A., Geers, A. E., Brenner, C., Altuna, D., & Gabbert, G. (2003). Factors associated with development of speech production skills in children implanted by age five. *Ear and Hearing, 24*(1 Suppl.), 36S–45S.

Total Communication–Beginnings. (2017). Retrieved from https://ncbegin.org/total-communication/

Uhler, K., Biever, A., & Gifford, R. H. (2016). Method of speech stimulus presentation impacts pediatric speech recognition: Monitored live voice versus recorded speech. *Otology and Neurotology, 37*(2), e70–e74.

Usami, S., Abe, S., Weston, M. D., Shinkawa, H., Van Camp, G., & Kimberling, W. J. (1999). Nonsyndromic hearing loss associated with enlarged vestibular aqueduct is caused by PDS mutations. *Human Genetics, 104*(2), 188–192.

Varga, L., Masindova, I., Huckova, M., Kabatova, Z., Gasperikova, D., Klimes, I., & Profant, M. (2014). Prevalence of DFNB1 mutations among cochlear implant users in Slovakia and its clinical implications. *European Archives of Otorhinolaryngology, 271*(6), 1401–1407.

Vermeulen, A. M., van Bon, W., Schreuder, R., Knoors, H., & Snik, A. (2007). Reading comprehension of deaf children with cochlear implants. *Journal of Deaf Studies and Deaf Education, 12*(3), 283–302.

Vesseur, A., Free, R., Langereis, M., Snels, C., Snik, A., Ravenswaaij-Arts, C., & Mylanus, E. (2016). Suggestions for a guideline for cochlear implantation in CHARGE syndrome. *Otology and Neurotology, 37*(9), 1275–1283.

Wakil, N., Fitzpatrick, E. M., Olds, J., Schramm, D., & Whittingham, J. (2014). Long-term outcome after cochlear implantation in children with additional developmental disabilities. *International Journal of Audiology, 53*(9), 587–594.

Walker, E. A., McCreery, R. W., Spratford, M., Oleson, J. J., Van Buren, J., Bentler, R., . . . Moeller, M. P. (2015). Trends and predictors of longitudinal hearing aid use for children who are hard of hearing. *Ear and Hearing, 36*(Suppl. 1), 38S–47S.

Walton, J., Gibson, W. P., Sanli, H., & Prelog, K. (2008). Predicting cochlear implant outcomes in children with auditory neuropathy. *Otology and Neurotology, 29*(3), 302–309.

Waltzman, S. B., Scalchunes, V., & Cohen, N. L. (2000). Performance of multiply handicapped children using cochlear implants. *American Journal of Otology, 21*(3), 329–335.

Wolfe, J., Baker, S., Caraway, T., Kasulis, H., Mears, A., Smith, J., . . . Wood, M. (2007). 1-year postactivation results for sequentially implanted bilateral cochlear implant users. *Otology and Neurotology, 28*(5), 589–596.

Wu, C. M., Ko, H. C., Tsou, Y. T., Lin, Y. H., Lin, J. L., Chen, C. K., . . . Wu, C. C. (2015). Long-term cochlear implant outcomes in children with GJB2 and SLC26A4 mutations. *PLoS One, 10*(9), e0138575.

Yan, D., & Liu, X. Z. (2010). Genetics and pathological mechanisms of Usher syndrome. *Journal of Human Genetics, 55*(6), 327–335.

Yoshida, H., Takahashi, H., Kanda, Y., & Chiba, K. (2017). PET-CT observations of cortical activity in pre-lingually deaf adolescent and adult patients with cochlear implantation. *Acta Otolaryngologica, 137*(5), 464–470.

Yoshida, H., Takahashi, H., Kanda, Y., Kitaoka, K., & Hara, M. (2017). Long-term outcomes of cochlear implantation in children with congenital cytomegalovirus infection. *Otology and Neurotology, 38*(7), e190–e194.

Young, N. M., Tournis, E., Sandy, J., Hoff, S. R., & Ryan, M. (2017). Outcomes and time to emergence of auditory skills after cochlear implantation of children with Charge syndrome. *Otology and Neurotology, 38*(8), 1085–1091.

Zeitler, D. M., Anwar, A., Green, J. E., Babb, J. S., Friedmann, D. R., Roland, J. T., Jr., & Waltzman, S. B. (2012). Cochlear implantation in prelingually deafened adolescents. *Archives of Pediatric Adolescent Medicine, 166*(1), 35–41.

23

Optimizing the Audiologic Management of Recipients of Cochlear Implants: Integrating Clinical Knowledge to Maximize Recipient Outcomes

Jace Wolfe

The previous chapters in this text addressed several elements pertaining to cochlear implants, including a review of hardware, technology, signal coding and processing, assessment of candidacy and outcomes, cochlear implant programming, objective measures used with cochlear implants, and factors that affect the outcomes recipients achieve with their cochlear implants. The objective of this chapter is to assimilate all of the aforementioned information into a practical guide intended to optimize the outcomes of cochlear implant recipients. General information also is provided on recipient counseling, habilitation/rehabilitation, and interdisciplinary teaming. Of note, this chapter will not provide detailed information pertaining to the procedures that an audiologist should use to determine a recipient's stimulation levels. Chapters 7, 14, and 18 provide a thorough discussion of the methods audiologists should use to determine a recipient's cochlear implant stimulation levels. Additionally, this chapter will not provide specific information pertaining to the use of objective measures for the purpose of cochlear implant estimating stimulation and guiding in the optimal management of a cochlear implant recipient. The interested reader is referred to Chapter 18 for a discussion on the use of objective measures to estimate stimulation levels and enhance the management of a cochlear implant recipient's outcome.

Collaboration with the Cochlear Implant Surgeon/Medical Evaluation

Prior to the initial activation of the sound processor, the audiologist should consult with the cochlear implant surgeon to determine if there are any relevant medical factors that may affect the cochlear implant programming process and/or the recipient's outcomes related to the cochlear implant. Preimplant imaging studies, such as computed tomography (CT) and magnetic resonance imaging (MRI), will reveal any abnormalities within the auditory system that may influence the management of the recipient. For instance, the presence of ossification or fibrous tissue growth in the cochlea, which may occur for patients who have a history of bacterial meningitis or otosclerosis, may prevent a full insertion of the electrode array into the cochlea, may increase the likelihood of nonauditory side effects such as facial nerve stimulation, may elevate the stimulation levels or the alter electrode coupling mode required to elicit a satisfactory auditory response, and may limit the recipient's hearing performance. Additionally, these imaging studies will reveal the presence of a common cavity cochlea or Mondini's dysplasia. These conditions may also complicate the insertion of the electrode array, may alter the selection of the electrode array for the recipient (e.g., a lateral wall electrode array with full-band electrode contacts may be preferred over a perimodiolar electrode array with half-band contacts for a recipient who has a common cavity cochlea, because the perimodiolar array may fold over in a common cavity and half-band electrode contacts may not be positioned toward the neural elements because of the lack of organized anatomy in the cochlea), and may also be associated with higher stimulation levels, fluctuating stimulation levels, and nonauditory side effects (i.e., facial nerve stimulation, tactile sensation, etc.).

Furthermore, an MRI will provide an indication of the status of the cochlear nerve. As previously mentioned, several studies have suggested that some children with congenital deafness are born with aplastic cochlear nerves (i.e., absent or severely deficient auditory nerves; Buchman et al., 2006; Rance, 2005), which would be expected to diminish the outcomes and success a child experiences with a cochlear implant. An a priori knowledge of cochlear nerve aplasia allows the audiologist to provide counsel to the family regarding the potential for a limited outcome. Although research has indicated that most children who receive cochlear implants achieve optimal spoken language outcomes when the family uses an auditory-oral mode of communication and forgoes the use of sign language (Ching & Dillon 2013; Geers et al,. 2003, 2007, 2011; Moog & Geers, 2003), children who have cochlear nerve aplasia are an exception and should be provided with access to spoken language and sign language to ensure that the child is exposed to a communication mode that will facilitate communication development during the critical period of language development (Peng et al., 2017). Moreover, an a priori knowledge of cochlear nerve aplasia is helpful for cochlear implant programming, because the audiologist will have an expectation that the recipient's requisite stimulation levels are likely to be higher than those of the typical recipient. However, it should also be noted that research has shown that many cases of cochlear nerve aplasia are unilateral (Buchman et al., 2006). Identification of unilateral aplasia would be critical in selecting the ideal ear for implantation. This information is obviously important to consider during the preimplant counseling process. Additionally, obtaining an MRI prior to surgery is desirable to evaluate the structural integrity of the cerebrum and brainstem, particularly given the fact that it may be difficult to obtain an MRI

of the head after cochlear implant surgery. The MRI identification may identify lesions in the cerebrum that may provide an explanation for a poor outcome (e.g., plaques on the brain of children with congenital CMV, lesions in the brain of children with a history of bacterial meningitis).

The audiologist should also inquire about postoperative imaging (e.g., x-rays, CT scan) that was conducted to evaluate the status of the electrode array insertion. Postoperative imaging is important as it indicates how many stimulating electrode contacts are inserted into the cochlea and any extracochlear electrode contacts that should be disabled. Furthermore, a postoperative CT scan may possibly indicate the scala in which the electrode array resides. Better outcomes are associated with cochlear implant electrode arrays that are entirely within the scala tympani (i.e., not located in the scala vestibuli or scala media) (Aschendorff, 2007; Finley et al., 2008; Holden et al., 2013; Wanna et al., 2015). Finally, the audiologist should query the cochlear implant surgeon about any other surgical/postsurgical complications that might influence the programming of the cochlear implant and/or the outcomes of the recipients. Recipients with complications may exhibit anxiety at the activation appointment and often will benefit from positive encouragement from the programming audiologist.

At the initial activation and all remaining appointments, the audiologist should visually inspect the incision and implant site to ensure that there are no signs of inflammation or distress. Also, the audiologist should conduct an otoscopic evaluation to rule out the presence of an external otitis and an otitis media. Additionally, the audiologist should consider removing cerumen for recipients who use electric-acoustic stimulation (EAS) so that the presence of the cerumen will not interfere with the appropriate function of the acoustic receiver. Cerumen should also be removed if the audiologist believes it may compromise the success of measuring the electrically evoked stapedial reflex.

Most clinics activate the sound processor two to four weeks after surgery to allow the incision site to heal and for the resolution of otitis media with serous effusion in the middle ear space, which is not uncommon beyond a few weeks postimplantation. The middle ear effusion often requires three to six weeks to resolve. This is a particularly important factor for recipients who had a considerable amount of low-frequency hearing prior to surgery and for whom an attempt has been made to preserve that low-frequency hearing to allow for EAS. For recipients who may benefit from EAS, it is imperative to measure air and bone conduction thresholds at all octave and inter-octave frequencies beginning at 125 Hz in order to effectively determine how to provide acoustic amplification. In the early stages in which a middle ear effusion may be present, the completion of bone conduction pure threshold assessment will assist in determining whether the recipient may benefit from acoustic amplification in the implanted ear once the middle ear effusion resolves and the hearing thresholds subsequently improve.

At the activation appointment, the audiologist should inspect the skin near the implant site to help determine the appropriate strength of the magnet in the external coil to facilitate adequate adherence without discomfort. Any swelling or inflammation at the implant site on the day of activation may necessitate a stronger magnet to facilitate adequate retention of the sound processor coil. However, when the magnet is too strong, it may restrict circulation of blood to the skin underneath the coil. Long-term use of a magnet that is too strong for the recipient may cause discomfort and in rare cases necrosis, which may lead to a skin flap breakdown requiring removal of the implant. The audiologist must closely monitor the implant site and magnet strength while any swelling/inflammation resolves in order to ensure that the magnet strength is appropriate. Often, as edema resolves, the strength of the recipient's magnet will need to be reduced. The audiologist should refer the recipient to the cochlear implant surgeon for otologic evaluation when there is evidence of significant trauma or inflammation at the incision site. Also, medical referral should be considered when there is persistent purulent otitis media or otitis media with serous effusion that persists beyond six weeks postactivation.

Programming Schedule

Two-Day Initial Activation Sessions

The optimal stimulation levels for an individual recipient normally change over the first few weeks or months of cochlear implant use. As a result, frequent programming appointments are necessary to ensure optimal stimulation levels as well as maximum performance and benefit. Frequent programming sessions throughout the first months of implant use are also beneficial, because they provide the audiologist with the opportunity to counsel the recipient and his/her family on proper care, use, and maintenance of the implants as well as on communication strategies that will optimize the recipient's outcome. After the first year of implant use, fewer appointments are necessary.

For most recipients, sound processor activation should be divided into two consecutive days. Table 23–1 provides a description of the components comprised by the two-day activation process. The obvious goals of the first day are to activate the recipient's cochlear implant(s), attempt to set stimulation levels that are comfortable and that provide consistent audibility for sounds across the speech frequency range, and assist the recipient in learning how to operate the cochlear implant. The second-day appointment provides the recipient with the opportunity to provide feedback to the audiologist about early listening experiences with the cochlear implant, and the audiologist can use this feedback to make adjustments and fine-tune the programming of the sound processor. The audiologist may also provide further counsel regarding the appropriate operation of and care for the cochlear implant system.

On day 1, after the physical examination of the ear and implant site, the audiologist should determine the appropriate magnet strength to support adherence of the external transmitting coil to the recipient's head. Young children and elderly recipients (especially elderly women) often have thin skin flaps, and as a result, they require relatively weak magnets. Middle-aged men and recipients who are obese, however, often have thick skin flaps and require strong magnets. Additionally, it can be difficult to obtain good coil adherence for recipients who have stiff, thick, and wiry hair. For users with very thick skin flaps and/or thick, stiff hair, it may be helpful to shave the hair directly underneath the transmitting coil. The audiologist should consider keeping disposable razors in the clinic to allow for shaving of the implant site if the presence of hair prevents coil retention or the delivery of a consistent signal. For very thin skin flaps, it may be helpful to place a layer of mole skin on the underneath side of the transmitting coil to provide cushion between the coil and skin. Cochlear also has produced coil spacers (a small plastic disk that clips to the underneath side of the coil) to alleviate signal interruptions that may occur with Nucleus users who have thin skin flaps.

TABLE 23–1. Overview of 2-Day Activation Appointments

Time Postsurgery	Duration	Basic Overview of Typical Procedures
2 to 4 weeks	2 hours	- Visual examination of incision site and otoscopy
		- Counsel caregiver to monitor incision site
		- Basic information: early expectations, use, care, volume control, and batteries
		- Determine processor magnet strength
		- Measure impedance at electrode contacts
		- Select signal coding strategy and base parameters
		- Determine T levels, USL, volume control
2 to 4 weeks	1.5 hours	- Visual examination of incision site and otoscopy
		- Additional information: proper use, care, habilitation/rehabilitation, and telephone use
		- Demonstrate mastery of basic processor functions
		- Adjust stimulation levels, measure ESRT* and ECAP
		- Frequency-specific programming
		- Adjust and fine-tune programming, restrict volume control

Note. * = if recipient will tolerate procedure; ECAP = electrically evoked compound action potential; ESRT = electrically evoked stapedius reflex threshold; T = threshold levels; USL = upper-stimulation levels.

Determination of the correct magnet will improve as the audiologist develops experience; however, the manufacturers provide guidelines on typical magnet strength for children and adults. Although the audiologist may be tempted to select a magnet strength that prevents the coil from ever falling off the recipient's head, it is normal for the coil to occasionally detach during rigorous physical activity (e.g., gymnastics, basketball, wrestling, or rough child's play). A magnet with an appropriate strength should be selected cautiously to avoid restriction of circulation to the skin near the internal site. If the audiologist can hold the external coil several inches from the side of the recipient's head and the transmitting coil is aggressively drawn to the internal magnet, then the coil is likely too strong. However, if the transmitting coil falls off the recipient's head several times during programming, the magnet is obviously too weak. For older children and adults, the audiologist can test the appropriateness of the strength of the external magnet by asking the recipient to raise his/her heels upward in order to stand up on his/her toes while in a standing position. Then, the recipient should drop back down to his/her heels. If the external coil dislodges from the recipient's head, then the magnet is most likely too weak. When the audiologist has doubt

when trying to select between two possible magnet strengths, he/she should most likely start with the weaker of the two magnets under consideration in an effort to avoid causing discomfort or injury to the implant site.

Regardless of the initial magnet strength, the audiologist visually should examine the skin flap at every clinical visit. If any sign of irritation occurs or a very prominent impression of the coil can be seen in the user's skin, the magnet strength should be reduced. Adult users may be advised of the signs of excessive magnet strength (e.g., discomfort near implant site, prominent impression of the coil in the skin when the coil is removed), and in some cases, they can be counseled on how to reduce their own magnet strength if they feel tightness or discomfort around the coil site. Caregivers of young recipients should be counseled to routinely monitor the status of the incision site. The caregiver should monitor the skin flap for several days after the child's implant is activated and again for several days after any time that the magnet strength is changed (e.g., upgrade to new sound processor, a switch to a stronger magnet). Also, if the child has a haircut that substantially changes the length of his/her hair, then caregivers should monitor the skin flap closely for the next several days.

A change in skin flap thickness may alter the power level required to deliver the signal without intermittency. This may occur when the recipient gains or loses a substantial amount of weight or when he/she has a substantial change in hair length or style. The Advanced Bionics implants use bidirectional telemetry to allow for continuous, real time measurement of the minimum power level needed to deliver the signal without intermittency, and as a result, changes in the skin flap do not affect signal continuity. For other recipients, it may be necessary to re-measure the requisite power level after a substantial change in skin flap thickness or hair length/style.

After the magnet is selected for the transmitting coil, the audiologist should connect the recipient's sound processor to the programming computer via a device-specific interface. Contemporary cochlear implant programming software contains several icons that inform the audiologist that the computer is connected to the programming interface and that the external sound processor and cochlear implant have been identified. These indicators are helpful in signifying that all equipment is engaged and prepared for the programming process. They are also helpful tools to use for the troubleshooting process to identify components that may be faulty (e.g., sound processor, coil, cable, cochlear implant). When the programming computer indicates successful communication with the recipient's internal device, the audiologist should measure the impedance of the stimulating and reference electrode contacts. The programmer must disable identified short or open electrode circuits. Then, the audiologist must select the appropriate signal coding strategy and initial parameters. Refer to Chapters 8, 15, 16, and 17 for direction on choosing signal coding strategies and various adjustable parameters for each implant system.

Next, the audiologist should remind the recipient about realistic expectations in the early stages of cochlear implant use. The audiologist may counsel the postlingually deafened adult recipient as follows: "Remember, when we turn your cochlear implant on today, you may not be entirely pleased with the sound you receive. In fact, you may leave here today thinking, 'I've made a big mistake.' Also, when we first turn on a cochlear implant, many people say that voices sound much different from what they remember from when they had better hearing. Some people say that voices sound cartoonish (e.g., like a chipmunk or Mickey Mouse), mechanical, or robotic. In some instances, recipients comment that speech sounds may even sound like beeps or noise.

Don't worry. As we've discussed before, it will take some time for the hearing centers of your brain to adjust to the new audio signal that you are receiving from your cochlear implant. You should notice considerable improvement in sound quality and speech understanding over the next few weeks and months. It will just take time and experience to reach that point. So, the main point today is to not panic or be concerned if the initial sound you receive is less than ideal. Our goal today is to simply provide you with sound across the speech range that is audible and comfortable."

For the caregivers of young children, the conversation immediately prior to activation will be different and may go as follows: "Remember, the initial response a young child shows to the audio signal from a cochlear implant varies widely from child to child. Some children may cry or become upset. We will be very conservative while activating your child's cochlear implant, so it is unlikely that the sound is uncomfortably loud; they are simply unsettled by the experience of being able hearing sounds they've never heard before. Other children may smile, wave, or point to their ear. However, in many cases, a child's first responses are subtle. For instance, they may stop playing with the toys, they may glance at you, me, or the programming audiologist or assistant, they may change their sucking pattern on their pacifier, or they may slightly change their facial expression. Finally, on occasion, children may exhibit very limited responses. Regardless of your child's initial response, remember that it is not at all indicative of how they will eventually perform with the cochlear implant. Also, please remember that your child's auditory skill level is similar to that of a newborn; therefore, sound will have little meaning today. It will take time for the brain to associate meaning with signals from the cochlear implant. As a result, the early responses may be very inconsistent and less than what you may have hoped. Take heart in the fact that we fully expect your child to benefit from the implant with time and experience."

After the recipient's expectations are established, the programming audiologist should determine the signal coding parameters and appropriate stimulation levels for the recipient. This is likely the most important component of the implant programming process, and research has suggested that a substantial degree of variability exists in the methods employed to create cochlear implant recipients' programs (Vaerenberg et al., 2014). Refer to Chapter 14 for a detailed description regarding the procedures audiologists should use to measure electrical threshold and upper-stimulation levels. During the first two days of activation, it may be difficult for the adult patient to respond to programming stimuli at threshold (i.e., T level) because of inexperience with the auditory sensation elicited by electrical stimulation and potential interference from constant tinnitus. For young, prelingually deafened children with limited to no experience with sound, initial thresholds are likely to be minimal response levels and suprathreshold in nature. As a result, the actual T levels are likely to be slightly lower than the measured minimal response levels. It is often necessary to provide a small global decrease in T levels from the values measured to programming stimuli. The child's T level responses to programming stimuli may include changes in sucking patterns and/or facial expressions, a time-locked head turn to the stimulus, a glance toward the parent, audiologist, or assistant, a change in play, smiling, pointing to his or her ear, crying, and so forth. The child's caregivers and the programming assistant should help the audiologist observe the child's behavior for signs of responsiveness to the signals being delivered from the cochlear implant.

As previously discussed in earlier chapters, it should be noted that some manufacturers do not recommend (e.g., default programming procedures of Advanced Bionics cochlear implants do not include measurement of T level) or even discourage the measurement of T level (e.g., MED-EL). This recommendation is supported by research that shows adequate access to low-level sounds for many recipients when T levels are estimated, particularly when mapping functions (e.g., maplaw) are optimized (Boyd, 2006). However, due to variability that exists in optimal stimulation levels across recipients, along with research that does suggest that T level measurement may improve the recipient's hearing performance (Holden et al., 2011), the author of this chapter routinely measures minimal response levels for all children and adults in order to establish the amount of stimulation that is necessary to provide audibility for the recipient. The measured T levels are included in the programs that are created for Nucleus and Advanced Bionics recipients. Based on the recommendation of the manufacturer, the author is more inclined to base T levels on the upper-stimulation levels for MED-EL recipients (i.e., set THR to 10% of MCL with the maplaw set to 1,000). However, the author does include measured T levels (i.e., THR) in the programs of some MED-EL recipients in order to optimize audibility for low-level sounds (e.g., pro-

vide sufficient access to low-level speech and environmental sounds, obtain sound-field warbled tone thresholds in the 20 to 30 dB HL range). In cases in which THR are manually measured for MED-EL recipients, the author measures THR levels and then globally decreases these measured values to a level at which there is a high degree of confidence that the recipient will not experience a continuous low-level buzzing/humming noise secondary to consistently audible, low-level electrical stimulation. Ultimately, the author's objective is to provide low-level stimulation that will result in sound-field detection thresholds that are no higher than 25 dB HL for children and 30 dB HL for adults. Fine tuning of T levels is conducted when sound-field detection thresholds do not meet these criteria.

For measurement of upper-stimulation levels, the programming audiologist should closely watch the child for signs of discomfort while the stimulation levels are increased. Ideally, the programming audiologist should also ask the programming assistant to closely observe for signs of discomfort and unease while stimulation levels are increased. If a child exhibits signs of unease, anxiety, uncertainty, nervousness, unrest, or discomfort, the audiologist should exercise caution with continued increases in stimulation with the goal of avoiding overstimulation. Excessively loud stimulation is unpleasant for adults, but it may particularly complicate the early stages of implant use for young children. Specifically, if the child associates the cochlear implant with an unwanted or unpleasant percept, he or she may refuse to wear it. Therefore, when initially activating the implant in live speech mode, threshold and upper-stimulation levels should be set at a low level and increased slowly as the programming audiologist, the programming assistant, or the child's caregivers talk to and observe the reaction of the young recipient. For young children, T levels are fixed at the initial-measurement level. However, after a response is obtained, increases to upper-stimulation levels should continue slowly while the child's response is observed.

The final upper-stimulation levels for children are based on numerous factors, including typical stimulation levels of the cochlear implant system, behavioral responses during programming, electrically evoked stapedial reflex thresholds (ESRT), and observations made while the child is listening through the cochlear implant in live speech mode. For instance, when activating young recipients who use the Nucleus cochlear implant system, the author of this chapter attempts to set the upper-stimulation levels to approximately 40 clinical units above the

T levels. However, if a child is uncomfortable with these levels, a reduced dynamic range is used for the initial program(s) in order to ensure that the auditory signal provided by the cochlear implant is comfortable. Over time, the audiologist should continue to seek to refine and perfect the child's stimulation levels with the goals of identifying stimulation levels that are comfortably loud, that provide consistent audibility of low-, average-, and high-level speech, that provide a representation of loudness growth that is reasonably similar to that which is experienced by persons with normal hearing, and that optimizes the child's ability to recognize and produce speech. This process of optimizing stimulation levels will be accomplished through a combination of behavioral (e.g., behavioral T level measurement, loudness scaling and balancing, feedback from caregivers and therapists, spoken language development) and objective (e.g., ESRT, electrically evoked compound action potential) measures. Remember, the primary goal of the activation appointment for a young child is to facilitate bonding with the implant by providing an audible and comfortable signal across the frequency range, not to create the perfect program. It can be said that the process of developing spoken language and auditory skills for a young cochlear implant recipient is not a sprint, but rather a marathon. Given the importance of consistent audibility during the critical period of language development, it is necessary to move quickly toward the optimal program for a child. However, the entire "26.2 miles of the marathon" need not be completed during the first day. Ideally, the audiologist will seek to achieve optimal stimulation levels by the one-month postactivation appointment. Once again, a detailed description of the determination of T levels and upper-stimulation levels may be found in Chapter 14.

For adult recipients, the audiologist must provide an expectation for how speech and environmental sounds likely will be perceived when the sound processor is initially activated in live speech mode. The following instructions may be provided to the recipient: "We are now ready to turn on your cochlear implant so you can hear speech and other environmental sounds. We will start at a very soft volume level, and you most likely will not hear anything at first. After that, we will very slowly increase the volume until you can hear. At first, you may hear a buzzing or ringing sound from the implant. Don't worry. This sound will stop after you wear the implant for a short time, your brain is able to acclimate to the new signal you receive from your cochlear implant,

and your program settings are optimized. As I slowly increase the volume level of the sound from your cochlear implant, please feel free to let me know if it becomes too loud for you."

When live speech first becomes audible, an adult may initially complain. To address this complaint, the audiologist may temporarily decrease upper-stimulation levels (or possibly T levels as well); however, it is best to leave the stimulation on. In many cases, the slow increases to the upper-stimulation levels will result in better sound quality. The adult recipient should be asked to indicate when the global upper-stimulation level elicits the most comfortable listening level. In the author's experience, the initial level at which the recipient reports the audio signal to be most comfortable is typically not the most ideal level; therefore, it may be more desirable to continue slowly increasing the stimulation level in small step sizes while asking the adult to indicate when the signal is too loud. The audiologist may tell the patient, "I am going to increase the 'volume' by a small amount to see if it makes your implant sound better. Often when we turn up the volume, it improves the clarity and quality of speech and environmental sounds. If the sound becomes too loud, then we will turn the 'volume' back down." From this point, the audiologist then may decrease the upper-stimulation levels by small increments (e.g., 2–5 CL/CU or 1–3% in MED-EL) and confirm that the sound quality is satisfactory. In many cases, recipients request an increase in stimulation levels after acclimating to the sound from the cochlear implant for a short while. In other cases, the user may report that certain sounds are too loud. If this occurs, the audiologist may decrease upper-stimulation levels in the corresponding frequency range or re-counsel the recipient about using the volume control. Furthermore, some users will report hearing some sounds (e.g., low-frequency sounds) but struggling to hear others (e.g., high-frequency sounds). In this case, the audiologist can make frequency-specific programming changes to alleviate the difficulties. Finally, at the end of every programming session, the audiologist may wish to ensure that the recipient can at least detect, if not discriminate, all six Ling sounds. This step ensures sufficient audibility for sounds throughout the speech frequency range (see Chapter 14). Upper-stimulation levels will likely increase throughout the first day and the next few weeks of implant use as the recipient becomes acclimated to hearing with the cochlear implant.

During the first few weeks of cochlear implant use, it is wise to provide a full range for the volume control, particularly for pediatric recipients. The provision of a wide volume control range allows the recipient or the recipient's caregivers to initially place the transmitting coil on the head with a minimal amount of stimulation and then gradually increase the stimulation to a desired listening level. A wider volume control range also provides the recipient with flexibility to adjust his/her stimulation levels to suit his/her needs as he/she acclimates to electrical hearing across a wide variety of environments. Access to a wide volume control range is especially important for the caregivers of young children. Specifically, the volume control can be set to the minimum position when the processor and coil are placed on the head, and over the course of several seconds, the volume control setting may be increased to the level that the audiologist deemed to be appropriate in the programming session. If the child reacts negatively to sound as the volume control is being increased, then the caregiver should be counseled to set the volume control to a level that is lower than what was prescribed at the programming session in order to facilitate comfort and full-time implant use. The caregiver should be counseled to attempt to increase the volume setting to the preferred setting throughout the first day or few days of implant use. However, the audiologist should also inform the caregiver that it is acceptable to remain at a volume control setting that is lower than what was recommended by the audiologist if the child exhibits signs of discomfort when the caregiver increases the volume control to the recommended setting. For children, the audiologist should always limit the volume control so that the upper-stimulation levels provided within a given program used during daily listening will not exceed what was considered appropriate in the programming session. For adults, the author of this chapter generally provides a little "headroom" beyond the volume control setting that was deemed to be most comfortable during the programming session so the recipient may access more stimulation if needed. Typically, the audiologist should provide about a 20 to 25% increase in headroom beyond the volume control setting used during the programming session. For example, the volume control of the Nucleus 7 sound processor ranges from 1 to 10 in one-unit steps. The audiologist should consider setting upper-stimulation levels so that a most comfortable listening level is established at a volume control setting of 6 with the volume control range set to 50%. With these settings, increasing the volume control from the setting of 6 to the maximum setting of 10 will result in a 20% increase in stimulation for

moderate to high-level sounds. To further clarify this concept, the reader is referred to Chapters 15 through 17 for a detailed discussion of the effect of the volume control setting for the contemporary processors offered by each implant manufacturer.

A common practice (particularly with pediatric recipients) during the early stages of cochlear implant use is to provide the recipient with multiple programs with successively greater stimulation levels (i.e., progressive programs/MAPs). This is especially helpful for people who exhibit significant tolerance problems during the first two days of activation. The audiologist should use his/her clinical insight when determining how many progressive programs to provide for a recipient and the increase in upper-stimulation level that will occur from one program to the next. A typical set of progressive programs may be generated within Cochlear's Custom Sound programming software. Once the audiologist has created the recipient's initial program, the audiologist may select the "Create Progressive MAP" button and three additional programs will be created with each one containing upper-stimulation levels that are five Clinical Units greater than its predecessor. The audiologist should encourage the recipient or the recipient's caregiver to try to progress through each of the four programs by the next programming session. Again, if the recipient exhibits signs of distress at any program, the previous program should be used. Furthermore, if program #1 is too loud for the recipient, the volume control setting can be reduced from the recommended setting. If the audiologist is satisfied with the stimulation levels that the recipient is using at the initial activation session, then it is not necessary to provide multiple (progressive) programs. In fact, in most cases, the author of this chapter finds it to be simpler to provide one program with a wide volume control range, which allows the recipient to access the desired amount of stimulation across a wide variety of environments. Situation-specific programs (e.g., noise, telephone, music) are not typically introduced until after the recipient has had at least one full week of cochlear implant use to allow for mastery of the more basic functions of the cochlear implant sound processor.

To aid in the determination of appropriate stimulation levels during the two-day activation process, the audiologist may choose to complete objective measures of cochlear implant function, including the ESRT and the electrically evoked compound action potential (ECAP). As previously mentioned, the ESRT is an excellent tool to establish appropriate upper-stimulation levels. However, due to the high level stimulus necessary to elicit the ESRT, some recipients (i.e., young children) may not tolerate this testing during the first two days of activation. During the first several sessions, the acoustic immittance probe should be placed in the ear contralateral to the cochlear implant. If the user received simultaneous bilateral cochlear implants, the audiologist should conduct otoscopy and tympanometry and place the immittance probe in the ear with the best admittance. If the ESRT is not obtained in the selected ear, it may be worthwhile to re-measure the ESRT in the opposite ear if it has reasonable admittance at the tympanic membrane.

The stimulus used for ECAP possesses a much lower stimulation rate than the stimuli used for programming and live speech. This lower rate results in a softer loudness percept at an equivalent level of stimulation (i.e., CL/clinical unit/charge unit) because of temporal summation. As a result, most recipients can tolerate the measurement of the ECAP on some (and typically all) channels during the first two days of use. The ECAP measurement system is referred to as Auditory Response Telemetry (ART), Neural Response Imaging (NRI), and Neural Response Telemetry (NRT) in the MED-EL, Advanced Bionics, and Cochlear Corporation systems, respectively. The clinical utility of the ECAP is discussed later in this chapter.

Finally, the audiologist must counsel the recipient and his or her family about care, use, and maintenance of the cochlear implant equipment. Recipients often become overwhelmed if every single aspect of the external equipment is discussed during the first day (e.g., accessories, warranty, implications for MRI). For this reason, the authors recommend discussing and reviewing the basics of implant use during the first two days and more advanced topics at subsequent programming sessions. It is helpful to have the recipient or a family member demonstrate mastery of the most basic functions, such as powering the processor on and off, adjusting the volume control, and changing the batteries.

Additionally, it is useful to discuss a wear schedule with the recipient. In most cases, the authors of this textbook subscribe to the philosophy of "eyes open, ears on." In other words, when a recipient is awake, she/he should be using the cochlear implant, even if the stimulation levels are lower than what was recommended by the audiologist. Some audiologists may suggest that recipients should gradually build up to using the cochlear implant during all waking hours. The authors of this book do not

agree with that opinion. When the implant is programmed appropriately, it should be used to enable audibility for speech and environmental sounds at every moment that the recipient is awake. Possible exceptions include when the recipient is experiencing considerable pain/discomfort or a nonauditory side effect that cannot be resolved with a change in the volume control setting. The recipient should be encouraged to contact the clinic if the implant cannot be worn during all waking hours.

Another exception to full-time use is when there is a chance that a nonwaterproof processor might be submerged in water. However, most manufacturers now provide solutions that enable sound processor use during activities that the processor may get wet. Implant use during all waking hours is especially imperative for pediatric recipients. Research has conclusively demonstrated that consistent audibility of intelligible speech is necessary for children to develop age-appropriate speech, language, and auditory abilities (Moog & Geers, 2003; Sharma, Dorman, & Spahr, 2002). Every moment that the implant is not used is a moment in which the child is deprived of stimulation that facilitates auditory brain development. The audiologist has an important responsibility to stress the importance of full-time cochlear implant use to families across multiple programming sessions. Of course, the adjustment that an adult will make to his/her cochlear implant is also expedited when the implant is used during all waking hours.

Some recipients inquire about whether they should use the implant while sleeping. The general recommendation is for the implant to be removed while the recipient sleeps. This provides the implant site an opportunity to be free from the pressure of the coil, and it gives the recipient an opportunity to charge the sound processor batteries. Some adult recipients insist on using their implant at night because they have to be able to hear important sounds while sleeping (e.g., a new mother needs to hear her baby). In these cases, the recipient is encouraged to closely monitor the coil site to ensure that there are no signs of irritation or inflammation. Some parents also report that their children refuse to remove the implant before going to bed. In these cases, the parents are counseled to allow the child to fall asleep with the implant, and then it may be removed once the child is asleep.

During waking hours, it is also important to encourage the recipient to explore the sounds in her/his environment. Parents are encouraged to take their child on a "listening walk" in which they create and point out common sounds around the house (e.g., the telephone ringing, the dog barking, a musical instrument, water running). Adults are also encouraged to actively explore the sounds of their environment and to ask a friend or loved one to identify the source of sounds with which they are unfamiliar.

Table 23–2 provides a suggested schedule for discussing various topics throughout the first few weeks of cochlear implant use. Furthermore, the manufacturers provide excellent literature and videos describing the use, care, and maintenance of the cochlear implant along with contraindications for medical procedures. Finally, it is beneficial to provide some basic aural habilitation/rehabilitation during the first two days of activation. Specific suggestions are provided later in this chapter.

TABLE 23–2. Suggested Clinician Discussion Topics the First Few Programming Sessions

Activation Appointment: Session 1
A. Basic Processor Operation: (1) Powering processor on/off, (2) Changing and recharging batteries, (3) Typical battery life, (4) Adjusting volume control, (5) Operation of remote control
B. Wear Schedule: (1) Importance of full-time use, (2) Recommended VC setting and program, (3) For children, instruct parent to decrease processor VC to minimum, place on child's head, then increase to recommended setting, (4) Progressive programs, if provided, (5) Importance of monitoring health of incision and coil sites
C. Listening Strategies: (1) Recommend age-appropriate listening strategies, (2) Creating ideal listening environment
D. Avoid Processor Damage: (1) Avoid excessive moisture and sources of static electricity
E. Misc: (1) Processor wearing/retention options, (2) Contact information; questions/problems
Activation Appointment: Session 2
A. Discuss Experiences: Counsel about reported experiences
B. Basic Processor Operation: Reiterate basic operation of processor-VC, battery life, etc.
C. Basic Care, Use, and Maintenance: (1) Use of dehumidifier, (2) Microphone care, (3) Integrity of various components/reducing strain on and replacing cables, (4) Warranty policies
D. Basic Troubleshooting and Contraindications: (1) MRI precautions, (2) Avoid monopolar cautery, (3) Avoid contact sports with risk of injury and scuba diving below 100 meters
1-Week Session
A. Discuss Experiences: Counsel about reported experiences
B. Basic Processor Operation and Accessories: (1) Inspect settings to ensure appropriate use, (2) Discuss basic operation as necessary, (3) For adults, discuss situations-specific programs, (4) Accessory cables-connecting to remote devices, (5) Monitoring earphones
C. Bacterial Meningitis Vaccination: Importance of vaccination with recommended schedule
D. Miscellaneous: (1) Rehabilitative/habilitative guidance, (2) Care of processor in extreme conditions (e.g., sports, exercise, working outside, toddlers)
1-Month Session
A. Discuss Experiences: Counsel about reported experiences
B. Basic Processor Functions: (1) Inspect settings to ensure appropriate use, (2) Discuss basic operation as necessary, (3) Importance of functional backup equipment loaded with current programs, bring to every subsequent appointment, (4) Protocol for replacing faulty equipment
C. Removing Barriers: (1) Hearing Assistance Technology, (2) Ensure adequate telephone abilities, (3) Introduce FM system if need additional assistance in challenging listening situations
D. Future Sessions: Discuss schedule for future programming appointments

One-Week Postactivation Appointment

Following the two-day activation appointment, children and adults should come back for a one-week postactivation appointment to adjust programming parameters. The weeklong experience with the cochlear implant will: (1) allow recipients to gather experiences with sound from the implant so that they may provide useful information to the audiologist to guide programming changes and (2) allow adults and older children to be more effective listeners when behavioral responses are required. Furthermore, recipients usually are able to tolerate higher levels of stimulation and objective measures after they have used the implant for a short time (i.e., ESRT, ECAP). The week 1 appointment and all subsequent appointments are scheduled for 60 to 90 minutes depending on the individual needs of the recipient as well as the objectives that the audiologist wants to accomplish within a session. Additional time is required for appointment sessions in which the audiologist chooses to complete outcomes assessment (e.g., warbled tone sound-field detection thresholds, speech recognition in quiet and/or in noise, questionnaires). Bilateral cochlear implant recipient appointments are scheduled for 90 to 120 minutes to accommodate for the additional time required to program two cochlear implant systems and to evaluate auditory function with each ear separately and in the bilateral condition. Bimodal recipients should also be scheduled for 90 to 120 minutes, particularly when auditory function has to be evaluated in each unilateral listening condition as well as in the bimodal condition and when the hearing aid needs to be fitted or fine-tuned (e.g., real-ear probe microphone measurements, cochlear dead region evaluation).

At the week 1 appointment, the audiologist should once again commence with otoscopy to rule out any external or middle ear pathology as well as with an inspection of the implant site to confirm the absence of complications. Then, for adult recipients and older children (5 years old and up), the audiologist should measure frequency-specific, sound-field detection thresholds to ensure adequate access to low-level sounds (i.e., ≤30 dB HL warble tones from 250 to 6000 Hz). When responses fall outside of the expected range, the audiologist should make programming adjustments to improve access to low-level sounds. In most cases, open-set speech recognition is not measured at the one-week appointment because the recipient is still acclimating to the cochlear implant and will likely find open-set speech recognition assessment to be difficult and an experience that may be discouraging. However, if the recipient is doing very well (e.g., reports conversing over the telephone, understanding speech in conversation with minimal effort, understanding speech over the television without closed caption), then the audiologist may choose to evaluate open-set speech recognition after sound-field warbled tone threshold assessment is completed. Audiometric sound-field assessment typically is not performed for young children (<5 years) at the one-week postactivation appointment given the likelihood that young children often have limited attention spans and may not participate in sound-field detection threshold assessment as well as remain cooperative for the cochlear implant programming session too. Instead, the audiologist should focus on optimization of the child's program with the goal of identifying ideal stimulation levels for the child. Once again, however, if the audiologist believes that the child's optimal stimulation levels were determined during the first two activation appointments, then the decision may be made to begin the one-week programming session with an evaluation of sound-field warbled tone thresholds to confirm that the child has excellent access to low-level sounds (i.e., 25 dB HL or better from 250 to 6000 Hz). When the physical examination and behavioral assessment are completed, the audiologist should measure the impedance of all of the electrode contacts. Impedance values likely will decrease substantially from the first day of activation and will begin to stabilize.

Next, the audiologist should measure T levels on as many channels as possible to adequately characterize the recipient's electrical threshold profile across the electrode array. Of note, the anecdotal experience of the author of this chapter suggests that it may be difficult to measure T levels for children with behavioral observation audiometry (BOA) or visual reinforcement audiometry (VRA) at the one-week checkup because the child has had experience with a variety of interesting sounds throughout the first week of implant use, and as a result, the programming stimuli are no longer novel and intriguing to the child. The child's caregivers may become concerned if the child does not appear to readily respond to the programming stimuli. However, the audiologist should consider informing the caregivers prior to the one-week programming session that the child may no longer be interested in the relatively mundane programming stimuli and may not produce a robust response during BOA or VRA assessment of T levels. Also, because the child has heard speech and environmental sounds with the implant for a week, it may be challenging to keep young children engaged during the programming session. In particular, pediatric recipients who achieve excellent outcomes with their cochlear implant(s) and who use their cochlear implants during all waking hours will often become reluctant to remove their cochlear implants for programming. They may also become distressed at the thought of their sound processor being connected by a cable to the programming computer. The audiologist should be prepared with engaging toys and distractors (e.g., light-up toys, spinners, cars, dolls, computer tablets) to facilitate the child's cooperation when the sound processor is removed for programming.

When the T level measurements are complete, the audiologist should optimize upper-stimulation levels. This should first be completed through the use of behavioral measures with adults and older children (see Chapter 14 for a detailed discussion pertaining to the procedures audiologists should use to determine upper-stimulation levels for both young children and adults). Again, it is prudent to stress how important it is for the audiologist to optimize stimulation levels and to achieve balanced loudness of upper-stimulation levels across the electrode array because the recipient's speech recognition abilities and overall hearing performance and experience (e.g., sound quality, listening comfort) are highly dependent upon the provision of optimal stimulation levels.

For younger children (7 years old and below) who are unlikely to be able to provide valid verbal feedback about the loudness of the stimulation they receive (i.e., younger children are unlikely to be able to participate in the loudness balancing task and are also less likely to provide valid feedback on loudness scaling tasks), the audiologist should attempt to measure the ESRT to assist in the determination of upper-stimulation levels. When ESRT cannot be measured for young children, upper-stimulation levels should be based on a combination of behavioral measures, the audiologist's observations of the child's reaction to stimulation, feedback the audiologist receives from the child's caregivers and therapists, and the audiologist's knowledge of what typically constitutes appropriate stimulation levels with the implant the child is using. Although the ECAP measurement is not strongly correlated to upper-stimulation levels, the audiologist may use it as another piece of information to guide in determination of appropriate upper-stim-

ulation levels (again, the reader is referred to Chapter 14 for a detailed discussion on the determination of stimulation levels for young children and Chapter 18 for information on the use of objective measures to set cochlear implant stimulation levels). Furthermore, the ESRT measure should also be attempted with adult recipients, even when the audiologist believes that the behavioral measures are valid, because the ESRT serves as an excellent cross-check to confirm the appropriateness of upper-stimulation levels. Additionally, the ECAP should be measured for electrodes that were not completed at previous sessions, so the audiologist may establish a record (i.e., a baseline) of the recipient's physiologic responses to electrical stimulation across the electrode array.

If an adult seems to understand the basic function of the sound processor and tolerates appropriate stimulation levels, the audiologist may introduce situation-specific programs (e.g., telephone, listening in noise, music; see Chapters 15, 16, and 17 for examples of environmentally specific programs that users might find to be beneficial with each cochlear implant system). However, for young children who cannot reliably switch to a program that will optimize their performance for a given listening environment, it is usually ideal to provide one program that is suitable across a variety of environments. If the caregiver reports that the child is still not tolerating appropriate stimulation levels, it may be necessary to continue providing multiple programs with increasing levels of stimulation. If the child is showing no aversion to appropriate stimulation levels and is able to initiate implant use at the recommended volume control setting, then the audiologist should reduce the range over which the volume control operates (i.e., reduce the volume control range so that a change from the maximum to minimum position only decreases upper-stimulation levels by 20% to 30% or possibly even disable the volume control altogether). This will result in more precise control of volume adjustment for the child or parent.

If time permits, the audiologist may demonstrate the use of accessory items (e.g., wireless hearing assistive technologies such as remote microphones, telephone/television streaming devices, personal audio cables, monitoring earphones, waterproof accessories) and review and expand on the proper care of the system (i.e., changing microphone cover, cleaning the sound processor, and using the dehumidifier). In particular, the audiologist should stress the importance of remote microphone technology (i.e., personal digital RF/FM system) in optimizing children's listening abilities and access to intelligible speech in real-world situations. The use of wireless remote microphone technology will optimize a child's access to intelligible speech, which is particularly useful in acoustically hostile situations and for young children who are developing language and are dependent on a robust model of intelligible speech. The reader is referred to Chapter 20 for additional discussion of the use of remote microphone technology with cochlear implants. Of note, third-party payers (e.g., health insurance companies, government funding of health care, etc.) may refuse to provide reimbursement for the time an audiologist spends counseling a recipient about the proper care, use, and maintenance of his/her cochlear implant hardware and hearing assistive technology, which is unfortunate considering the vital importance of properly functioning equipment on the outcome of the recipient. The cochlear implant program may consider assigning poorly reimbursed tasks to audiology assistants in order to minimize the cost of providing these services.

If at this point, appropriate stimulation levels still have not been determined for a child at the conclusion of the appointment, then the child should be scheduled for another programming session within a week. Otherwise, the recipient should return in three weeks for a one-month, postactivation checkup. A summary of the procedures in typical one- and three-week appointments are provided in Table 23–3.

One-Month Postactivation Programming Session

By the one-month appointment, the recipient should begin to develop a strong bond with the cochlear implant. The recipient and family usually are able to provide substantial feedback about the recipient's progress and experiences with speech and other environmental sounds in order to guide the audiologist in any programming changes that are necessary to further optimize hearing performance. Typically, postlingually deafened adult recipients will report significant improvements in their ability to understand speech. As a result, aided sound-field detection thresholds and speech recognition should be evaluated at the beginning of the one-month postactivation session. For users of bilateral implants, thresholds and speech recognition should be measured for each ear. These thresholds and scores contribute to necessary program changes. For example, if warbled tone detection thresholds are elevated in the high-frequency range (e.g., >25 dB HL, 2000 to 6000 Hz), the audiologist should focus on programming adjustments to improve access to high-frequency, low-level sounds.

At this point, children should be using their cochlear implant during all waking hours. If the parent reports situations (other than bath time or swimming or other situations in which the cochlear implant should be removed to avoid damage) in which the cochlear implant is not used, the audiologist should counsel the family about the importance of full-time

TABLE 23–3. Overview of 1-Week and Optional 3-Week Postactivation Appointments

Time Postactivation	Duration	Basic Overview of Typical Procedures
1 week	1 hour	- Visual examination of incision site, otoscopy, impedances - Measure T levels, ESRT, and ECAP for remaining electrodes - Adjustments to USL in live speech mode - Child: provide one program - Adult: aided sound-field thresholds; situation-specific programs - Reduce volume control range - Discuss care in greater detail and demonstrate accessories
3-week interim	1 hour	- Only necessary when T and USL levels not yet determined - Visual examination of incision site and otoscopy - Protocol similar to 1-week appointment

Note. ECAP = electrically evoked compound action potential; ESRT = electrically evoked stapedius reflex threshold; T = threshold levels; USL = upper-stimulation levels.

implant use. The child's language development is dependent upon the full-time use of properly functioning cochlear implant technology so that he/she may have exposure to a language-rich listening environment full of intelligible speech. Failure to ensure that the child is using his/her cochlear implant(s) during all waking hours is neglect, because insufficient exposure to intelligible speech during the critical period of language development (i.e., the first three years of life) will have an irreparable negative impact on the child's ability to develop a method to communicate, a fact that will have lifelong unfortunate consequences for the child. The audiologist should remember that the family may not be privy to the importance of exposure to a language-rich listening environment during the formative years of brain and language development. The family may be under the impression that they have the luxury of gradually building up toward full-time use of the cochlear implant. They may erroneously believe that their child will suffer no detrimental consequences from part-time implant use, and they may believe that there is no problem with waiting until the child is older to commence with full-time implant use. The audiologist is responsible for informing the family of the importance of implant use during all waking hours. It is also the audiologist's responsibility to advocate for the child if the caregivers are not assisting the child in attaining full-time cochlear implant use from the earliest stages. The audiologist should inspect the results of data logging, when available, to ensure that full-time implant use is occurring and that the child is exposed to environments with speech present. Additionally, sound-field detection thresholds should be evaluated at the beginning of the appointment and should be no poorer than 30 dB HL in the low frequencies and 25 dB HL in the mid to high frequencies. If the child does not have consistent access to low-level sounds, the audiologist must make programming changes to optimize the audibility of soft sounds. When possible, the audiologist should consider evaluating the child's speech recognition abilities with use of the cochlear implant. The reader is referred to Chapter 6 for information on the speech recognition measures to use for the assessment of young children.

The remainder of the one-month appointment involves the same measures conducted at previous appointments. The audiologist should conduct otoscopy and an examination of the implant site as well as complete a visual inspection of the sound pro-cessor (i.e., signs of wear, tear, or damage). When possible, the audiologist should perform a biologic listening check with monitor earphones to evaluate the status of the sound processor microphone. The audiologist should ensure that the microphone covers are clean. Next, the audiologist should complete electrode impedance measures and measure T levels and upper-stimulation levels. Ideally, the audiologist should complete multiple T level measurements at several channels in an effort to determine the T level profile across the electrode array. If T levels are relatively constant across the array, they will be measured on only a few electrodes and the remaining values may be interpolated. However, substantial T level variability from one measured channel to the next warrants measurements on a greater number of channels. Next, the audiologist should optimize upper-stimulation levels using previously discussed procedures, and the ESRT should be measured on several channels across the electrode array. For adults, the volume control range should allow for only a small change in stimulation levels when the volume control is adjusted from the maximum to the minimum position (e.g., −30%/+15% of the dynamic range). In children, the upper end of the volume control should not exceed the upper-stimulation levels set in the program in order to avoid stimulation levels that may be uncomfortable for the child during everyday use. The lower end of the volume control range is dependent upon the child's tolerance for stimulation. If no tolerance problems exist, the volume control should be disabled or should only allow for minimal decreases in volume (e.g., −20% of the dynamic range or less). However, if the child does exhibit evidence of loudness tolerance problems, the volume control should allow for substantial decreases (i.e., 50% or greater of the dynamic range).

If an adult subject is struggling substantially, it may be worthwhile to trial different signal coding strategies and/or stimulation rates in an effort to provide better sound quality and/or performance. The default signal coding strategies recommended in this book will allow most recipients to achieve satisfactory levels of hearing performance. However, when a recipient experiences early difficulty adjusting to the signal from the cochlear implant, the audiologist should take advantage of the various options in signal coding that the manufacturers offer. When switching to an alternative signal coding strategy, the audiologist should re-measure stimulation levels with the new signal coding strategy. For recipients who are elderly, who have a long duration of deafness, or who have evidence of potential neural deficits (e.g., ANSD, multiple sclerosis, cochlear nerve aplasia), the audiologist should consider decreasing the stimulation rate. For other recipients who are struggling to hear well with the stimulation rates recommended in this book, the audiologist may consider creating programs with slower and faster stimulation rates in an effort to determine the optimal stimulation rate for the recipient. Again, when stimulation rates are changed, the audiologist will most likely need to re-measure stimulation levels.

Also at the one-month appointment, the audiologist should provide an introduction of situation-specific programs if not yet completed at the previous session. Additionally, the audiologist or audiology assistant should once again discuss the proper care, use, and maintenance of the cochlear implant system and provide the recipient with an opportunity to ask any questions that he/she may have about proper use of the cochlear implant. Moreover, the audiologist (or audiology assistant) should revisit the use of hearing assistive technology to ensure that the recipient is aware of accessory technologies that are available to optimize hearing performance across a range of listening environments.

Remainder of Programming Schedule

After the one-month appointment, programming schedules differ between adults and children but involve similar procedures and mirror those described for the one-month session. A summary of the steps included in the one- and three-month postactivation appointments is shown in Table 23–4. For children younger than 7 years, two- and three-month postactivation appointments are scheduled to ensure optimal access to low-level sounds and appropriate program settings. Following the three-month appointment, the child should return every three months for assessment of auditory skills, verification of cochlear implant function, and programming. In most cases, minimal programming changes are necessary at these appointments. Nonetheless, the appointments are very essential to ensure that the child's performance is satisfactory in the audiology test booth and to evaluate the physical integrity of the implant site as well as the child's external and middle ear status. Furthermore, the audiologist may ensure that the implant equipment is all functioning appropriately and that the implant is being used effectively during all waking hours. These appointments also provide the audiologist with the opportunity to provide

TABLE 23–4. Overview of 1-Month and 3-Month Postactivation Appointments

Time Postactivation	Duration	Basic Overview of Typical Procedures
1 mo	1 hour	- Visual examination of incision site and otoscopy
		- Feedback about progress and discuss duration of implant use
		- Aided sound-field thresholds and speech recognition
		- Visual exam and biologic listening check on processor
		- Measure electrode impedances and T levels
		- Optimize USL; measure ESRT
		- Reduce volume control range or disable
		- Provide situation-specific programs
2/3 mo	1 hour	- Visual examination of incision site and otoscopy
		- Sound-field detection thresholds and speech recognition
		- Similar procedures as 1-month session
		- Child: Ensure access to soft sounds; determine if program levels and settings appropriate
		- Adult: seen at 2 mo if struggling; otherwise, seen at 3 mo

Note. ESRT = electrically evoked stapedius reflex threshold; mo = months; T = threshold levels; USL = upper-stimulation levels.

continual counsel to the family in an effort to optimize the recipient's communication performance and development.

In addition, young children with cochlear implants should receive intensive audition-based therapy/habilitation to optimize auditory and spoken language development. The audiologist should collaborate with the Listening and Spoken Language Specialist (LSLS) or speech-language pathologist to ensure that the child's speech and language is developing appropriately. If concerns arise, more frequent audiologic evaluations and implant-programming sessions may be warranted. When the child reaches 7 years of age and has at least two years of cochlear implant experience, audiologic assessment and programming should be conducted every six months.

Following the one-month postactivation appointment, adults typically return for a three-month programming session. However, if an adult is struggling at the one-month appointment, he or she should be seen for a two-month postactivation appointment. Following the three-month appointment, adults should be seen every three months for audiologic assessment and a cochlear implant checkup/programming through the first year of implant use and

on a biannual or annual basis thereafter. A summary of the appointments following the three-month postactivation session is outlined in Table 23–5.

Additional Habilitative/Rehabilitative Considerations

Developing an ideal cochlear implant program with optimal stimulation levels is certainly important for success with a cochlear implant, but receiving specialized audition-based therapy or aural rehabilitation is, in many cases, equally important to promoting a successful outcome. This specialized therapy or rehabilitation facilitates maximal performance with the device for two reasons. First, the electrical signal from a cochlear implant is much different than the acoustic signal from a hearing aid. Second, auditory skills acquired with cochlear implants are very impressive but still do not match those of a person with normal-hearing sensitivity. Therefore, to enhance satisfaction, performance, and benefit, aural rehabilitation for adult recipients is recommended during the first few weeks or months of cochlear implant use. Auditory-

TABLE 23–5. Appointment Schedule Following the 3-Month Postactivation Session

Time Postactivation	Duration	Basic Overview of Typical Procedures
Every 3 months	1 hour	- Visual examination of incision site and otoscopy - Sound-field detection thresholds and speech recognition - Visual exam and biologic listening check on processor - Measure electrode impedances and ESRT - Adjust T levels, USL, parameters, and programs - Child: assess auditory skills; clinician collaborate with LSLS
Child: Every 6 months	1 hour	- For child 7 years or older with 2 years of implant experience - Visual examination of incision site and otoscopy - Sound-field detection thresholds and speech recognition - Procedures similar to 3-month session
Adult: Biannual or Annual	1 hour	- For adult after 1 year of implant use; dependent on needs - Visual examination of incision site and otoscopy - Sound-field detection thresholds and speech recognition - Perform procedures similar to 3-month session

Note. ESRT = electrically evoked stapedius reflex threshold; LSLS = language and spoken language specialist; T = threshold levels; USL = upper-stimulation levels.

Verbal therapy is recommended for children throughout the first few years of life and until it is established that the child's speech, language, and auditory abilities are consistent with their normal-hearing peers who have a similar nonverbal IQ and that the child is developing complex spoken language abilities.

Aural Rehabilitation for Adult Cochlear Implant Recipients

The rehabilitation program should be directed by an LSLS or by an audiologist with experience in aural rehabilitation for adults with severe to profound deafness. In addition, the cochlear implant manufacturers have developed very effective training exercises and computer-based aural rehabilitation programs, which are available on their websites, online video-sharing sites (e.g., YouTube), and/or compact disc (CD-ROM). These manufacturer-designed programs are often critical for adults who do not have access to individualized aural therapy but also supplement rehabilitation of adults enrolled in formal programs. In cases in which more intensive home-based aural rehabilitation is needed, the audiologist should consider evidence-based, computer facilitated programs, such as LACE (Listening and Communication Enhancement), which have been designed to facilitate auditory skill development in adults with hearing loss (Ferguson & Henshaw, 2015). Home-based aural rehabilitation programs and activities are particularly important for elderly recipients who live alone and have limited social and occupational activity. These recipients often have sparse exposure to spoken language, and as a result their auditory systems are not consistently subjected to the intelligible speech necessary to facilitate the auditory nervous system's acclimatization to the signal from the cochlear implant.

The programming audiologist also should be equipped with several rehabilitative tools to facilitate early success with the cochlear implant. For example, when the implant initially is activated in live speech mode, the audiologist may ask the recipient to listen as the former says the days of the week or months of the year. In this task, the audiologist should stop on a given day or month and ask the recipient to say the following day/month (e.g., the audiologist says, "Monday, Tuesday, Wednesday, Thursday" and stops, and then the recipient says, "Friday"). In this example, the recipient's auditory memory is used to support the auditory input received from the cochlear

implant. Most recipients can accomplish this exercise, which helps them associate meaning to the sound they receive from their cochlear implant. For recipients who may struggle to hear well at the activation of their implant (e.g., long-term deafened recipients, elderly), the audiologist may choose to say the days of the week slowly in order to allow the recipient to follow along. For recipients who are performing at a higher level, the audiologist may choose the speed of the pace of the task and switch from days of the week to months of the year. Then, the audiologist may choose to switch back to the days of the week without prompting the recipient or switch without notice to numbers or another task with a familiar sequence. This simple listening task serves as an excellent confidence builder because it allows the recipient to realize the potential benefit of the signal he/she is receiving from the new implant. The audiologist should also encourage adult recipients to seek out sounds during the first few weeks of cochlear implant use. For example, they can turn on the water faucet to associate meaning to the sound it generates or listen to the sounds of the ringer and/or alarms on their smartphone. The audiologist should also encourage recipients to seek out sounds that they cannot readily identify (e.g., if they hear a new rhythmic sound, they should explore for the source, which they may for example determine to be a ticking clock). If the recipient cannot identify the source of a sound, then the audiologist should encourage the former to ask family members or friends to provide assistance in identifying its source (e.g., the rhythmic sound heard in an automobile may turn out to be the turn indicator).

Auditory/visual tracking is another effective rehabilitation activity in the early stages of implant use. In this exercise, the recipient listens and follows along visually as the audiologist reads aloud from a book, magazine, or newspaper. When the audiologist stops reading somewhere within the passage, the recipient's task is to say the next word in the passage. In the auditory/visual tracking task, the recipient is able to rely on visual input to support the auditory signal he/she is receiving from the cochlear implant, and as a result, the tracking exercise should help the recipient associate specific words on the page to words that are heard with use of the implant. The audiologist should recommend that family members conduct this tracking exercise with the recipient at home. If the recipient lives alone or is unable (or does not want) to practice tracking with a family member, then he/she may still engage in the tracking exercise by obtaining an unabridged version of an audio book recording (MP3/digital audio file, audio streaming, compact disc, etc.) as well as the paper version of the book. The recipient can follow along visually in the book while listening to the audio recording. Many public libraries carry unabridged recorded audio copies of the paper books they have on their shelves.

Familiar phrase cards are also beneficial during initial stages of implant use. For the familiar phrase task, the audiologist places two to four cards on a table and the audiologist reads the phrase or words on one of the cards aloud. The recipient is tasked with selecting the card that was read. This task can begin at the level of pattern perception (i.e., cards having words with different syllable length) and progress to closed-set word identification. Although the previously mentioned exercises seem somewhat elementary, they help to build confidence and auditory skill level at the initial activation sessions. The aforementioned exercises do not represent a comprehensive aural rehabilitation program for the adult patient. Again, if the programming audiologist is not well versed in audiologic rehabilitation, he/she should consider referring the recipient to a hearing health care professional who specializes in providing aural rehabilitation for cochlear implant recipients. Of note, lengthy aural rehabilitation programs are not necessary for most adult recipients, but such programs may be beneficial for recipients who struggle to acclimate to the implant, especially when the audiologist has optimized the recipient's hearing technology. Aural rehabilitation is most likely to be useful for recipients who have long durations of deafness, those who are elderly, and those who may have additional disabilities.

Audition-based habilitation/rehabilitation is absolutely critical for young children with a cochlear implant. Although the programming audiologist can provide support, all children should be managed closely by an LSLS who will guide the child and family toward optimal development of speech, language, and auditory skills. As previously stated, the audiologist should correspond closely with the LSLS to ensure the child is making satisfactory progress in speech, spoken language, and auditory skill development. At the initial activation appointment, the programming audiologist must ensure that the child's caregivers have a thorough understanding of the use, care, and maintenance of the cochlear implant system as well as the importance of using it during all waking hours. Oral and written instruction should

be provided at the initial session, and the audiologist should revisit the basics of implant use at subsequent appointments. In addition, the audiologist and family should determine the most appropriate wearing option for retention of the sound processor to the child's head to body.

On the first day of cochlear implant use, families should be encouraged to walk around the home and point out the different sounds they encounter. For instance, they can knock on the door, point to their ear, and say, "I heard that." The LSLS often refers to this activity as a "listening walk," which helps children associate meaning to new sounds. Other examples of sounds on a listening walk include speech, laughing, and/or music from a parent or sibling, ringing from the telephone, running water, a door shutting, a dog barking, leaves blowing in the wind, sounds from toys, etc. If the child appears to respond to speech or an environmental sound, the caregiver should provide enthusiastic positive reinforcement while pointing to her own ear and saying, "I heard that!"

Parents should also be encouraged to provide an oral description of even the most mundane events of life. For example, when walking into a room, the parent should say, "Okay, we're walking into the room, and now we're going to turn on the light. Oh, the light came on." Joanna Smith and Teresa Caraway, Listening and Spoken Language Specialists, encourage caregivers to be "sports radio play-by-play announcers" who provide a verbose description of all of the mundane activities that occur throughout the child's day. Consistent verbal descriptions of daily activities provide the child with a listening-rich model of speech and language development. Another wonderful exercise to recommend for auditory skill development in young children is the simple act of reading books. Reading aloud to children serves as an excellent model for language and literacy development. Carol Flexer, audiologist and Listening and Spoken Language Specialist, suggests that caregivers should read at least 10 books a day to children with hearing loss.

Finally, caregivers should attempt to optimize the acoustics in the home. For example, if no one is watching the television, it should be turned off to reduce competing noise. Hardwood and tile floors can be covered with rugs, windows can be covered with drapes, and furniture can be outfitted with soft covers to reduce reverberation. Also, to provide a good signal-to-noise ratio during the early stages of implant use, the parent should attempt to remain in close proximity to the child and direct speech to the side of the implant when communicating. Obviously, the aforementioned suggestions are not exhaustive and only introduce a few ideas for building an "auditory lifestyle." However, audiologists should ensure that young children who receive cochlear implants have access to Auditory-Verbal therapy in order to optimize the child's listening and spoken language abilities. For more information on Auditory-Verbal therapy for children with cochlear implants, the interested reader is referred to *Auditory Verbal Therapy: For Young Children with Hearing Loss and Their Families, and the Practitioners Who Guide Them*, Warren Estabrooks, Karen MacIver-Lux, and Ellen A. Rhoades (Plural Publishing, Inc.).

Patient Complaints and Complications

Advances in cochlear implant technology and clinical procedures, expansion of candidacy, and earlier identification of hearing loss in children have resulted in considerable benefit for the overwhelming majority of recipients. In some instances, however, children with cochlear implants do not develop age-appropriate speech and language skills, and adults do not achieve excellent open-set speech recognition. Although these undesirable outcomes may be attributed to factors outside of the audiologist's control (e.g., low nonverbal IQ, additional disabilities, poor familial support, abnormal anatomy), it is also possible that poor outcomes may be related to a suboptimal program/MAP that fails to meet the recipient's needs. The interested reader is referred to Chapters 21 and 22, which highlight factors associated with cochlear implant outcomes for adults and children, respectively.

Some recipients experience initial difficulties with their cochlear implants, but after adept management by the programming audiologist, they achieve substantial benefit. It is fairly common for even the most successful recipients to experience temporary setbacks, which may be attributed to faulty external equipment or minor programming needs. These issues typically are addressed efficiently and effectively by the seasoned programming audiologist. The goal of the proceeding sections is to discuss the audiologic management of recipients who experience suboptimal outcomes, complications, and temporary and chronic difficulties. Suggestions also are provided for the management of difficult-to-program recipients.

Managing Recipients Who Experience Disappointing Outcomes

Numerous factors may be responsible for deficient performance with a cochlear implant, but a poor outcome is often related to patient characteristics (see Chapters 21 and 22). In other cases, unsatisfactory performance or temporary difficulty may be attributed to an extrinsic factor (e.g., faulty hardware, poor program). Therefore, the following potential extrinsic causes should be evaluated.

External Hardware

Although the reliability and durability of external hardware is exceptionally good, malfunction of the external sound processor and its components (e.g., cable, transmitting coil) should always be considered as a potential cause for poor or limited performance. Cochlear implant recipients typically use their sound processors during all waking hours, and as a result, the external hardware is frequently subjected to adverse elements, such as heat, body oil, moisture (from perspiration, humidity, rain, bathing, swimming pools, etc.), and being dropped on hard surfaces. The audiologist should routinely conduct an examination of the function of a recipient's external hardware. This should take place at least every three months for children and one to two times a year for adults. The examination should include the following components.

First, a visual examination of the external hardware should be conducted to check for signs of wear or faults. It is especially important to inspect the transmitting cable(s) for evidence of anomalies as the wires inside the cable often are susceptible to breakage. In fact, the transmitting cable is typically the weakest of all of the external components, and as a result, when recipients present with no sound or an intermittent signal from their implant system, the most likely cause is a faulty transmitting cable. When the function of the transmitting cables is in doubt, the audiologist should switch to a clinic loaner cable or the recipient's backup cable, or if troubleshooting over the telephone, then the recipient should be directed to switch to his/her backup cable. The audiologist can confirm that the transmitting coil is sending and receiving signals to the internal device using a signal-check wand, a diagnostic remote control, or a telemetry measure via the computer programming software interface. For young children who cannot report on the integrity of the signal, the transmitting cables should be replaced every six months.

Next, the audiologist visually should assess the appearance of the sound processor's microphone port(s) or covers. The microphone covers should be clean and free of debris and should also be periodically replaced. For infants and children, active recipients, and those living in humid/tropical environments, the covers should be replaced every two to three months. At a minimum, the covers should be replaced every four to six months (e.g., inactive recipients or those living in arid or relatively dry environments).

When possible, the audiologist should also assess the microphone function with a listening check (i.e., Cochlear monitor earphones/Advanced Bionics listening check/MED-EL microphone test device) or with the remote control if applicable. Additionally, as previously discussed, it is imperative to measure sound-field detection thresholds to ensure that the sensitivity of the microphone allows for access to low-level sounds across the speech-frequency range (i.e., 250–6000 Hz). In the initial stages of microphone deterioration, sound-field thresholds often increase in the high frequencies.

The audiologist should also inspect the sound processor batteries and battery contacts for signs of corrosion or faults. Furthermore, the audiologist should verify that all controls and indicators are functioning properly and that adjustable controls, such as the volume and sensitivity controls, are set to the appropriate setting. Moreover, the audiologist should ensure that the recipient is using the correct program and that the telecoil, hearing assistive technologies, and other auxiliary sound input sources are functioning properly. Finally, most recipients own a backup sound processor for troubleshooting purposes, and in the event that performance and progress are poor, the audiologist should always remember to ask the recipient to switch to the backup external equipment. If the problem is addressed, then the audiologist should systematically replace each of the sound processor components one by one in order to identify the faulty link. If the recipient does not have a backup processor, then the clinic's loaner equipment should be used for troubleshooting.

With regard to ensuring optimal function of external hardware, the audiologist and recipient will both benefit from the old adage that "an ounce of prevention is worth a pound of cure." As previously suggested, the recipient should be counseled to routinely replace the microphone covers on schedule as recommended by the audiologist. Also, the audiologist should counsel the recipient about the frailty of the transmitting cable to encourage the recipient to exercise caution when removing the coil from the head (i.e., do not pull the processor off the head by grabbing the coil). The recipient should be provided with a thorough understanding of the water resistance of his/her sound processor as well as suggestions for facilitating reliable sound processor function when in the presence of water. Regardless of the water resistance rating of the sound processor, the recipient should be counseled to place the sound processor in a dehumidifier every night. Routine use of a dehumidifier will markedly improve the reliability and function of sound processors, even for those that are waterproof. Furthermore, audiologists should ask the recipient to hold the sound processor a short distance over a soft surface (if possible) when the processor is being handled (e.g., changing batteries, adjusting controls). This will reduce the likelihood that the processor falls from a high distance onto a hard surface. Finally, the audiologist should assist the recipient in identifying the necessary means for ensuring that the processor securely adheres the recipient's ear/head. Many older children and adults can simply wear the processor on the ear without concern of it falling off. However, active recipients (e.g., sports, manual labor) may need assistance in identifying accessories (e.g., Snugfit, earmold, double-sided tape, Ear Gear, retention cords) or special wearing configurations (e.g., body-worn configurations) that will facilitate adequate retention during periods of strenuous activity.

Determine Wear Schedule and Facilitate an Auditory Lifestyle

To achieve their full potential with a cochlear implant, young children must use the device during all waking hours ("eyes open, ears on"), and the family must provide a listening-rich model for speech, language, and auditory development. Children in families that enforce only sporadic use of the implant achieve fair progress at best. In addition, children in families that do not stress audition and have limited expectations for spoken language typically will lag far behind the development of their peers with normal hearing.

When inquiring about a wear schedule and the communication lifestyle at home, questions should be worded carefully to elicit a forthright response. If the audiologist asks whether the child wears the cochlear implant during all waking hours, the caregiver likely will answer affirmatively, as the question implies that the objective is full-time use. In contrast, an inquiry about the number of times or hours the child wears the implant or "takes a break" from the implant is likely to yield a more accurate estimate from the caregiver. The audiologist should gently and tactfully reinforce the importance of full-time cochlear implant use. Modern sound processors feature data logging that indicates the number of hours the sound processor is used per day as well as the number of hours the child is exposed to speech. This information can be critically important when a young child is making undesirable progress. The audiologist must have a frank discussion with the child's caregivers to strongly recommend implant use during all waking hours as well as to provide a sufficient model of intelligible speech. When a family decides that the child will use spoken language as his/her mode of communication (either by way of an Auditory Oral, Auditory Verbal, or Total Communication approach) anything short of implant use during all waking hours is neglect of the child's development.

Likewise, the audiologist should inquire about the number and types of visual supports used to assist communication. If the family relies heavily on visual input, the audiologist may provide some suggestions for supporting communication through audition-based strategies. The family is entitled to use the method(s) they want to use to communicate with their child. However, the audiologist should inform the family that research suggests that children who have cochlear implants achieve better spoken language abilities when they communicate via listening and spoken language rather than through visual communication, such as sign language (Ching & Dillon, 2013; Chu et al., 2017; Dettman et al., 2016; Geers et al., 2003, 2011, 2017; Nelson et al., 2017). Finally, the audiologist should correspond with the child's LSLS or speech-language pathologist to ensure that the family is equipped with effective strategies to facilitate listening at home.

For the elderly adult who lives alone, it may be difficult to establish consistent social interaction with friends or loved ones. As previously mentioned, a new recipient requires a period of time to adjust to the new signal. If the user is unable to practice listening and have routine conversations, the progress will be slow and the adjustment of the central auditory system to novel signal from the implant will be delayed. For those with limited social interaction, the audiologist should suggest activities or structured therapy to facilitate adjustment to the device.

Evaluate the Appropriateness of the Cochlear Implant Program

When the external equipment is functioning normally and the recipient is using the device properly, the audiologist should reevaluate the appropriateness of the user's program. Electrode impedances should be within normal limits, have unremarkable morphology (e.g., no large variability in impedance between contacts), and be similar to previous measurements. Next, the audiologist should confirm that threshold (T) levels and upper-stimulation levels are set accurately. Of all adjustable program parameters, the threshold and upper-stimulation levels will have the greatest influence on patient performance and sound quality. Again, the electrically evoked stapedial reflex threshold (ESRT) serves as the best indicator of appropriate upper-stimulation levels (see Chapter 18).

If the stimulation levels are set appropriately, the audiologist may consider revising the signal coding strategy or adjustable program parameters, such as stimulation rate, maxima, and input dynamic range (see Chapters 7, 14, 15, 16, and 17). Finally, the audiologist should obtain objective measures of auditory function (e.g., ECAP) and compare them with previous results to identify any unwanted changes. If degradation is observed, the audiologist should schedule a medical evaluation and an integrity assessment of the internal device. As mentioned in Chapter 18, the audiologist should also be concerned when upper-stimulation levels are substantially lower or higher than the recipient's ECAP threshold. When adjustments of the aforementioned parameters are successful, the programming audiologist, recipient, family, and LSLS should notice considerable improvement in performance immediately, but definitely no later than three months.

Assessment of Internal Hardware

When all other factors are ruled out as potential causes of poor progress, the audiologist should scrutinize and assess the function of the internal device. All three manufacturers offer technical support in providing relatively thorough assessments of internal device integrity. Many faults are identified successfully with these assessments, but some recipients will have "normal" findings with a faulty internal device.

The audiologist also may consult with the cochlear implant surgeon to determine whether another postoperative plain film x-ray is necessary to confirm that the internal device has not migrated or moved from its original position. This recommendation is especially warranted for sudden changes in stimulation levels or electrode impedance values. The cochlear implant surgeon will determine whether shifts in internal device placement may be responsible for the negative changes in a recipient's performance.

Finally, recent evidence suggests that more advanced imaging procedures, such as computerized rotational tomography and 64-slice computerized tomography scan imaging, may provide valuable information about electrode array placement and the cochlea's condition after implantation. Specifically, research shows this imaging can be used to determine whether the electrode array has remained in the scala tympani or has dislocated to other chambers within the cochlea (Holden et al., 2013; Lane, Driscoll, Witte, Primak, & Lindell, 2007; Postnov et al., 2006). Research suggests that recipient performance is related inversely to the number of electrodes outside the scala tympani (Finley et al., 2008; Holden et al., 2013). This imaging also may be used to identify the presence of fibrous tissue growth or ossification after implantation.

Identifying "Red Flags"

Amy McConkey Robbins introduced the term "red flag" as an indicator of an implant recipient's slow or limited progress (Robbins, 2005). A red flag occurs when a certain skill lags behind the development of normal-hearing peers or below expectations for a given time period after activation. A red flag signifies the need for more proactive monitoring of pediatric recipient performance, but it is also applicable to adult recipients.

In order to identify a possible red flag, the audiologist must be aware of typical progress with a cochlear implant and normal speech and language development. The most desirable objective of cochlear implantation is to allow for communication via spoken language across a variety of listening environments, and this goal is achieved for most recipients. Most children who receive a cochlear implant at a relatively young age (≤3 years) and have normal cognitive and neurological function develop some speech, language, and auditory skills within one year of implant use. This goal also should apply to children who received considerable benefit from hearing aids and received a cochlear implant at a later age. When a child's progress does not meet this bench-

mark, the cochlear implant team should explore the reason(s) for the limited benefit.

Most adults with postlingual deafness and a limited duration of deafness (i.e., <20 years) develop good-to-excellent open-set speech recognition and spoken language skills. In fact, the vast majority of adults who use recent technology and obtain regular audiology services should be able to converse over the phone and achieve ceiling performance (i.e., 100% correct) on open-set sentence-recognition tests after three months of implant use. Certainly, the adult's performance should be significantly better than that obtained with hearing aids immediately prior to implantation. Once again, if these goals are not met, the cochlear implant team actively should explore the reasons for limited progress and suggest means for improved performance.

Key Concepts

After reading this chapter, the reader should recognize concepts associated with the following topics:
- The audiologist should consult with the surgeon about the pre- and postimplantation imaging results and other medical needs.
- The cochlear implant activation appointment should be scheduled on two separate days to complete the necessary measurements and assessments.
- The one-week and one-month postactivation appointments should be followed by different appointment schedules for adults and for children.
  - Although behavioral stimulation levels typically facilitate excellent performance when they are measured in a reliable and valid manner, the audiologist should also use objective measures as a cross-check to behavioral cochlear implant program levels.
  - In the cases of young children and other recipients who cannot provide reliable feedback about the signals they receive from their cochlear implant, the audiologist may have to rely on a combination of objective and behavioral measures to create a functional cochlear implant program. However, the ECAP threshold should never be used as the primary tool to determine stimulation levels when valid behavioral levels and other objective measures (and in the case of upper-stimulation levels, the ESRT) can be obtained.

- Habilitation/rehabilitation is necessary for adults and children to achieve their full potentials with the cochlear implant.

References

Aschendorff, A., Kromeier, J., Klenzner, T., & Laszig, R. (2007). Quality control after insertion of the Nucleus contour and contour advance electrode in adults. *Ear and Hearing, 28*(2 Suppl), 75S–79S.

Boyd, P. J. (2006). Effects of programming threshold and maplaw settings on acoustic thresholds and speech discrimination with the MED-EL COMBI 40+ cochlear implant. *Ear and Hearing, 27*(6), 608–618.

Buchman, C. A., Roush, P. A., Teagle, H. F., Brown, C. J., Zdanski, C. J., & Grose, J. H. (2006). Auditory neuropathy characteristics in children with cochlear nerve deficiency. *Ear and Hearing, 27*(4), 399–408.

Ching, T. Y., & Dillon, H. (2013). Major findings of the LOCHI study on children at 3 years of age and implications for audiological management. *International Journal of Audiology, 52*(Suppl . 2, S65–68.

Chu, C., Choo, D., Dettman, S., Leigh, J., Traeger, G., Lettieri, G., , , , Dowell, R. (2016, May 22–25). *Early intervention and communication development in children using cochlear implants: The impact of service delivery practices and family factors.* Presented at Audiology Australia National Conference 2016,Melbourne, Australia.

Dettman, S. J., Dowell, R. C., Choo, D., Arnott, W., Abrahams, Y., Davis, A., . . . Briggs, R. J. (2016). Long-term communication outcomes for children receiving cochlear implants younger than 12 months: A multicenter study. *Otology and Neurotology, 37*(2), e82–e95.

Estabrooks, W., MacIver-Lux, K., & Rhoades, E. A. (2016). *Auditory-verbal therapy: For young children with hearing loss and their families, and the practitioners who guide them.* San Diego, CA: Plural.

Ferguson, M. A., & Henshaw, H. (2015). Auditory training can improve working memory, attention, and communication in adverse conditions for adults with hearing loss. *Frontiers in Psychology, 6*, 556.

Finley, C. C., Holden, T. A., Holden, L. K., Whiting, B. R., Chole, R. A., Neely, G. J., . . . Skinner, M. W. (2008). Role of electrode placement as a contributor to variability in cochlear implant outcomes. *Otology and Neurotology, 29*(7), 920–928.

Geers, A. E., Mitchell, C. M., Warner-Czyz, A., Wang, N. Y., Eisenberg, L. S., & Team, C. DaCI Investigative. (2017). Early sign language exposure and cochlear implantation benefits. *Pediatrics, 140*(1).

Geers, A. E., Nicholas, J. G., & Sedey, A. L. (2003). Language skills of children with early cochlear implantation. *Ear and Hearing, 24*(1 Suppl.), 46S–58S.

Geers, A. E., Strube, M. J., Tobey, E. A., Pisoni, D. B., & Moog, J. S. (2011). Epilogue: Factors contributing to long-term outcomes of cochlear implantation in early childhood. *Ear and Hearing, 32*(1, Suppl), 84S–92S.

Holden, L. K., Brenner, C., Reeder, R. M., & Firszt, J. B. (2013). Postlingual adult performance in noise with HiRes 120 and ClearVoice Low, Medium, and High. *Cochlear Implants International, 14*(5), 276–286.

Holden, L. K., Finley, C. C., Firszt, J. B., Holden, T. A., Brenner, C., Potts, L. G., . . . Skinner, M. W. (2013). Factors affecting open-set word recognition in adults with cochlear implants. *Ear and Hearing, 34*(3), 342–360.

Holden, L. K., Reeder, R. M., Firszt, J. B., & Finley, C. C. (2011). Optimizing the perception of soft speech and speech in noise with the Advanced Bionics cochlear implant system. *International Journal of Audiology, 50*(4), 255–269.

Lane, J. I., Driscoll, C. L., Witte, R. J., Primak, A., & Lindell, E. P. (2007). Scalar localization of the electrode array after cochlear implantation: A cadaveric validation study comparing 64-slice multidetector computed tomography with microcomputed tomography. *Otology and Neurotology, 28*(2), 191–194.

Moog, J. S., & Geers, A. E. (2003). Epilogue: Major findings, conclusions and implications for deaf education. *Ear and Hearing, 24*(1 Suppl), 121S–125S.

Nelson, L. H., Herde, L., Munoz, K., White, K. R., & Page, M. D. (2017). Parent perceptions of their child's communication and academic experiences with cochlear implants. *International Journal of Audiology, 56*(3), 164–173.

Peng, K. A., Kuan, E. C., Hagan, S., Wilkinson, E. P., & Miller, M. E. (2017). Cochlear nerve aplasia and hypoplasia: Predictors of cochlear implant success. *Otolaryngology–Head and Neck Surgery, 157*(3), 392–400.

Postnov, A., Zarowski, A., De Clerck, N., Vanpoucke, F., Offeciers, F. E., Van Dyck, D., & Peeters, S. (2006). High resolution micro-CT scanning as an innovative tool for evaluation of the surgical positioning of cochlear implant electrodes. *Acta Otolaryngologica, 126*(5), 467–474.

Rance, G. (2005). Auditory neuropathy/dys-synchrony and its perceptual consequences. *Trends in Amplification, 9*(1), 1–43.

Robbins, A. M. (2005). Clinical red flags for slow progress in children with cochlear implants. *Loud and Clear, 1* 1–8. Retrieved from http://www.bionicear.com

Sharma, A., Dorman, M. F., & Spahr, A. J. (2002). A sensitive period for the development of the central auditory system in children with cochlear implants: Implications for age of implantation. *Ear and Hearing, 23*(6), 532–539.

Vaerenberg, B., Smits, C., De Ceulaer, G., Zir, E., Harman, S., Jaspers, N., . . . Govaerts, P. J. (2014). Cochlear implant programming: A global survey on the state of the art. *Scientific World Journal, 2014*, 501738.

Wanna, G. B., Noble, J. H., Gifford, R. H., Dietrich, M. S., Sweeney, A. D., Zhang, D., . . . Labadie, R. F. (2015). Impact of intrascalar electrode location, electrode type, and angular insertion depth on residual hearing in cochlear implant patients: Preliminary results. *Otology and Neurotology, 36*(8), 1343–1348.

24

Hearing Preservation After Cochlear Implantation, Electric-Acoustic Stimulation, and Hybrid Cochlear Implants

Jace Wolfe

Introduction

Research has shown that hearing aids often provide limited benefit for persons with severe to profound high-frequency hearing loss (Ching, Dillon, & Byrne, 1998; Cox et al., 2011; Cox, Johnson, & Alexander, 2012; Hogan & Turner, 1998; Hornsby & Ricketts, 2006; Moore, 2001; Stelmachowicz, Pittman, Hoover, Lewis, & Moeller, 2007; Zhang et al., 2014). Moreover, several studies have shown that the aided word speech recognition of listeners who have severe to profound high-frequency hearing loss is often fair to poor with the use of high-frequency amplification (Glista et al., 2009; Moore, 2001; Simpson, McDermott, & Dowell, 2005; Simpson, Hersbach, & McDermott, 2006; Summers, 2004; Zhang et al., 2014). Cochlear implantation may provide better access to high-frequency audio signals and, as a result, an improvement in speech recognition. Historically, however, cochlear implantation typically resulted in a loss of the recipient's natural acoustic hearing. The loss of a recipient's low-frequency acoustic hearing may diminish his/her ability to distinguish pitch, to differentiate between two talkers, to understand speech in noise, to recognize melody and enjoy music, to localize sounds, etc. Individuals who have severe to profound hearing loss in the high-frequency regions, better residual hearing in the low-frequency regions, and difficulty communicating with hearing aids may be candidates for combined electric-acoustic stimulation (EAS). EAS provides access to high-frequency sounds via electrical stimulation from a cochlear implant while providing acoustic stimulation for low-frequency sounds. In order for a cochlear implant recipient to benefit from EAS, at least some of his/her low-frequency acoustic hearing must be preserved after the cochlear implant surgery (i.e., hearing preservation). The term "hybrid cochlear implant" is often associated with EAS and hearing preservation. A hybrid cochlear implant describes a cochlear implant system that is designed to preserve low-frequency acoustic hearing in order to provide high-frequency electrical stimulation and low-frequency acoustical stimulation. Over the past two decades, several researchers, surgeons, and audiologists have explored the potential benefits of EAS and hybrid cochlear implantation. This chapter provides a review of hearing preservation after implantation, EAS, and hybrid cochlear implantation. The chapter will provide a brief overview of hybrid cochlear implant fundamentals and hardware, will provide a review of recent research addressing performance of recipients who use EAS and the factors that influence outcomes with EAS, and will discuss recommended procedures for the programming and fitting of EAS devices. For a more in-depth view of the development of EAS, the reader is referred to several reviews addressing the topic (Mowry, Woodson, &

Gantz, 2012; Turner, Reiss, & Gantz, 2008; von Ilberg, Baumann, Kiefer, Tillein, & Adunka, 2011; Woodson, Reiss, Turner, Gfeller, & Gantz, 2011).

Fundamentals of Hearing Preservation, EAS, and Hybrid Cochlear Implantation

The primary premise of a hybrid cochlear implant is to provide electrical stimulation to the cochlear nerve for mid- to high-frequency audio inputs. Additional objectives of hybrid cochlear implantation include the preservation of low-frequency acoustic hearing for recipients who have functional low-frequency hearing (i.e., normal to moderate hearing loss from 125 Hz to at least 500 Hz). For hybrid recipients who have a mild to moderate low-frequency hearing loss after implantation, a hybrid cochlear implant system provides low-frequency acoustic amplification to enhance the user's ability to hear low-frequency inputs.

In general, hybrid cochlear implants differ from conventional cochlear implants in several respects. First, a hybrid cochlear implant typically contains an electrode array that differs in many ways from a conventional electrode array. Hybrid cochlear implant electrode arrays are typically shorter in length and narrower in diameter than conventional electrode arrays (see Figures 24–1 and 24–2). Of note, the exact length of a hybrid cochlear implant electrode array differs across manufacturers, a point that will be further discussed later in this chapter. Addition-ally, a hybrid implant electrode array is more flexible/flaccid (i.e., less stiff) than a conventional electrode array and is designed for lateral wall placement (rather than perimodiolar placement); the flaccidity and the lateral wall location of a hybrid electrode array are intended to minimize cochlear trauma during electrode array insertion and to avoid the delicate cochlear structures of the organ of Corti. It should be noted, however, that some reports describe almost complete preservation of low-frequency hearing for some recipients who have received conventional, long electrode arrays and/or perimodiolar electrode arrays (James et al., 2005; Kiefer et al., 2004; Prentiss, Sykes, & Staecker, 2010). In short, although hearing preservation is probably more likely with shorter, lateral wall electrode arrays, these do not appear to be requisite characteristics for hearing preservation for some recipients. Considering the fact that hearing preservation can be achieved with conventional electrode arrays, it is important to point out the fact that hybrid cochlear implantation is not entirely synonymous with hearing preservation and EAS. Hearing preservation and the use of EAS are objectives of hybrid cochlear implantation, but some recipients of conventional electrode arrays have functional low-frequency hearing after implant surgery and benefit from EAS. The different factors associated with the preservation of low-frequency hearing in cochlear implant recipients will be described in more detail later in this chapter.

The external sound processor of a hybrid implant system is similar to a conventional cochlear implant

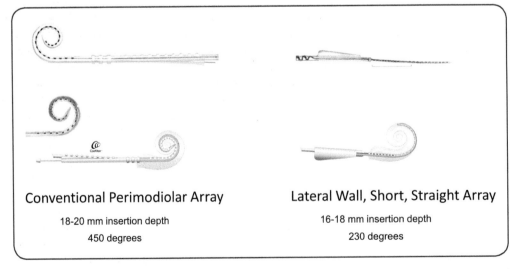

Conventional Perimodiolar Array

18-20 mm insertion depth

450 degrees

Lateral Wall, Short, Straight Array

16-18 mm insertion depth

230 degrees

FIGURE 24–1. Examples of perimodiolar and lateral wall electrode arrays. Image provided courtesy of Cochlear Americas, ©2018.

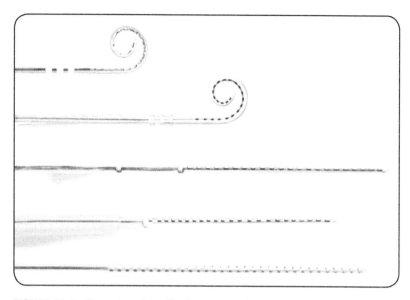

FIGURE 24–2. Examples of the Nucleus electrode array portfolio which features perimodiolar and lateral wall electrode arrays as well as electrode arrays with thin and conventional cross-sectional diameters. Image provided courtesy of Cochlear Americas, ©2018.

sound processor, but it also contains an acoustic component (i.e., an acoustic receiver) that is used to deliver low-frequency amplification. As shown in Figure 24–3, the acoustic component may be coupled to the sound processor with a thin cable or it may be housed within the apex of the sound processor and coupled to an acoustic tube that leads to an earmold. Additionally, some recipients may have normal to near-normal low-frequency hearing sensitivity after implant surgery, and as a result, they are able to hear low-frequency sounds as they naturally pass through their open external auditory meatus while they hear mid- to high-frequency sounds via electric stimulation from the cochlear implant. Prior to the commercial availability of hybrid sound processors, some EAS users wore both a custom in-the-ear hearing aid and a conventional cochlear implant to provide low-frequency acoustic stimulation and high-frequency electric stimulation, respectively.

Surgical Considerations

To aid in hearing preservation, cochlear implant surgeons developed surgical techniques and strategies designed to reduce cochlear trauma during these hybrid electrode array insertions. Initially, surgical methods intended to preserve the low-frequency acoustic hearing of hybrid implant recipients were described as "soft" surgical techniques. Now, however, it is widely recognized that preservation of the delicate cochlear structures is likely to benefit recipients of both hybrid and conventional electrode arrays (Rau et al., 2016), regardless of whether low-frequency hearing preservation is a goal. As a result, the surgical techniques developed to reduce cochlear trauma are commonplace regardless of whether the surgeon is attempting to preserve low-frequency acoustic hearing. The exact surgical techniques used for hybrid cochlear implant surgery have differed as described in published reports (Woodson, Reiss, Turner, Gfeller, & Gantz, 2011). Some surgeons prefer to insert the electrode array via cochleostomy, whereas others prefer to enter the scala tympani through the round window (Nguyen et al., 2013). When a cochleostomy approach is used, the surgeon selects a small (e.g., 1 mm) diamond burr and slow drill speed (e.g., 5,000–10,000 revolutions per minute) to access the cochlea. Bone is carefully excavated to expose the endosteum, which is then gently opened using a metal pick. With a round window approach, the surgeon will often remove the bony overhang near the round window to visualize the round window membrane. Then, a pick is used to enter the round window membrane.

With either a round window or cochleostomy technique, the surgeon uses copious amounts of irrigation and suction prior to making the cochleostomy or entering the round window in order to ensure

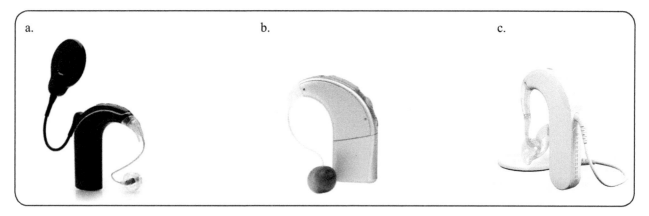

FIGURE 24–3. A. Cochlear Nucleus 7 EAS sound processor. Image provided courtesy of Cochlear Americas, ©2018. **B.** Advanced Bionics Naída CI Q90 EAS sound processor. Image provided courtesy of Advanced Bionics, LLC. **C.** MED-EL SONNET EAS sound processor. Image provided courtesy of MED-EL Corporation.

that blood, bone, and other debris do not enter the cochlea. Suction is typically avoided once the cochlea is opened in an attempt to reduce the possibility of a noise-induced hearing loss and disturbance of cochlear fluids. Finally, most surgeons prescribe anti-inflammatory steroids prior to cochlear implant surgery and/or administer a steroid intraoperatively in an attempt to reduce cochlear inflammation, which may increase the likelihood of cochlear damage and hearing loss.

Theoretical Benefits of EAS

Theoretically, the use of low-frequency acoustic hearing could provide the user with better speech-recognition performance in quiet and especially in noise, improvements in temporal processing (e.g., fine temporal structure), enhanced spectral resolution, improvements in localization of sound, and better music appreciation/perception compared with a traditional, long-electrode cochlear implant. The importance of access to fine temporal structural cues was discussed in Chapter 3. Fine temporal structure has been shown to be the dominant cue that listeners use to recognize melody in music and the pitch of the human voice and environmental sounds (Smith, Delgutte, & Oxenham, 2002). Smith et al. (2002) have also shown that access to acoustic fine structure is critical for localization. Additionally, the provision of fine structural cues improves speech recognition in noise (Moore, 2008). As discussed in Chapter 3, the fine temporal structure of audio signals cannot be faithfully processed by the cochlear nerve in response

to the brief pulsatile electrical signal delivered by a cochlear implant. Preservation of low-frequency acoustic hearing potentially allows the EAS user to access important low-frequency fine structural cues via the amplified acoustic signal of the EAS sound processor. Indeed, research has shown that recipients achieve better speech recognition in quiet and in noise, better melody recognition and music appreciation, better localization, and better pitch recognition in the EAS listening condition compared with the electric-only condition (Dorman & Gifford, 2010, 2017; Dorman et al,. 2013; Dunn et al., 2010; Gifford, Dorman, & Brown, 2012; Gifford et al., 2014; Sheffield, Jahn, & Gifford, 2015).

It should be noted that some patients who receive hybrid implants lose their low-frequency acoustic hearing (Fitzgerald et al., 2008; Gantz et al., 2009; Gstoettner et al., 2009; Reiss, Perreau, & Turner, 2012; Skarzyński, Lorens, Piotrowska, & Anderson, 2007). However, these recipients typically achieve better speech recognition with the use of their hybrid cochlear implant, particularly when used in concert with a contralateral hearing aid, compared with preimplant performance with binaural hearing aids (Roland et al., 2016).

Electrode Array Location and Place of Stimulation

Prior to a discussion of hybrid cochlear implant hardware, it is important to review the relationship between electrode array location, the site of stimulation in the cochlea, and the frequency of maximum stimulation. The relationship between cochlear place of stimulation and frequency is well established (Greenwood, 1961, 1990; Kawano et al., 1996; Stakhovskaya, Sridhar, Bonham, & Leake, 2007). The Greenwood function assigns a characteristic response frequency to a particular location in the organ of Corti of the cochlea (Greenwood, 1961, 1990). It essentially serves as a map of tonotopic organization along the basilar membrane and has often been used to estimate the frequency range that should be allocated to an electrode located at a specific site (Kiefer et al., 2005; Skarzyński et al., 2007).

However, for multiple reasons, the Greenwood function does not entirely explain the relationship between electrode location and frequency of neural stimulation (the reader is referred to Chapter 3 for a summary of the Greenwood function and the work of Stakhovska and colleagues [2007] along with an explanation of the relationship between the location of cochlear implant stimulation and the frequency of neural stimulation). For instance, this relationship is substantially influenced by whether the electrode array is designed for lateral wall or perimodiolar placement. Theoretically, perimodiolar electrodes are more inclined to deliver stimulation directly to the spiral ganglion bodies of the auditory nerve, so the Greenwood function may not serve as a precise estimate of the frequency that is stimulated by the implant. Lateral wall electrodes are theoretically more inclined to deliver stimulation to a location that is more proximal to the radial nerve fibers innervating the organ of Corti (i.e., the cochlear nerve dendrites adjacent to the basilar membrane), and as a result, the Greenwood function may provide a closer approximation of the frequency place of stimulation.

The pioneering work of Stakhovskaya and colleagues showed that the length of the organ of Corti is much longer (30.5 to 36.87 mm) than the length of the spiral ganglion measured at the center of Rosenthal's canal (12.54 to 14.62 mm) (Stakhovskaya et al., 2007). As a result, a perimodiolar electrode array does not need to be inserted nearly as deep as a lateral wall electrode in order to elicit a particular frequency of neural stimulation. For example, Stakhovskaya and colleagues estimated that a lateral wall electrode array would have to be inserted about 20 mm into the scala tympani to elicit an auditory neural response at 1000 Hz, but in contrast, a perimodiolar electrode array would only have to be inserted about 14 mm into the scala tympani to evoke the same frequency of stimulation. Although the two different types of elec-

trode arrays differ in length, they have both reached approximately the same depth of about 360 degrees (a reference point of 0 degrees at the round window). In other words, given a starting place of the round window (which corresponds to 0 degrees), each electrode array has been inserted to a depth that results in the completion of one full circle (i.e., the tip of the electrode resides at a location that is adjacent to the round window; Figure 24–4).

Given the discussion above, cochlear implant insertion depth may be described in two ways, by the linear distance of the electrode array insertion or by the angular insertion depth (Verbist et al., 2010). The linear insertion depth refers to the distance (in millimeters) that the electrode array is inserted into the cochlea, whereas angular insertion depth (measured in degrees) refers to the degrees of rotation relative to the starting point of the insertion (e.g., the round window) (see Figure 24–4). It is important

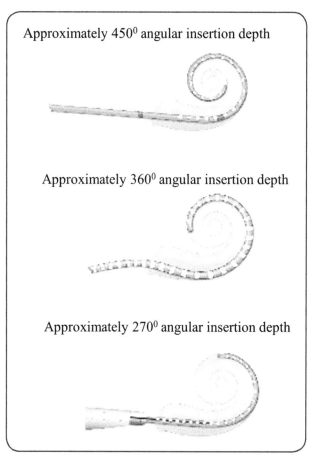

FIGURE 24–4. A visual example lateral wall electrode arrays inserted to various angular insertion depths. Image provided courtesy of Cochlear Americas, ©2018.

to note that Stakhovskava and colleagues (2007) reported that significant intersubject variability exists in the length of the organ of Corti and spiral ganglion. Additionally, researchers have noted that the final resting location of the tip of an electrode array will depend on whether the electrode array is located near the medial (i.e., perimodiolar array) or outside wall (i.e., lateral wall array) of the scala tympani (O'Connell et al., 2016; Verbist et al., 2010). Again, as discussed above, a perimodiolar electrode array must be inserted approximately 14 mm into the cochlea to achieve an angular insertion depth of 360 degrees, whereas a lateral wall electrode array must be inserted approximately 20 mm to achieve an angular insertion depth of 360 degrees. A good analogy of the relationship of angular insertion depth and electrode array type (e.g., lateral wall vs. perimodiolar) may be found in the staggered starts that occur in the 400 meter race that is run in track and field events. Runners in the inside lane of the track have a shorter distance to run one full lap of the 400-meter track than runners in the outside lane (i.e., completion of one full lap in the inside lane covers 400 meters, whereas completion of one full lap in the outside lane covers 453.66 meters). As a result, the runners in the outside lanes start the race at a farther distance up the track (by 53.66 meters) to account for the fact that running in the outside lane requires a longer distance to complete one full lap of the track. With this fact in mind, the use of angular insertion depth is generally recommended as the metric of choice for describing the depth of cochlear implant electrode array insertion. The interested reader is referred to the publication by Stakhovskava and colleagues (2007) for the estimated frequency of stimulation for various angular insertion depths.

It is also important to note that the exact frequency that is stimulated in the auditory system is likely dependent upon the extent of degeneration of cochlear nerve fibers, particularly in the case of lateral wall electrodes. Research has suggested that radial dendrites often degenerate secondary to severe to profound deafness (McMullen & Glaser, 1988; McMullen, Goldberger, Suter, & Glaser, 1988), and as a result, electrical current may have to spread to the spiral ganglion fibers to elicit an auditory response. In such an event, the Stakhovskava et al. (2007) data correlating frequency to spiral ganglion length may be a better predictor of the frequency of stimulation than the Greenwood function. Additionally, innervation of the cochlea becomes more complex and variable at the apical end, so it is more difficult to predict the frequency of the response. Also, cross-turn stimulation (i.e., the spread of electrical current from one turn of the cochlea to a neighboring turn) may elicit complex frequency responses/pitch percepts (Briaire & Frijns, 2006). Furthermore, the stimulation of neighboring neural elements may be influenced in complex fashions by the growth of fibrous tissue and/or bone in the cochlea following surgery (Richter et al., 2001). In short, predicting the characteristic frequency of stimulation at a specific electrode contact location in the cochlea is quite complicated, is dependent on a number of factors related to the design/configuration of the electrode array and the anatomy of the peripheral auditory system, and is likely to be variable across recipients.

Current Devices

Two implant manufacturers, Cochlear and MED-EL, have commercially available hybrid devices. The Cochlear™ Nucleus® Hybrid™ Implant System was approved for commercial use by the U.S. Food and Drug Administration (FDA) in 2015. The MED-EL FLEX²⁴ cochlear implant electrode array, which was originally known as the FLEX^EAS electrode array, was approved for commercial use in the United States in 2012. Although the MED-EL FLEX²⁴ is designed to facilitate low-frequency hearing preservation, the FDA had not yet approved the commercial use of an electric-acoustic sound processor when the FLEX²⁴ electrode array was introduced into the U.S. market. However, a multicenter clinical trial examining the outcomes of recipients of the MED-EL EAS implant indicated that 90% of participants were satisfied overall with the device. In 2016, the FDA approved the MED-EL SYNCHRONY EAS Hearing Implant System for commercial use in the United States. In the following paragraphs, a review will be provided of all of the hybrid cochlear implant technology developed by Cochlear and MED-EL for use in clinical trials or for commercial use either in the United States or in Europe. A brief description of the Advanced Bionics EAS sound processor will also be provided.

Cochlear Hybrid Implant Technology

In the late 1990s, Cochlear Ltd. began a collaboration with Bruce Gantz and colleagues at the University of Iowa to develop a hybrid (EAS) cochlear implant system. The initial device developed from this partnership was known as the Nucleus Hybrid S8 implant and possessed six intracochlear stimulating contacts and two extracochlear reference electrodes. The S8 electrode array is very thin with a cross-sectional diameter of 0.4 × 0.25 mm. The six intracochlear electrode contacts were housed on a 10-mm long straight electrode array that was coupled to the Nucleus CI24M receiver/stimulator. A later version was coupled to the Freedom-based receiver/stimulator. Recipients used the cochlear implant along with a custom in-the-ear hearing aid along with the most contemporary Nucleus sound processor to achieve EAS.

In a U.S. clinical trial, a total of 87 subjects were implanted with the 10 mm Hybrid S8 cochlear implant. Reports suggested that use of the Hybrid S8 implant was associated with an impressive rate of preservation of residual hearing (about 90% experienced some preservation of their residual hearing), and the majority of subjects achieved significant improvement in monosyllabic word recognition and sentence recognition in quiet and in noise (Gantz & Turner, 2004; Gantz, Turner, & Gfeller, 2004; Gantz, Turner, Gfeller, & Lowder, 2005). However, some of these recipients did lose their residual hearing, and although most performed better in the bimodal condition (i.e., electrical stimulation with short array in the implanted ear and acoustic stimulation from hearing aid in the opposite ear) than they did preoperatively with binaural hearing aids, 17 subjects were re-implanted with longer electrode arrays (presumably because their performance in the implanted ear was poorer than desired with use of such a short electrode array).

Cochlear also developed and conducted clinical trials with the Nucleus Hybrid S12 implant, which contained 10 intracochlear electrode contacts positioned along a 10-mm straight electrode array with the same cross-sectional dimensions as the Hybrid S8. In the United States, 24 subjects were implanted with the Hybrid S12 device, and like the S8 study, these subjects typically experienced improvements in speech recognition with the S12 device relative to their preimplant performance (Gantz & Turner, 2011; Gantz, Turner, & Gfeller, 2006; Gantz et al., 2009). However, approximately 30% of the subjects experienced at least a 30 dB shift in their low-frequency residual hearing, and as with the S8 device, the shallower insertion depth of the S12 array may have limited overall performance for these subjects. Once again, the merits and limitations of 10-mm electrode arrays are still being evaluated and reported in peer-reviewed literature (Gantz et al., 2017). Investigators will continue to weigh the benefits of a potentially higher likelihood of hearing preservation associated with a shorter array against the potential limitations of reduced performance that may arise if acoustic hearing is lost and the recipient is forced to rely on coding the entire speech frequency range with a 10-mm electrode array.

In an effort to balance the goals of providing adequate mid-to-high-frequency electrical coverage along with a relatively high likelihood of preservation of low-frequency residual hearing, Cochlear developed the Nucleus Hybrid L24 cochlear implant (Figure 24–5), which was approved for commercial use by the U.S. FDA in 2014. The commercial name of the Nucleus Hybrid L24 device is the Nucleus Hybrid Implant System. However, in this chapter, the FDA-approved device will be referred to as the Nucleus

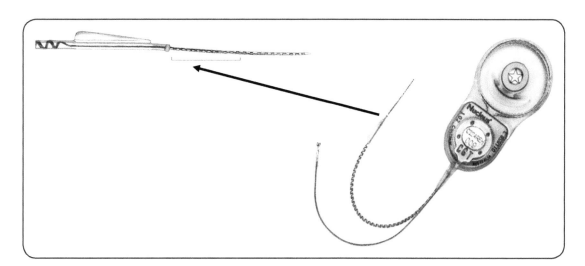

FIGURE 24–5. The Cochlear Nucleus L24 Hybrid cochlear implant. Image provided courtesy of Cochlear Americas, ©2018.

Hybrid L24 device in order to prevent confusion with the earlier model Nucleus hybrid cochlear implants. The Nucleus Hybrid L24 implant contains the Nucleus Freedom receiver/stimulator, which is coupled to a thin electrode array designed to be inserted approximately 16 mm into the cochlea. The L24 electrode array has a cross-sectional diameter of 0.25 by 0.35 mm at the apical end of the array and 0.4 by 0.55 mm at the basal end of the array. The thin diameter of this array makes it ideal for round window or cochleostomy insertion. Furthermore, the L24 electrode array possesses 22 half-banded electrode contacts, which are distributed over 15 mm and are designed to point toward the modiolus. Use of half-banded electrode contacts, rather than full ring electrodes, allows for a thinner array carrier and results in a smooth surface, which may reduce resistance during insertion and promote hearing preservation.

The L24 array is intended to be inserted along the lateral wall of the scala tympani, and like the S8 and S12 devices, it possesses a "stopper" that prevents insertion beyond a desired depth, which in the case of the L24 is 16 mm (i.e., the medial end of the stopper is 16 mm from the tip of the array), which corresponds to an angular insertion depth of about 235 or 270 degrees for a typical round window or cochleostomy insertion, respectively. It also features a fan-shaped handle at the base of the array that is intended to facilitate ease of insertion. Finally, the electrode lead wires are 20 micrometers in diameter, and as a result, the array is quite flexible at the apical end and relatively stiff at the basal end. This charac-

teristic is intended to reduce trauma during insertion, while also enhancing the surgeon's ease of handling.

Although it is not formally considered as a hybrid cochlear implant, the Nucleus CI522 implant (e.g., Slim research array—see Figure 24–6) was designed to be an atraumatic array and has also been considered as an EAS device (Skarzyński et al., 2012, 2014). The CI522 device has a straight array designed for lateral wall insertion. It possesses a cross-sectional diameter of 0.3 × 0.35 mm and 0.5 × 0.6 mm at the apical and basal ends, respectively, which makes it relatively narrow in comparison to the Contour Advance perimodiolar array. Additionally, the CI522 possesses two "markers" to guide the surgeon in achieving an insertion depth of approximately 20 or 25 mm. A 20-mm insertion depth for a lateral wall electrode generally results in about a 330 to 360 angular degree insertion depth, whereas a 25-mm insertion depth results in a 430 to 480 angular degree insertion depth, depending on insertion technique and the recipient's cochlear anatomy.

The L24 Hybrid implant system initially included the Nucleus Freedom hybrid sound processor (Figure 24–7). In 2013, the Nucleus 6 sound processor was introduced as the EAS sound processor for use with the Nucleus L24 Hybrid implant. In 2017, Cochlear received FDA approval to commercially distribute the Nucleus 7 sound processor (Figure 24–8), which at the time of this writing is the most modern Nucleus EAS sound processor. The Nucleus 7 sound processor is described in detail in Chapter 10. Like the Freedom and Nucleus 6 EAS sound processors,

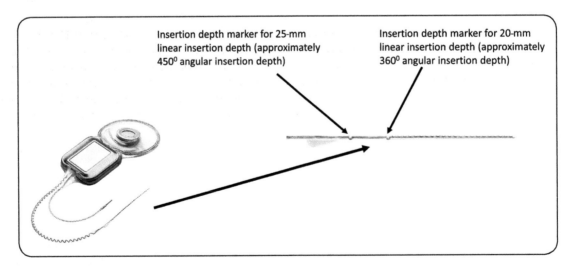

FIGURE 24–6. The Cochlear Nucleus CI522 cochlear implant with the Slim Straight electrode array. Image provided courtesy of Cochlear Americas, ©2018.

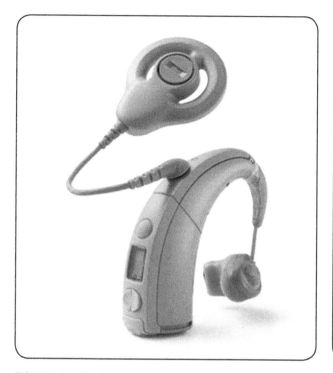

FIGURE 24–7. The Cochlear Nucleus Freedom EAS sound processor. Image provided courtesy of Cochlear Americas, ©2018.

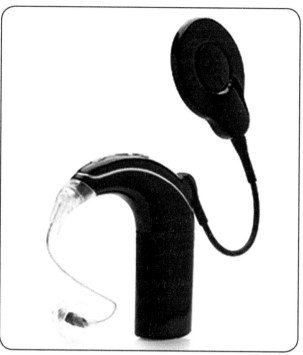

FIGURE 24–8. The Cochlear Nucleus 7 EAS sound processor. Image provided courtesy of Cochlear Americas, ©2018.

the Nucleus 7 sound processor possesses an acoustic driver, which may be coupled to a thin wire that connects to an acoustic receiver. Three acoustic receiver options are available: 60, 85, and 100. The three different receivers (60, 85, and 100) are supposed to provide sufficient output for a 60, 85, and 100 dB HL hearing loss, respectively. The acoustic receiver may be coupled to a generic dome (a variety of which are available) or to a custom shell, which may be ordered from an earmold laboratory. The electroacoustic specifications of the Nucleus 7 receivers are shown in Figure 24–9. The acoustic receivers of the Nucleus 7 sound processor are smaller than the acoustic receivers available for the Nucleus Freedom and Nucleus 6 sound processors. Also, the "100" receiver of the Nucleus 7 receiver provides a higher gain and output level than the Nucleus Freedom and Nucleus 6 acoustic receivers.

Custom Sound Software Options for Programming Nucleus EAS Devices

The audiologist may adjust several programmable parameters for the acoustic component of Nucleus EAS sound processors (Figure 24–10). The audiologist must first enter the recipient's air conduction pure-tone thresholds. Ideally, the pure tone threshold at 125 Hz should be measured and entered. The Custom Sound programming software provides acoustic amplification from 125 Hz up to the first frequency (i.e., the lowest frequency), which has an air conduction pure-tone threshold that is poorer than 70 dB HL.

Three different prescriptive gain methods are available to assign gain and output based on the recipient's hearing loss: (1) Cochlear Hybrid Prescription (CHP), (2) Desired Sensation Level (DSL), and (3) National Acoustic Laboratories–Revised Profound (NAL). Additionally, the audiologist must determine whether the gain of acoustic amplification will be delivered in a nonlinear (i.e., wide dynamic range compression [WDRC]) or linear manner. Furthermore, the audiologist must indicate which acoustic receiver is being used (60, 85, or 100) as well as the type of mold to which the acoustic receiver is being coupled (closed dome, open dome, or custom earmold). If a custom earmold is selected, the audiologist is prompted to indicate the size of the vent included in the earmold. The choices of fitting method (CHP, DSL, NAL-RP), receiver type, and earmold option all influence the gain/output assigned by the Custom Sound software.

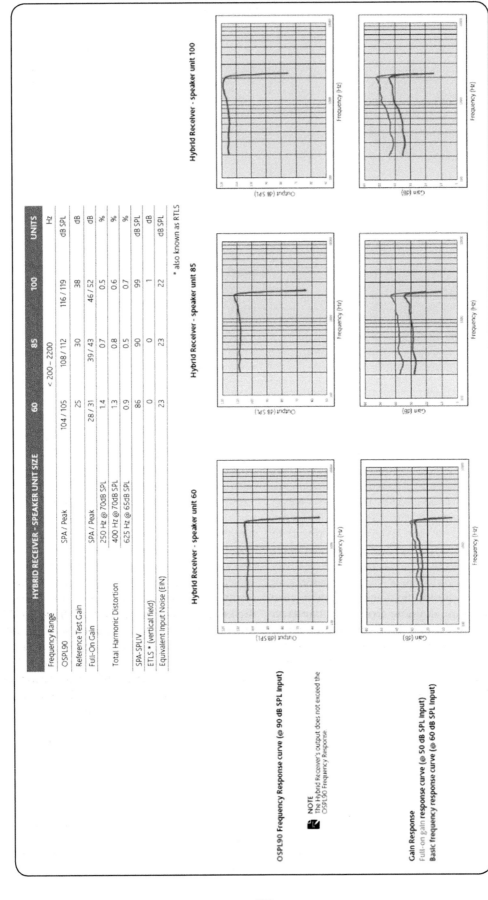

HYBRID RECEIVER - SPEAKER UNIT SIZE		60	85	100	UNITS
Frequency Range		< 200 - 2200			Hz
OSPL90	SPA / Peak	104 / 105	108 / 112	116 / 119	dB SPL
Reference Test Gain		25	30	38	dB
Full-On Gain	SPA / Peak	28 / 31	39 / 43	46 / 52	dB
Total Harmonic Distortion	250 Hz @ 70dB SPL	1.4	0.7	0.5	%
	400 Hz @ 70dB SPL	1.3	0.8	0.6	%
	625 Hz @ 65dB SPL	0.9	0.5	0.7	%
SPA-SPLIV		86	90	99	dB SPL
ETLS * (vertical field)		0	0	1	dB
Equivalent Input Noise (EIN)		23	23	22	dB SPL

* also known as RTLS

Hybrid Receiver - speaker unit 60

Hybrid Receiver - speaker unit 85

Hybrid Receiver - speaker unit 100

OSPL90 Frequency Response curve (@ 90 dB SPL Input)

NOTE
The Hybrid Receiver's output does not exceed the OSPL90 Frequency Response

Gain Response
Full-on gain response curve (@ 50 dB SPL Input)
Basic frequency response curve (@ 60 dB SPL Input)

FIGURE 24–9. Electroacoustic specifications of the Nucleus 7 EAS 60, 85, and 100 acoustic receivers. Image provided courtesy of Cochlear Americas, ©2018.

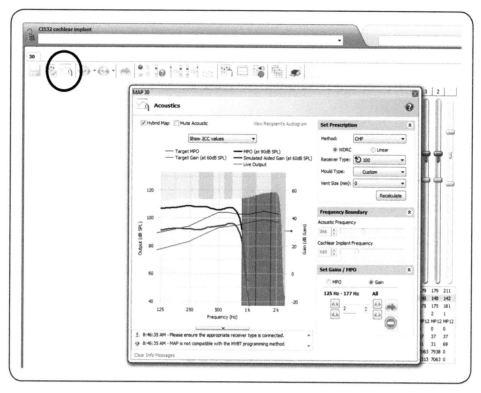

FIGURE 24–10. Accessing the electric-acoustic programming parameters in Custom Sound. Image provided courtesy of Cochlear Americas, ©2018.

Within the "Acoustics" menu used to program Nucleus EAS processors, the audiologist may also adjust the range over which acoustic and electrical stimulations are provided. Optimizing the provision of acoustic and electrical stimulation for EAS users is a topic that is covered later in this chapter. In the "Set Gains/MPO" section of the "Acoustics" menu, the audiologist may adjust multiple frequency bands to allow for precise shaping of the low- to mid-frequency response (up to nine adjustable bands). Specifically, the audiologist may adjust overall maximum power output (MPO) and gain and may also adjust these two parameters within each of the nine frequency bands.

MED-EL EAS Technology

European surgeons working with MED-EL implants pioneered the concept of EAS (Kiefer et al., 2004; Skarżyński et al., 2002). Some of the earliest attempts to provide EAS were with the MED-EL COMBI 40+ implant with the STANDARD electrode array (31.5 mm in length) (Kiefer et al., 2004; Skarżyński et al., 2002). For instance, Skarżyński et al. (2002) found preser-

vation of at least some low-frequency residual hearing in 21 of 26 recipients who were implanted with a deeply inserted MED-EL COMBI 40+ STANDARD array using surgical techniques that intended to reduce trauma to the cochlea. Kiefer and colleagues (2004) also reported impressive hearing preservation results with the MED-EL COMBI 40+ Standard array. Kiefer et al. (2004) inserted the MED-EL COMBI 40+ STANDARD array and a modified version of the STANDARD array at a shallower depth (19–24 mm) in 14 adults with air conduction thresholds in the 20 to 60 dB HL range from 125 to 500 Hz. Some low-frequency hearing was preserved in 12 of 14 recipients, and the mean decrease in air conduction thresholds were 10, 15, 17.5, and 5 dB at 125, 250, 500, and 1000 Hz, respectively. The results of the Kiefer et al. (2004) study elicited interest in the concept of providing a shallower insertion (18–24 mm) to better facilitate hearing preservation, and as a result, surgeons began to turn their focus toward the use of shorter insertion depths for cases in which hearing preservation was a desirable goal.

At that time, MED-EL also offered the MEDIUM electrode array, which was developed for cases in which a sufficient insertion of the STANDARD array could not be achieved (i.e., the recipient had a shorter cochlea than normal; the recipient was receiving a MED-EL implant as a replacement for a faulty competitor's implant which had an electrode array that was shorter than the MED-EL STANDARD array; or the recipient had fibrous tissue growth preventing a full insertion with the STANDARD array). The distance between the most basal electrode and the tip of the MEDIUM array is approximately 22 mm, which is considerably shorter than for the STANDARD array (approximately 28 mm). The STANDARD and MEDIUM electrode arrays each include 12 electrode contacts, but the distance between electrode contacts is shorter for the MEDIUM array (1.9 mm) than for the STANDARD array (2.4 mm). European surgeons who were exploring the feasibility of EAS logically began to use the MEDIUM array to achieve a shallower insertion for recipients who had a substantial amount of functional low-frequency hearing (Gstoettner et al., 2008). Insertion of a lateral wall electrode to a depth of 20 mm results in a 360-degree angular insertion depth in the typical cochlea which would reach to the 1000 Hz place in the cochlea. One research study has suggested that a significant reduction in cochlear trauma is possible with angular insertion depths of 360 degrees and less (Adunka & Kiefer, 2006).

Gstoettner et al. (2008) reported on results from a multicenter study in which the MEDIUM array was implanted in 18 adults with considerable low-frequency hearing and profound high-frequency hearing loss. The MEDIUM array was inserted 18 to 22 mm into the cochlea, and steroids were administered to decrease cochlear inflammation and to increase the likelihood of hearing preservation. Gstoettner and colleagues (2008) attempted to provide acoustic amplification at all frequencies with an air conduction threshold of 80 dB HL or better. Three subjects lost all of their residual hearing following the surgery. Another three subjects had some hearing preservation, but their postoperative hearing loss was too severe to consider the provision of low-frequency amplification. Twelve of the 18 subjects (66.6%) did have sufficient postoperative low-frequency hearing to warrant consideration of amplification, but six of these subjects felt that use of the acoustic amplification was detrimental or provided no benefit. The authors noted that the subjects had to use a separate hearing aid with their cochlear implant sound processor, and many may have rejected EAS because use

of two devices was cumbersome and inconvenient. Indeed, much like the first subjects in the Gantz Nucleus Hybrid short array studies, the earliest MED-EL EAS recipients typically used the TEMPO+ sound processor with an in-the-ear hearing aid to achieve EAS. In response to this limitation, MED-EL developed the DUET EAS/Hybrid processor. Gstoettner et al. (2008) reported significant improvement in performance for the six EAS users relative to their preoperative performance, but performance with EAS was not compared with that of electric-only stimulation.

Early experiences with the STANDARD and MEDIUM arrays proved that hearing preservation was possible with MED-EL electrode arrays. However, surgeons and MED-EL scientists, engineers, and researchers realized that the potential of hearing preservation could be further improved with the development of an electrode array that is specifically designed to promote atraumaticity and hearing preservation. In response to these early reports of the benefits of EAS, MED-EL developed the FLEX electrode array technology, which possesses several features that are specifically intended to facilitate reduction of cochlear trauma and enhance the potential of hearing preservation (Figures 24–11 through 24–15). The unique features of FLEX arrays are as follows:

1. In contrast to conventional MED-EL electrode arrays that pair two electrode contacts to create a stimulation site, the five most apical stimulation sites of the FLEX array consist of single electrode contacts, a design characteristic which reduces the diameter and increases the flexibility/flaccidity of the apical end of the array. The reduction in the diameter of the apical end of the array (i.e., tapering) is important, because the scala tympani becomes narrower as it courses from the basal end to the apex. A smaller apical diameter reduces the chance that the electrode will come in contact with the delicate structures of the organ of Corti. Also, the enhanced flexibility of the apical end reduces the likelihood of cochlear trauma during the insertion process. It should be noted that the seven most basal stimulation sites each comprise two oval-shaped electrode contacts, which is similar to what is found for all 12 stimulation sites of the Standard array.

2. The diameter of the FLEX electrode arrays is narrower at the apical tip of the array and increases at the basal end where the electrode array resides in the round window or cochleostomy. The nar-

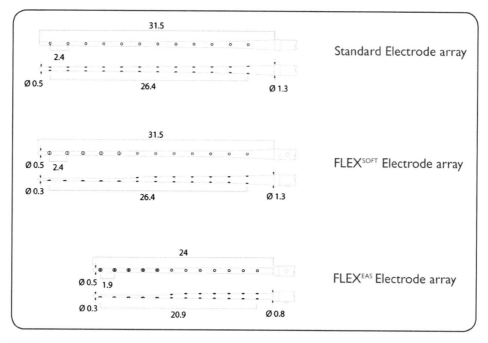

FIGURE 24–11. MED-EL electrode arrays. Image provided courtesy of MED-EL Corporation.

row diameter at the tip of the FLEX electrode array compare favorably to other electrode arrays available for commercial use at the time of this writing. The tapered design of the FLEX array, which is shown in Figure 24–13, allows for increased mechanical flexibility at the tip of the array, insertion into the narrow lumen of the most apical region of the scala tympani, and ease of handing at the basal end on the part of the surgeon.

3. The wires (e.g., electrode leads) in the FLEX series of MED-EL electrode arrays are configured in a wave-shaped pattern, which further enhances the electrode array's flexibility, which promotes atraumaticity.

At the time of this writing, the FLEX[24] and FLEX[28] electrode arrays were both available for commercial distribution in the United States. The FLEX[24] is a 24-mm-long electrode array (from the round window/cochleostomy marker to the tip of the array) with 12 intracochlear stimulating sites. The distance between the most basal electrode contacts and the tip of the FLEX[24] array is 20.9 mm. The cross-sectional diameter of the array ranges from 0.3 to 0.49 mm at the apex to 0.8 at the basal end near the cochleostomy. The FLEX[24] array is designed to be inserted along the lateral wall of the cochlea. Reports have

suggested a higher likelihood of hearing preservation with the FLEX[24] when it is inserted in the round window rather than a cochleostomy (Adunka et al., 2004; Gstoettner et al., 2004).

MED-EL also offers the FLEX technology in the FLEX[28] electrode array and the FLEX[SOFT] array. The FLEX[28] is available for use in the United States, whereas the FLEX[28] and FLEX[SOFT] are both available in most other parts of the world. The FLEX[28] and FLEX[SOFT] electrodes are longer, but they do contain the FLEX technology to promote cochlear atraumaticity and hearing preservation. The reader is referred to Chapter ## for a detailed description of the FLEX[28] and FLEX[SOFT] arrays. It should also be noted that MED-EL offers the FLEX[20] electrode array, which features the FLEX technology but is 20 mm in length with the 12 stimulation sites spaced across 15.4 mm. At the time of this writing, the MED-EL FLEX[20] electrode array was not approved by the FDA for use in the United States.

At this time, there is no clear consensus as to what the ideal insertion depth is to promote hearing preservation and optimize speech recognition for MED-EL EAS users. Prentiss et al. (2010) evaluated hearing preservation in 18 recipients implanted with the MED-EL PULSAR CI[100] with STANDARD or MEDIUM arrays inserted to varying depths ranging from 20 to 28 mm.

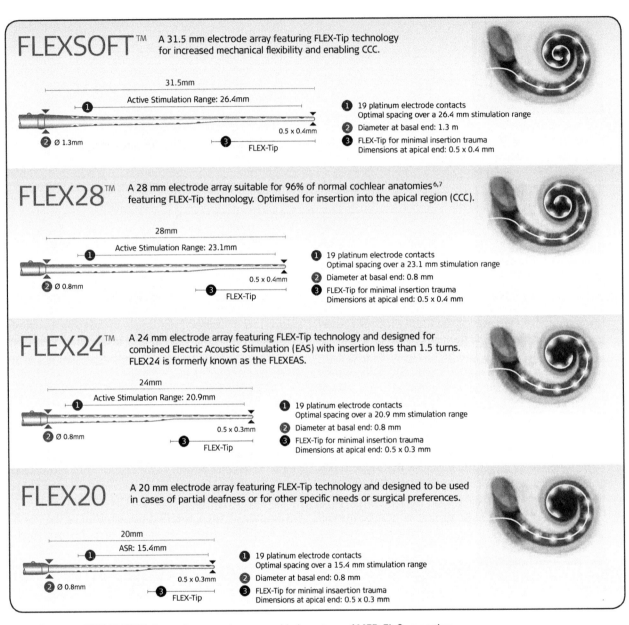

FLEXSOFT™ A 31.5 mm electrode array featuring FLEX-Tip technology for increased mechanical flexibility and enabling CCC.

31.5mm
Active Stimulation Range: 26.4mm
①
② Ø 1.3mm
0.5 x 0.4mm
③ FLEX-Tip

① 19 platinum electrode contacts
Optimal spacing over a 26.4 mm stimulation range
② Diameter at basal end: 1.3 m
③ FLEX-Tip for minimal insertion trauma
Dimensions at apical end: 0.5 x 0.4 mm

FLEX28™ A 28 mm electrode array suitable for 96% of normal cochlear anatomies[6,7] featuring FLEX-Tip technology. Optimised for insertion into the apical region (CCC).

28mm
Active Stimulation Range: 23.1mm
①
② Ø 0.8mm
0.5 x 0.4mm
③ FLEX-Tip

① 19 platinum electrode contacts
Optimal spacing over a 23.1 mm stimulation range
② Diameter at basal end: 0.8 mm
③ FLEX-Tip for minimal insertion trauma
Dimensions at apical end: 0.5 x 0.4 mm

FLEX24™ A 24 mm electrode array featuring FLEX-Tip technology and designed for combined Electric Acoustic Stimulation (EAS) with insertion less than 1.5 turns. FLEX24 is formerly known as the FLEXEAS.

24mm
Active Stimulation Range: 20.9mm
①
② Ø 0.8mm
0.5 x 0.3mm
③ FLEX-Tip

① 19 platinum electrode contacts
Optimal spacing over a 20.9 mm stimulation range
② Diameter at basal end: 0.8 mm
③ FLEX-Tip for minimal insertion trauma
Dimensions at apical end: 0.5 x 0.3 mm

FLEX20 A 20 mm electrode array featuring FLEX-Tip technology and designed to be used in cases of partial deafness or for other specific needs or surgical preferences.

20mm
ASR: 15.4mm
①
② Ø 0.8mm
0.5 x 0.3mm
③ FLEX-Tip

① 19 platinum electrode contacts
Optimal spacing over a 15.4 mm stimulation range
② Diameter at basal end: 0.8 mm
③ FLEX-Tip for minimal insaertion trauma
Dimensions at apical end: 0.5 x 0.3 mm

FIGURE 24–12. MED-EL FLEX electrode arrays. Image provided courtesy of MED-EL Corporation.

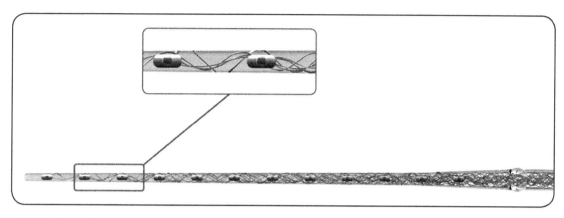

FIGURE 24–13. The wave-shaped electrode leads (i.e., wires) of the MED-EL FLEX electrode array. Image provided courtesy of MED-EL Corporation.

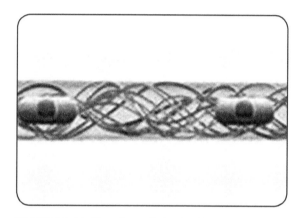

FIGURE 24–14. The electrode leads of the MED-EL FLEX electrode array are arranged in a zig-zag pattern to promote greater flexibility which reduces insertion forces and trauma. Image provided courtesy of MED-EL Corporation.

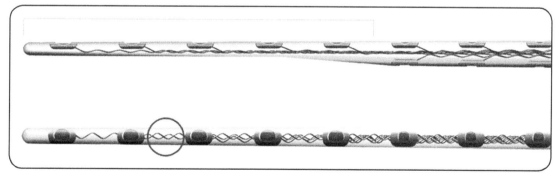

FIGURE 24–15. The MED-EL FLEX electrode array contains a tapered apical end to reduce cochlear trauma. Image provided courtesy of MED-EL Corporation.

The examiners employed surgical techniques that were designed to facilitate hearing preservation. All subjects were implanted with a round window insertion. Some residual hearing was preserved in all 18 subjects, and no clear relationship was observed between the insertion depth and the degree of hearing preservation. As a result, the authors suggested that soft surgical techniques may be a primary factor responsible for hearing preservation, and reasonable hearing preservation may be achieved with deep insertions if soft surgical techniques are employed.

Baumgartner et al. (2007) reported on hearing preservation outcomes for 23 adults who had severe to profound hearing loss and were implanted with the FLEX[SOFT] array. The array was inserted 31.5 mm into the cochlea for 19 of 23 subjects. Shorter insertions occurred for other subjects, because the full insertion could not be achieved. At 1-month postactivation, hearing preservation was found in half of the subjects who had measurable preoperative hearing. At 1-year postactivation, hearing preservation was achieved in one-fourth of the subjects who had measurable preoperative hearing. Taken collectively, the results of the Prentiss et al. (2010) and Baumgartner et al. (2007) studies indicate that hearing preservation is possible with deeply inserted electrodes, particularly when soft surgical techniques are employed and the electrode array is designed to facilitate hearing preservation. Additional research is needed to further clarify the relationship between insertion depth and hearing preservation.

The MED-EL FLEX electrode arrays (including the FLEX[24] and FLEX[20]) are used with the MED-EL SYNCHRONY cochlear implant.

The DUET and DUET 2 sound processors were the first sound processors MED-EL developed for EAS (the DUET 2 sound processor is pictured in Figure 24–16). Each possessed an acoustic receiver, which was acoustically coupled to an earhook that may be attached to a custom-made earmold. In 2016, the FDA approved commercial distribution of the MED-EL SYNCHRONY Hearing Implant System, which included the SYNCHRONY implant coupled to the electrode array selected for hearing preservation and the SONNET EAS sound processor (Figure 24–17). The SONNET sound processor contains an acoustic receiver located at the apex of the sound processor essentially in the same location that the receiver is located in a behind-the-ear hearing aid. In EAS mode, an acoustic earhook may be connected to the SONNET sound processor to deliver the amplified signal to an acoustic earmold.

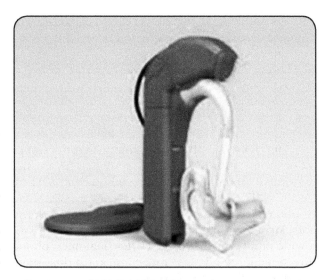

FIGURE 24–16. MED-EL DUET 2 EAS sound processor. Image provided courtesy of MED-EL Corporation.

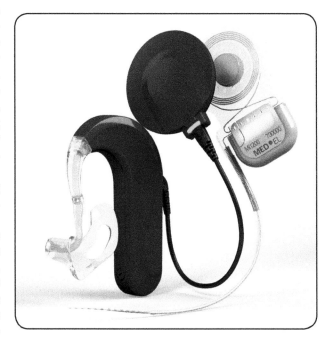

FIGURE 24–17. MED-EL SONNET EAS sound processor. Image provided courtesy of MED-EL Corporation.

The hearing aid portion of the SONNET sound processor provides approximately 48 dB of gain from approximately 125 Hz to 2000 Hz. The maximum power output of the SONNET sound processor is 118 dB SPL. The acoustic component of the SONNET sound processor is controlled by a digital signal processor and contains six channels. The acoustic settings are programmable, allowing the audiologist to adjust several parameters, including but not limited to frequency-specific gain across the six channels and maximum output. The acoustic-electric crossover is set to the lowest frequency at which the unaided pure tone threshold crosses 65 dB HL. The audiologist may change the acoustic-electric crossover frequency within the acoustic fitting tab (Figure 24–18).

The SONNET processor offers electrical stimulation from 70 to 8500 Hz, with adjustment for the low-frequency boundary to accommodate EAS users. The SONNET sound processor also contains the same front-end processing available on all MED-EL processors, including Automatic Sound Management (ASM), a wide input dynamic range (IDR), dual-microphone directionality, wind noise reduction, and a dual-stage automatic gain control (AGC).

Advanced Bionics EAS

Advanced Bionics also has developed an EAS sound processor. The Naída CI Q90 sound processor may be coupled to the to the Naída CI Q90 Acoustic Earhook, which consists of the Phonak xP Receiver that is connected to the top Naída CI Q90 sound pro-

cessor after the conventional earhook or T-Mic™ 2 has been removed (Figure 24–19). The Naída EAS technology was approved by the FDA in 2018 for use in the United States. Advanced Bionics has not developed a hybrid electrode array. However, the Advanced Bionics HiFocus Mid-Scala electrode array was developed to minimize cochlear trauma, which obviously would enhance the possibility of hearing preservation. Boyle (2016) reported on 94 recipients of the Advanced Bionics Mid-Scala array and indicated that "aidable hearing" was measured in 81% of the recipients with a mean loss of 12 dB across 250, 500, and 1000 Hz at 12 months postactivation. Hunter et al. (2016) evaluated hearing preservation in 39 ears of individuals who had preoperative low-frequency hearing (air conduction pure-tone no worse than 85 dB HL at 250 Hz) and received the Mid-Scala electrode array. Hunter and colleagues reported that 30.8% of the recipients had aidable low-frequency hearing at the one-year postsurgery appointment. The mean elevation of the participants' low-frequency pure-tone hearing (averaged at 125, 250, and 500 Hz) was 20.2 dB after surgery. Advanced Bionics also offers the HiFocus SlimJ electrode array, which is a thin, lateral wall array designed to preserve cochlear structures (Advanced Bionics, 2018).

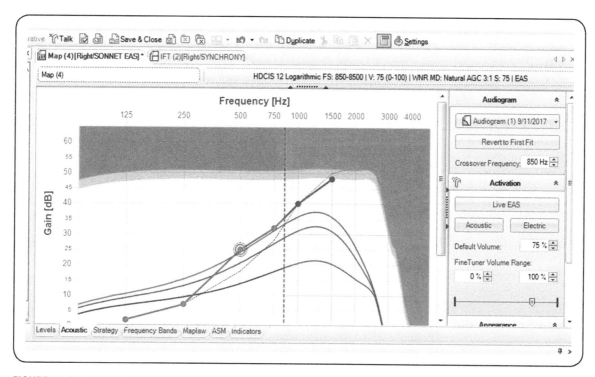

FIGURE 24–18. MED-EL MAESTRO EAS programming screen. Image provided courtesy of MED-EL Corporation.

The Naída CI90 Acoustic Earhook can provide up to 53 dB of acoustic amplification with a frequency response that extends to 1600 Hz. To program the Naída CI 90Q sound processor for EAS use,

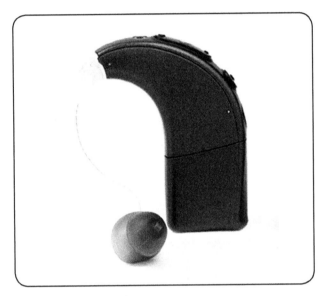

FIGURE 24–19. Advanced Bionics Naída CI Q90 EAS sound processor. Image provided courtesy of Advanced Bionics, LLC.

the audiologist must enable the "Acoustic Mode" in the "Implant" menu of the SoundWave fitting software (Figure 24–20). Then, the audiologist must enter the recipient's pure tone unaided air conduction thresholds into the "Acoustic Parameters" tab of the Patient File section of SoundWave (Figure 24–21). The audiologist may choose from one of three prescriptive fitting methods to be used to assign gain and output based upon the recipient's unaided hearing thresholds: (1) the proprietary AB-Phonak Fitting Formula (default fitting method), (2) NAL-RP, and (3) DSL v5. Advanced Bionics and Phonak designed the AB-Phonak Fitting Formula to align the acoustic and electric signals delivered to the implanted ear as well as to align the loudness and dynamic behavior of the acoustic signal delivered to the implanted ear with the acoustic signal of a Phonak hearing aid fitted to the nonimplanted ear (i.e., Phonak Naída Link behind-the-ear hearing aid for the nonimplanted ear—bimodal).

To create an EAS program, the audiologist must enable the "Acoustic Mode" option in the lower panel of the SoundWave program screen. Within this "Acoustic Mode" pane, the audiologist may also change the prescriptive fitting method used to assign gain to the acoustic receiver, adjust both the acoustic and electric

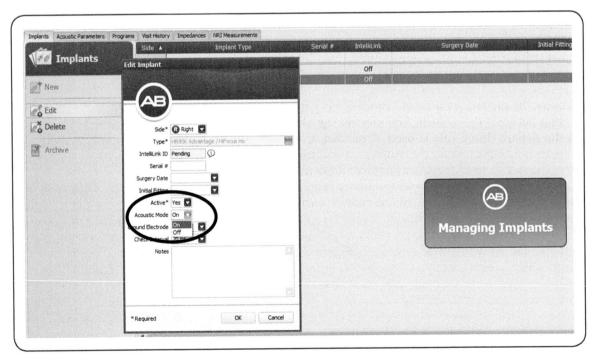

FIGURE 24–20. Enabling EAS programming in the Advanced Bionics SoundWave software. Image provided courtesy of Advanced Bionics, LLC.

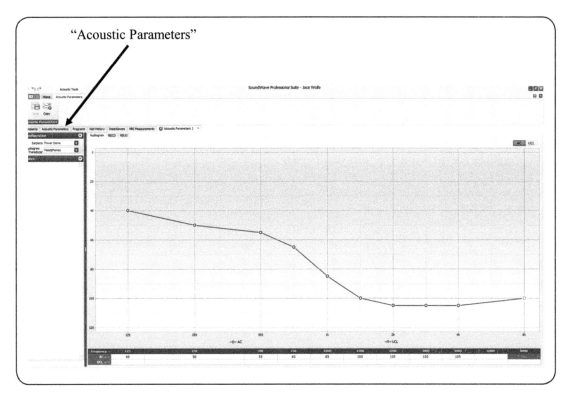

FIGURE 24–21. Advanced Bionics SoundWave EAS programming screen. Image provided courtesy of Advanced Bionics, LLC.

cutoff frequencies, adjust the range over which the volume control provides a change in level (dB), and provide adjustments in the overall gain of the acoustic signal (Figure 24–22). The SoundWave default fitting rule is to place the acoustic and electrical cutoff frequencies at the point at which the acoustic threshold crosses 70 dB HL. As a result, there is no gap or overlap between the acoustic and electric signals when the default fitting rule is used. If needed, the audiologist may adjust either the acoustic or electric cutoff frequency to provide acoustic or electric stimulation across a narrower or broader frequency range. For the Naída CI Q90 processor volume control, each button push provides a 1 dB change in the acoustic gain and a 4 CU change in electrical stimulation. The audiologist may make frequency-specific adjustments to the acoustic gain by selecting the "Acoustic" tab at the top corner of the programming screen. Once inside the "Acoustic" menu, the audiologist may make frequency-specific adjustments to the acoustic gain for three different input levels ("soft, medium, and loud") and to the maximum power output (see Figure 24–22). The audiologist saves EAS programs to the Naída CI Q90 sound processor using the same "click-

and-drag" procedure used to program the Naída CI processor for electric-only recipients (see Chapter 9). Of note, however, when used as an EAS sound processor, the Naída CI 90Q must be initialized for either the right or left ear.

Performance with Hybrid or Minimally Invasive Cochlear Implants

Studies on the efficacy of EAS suggest significantly better postimplant outcomes compared with performance with traditional acoustic hearing aids alone and in most cases also compared with the cochlear implant alone (Büchner et al., 2009; Fraysse et al., 2006; Gantz, Turner, & Gfeller, 2004; Gantz, Turner, Gfeller, & Lowder, 2005; Gantz et al., 2009; Kiefer et al., 2005; Lenarz et al., 2013; Luetje, Thedinger, Buckler, Dawson, & Lisbona, 2007). For example, Kiefer et al. (2005) reported an average improvement of 8% for word and sentence recognition in a quiet condition with EAS compared with the cochlear implant alone in 13 individuals after using MED-EL implants for

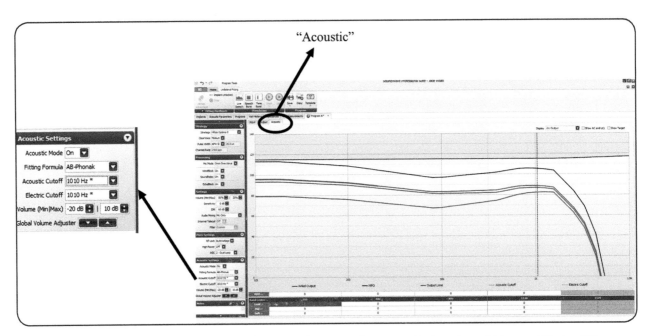

FIGURE 24–22. Advanced Bionics SoundWave EAS programming screen. Image provided courtesy of Advanced Bionics, LLC.

1 year. In these same participants, sentence recognition in background noise at a +10 signal-to-noise ratio (SNR) improved by 23% in the EAS condition versus the cochlear implant alone condition. In another study, Büchner et al. (2009) examined sentence-recognition thresholds in the presence of a single competing talker in 22 patients using the Nucleus Hybrid L implant. The best thresholds (lowest) were obtained with the combined cochlear implant and hearing aid (3.9 dB) compared with the cochlear implant alone (10.8 dB) or hearing aid alone (15.9 dB).

In a clinical trial, Gantz et al. (2009) reported results from 85 patients implanted with the Cochlear Hybrid 10 device and revealed that 91% of these patients maintained some usable residual hearing. Improvements in word recognition in quiet and sentence-in-noise thresholds were obtained by half of the patients when using EAS over preoperative hearing aids alone. Interestingly, 91% of the variance in the performance of patients ($n = 16$) who did not benefit from EAS over hearing aids alone was explained by the preoperative word-recognition performance and duration of deafness in the high-frequency region (i.e., poorer EAS benefit was associated with poorer preoperative word recognition performance and a longer duration of high-frequency deafness—greater than 30 years).

Lenarz et al. (2013) examined behavioral and subjective performance in 66 adults who received Nucleus Hybrid L24 implants. Eighty-eight percent of the participants maintained residual low-frequency hearing after surgery, and 88% continued to use the hybrid devices 1 year following surgery. On average, 65% of these participants realized an increase in speech recognition in quiet, whereas 74% improved in noise. Subjective questionnaires yielded significant improvements in ratings of speech understanding, spatial aspects of hearing speech, and the quality of speech.

Hybrid implants are also reported to improve localization abilities and subjective performance. In one study, Dunn, Perreau, Gantz, and Tyler (2010) reported that, when combining the use of a hybrid implant in one ear (implant plus hearing aid) with an acoustic hearing aid on the nonimplanted ear, 11 patients with Nucleus Hybrid 10 implants displayed significantly better speech recognition in noise and localization than they achieved with the Hybrid implant alone or a bimodal arrangement (traditional cochlear implant plus contralateral hearing aid). In a study focused on the potential subjective benefits of EAS, Gstoettner et al. (2011) asked 23 patients with MED-EL devices to rate their percentage of difficulty hearing in various listening situations. Compared with the global average preoperative rating of 74% with their hearing aids alone, the patients reported a significant decrease in global hearing difficulty with a rating of 45% when using EAS for 3 months.

Another substantial benefit of hybrid implantation is the preservation of low-frequency hearing in both ears to allow the recipient to capitalize on interaural timing cues to better understand speech in noise when spatial separation exists between the speech and noise signals. Gifford et al. (2013) evaluated speech recognition in noise for 38 subjects who used electroacoustic stimulation in one ear and a hearing aid in the opposite ear. Speech recognition was assessed using an eight-loudspeaker array (each loudspeaker separated by 45 degrees), with the signal of interest presented from the loudspeaker located directly in front of the subject and the noise presented from each of the eight loudspeakers. The noise was presented at 72 dBA, and speech recognition was assessed at fixed SNRs of +2 and +6 dB. Also, speech recognition was evaluated adaptively to determine the SNR necessary for 50% correct performance. Furthermore, the testing was completed in a sound-treated audiometric test booth with minimal reverberation as well as with a simulated reverberation time of 0.6 seconds. For the aforementioned conditions, performance was assessed in several conditions: (1) bimodal—use of the hearing aid for the nonimplanted ear along with electrical stimulation only for the implanted ear, (2) combined—use of the hearing aid for the nonimplanted ear along with electroacoustic stimulation for the implanted ear, and (3) binaurally aided—acoustic only stimulation for each ear.

Gifford and colleagues (2013) found that electrical stimulation provided significantly better performance than the binaural hearing aid condition. Additionally, the best performance was obtained when the subjects used the combined mode of stimulation (i.e., electroacoustic stimulation for the implanted ear along with the hearing aid for the opposite ear). Compared with the bimodal condition, use of the combined mode of stimulation resulted in a 6 to 10-percentage point improvement in speech recognition at the fixed SNR and a 1.8 dB improvement in the SNR needed for 50% correct performance. They also reported that benefit from combined use was correlated with the degree of postoperative low-frequency hearing and the interaural time difference threshold. Gifford et al. (2013) concluded that the availability of binaural low-frequency hearing secondary to the preservation of low-frequency hearing in the implanted ear allowed the subjects to take advantage of interaural timing cues to capitalize on the squelch effect to understand speech better in the presence of spatially separated noise.

As previously discussed, the U.S. FDA approved the Nucleus L24 Hybrid cochlear implant for commercial use in March of 2014. This approval followed a Cochlear-sponsored clinical trial of the L24 device that was designed to evaluate recipient outcomes to justify the manufacturer's proposed labeling for clinical use in the United States. Fifty adult recipients participated in this trial at 10 different cochlear implant centers in the United States. Subjects met the following audiometric inclusion criteria for participation in the study:

1. Severe to profound sensorineural hearing loss (an air conduction pure-tone threshold average at 2000, 3000, and 4000 Hz equal to or poorer than 75 dB HL) for frequencies greater than 1500 Hz along with low frequency at 500 Hz and below of 60 dB HL or better.
2. Consonant-Nucleus-Consonant (CNC) monosyllabic word recognition scores equal to or better than 10 but no better than 60% correct in the ear to be implanted.
3. CNC word scores in the contralateral ear equal to or better than the implanted ear but no better than 80% correct.
4. No conductive hearing loss.
5. The duration of severe to profound hearing loss cannot exceed 30 years.

These subjects were fitted with the Nucleus Freedom hybrid sound processor. Postoperative air conduction and bone conduction thresholds were measured bilaterally at every octave and inter-octave frequency from 125 to 8000 Hz. Acoustic amplification was provided at all frequencies possessing an air conduction threshold better than 90 dB HL. The output of the acoustic component was fitted to the NAL prescriptive target across the low-frequency range. The low-frequency boundary of electrical stimulation was set at a frequency at which the unaided audiometric threshold of the implanted ear was 90 dB HL or poorer.

The participants in the study performed significantly better with their L24 hybrid cochlear implant system than they did preoperatively with binaural hearing aids. Specifically, they achieved an average improvement of 37% on CNC word testing at 60 dBA and 36% on AzBio sentences in noise (+5 dB SNR). Additionally, the subjects performed better in the EAS mode than they did in both the acoustic and electric-only conditions. This study included a relatively large number of subjects with an EAS device that is now commercially available. The favorable results obtained by the study subjects lend credibility to the procedures used to program the acoustic and electrical stimulation levels of the Nucleus Freedom hybrid sound processor (Roland et al., 2016).

Some studies have shown that the benefits of low-frequency hearing preservation after implantation are most prevalent in complex listening environments. For example, Sheffield, Jahn, and Gifford (2015) reported that speech recognition in quiet and in the presence of spatially coincident noise (i.e., speech and noise presented from same location) was similar between the bimodal condition (i.e., electric-only for implanted ear with acoustic amplification for nonimplanted ear) and the condition in which the listener used the cochlear implant along with low-frequency amplification in each ear. However, when speech was presented from one location and noise from various locations, speech recognition was better in the condition in which the recipient had access to electric hearing in the implanted ear and acoustic hearing in both ears compared with either the bimodal condition or the ipsilateral EAS condition. In short, the availability of low-frequency acoustic hearing in each ear allowed for better speech recognition in noise in an environment with diffuse noise sources. Additionally, Gifford et al. (2017) evaluated speech recognition in a diffuse noise environment and found that the best performance was obtained when the participants were able to use EAS in the implanted ear and a hearing aid for the nonimplanted ear. Also of note, Gifford et al. (2015) reported similar results for a small group of three recipients who had bilateral cochlear implants with hearing preservation in each ear. The best speech recognition in noise was obtained when the listeners were able to use EAS in each ear. Ideally, for persons who have precipitously sloping severe to profound high-frequency hearing loss, optimal speech recognition in a diffuse noise environment will be obtained with the use of bilateral EAS with symmetrical low-frequency hearing preservation (Dorman et al., 2013).

Research has also explored the benefits of hearing preservation for sound localization. In general, studies have shown that hearing preservation and the use of EAS improve sound localization compared with the electric-only or bimodal conditions (Dunn et al., 2010; Gifford et al., 2014; Loiselle et al., 2015). However, localization is generally poorer for recipients with asymmetric low-frequency hearing compared with recipients who have symmetric low-frequency hearing after surgery (Dunn et al., 2010; Loiselle et al.,

2010). Consequently, EAS candidates should be counseled that their localization abilities may be impaired if they lose a significant amount of low-frequency hearing after implantation. Of note, Loiselle et al. (2015) found that the use of amplification in the poorer ear of EAS recipients who have asymmetrical low-frequency hearing resulted in poorer localization of wideband stimuli compared with the unaided condition. Loiselle and colleagues attributed this finding to the possibility that cochlear dead regions in the poorer ear may result in distortion that impairs aided localization abilities. As a result, audiologists should be careful to not provide too much amplification in frequencies at which dead regions may exist.

In another study, Loiselle et al. (2016) evaluated the localization abilities of two groups, one with bilateral conventional cochlear implants (without hearing preservation) and another with EAS for the implanted ear and a hearing aid for the nonimplanted ear. Localization abilities were evaluated with three different stimuli, a low-pass noise, a high-pass noise, and a wideband noise. The bilateral CI group had good localization abilities for the high-pass stimulus but relatively poor localization of the low-pass stimulus, whereas the EAS/hearing aid group had good localization for the low-pass stimulus and relatively poor localization of the high-pass stimulus. The bilateral CI group presumably struggled to localize the low-pass noise, because interaural timing cues are often difficult to process via electric-only hearing (Salloum et al., 2010). The EAS group struggled to localize the high-frequency noise, because the participants did not have access to high-frequency audio information in the nonimplanted ear because of their severe to profound high-frequency hearing loss. The two groups had similar localization performance for the wideband noise, but they likely used different cues to localize the wideband signal. In short, optimal localization of everyday sounds is likely dependent on the ability to process low-frequency timing cues and high-frequency level cues. For individuals with precipitously sloping severe to propound high-frequency hearing loss, localization abilities will most likely be optimized with bilateral EAS as long as low-frequency hearing is preserved for each ear and is symmetrical (Dorman et al., 2013).

Other studies compared performance of patients using hybrid implants to patients with traditional cochlear implants with long-electrode arrays (Dorman et al., 2009; Golub, Wan, Drennan, Worman, & Rubinstein, 2012). For example, Dorman et al. (2009) compared word-recognition performance in 22 patients with the 10-mm Cochlear Nucleus Hybrid implants (EAS) with 25 patients using Cochlear or Advanced Bionics implants with conventional (long) electrode arrays. Although both groups showed significant improvements relative to preoperative performance with hearing aids, the patients using conventional electrode arrays had significantly better performance than the patients using Hybrid implants, which the author related to the broader band stimulation from the conventional versus the hybrid implants. It is important to note that the hybrid recipients in the Dorman et al. (2009) study were implanted with the 10 mm Nucleus hybrid array, which is substantially shorter than any other electrode that is commercially available and used for EAS application (i.e., Nucleus [L24] Hybrid, Nucleus CI422, MED-EL FLEX[24]). As a result, the findings of the Dorman et al. (2009) study do not necessarily apply to the experience one would expect for the typical EAS recipient seen in clinical environments.

Selecting Electrode Arrays for Hearing Preservation

At this point, the reader may be wondering which linear length/angular insertion depth is ideal for optimizing hearing preservation and performance. Although research has yet to suggest a fail-proof protocol for electrode selection and depth for recipients with residual low-frequency hearing, there are some study findings that may offer audiologists some guidance in this decision-making process. Although hearing preservation has been demonstrated with long and periomodiolar arrays (Mick et al., 2014; Stanisławek-Sut, Morawski, & Niemczyk, 2013), conventional wisdom as well as some studies suggest that the likelihood of hearing preservation is better with electrode arrays that are shorter, thinner in diameter, and designed for lateral wall placement (Gantz et al., 2009; Mick et al., 2014; O'Connell et al., 2016; Sweeney et al., 2016). Indeed, temporal bone studies have demonstrated that electrode insertions that extend deeper than 360 degrees (about 20 mm for a lateral wall insertion) are more likely to cause damage to delicate cochlear structures (Adunka & Kiefer, 2006). However, other studies have suggested that angular insertion depth and electrode type are not predictors of hearing preservation (Erixon, Kobler, & Rask-Anderson, 2012; Skarzynski et al., 2009; Wanna et al., 2015). The following section reviews several studies

that explore factors that affect hearing preservation after cochlear implantation.

Skarzyński and colleagues (2014) examined low-frequency hearing preservation for a group of 35 recipients of the Cochlear Nucleus CI422 implant. The researchers divided the subjects into three groups on the basis of their preoperative air conduction threshold at 500 Hz: (1) better than or equal to 50 dB HL, (2) poorer than 50 dB HL but better than 80 dB HL, and (3) equal to or poorer than 80 dB HL. They reported several interesting findings. First, the vast majority of subjects achieved significant improvements in speech recognition in quiet and in noise with their cochlear implant relative to their preoperative binaural hearing aid performance. However, subjects with better preoperative hearing generally achieved better speech recognition in quiet and in noise with their implant compared with the subjects with poorer preoperative hearing. In contrast, the subjects with better preoperative low-frequency hearing thresholds tended to suffer a greater amount of low-frequency hearing loss after surgery than subjects with poorer preoperative hearing (most likely because they had more functional low frequency to lose).

Skarzyński and colleagues (2014) provided a compelling explanation for the greater change in hearing loss suffered by the group with better preoperative hearing thresholds. In short, they contended that the group with better preoperative low- to mid-frequency hearing thresholds (in the normal to mild hearing loss range) was more likely to possess functioning outer hair cells that enhanced hearing sensitivity in the apical region of the cochlea via the cochlear amplifier. Furthermore, they theorized that the presence of the electrode array may impair the active process of the cochlear amplifier, leading to a decrease in outer hair gain and subsequently to a loss of hearing sensitivity. More specifically, Skarzynski et al. (2014) hypothesized that greater impairment of outer hair cell function would occur as the electrode array was inserted closer to the location of the functioning outer hair cells, resulting in hearing loss at a given characteristic frequency corresponding to that location. The researchers evaluated their theory by examining the relationship between hearing threshold shift at different frequencies across the low-frequency octaves and the location of the electrode array as indicated by postoperative spiral CT scans. The estimated characteristic frequency at a specific location was estimated based on the angular insertion depth of the electrode array relative to the Greenwood function. Indeed, Skarzyński and colleagues

(2014) found a much higher potential for significant decreases in hearing thresholds at estimated characteristic frequencies that were within 135 degrees of the tip of the electrode array. They attributed this degradation in threshold to a change in cochlear mechanics and to altered cochlear function and basilar membrane movement associated with the physical presence of the array.

Based on their findings, Skarzyński et al. (2014) provided the following clinical suggestions. If an electrode is inserted 360 degrees (one full turn along the lateral wall) into the cochlea (e.g., the CI522 inserted to 20 mm), then one would expect a higher chance of impairing outer hair cell function at 1000 Hz and causing a decrease in hearing sensitivity at that frequency (because an angular insertion depth of 360 degrees corresponds with the 1000 Hz location of the cochlea). Based on this line of thinking, a shorter array, like the Nucleus L24 Hybrid device, is likely to be more appropriate for recipients with useful residual hearing sensitivity (e.g., 65 dB HL or better) at 1000 Hz. However, if the goal is to preserve useful residual hearing at 500 Hz and below (because hearing sensitivity at higher frequencies is too poor to expect benefit from amplification), then an electrode array that is inserted to 360 degrees is appropriate.

A few additional points are worth discussing. First, there are some reports that suggest that implants with arrays inserted to an angular insertion depth of 360 degrees provide similar speech recognition in the electric-only mode compared with performance obtained by users with electrode arrays of a conventional length (Balkany et al., 2007; Roland et al., 2016). For instance, 50 subjects in the U.S. FDA clinical trial of the Nucleus L24 Hybrid cochlear implant achieved similar mean monosyllabic word recognition as subjects who received the Freedom implant with the Contour Advance electrode array with a typical angular insertion depth of 430 degrees (Balkany et al., 2007; Roland et al., 2016). Of course, one might contend that the recipients in the L24 clinical trial possessed preoperative otologic histories that were more favorable than the recipients who participated in the Freedom Contour Advance trial, and as a result, their speech recognition should have been better. Although that may be true, Adunka et al. (2010) also found similar speech recognition for a group of users of the MED-EL FLEX²⁴ (formerly FLEXᴱᴬˢ) with an insertion depth of approximately 20 mm (360 degrees) compared with a group of MED-EL recipients with STANDARD arrays (e.g., 31-mm insertion depth). The two groups were matched on several variables, including preoperative pure-tone air conduction thresholds and aided word recognition. Both groups achieved about 50% monosyllabic word recognition in the ipsilateral electric-only condition six months after implant activation, but the hybrid group achieved a mean score of 69% correct on monosyllabic word recognition in the EAS condition.

Likewise, Helbig, Helbig, Rader, Mack, and Baumann (2009) compared speech recognition for subjects who underwent re-implantation with a longer electrode array after experiencing a significant decrease in residual hearing following hybrid cochlear implant surgery. Based on their findings (with lateral wall electrode arrays), these researchers concluded that a minimum electrode array length of 18 mm is needed to provide adequate performance via electric-only stimulation.

In contrast, research has suggested that conventional-length electrode arrays are likely most appropriate for persons with severe to profound hearing loss across the electrode array (Dorman, Loizou, & Rainey, 1997; Stakhovskaya et al., 2007). Additionally, there are several studies that demonstrate the benefits of perimodiolar electrode array placement, which is designed to be inserted in close proximity to the modiolus and the target spiral ganglion cell bodies. Theoretical advantages of a perimodiolar electrode array over a lateral wall array include a need for lower stimulation levels to elicit a given psychophysical percept, better battery life, and reduced channel interaction (Balkany, Eshraghi, & Yang, 2002; O'Leary, Richardson, & McDermott, 2009; Wackym et al., 2004). Indeed, several researchers have reported lower stimulation thresholds for perimodiolar arrays than straight arrays (Cohen et al., 2001; Gordin et al. 2009; Jeong et al., 2015; Muller et al., 2015; Runge-Samuelson et al., 2009). Other researchers have found reduced channel interaction with the use of perimodiolar arrays (Hughes & Abbas, 2006; Hughes & Stille, 2010). A reduction in channel interaction may improve spectral resolution, which may improve speech recognition. Holden and colleagues (2013) found that better speech recognition was associated with closer proximity of the electrode array to the modiolus. Likewise, Esquia Medina et al. (2013) reported that better word recognition was associated with close proximity of the electrode contacts to the modiolous. Given the collective results of these studies, conventional length electrode arrays and perimodiolar electrode arrays are still likely to be beneficial for candidates with severe to profound hearing loss across the audiometric frequency range.

In short, more research is needed to clarify the benefits and limitations of short versus long electrodes for persons with precipitously sloping high-frequency hearing loss.

A number of other researchers have explored various factors that may influence the potential to preserve hearing after cochlear implant surgery. For example, a group of surgeons and researchers at Vanderbilt University have published a series of peer-reviewed papers describing studies that have explored factors that influence hearing preservation of cochlear implant recipients. Wanna et al. (2015) evaluated the impact of intrascalar electrode location (i.e., did the electrode array remain in the scala tympani as desired or did it translocate to the scala media and/or scala vestibuli?), electrode type (e.g., lateral wall, mid-scala, perimodiolar), and angular insertion depth on the residual hearing of 45 ears (36 recipients with 9 receiving bilateral cochlear implants). Intrascalar location was determined by a postoperative CT scan. Thirty-eight of the 45 electrode arrays were located fully within the scala tympani. Six of the electrode arrays had translocated from the scala tympani to the scala vestibuli, whereas 1 electrode was inserted fully into the scala vestibuli. Almost 58% of the recipients with full scala tympani insertions maintained residual hearing after surgery, whereas none of the 7 recipients with electrode arrays in the scala vestibuli had residual hearing after surgery. Recipients with round window insertions had a higher likelihood of the electrode array being fully located in the scala tympani than recipients whose electrode arrays were inserted into a cochleostomy. It is important to note that for the recipients who had full scala tympani insertions, the type of electrode array (lateral wall vs. perimodiolar) did not influence postoperative residual hearing. Also, angular insertion depth did not influence postoperative residual hearing for recipients with full scala tympani insertions. Wanna and colleagues (2015) acknowledged that the relatively small number of participants in their study limits the conviction with which they can draw conclusions, but they did stress the importance of a full insertion in the scala tympani as a factor that enhances the likelihood of hearing preservation after implantation, regardless of the type of electrode or angular insertion depth. Additionally, they noted that dislocation of the electrode array from the scala tympani to the scala vestibuli may cause damage to cochlear structures, which would obviously lead to a higher chance of hearing loss. Moreover, they noted that dislocation from the scala tympani may result in damage to the vascular structures of the cochlea. However, they also recognized that over 40% of the recipients with full scala tympani insertions still lost their hearing during or shortly after surgery, a fact that they attributed to cochlear inflammation and/or vascular injury.

O'Connell et al. (2016) also demonstrated the importance of a complete scala tympani insertion in a study in which they examined outcomes associated with 56 implant surgeries, 36 with perimodiolar electrode arrays and 20 with lateral wall electrode arrays. Ninety percent of the lateral wall electrodes were inserted entirely within the scala tympani, whereas a complete scala tympani insertion was only achieved with 47% of the perimodiolar electrode arrays. However, when CNC word recognition was evaluated only for recipients whose electrodes were entirely located within the scala tympani, there was not a statistically significant difference in performance between recipients with lateral wall and perimodiolar electrode arrays.

It is important to note that the Nucleus Contour Advance was the two perimodiolar electrode arrays used in this study. Since that time, Cochlear has released the CI532 with the Slim Modiolar electrode array, which is substantially thinner than the Contour Advance. Aschendorff et al. (2017) examined the position of the Nucleus 532 electrode array after it was inserted in 44 adult recipients by 11 different surgeons who had completed a training workshop prior to implantation. Postoperative imaging indicated that the perimodiolar electrode array was located entirely within the scala tympani for all 44 recipients, a finding that Aschendorff and colleagues attributed to several findings. First, they noted that "successful scala tympani insertion appears to depend on surgical technique to a significant degree." Consistent with this idea, Aschendorff et al. noted that the surgical technique employed to insert the Slim Modiolar array was most likely a factor in the consistent attainment of complete scala tympani insertions. Additionally, Aschendorff and colleagues noted that the cross-sectional diameter of the Slim Modiolar electrode array is 40% less than the Contour Advance. It is possible that the thinner dimensions of the Slim Modiolar array further enhanced the likelihood of a full scala tympani insertion. However, it should be noted that in an earlier study, Aschendorff et al. (2007) evaluated the final position of the Contour Advance electrode array. When the surgeon created a cochleostomy in the scala tympani (i.e., the electrode array was initially inserted into the scala tympani rather than the scala vestibuli) and employed the recommended Contour Advance insertion procedure, the Contour Advance electrode array was located entirely within the scala tympani in 85% of the cases. Again, Aschendorff et al. (2007) stressed the importance of the surgical technique in achieving a full scala tympani insertion with a perimodiolar electrode array. Considering the results of the Aschendorff et al. studies (2007, 2017), with use of recommended surgical technique and modern electrode array technologies, it is possible (and even probable) to consistently achieve a complete scala tympani insertion with perimodiolar electrode arrays. According to the work of Wanna et al. (2015) and O'Connell et al. (2016), hearing preservation after implantation does appear to depend on a complete scala tympani insertion.

Wanna and colleagues (2017) also examined short-term (measured two to three weeks after surgery) and long-term (one year after surgery) hearing preservation for 196 recipients (225 implants) who received conventional-length electrode arrays. All recipients had an air conduction pure-tone hearing threshold of 80 dB HL or better at 250 Hz prior to implantation. Short-term functional hearing preservation (i.e., 80 dB HL or better at 250 Hz) was achieved in 38% of ears, and long-term functional hearing preservation was achieved in 18% of ears. Better hearing preservation was associated with a round window insertion, postoperative treatment with anti-inflammatory steroids, and use of a lateral wall electrode array. The location of the electrode array in the cochlea was not measured in this study, so transcalar dislocation cannot be determined as a cause of loss of residual hearing after implantation. The findings of this study indicate that many recipients may have functional hearing shortly after implant surgery but lose hearing over the next few months. More research is needed to determine whether the use of steroids and/or other pharmacologic agents may reduce cochlear inflammation, the formation of fibrous scar tissue, and the likelihood of long-term hearing loss. The incidence of hearing preservation in this study is not as good as what has been reported with shorter electrode arrays (Gantz et al., 2009; Lenarz et al., 2009; Roland et al., 2016), suggesting that shorter (hybrid) electrode array may be desirable in cases in which hearing preservation is of high importance. Finally, Wanna et al. (2017) reported that age and gender did not influence hearing preservation. There is no consensus in previous research regarding the effect of age and gender on hearing preservation. Some studies have shown better hearing preservation

in women and younger recipients (Anagiotos et al., 2015; Cosetti et al., 2013; Kopelovich et al. 2014), whereas others have found no such relationship (Eshraghi et al., 2017; Sweeney et al., 2016; Zanetti, Nassif, & Redaelli de Zinis, 2015).

How Much Hearing Is Worth Preserving?

It should be noted that at the time of this writing, there is limited evidence to indicate the maximum amount of low-frequency hearing loss for which a recipient may have and still received benefit from low-frequency amplification. A number of research studies have suggested that the benefits of acoustic amplification are limited when hearing thresholds exceed 70 dB HL (Ching et al., 1998; Hogan et al., 1998; Hornsby et al., 2003, 2006, 2007; Turner et al., 1999; Vickers et al., 2001; Zhang et al., 2014). However, it is important to note that most studies examining the potential benefit for amplification for individuals with severe hearing loss have focused on the provision of high-frequency amplification (Hogan et al., 1998; Simpson & McDermott, 2005; Turner, 2006). The original version of the fitting software for the Cochlear L24 Hybrid implant assigned acoustic stimulation for low frequencies with hearing thresholds up to 90 dB HL. Gifford et al. (2017) evaluated the low-frequency cutoff of electrical stimulation (i.e., the lowest frequency at which electrical stimulation was provided) for 11 EAS recipients. Sentence recognition in noise was evaluated at each of seven different cutoff frequencies beginning at 188 Hz and increasing in 125 Hz steps to 938 Hz. Gifford and colleagues reported that sentence recognition in noise was better when the electrical cutoff was set to a frequency at which the unaided audiometric threshold exceeded 70 dB compared with performance obtained with the electrical cutoff set to a frequency at which the unaided audiometric threshold exceeded 90 dB HL. In short, the results of the Gifford et al. (2017) study suggest that the benefit of low-frequency acoustic amplification becomes diminished when audiometric threshold exceeds 70 dB HL, and as a result, the recipient performs better with the provision of electrical stimulation within that frequency range. Of note, however, many of the Vanderbilt studies (Dr. Gifford is affiliated with the Vanderbilt Cochlear Implant Program) suggest that functional low-frequency residual hearing exists if the unaided pure-tone audiometric threshold is better than 80 dB HL. In summary, more research is needed to determine the audiometric threshold at which low-frequency residual hearing is no longer likely to benefit the EAS recipient. However, based on preliminary findings, the audiologist should consider providing acoustic amplification at low frequencies with unaided air conduction pure-tone thresholds of better than 75 to 80 dB HL. As previously discussed, low-frequency amplification may be detrimental for persons who have asymmetric low-frequency hearing sensitivity with severe low-frequency hearing loss on the poorer ear. The audiologist should proceed cautiously with amplification under such circumstances. Also of note, although Wolfe and colleagues have shown that children can achieve better speech recognition with EAS compared with the electric-only and bimodal conditions, there is little to no evidence exploring how much residual low-frequency hearing children may need to potentially benefit from EAS.

Sheffield, Jahn, and Gifford (2015) did systematically evaluate the effect of the bandwidth of low-frequency amplification on speech recognition in quiet and in noise of seven adult EAS users. Word recognition in quiet in the EAS condition was not significantly better than the electric-only condition when acoustic amplification was provided to up to 250 Hz. However, word recognition in quiet was better in the EAS condition relative to the electric-only condition when acoustic audibility was provided up to 500 Hz. Further increases in the acoustic bandwidth resulted in additional improvement in word recognition in quiet in the EAS condition. Word recognition in noise was significantly better in the EAS condition compared with the electric-only condition, even when acoustic audibility was only made available up to 125 Hz. Increasing the acoustic bandwidth up to 750 Hz resulted in further improvements in word recognition in noise in the EAS condition. In summary, EAS users may achieve better speech recognition in noise with the provision of an acoustic signal with a bandwidth as low as 125 Hz. Extending the bandwidth even further allows for even better speech recognition in noise. The acoustic bandwidth must extend to at least 500 Hz in order to improve word recognition in quiet beyond the electric-only condition.

Optimizing the EAS Fitting

There are several considerations to take into account when programming EAS devices. Some of the more basic considerations include: (1) prescriptive fitting strategy to determine the gain and maximum power

output of the hearing aid portion of the device, (2) cutoff frequency for acoustic amplification, and (3) the frequency range over which electrical stimulation will be allocated. Additional considerations include: (1) taking into account the potential differences in compression parameters associated with the acoustic and electric signals, (2) managing contrasting delays that may exist in the delivery of the acoustic and electric signals, and (3) attempting to use pitch and/or loudness scaling to optimize the allocation of the acoustic and electric signals. Pitch or loudness scaling may be necessary to balance the loudness of the acoustic and electric signals provided from the EAS sound processor and to balance the loudness of the signals provided by the EAS sound processor and the contralateral hearing aid.

In the following paragraphs, we will discuss the results of research studies that have examined the aforementioned considerations. At this point in time, it is important to note that there is a paucity of research examining the effects of advanced parameters, such as delay times between the electric and acoustic signals along with signal processing characteristics (i.e., compression time constants) or loudness balancing between acoustic and electric signals, on recipient performance. As a result, those parameters will not be discussed in detail in this chapter. Following the review of existing research pertaining to the programming of EAS devices, a clinical protocol for the programming of hybrid cochlear implants (e.g., EAS) will be provided.

Frequency Allocation of Acoustic and Electric Stimulation

As indicated in earlier chapters in this book, a conventional cochlear implant provides electric stimulation to convey the entire speech frequency range. In contrast, an EAS device provides acoustical stimulation for low-frequency inputs and electric stimulation for high-frequency inputs. With an EAS device, the audiologist is faced with the task of determining how acoustic and electric stimulation should be allocated for sound inputs across the speech frequency range. A number of studies have sought to determine how acoustic inputs should be allocated in the acoustic and frequency stimulation modes, and the following section will briefly describe these studies.

Kiefer et al. (2005) examined performance of 13 recipients who had air conduction thresholds better than 60 dB HL below 1000 Hz and who received the MED-EL COMBI 40+. During the course of the study, the electrode array of the COMBI 40+ that was conventionally provided at the time of the study was modified so that the distance from the tip to the most basal intracochlear stimulating electrode contact was 21.9 mm (as opposed to a typical distance of 27.4 mm). This resulted in a reduction of the distance between intracochlear electrode contacts from 2.4 to 1.9 mm, which allowed for a larger number of electrode contacts to be inserted into the cochlea. Regardless of which electrode array was inserted, the typical insertion electrode array depth achieved in the study was about 20 mm. Two of the recipients lost their low-frequency residual hearing, so EAS results are available for 11 of the 13 participants. These subjects were fitted with digital in-the-ear hearing aids in order to receive EAS. The hearing aids were set with the gain of low-frequency amplification to half of the air conduction threshold (e.g., 30 dB of gain at 500 Hz if the air conduction threshold at that frequency was 60 dB HL—"½-gain rule"). Real ear measures were not conducted to measure the in situ output of the ipsilateral hearing aid.

During word- and sentence-recognition testing in quiet, participants used three frequency allocations for electrical stimulation: full frequency range (300–5500 Hz), 650 Hz low-frequency boundary (650–5500 Hz), and 1000 Hz low-frequency boundary (1000–5500 Hz). In all but one participant, the best performance and subjective benefit was obtained with the full frequency range of electrical stimulation in combination with the hearing aid. The remaining patient performed best with the 650 Hz low-frequency boundary. It should be noted that only 4 of the 11 EAS subjects possessed an air conduction threshold better than 90 dB HL at 500 Hz; therefore, the group's benefit from acoustic stimulation above 500 Hz was likely limited. Because of that and the fact that verification measures were not conducted to ensure in situ audibility for low-frequency speech inputs, the results of this study may not apply to the typical EAS recipient seen in clinical settings.

In another study, Fraysse et al. (2006) evaluated speech recognition in 27 recipients of the Cochlear Nucleus 24 implant with the Contour Advance electrode array. Soft surgical techniques were employed and low-frequency hearing, which was defined as air conduction thresholds of 80 dB HL or better at 125 and 250 Hz and 90 dB HL or better at 500 Hz, was preserved in 9 recipients. These 9 recipients were fitted in the implanted ear with custom hearing aids with the gain set to the Desired Sensation Level (Input/Output) prescriptive method. Two implant programs, which differed in the way in which electrical stimulation was frequency allocated, were created for the subjects using EAS. One program provided electrical stimulation across the entire speech frequency range, which presumably resulted in some overlap between acoustic and electric stimulation provided for low-frequency inputs. In the second program, the only acoustic stimulation was provided for low-frequency inputs, and electrical stimulation was only provided for the high-frequency inputs. The exact cutoff between low- and high-frequency inputs was not defined in this study, nor was the method used to determine the cutoff between acoustic and electric stimulation for the second program. The researchers reported that 7 of 9 subjects preferred the program without overlap between the acoustic and electric stimulation, whereas two subjects preferred the program with overlapping stimulation. There was no difference in word recognition in quiet between the two programs, but there was a trend toward better sentence recognition in noise with use of the non-overlapping program. However, there were insufficient data to allow for a formal statistical analysis. It is possible that the trend toward poorer speech recognition in noise with the overlapping program may have been attributed to masking of the low-frequency acoustic signal by the low-frequency electrical stimulation.

Simpson, McDermott, Dowell, Sucher, and Briggs (2009) compared behavioral performance of five users of the Nucleus Freedom Contour Advance electrode array when using: (1) only high-frequency electrical stimulation paired with the hearing aid providing low-frequency information below a specified cutoff versus and (2) a map with the full frequency range plus the hearing aid proving the same low-frequency input. With both maps, participants showed significantly better speech-recognition performance in quiet relative to preoperative performance with hearing aids alone, but no significant differences in performance were detected between the two maps for speech recognition in quiet and in noise.

Most recently, Karsten and colleagues (2013) at the University of Iowa examined the effect of varying frequency allocations in 10 users of the Cochlear Nucleus Hybrid (S8 or S12) device with a 10-mm electrode array. All subjects used the Nucleus Freedom hybrid sound processor. The Audioscan Verifit real-ear measurement system was used to evaluate the output of the acoustic component, which was programmed to provide an output that matched (±7 dB) the National Acoustics Laboratories Non-Linear 1 (NAL-NL1) prescriptive target for a 65 dB SPL calibrated speech signal. The upper edge of acoustic amplification was defined as the highest frequency that was within 7 dB of the NAL-NL1 target. Acoustic channels above this frequency were disabled. Three programs with differing cutoff frequencies for electric stimulation were created: (1) the "meet" program aimed to set the cutoff frequency of electrical stimulation to match the upper edge of acoustic amplification, (2) the "overlap" program, which set the lower end of the electrical range so that it was less than 50% of the upper edge of the acoustic amplification, and (3) the "gap" program, which set the lower end of the electrical range to be 50% higher than the upper edge of acoustic amplification. Figure 24–23 provides an example of acoustic-electric allocation with use of the "meet," "overlap," and "gap" approaches.

Speech recognition in quiet and in noise as well as subjective preference were compared across the three different programs. Although there was a trend toward better speech recognition in quiet with the "meet" program, there was not a statistically significant difference in speech recognition in quiet across the three programs. However, recognition of spondees in noise was significantly better in the "meet" condition compared with the "overlap" condition. Additionally, subjective results yielded better ratings for the "meet" condition over the remaining two frequency allocation conditions. Overall, the authors theorized that, because acoustic hearing provides better frequency resolution than electric hearing, the "overlap" program may have impaired speech recognition in noise by allowing for electric masking of the acoustic signal. The authors also concluded that the "meet" program generally provided better overall performance than the "overlap" program. Finally, it should be noted that this study included subjects with a 10 mm hybrid electrode array. A 10-mm electrode array typically extends to the 4000 Hz place in the cochlea, and as a result, the likelihood of physical interaction between the electric signal and the low-frequency acoustic signal is reduced. In contrast, commercially available EAS implants (e.g., Cochlear Nucleus L24 Hybrid, MED-EL FLEX[24]) are longer; thus, a higher likelihood of physical interaction may exist.

Vermiere and colleagues (2008) conducted a smaller study (e.g., four subjects) to examine how EAS stimulation should be frequency allocated in both the acoustic and electric domains. This study included recipients of the MED-EL COMBI 40+ Medium electrode array, which was inserted to a depth of 18 mm. The subjects' postoperative air conduction hearing threshold at 500 Hz ranged from 65 to 100 dB HL at the time of the ipsilateral hearing aid. Acoustic stimulation was allocated in two different ways: (1) no amplification was provided at frequencies in which the air conduction threshold exceeded 85 dB HL, and (2) acoustic amplification was allocated for all frequencies with air conduction thresholds better than 120 dB HL. The latter strategy was more likely to allow for amplification of frequency regions often associated with cochlear dead regions (Moore, Vickers, Glasberg, & Baer, 1997). Some studies have suggested that it may be beneficial to amplify one octave into a dead region for subjects with precipitously sloping hearing loss (Baer, Moore, & Kluk, 2002). The output of an Oticon Adapto P in-the-ear (ITE) hearing aid was measured with in situ real ear probe microphone measures to ensure it was appropriate at the frequencies over which acoustic amplification was provided. Electric stimulation was also allocated in two different manners: (1) the "full" range of electrical stimulation was provided as with the conventional MED-EL TEMPO+ processor, and (2) electrical stimulation began at the first air conduction frequency exceeding 65 dB HL. Sentence recognition in noise and subjective ease of listening were evaluated across all conditions. The subjects generally performed better when electric allocation was limited to the mid- to high-frequencies (i.e., reduced electrical overlap). However, the subjects typically achieved better speech recognition and expressed a

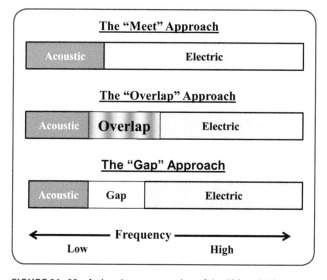

FIGURE 24–23. A visual representation of the "Meet," "Overlap," and "Gap" EAS allocation approaches.

greater preference for the program with the broader acoustic allocation (Vermiere et al., 2008). It should be noted that the findings of this study are limited by the small number of study participants as well as by the fact that postoperative, low-frequency residual hearing was relatively poor.

Turner, Reiss, and Gantz (2008) compared speech recognition of seven Nucleus S8 (10-mm insertion) hybrid recipients with two different programs: (1) electrical stimulation allocated from 750 to 8000 Hz and acoustic allocation from 750 Hz and below, and (2) electrical allocation from 2000 to 5000 Hz and acoustic allocation from 750 Hz and below. It should be noted that allocating electrical stimulation from 2000 to 5000 Hz closely corresponds to the typical frequency place of stimulation in the cochlea where the 10-mm-long electrode array resides. The researchers measured speech recognition in quiet with the two different programs and found mixed results. Three of the seven subjects performed better with the program with the wider range of electrical allocation, whereas one subject performed better with the program with the reduced range of electrical allocation. There was no difference in the mean performance between the two programs. The authors noted the fact that most of the subjects performed relatively well with the wide range of frequencies allocated electrically over a 10-mm span in the basal region of the cochlea, a finding they suggested as evidence of the plasticity of the auditory system with its capability to acclimate to a signal that is significantly shifted/distorted in the frequency domain. Again, the results of this study may not be completely applicable to the typical contemporary clinical experience, as current commercially available EAS devices across the world customarily incorporate longer electrode arrays with deeper insertion depths.

In a similar study with three Nucleus S8 (10-mm electrode array with six intracochlear electrode contacts) hybrid recipients, Reiss, Perreau, and Turner (2012) compared speech recognition and pitch perception for two different programs: (1) electrical stimulation allocated from 688 to 7938 Hz, and (2) electrical stimulation allocated from 188 to 7938 Hz. All three subjects lost their low-frequency hearing within the first year following implant surgery, so they discontinued ipsilateral hearing aid use. On the opposite ear, they did use a hearing aid, which was fitted to the NAL-NL1 prescriptive target for a 65 dB SPL speech signal. Word recognition in quiet and sentence recognition in noise was measured with the two programs. Pitch matching relative to

the contralateral ear was also compared across the two programs. The authors noted that the subjects generally realized no improvement in speech recognition in quiet or in noise with the wider allocation of electrical stimulation. However, the subjects did demonstrate changes in pitch perception associated with the changes in frequency allocation. This finding, again, demonstrates the ability of the auditory system to acclimate to a frequency-shifted signal.

Several studies have set the high-frequency cutoff of the hearing aid based on the first frequency at which the air conduction pure tone threshold reaches the profound range. In general, this approach places the high-frequency cutoff of amplification at the edge of usable residual hearing in the low frequencies. Specifically, several research groups recommend a cutoff frequency where pure-tone hearing thresholds exceeded 90 dB HL (Gantz et al., 2009; Golub et al., 2012; Lenarz et al., 2013). To examine the potential effects of hearing aid cutoff frequency Büchner et al. (2009) compared sentence recognition in noise across three cutoff frequencies (300, 500, 700 Hz cutoffs) in eight participants using the Nucleus Hybrid L24 device with a full frequency range for electrical stimulation (i.e., acoustic-electric overlap). The speech recognition results suggested that increasing the cutoff beyond 300 Hz did not significantly improve performance. It should be noted that the subjects in the Büchner study generally had a substantial amount of low-frequency hearing loss, so it is possible that the limited benefit of low-frequency amplification was due to the subjects' poor auditory function across the frequency range under study.

Dillon and colleagues (2014) evaluated the effect of the acoustic settings on the speech recognition of nine MED-EL EAS users. CNC word recognition and AzBio sentence recognition in noise (+10 dB SNR) were evaluated with each of two programs, one with the acoustic settings based on the manufacturer's default settings and one with the acoustic settings based on the NAL-NL1 prescriptive method. Electric stimulation began at the frequency at which the unaided air conduction threshold in the implanted ear met or exceeded 65 dB HL. CNC word recognition and AzBio sentence recognition in noise were both significantly better with the acoustic settings based on the NAL-NL1 prescriptive method. In short, Dillon et al. (2014) recommended the use of an evidence-based prescriptive method to determine the output of the acoustic receiver for EAS recipients.

As previously discussed in the review of functional hearing preservation in this chapter, Gifford and colleagues (2017) sought to determine the optimal low-frequency cutoff for electrical stimulation for 11 experienced EAS users. Gifford et al. found that the electrical low-frequency cutoff should be set to the frequency at which the unaided audiometric threshold met or exceeded 70 dB HL, which typically occurred around 313 to 438 Hz for the participant in the study. The manufacturer's software default at the time of the study set the electrical low-frequency cutoff at the unaided audiometric frequency that met or exceeded 90 dB HL. Gifford hypothesized that use of the lower audiologic criterion of 70 dB HL resulted in better speech recognition because the participants were unable to effectively process cues via acoustic amplification alone in frequency regions with severe to profound hearing loss. Gifford also hypothesized that the lower electrical cutoff frequency (e.g., 438 Hz) allowed for the provision of first formant speech information via the cochlear implant and the hearing aid, which may offer the listener redundant cues that may be used to improve speech recognition. Gifford acknowledged the fact that the participants in the study all used cochlear implants with conventional-length Nucleus electrode arrays. Further research is needed to determine whether the results of the Gifford et al. (2017) study also apply to shorter electrode arrays (i.e., Cochlear Nucleus Hybrid) and to longer electrode arrays (i.e., MED-EL). Additionally, more research is required to determine whether the optimal acoustic-electrical allocation settings vary by electrode array type (e.g., perimodiolar vs. mid-modiolar vs. lateral wall).

Overall, there is a paucity of published studies that have systematically examined the cutoff frequency to determine the optimal frequency range over which acoustic amplification should be provided to maximize the performance of recipients using modern EAS devices. Furthermore, research has yet to reveal the maximum threshold (in dB HL) at each octave and inter-octave audiometric low frequency at which acoustic amplification is likely to no longer be beneficial. Furthermore, additional research is needed to further clarify the optimal electrical cutoff frequency as a function of electrode array type and low-frequency residual hearing. Moreover, research is needed to determine the merits and limitations associated with overlap of acoustic and electric stimulation.

Until future research determines a more appropriate fitting model, evidence-based prescriptive fitting strategies along with real-ear measures are recommended for determining the appropriate hearing aid gain below the low-frequency cutoff for acoustic

amplification. Many researchers who have completed studies with hybrid implants reported use of the NAL NL-1 (Byrne et al., 2001) or the Desired Sensation Level (DSL) v5 (Scollie et al., 2005) prescriptive fitting strategies as a starting point for gain in the lower-frequency regions (Dillon et al., 2014; Dorman et al., 2009; Gantz et al., 2009; Golub et al., 2012; Karsten et al., 2013; Lenarz et al., 2013), and use of these prescriptive strategies resulted in good to excellent speech recognition performance for many of the patients in these studies. In one study, investigators used the half-gain rule along with the nonlinear compression model to determine appropriate gain for frequencies ranging from 125 to 1000 Hz (Kiefer et al., 2005).

Of note, some researchers have explored the use of pitch scaling and matching as a tool to determine acoustic/electric allocation for EAS users (Baumann, Rader, Helbig, & Bahmer, 2011; Simpson et al., 2009). Simpson and colleagues (2009) determined the acoustic frequency corresponding to electric stimulation (pulse train at 900 pps) on the most apical electrode (electrode 22) for a group of five Nucleus Freedom Contour Advance recipients with residual hearing in the ipsilateral or contralateral ear. Soft surgical techniques were employed, and the Contour Advance electrode array was inserted approximately 17 mm into the cochlea. The pitch matching was completed in the ipsilateral ear for two subjects who had residual hearing in the implanted ear and in the opposite ear for three subjects who had no postoperative residual hearing. Speech recognition in quiet and in noise was compared with two programs: (1) a conventional program with electrical stimulation allocated across the entire speech frequency range (188 to 7938 Hz) and (2) the lowest frequency of electrical stimulation based on the acoustic frequency that yielded a pitch match to electrical stimulation on electrode 22. Subjects were tested in the electric-only condition as well as while they used a hearing aid. Subjects with residual hearing in the implanted ear used a hearing aid in the ipsilateral and contralateral ears. The output of the hearing aid was matched to NAL-NL1 prescriptive targets. For the two subjects with ipsilateral residual hearing, the cutoff frequency of amplification was set to the highest frequency possessing an air conduction pure-tone threshold better than 90 dB HL. The researchers reported that the subjects performed better with EAS stimulation than they did with the hearing aids or cochlear implant alone. This finding supports the use of hearing aids programmed to an evidence-based prescriptive target to improve speech recognition relative to the use of electric stimulation alone. However, Simpson and colleagues (2009) found no difference in speech recognition between the two cochlear implant programs. The small number of subjects in this study, particularly those with residual hearing in the implanted ear, limits its application to the clinical management of EAS users.

Baumann and colleagues (2009) conducted pitch matching with eight EAS users who had residual low-frequency hearing in their ipsilateral and contralateral ears. These subjects used MED-EL PULSARCI[100] or PULSAR SONATA TI[100] implants. Four of these recipients were implanted with the MED-EL FLEX[24] electrode array, whereas the other four were implanted with the MED-EL STANDARD array (31.5 mm in length). The subjects listened to an 800 pps pulse train presented to a single electrode and adjusted the frequency of an acoustic pure tone to match the pitch of the electrical signal. This assessment was conducted on two to four of the most apical electrodes and was completed for the ipsilateral and contralateral ears.

Baummann et al. (2009) discovered that the difference in pitch matching between the ipsilateral and contralateral ears was quite small (the mean average was 14 Hz). They also reported that the FLEX[24] recipients matched the electrical signal on electrode 1 (the most apical electrode) to an acoustic pure tone frequency of 583 Hz, whereas the recipients with STANDARD electrode arrays matched their most apical electrode to a mean frequency below 250 Hz. As expected, electrodes positioned at a deeper angular insertion depth were associated with a lower pitch percept. Of significant note, these researchers noted a large amount of intersubject variability for pitch matching as a function of electrode location. Also, this study did show the potential of using pitch matching to determine the crossover frequency between acoustic and electric hearing. Considering the relatively small number of subjects in this study along with the significant amount of intersubject variability, additional research is needed in order to determine how pitch matching may be implemented in the clinical programming of EAS devices.

Clinical Protocol for Programming EAS Devices

The following protocol is based on the aforementioned research studies as well as the author's clinical experiences with programming EAS devices. The first step involved with the programming of EAS devices is to obtain a pure tone air conduction and bone conduction audiogram for the implanted ear. It is important to measure 125 Hz as well as every octave and interoctave frequency thereafter. Sheffield, Jahn, and Gifford (2015) have demonstrated that functional acoustic hearing at 125 Hz is sufficient to improve speech recognition in noise. Bone conduction audiometry should be completed to identify the presence of a potential conductive component. Conductive hearing loss is commonplace during the first several weeks after cochlear implant surgery due to the presence of middle ear effusion. The author generally waits about 4 weeks following surgery to activate the sound processor of EAS recipients in order to allow for the resolution of a potential middle ear effusion. The middle ear is typically free of effusion related to the surgery by 6 to 8 weeks. However, a conductive hearing loss can persist. Chole, Hullar, and Potts (2014) reported on the presence of a persistent air–bone gap after cochlear implantation for four recipients who had hearing preservation after surgery. Chole and colleagues attributed the presence of the air–bone gaps to changes in cochlear mechanics related to the cochlear implant surgery or to the presence of the electrode array. Middle ear measurements (e.g., tympanometry) can assist the audiologist in determining whether the conductive component is likely to be temporary because it is related to middle ear dysfunction or possibly permanent. Of course, the audiologist should complete an otoscopic evaluation prior to the audiometric assessment to ensure there are no contraindications to the placement of the earphone or hybrid acoustic component as well as to evaluate middle ear status. The audiologist should also evaluate the implant site to determine whether problems may arise when the sound processor is placed near the incision.

Figures 24–24 and 24–25 provide examples of a recipient's preoperative and postoperative audiometric profile. This recipient received a Nucleus CI532 cochlear implant with the Slim Modiolar electrode array for his right ear. As shown in these figures, a significant amount of low-frequency residual hearing remained after receiving each cochlear implant. The remainder of this example will illustrate how the Nucleus 7 sound processor was programmed for his right ear.

After completion of the audiometric assessment, the audiologist must determine how acoustic and electrical stimulation will be allocated for the recipient. Recent research suggests that it may be worthwhile to amplify low-frequency inputs at fre-

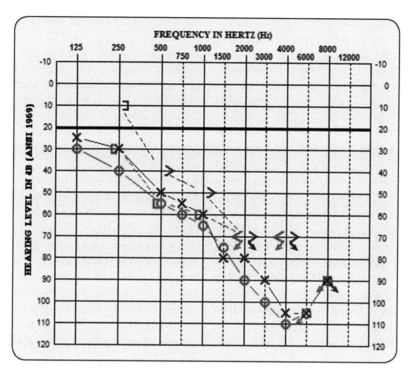

FIGURE 24–24. An example of a preoperative audiogram.

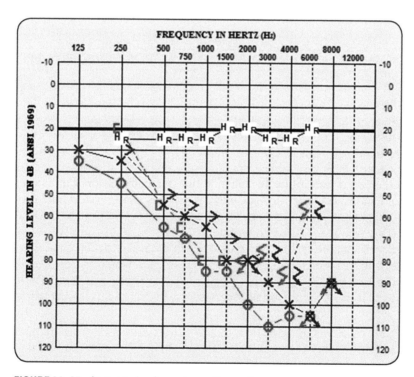

FIGURE 24–25. An example of a postoperative audiogram.

quencies with air conduction thresholds of 75 to 80 dB HL or better (Gifford et al., 2013; Wanna et al., 2015, 2017). The author recommends conducting in situ real ear probe microphone measures to evaluate the output of the acoustic component of the EAS device. The recipient's real-ear-to-coupler difference should be evaluated prior to in situ real-ear measurement so that the impact of the acoustics of the recipient's external and middle ear can be accounted for in the unaided thresholds used for device programming and real-ear measurement. Next, the author recommends programming the acoustic component so that the output is matched (±5 dB) to an evidence-based prescriptive target (e.g., DSL v5.0 Adult, DSL v5.0 Child, NAL-NL2). The author typically matches the output of the acoustic component to the NAL-NL2 prescriptive target at frequencies with audiometric thresholds of 75 dB HL and better. Also, it is likely most important that the slope of the acoustic response approximates the slope that is prescribed by the evidence-based generic prescriptive target. Ideally, the output should be measured for calibrated speech signals presented at 55, 65, and 75 dB SPL. Then, a high-level (85–90 dB SPL) swept pure tone should be presented to ensure that the MPO is appropriate (i.e., the maximum power output is set high enough to maximize usable headroom without exceeding the recommended maximum output of the prescriptive method). Figure 24–26 provides an example of real-ear probe microphone results for the EAS user with

the audiogram shown in Figure 24–25. The author does not typically provide acoustic amplification for frequencies with pure-tone thresholds of 80 to 85 dB HL or higher. However, some researchers (Baer, Moore, & Kluk, 2002) have suggested that it may be beneficial to provide amplification up to one octave above the start frequency of a dead region. With that in mind, some subjects may benefit from a wider acoustic bandwidth than is suggested in this text. The audiologist should consider evaluating for the presence of cochlear dead regions to determine whether audible amplification should be provided at a frequency at which the hearing loss is in the severe range (i.e., 75 dB HL or poorer).

After the fitting of the acoustic component, the author recommends determining the low-frequency boundary of the electrical signal by noting the last acoustic frequency that meets each of the following criteria: (1) the output of the acoustic component meets the prescriptive target for the 65 dB SPL speech signal, and (2) the frequency possesses an air conduction threshold of 75 dB HL or better. Electrical allocation should be provided at the lowest frequency at which the output of the acoustic component does

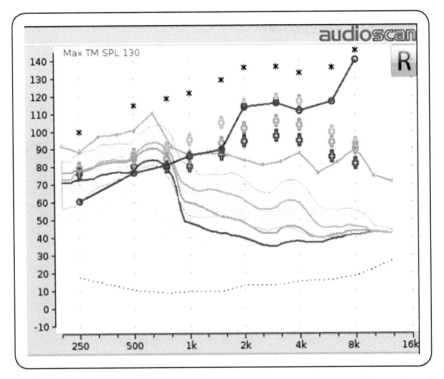

FIGURE 24–26. An example real-ear probe microphone measurements with matching of the output of the EAS sound processor's acoustic receiver to evidence-based prescriptive targets.

not match the evidence-based prescriptive target (i.e., minimizing EAS gap and overlap by implementing **the "meet" approach**). Figure 24–27 provides an example of electrical allocation based on the results of the real-ear probe microphone testing shown in Figure 24–26.

Next, electrical threshold levels (i.e., T levels) will need to be measured for all functional intra-cochlear electrode contacts in the same manner as T-level measurements are made with a conventional cochlear implant recipient. Then, upper-stimulation levels are also determined in the electric-only mode in the same manner that upper-stimulation levels are optimized with a conventional cochlear implant recipient. Specifically, upper-stimulation levels can be adjusted globally to the recipient's most comfortable listening level with the volume control set at a level that allows the recipient ample headroom so that she/he may increase or decrease stimulation as needed in real world use. The audiologist should then balance upper-stimulation levels in loudness across the electrode array. Following loudness balancing, the audiologist can once again adjust the upper-stimulation levels globally to the recipient's most comfort-

able listening level (MCL) at a volume control setting that provides for both an increase or decrease in stimulation during real world use. Furthermore, the audiologist should alternate between the ipsilateral acoustic only and electric only conditions to ensure that the loudness is balanced between the two modes of stimulation. Finally, the audiologist will need to ensure that the loudness of the signal provided via the EAS device is similar to the loudness provided by the hearing technology used on the opposite ear.

As previously mentioned, additional research is needed to precisely determine how acoustic and electric allocation should be optimized for EAS users. For recipients who are struggling to perform well with EAS settings that are based on the fitting protocol mentioned above, the audiologist should ensure that electrical stimulation levels are optimized. Ideally, sound-field warbled tone thresholds should be obtained in the 20 to 25 dB HL range with use of the EAS device. If sound-field thresholds are elevated, then the audiologist may need to adjust the electric or acoustic settings depending on the frequency range at which the recipient's thresholds are elevated. If the audiologist is convinced that stimulation levels

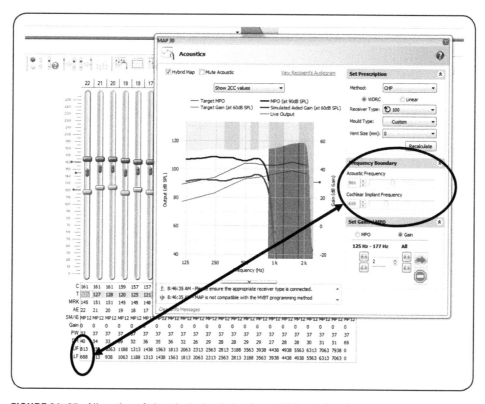

FIGURE 24–27. Allocation of electrical stimulation for an EAS recipient. Image provided courtesy of Cochlear Americas, ©2018.

are optimized, then attention should be directed toward optimizing the acoustic-electric allocation. Given the Gifford et al. (2017) study that suggested that many EAS recipients who used conventional-length electrode arrays benefited from electrical allocation down to 438 Hz, the audiologist may consider lowering the electric cutoff frequency for recipients who have conventional-length electrode arrays and whose electrical cutoff frequency is set to a higher frequency based on probe microphone results and the "Meet" strategy. The audiologist may also choose to measure for cochlear dead regions to determine whether acoustic amplification may be causing distortion due to being delivered to a nonfunctional area of the cochlea.

The Future of EAS

Additional research will need to be conducted to continue to examine the behavioral and subjective benefit of EAS with hybrid implants as well as the optimal programming parameters for the electrical stimulation from the implant and acoustic gain from the hearing aid. It is likely that the clinical protocol suggested in this chapter will evolve and change as more knowledge pertaining to the management of EAS devices is acquired. Additionally, more research is needed to identify electrode array technologies, surgical techniques, and pharmaceutical developments that may enhance the likelihood of hearing preservation after cochlear implantation.

Key Concepts

The reader should understand the potential benefits of EAS, programming considerations for hybrid implants, and the following key concepts:

- Hybrid implants are currently commercially distributed in the United States, and each manufacturer offers an implant array that is designed to enhance the likelihood of low-frequency hearing preservation. Hearing preservation is possible with hybrid electrode arrays as well as with long and perimodiolar electrode arrays. Advanced Bionics, Cochlear, and MED-EL all distribute an EAS processor.

- On average, EAS provides superior behavioral and subjective performance over the preoperative condition with hearing aids, the electric-only condition, and the hearing aid alone condition. The benefits of EAS are most prominent in acoustically complex environments. Individuals with precipitously sloping severe to profound high-frequency hearing loss are likely to achieve optimal performance with the use of bilateral EAS.

- When programming hybrid implants, the audiologist will need to consider the frequency range for the electrical stimulation, the prescriptive fitting strategy for the hearing aid, and the cutoff frequency for the hearing aid. Real-ear probe microphone measurements should be completed to determine the gain and output of the acoustic receiver of the EAS sound processor.

References

Adunka, O., & Kiefer, J. (2006). Impact of electrode insertion depth on intracochlear trauma. *Otolaryngology–Head and Neck Surgery, 135*(3), 374–382.

Adunka, O., Kiefer, J., Unkelbach, M. H., Lehnert, T., & Gstoettner, W. (2004). Development and evaluation of an improved cochlear implant electrode design for electric acoustic stimulation. *Laryngoscope, 114*(7), 1237–1241.

Adunka, O. F., Pillsbury, H. C., Adunka, M. C., & Buchman, C. A. (2010). Is electric acoustic stimulation better than conventional cochlear implantation for speech perception in quiet? *Otology and Neurotology, 31*(7), 1049–1054.

Advanced Bionics. (2018). *The foundation of better hearing: AB implantable technology.* Retrieved from https://www.advancedbionics.com/content/dam/advancedbionics/Documents/Global/en_ce/Products/HiRes-Ultra/HiRes-Ultra-Brochure.pdf

Anagiotos, A., Hamdan, N., Lang-Roth, R., Gostian, A. O., Luers, J. C., Huttenbrink, K. B., & Beutner, D. (2015). Young age is a positive prognostic factor for residual hearing preservation in conventional cochlear implantation. *Otology and Neurotology, 36*(1), 28–33.

Aschendorff, A., Briggs, R., Brademann, G., Helbig, S., Hornung, J., Lenarz, T., . . . James, C. J. (2017). Clinical investigation of the Nucleus Slim Modiolar Electrode. *Audiology and Neurotology, 22*(3), 169–179.

Aschendorff, A., Kromeier, J., Klenzner, T., & Laszig, R. (2007). Quality control after insertion of the Nucleus contour and contour advance electrode in adults. *Ear and Hearing, 28*(2 Suppl), 75S–79S.

Baer, T., Moore, B. C., & Kluk, K. (2002). Effects of low pass filtering on the intelligibility of speech in noise for people with and without dead regions at high frequencies. *Journal of the Acoustical Society of America, 112*(3 Pt. 1), 1133–1144.

Balkany, T. J., Eshraghi, A. A., & Yang, N. (2002). Modiolar proximity of three perimodiolar cochlear implant electrodes. *Acta Otolaryngologica, 122*(4), 363–369.

Balkany, T., Hodges, A., Menapace, C., Hazard, L., Driscoll, C., Gantz, B., . . . Payne, S. (2007). Nucleus Freedom North American clinical trial. *Otolaryngology–Head and Neck Surgery, 136*(5), 757–762.

Baumann, U., & Helbig, S. (2009). [Hearing with combined electric acoustic stimulation]. *HNO, 57*(6), 542–550.

Baumann, U., Rader, T., Helbig, S., & Bahmer, A. (2011). Pitch matching psychometrics in electric acoustic stimulation. *Ear and Hearing, 32*(5), 656–662.

Baumgartner, W. D., Jappel, A., Morera, C., Gstottner, W., Muller, J., Kiefer, J., . . . Nielsen, S. B. (2007). Outcomes in adults implanted with the FLEX^soft electrode. *Acta Otolaryngologica, 127*(6), 579–586.

Boyle, P. J. (2016). The rationale for a mid-scala electrode array. *European Annals of Otorhinolaryngology, Head and Neck Disorders, 133*(Suppl. 1), S61–S62.

Briaire, J. J., & Frijns, J. H. (2006). The consequences of neural degeneration regarding optimal cochlear implant position in scala tympani: A model approach. *Hearing Research, 214*(1–2), 17–27.

Buchner, A., Schussler, M., Battmer, R. D., Stover, T., Lesinski-Schiedat, A., & Lenarz, T. (2009). Impact of low-frequency hearing. *Audiology and Neurotology, 14*(Suppl. 1), 8–13.

Byrne, D., Dillon, H., Ching, T., Katsch, R., & Keidser, G. (2001). NAL-NL1 procedure for fitting nonlinear hearing aids: Characteristics and comparisons with other procedures. *Journal of the American Academy of Audiology, 12*, 37–51.

Ching, T. Y., Dillon, H., & Byrne, D. (1998). Speech recognition of hearing-impaired listeners: Predictions from audibility and the limited role of high-frequency amplification. *Journal of the Acoustical Society of America, 103*(2), 1128–1140.

Chole, R. A., Hullar, T. E., & Potts, L. G. (2014). Conductive component after cochlear implantation in patients with residual hearing conservation. *American Journal of Audiology, 23*(4), 359–364.

Cohen, L. T., Saunders, E., & Clark, G. M. (2001). Psychophysics of a prototype perimodiolar cochlear implant electrode array. *Hearing Research, 155*(1–2), 63–81.

Cosetti, M. K., Friedmann, D. R., Zhu, B. Z., Heman-Ackah, S. E., Fang, Y., Keller, R. G., . . . Waltzman, S. B. (2013). The effects of residual hearing in traditional cochlear implant candidates after implantation with a conventional electrode. *Otology and Neurotology, 34*(3), 516–521.

Cox, R. M., Alexander, G. C., Johnson, J., & Rivera, I. (2011). Cochlear dead regions in typical hearing aid candidates: Prevalence and implications for use of high-frequency speech cues. *Ear and Hearing, 32*(3), 339–348.

Cox, R. M., Johnson, J. A., & Alexander, G. C. (2012). Implications of high-frequency cochlear dead regions for fitting hearing aids to adults with mild to moderately severe hearing loss. *Ear and Hearing, 33*(5), 573–587.

Dillon, M. T., Buss, E., Pillsbury, H. C., Adunka, O. F., Buchman, C. A., & Adunka, M. C. (2014). Effects of hearing aid settings for electric-acoustic stimulation. *Journal of the American Academy of Audiology, 25*(2), 133–140.

Dorman, M. F., & Gifford, R. H. (2010). Combining acoustic and electric stimulation in the service of speech recognition. *International Journal of Audiology, 49*(12), 912–919.

Dorman, M. F., & Gifford, R. H. (2017). Speech understanding in complex listening environments by listeners fit with cochlear implants. *Journal of Speech, Language, and Hearing Research, 60*(10), 3019–3026.

Dorman, M. F., Gifford, R., Lewis, K., McKarns, S., Ratigan, J., Spahr, A., . . . Loiselle, L. (2009). Word recognition following implantation of conventional and 10-mm hybrid electrodes. *Audiology and Neurotology, 14*(3), 181–189.

Dorman, M. F., Loizou, P. C., & Rainey, D. (1997). Simulating the effect of cochlear-implant electrode insertion depth on speech understanding. *Journal of the Acoustical Society of America, 102*(5 Pt. 1), 2993–2996.

Dorman, M. F., Spahr, A. J., Loiselle, L., Zhang, T., Cook, S., Brown, C., & Yost, W. (2013). Localization and speech understanding by a patient with bilateral cochlear implants and bilateral hearing preservation. *Ear and Hearing, 34*(2), 245–248.

Dunn, C. C., Perreau, A., Gantz, B., & Tyler, R. S. (2010). Benefits of localization and speech perception with multiple noise sources in listeners with a short-electrode cochlear implant. *Journal of the American Academy of Audiology, 21*(1), 44–51.

Erixon, E., Kobler, S., & Rask-Andersen, H. (2012). Cochlear implantation and hearing preservation: Results in 21 consecutively operated patients using the round window approach. *Acta Otolaryngologica, 132*(9), 923–931.

Eshraghi, A. A., Ahmed, J., Krysiak, E., Ila, K., Ashman, P., Telischi, F. F., . . . Valendia, S. (2017). Clinical, surgical, and electrical factors impacting residual hearing in cochlear implant surgery. *Acta Otolaryngologica, 137*(4), 384–388.

Esquia Medina, G. N., Borel, S., Nguyen, Y., Ambert-Dahan, E., Ferrary, E., Sterkers, O., & Grayeli, A. B. (2013). Is electrode-modiolus distance a prognostic factor for hearing performances after cochlear implant surgery? *Audiology and Neurotology, 18*(6), 406–413.

Fitzgerald, M. B., Sagi, E., Jackson, M., Shapiro, W. H., Roland, J. T., Jr., Waltzman, S. B., & Svirsky, M. A. (2008). Reimplantation of hybrid cochlear implant users with a full-length electrode after loss of residual hearing. *Otology and Neurotology, 29*(2), 168–173.

Fraysse, B., Macias, A. R., Sterkers, O., Burdo, S., Ramsden, R., Deguine, O., . . . James, C. (2006). Residual hearing conservation and electroacoustic stimulation with the Nucleus 24 contour advance cochlear implant. *Otology and Neurotology, 27*(5), 624–633.

Gantz, B. J., Dunn, C. C., Oleson, J., & Hansen, M. R. (2018). Acoustic plus electric speech processing: Long-term results. *Laryngoscope, 128*(2), 473–481.

Gantz, B. J., Hansen, M. R., Turner, C. W., Oleson, J. J., Reiss, L. A., & Parkinson, A. J. (2009). Hybrid 10 clinical trial: Preliminary results. *Audiology and Neurotology, 14*(Suppl. 1), 32–38.

Gantz, B. J., & Turner, C. (2004). Combining acoustic and electrical speech processing: Iowa/Nucleus hybrid implant. *Acta Otolaryngologica, 124*(4), 344–347.

Gantz, B., & Turner, C. (2011). *Combining acoustic and electric hearing.* New York, NY: Springer.

Gantz, B. J., Turner, C., & Gfeller, K. (2004). Expanding cochlear implant technology: Combined electrical and acoustical speech processing. *Cochlear Implants International, 5*(Suppl. 1), 8–14.

Gantz, B. J., Turner, C., & Gfeller, K. E. (2006). Acoustic plus electric speech processing: Preliminary results of a multicenter clinical trial of the Iowa/Nucleus Hybrid implant. *Audiology and Neurotology, 11*(Suppl. 1), 63–68.

Gantz, B. J., Turner, C., Gfeller, K. E., & Lowder, M. W. (2005). Preservation of hearing in cochlear implant surgery: Advantages of combined electrical and acoustical speech processing. *Laryngoscope, 115*(5), 796–802.

Gifford, R. H., Davis, T. J., Sunderhaus, L. W., Menapace, C., Buck, B., Crosson, J., . . . Segel, P. (2017). Combined electric and acoustic stimulation with hearing preservation: Effect of cochlear implant low-frequency cutoff on speech understanding and perceived listening difficulty. *Ear and Hearing, 38*(5), 539–553.

Gifford, R. H., Dorman, M. F., Brown, C., & Spahr, A. J. (2012). Hearing, psychophysics, and cochlear implantation: Experiences of older individuals with mild sloping to profound sensory hearing loss. *Journal of Hearing Science, 2*(4), 9–17.

Gifford, R. H., Dorman, M. F., Sheffield, S. W., Teece, K., & Olund, A. P. (2014). Availability of binaural cues for bilateral implant recipients and bimodal listeners with and without preserved hearing in the implanted ear. *Audiology and Neurotology, 19*(1), 57–71.

Gifford, R. H., Dorman, M. F., Skarzynski, H., Lorens, A., Polak, M., Driscoll, C. L., . . . Buchman, C. A. (2013). Cochlear implantation with hearing preservation yields significant benefit for speech recognition in complex listening environments. *Ear and Hearing, 34*(4), 413–425.

Gifford, R. H., Driscoll, C. L., Davis, T. J., Fiebig, P., Micco, A., & Dorman, M. F. (2015). A Within-subject comparison of bimodal hearing, bilateral cochlear implantation, and bilateral cochlear implantation with bilateral hearing preservation: High-performing patients. *Otology and Neurotology, 36*(8), 1331–1337.

Gifford, R. H., Grantham, D. W., Sheffield, S. W., Davis, T. J., Dwyer, R., & Dorman, M. F. (2014). Localization and interaural time difference (ITD) thresholds for cochlear implant recipients with preserved acoustic hearing in the implanted ear. *Hearing Research, 312*, 28–37.

Glista, D., Scollie, S., Bagatto, M., Seewald, R., Parsa, V., & Johnson, A. (2009). Evaluation of nonlinear frequency compression: Clinical outcomes. *International Journal of Audiology, 48*(9), 632–644.

Golub, J. S., Won, J. H., Drennan, W. R., Worman, T. D., & Rubinstein, J. T. (2012). Spectral and temporal measures in hybrid cochlear implant users: On the mechanism of electroacoustic hearing benefits. *Otology and Neurotology, 33*(2), 147–153.

Gordin, A., Papsin, B., James, A., & Gordon, K. (2009). Evolution of cochlear implant arrays result in changes in behavioral and physiological responses in children. *Otology and Neurotology, 30*(7), 908–915.

Greenwood, D. D. (1961). Critical bandwidth and the frequency coordinates of the basilar membrane. *Journal of the Acoustical Society of America, 33*, 1344–1356.

Greenwood, D. D. (1990). A cochlear frequency-position function for several species—29 years later. *Journal of the Acoustical Society of America, 87*(6), 2592–2605.

Gstoettner, W., & Arnoldner, C. (2008). Re: Reimplantation of hybrid cochlear implant users with a full-length electrode after loss of residual hearing. *Otology and Neurotology, 29*(6), 881; author reply 881–882.

Gstoettner, W., Kiefer, J., Baumgartner, W. D., Pok, S., Peters, S., & Adunka, O. (2004). Hearing preservation in cochlear implantation for electric acoustic stimulation. *Acta Otolaryngologica, 124*(4), 348–352.

Gstoettner, W. K., Van de Heyning, P., O'Connor, A. F., Kiefer, J., Morera, C., Sainz, M., . . . Helbig, S. (2011). Assessment of the subjective benefit of electric acoustic stimulation with the abbreviated profile of hearing aid benefit. *ORL Journal of Otorhinolaryngology and Related Specialties, 73*(6), 321–329.

Gstoettner, W. K., van de Heyning, P., O'Connor, A. F., Morera, C., Sainz, M., Vermeire, K., . . . Adunka, O. F. (2008). Electric acoustic stimulation of the auditory system: Results of a multicentre investigation. *Acta Otolaryngologica, 128*(9), 968–975.

Helbig, S., Helbig, M., Rader, T., Mack, M., & Baumann, U. (2009). Cochlear reimplantation after surgery for electric-acoustic stimulation. *ORL Journal of Otorhinolaryngology and Related Specialties, 71*(3), 172–178.

Hogan, C. A., & Turner, C. W. (1998). High-frequency audibility: Benefits for hearing-impaired listeners. *Journal of the Acoustical Society of America, 104*(1), 432–441.

Holden, L. K., Finley, C. C., Firszt, J. B., Holden, T. A., Brenner, C., Potts, L. G., . . . Skinner, M. W. (2013). Factors affecting open-set word recognition in adults with cochlear implants. *Ear and Hearing, 34*(3), 342–360.

Hornsby, B. W., & Ricketts, T. A. (2003). The effects of hearing loss on the contribution of high- and low-frequency speech information to speech understanding. *Journal of the Acoustical Society of America, 113*(3), 1706–1717.

Hornsby, B. W., & Ricketts, T. A. (2006). The effects of hearing loss on the contribution of high- and low-frequency speech information to speech understanding. II. Sloping hearing loss. *Journal of the Acoustical Society of America, 119*(3), 1752–1763.

Hornsby, B. W., & Ricketts, T. A. (2007). Effects of noise source configuration on directional benefit using symmetric and asymmetric directional hearing aid fittings. *Ear and Hearing, 28*(2), 177–186.

Hughes, M. L., & Abbas, P. J. (2006). Electrophysiologic channel interaction, electrode pitch ranking, and behavioral threshold in straight versus perimodiolar cochlear implant electrode arrays. *Journal of the Acoustical Society of America, 119*(3), 1538–1547.

Hughes, M. L., & Stille, L. J. (2010). Effect of stimulus and recording parameters on spatial spread of excitation and masking patterns obtained with the electrically evoked compound action potential in cochlear implants. *Ear and Hearing, 31*(5), 679–692.

Hunter, J. B., Gifford, R. H., Wanna, G. B., Labadie, R. F., Bennett, M. L., Haynes, D. S., & Rivas, A. (2016). Hearing preservation outcomes with a mid-scala electrode in cochlear implantation. *Otology and Neurotology, 37*(3), 235–240.

James, C., Albegger, K., Battmer, R., Burdo, S., Deggouj, N., Deguine, O., . . . Fraysse, B. (2005). Preservation of residual hearing with cochlear implantation: How and why. *Acta Otolaryngologica, 125*(5), 481–491.

Jeong, J., Kim, M., Heo, J. H., Bang, M. Y., Bae, M. R., Kim, J., & Choi, J. Y. (2015). Intraindividual comparison of psychophysical parameters between perimodiolar and lateral-type electrode arrays in patients with bilateral cochlear implants. *Otology and Neurotology, 36*(2), 228–234.

Karsten, S. A., Turner, C. W., Brown, C. J., Jeon, E. K., Abbas, P. J., & Gantz, B. J. (2013). Optimizing the combination of acoustic and electric hearing in the implanted ear. *Ear and Hearing, 34*(2), 142–150.

Kawano, A., Seldon, H. L., & Clark, G. M. (1996). Computer-aided three-dimensional reconstruction in human cochlear maps: Measurement of the lengths of organ of Corti, outer wall, inner wall, and Rosenthal's canal. *Annals of Otology, Rhinology, and Laryngology, 105*(9), 701–709.

Kiefer, J., Gstoettner, W., Baumgartner, W., Pok, S. M., Tillein, J., Ye, Q., & von Ilberg, C. (2004). Conservation of low-frequency hearing in cochlear implantation. *Acta Otolaryngologica, 124*(3), 272–280.

Kiefer, J., Pok, M., Adunka, O., Sturzebecher, E., Baumgartner, W., Schmidt, M., . . . Gstoettner, W. (2005). Combined electric and acoustic stimulation of the auditory system: Results of a clinical study. *Audiology and Neurotology, 10*(3), 134–144.

Kopelovich, J. C., Reiss, L. A., Oleson, J. J., Lundt, E. S., Gantz, B. J., & Hansen, M. R. (2014). Risk factors for loss of ipsilateral residual hearing after hybrid cochlear implantation. *Otology and Neurotology, 35*(8), 1403–1408.

Lenarz, T., James, C., Cuda, D., Fitzgerald O'Connor, A., Frachet, B., Frijns, J. H., . . . Uziel, A. (2013). European multi-centre study of the Nucleus Hybrid L24 cochlear implant. *International Journal of Audiology, 52*(12), 838–848.

Lenarz, T., Stover, T., Buechner, A., Lesinski-Schiedat, A., Patrick, J., & Pesch, J. (2009). Hearing conservation surgery using the Hybrid-L electrode. Results from the first clinical trial at the Medical University of Hannover. *Audiology and Neurotology, 14*(Suppl. 1), 22–31.

Lenarz, T., Zwartenkot, J. W., Stieger, C., Schwab, B., Mylanus, E. A., Caversaccio, M., . . . Mojallal, H. (2013). Multicenter study with a direct acoustic cochlear implant. *Otology and Neurotology, 34*(7), 1215–1225.

Loiselle, L. H., Dorman, M. F., Yost, W. A., Cook, S. J., & Gifford, R. H. (2016). Using ILD or ITD cues for sound source localization and speech understanding in a complex listening environment by listeners with bilateral and with hearing-preservation cochlear implants. *Journal of Speech, Language, and Hearing Research, 59*(4), 810–818.

Loiselle, L. H., Dorman, M. F., Yost, W. A., & Gifford, R. H. (2015). Sound source localization by hearing preservation patients with and without symmetrical low-frequency acoustic hearing. *Audiology and Neurotology, 20*(3), 166–171.

Luetje, C. M., Thedinger, B. S., Buckler, L. R., Dawson, K. L., & Lisbona, K. L. (2007). Hybrid cochlear implantation: Clinical results and critical review in 13 cases. *Otology and Neurotology, 28*(4), 473–478.

McMullen, N. T., & Glaser, E. M. (1988). Auditory cortical responses to neonatal deafening: pyramidal neuron spine loss without changes in growth or orientation. *Experimental Brain Research, 72*(1), 195–200.

McMullen, N. T., Goldberger, B., Suter, C. M., & Glaser, E. M. (1988). Neonatal deafening alters nonpyramidal dendrite orientation in auditory cortex: A computer microscope study in the rabbit. *Journal of Computational Neurology, 267*(1), 92–106.

Mick, P., Amoodi, H., Shipp, D., Friesen, L., Symons, S., Lin, V., . . . Chen, J. (2014). Hearing preservation with full insertion of the FLEX^soft electrode. *Otology and Neurotology, 35*(1),e40–e44.

Moore, B. C. (2001). Dead regions in the cochlea: Diagnosis, perceptual consequences, and implications for the fitting of hearing aids. *Trends in Amplification, 5*(1), 1–34.

Moore, B. C. (2008). The role of temporal fine structure processing in pitch perception, masking, and speech perception for normal-hearing and hearing-impaired people. *Journal of Associated Research in Otolaryngology, 9*(4), 399–406.

Moore, B. C., Vickers, D. A., Glasberg, B. R., & Baer, T. (1997). Comparison of real and simulated hearing impairment in subjects with unilateral and bilateral cochlear hearing loss. *British Journal of Audiology, 31*(4), 227–245.

Mowry, S. E., Woodson, E., & Gantz, B. J. (2012). New frontiers in cochlear implantation: acoustic plus electric hearing, hearing preservation, and more. *Otolaryngology Clinics of North America, 45*(1), 187–203.

Muller, A., Hocke, T., & Mir-Salim, P. (2015). Intraoperative findings on ECAP-measurement: Normal or special case? *International Journal of Audiology, 54*(4), 257–264.

Nguyen, Y., Mosnier, I., Borel, S., Ambert-Dahan, E., Bouccara, D., Bozorg-Grayeli, A., . . . Sterkers, O. (2013). Evolution of electrode array diameter for hearing preservation in cochlear implantation. *Acta Otolaryngologica, 133*(2), 116–122.

O'Connell, B. P., Cakir, A., Hunter, J. B., Francis, D. O., Noble, J. H., Labadie, R. F., . . . Wanna, G. B. (2016). Electrode location and angular insertion depth are predictors of audiologic outcomes in cochlear implantation. *Otology and Neurotology, 37*(8), 1016–1023.

O'Connell, B. P., Hunter, J. B., Gifford, R. H., Rivas, A., Haynes, D. S., Noble, J. H., & Wanna, G. B. (2016). Electrode location and audiologic performance after cochlear implantation: A comparative study between Nucleus CI422 and CI512 electrode arrays. *Otology and Neurotology, 37*(8), 1032–1035.

O'Connell, B. P., Hunter, J. B., & Wanna, G. B. (2016). The importance of electrode location in cochlear implantation. *Laryngoscope Investigative Otolaryngology, 1*(6), 169–174.

O'Leary, S. J., Richardson, R. R., & McDermott, H. J. (2009). Principles of design and biological approaches for improving the selectivity of cochlear implant electrodes. *Journal of Neural Engineering, 6*(5), 055002.

Prentiss, S., Sykes, K., & Staecker, H. (2010). Partial deafness cochlear implantation at the University of Kansas: Techniques and outcomes. *Journal of the American Academy of Audiology, 21*(3), 197–203.

Rau, T. S., Harbach, L., Pawsey, N., Kluge, M., Erfurt, P., Lenarz, T., & Majdani, O. (2016). Insertion trauma of a cochlear implant electrode array with Nitinol inlay. *European Archives of Otorhinolaryngology, 273*(11), 3573–3585.

Reiss, L. A., Perreau, A. E., & Turner, C. W. (2012). Effects of lower frequency-to-electrode allocations on speech and pitch perception with the hybrid short-electrode cochlear implant. *Audiology and Neurotology, 17*(6), 357–372.

Richter, B., Jaekel, K., Aschendorff, A., Marangos, N., & Laszig, R. (2001). Cochlear structures after implantation of a perimodiolar electrode array. *Laryngoscope, 111*(5), 837–843.

Roland, J. T., Jr., Gantz, B. J., Waltzman, S. B., Parkinson, A. J., & Multicenter Clinical Trial, G. (2016). United States multicenter clinical trial of the cochlear Nucleus hybrid implant system. *Laryngoscope, 126*(1), 175–181.

Runge-Samuelson, C., Firszt, J. B., Gaggl, W., & Wackym, P. A. (2009). Electrically evoked auditory brainstem responses in adults and children: effects of lateral to medial placement of the Nucleus 24 contour electrode array. *Otology and Neurotology, 30*(4), 464–470.

Salloum, C. A., Valero, J., Wong, D. D., Papsin, B. C., van Hoesel, R., & Gordon, K. A. (2010). Lateralization of interimplant timing and level differences in children who use bilateral cochlear implants. *Ear and Hearing, 31*(4), 441–456.

Scollie, S., Seewald, R., Cornelisse, L., Moodie, S., Bagatto, M., Laurnagaray, D., . . . Pumford, J. (2005). The desired sensation level multistage input/output algorithm. *Trends in Amplification, 4*(9), 159–197.

Sheffield, S. W., Jahn, K., & Gifford, R. H. (2015). Preserved acoustic hearing in cochlear implantation improves speech perception. *Journal of the American Academy of Audiology, 26*(2), 145–154.

Simpson, A., Hersbach, A. A., & McDermott, H. J. (2006). Frequency-compression outcomes in listeners with steeply sloping audiograms. *International Journal of Audiology, 45*(11), 619–629.

Simpson, A., McDermott, H. J., & Dowell, R. C. (2005). Benefits of audibility for listeners with severe high-frequency hearing loss. *Hearing Research, 210*(1–2), 42–52.

Simpson, A., McDermott, H. J., Dowell, R. C., Sucher, C., & Briggs, R. J. (2009). Comparison of two frequency-to-electrode maps for acoustic-electric stimulation. *International Journal of Audiology, 48*(2), 63–73.

Skarzyński, H., Lorens, A., D'Haese, P., Walkowiak, A., Piotrowska, A., Sliwa, L., . . . Anderson, I. (2002). Preservation of residual hearing in children and post-lingually deafened adults after cochlear implantation: An initial study. *ORL: Journal for Otorhinolaryngology and Its Related Specialties, 64*(4), 247–253.

Skarzyński, H., Lorens, A., Matusiak, M., Porowski, M., Skarzynski, P. H., & James, C. J. (2012). Partial deafness treatment with the nucleus straight research array cochlear implant. *Audiology and Neurotology, 17*(2), 82–91.

Skarzyński, H., Lorens, A., Matusiak, M., Porowski, M., Skarzynski, P. H., & James, C. J. (2014). Cochlear implantation with the Nucleus slim straight electrode in subjects with residual low-frequency hearing. *Ear and Hearing, 35*(2), e33–e43.

Skarzyński, H., Lorens, A., Piotrowska, A., & Anderson, I. (2007). Preservation of low-frequency hearing in partial deafness cochlear implantation (PDCI) using the round window surgical approach. *Acta Otolaryngologica, 127*(1), 41–48.

Skarzyński, H., Lorens, A., Piotrowska, A., & Podskarbi-Fayette, R. (2009). Results of partial deafness cochlear implantation using various electrode designs. *Audiology and Neurotology, 14*(Suppl. 1), 39–45.

Smith, Z. M., Delgutte, B., & Oxenham, A. J. (2002). Chimaeric sounds reveal dichotomies in auditory perception. *Nature, 416*(6876), 87–90.

Stanislawek-Sut, O., Morawski, K., & Niemczyk, K. (2013). Hearing preservation results after cochlear implantation in short-term and long-term observation. *Otolaryngologia Polska, 67*(3), 135–138.

Stakhovskaya, O., Sridhar, D., Bonham, B. H., & Leake, P. A. (2007). Frequency map for the human cochlear spiral ganglion: Implications for cochlear implants. *Journal of Assocaited Research in Otolaryngology, 8*(2), 220–233.

Stelmachowicz, P. G., Lewis, D. E., Choi, S., & Hoover, B. (2007). Effect of stimulus bandwidth on auditory skills in normal-hearing and hearing-impaired children. *Ear and Hearing, 28*(4), 483–494.

Summers, V. (2004). Do tests for cochlear dead regions provide important information for fitting hearing aids? *Journal of the Acoustical Society of America, 115*(4), 1420–1423.

Sweeney, A. D., Hunter, J. B., Carlson, M. L., Rivas, A., Bennett, M. L., Gifford, R. H., . . . Wanna, G. B. (2016). Durability of hearing preservation after cochlear implantation with conventional-length electrodes and scala tympani insertion. *Otolaryngology–Head and Neck Surgery, 154*(5), 907–913.

Turner, C. W. (2006). Hearing loss and the limits of amplification. *Audiology and Neurotology, 11*(Suppl. 1), 2–5.

Turner, C. W., & Cummings, K. J. (1999). Speech audibility for listeners with high-frequency hearing loss. *American Journal of Audiology, 8*(1), 47–56.

Turner, C. W., Reiss, L. A., & Gantz, B. J. (2008). Combined acoustic and electric hearing: Preserving residual acoustic hearing. *Hearing Research, 242*(1–2), 164–171.

Verbist, B. M., Joemai, R. M., Briaire, J. J., Teeuwisse, W. M., Veldkamp, W. J., & Frijns, J. H. (2010). Cochlear coordinates in regard to cochlear implantation: A clinically individually applicable 3-dimensional CT-based method. *Otology and Neurotology, 31*(5), 738–744.

Vermeire, K., Anderson, I., Flynn, M., & Van de Heyning, P. (2008). The influence of different speech processor and hearing aid settings on speech perception outcomes in electric acoustic stimulation patients. *Ear and Hearing, 29*(1), 76–86.

Vickers, D. A., Moore, B. C., & Baer, T. (2001). Effects of low-pass filtering on the intelligibility of speech in quiet for people with and without dead regions at high frequencies. *Journal of the Acoustical Society of America, 110*(2), 1164–1175.

von Ilberg, C. A., Baumann, U., Kiefer, J., Tillein, J., & Adunka, O. F. (2011). Electric-acoustic stimulation of the auditory system: A review of the first decade. *Audiology and Neurotology, 16*(Suppl. 2), 1–30.

Wackym, P. A., Firszt, J. B., Gaggl, W., Runge-Samuelson, C. L., Reeder, R. M., & Raulie, J. C. (2004). Electrophysiologic effects of placing cochlear implant electrodes in a perimodiolar position in young children. *Laryngoscope, 114*(1), 71–76.

Wanna, G. B., Noble, J. H., Gifford, R. H., Dietrich, M. S., Sweeney, A. D., Zhang, D., . . . Labadie, R. F. (2015). Impact of intrascalar electrode location, electrode type, and angular insertion depth on residual hearing in cochlear implant patients: Preliminary results. *Otology and Neurotology, 36*(8), 1343–1348.

Wanna, G. B., O'Connell, B. P., Francis, D. O., Gifford, R. H., Hunter, J. B., Holder, J. T., . . . Haynes, D. S. (2018). Predictive factors for short- and long-term hearing preservation in cochlear implantation with conventional-length electrodes. *Laryngoscope, 128*(2), 482–489.

Woodson, E. A., Reiss, L. A., Turner, C. W., Gfeller, K., & Gantz, B. J. (2011). The Hybrid cochlear implant: A review. *Advances in Otorhinolaryngology, 67*, 125–134.

Zanetti, D., Nassif, N., & Redaelli de Zinis, L. O. (2015). Factors affecting residual hearing preservation in cochlear implantation. *Acta Otorhinolaryngologica Italica, 35*(6), 433–441.

Zhang, T., Dorman, M. F., Gifford, R., & Moore, B. C. (2014). Cochlear dead regions constrain the benefit of combining acoustic stimulation with electric stimulation. *Ear and Hearing, 35*(4), 410–417.

Auditory Brainstem Implants

Jace Wolfe

As discussed in detail in previous chapters in this textbook, the cochlear implant is the most successful sensory prosthetic device in medicine and has been used to provide impressive open-set speech recognition capacity and hearing performance in hundreds of thousands of persons with severe to profound hearing loss. However, there exists a minority of persons who have severe to profound hearing loss and who cannot derive useful benefit from a cochlear implant. For instance, neurofibromatosis type 2 is a genetic disorder that causes a proliferation of benign tumor growth, with the most common type of tumors being vestibular schwannomas. Acoustic neuroma may also form in individuals who have neurofibromatosis type 2 syndrome. These tumors can be life-threatening because they compress the brainstem as well as surround cranial nerves and vascular structures. As a result, neurosurgeons must remove these tumors, and during resection, the cochlear nerve is often injured. Additionally, the proliferation of tumor growth may cause considerable degeneration of the cochlear nerve. Consequently, most individuals who lose their hearing because of neurofibromatosis do not receive benefit from cochlear implantation. Other disorders that preclude benefit from cochlear implants include a severed cochlear nerve from a temporal bone fracture, congenital cochlear nerve aplasia, cochlear aplasia, and cochlear ossification.

Auditory brainstem implants may be considered for persons who have severe to profound hearing loss with cochlear or cochlear nerve anatomy that is not conducive to cochlear implantation. The Cochlear Nucleus ABI541 auditory brainstem implant is shown in Figure 25–1. Auditory brainstem implants function similarly to cochlear implants, but instead of containing an electrode array that is housed on a wire that is inserted into the cochlear, the electrode contacts of an auditory brainstem implant are typically housed on a layer of silicone that resembles a paddle. The auditory brainstem implant system contains two components, an external sound processor and the auditory brainstem implant. The external sound processor typically contains an ear-level sound processor that is coupled to an external transmitting coil that surrounds a magnet. The auditory brainstem implant contains an internal receiving coil that also surrounds a magnet, the internal processor/stimulator (current generator), an electrode lead, and an electrode array.

The electrode array is typically placed over the cochlear nucleus and held in place with a mesh backing. The magnet of the external coil allows adherence to and alignment with the magnet of the internal coil. However, the magnet of an auditory brainstem implant may be removed and the external coil may be held in place with an adhesive disk or a headband so that the recipient may undergo serial MRI assessment after implantation, which is of particular importance to individuals with neurofibromatosis. The audio signal is captured by the microphones of the sound processor and delivered to the digital signal processor for analysis. The processed electrical signal is then delivered to the external coil, where

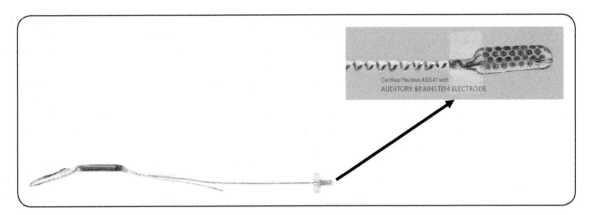

FIGURE 25–1. The Cochlear Nucleus ABI541 auditory brainstem implant. Image provided courtesy of Cochlear Americas, ©2018.

it is converted to an electromagnetic signal that is transmitted to the internal coil of the implant via short-range radio frequency transmission. The signal received by the internal coil is converted to an electrical current that is delivered to the implant's processor, where it is analyzed and converted to electrical pulses. The electrical pulses are then delivered to the electrode contacts on the paddle that resides on the cochlear nucleus.

In 1979, William House, M.D., an otologic surgeon who was one of the pioneers of cochlear implant technology, and colleagues placed a single ball electrode on the cochlear nucleus of a patient who had a severed cochlear nerve secondary to neurofibromatosis type 2 syndrome (Hitselberger et al., 1984). The patient was able to experience auditory sensations from the auditory brainstem implant and used the device for over three decades. Because of this success, Dr. House and colleagues collaborated with Cochlear Ltd. to develop a multiple-channel auditory brainstem implant. In the 1990s and early 2000s, MED-EL and Advanced Bionics also developed auditory brainstem implants.

Assessment of Candidacy for Auditory Brainstem Implants

The U.S. FDA has approved the Cochlear Nucleus ABI541 and the Cochlear Nucleus ABI24M for use in individuals who are 12 years of age and older and who have lost their hearing because of neurofibromatosis type 2 syndrome. There are no specific audiometric criteria listed in the FDA-approved indications

for use for the Cochlear Nucleus auditory brainstem implants. However, an auditory brainstem implant is often implanted during the same surgical procedure in which tumors are resected and the cochlear nerve is severed. Although it is not approved by the FDA in the United States, the auditory brainstem implant may also be considered for adults and children who have lost their hearing because of cochlear nerve injury secondary to a temporal bone fracture and for individuals who have suffered cochlear ossification secondary to bacterial meningitis. Individuals who have lost their hearing after contracting bacterial meningitis are typically provided with a cochlear implant prior to consideration of an auditory brainstem implant. Additionally, auditory brainstem implants may be considered for persons who have cochlear ossification from otosclerosis and for individuals who had a cochlear implant that failed but a replacement cannot be provided because of fibrous tissue growth in the cochlea.

Auditory brainstem implants may also be considered for children who have congenital hearing loss and who meet the following criteria:

- Congenital cochlear nerve aplasia and/or cochlear aplasia (i.e., no cochlea)
- Bilateral profound hearing loss
- 18 months to 5 years of age
- Strong family support with a commitment to postoperative habilitation and realistic expectations regarding outcomes following implantation

Children who are being considered for an auditory brainstem implant should typically undergo a failed trial with a cochlear implant. Although an MRI assessment may suggest cochlear nerve aplasia, cochlear implantation should still be pursued to determine whether an auditory response may be elicited with use of a cochlear implant. An auditory brainstem implant may be considered if an auditory response cannot be obtained with stimulation from a cochlear implant. Delaying the provision of an auditory brainstem implant until 18 months of age allows for the completion of a cochlear implant trial. Additionally, children under the age of 12 months present a greater risk for complication during auditory brainstem implant surgery. The child's family should be informed that the outcomes obtained with an auditory brainstem implant are poorer than outcomes obtained with cochlear implants and that their child may not develop open-set speech recognition and spoken language with use of the auditory brainstem implant. Most children who receive cochlear implants are able to develop spoken language without the need for sign language (in fact, children who have cochlear implants and do not use sign language typically develop better spoken language abilities than children who use sign language). However, sign language should be used with children who receive auditory brainstem implants to ensure that the child has access to a usable method of communication to allow for language development.

The auditory brainstem implant assessment team should include an otologic surgeon, a neurosurgeon, a neuroradiologist, an audiologist, an electrophysiologist, and in many cases, a speech-language pathologist. A psychologist may also be included if the team has concerns about the candidate's psychosocial-emotional status. Candidates typically undergo a comprehensive audiometric assessment to evaluate air- and bone-conduction thresholds and speech recognition ability with use of appropriately fitted hearing aids. Auditory brainstem assessment will likely need to be conducted along with behavioral audiometric measures with infants and young children to confirm the degree and configuration of hearing status. Imaging assessment is a vital component of the auditory brainstem implant assessment. Specifically, an MRI is completed to evaluate the anatomy of the cochlear nerve as well as the cerebrum, brainstem, and cranial nerves. The surgeon will likely also want to review a CT scan to evaluate bony anatomy in preparation for the surgery. Counseling is also a critical part of the assessment process. The auditory brainstem implant team must ensure that the candidate and his/her family members are aware that

many auditory brainstem recipients do not acquire open-set speech recognition after implantation. Instead, the auditory brainstem implant may merely provide awareness of sound and may serve as an aid to improve the recipient's speech reading ability. The team should also discuss the likely need for the recipient to rely on visual forms of communication, including sign language, text and closed caption, and so forth.

Auditory brainstem implant surgery requires the surgeon to perform a craniotomy (i.e., removal of part of the skull) so that the implant's electrode array can be inserted through the fourth ventricle and onto the surface of the cochlear nucleus. Two basic surgical approaches are used to gain access to the cochlear nucleus, the translabyrinthine approach and the retrosigmoid approach. The translabyrinthine approach involves removal of the mastoid bone behind the auricle as well as the semicircular canals of the inner ear. The translabyrinthine approach generally eliminates the possibility of preserving residual hearing, and as a result, it is not used if the surgeon desires to attempt to preserve any residual hearing that the patient may have. The translabyrinthine approach is desirable for auditory brainstem implantation because it provides good visualization of the lateral recess of the fourth ventricle (Cole et al., 2015). Moreover, the translabyrinthine approach does not require retraction of the cerebellum and provides good visualization of the facial nerve. The retrosigmoid approach is less invasive and involves an incision made behind the auricle and accessing the brainstem and cerebellum through a small opening (i.e., "keyhole" opening) that is made near the base of the skull. The retrosigmoid approach requires retraction of the cerebellum and does not provide complete visualization of the facial nerve. However, the retrosigmoid approach does enable removal of skull-based tumors and provides improved visualization of the cochlear nerve, which enhances the likelihood of preserving residual hearing (Cole et al., 2015). Consequently, the retrosigmoid approach may be used to remove tumors from patients who have neurofibromatosis type 2 and some functional hearing that is desirable to preserve. If intraoperative auditory brainstem response assessment indicates preservation of auditory function after tumor removal, then the auditory brainstem implant would not be provided. In short, the choice of whether to proceed with a translabyrinthine or retrosigmoid approach is dependent on several factors, including the surgeon's preference.

Auditory brainstem implant surgery is completed while the recipient is under general anesthesia. The objective of cochlear implant electrode array insertion is quite clear. The surgeon attempts to insert the electrode array into the scala tympani to a predetermined depth. In contrast, the optimal location of the electrode array is less clear during auditory brainstem implantation. Because the recipient is unconscious during the procedure, an audiologist is typically present to complete electrically evoked auditory brainstem response measurements with stimuli delivered from the electrode contacts of the implant. The surgeon's objective is to place the electrode array at a location that will generate a robust auditory brainstem response from the largest number of electrodes. Because the signal is not passing through the peripheral auditory system, wave V of the electrically evoked auditory brainstem response typically occurs between 2 and 3 msec (Waring, 1995). The relatively short latency of the electrically evoked auditory brainstem response allows the audiologist to differentiate the auditory response from responses of other nearby cranial nerves or neural structures, which are likely to have slightly longer latency responses. During auditory brainstem implant surgery, an electrophysiologist should be present to evaluate the integrity and function of nearby cranial nerves V, VII, VIII (if it is not already being monitored by the audiologist), IX, and XI. The auditory brainstem implant surgery is likely to take substantially longer to complete than a cochlear implant surgery, particularly for patients who have neurofibromatosis type 2 and require tumor removal. Additionally, cochlear implantation is usually an outpatient procedure, whereas auditory brainstem recipients are usually hospitalized for several days to allow for recovery from the more invasive procedure.

Postoperative Management of Recipients of Auditory Brainstem Implants

Auditory brainstem implant recipients typically return in four to eight weeks for device activation. The programming of an auditory brainstem implant contains both some similarities to and some differences from the programming of a cochlear implant. As with a cochlear implant, the audiologist must determine electrical threshold and upper-stimulation levels for each electrode contact. There are, however, many tasks that are central to the programming of an auditory brainstem implant but only performed in exceptional cases of cochlear implant programming. For example, the likelihood of eliciting a non-auditory side effect with stimulation from an auditory brainstem is much higher than with a cochlear implant. The electrode array of an auditory brainstem implant is in close proximity to several neural structures other than the cochlear nucleus, and as a result, it is fairly common to facilitate non-auditory responses. Examples of non-auditory responses include a tingling sensation that may occur throughout the ipsilateral side of the body (e.g., face, shoulder arm, torso, leg) (Colletti, Shannon, & Colletti, 2012). These tingling tactile sensations are likely caused by electrical stimulation of the cerebellar peduncle. The recipient may also report dizziness and experience nystagmus from electrical stimulation of the cerebellar flocculus or vestibular system (Colletti, Shannon, & Colletti, 2012). Facial nerve stimulation is another possible side effect. Additionally, the audiologist should be aware of the possibility of eliciting a response from the cardiac system by electrically stimulating the vasoactive centers of the brainstem (e.g., cranial nerve X). The threat of eliciting an adverse cardiac or respiratory response via stimulation for an auditory brainstem response is rare, but most auditory brainstem implant teams take precautions to ensure the safety of the recipient during activation. Specifically, programming during initial activation usually takes place within close proximity to emergency medical services. In many cases, the programming audiologist will disable electrodes that produce non-auditory side effects. However, if the side effect is minor (e.g., subtle tingling), the audiologist may attempt to increase the pulse width of the electrical pulse or change the electrode coupling mode (e.g., switch to a more narrow bipolar mode) to avoid the nonauditory side effect.

After the audiologist identifies the electrodes that facilitate an auditory response, he/she can commence with measuring electrical threshold and upper-stimulation level for all active electrodes. Then, the audiologist should attempt to ensure that the pitch changes in an orderly and expected manner across the active electrodes. Unlike the cochlea, which is tonotopically organized in a predictable manner from base to apex, the tonotopic organization of the cochlear nucleus is quite variable. Furthermore, the cochlear nucleus is not necessarily tonotopically organized along its surface, but instead, it is organized in a complex manner with low-frequency sounds primarily being processed at the ventrolateral region of the cochlear nucleus and high-frequency sounds processed in the dorsomedial region (Sando, 1965; Webster, 1971). As a result, the audiologist must complete pitch-scaling and arrange the channel-to-electrode relationship so that stimulation of low-frequency channels elicit a low pitch and high-frequency channels elicit a high pitch and so that the pitch progresses as expected across the multiple channels within the device. Obviously, most infants and young children will be unable to complete the pitch-scaling task. After pitch-scaling is completed, the audiologist should ensure that loudness is balanced at upper-stimulation level across the electrode array. Finally, upper-stimulation levels should be globally adjusted in live speech mode to the recipient's most comfortable listening level. Again, the audiologist should identify any non-auditory side effects and/or aversive effects that occur during live speech mode. If an issue is identified, the audiologist should sweep stimulation at upper-stimulation level across the electrode array in an attempt to identify the offensive electrode.

The auditory brainstem recipient should be seen for audiologic follow-up several times during the first few months of device use and at least twice a year after the first year of use. Young children should likely be seen at least quarterly for the first several years after implantation to ensure that progress is optimized. Because speech recognition outcomes with auditory brainstem implants are typically not as good as what occurs with cochlear implants, the audiologist will need to be prepared to administer closed-set speech recognition tests, such as the Early Speech Perception (ESP) Test (Moog & Geers, 1990), Children's Perception of Speech (NU-CHIPS) (Elliott & Katz, 1980), and the like, to evaluate speech perception. For recipients who do develop some open-set speech recognition capacity, open-set measures

of speech recognition, such as the CNC monosyllabic word test, Central Institute for the Deaf Overlearned Sentences, Hearing In Noise Test (HINT) administered in quiet (Nilsson, Soli, & Sullivan, 1994), and so forth, should be administered to determine the extent of the recipient's speech perception ability. Warbled tone sound-field detection thresholds should be measured with the objective of providing satisfactory audibility for low-level sounds.

Cochlear Nucleus ABI24M and ABI541 Auditory Brainstem Implants

The Cochlear Nucleus ABI24M auditory brainstem implant (Figure 25–2) was the first auditory brainstem implant approved by the FDA (in 2000) for commercial distribution in the United States. The Nucleus ABI24M is also used in other parts of the world, including Europe and Australia. The ABI24M is similar to the Cochlear Nucleus 24 cochlear implant but includes 21 platinum electrode contacts that are housed on a flexible silicone paddle with a Dacron mesh backing that is used to adhere the electrode array to the auditory structures of the brainstem. The ABI24M contains a removable magnet in the center of the internal receiving coil. The magnet will likely be left in place for recipients who do not have a history of tumor growth (e.g., severed cochlear nerve from temporal bone fracture, aplastic cochlear nerve), but for patients with neurofibromatosis type 2 syndrome, the magnet should be removed, and the external coil of the sound processor will be held in place by an

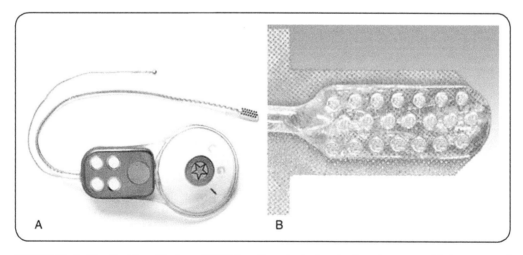

FIGURE 25–2. The Cochlear Nucleus ABI24M auditory brainstem implant. Image provided courtesy of Cochlear Americas, ©2018.

adhesive disc. Removal of the magnet allows for serial MRI assessment after implantation.

At the time of this writing, the Nucleus 6 is the latest processor that is compatible for use with the Nucleus ABI24M implant. The same signal coding strategies used with Nucleus cochlear implants are available for use with the Nucleus auditory brainstem implant. Although the Nucleus ABI24M implant is capable of operating the Advanced Combination Encoder (ACE) and Continuous Interleaved Sampling (CIS) signal coding strategies, only the SPEAK signal coding strategy is approved for use by the FDA. The Nucleus ABI24M is programmed by the audiologist using the same Custom Sound programming software used to program Nucleus cochlear implants. As with Nucleus cochlear implants, a fundamental

component of the ABI24M programming process is the measurement of T and C levels. In contrast to programming Nucleus cochlear implants, when activating a Nucleus ABI24M, the audiologist must spend a relatively considerable amount of time completing pitch scaling measurements and allocating the channel-to-electrode relationship so that the pitch changes in an orderly and expected manner from low- to high-frequency channels. The channel-to-electrode relationship is adjusted by changing the active electrode ("AE") associated with each channel (Figure 25–3). Electrodes that do not elicit an auditory response or that elicit a non-auditory side effect may be disabled by right clicking on the channel corresponding to the electrode in question and selecting "Disable Channel."

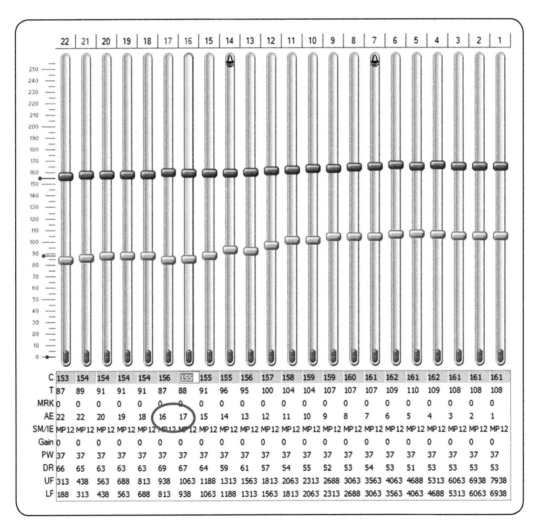

FIGURE 25–3. Adjusting the channel-to-electrode relationship in the Custom Sound programming software. Image provided courtesy of Cochlear Americas, ©2018.

The FDA has also approved the Nucleus Profile ABI541 auditory brainstem implant (see Figure 25–1). The Nucleus ABI541 contains the same case and electronics as the Nucleus 500 series cochlear implant. As a result, the ABI541 is much thinner than its predecessor, the ABI24M implant. The Nucleus ABI541 uses a paddle-shaped electrode array similar to what I used with the ABI24M implant. Moreover, the Nucleus ABI541 implant is compatible with the Nucleus 7 sound processor and may be used with the ACE signal coding strategy.

MED-EL Auditory Brainstem Implant

MED-EL manufactures an auditory brainstem implant that is not approved by the FDA for use in the United States but is approved for commercial distribution in Europe and in other countries around the world. The MED-EL auditory brainstem implant contains 12 electrode contacts that are housed on a paddle-shaped layer of silicone which is held on the brainstem with surgical mesh. At the time of this writing, the MED-EL auditory brainstem implant electrode array is coupled to the CONCERTO (Mi1000) implant receiver/body/stimulator. The magnet of the CONCERTO implant may be removed for recipients who are likely to require serial MRI assessments following implantation. Of note, the MED-EL auditory brainstem implant array has also been used with the MED-EL SYNCHRONY implant, which has a magnet that is compatible with MRI assessments of 3.0 tesla and less (Shew et al., 2017). As a result, the recipient of a MED-EL SYNCHRONY auditory brainstem implant may undergo MRI assessment with the magnet in place. The MED-EL CONCERTO auditory brainstem implant may be used with the OPUS 2 sound processor. The CIS signal coding strategy with monopolar stimulation is used with MED-EL auditory brainstem implants.

Advanced Bionics

Advanced Bionics developed an auditory brainstem implant that never received FDA approval for commercial distribution in the United States. Like its cochlear implants, the Advanced Bionics auditory brainstem implant had 16 electrode contacts which were housed on a paddle-shaped layer of silicone. Advanced Bionics no longer produces auditory brainstem implants.

Outcomes with Auditory Brainstem Implants

Outcomes with auditory brainstem implants are quite variable and are likely to be dependent upon several factors, including the etiology of the hearing loss, the extent of neural degeneration in the brainstem, the location of the electrode array relative to the auditory neural structures of the brainstem, the duration of deafness, the age at implantation, the recipient's neuro-cognitive status, and so forth. In short, research has clearly shown that individuals who do not have neurofibromatosis type 2 syndrome typically achieve a better outcome with auditory brainstem implants compared with recipients who have neurofibromatosis type 2 disorder. Otto and colleagues (2002) reported on the outcomes of 61 adults who had received auditory brainstem implants at the House Ear Institute. These recipients were typically able to perform slightly above chance levels on a test that evaluated their ability to recognize common environmental sounds. When speech recognition was evaluated in the audio+visual condition (i.e., sentences presented via video laser disc so that the talker could be seen on a video screen while producing the sentences), use of the auditory brainstem implant improved the recipients' ability to understand speech by an average of 26 percentage points compared with the visual-only condition. In short, the auditory brainstem implant served as an aid to improve communication when speechreading cues were available. However, only 4 out of the 61 recipients scored above 20% correct on open-set sentence recognition assessment in the audio-only condition, although one recipient did score above 60%. The mean open-set speech recognition score was less than 10% correct.

Vittorio Colletti is a neurotologic surgeon who has likely performed more auditory brainstem implant surgeries than anyone else in the world. Colletti and colleagues (2009) reported on the outcomes of 80 auditory brainstem recipients. Thirty-two of these recipients had a history of neurofibromatosis type 2 syndrome, whereas the other 48 recipients had a "non-tumor" history. Mean open-set speech recognition performance of the group with the neurofibromatosis type 2 history was 10% correct. In contrast, recipients who had a diagnosis of cochlear nerve aplasia or a severed nerve due to a temporal bone fracture achieved a mean score of almost 60% correct. Some recipients with cochlear nerve aplasia scored 100% on measures of open-set sentence recognition. Colletti et al. (2009) attributed the poor performance of recipients with neurofibromatosis type 2 syndrome to neural degeneration in the brainstem secondary to the proliferation of tumor growth.

In recognition of the relatively poor outcomes that individuals with neurofibromatosis type 2 syndrome achieve with auditory brainstem implants (along with recognition of the relatively poor outcomes of auditory brainstem recipients compared with cochlear implant recipients), researchers have explored novel ways to improve the hearing performance obtained with auditory brainstem implants. For instance, some groups have placed the electrode array of the auditory brainstem implant on the inferior colliculus (i.e., auditory nuclei of the midbrain) of individuals with neurofibromatosis type 2 syndrome (Colletti et al., 2006; Lenarz et al., 2006; Lim & Anderson, 2007a, 2007b; Lim & Lenarz, 2015; Lim, Lenarz, & Lenarz, 2009; Samii et al., 2006). The objective of auditory midbrain placement is to avoid the damaged neurons in the cochlear nucleus. Unfortunately,

studies evaluating the outcomes of individuals who had neurofibromatosis and who received an auditory midbrain implant have shown similar speech recognition results as have been obtained with electrode array placement on the cochlear nucleus (Colletti et al., 2006; Lim & Lenarz, 2015). Additional work is under way to explore methods to improve outcomes obtained with auditory midbrain implants (Lim & Lenarz, 2015).

Researchers have also explored the use of a penetrating electrode array which contains electrode contacts that are arranged as pins of various lengths and are designed to be inserted into the cochlear nucleus (Otto et al., 2008). The use of multiple-length electrode pins is intended to access multiple frequencies because the cochlear nucleus is tonotopically organized from the surface (low-frequency sounds) toward the center (high-frequency sounds) (Figure 25–4; Graham-Rowe, 2004). Otto and colleagues (2008) reported on the outcomes of 10 adults who

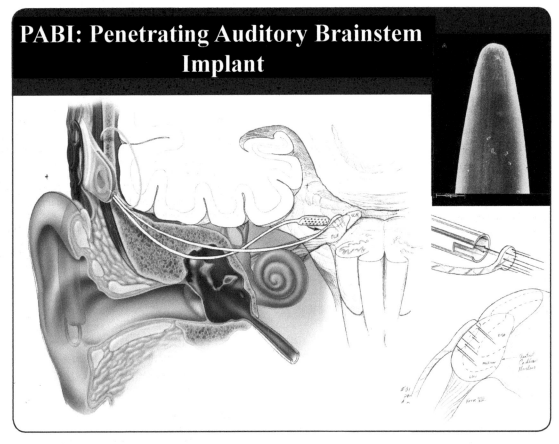

FIGURE 25–4. A visual illustration of an auditory brainstem implant with a penetrating electrode array. Image provided courtesy of Robert Shannon, PhD and the House Ear Institute.

received auditory brainstem implants with a penetrating electrode array. Although these recipients were able to obtain auditory sensation with use of the penetrating electrode array, there was no improvement in speech recognition compared with the outcomes typically obtained with an auditory brainstem implant with a surface electrode (Otto et al., 2008). Again, research is ongoing to explore new electrode arrays, signal coding strategies, and surgical techniques to improve the outcomes of auditory brainstem implant recipients (Lim & Lenarz, 2015).

Key Concepts

- Auditory brainstem implants may be considered for children and adults who have a site-of-lesion at the cochlear nerve and who consequently have failed to receive benefit from a cochlear implant.
- The Cochlear Nucleus auditory brainstem implant is approved by the FDA for use in individuals who are at least 12 years old and who have neurofibromatosis type 2 disorder.
- Auditory brainstem implants have been shown to improve sound detection/awareness for most recipients as well as to serve as an aid for speech reading. Some auditory brainstem recipients do obtain open-set speech recognition after implantation. Better outcomes are typically obtained for recipients who do not have a history of neurofibromatosis type 2 disorder or additional disabilities.
- An interdisciplinary health care professional must be available to provide the necessary services required for recipients of auditory brainstem implants to reach their full potential with the implant.

References

Cole, T., Veeravagu, A., Zhang, M., Azad, T., Swinney, C., Li, G. H., . . . Giannotta, S. L. (2015). Retrosigmoid versus translabyrinthine approach for acoustic neuroma resection: An assessment of complications and payments in a longitudinal administrative database. *Cureus, 7*(10), e369.

Colletti, L., Shannon, R., & Colletti, V. (2012). Auditory brainstem implants for neurofibromatosis type 2. *Current Opinion Otolaryngology–Head and Neck Surgery, 20*(5), 353–357.

Colletti, V., Shannon, R., Carner, M., Sacchetto, L., Turazzi, S., Masotto, B., & Colletti, L. (2006). The first successful case of hearing produced by electrical stimulation of the human midbrain. *Otology and Neurotology, 28*(1), 39–43.

Colletti, V., Shannon, R., Carner, M., Veronese, S., & Colletti, L. (2009). Outcomes in non-tumor adults fitted with the auditory brainstem implant: 10 years' experience. *Otology and Neurotology, 30*(5), 614–618.

Elliott, L.L., & Katz, D. (1980). *Development of a new children's test of speech discrimination* (Technical manual). St. Louis, MO: Audiotec.

Graham-Rowe, D. (2004, January 7). First brainstem implants aim to tackle deafness. *New Scientist.* Retrieved from https://www.newscientist.com/article/dn4540-first-brainstem-implants-aim-to-tackle-deafness/

Hitselberger, W. E., House, W. F., Edgerton, B. J., & Whitaker, S. (1984). Cochlear nucleus implants. *Otolaryngology–Head and Neck Surgery, 92*(1), 52–54.

Lenarz, T., Lim, H. H., Reuter, G., Patrick, J. F., & Lenarz, M. (2006). The auditory midbrain implant: A new auditory prosthesis for neural deafness-concept and device description. *Otology and Neurotology, 27*(6), 838–843.

Lim, H. H., & Anderson, D. J. (2007a). Spatially distinct functional output regions within the central nucleus of the inferior colliculus: Implications for an auditory midbrain implant. *Journal of Neuroscience, 27*(32), 8733–8743.

Lim, H. H., & Anderson, D. J. (2007b). Antidromic activation reveals tonotopically organized projections from primary auditory cortex to the central nucleus of the inferior colliculus in guinea pig. *Journal of Neurophysiology, 97*(2), 1413–1427.

Lim, H. H., Lenarz, M., & Lenarz, T. (2009). Auditory midbrain implant: A review. *Trends in Amplification, 13*(3), 149–180.

Lim, H. H., & Lenarz, T. (2015). Auditory midbrain implant: Research and development towards a second clinical trial. *Hearing Research, 322*, 212–223.

Moog, J. S., & Geers, A. E. (1990). *Early speech perception test for profoundly hearing-impaired children.* St. Louis, MO: Central Institute for the Deaf.

Otto, S. R., Brackmann, D. E., Hitselberger, W. E., Shannon, R. V., & Kuchta, J. (2002). Multichannel auditory brainstem implant: Update on performance in 61 patients. *Journal of Neurosurgery, 96*(6), 1063–1071.

Otto, S. R., Shannon, R. V., Wilkinson, E. P., Hitselberger, W. E., McCreery, D. B., Moore, J. K., & Brackmann, D. E. (2008). Audiologic outcomes with the penetrating electrode auditory brainstem implant. *Otology and Neurotology, 29*(8), 1147–1154.

Peterson, G. E., & Lehiste, I. (1962). Revised CNC lists for auditory tests. *Journal of Speech and Hearing Disorders, 27*, 62–70.

Samii, A., Lenarz, M., Majdani, O., Lim, H. H., Samii, M., & Lenarz, T. (2007). Auditory midbrain implant: A combined approach for vestibular schwannoma surgery and device implantation. *Otology and Neurotology, 28*(1), 31–38.

Sando, I. (1965). The anatomical interrelationships of the cochlear nerve fibers. *Acta Otolaryngologica, 59*, 417–436.

Shew, M., Bertsch, J., Camarata, P., & Staecker, H. (2017). Magnetic resonance imaging in a neurofibromatosis type 2 patient with a novel MRI-compatible auditory brainstem implant. *Journal of Neurological Surgery Reports, 78*(1), e12–e14.

Webster, D. B. (1971). Projection of the cochlea to cochlear nuclei in Merriam's kangaroo rat. *Journal of Computational Neurology, 143*(3), 323–340.

Waring, M. D. (1995). Intraoperative electrophysiologic monitoring to assist placement of auditory brainstem implant. *Annals of Otology, Rhinology, and Laryngology Supplement, 166*, 33–36.

26

Implantable Bone Conduction Hearing Devices

Jace Wolfe

Introduction

This chapter provides an introduction to osseointe-grated bone conduction hearing devices and other implantable bone conduction implants. The basic concept of implantable bone conduction hearing devices will be discussed along with a description of the candidacy criteria for implantable bone conduction hearing devices and other implantable bone conduction hearing devices. Additionally, the theoretical advantages and limitations of bone conduction hearing devices will be reviewed. Furthermore, modern bone conduction hearing devices will be described, as will the audiologic management of modern implantable bone conduction hearing devices. The medical aspects surrounding implantable bone conduction hearing devices will be discussed in Chapter 27.

Implantable Bone Conduction Hearing Device

Implantable bone conduction hearing devices contain two components, (1) an external sound processor that captures acoustic signals, converts the acoustic signal to analogous mechanical vibrations, and delivers the mechanical vibrations to and (2) a titanium component that is surgically implanted in the skull and used to deliver the mechanical vibrations to the cochlea via bone conduction (Figure 26–1). Many bone conduction implants deliver mechanical vibrations to a component that is coupled to the skull via osseointegration. Mavrogenis et al. (2009) define **osseointegration** as "a direct structural and functional connection between ordered, living bone and the surface of a load-carrying implant." Quite simply, osseointegration refers to the process in which bone cells attach/adhere to the surface of a metal (titanium) surface. Specifically, the osteoblasts and supporting tissues (such as collagen) of bone can connect to the pores and/or grooves within the implant surface (Stanford & Keller, 1991). However, osseointegration is not a requirement of bone conduction implants, a fact that will be discussed further below.

The external sound processor of the implantable bone conduction system generally contains an **electromagnetic transducer** that converts an electrical current into mechanical energy. A visual description of a basic electromagnetic bone conduction oscillator is shown in Figure 26–2. The typical electromagnetic transducer of a bone conduction sound processor contains two components that are made of ferrite and separated by small air spaces. Ferrite is a ceramic material that is formed by combining multiple metal oxides into one substance. Soft ferrite material is made up of metal oxides that contain an electron structure that allows the ferrite material to be magnetized or demagnetized when exposed to an electromagnetic field (i.e., the electrons within the soft ferrite material may be aligned and nonaligned depending on the polarity of the lines of flux from

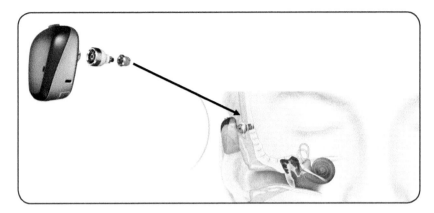

FIGURE 26–1. A visual example of a percutaneous implantable bone conduction implant. Image provided courtesy of Cochlear Americas, ©2018.

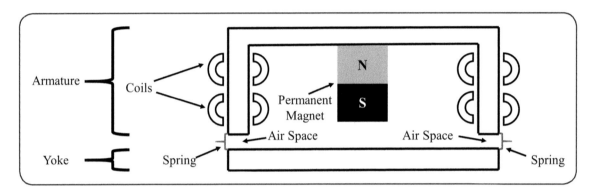

FIGURE 26–2. A visual illustration of an electromagnetic bone conduction transducer.

the electromagnetic field; the change in electron alignment alters the magnetic state of the soft ferrite). One of the ferrite components of the electromagnetic bone conduction transducer is surrounded by wired coils and is typically known as the armature, whereas the other ferrite component is known as the yoke. The armature is the component that is capable of movement when stimulated, whereas the yoke is fixed in place. The armature also contains a permanent magnet (or magnets) that creates a static (i.e., nonchanging) magnetic field between the two ferrite components. Additionally, small springs connect the two ferrite components and create a suspension system that serves to prevent the two components from making physical contact. The static magnetic field created by the permanent magnet, the suspension from the springs, and the air spaces between the ferrite components combine to create a "balance" between the two ferrite components when the system is at rest.

When an electrical current is delivered through the coils surrounding the armature, a magnetic field is generated in the underlying ferrite material. As the electrical current fluctuates in frequency and intensity as it passes through the coil, an oscillating magnetic field is created that serves to alter the magnetic field between the two ferrite components, which alternately attracts and repels the armature to and from the yoke. The movement of the armature relative to the yoke creates mechanical energy (i.e., vibration) in the transducer that may be transmitted to the skull when the sound processor is coupled to the head.

The transducers in modern bone conduction sound processors contain a complex series of springs, air spaces, and permanent magnets that are arranged in a manner to optimize the gain, maximum output, and frequency response of the device while also minimizing distortion (Flynn, 2015). In short, the bone conduction transducers of modern bone conduction sound processors are far more complex than the example shown in Figure 26–2. Of note, bone conduction oscillators can be created with piezoelectric or magnetostrictive transducers, but each of these types of transducers produces a relatively poor low-frequency output compared with an electromagnetic transducer (Hakansson, 2003).

Implantable bone conduction hearing devices are primarily intended for use with two applications, (1) for persons with conductive hearing loss, particularly when air conduction hearing aids are not an appropriate solution (e.g., aural atresia, chronically draining middle ear, chronic external otitis), and (2) single-sided deafness. Implantable bone conduction hearing devices are especially well suited for persons with conductive hearing loss, because the compromised air conduction route may be bypassed, and the signal of interest may be transmitted to the intact cochlea via bone conduction. Implantable bone conduction hearing devices are ideal for persons with normal or near-normal bone conduction hearing thresholds but are also recommended for some persons with bone conduction hearing thresholds in the mild to moderate hearing loss range. For persons with single-sided deafness, implantable bone conduction hearing devices essentially function similarly to

a contralateral-routing-of-signal (CROS) hearing aid. The sound processor of the implantable bone conduction hearing system is worn on the side of the poorer hearing ear and is used to transmit the audio signal from the side of the poorer ear to the better hearing ear via bone conduction.

Percutaneous and Transcutaneous Implantable Bone Conduction Hearing Devices

Implantable bone conduction hearing devices are available in two basic forms, (1) percutaneous systems and (2) transcutaneous systems. With **percutaneous** implantable bone conduction hearing devices (Figure 26–3), a titanium fixture is surgically implanted into the skull and osseointegration creates an intimate adherence to the skull bone. The fixture possesses the appearance of a screw, and the threads of the fixture play a prominent role in facilitating adherence and osseointegration to the skull. The fixture protrudes from the skull and through the skin (hence the preface "per," which refers to "through" the skin). Above the skin, the superior end of the fixture contains a threaded hole to which the abutment of the percutaneous may be mounted (i.e., screwed

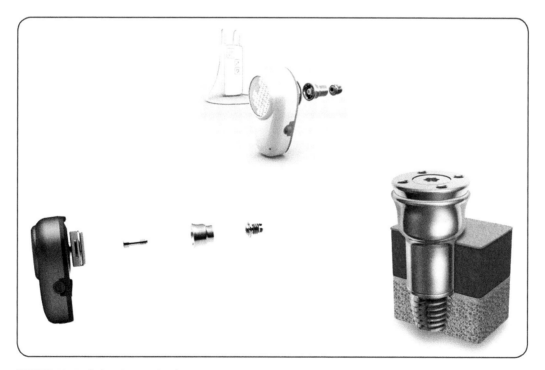

FIGURE 26–3. A visual example of a percutaneous implantable bone conduction implant. Image provided courtesy of Oticon Medical.

or threaded into or out of the threaded hole at the top of the fixture). In most cases, the abutment is premounted to the fixture, but in the case of a two-stage surgical procedure, the abutment is unscrewed from the fixture so that the fixture may be implanted into the skull alone. The abutment is then mounted to the fixture in a second surgery that typically takes place three to six months after the first surgical procedure. The superior end of the abutment contains a connector that may be coupled to the "snap coupling" post of the sound processor. The sound processor oscillates in response to sound stimulation, and the vibrations from the sound processor are transmitted to the abutment and then to the fixture. Finally, the vibrations transmitted to the fixture radiate throughout the skull and to both cochleae (i.e., via bone conduction transmission).

An example of a transcutaneous implantable bone conduction hearing device is shown in Figure 26–4. With a **transcutaneous** implantable bone conduction hearing device, the titanium component that is implanted into the skull is coupled to a magnetic plate that rests on the top of the skull at the mastoid bone just behind the auricle. The snap coupling of the bone conduction sound processor is connected to a magnetic plate that adheres to the head by way of the magnetic attraction between the external and internal magnets. The sound processor oscillates in response to sound stimulation, and the vibrations from the sound processor are transmitted across the skin ("trans" = across, hence, the name transcutaneous) to the external magnet coupled to the processor and then across the skin and to the magnetic plate that is attached to the fixture. Finally, the vibrations transmitted to the fixture radiate throughout the skull and to both cochleae (i.e., via bone conduction transmission). As previously noted, osseointegration is not necessarily a critical component of transcutaneous devices. For example, the mechanical vibrations from the Medtronic Sophono sound processor are delivered through the skin to the titanium body of the implant, which is seated into pockets that the surgeon creates in the skull. Then, the mechanical vibrations radiate through the titanium implant to the skull.

Advantages and Limitations of Percutaneous and Transcutaneous Implantable Bone Conduction Hearing Devices

There are several advantages inherent with transcutaneous implantable bone conduction hearing devices:

- There is a lower rate of complications at and around the incision site (Godbehere et al., 2017; Iseri et al., 2015).

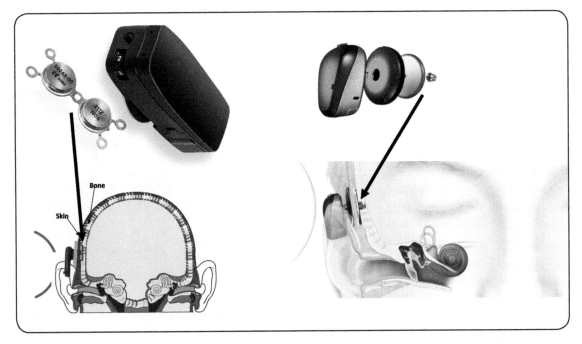

FIGURE 26–4. A visual example of a transcutaneous implantable bone conduction implant. Images provided courtesy of Medtronic Sophono and Cochlear Americas, ©2018.

- Minimal wound care is required; recipients do not have to clean around the abutment site to remove dead skin tissue; however, recipients do need to ensure an appropriate magnet strength, as skin necrosis is possible if the magnet is too strong (Chen, Mancuso, & Lalwani, 2017); a soft pad may be worn underneath the external magnet to promote comfort and a healthy implant site.
- Some may consider a transcutaneous device to have superior aesthetics because there is no abutment present, and as a result, the implant is invisible when the sound processor is removed.
- Some recipients may find attachment and removal of a transcutaneous device to be simpler than a percutaneous device.
- There may be less risk of trauma to the implant (e.g., a blow to the side of the head is less likely to damage the fixture).
- The U.S. Food and Drug Administration (FDA) has approved activation of the sound processor within four weeks of surgery for a transcutaneous device.

The relative limitation inherent in transcutaneous implantable bone conduction hearing devices include:

- An attenuation of 10 to 15 dB occurs when mechanical oscillations are delivered across the skin rather than directly to bone (Hakansson, Tjellstrom, & Carlsson, 1990). The attenuation is frequency specific and is greater in the high-frequency portion of the speech band (i.e., 3000 to 8000 Hz). As a result, transcutaneous devices may provide insufficient power for persons with bone conduction pure-tone thresholds in the mild to moderate hearing loss range.
- Not approved for MRI with a strength greater than 1.5 tesla (T). Additionally, the presence of the implantable magnetic plate will cast a large artifact/shadow in and around the implant.
- Pressure from magnet may aggravate the skin of recipients who have problems with the soft tissue of the scalp (e.g., thin skin, chronic necrosis, poor vascularity).

The relative advantages inherent with percutaneous implantable bone conduction hearing devices include:

- Transmission of mechanical oscillations directly to the skull results in optimal delivery of the signal. As a result, percutaneous systems offer

maximum performance, particularly for recipients who have elevated bone conduction thresholds. Kurz et al. (2014) reported that the aided warbled tone thresholds obtained with percutaneous devices were about 5 to 10 dB better than what was obtained with transcutaneous devices at 1000 to 2000 Hz and 10 to 25 dB better from 4000 to 8000 Hz. Additionally, Kurz et al. (2014) found significantly better monosyllabic word recognition with use of a percutaneous device relative to use of a transcutaneous device.
- May be preferable for recipients who have issues with skin (e.g., thin skin, chronic necrosis, poor vascularity) that may be aggravated by the pressure from the magnetic plate of a transcutaneous device.
- Excellent retention for active recipients.
- Approved for MRI with strength up to 3T. Additionally, implant-related artifact/shadow is minimized with the use of only a fixture and not the implantable magnet.

The relative limitations inherent in percutaneous implantable bone conduction hearing devices include:

- Increased risk for complications near and around the abutment, including fixture extrusion, overgrowth of skin over the abutment, infection at the abutment, development of granulation tissue, and so forth.
- Need to maintain hygiene at abutment.
- U.S. FDA indicates a 3 to 6 month waiting period between surgery and coupling of processor to abutment in order to allow for osseointegration to occur.
- Some recipients may consider the protruding abutment to be aesthetically displeasing.
- Recipients with dexterity problems may find it difficult to attach and remove the sound processor to and from the abutment.
- Relative to a transcutaneous implant, a percutaneous implant is at higher risk for loss due to head trauma (e.g., a blow to the side of the head).

Indications for Use

Implantable bone conduction hearing devices are regulated by each country's department or organization that oversees medical technology and devices. Chapter 2 of this textbook provides a discussion of the medical regulatory process with an emphasis on the process by which the FDA approves drugs and medical devices for use with humans. The FDA classifies implantable bone conduction hearing devices as a Class II medical device. As a result, the manufacturers of implantable bone conduction hearing devices must adhere to all of the commercial and manufacturing practices and policies reviewed for Class II medical devices in Chapter 2.

As with cochlear implants, manufacturers propose to the FDA (or the respective regulatory body of a country outside of the United States) indications of use for implantable bone conduction hearing devices. These indications for use are supported by previous research and performance standards and are approved by the regulatory body for each particular make and model of implantable bone conduction hearing device. As mentioned in Chapter 2, slight differences exist in the FDA-approved indications for use of the cochlear implants that are commercially offered by the various manufacturers. In contrast, the indications for use for implantable bone conduction hearing devices are quite similar across manufacturers.

Indications for Use of Percutaneous Implantable Bone Conduction Hearing Devices

Percutaneous implantable bone conduction hearing devices are considered to be appropriate for persons who meet the following criteria:

- At least 5 years old to allow for maturation of the mastoid bone; children who are younger than 5 years old are likely to have insufficient skull thickness, and as a result, fixture extrusion is more likely. Children younger than 5 years are typically fitted with a bone conduction processor that is worn on a headband. Of specific note, children should have a skull thickness of at least 2.5 mm to accommodate an implantable bone conduction implant (Davids et al., 2007; Tjellstrom, Hakansson, & Granstrom, 2001).
- Persons with **conductive hearing loss** (unilateral or bilateral) are ideal candidates for implantable bone conduction hearing devices. In particular, implantable bone conduction hearing devices are ideal for persons who have conditions that complicate/contraindicate the use of conventional air conduction hearing aids such as aural atresia (or other congenital ear malformations), stenosis of the external auditory meatus, skin allergies that are aggravated by the presence

of a conventional air conduction hearing aid, chronically draining middle ear, chronic external otitis, previous surgeries that complicate effective hearing aid use (e.g., mastoidectomy, canal wall down), etc. Of note, studies have suggested that persons who have an **air–bone gap exceeding 30 to 35 dB** (pure-tone average) will achieve better auditory outcomes with implantable bone conduction hearing devices relative to their performance with air conduction hearing aids (De Wolf et al., 2011; Hol et al., 2005; McDermott et al., 2002; Snik et al., 2005).

- Persons with **mixed hearing loss** (unilateral or bilateral) may also be good candidates for implantable bone conduction hearing devices. Indications for use state that implantable bone conduction hearing devices are appropriate for consideration for persons with a **mild-to-moderate sensorineural** component. Specifically, percutaneous bone conduction implants may be appropriate for persons with **bone conduction thresholds of 65 dB HL or better** (averaged at 500, 1000, 2000, and 3000 Hz). In general, the benefit derived from implantable bone conduction hearing devices begins to become limited when bone conduction thresholds exceed 40 to 45 dB HL. Of note, persons with poorer bone conduction thresholds (i.e., 30 dB HL and worse) should ideally be fitted with sound processors that allow for separation of the sound processor microphone and the oscillating/vibrating transducer in order to prevent acoustic feedback (e.g., **body-worn sound processor, ear-level processor/microphone** with cable connected to the vibrator that is coupled to the abutment). Again, persons with mixed hearing loss are more likely to derive benefit from implantable bone conduction hearing devices when the **air–bone gap is 30 to 35 dB or greater** (De Wolf et al., 2011; Hol et al., 2005; McDermott et al., 2002; Snik et al., 2005).
- Persons with **single-sided deafness (SSD)** are also candidates for implantable bone conduction hearing devices. When used with persons with SSD, implantable bone conduction hearing devices essentially operate as a contralateral routing-of-signal (CROS) device. The implant is placed on the side of the poorer ear so that the sound processor may capture sound near the poorer hearing ear and relay that sound to the better hearing ear via bone conduction. Ideally, the better hearing ear should have

bone conduction thresholds of 20 dB HL or better. However, percutaneous bone conduction implants are generally able to provide enough stimulation that will allow for transfer of the bone conducted signal to the better hearing ear with thresholds in the mild hearing loss range. Use of implantable bone conduction hearing devices will provide access to sound on the side of the poorer hearing ear (overcoming the head shadow effect) and will improve speech recognition in noise when the signal of interest originates from the side of the poorer hearing ear. For persons with SSD, implantable bone conduction hearing devices do not restore hearing in the poorer hearing ear, and generally do not improve localization or speech recognition in noise when the signal arrives from the front or from the side of the better hearing ear. Compared with conventional CROS air conduction hearing aids, implantable bone conduction hearing devices do not occlude the better hearing ear and do not require the recipient to wear hearing devices on each ear.

Indications for Use of Transcutaneous Implantable Bone Conduction Hearing Devices

Transcutaneous implantable bone conduction hearing devices are also appropriate for use by persons with conductive hearing loss, mixed hearing loss, and SSD. In fact, the indications for use of transcutaneous implantable bone conduction hearing devices are similar to the indications for use of percutaneous implantable bone conduction hearing devices save one important exception.

- As with percutaneous implants, the child should be at least 5 years old to allow for maturation of the mastoid bone; of specific note, children should have a skull thickness of at least 2.5 mm to accommodate an implantable bone conduction implant (Davids et al., 2007; Tjellstrom, Hakansson, & Granstrom, 2001). Additionally, a skin thickness of at least 3 mm is required to accommodate the presence of the transcutaneous implant's magnetic plate that is located underneath the skin (Cochlear Baha 4 Systems Candidate Selection Guide, 2014).
- Transcutaneous implantable bone conduction hearing devices are considered for persons with bone conduction thresholds of 45 dB HL or better. As previously indicated, percutaneous

implantable bone conduction hearing devices may be considered for persons with bone conduction thresholds of 65 dB HL or better. The more conservative bone conduction threshold criterion for use with transcutaneous implantable bone conduction hearing devices is attributed to the attenuation of the signal that occurs when the sound-related vibrations travel across the skin from the sound processor to the implant (Kurz et al., 2014; Tjellstrom et al., 1990; Verstraeten et al., 2009). Of note, transcutaneous devices are most likely to be successful for persons with no more than a mild sensorineural hearing loss. Hence, the candidacy guide for the Sophono transcutaneous device states that the Sophono is FDA approved for cochlear hearing loss up 45 dB "with ideal candidacy up to 35 dB HL."
- Transcutaneous implantable bone conduction hearing devices are considered to be especially suitable for persons who have conductive hearing loss with normal bone conduction thresholds or SSD with normal bone conduction thresholds in the better hearing ear, because the excellent cochlear hearing sensitivity allows for sufficient audibility in spite of the attenuation that occurs as the sound vibrations travel across the skin.

Assessment of Candidacy Implantable Bone Conduction Devices

The audiometric evaluation is fairly straightforward to determine candidacy for implantable bone conduction devices. Most importantly, bone conduction pure-tone thresholds should be obtained at 250, 500, 1000, 1500, 2000, 3000, and 4000 Hz (**500, 1000, 2000, and 3000 Hz** at a minimum). When possible, masked bone conduction thresholds should be obtained for each ear. Also when possible, air conduction pure-tone thresholds should be measured for each ear from 250 to 8000 Hz. Ideally, speech recognition should also be assessed for each ear. Although speech recognition scores are not included in the audiologic criteria that determine indications for use, the audiologist should attempt to understand the speech recognition capacity of each ear to determine the potential for benefit from an implantable bone conduction device.

Older children and adults should be given the opportunity to undergo a listening test with the bone conduction sound processor. Preoperative listening tests may be conducted with the sound processor coupled to a soft headband, a metal headband, a testband, a test rod, or a proprietary head-worn coupler (Figure 26–5). The audiologist should keep in mind that the listener's experience and performance obtained during a listening test may be poorer than what would be obtained with an implantable bone conduction device, because the coupling of the signal to the skull will not be as good as what will likely be obtained with an implantable device, particularly compared with percutaneous implants. However, a listening test can provide a reasonable expectation of the benefit that can be derived from an implantable bone conduction device. A formal listening test comprises the completion of sound-field audiometric assessment to determine the performance the listener may achieve with a bone conduction device. A formal listening test may include sound-field warbled tone detection thresholds and aided sound-field speech recognition assessment. Aided warbled tone assessment provides an indication of the extent to which an implantable bone conduction device will provide audibility for the eventual recipient. It should be noted that aided warbled tone thresholds obtained during a formal listening test are likely to be an excellent indicator of the aided thresholds that a recipient would obtain with a transcutaneous implantable

bone conduction device. However, the aided warbled tone thresholds obtained with a test-band or test rod are likely to be poorer than what might be obtained with a percutaneous implantable bone conduction device. Kurz et al. (2014) reported that a percutaneous implantable bone conduction device provided warbled tone thresholds that were about 5 to 10 dB better than a transcutaneous device at 1000 and 2000 Hz and about 10 to 25 dB better from 4000 to 8000 Hz.

Aided sound-field speech recognition should be conducted with and without the use of the bone conduction sound processor. For persons with conductive and mixed hearing loss, word recognition assessment should be completed in the sound-field at a presentation level consistent with average conversational level speech (i.e., 60 dBA) and possibly also at a presentation level consistent with soft speech (i.e., 50 dBA). Comparisons can be made between performance obtained in the unaided and aided conditions as well as between the air conduction hearing aid and bone conduction conditions. The audiologist may also choose to evaluate sentence recognition in noise as time allows.

A formal listening test should be modified for a candidate who has SSD. Because of the normal auditory function in the better hearing ear, word recog-

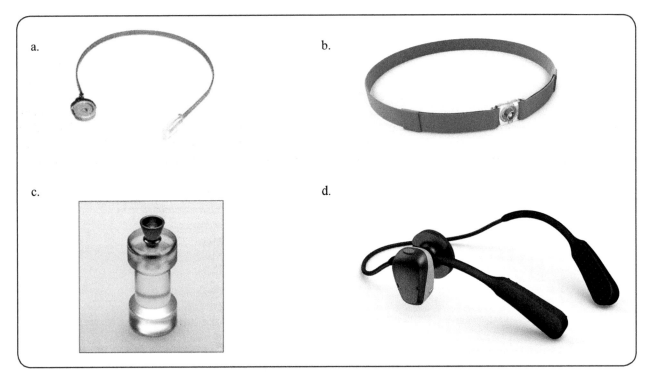

FIGURE 26–5. An example of options that may be used to deliver a signal from a bone conduction sound processor to the user who has not undergone bone conduction implant surgery. Images provided courtesy of Cochlear Americas, ©2018 and Oticon Medical.

nition is unlikely to differ between the unaided and aided conditions. As a result, sentence recognition in noise should be completed with and without the bone conduction sound processor. Specifically, the listener should be positioned with one loudspeaker located at 90 degrees azimuth and the other at 270 degrees azimuth (Figure 26–6). The speech signal of interest should be presented from the loudspeaker adjacent to the poorer hearing ear, whereas the competing noise signal should be presented from the loudspeaker adjacent to the better hearing ear. The simplest way to demonstrate benefit of a bone conduction device for a listener with SSD is to use an adaptive speech-recognition-in-noise task (e.g., BKB-SIN, QuickSIN, HINT). The difference in the signal-to-noise ratio (SNR) required for 50% correct performance between the unaided and aided conditions should serve as a predictor of the benefit a bone conduction device may provide for a candidate with SSD when the signal of interest arrives at the side of the poorer ear in a noisy environment. Alternatively, the audiologist can adjust the level of the competing noise signal to determine the presentation level necessary for 50% correct performance in the unaided condition. Then, testing in the unaided and aided conditions may be repeated at the same fixed SNR. The improvement in the SNR in the aided condition once again serves as a predictor of potential benefit in noise.

Special Considerations for the Assessment of Implantable Bone Conduction Devices for Children

Audiologists may be unable to complete behavioral assessment to determine air and bone conduction pure-tone thresholds in infants and young children. Consequently, determination of candidacy for a bone conduction device must be made with the use of audi-tory evoked response measurements. Specifically, the tone burst–elicited auditory brainstem response (ABR) is the gold standard measurement for estimating frequency-specific thresholds in infants and young children. As with adults, a child's bone conduction hearing sensitivity is the most relevant factor in an audiologic assessment to determine candidacy for a bone conduction device. Numerous studies have proven that the tone burst ABR may be used to estimate pure-tone bone conduction thresholds in infants (Cone-Wesson, 1995; Foxe & Stapells, 1993; Hatton, Janssen, & Stepells, 2012; Valeriote & Small, 2015). A full description of tone-burst ABR assessment is far beyond the scope of this text, so the reader who is interested in learning more is referred to several excellent resources addressing the topic (OIHP Guideline, 2008; Small & Stapells, 2017; Stevens et al., 2013).

When possible, masked bone conduction thresholds should be obtained to determine the ear that is producing the response (Sutton, 2013). However, masking cannot be used to isolate the responding cochlea in some cases. For instance, air conduction masking cannot be used with children who have bilateral aural atresia. Additionally, because of the threat of overmasking (i.e., the masking signal presented to the nontest ear crosses over the skull and masks the test signal presented to the test ear), the masking dilemma does not allow for the use of air conduction masking during the bone conduction assessment of any child who presumably has a bilateral conductive hearing loss in the moderate hearing loss range or worse (Naunton, 1960). When it is not possible to use air conduction masking to obtain ear-specific bone conduction thresholds, the audiologist may consider the use of a two-channel ABR recording to determine the cochlea that is producing the ABR. With a two-channel ABR recording, the noninverting electrode is

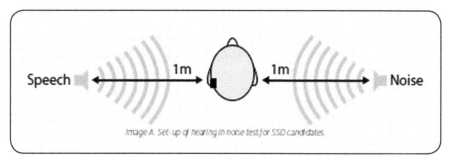

Image A. Set-up of hearing in noise test for SSD candidates

FIGURE 26–6. An illustration of a test setup for evaluating the speech recognition of persons who have single-sided deafness and are considering an implantable bone conduction implant. Image provided courtesy of Cochlear Americas, ©2018.

placed at the high forehead or Cz location, whereas the two inverting electrodes are placed at each mastoid or on each earlobe (placement of the inverting electrode on the earlobe may reduce the magnitude of stimulus-related artifact that can be problematic during bone conduction auditory evoked response measurement. The ground electrode may be placed anywhere else (e.g., low forehead, cheek, shoulder). Two-channel ABR assessment with the aforementioned electrode montage allows the audiologist to compare ipsilateral and contralateral ABR responses to surmise the ear that is producing the response. The presence of a wave I in the ipsilateral channel is a biological marker that the ABR is being produced by the ear that is being stimulated (i.e., the ear nearest to the bone conduction transducer) (Hall & Swanepoel, 2010). Additionally, the latency of wave V may be compared in the ipsilateral and contralateral channels. If the loss is a conductive hearing loss, the latency of wave V will be slightly shorter in the ipsilateral channel relative to the wave V latency recorded in the contralateral channel (Edwards, Durieux-Smith, & Picton, 1985; Foxe & Stapells, 1993; Stapells, 1989; Stapells & Mosseri, 1991). Visual reinforcement audiometry (VRA) may typically be used to obtain frequency-specific threshold responses when a child is as young as 6 to 9 months up to 24 to 30 months (Gravel & Traquina, 1992; Jerger, 1984; Madell & Flexor, 2008; Thompson & Folsom, 1985). Conditioned play audiometry is the ideal approach to determine frequency-specific thresholds from 2 years old through the early elementary years. Behavioral observation audiometry (BOA) is not a reliable technique to obtain threshold-level responses in infants and young children (Gravel & Traquina, 1992; Jerger, 1984; Madell & Flexor, 2008; Thompson & Folsom, 1985). Of course, middle ear measurements (e.g., tympanometry, stapedial reflex thresholds, wideband reflectance) should also be routinely completed with children being evaluated for bone conduction devices.

Preoperative Counseling for Recipients of Implantable Bone Conduction Devices

The audiologist must complete thorough preoperative counseling with the implantable bone conduction device candidate and his/her family. The preoperative counseling session should include:

- A discussion of the potential benefits of implantable bone conduction devices relative to the recipient's individual needs

- The comprehensive intervention process pertaining to an implantable bone conduction device including the surgical procedure, the time required for healing and osseointegration between the surgery and activation of the sound processor, aftercare required to maintain health of the implant site and proper function of the implantable bone conduction system (of note, the surgeon is primarily responsible for discussing details pertaining to implantation), and audiologic intervention including sound processor programming and postoperative assessment
- Cost and payment logistics

Potential Benefits of Implantable Bone Conduction Devices. The potential benefits of implantable bone conduction devices are dependent on the audiometric characteristics and listening needs of the candidate. Specifically, the potential benefit varies depending on whether the candidate has a conductive/mixed hearing loss or a single-sided (sensorineural) deafness. Use of an implantable bone conduction device will generally provide a substantial improvement in audibility (relative to the unaided condition) in an ear with conductive hearing loss or with mixed hearing loss with bone conduction thresholds in the mild hearing loss range. Candidates who have poorer bone conduction thresholds are less likely to have desirable audibility with an implantable bone conduction device. Again, with candidates who have poorer bone conduction, it is particularly important to complete preoperative assessment with a bone conduction sound processor on a testband or softband to predict audibility that will be provided by an implantable bone conduction implant.

Unilateral Conductive Hearing Loss. Persons with unilateral conductive hearing loss generally have adequate access to conversational speech via the good ear. As previously discussed, the head shadow effect may hinder audibility for high-frequency speech sounds (i.e., greater than 1500 Hz) when the signal of interest arrives at the side of the poorer ear. As a result, persons with unilateral conductive hearing loss will likely experience an improvement in speech recognition in quiet when the signal of interest arrives from the side of the poorer ear. Of note, Snik, Mylanus, and Cremers (2002) measured the speech recognition threshold (SRT) in quiet for eight participants who had unilateral conductive hearing loss and who listened to speech stimuli presented from a loudspeaker located at 0 degrees azimuth. Four of the eight participants achieved a statistically significant improvement in their SRT in quiet with use of the bone conduction implant relative to the condition in which they listened with their better ear alone. Likewise, Kunst et al. (2008) reported that four of ten participants with unilateral conductive hearing loss achieved a statistically significant improvement in their SRT in quiet with use of their bone conduction sound processor relative to the unaided condition. Neither the Snik nor the Kunst study found a statistically significant improvement in speech recognition in quiet for the group of subjects.

Research results are variable for studies examining the potential improvement in speech recognition in noise provided by implantable bone conduction implants for persons who have unilateral conductive hearing loss. Of note, Danhauer et al. (2010) surveyed the peer-reviewed literature pertaining to use of implantable bone conduction implants for persons with unilateral conductive hearing loss and concluded that there is a paucity of strong evidence demonstrating the audiologic benefits of implantable bone conduction devices for persons with unilateral hearing loss. Hol et al. (2005) and Priwin et al. (2007) evaluated the potential benefits of implantable bone conduction implants for persons with unilateral conductive hearing loss and concluded that the bone conduction implant was beneficial for this population, particularly when the air–bone gap was 50 dB or greater.

Snik and colleagues (2002) evaluated speech recognition in noise with the speech signal presented from 0 degrees azimuth and the noise presented from the side of the poorer ear in one condition and from the side of the better ear in another condition. No change in speech recognition in noise was observed when the noise was presented from the side of the poorer ear. However, a significant improvement in speech recognition in noise was achieved with use of an implantable bone conduction device by 7 of 8 participants when the noise was presented from the side of the better hearing ear. Kunst et al. (2008) also reported no change in speech recognition in noise with use of an implantable bone conduction device when the competing noise was presented from the side of the poorer ear. Of note, only 4 of the 10 participants in the Kunst study achieved a significant improvement in speech recognition in noise when the noise was presented from the side of the better ear, and use of an implantable bone conduction implant did not result in a statistically significant improvement

in the group mean performance. To briefly summarize, for persons with unilateral conductive hearing loss, use of an implantable bone conduction implant is likely to provide an improvement in speech recognition in noise when the signal of interest arrives from the side of the poorer ear. When the signal of interest arrives from the front, use of an implantable bone conduction implant is likely to result in no change in speech recognition in noise when the noise is located at the side of the poorer ear or when the speech and noise are spatially coincident (i.e., arrive from the same location). Use of an implantable bone conduction implant may provide an improvement in speech recognition in noise when the speech arrives from the front and the noise is primarily located at the side of the better hearing ear.

Of note, results are also variable in research studies examining the potential improvement in localization provided by use of an implantable bone conduction implant by persons with unilateral conductive hearing loss. Five of the 8 participants in the Snik et al. (2002) study achieved a significant improvement in localization with use of an implantable bone conduction implant (with some achieving improvements ranging from 30 to 60 degrees in mean absolute error). In contrast, Kunst and colleagues (2008) found no statistically significant improvement in the mean localization abilities of 20 participants who had unilateral conductive hearing loss and received an implantable bone conduction implant. To summarize, use of an implantable bone conduction implant may improve localization abilities for some, but not all, recipients who have unilateral conductive hearing loss. Peer-reviewed research has failed to identify variables that predict candidates who are most likely to obtain benefit from an implantable bone conduction implant.

Bilateral Conductive Hearing Loss. The improvement in audibility provided by an implantable bone conduction device is especially dramatic for persons with bilateral conductive hearing loss. Relative to the unaided condition, implantable bone conduction implants have been shown to provide significant improvements in warbled tone sound-field thresholds and in speech recognition in quiet. Of note, aided warbled tone sound-field thresholds should be restored to 20 to 25 dB HL for persons with normal bone conduction thresholds and to a level similar to the bone conduction thresholds for recipients who have bone conduction pure-tone thresholds in the mild to moderate hearing loss range. Because of the improvement in audibility, speech recognition in quiet should improve with use of the implantable bone conduction implant, particularly when the speech originates from the front or from the side of the implanted ear. The head shadow effect may hinder the speech recognition unilateral implantable bone conduction implant recipients when the speech signal arrives from the side of the nonimplanted ear. As a result, bilateral implantable bone conduction implantation is a worthy consideration for persons with bilateral conductive hearing loss.

Use of an implantable bone conduction device will certainly provide improvement in speech recognition in noise for persons with bilateral conductive hearing loss when the speech signal arrives from the side of the implanted ear. Additionally, persons with significant conductive or mixed hearing loss (i.e., air conduction hearing thresholds poorer than 40 dB HL) will almost certainly experience an improvement in speech recognition in noise with use of an implantable bone conduction device because of the improvement in audibility provided by the implant. Research does show that use of bilateral implantable bone conduction implants improves the SRT in quiet; Priwin et al. (2004) found a 5.8 dB improvement in the SRT in quiet with bilateral bone conduction implant use relative to unilateral use. Research also shows that the use of bilateral implantable bone conduction devices improves speech recognition in noise compared with the unilateral implantable bone conduction device condition when speech arrives from the front or from the side of the better-hearing ear and the noise surrounds the listener (Bosman et al., 2001; Colquit et al., 2011; Janssen, Hong, & Chadha, 2012; Priwin et al., 2004; van der Pouw, Snik, & Cremers, 1998). For instance, Priwin and colleagues (2004) reported a 2.8 dB improvement in the SNR for 50% correct performance in noise in the bilateral bone conduction condition relative to the unilateral condition. However, research has also indicated that use of bilateral implantable bone conduction implants can result in a small deterioration in speech recognition in noise (relative to the unilateral condition) when the competing noise is presented from the side of the better hearing ear (Janssen, Hong, & Chadha, 2012; Priwin et al., 2004). Of note, the majority of studies examining speech recognition in noise with use of implantable bone conduction implants have been conducted with sound processors containing omnidirectional microphones. Recent research has suggested that modern sound processors containing directional microphone technology are more likely to

offer an improvement in speech recognition in noise when the signal of interest arrives from the front (Krempaska et al., 2014).

Numerous studies have also examined localization in persons with bilateral conductive hearing loss and have generally concluded that use of bilateral implantable bone conduction implants provides a significant improvement in spatial hearing ability relative to the unilateral condition (Bosman et al., 2001; Colquit et al., 2011; Janssen, Hong, & Chadha, 2012; Priwin et al., 2004; van der Pouw, Snik, & Cremers, 1998). In short, for persons with bilateral conductive hearing loss, use of an implantable bone conduction implant will likely improve audibility as well as speech recognition in quiet and in noise, particularly for persons with significant conductive hearing loss and for situations where the signal of interest arrives from the side of the implanted ear. Moreover, use of bilateral implantable bone conduction implants will likely provide better audibility, speech recognition in quiet and in noise, and localization compared with the unilateral bone conduction implant condition.

Single-Sided Sensorineural Deafness. The primary benefit of an implantable bone conduction device for persons with single-sided sensorineural deafness is the alleviation of the head shadow effect. When speech arrives from the side of the poorer hearing ear, use of an implantable bone conduction device will likely improve speech recognition in quiet and in noise (Bosman, Hol, & Mylanus, 2003; Hol et al., 2004; Lin et al., 2006; Wazen et al., 2003). However, when speech arrives from the front and noise is diffuse, use of an implantable bone conduction implant does not improve speech recognition in noise. Furthermore, when the speech signal arrives from the side of the better hearing ear or from the front and the competing noise primarily arrives from the side of the poorer ear, use of an implantable bone conduction device may cause a decrease in speech recognition in noise (Bosman, Hol, & Mylanus, 2003; Hol et al., 2004; Lin et al., 2006; Wazen et al., 2003). Studies examining localization have generally shown that use of an implantable bone conduction device offers no improvement in spatial hearing ability for persons who have single-sided deafness (Bosman, Hol, & Mylanus, 2003; Hol et al., 2004; Lin et al., 2006; Saroul et al., 2013). Of note, Saroul and colleagues (2013) investigated long-term satisfaction and performance of 36 persons who had single-sided deafness and who had received an implantable bone conduction device. They reported that approximately 64% of the participants used their bone conduction sound processor for more than 8 hours per day, and 82% used their processor for more than four hours per day. Additionally, in spite of the fact that localization did not improve and only modest improvements were seen in speech recognition in noise, the participants generally reported their bone conduction implants to be beneficial in real world use. In short, use of an implantable bone conduction device will alleviate the head shadow effect for persons with single-sided deafness but is likely to provide limited to no improvement in spatial hearing abilities and speech recognition in noise. However, patients who respond favorably to a preoperative trial with a bone conduction sound processor worn on a test band or soft band are likely to realize benefit from use of an implantable bone conduction device in real world situations.

Selecting the Implantable Bone Conduction Device That Meets the Individual Needs of the Candidate

As with cochlear implants, the audiologist should work with the implantable bone conduction candidate to identify the specific bone conduction implant that best meets the unique needs of the candidate. The audiologist must be familiar with the specific features of the implant and of the sound processors of each implantable bone conduction implant manufacturer in order to effectively assist the candidate in selecting the ideal system to meet his/her individual needs.

Additionally, the audiologist should assist the candidate in selecting between a percutaneous and transcutaneous implantable bone conduction implant as well as in selecting a particular model of sound processor. Selection of a particular implant and sound processor may be guided by the results of the listening evaluation. For example, in situ bone conduction thresholds may be measured with a bone conduction sound processor coupled to a test band or soft band. If the in situ thresholds are obtained in the fitting range of the sound processor, then a formal listening evaluation may be completed. If the results of the formal listening evaluation are favorable, then the candidate will likely benefit from a transcutaneous implant with the sound processor used during the listening evaluation. If results are unfavorable, then the audiologist may choose to repeat the assessment with a more powerful sound processor. If in situ thresholds cannot be obtained in the fitting range of the sound processor and/or if the results of the listening evaluation are unfavorable with the range of sound processors available, then the audiologist should rec-

ommend use of a percutaneous implantable implant. Of note, transcutaneous implantable bone conduction implants are typically unsuitable for persons with mild to moderate sensorineural hearing loss. The pros and cons of percutaneous and transcutaneous implants were described earlier in this chapter and should be considered during the selection process. Also of note, an ear-level or body-worn sound processor may be the most appropriate option for persons with moderate bone conduction thresholds.

Cost and Reimbursement for Implantable Bone Conduction Devices

A comprehensive discussion pertaining to the cost of and reimbursement for implantable bone conduction implants is beyond the scope of this book. The cost of the devices is variable across different regions of the world (as well as within regions based on whether the device is being purchased directly by the patient or through medical insurance) and changes with advances in technology. Additionally, the reimbursement that third-party payers provide for implantable devices is even more variable depending on the economics of the health care system in which the device is provided. It should be noted that most third-party payers do provide coverage for implantable bone conduction implants. All of the major manufacturers of implantable bone conduction devices contain departments that specialize in matters pertaining to cost, reimbursement, insurance benefits, and so forth. regarding implantable implants. The hearing health care provider or bone conduction implant candidate should contact the manufacturer as needed to pursue assistance with matters related to cost of and reimbursement for implantable bone conduction devices.

Postoperative Management of Recipients of Implantable Bone Conduction Devices

The medical and surgical aspects pertaining to implantable bone conduction devices are discussed in Chapter 27. The following sections describe the audiologic components of postoperative management of recipients of implantable bone conduction devices.

Attaching and Removing the Sound Processor

The audiologist must assist the recipient in learning how to properly attach and remove the bone conduction sound processor. Recipients of transcutaneous implantable bone conduction implants will need to be initially assisted with identifying where the internal magnet is located. Once the recipient becomes familiar with the location of the internal magnet, he/she usually becomes pretty adept at locating the spot on the head to place the sound processor. If the magnet strength is appropriately selected, a modest magnetic attraction should exist as the sound processor is placed near the implant site. The audiologist should select a magnet strength that facilitates adequate retention without eliciting discomfort or irritation of the implant site. To test whether the magnet strength is appropriate, the audiologist may ask older children and adults to stand on their toes and then drop to their heels. If the sound processor dislodges when the recipient moves from a toe stand to a heel drop, the audiologist may want to consider increasing the magnet strength.

Some transcutaneous sound processors may be fitted with a cushioned pad that may be adhered to the underneath side of the sound processor's magnet. Use of these cushioned pads is particularly essential for recipients who have thin skin (i.e., less than 4 mm). However, all recipients may use the cushioned pads if the use of the sound processor and magnet causes discomfort. Regardless of the magnetic strength that is selected or whether the recipient uses a cushioned pad, the audiologist should inspect the implant site at each checkup appointment and advise the recipient's caregivers or significant other to routinely inspect the implant site for signs of irritation. Also, the magnet strength may need to be reduced if the recipient develops discomfort around the implant site. Table 26–1 provides an example of magnet recommendations for different skin flap thicknesses and retention needs for the Cochlear Attract transcutaneous implantable bone conduction device.

The audiologist must also provide careful counsel to guide recipients of percutaneous implantable bone conduction devices in the proper attachment and removal of the sound processor. Ideally, the audiologist should counsel the recipient to use the "tilt technique" when connecting and disconnecting the sound processor to and from the abutment. Figure 26–7 provides a visual illustration of the tilt technique, which involves tilting the bottom side of the processor away from the head when connecting the snap coupling to the abutment. Also, the recipient should rotate the sound processor while attaching and removing the sound processor. While attaching the sound processor to the abutment, the recipient should leave the bottom side of the sound processor tilted away from the

TABLE 26–1. Recommendations for Magnet Strength for Cochlear Baha Attract Users as a Function of the Thickness of the Skin at the Implant Site

Sound Processor Magnet	Soft Tissue Thickness, mm			
	3	4	5	6
No. 6				Extra
No. 5			Extra	Normal
No. 4		Extra	Normal	Start
No. 3	Extra	Normal	Start	Low
No. 2	Normal	Start	Low	Low
No. 1	Start	Low	Low	Low
No. 2 with 2 SoftWear Pads	Low			
No. 1 with 2 SoftWear Pads	Low			

Source: Provided courtesy of Cochlear Americas, ©2018.

head while initially making contact with the abutment. While pressing into the abutment, the recipient should simultaneously tilt the bottom of the sound processor toward the head and rotate the sound processor toward the back of the head. To remove the sound processor, the recipient should place one finger on the top of the sound processor and another at the base of the processor. Then, the recipient should simultaneously tilt the bottom of the sound processor away while rotating the sound processor toward the auricle. Of note, for both transcutaneous and percutaneous implantable bone conduction devices, the microphone ports of the sound processor should be aligned in the horizontal plane so that the directional microphone system focuses on sounds arriving from the front.

Caring for the Implant Site

The audiologist must provide a thorough description of proper care of the implant site, particularly for recipients of percutaneous implantable bone conduction implants. Excellent hygiene is imperative in order to maintain the integrity of the implant and of the soft tissue surrounding the implant. After the surgical dressing has been removed from the implant site, the recipient should gently wash his/her hair to avoid skin overgrowth and the development of an infection at the abutment site during the healing

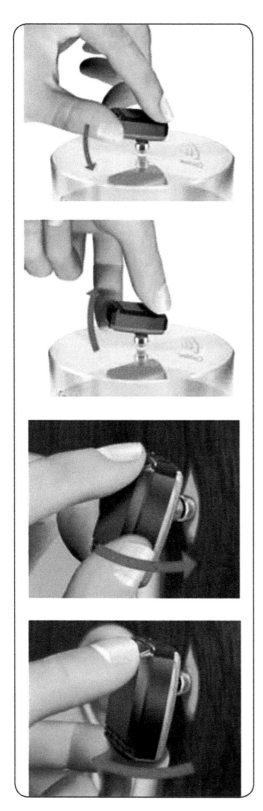

FIGURE 26–7. An illustration of the proper technique to connect and remove a bone conduction processor to and from the abutment. Image provided courtesy of Cochlear Americas, ©2018.

period. Also, an alcohol-free cleaning wipe should be used to keep the skin clean around the abutment.

After the first few weeks following surgery, the recipient should clean the outside of the abutment with warm water and mild soap on a daily basis. Again, a cleaning wipe should be used to wipe around the base of the abutment and the abutment itself. The recipient should understand that the primary objective should be to remove any crust or debris that forms around the base of the abutment. Once the abutment is cleaned, the recipient should gently dry the area around the abutment. It is important to avoid overheating the abutment area.

After the healing period (4 to 8 weeks), the area around the abutment should be cleaned with the brush provided with the implantable system. It is important that the recipient only uses a brush with very soft bristles. The brush may be used to remove debris from the abutment site as well as from inside the abutment. After cleaning, the brush should also be cleaned with mild soap and warm water and left in a well-ventilated space to air dry. Furthermore, the brush should be replaced every three months. Bilateral recipients should use a separate cleaning brush for each ear to avoid transmitting potential infection from one ear to the other.

If redness or soreness arises around the implant site, the recipient should clean the site and apply an antibiotic cream at the implant site. If the recipient has any concerns or doubts about the integrity of the implant site, he/she should see the audiologist or surgeon for assessment. If skin overgrowth occurs at the abutment site, the recipient should see the surgeon. Most likely the surgeon will recommend use of a topical steroid cream. It may also be necessary to try to switch to a longer abutment if the problem persists.

A practical advantage of transcutaneous implantable implants is the fact that complications are less likely at the implant site compared with transcutaneous devices. The most important aspect of care is to select an appropriate magnet strength, a process which was described in detail earlier in this chapter. Some recipients may need a cushioned pad to wear between the external magnet and the skin to prevent skin irritation. If discomfort or irritation does arise, the recipient should see the audiologist to determine the adjustments that need to occur.

Many recipients of implantable bone conduction implants will have to undergo MRI assessment for a medical purpose unrelated to the implant. The MRI compatibility of an implantable bone conduction implant varies by the make and model of the implant.

Recipients should consult with their implant surgeon prior to undergoing MRI. Hearing health care professionals should be familiar with the recommendations of the manufacturers in order to provide appropriate counsel to recipients regarding the steps that must be taken to ensure that the implant is not damaged and that the patient is free of harm during an MRI procedure.

Modern Implantable Bone Conduction Devices

Four major manufacturers produce commercially available implantable bone conduction devices. Although there are similarities in the implantable bone conduction technologies offered by each manufacturer, there are also several unique features of the various makes and models of modern implantable bone conduction implant systems. This chapter provides a general review of the latest technologies available from four commercial manufacturers of implantable bone conduction implant systems, (1) Cochlear Baha, (2) Oticon Ponto, (3) MED-EL BONEBRIDGE, and (4) Medtronic Sophono.

Cochlear Baha

The latest implantable bone conduction implant system of Cochlear Ltd. is the Baha 5 system. The Cochlear Baha osseointegrated bone conduction system contains two different types of osseointegrated implants, the percutaneous Baha Connect and the transcutaneous Baha Attract (Figure 26–8). The latest portfolio of Cochlear Baha sound processors contains three different sound processors, the Cochlear Baha 5, the Cochlear Baha 5 Power, and the Cochlear Baha 5 SuperPower (Figure 26–9).

Cochlear Baha Connect. The Cochlear Baha Connect implant features the BI300 implant fixture. The BI300 fixture possesses a wide diameter of 4.5 mm, which is intended to enhance stability with the skull. The BI300 is available in two lengths, 3 and 4 mm. The threads of the BI300 are smaller than its predecessor, a change that is designed to improve load distribution throughout the implant during use and to increase bone contact to the fixture by creating more contact points. Additionally, the BI300 features the TiOblast™ surface, a moderately roughened surface (with grooves and pores) which is designed to facilitate rapid osseointegration by allowing osteoblasts and supporting connective tissue to migrate into the small gaps in the roughened surface. The BI300 has an FDA-approved MRI compatibility of up to 3 tesla.

The Cochlear Baha Connect also includes the BA400 Dermalock Abutment, which is coupled to the BI300 implant fixture. The BA400 abutment is avail-

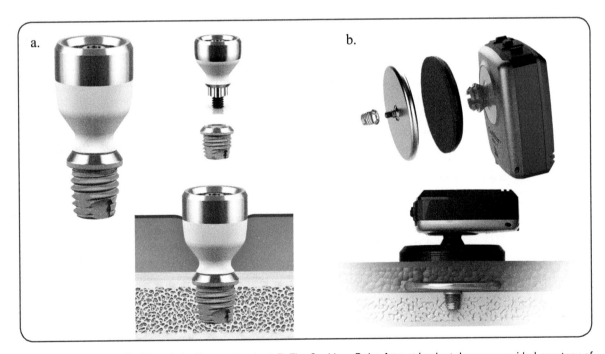

FIGURE 26–8. A. The Cochlear Baha Connect implant. **B.** The Cochlear Baha Attract implant. Images provided courtesy of Cochlear Americas, ©2018.

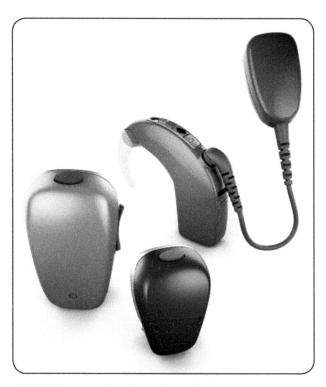

FIGURE 26–9. Cochlear Baha 5 sound processors. Image provided courtesy of Cochlear Americas, ©2018.

able in five different lengths, 6, 8, 10, 12, and 14 mm. The surface of the BA400 Dermalock Abutment is coated with a hydroxyapatite coating (i.e., Dermalock surface coating; the white surface at the base of the abutment) that is intended to promote the integration of the skin with the abutment by allowing the epithelial cells to bind to the surface more effectively than can occur with a titanium surface. The primary purpose of the Dermalock coating is to prevent the formation of pockets (i.e., spaces or gaps) between the abutment and the surrounding skin, because small pockets provide a place for bacteria and debris to collect (Kilpadi, Chang, & Bellis, 2001). Indeed, research has suggested a lower rate of complications, such as infections and irritation, with the use of the Dermalock hydroxyapatite coating (Nelissen et al., 2014). Furthermore, the BA400 abutment possesses a concave shape which is also designed to facilitate integration of the skin to the abutment. Research has suggested that a concave shape will provide a space for blood clots to form during the healing process (Rompen et al., 2007). The formation of blood clots is a precursor to soft tissue regeneration. The enhancement of skin growth results in a thickening of soft tissue around the curved shape of the abutment, which promotes better soft tissue stability with the implant.

The BI300 implant and BA400 Dermalock Abutment have an FDA-approved MRI compatibility of up to 3 tesla. The FDA has approved guidelines that state that 12 weeks should pass between implantation of the BI300/BA400 and connection to a Cochlear Baha sound processor. However, because of the design enhancements that are intended to facilitate quick osseointegration and soft tissue integration, many audiologists are activating the Baha sound processor with favorable results and a low rate of complications within four to six weeks of surgery (Nelissen et al., 2014). Additionally, a consensus report by Snik et al. (2005) stated that implantable bone conduction implants with a 3.75-mm diameter could be activated/loaded four to six weeks after surgery, but significantly longer healing periods are typically allowed for children and recipients with compromised bone. Faster osseointegration is expected to occur with 4.5-mm diameter implants with treated surfaces. Indeed, Nelisson and colleagues (2016) reported favorable osseointegration, implant stability, survival rates, and complication rates in a group of 30 adult recipients whose Baha BI300 implants were activated three weeks after surgery.

Cochlear Baha Attract. The Cochlear Baha Attract transcutaneous implant is also coupled to the BI300 fixture. After the BI300 is implanted securely into the skull, the surgeon may connect the implant magnet to the fixture with a cover screw. The Baha Attract has an FDA-approved MRI compatibility of up to 1.5 tesla. The FDA has approved guidelines that state that four weeks should pass between implantation of the Baha Attract and the fitting of a Cochlear Baha sound processor with an external magnet.

Cochlear Baha Sound Processors. The Cochlear Baha 5 sound processor portfolio includes three unique models, the Baha 5, the Baha 5 Power, and the Baha 5 SuperPower.

Cochlear Baha 5 Sound Processor. At the time of this writing, the Baha 5 sound processor is the smallest implantable bone conduction sound processor. Cochlear indicates that it may be considered for recipients who have bone conduction thresholds (average at 500, 1000, 2000, and 3000 Hz) of up to 45 dB HL (see Figure 26–10 for information regarding the maximum output level available from each Baha 5 sound processor). Relative to its predecessor, the Baha 5 contains a symmetric transducer (i.e., the BCDrive™ transducer) that is smaller than previous Baha transducers and is designed to provide adequate power

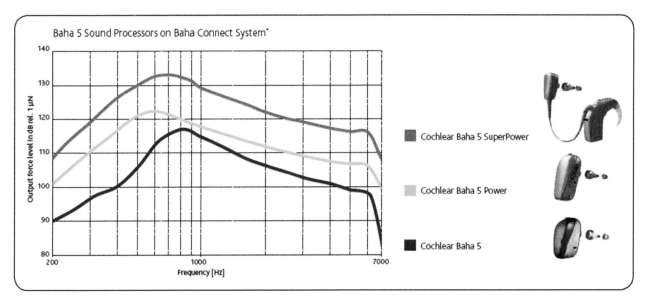

FIGURE 26–10. Maximum output force levels of the Baha 5 sound processors. Image provided courtesy of Cochlear Americas, ©2018.

with minimal distortion. The **BCDrive** transducer, which is depicted in Figure 26–11, contains a magnet that is coupled to two springs, each of which are connected to the case of the transducer. The use of two springs reduces distortion by creating symmetry in the forces provided by the springs and the magnet. The reduction in distortion results in clearer sound compared with a traditional asymmetric transducer (Flynn, 2015). Because of this design change, the Baha 5 is much smaller than the Baha 4 sound processor but is still able to generate similar output (Figure 26–12).

The Baha 5 also contains several features designed to enhance the user's listening performance. The Baha 5 contains a 17-channel-wide dynamic range compression system that is designed to deliver a wide range of acoustic inputs into the recipient's dynamic range of bone conduction hearing. The 17-channel processor allows for advanced processing features (such as adaptive noise reduction, feedback cancellation, adaptive directionality, etc.) to be implemented with excellent precision in a frequency-specific manner. For instance, gain may be reduced in a specific frequency region to reduce incoming noise or to quickly eliminate feedback without compromising the entire speech frequency range. The signal processing features within the Baha 5 operate on a platform on what is commercially referred to as the Ardium™ Smart platform.

Additionally, the Baha 5 contains two omnidirectional microphones that work in tandem to provide

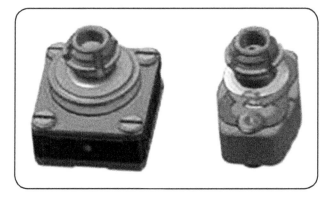

FIGURE 26–11. The Cochlear Baha BCDrive transducer. Image provided courtesy of Cochlear Americas, ©2018.

adaptive beamforming to improve speech recognition in noise. Three different microphone modes are available: (1) omnidirectional, (2) fixed directional —the microphone response provides significant attenuation for sounds arriving from behind (i.e., hypercardioid polar plot pattern) in all environments and at all times, and (3) adaptive directionality ("Auto")—the microphone response essentially functions in omnidirectional mode in quiet environments (with a slight bias toward sounds that arrive from the front much like the directivity of the unaided auricle), but in environments with moderate- to high-level noise, the microphone response automatically switches to a directional response with an adaptive polar plot pattern that provides significant attenuation for sounds arriving from a location in the rear hemisphere from which the most intense noise is arriving. A feature that is commercially referred to as "Active Balanced Directionality II" seamlessly blends between the omnidirectional and directional microphone response as the acoustical characteristics of the environment change (Figure 26–13). Omnidirectional is the default microphone mode for children,

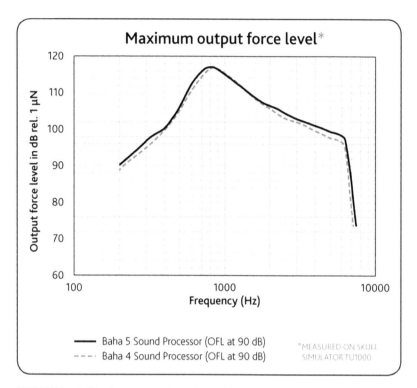

FIGURE 26–12. Maximum output force levels of the Baha 4 and Baha 5 sound processors. Image provided courtesy of Cochlear Americas, ©2018.

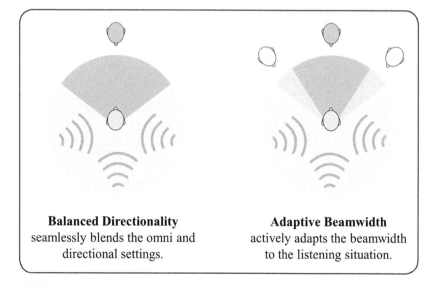

FIGURE 26–13. A visual representation of adaptive directional microphone system of the Baha 5 sound processor. Image provided courtesy of Cochlear Americas, ©2018.

whereas the automatic adaptive directional mode is the default microphone option for adults during everyday use.

Of note, a feature called "**Position Compensation**" serves to adjust the microphone response to provide modest directionality in order to focus on sounds arriving from the front much like the unaided auricle. Figure 26–14 provides a visual illustration of the microphone response with "Position Compensation" enabled and disabled. The use of "Position Compensation" prevents the microphones from being most sensitive to sounds arriving from the side and behind the listener (particularly for high-frequency sounds), which is a natural effect of locating a microphone toward the side and the back of the head (i.e., behind the auricle). Of note, it is imperative for the audiologist to program the Baha 5 sound processor for the ear on which it will be used (i.e., as a right or left ear sound processor) so that the dual-microphone beamformer may be used to focus on sounds arriving

from the front while in directional mode or when "Position Compensation" is active. Position Compensation should be enabled when the sound processor is worn on an abutment or with the Attract implant. Position Compensation is also enabled for adults who use a Soft Band. However, Position Compensation is disabled in the default mode when the Baha 5 is worn by children on a Soft Band, because the sound processor may not always be worn behind the ear or it may be switched between the right and left ears. Of note, in the test/demonstration mode, the microphone mode is set to the fixed-directional option.

The Baha 5 also contains adaptive noise reduction (commercially referred to as the Noise Manager II) (Figure 26–15). The noise reduction processing uses spectral subtraction processing to reduce the gain in channels that primarily contain noise while leaving the signal intact in channels that contain speech. The primary objective of the noise reduction technology is to improve listening comfort while preserving

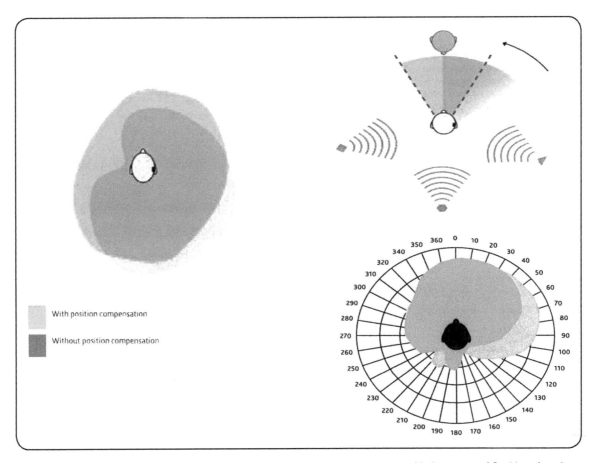

FIGURE 26–14. A visual description of microphone position compensation. Image provided courtesy of Cochlear Americas, ©2018.

speech recognition in noise. Furthermore, the Baha 5 contains active feedback cancellation. In implantable bone conduction systems, acoustic feedback has two primary origins. The mechanical vibration of the sound processor may produce an acoustic signal that travels back to the microphones of the sound processor, where it is processed again, creating a feedback loop. Also, the oscillation of the skull can create an acoustic signal that travels back to the microphones of the sound processor and creates a feedback loop. The feedback cancellation system uses two approaches to eliminate feedback. First, when acoustic feedback is detected, the gain in the channel corresponding to the frequency of the acoustic feedback is rapidly reduced to quickly eliminate the feedback sound. Secondly, the Baha 5 sound processor produces a signal that is

180 degrees out of phase with the acoustic signal in an attempt to cancel it. The audiologist may complete an acoustic feedback measurement during the fitting of the Baha 5 in order to optimize the function of the feedback cancellation system.

The Baha 5 sound processor contains SmartSound iQ processing, which is an acoustic scene classifier (Scene Classifier II) that analyzes the acoustic characteristics of the recipient's environment and classifies the listening condition into one of seven categories: (1) quiet, (2) soft speech, (3) loud speech, (4) speech in soft noise, (5) speech in loud noise, (6) soft noise, and (7) loud noise (Figure 26–16). Noise Manager II noise reduction is automatically enabled in environments containing noise, whereas Active Balanced Directionality II adaptive beam-forming is enabled in

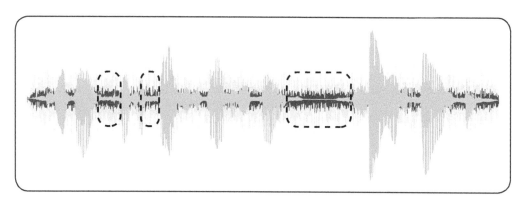

FIGURE 26–15. A visual depiction of the Baha 5 adaptive noise reduction (commercially referred to as the Noise Manager II). Image provided courtesy of Cochlear Americas, ©2018.

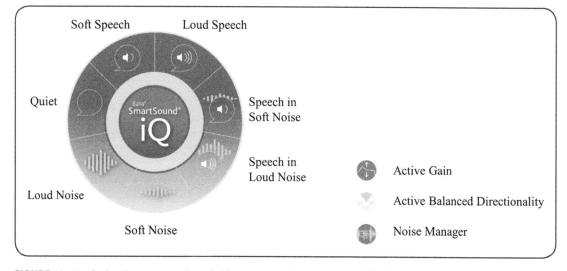

FIGURE 26–16. A visual representation of different types of processing within the Baha SmartSound iQ processing technology. Image provided courtesy of Cochlear Americas, ©2018.

environments containing speech in noise. The overall objective of the SmartSound iQ Scene Classifier II is to automatically select signal processing features that optimize comfort and hearing performance across a wide range of listening conditions without the need for the recipient to make an adjustment. A feature called "Active Gain" allows the audiologist to adjust the gain in each of the seven scenes in an attempt to provide an amplification level that matches the recipient's unique needs across different listening situations (e.g., increase the gain by 3 dB for soft speech if the recipient complains that soft speech is unclear).

Another unique feature of the Baha 5 sound processor is the inclusion of the same 2.4 GHz wireless hearing assistive technology that is in the Nucleus 6 and 7 cochlear implant sound processors (i.e., ReSound's proprietary wireless technology). The Baha 5 contains a 2.4 GHz wireless radio antenna that may be used to receive signals from the Cochlear Mini Mic 2 and 2+ remote microphones, the Cochlear Phone Clip, and the Cochlear TV Streamer (Figure 26–17). Additionally, the Baha 5 contains "Made-for-iPhone" (MiFi) compatibility that allows it to receive audio signals directly from Apple iPhone, iPod Touch, and iPad devices via wireless streaming. Furthermore, the Baha 5 Smart app may be used on the iPhone, iPod Touch, or iPad to control processor settings (e.g., volume control, program), control the operation of wireless accessories, locate a missing Baha 5 processor, examine device use via data logging, and troubleshoot the operation of the Baha processor (Figure 26–18). Also, the Baha 5 sound processor may be used with the Baha Remote Control 2 to allow the user to make adjustments to the volume control, program, audio streaming, and so forth.

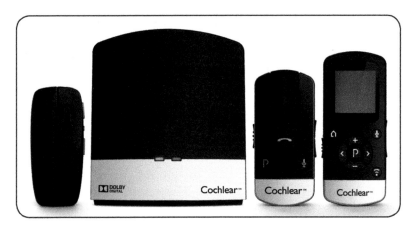

FIGURE 26–17. The Cochlear wireless hearing assistive technologies that may be used with the Baha 5 sound processor. Image provided courtesy of Cochlear Americas, ©2018.

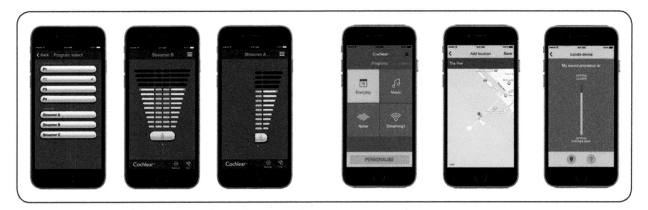

FIGURE 26–18. The Baha 5 Smart app. Image provided courtesy of Cochlear Americas, ©2018.

The Baha 5 sound processor is powered by a zinc-air 312 disposable battery that provides 60 to 80 hours per use for the typical recipient. The battery door may be configured to be tamper-proof. The Baha 5 processor contains a program push button that may be used to change the recipient's program and to enable/disable wireless streaming. The Baha 5 sound processor allows for use of up to four different user programs. The Baha 5 sound processor does not contain a manual volume control or an LED light.

Cochlear Baha 5 Power Sound Processor.

The Baha 5 Power sound processor contains all of the same technology features previously mentioned in the description of the Baha 5 sound processor. The Baha 5 Power processor is larger than the Baha 5 processor and is capable of generating a greater output level (see Figure 26–10). Cochlear suggests that the Baha 5 Power sound processor may be used for recipients with bone conduction thresholds (average at 500, 1000, 2000, and 3000 Hz) up to 55 dB HL. However, it should be noted that it may be difficult to provide adequate audibility before encountering acoustic feedback for recipients with bone conduction thresholds outside of the mild hearing loss range. Addition-

ally, unlike the Baha 5 processor, the Baha 5 Power contains a manual volume control and an LED light. Furthermore, the Baha 5 Power processor is powered by a zinc-air 675 (power) disposable battery, which should provide 135 to 220 hours of use for the typical recipient. The Baha 5 Power processor has a built-in tamper-proof door.

Cochlear Baha 5 Super Power Sound Processor.

The Baha 5 Super Power sound processor is a departure from the single-unit configuration that is common among implantable bone conduction sound processors. The Baha 5 Super Power sound processor contains two components, an ear-level worn processor (which is the same body form factor as the Nucleus 6 sound processor) and an Actuator unit. The rationale behind the two-component system is to allow for greater separation between the microphone of the sound processor and the oscillating transducer (i.e., Actuator). The greater separation is intended to allow for greater output before acoustic feedback occurs. Numerous wearing options are available with the Baha 5 Super Power processor (Figure 26–19). The recipient may wear the processor in the behind-the-ear position on the auricle at the side of the implant

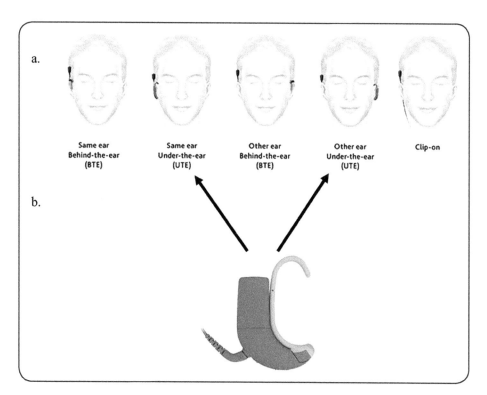

FIGURE 26–19. Wearing options for the Cochlear Baha 5 SuperPower sound processor. Image provided courtesy of Cochlear Americas, ©2018.

or on the contralateral auricle with use of a longer Actuator cable. Wearing the sound processor at the contralateral auricle creates more separation between the microphones and the Actuator, which may provide greater output level prior to acoustic feedback. The Baha 5 Super Power may also be worn with a special "Snugfit" loop in the "under-the-ear" position on the ipsilateral or contralateral auricle. Wearing the processor in the under-the-ear position places the microphones away from the skull and next to the fleshy part of the neck, which reduces the likelihood that bone-conducted oscillations from the skull will radiate to the microphones. Finally, a larger Actuator cable may be used to allow for the sound processor to be clipped to the recipient's clothes. The under-the-ear and body-worn positions are likely to be necessary to optimize audibility for recipients who have bone conduction thresholds in the moderate hearing loss range. Cochlear suggests that the Baha 5 Super Power sound processor may be used with recipients who have bone conduction thresholds (average at 500, 1000, 2000, and 3000 Hz) up to 65 dB HL.

The Baha 5 Super Power processor contains two push buttons that allow the recipient to change programs, enable/disable wireless streaming, and adjust the volume setting. The Baha 5 Super Power also contains an LED light, and it may be powered by two different sizes of rechargeable batteries (which provide 40 to 60 hours of use per charge for the typical user) or two zinc-air 675 (power) disposable batteries. The microphones of the Baha 5 Super Power Processor are protected by two microphone covers that should be replaced every two to three months. All of the signal processing features that are available in the Baha 5 and Baha 5 Power processors are also available in the Baha 5 Super Power processor.

Baha 5 Softband and SoundArc

The Baha 5 Softband is available for recipients who have yet to have surgery to receive a Baha implant. The Baha 5 Softband is a soft headband that is adjustable in size to fit a variety of head circumferences. The Baha 5 Softband contains a connector to which the Baha 5 sound processor may be attached. The underneath side of the connector contains the Baha SoftWear Pad, which is designed to improve comfort and signal transmission (Figure 26–20). The SoftWear Pad contains memory foam that adapts to the contours of the skin in order to distribute pressure across the skin and maximize the contact surface area to which the signal is delivered. The surface area of the underneath side of the Baha 5 connector is larger than the surface area of the connector used with the

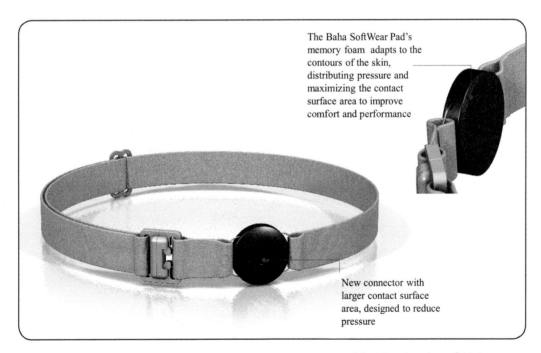

The Baha SoftWear Pad's memory foam adapts to the contours of the skin, distributing pressure and maximizing the contact surface area to improve comfort and performance

New connector with larger contact surface area, designed to reduce pressure

FIGURE 26–20. The Cochlear Baha Softband. Image provided courtesy of Cochlear Americas, ©2018.

Baha 4 Softband. The audiologist should indicate the coupling mechanism when a Baha 5 sound processor is used with the Baha 5 Softband so that the programming software can account for the attenuation that occurs when mechanical vibrations are transmitted across the skin to the skull rather than via an osseointegrated implant. Specifically, the programming software will provide a gain increase for Softband fittings (primarily in the high-frequency range) and the omnidirectional microphone mode will be selected with microphone position compensation disabled.

The Baha SoundArc is another nonsurgical option for Baha 5 users who do not have the Connect or Attract implant (Figure 26–21). The Baha SoundArc is a behind-the-head headband that is designed to provide similar performance as the Baha Softband. The SoundArc is available in several sizes and colors and is adaptable to accommodate different head shapes.

Oticon Medical Ponto

The Ponto BHX Implant is Oticon Medical's latest implantable bone conduction implant. The Ponto BHX Implant has a 4.5-mm-wide diameter and is available in lengths of 3 and 4 mm (Figure 26–22). The Oticon BHX Implant features OptiGrip geometry technology, which refers to the shape and size of the fixture, a design which is intended to provide a large surface for which bone may adhere (Figure 26–23). The increased surface in contact with bone is achieved by a combination of the geometry (i.e., shape) of the implant as well as by the increased threaded area, which extends throughout the full length of the implant. Oticon Medical reports that the greater bone surface contact area of the Ponto BHX implant allows for a better **implant stability quotient** relative to other percutaneous implants (Westerkull & Jinton,

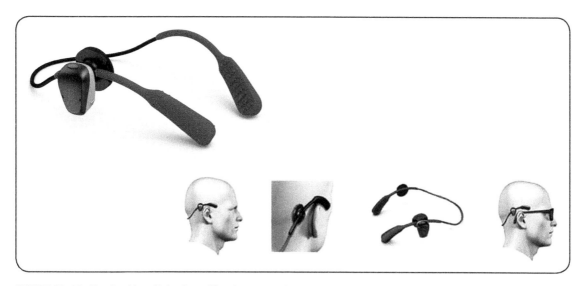

FIGURE 26–21. The Cochlear Baha SoundArc. Image provided courtesy of Cochlear Americas, ©2018.

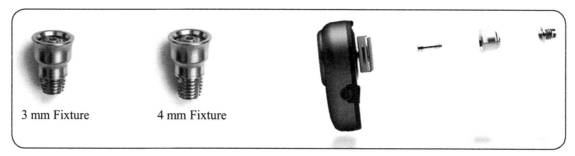

3 mm Fixture   4 mm Fixture

FIGURE 26–22. The Oticon Medical Ponto implant. Image provided courtesy of Oticon Medical.

Oticon Medical White Paper). The larger bone surface contact area is also supposed to facilitate more expeditious osseointegration and decrease implant mobility during the period in which osseointegration is occurring. Because of the large bone contact surface provided by the Oticon OptiGrip design, the Oticon BHX implant may be used with abutments rang-

ing from 6 mm to as long as 14 mm (Figure 26–24). The longer abutments may be especially suitable for persons with thick scalps and for the Oticon Minimally Invasive Ponto Surgery (MIPS). The abutments are coupled to the fixture by a coupling screw (Figure 26–25). Of note, the geometry of the OptiGrip design allows for a smaller hole to be drilled to

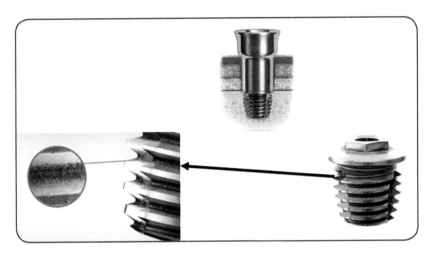

FIGURE 26–23. Oticon Medical BHX Implant features OptiGrip technology. Image provided courtesy of Oticon Medical.

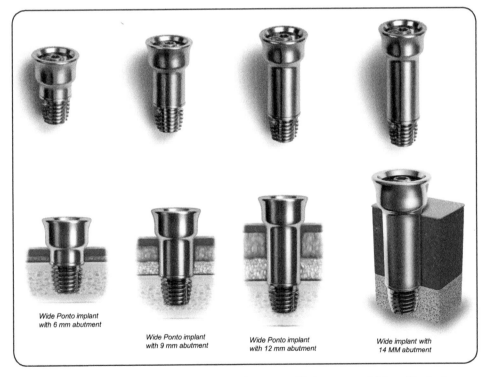

Wide Ponto implant with 6 mm abutment

Wide Ponto implant with 9 mm abutment

Wide Ponto implant with 12 mm abutment

Wide implant with 14 MM abutment

FIGURE 26–24. Oticon Medical Ponto abutments. Image provided courtesy of Oticon Medical.

accommodate the implant relative to other implants with a 4.5-mm diameter. Also, the shape of the cutting edge of threads is designed to reduce tissue pressure and friction between the cutting edge of the implant and the bone.

The Oticon Ponto BHX implant also includes a Biohelix™ surface, which is designed to facilitate osseointegration with the implant. The Biohelix sur-

face is created with the use of laser ablation technology that melts and heats the titanium at the base of the thread, resulting in the creation of three distinct layers at the surface, a macro, micro, and nano surface (Figure 26–26). The three different sizes of layers creates a complex roughened surface that may bond with the various and diverse topography of the surrounding bone. Research suggests that the Biohelix

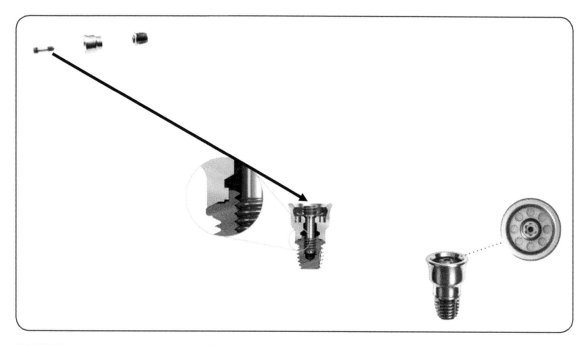

FIGURE 26–25. A visual representation of the screw that is used to couple the abutment to the fixture of the Oticon Ponto implant. Image provided courtesy of Oticon Medical.

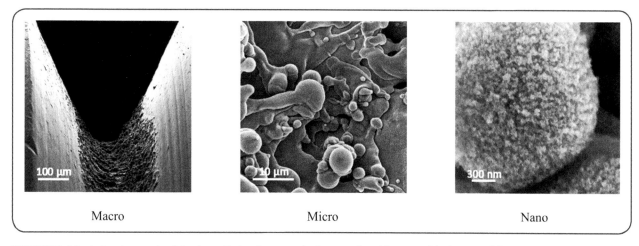

Macro   Micro   Nano

FIGURE 26–26. A visual example of the three distinct layers at the bone surface (1) macro, (2) micro, and (3) nano layers. Image provided courtesy of Oticon Medical.

surface may increase the strength of the bone-to-implant interface by more than 150% (Johansson et al., 2015).

The Oticon Medical Ponto OptiFit™ abutments have a smooth, machined titanium to facilitate a smooth interface between the skin and the abutment. The smooth surface is designed to prevent pockets for bacteria to be trapped, resulting in soft tissue inflammation and infection (Figure 26–27). A tight, conical seal exists between the implant and the abutment to prevent bacteria from migrating between the abutment and implant. The abutment possesses a gradually widening from the base to the shoulder to allow for effective integration of the skin to the abutment. Oticon Medical provides an array of abutment lengths to accommodate the variability in different scalp thicknesses that occurs across recipients. Oticon Medical also offers an angled abutment (10° angle) to allow for comfortable use of the sound processor for recipients who have unusual bone surfaces and/or for situations in which the implant cannot be inserted perpendicular to the skull surface. For these situations, the angled abutment may allow for a more cosmetically appealing fit of the sound processor and may reduce acoustic feedback.

Oticon Medical has developed the **Minimally Invasive Ponto Surgery** (MIPS) in an effort to mini-mize surgical trauma to the soft tissue and bone. The MIPS contains five steps:

1. A biopsy punch is used to make an incision hole in the skin.
2. A cannula (Figure 26–28) is placed in the hole in the skin until the cannula stops at the bone. The cannula serves to protect the skin during the drilling process.
3. A guide drill is inserted into the cannula and used to create a hole in the skull for the insertion of the implant. Then, a widening drill is used to

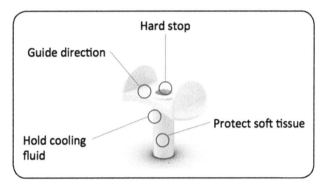

FIGURE 26–28. The Oticon Medical Ponto cannula. Image provided courtesy of Oticon Medical.

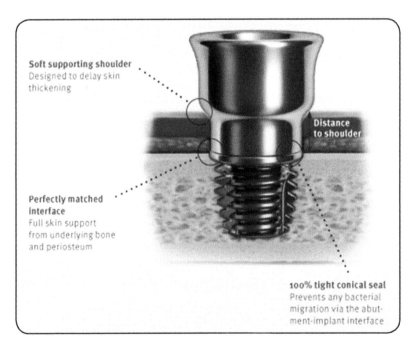

FIGURE 26–27. The Oticon Medical Ponto implant osseointegrated into the skull. Image provided courtesy of Oticon Medical.

widen the hole in the skull and prepare the bone for insertion of the implant. Irrigation is applied in the cannula throughout the drilling process to avoid overheating of the bone.

4. Next, a specialized drill with a low speed and automatic torque control is used to insert the implant in the bone.

5. Finally, a soft healing cap is placed onto the abutment, and medicated ribbon gauze is wrapped around the abutment.

The MIPS procedure generally takes 10 to 20 minutes to complete. The complication rate associated with the MIPS has been very favorable (Johansson et al., 2017).

Oticon Medical Ponto 3 Series Sound Processor

The Ponto 3 series is the latest generation of the Oticon Medical sound processor. The Ponto 3 sound processor portfolio includes three unique models, the Ponto 3, the Ponto 3 Power, and the Ponto 3 SuperPower.

Oticon Medical Ponto 3. The portfolio of Oticon Medical Ponto 3 sound processors is pictured in Figure 26–29 and includes the Ponto 3, the Ponto 3 Power, and the Ponto 3 SuperPower. The primary differences that exist between the different Ponto 3 sound processors is in maximum gain and output level and in size. Oticon Medical indicates that the Ponto 3 processor may be considered for recipients who have bone conduction thresholds (average at 500, 1000, 2000, and 3000 Hz) of up to 45 dB HL. Figure 26–30 provides

information regarding the electroacoustics characteristics of the portfolio of Oticon Ponto 3 processors. Relative to its predecessor, the Ponto Pro, the Ponto 3 is capable of generating a higher output level, particularly from 1000 to 10,000 Hz (Figure 26–31). In fact, the Ponto 3 is capable of generating the highest output level of any bone conduction processor worn directly on the abutment. Also, the bandwidth of the Ponto 3 extends to 9500 Hz, which is the widest frequency response of any bone conduction sound processor.

The Oticon Ponto 3 contains several technological features designed to improve the recipient's hearing performance across a variety of listening situations. The Ponto 3 contains the Inium processing platform, which is the same sophisticated signal processing platform that is available in modern Oticon air conduction hearing aids. The Ponto 3 contains a 15-channel wide dynamic range compression system and allows for the frequency response to be altered via 10 adjustable bands. The time constants of the wide dynamic range compression system are controlled by Oticon's Speech Guard technology, which adaptively transitions from slow to fast time constants with the goal of preserving the temporal properties of speech that are important for recognition. The Ponto 3 offers the Oticon Inium Sense feedback reduction system (Figure 26–32), which provides multi-stage feedback control with rapid, frequency-specific gain reduction as needed and feedback cancellation through the creation of a signal inverted in phase with the acoustic feedback sound. The Inium Sense feedback system also uses frequency shifting (by 10 Hz) to create a difference between the input and output signal with the objective of eliminating acoustic feedback.

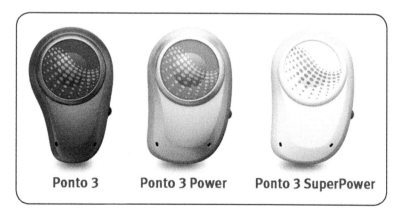

FIGURE 26–29. Oticon Medical Ponto 3 sound processors. Image provided courtesy of Oticon Medical.

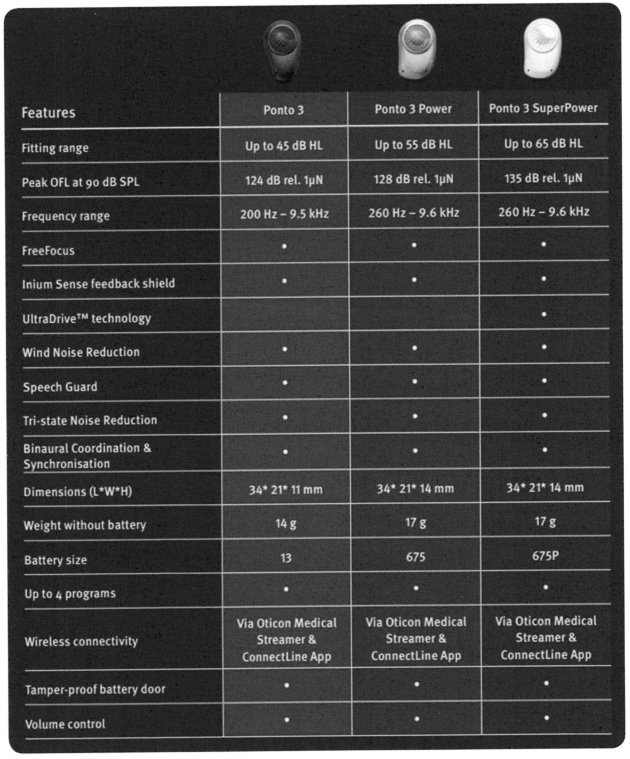

Features	Ponto 3	Ponto 3 Power	Ponto 3 SuperPower
Fitting range	Up to 45 dB HL	Up to 55 dB HL	Up to 65 dB HL
Peak OFL at 90 dB SPL	124 dB rel. 1µN	128 dB rel. 1µN	135 dB rel. 1µN
Frequency range	200 Hz – 9.5 kHz	260 Hz – 9.6 kHz	260 Hz – 9.6 kHz
FreeFocus	•	•	•
Inium Sense feedback shield	•	•	•
UltraDrive™ technology			•
Wind Noise Reduction	•	•	•
Speech Guard	•	•	•
Tri-state Noise Reduction	•	•	•
Binaural Coordination & Synchronisation	•	•	•
Dimensions (L*W*H)	34* 21* 11 mm	34* 21* 14 mm	34* 21* 14 mm
Weight without battery	14 g	17 g	17 g
Battery size	13	675	675P
Up to 4 programs	•	•	•
Wireless connectivity	Via Oticon Medical Streamer & ConnectLine App	Via Oticon Medical Streamer & ConnectLine App	Via Oticon Medical Streamer & ConnectLine App
Tamper-proof battery door	•	•	•
Volume control	•	•	•

FIGURE 26–30. Features and specifications of the Oticon Medical Ponto 3 sound processors. Image provided courtesy of Oticon Medical.

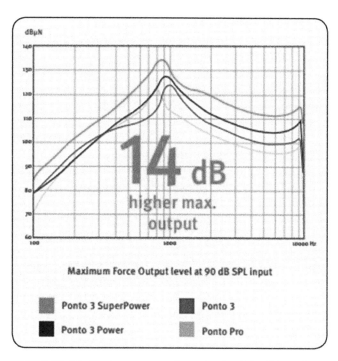

FIGURE 26–31. Maximum output force levels of the Oticon Ponto sound processors. Image provided courtesy of Oticon Medical.

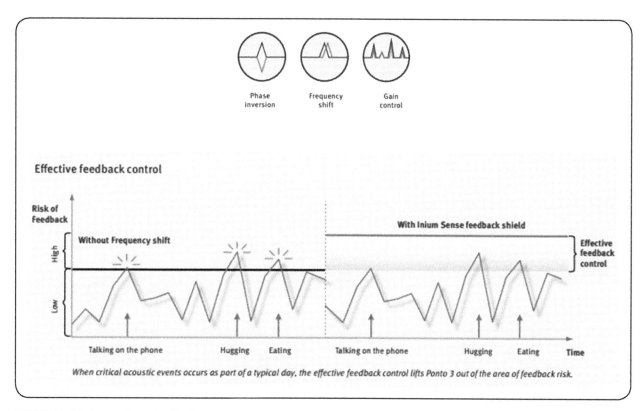

FIGURE 26–32. Oticon Ponto feedback management technology. Image provided courtesy of Oticon Medical.

The Oticon Ponto 3 contains two omnidirectional microphones that may be used to provide fully adaptive beam-forming to improve speech recognition in noise. The "FreeFocus" directional system is an adaptive directional beamformer that automatically switches the directionality of the microphone depending upon the environment. The FreeFocus contains four unique directional patterns: (1) optimized omnidirectional—essentially mimics the directivity provided by the unaided auricle, (2) speech focused—offers attenuation of sound arriving from 135 to 225 degrees in the horizontal plane, (3) split directional—provides a forward-facing directional response for high-frequency sounds while remaining in omnidirectional mode in the low-frequency range, and (4) full directional—primarily focuses on sounds arriving from 315 to 45 degrees in the horizontal plane. The primary objective of FreeFocus is to attempt to improve the SNR for the user when speech is present in noisy environments but to remain in omnidirectional mode in quiet environments or when speech is not present.

Additionally, the Oticon Ponto 3 processor contains Oticon's proprietary Tri-state Noise Reduction system, which uses modulation detection and analysis of the spectrum and level of the incoming signal to determine when noise is present. It also uses a proprietary analysis technology commercially known as VoiceFinder to determine whether speech is present. Aggressive noise reduction is provided when the input signal comprises primarily noise, particularly when the input level is high. However, noise reduction is minimized when speech is detected to avoid sacrificing audibility for important speech sounds. Moreover, the Tri-state Noise Reduction technology also contains Oticon proprietary wind noise reduction processing. The magnitude of gain reduction provided in windy environments is proportional to the wind noise level. Furthermore, the sound processor switches to an omnidirectional mode in windy situations to reduce the noise level generated by the wind.

Also, the Oticon Ponto 3 contains Binaural Processing, which is designed to improve hearing performance of and convenience for bilateral Ponto users. Binaural Synchronization synchronizes the noise reduction and directional systems between the two sound processors to ensure that both devices are in the same mode. Binaural Coordination technology allows the user to adjust a setting on one sound processor and have the same adjustment automatically made to the processor on the opposite ear. Binaural

Coordination applies to changes to the volume control, user program, and mute function.

The Oticon Ponto 3 sound processor allows for wireless audio streaming via the Oticon Medical Streamer, a neckworn device that receives digital radio signals (e.g., Bluetooth) from commercial audio devices (e.g., smartphone, MP3 player, tablet) or Oticon hearing assistive technologies (e.g., TV accessory) and transmits the signal to the sound processor via nearfield magnetic induction (Figure 26–33). Auxiliary audio cables (3.5-mm phone plug) and remote microphone receivers with Europlug connectors may also be connected to the Oticon Medical Streamer. The Oticon ConnectLine app may be used from a smartphone or tablet to adjust sound processor settings and to control the function of wireless devices used with the Oticon Medical Streamer.

The Oticon Ponto 3 sound processor contains a push button to allow the user to select up to four different user programs. The Ponto 3 also contains a digital rotary volume control, a hole to which a retention line may be attached, and a battery door that may be converted to be tamper resistant. The Oticon 3 processor is powered by a size 13 zinc-air disposable battery.

Oticon Medical Ponto 3 Power. The Oticon Ponto 3 Power is slightly larger than the Ponto 3 and produces a higher output level (see Figure 26–30). Oticon indicates that the Ponto 3 Power processor may

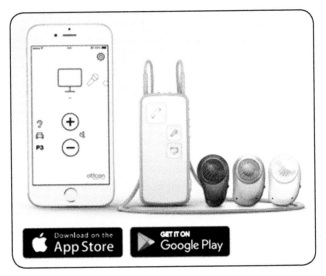

FIGURE 26–33. Oticon Medical Streamer. Image provided courtesy of Oticon Medical.

be considered for recipients who have bone conduction thresholds (average at 500, 1000, 2000, and 3000 Hz) of up to 55 dB HL. The Oticon Ponto 3 Power processor is powered by a zinc-air 675 disposable battery. The Ponto 3 Power sound processor contains the same technological features as described above for the Ponto 3 sound processor.

Oticon Medical Ponto 3 SuperPower. The Oticon Ponto 3 SuperPower is similar in size to the Ponto 3 Power but produces a higher output level (see Figure 26–30). The higher power level of the Ponto 3 SuperPower may be attributed to its unique, proprietary electromagnetic transducer, which was designed to provide greater gain and output ("UltraDrive" technology). Oticon indicates that the Ponto 3 Super Power processor may be considered for recipients who have bone conduction thresholds (average at 500, 1000, 2000, and 3000 Hz) of up to 65 dB HL. The Oticon Ponto 3 SuperPower processor is powered by a zinc-air 675 Power disposable battery. The Ponto 3 SuperPower sound processor contains the same technological features as described above for the Ponto 3 and Ponto 3 Power sound processors.

Medtronic Sophono Implantable Bone Conduction Implant System

The Medtronic Sophono implantable bone conduction implant system was the first implantable transcutaneous bone conduction implant to receive FDA approval for commercial use in the United States (in June of 2011). Sophono began manufacturing transcutaneous implantable bone conduction implants in Boulder, Colorado in 2010. Medtronic, one of the largest manufacturers of medical devices in the world, acquired Sophono in the summer of 2016. The Sophono implant is the latest Medtronic implantable bone conduction implant, whereas the Sophono Alpha 2 MPO is the latest Medtronic bone conduction sound processor (Figure 26–34).

Medtronic Sophono Implant. The Sophono implant contains two samarium cobalt magnets (about the size of a medium-sized coin; 10-mm diameter), which are housed in a titanium case (Figure 26–35), and is designed to be implanted in a single-stage procedure. The surgeon creates two beds in the skull to accommodate the magnets. The implant is held in place by five titanium screws that are inserted into the skull. Of note, however, the mechanical oscillations from the Sophono sound processor are primarily delivered to the two magnets (rather than to the screws), which are embedded into the bone beds created in the skull. The Sophono is a low-profile implant (2.6 mm) that follows the contour of the skull, which facilitates a snug fit to the bone and reduces the likelihood of complications. The dimensions of the Sophono are as follows: 39 mm length × 16 mm width × 2.6 mm height with a weight of 3.5 grams (Table 26–2).

Because the Sophono implant is a transcutaneous device that is not dependent on osseointegration to a fixture, the Sophono implant is FDA approved for activation one month following surgery. The Sophono implant procedure is typically performed under general anesthesia and typically requires less than to 45 minutes to complete. The Sophono is approved by the FDA for MRI up to 3 tesla. It casts an MRI shadow of 5 cm around the implant, which is relatively small for a magnet-containing implant.

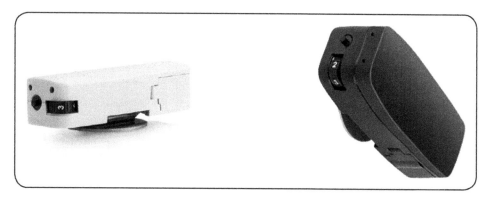

FIGURE 26–34. The Medtronic Sophono Alpha 2 MPO sound processor. Image provided courtesy of Medtronic Sophono.

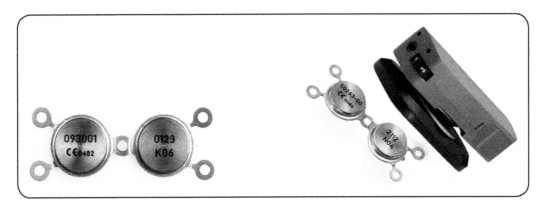

FIGURE 26–35. Medtronic Sophono implantable bone conduction implant. Image provided courtesy of Medtronic Sophono.

TABLE 26–2. Dimensions and Specifications of the Medtronic Sophono Implantable Bone Conduction Implant

Feature Details	Samarium Cobalt magnets sealed in titanium
Dimensions	39 mm L × 16 mm W × 2.6 mm H × 10 mm D
Weight	3.5 grams
Abutment free	Yes, implant technique under the skin
Low profile	Yes, 2.6-mm height
MRI shadow	5 cm, smallest MRI shadow
MRI conditional	Yes, static magnetic field of 3 tesla or less
MRI gradient field	Yes, spatial gradient field 720 gauss/cm or less
Implant kit	Sterile double blistered package containing implant, implant template, surgical template
Standard mastoidectomy tools	Yes, no special tools required
Surgical steps	Seven
Implant frame	Biocompatible titanium case
Configuration	Follows the contour of the skull
Warranty	2 years (industry standard)

Source: Provided courtesy of Medtronic Sophono.

***Medtronic Alpha 2 MPO ePlus*™.** The Medtronic Alpha 2 MPO ePlus™ is the latest sound processor designed for the Medtronic Sophono implant. Medtronic indicates that the Alpha 2 MPO may be considered for recipients who have conductive/mixed hearing loss with bone conduction thresholds (average at 500, 1000, 2000, and 3000 Hz) of up to 45 dB HL and for persons with single-sided deafness with normal hearing (bone conduction thresholds no poorer than 20 dB HL) in the opposite ear. Table 26–3 provides information regarding the electroacoustic characteristics. The transducer of the Alpha 2 MPO ePlus allows for up to 45 dB of gain (for the 60 dB SPL input) and a peak output force level of 121 dB SPL. Relative to its pre-

TABLE 26–3. Dimensions and Specifications of the Medtronic Sophono Alpha 2 MPO Sound Processor

Feature Details	Alpha 2 MPO processor
Placement	Either side, with ergonomic grip design
Headband configuration	Yes
Softband configuration	Yes
Abutment free	Yes
Digital signal processor	Yes
Data logging	Yes
Programs/memories	4
Microphone	Two microphones in an isolated compartment with omni- and directional modalities
Direct audio input	Standard Europlug
Retention clip and lanyard	Standard
Auto noise reduction	Yes
Auto feedback suppression	Yes
Frequency range	125–8000 Hz
Processor	16-band, 8-channel WDRC
Power supply	Type 13 zinc-air battery
Battery life	Up to 320 hrs
Peak output force level at 90 dB SPL re 1µN	115 dB
Output force level at 60 dB SPL re 1µN	105 dB
Audible warning tones	Yes
Colors	Anthracite, brown, champagne, silver
Skinit decal	Gift card for one pair included

Source: Provided courtesy of Medtronic Sophono.

decessor (the Alpha 2 MPO), the Alpha 2 MPO ePlus provides 6 to 10 dB more output from 1000 to 6000 Hz. The Alpha 2 MPO ePlus contains Medtronic's proprietary Transcutaneous Energy Transfer (TET) technology, which is deigned to optimize the delivery of high-frequency mechanical oscillations across the skin. Indeed, a study by Darius Kohan, M.D. (2015), with 15 recipients of implantable bone conduction implants found an average of almost 6 dB of greater gain with the Medtronic Alpha 2 MPO ePlus relative to competitive transcutaneous bone conduction implant systems.

The Alpha 2 MPO ePlus also contains several features designed to enhance the user's listening performance. The Alpha 2 MPO ePlus contains a 16-band, 8-channel-wide dynamic range compression system that is designed to deliver a wide range of acoustic inputs into the recipient's dynamic range of bone conduction hearing. Additionally, the Alpha 2 MPO ePlus™ contains two omnidirectional microphones that work in tandem to provide the option of omnidirectional microphone mode or adaptive beam-forming to improve speech recognition in noise. Three different microphone modes are available: (1) Omnidirectional Plus—which mimics the directivity of the unaided ear, (2) Adaptive Directional—in environments with moderate- to high-level noise, the microphone response automatically switches to a directional response with an adaptive polar plot pattern that provides significant attenuation for sounds arriving from a location in the rear hemisphere from which the most intense noise is arriving. Moreover, the Alpha 2 MPO ePlus contains adaptive noise reduction automatic feedback suppression. In implantable bone conduction systems, acoustic feedback has two primary origins. The mechanical vibration of the sound processor may produce an acoustic signal that travels back to the microphones of the sound processor, where it is processed again, creating a feedback loop. Also, the oscillation of the skull can create an acoustic signal that travels back to the microphones of the sound processor and creates a feedback loop. The feedback cancellation system uses two approaches to eliminate feedback. First, when acoustic feedback is detected, the gain in the channel corresponding to the frequency of the acoustic feedback is rapidly reduced to quickly eliminate the feedback sound. Secondly, the Baha 5 sound processor produces a signal that is 180 degrees out of phase with the acoustic signal in an attempt to cancel it. The audiologist may complete an acoustic feedback measurement during the fitting of the Baha 5 in order to optimize the function of the feedback cancellation system. Furthermore, up to four user programs may be loaded onto the Alpha 2 MPO ePlus.

A unique feature of the Alpha 2 MPO ePlus is the availability of a lithium ion rechargeable battery (the ZPower battery). With use of the ZPower rechargeable battery, the Alpha 2 MPO ePlus processor may be charged in the Medtronic battery charger for one full-day of processor use. The Alpha 2 MPO ePlus may also be powered by a zinc-air 13 disposable battery that provides up to 250 hours per use. The battery door may be configured to be tamperproof. The Alpha 2 MPO ePlus processor contains a program push button and a digital rotary volume control. It also contains a Europort for connection to remote microphone receivers and a programming port for connection to the programming interface.

MED-EL ADHEAR and BONEBRIDGE

MED-EL manufactures two unique types of bone conduction devices, the MED-EL BONEBRIDGE and the MED-EL ADHEAR. At the time of this writing, both of these devices were recently approved by the FDA

for commercial use in the United States; however, neither device was available for clinical use, and as a result, the author did not have access to detailed materials discussing these devices and the audiologic management of MED-EL bone conduction devices. Of note, basic information pertaining to these devices may be retrieved from MED-EL's website. The MED-EL BONEBRIDGE (BCI 601) contains four general components (Figure 26–36): (1) a coil to receive electromagnetic signals from an external sound processor (the coil is essentially identical to the receiving coil of a cochlear implant), (2) a magnet that is housed in a Silastic silicone sleeve in the center of the coil, (3) a processor that is housed in a titanium case and used to analyze the signal and determine the stimulation that should be delivered for the recipient, and (4) a bone conduction floating mass transducer (BC-FMT) that receives signals from the implant's processor and converts the signal to mechanical oscillations that are delivered to the skull. The surgeon creates a bed in the skull bone and places the BC-FMT inside the bed. The BC-FMT contains two receptacles on each side of the transducer to allow the surgeon to fix the implant to the skull with two titanium screws. The BC-FMT essentially operates as a bone conduction oscillator and delivers vibrations directly to the skull.

The recipient wears the SAMBA sound processor on the head just behind and above the auricle. The SAMBA sound processor contains a magnet that allows it to adhere to the head via the attraction to the magnet that is located inside of the coil of the BONEBRIDGE implant (Figure 26–37). The SAMBA sound processor contains two omnidirectional microphones that capture outside sounds and delivers the

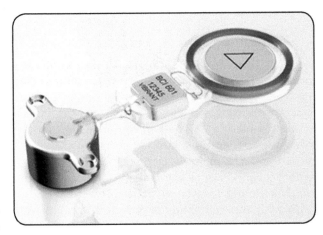

FIGURE 26–36. MED-EL BONEBRIDGE implantable bone conduction implant. Image provided courtesy of MED-EL Corporation.

signal to the processor for analysis. The processed signal is then delivered to a transmitting coil located at the periphery of the SAMBA. The transmitting coil

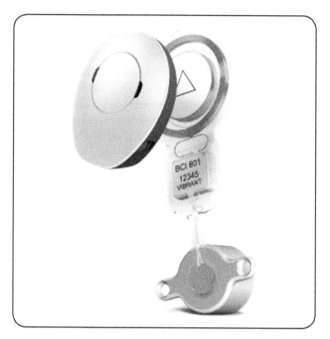

FIGURE 26–37. MED-EL BONEBRIDGE implantable bone conduction implant with the SAMBA sound processor. Image provided courtesy of MED-EL Corporation.

converts the signal to an electromagnetic signal that is transmitted across the skin and received by the internal coil of the BONEBRIDGE implant (similar to the telemetry used by a cochlear implant). As a result, the implant is housed entirely underneath the skin, but the mechanical stimulation is provided directly to the bone. In effect, the BONEBRIDGE provides advantages of a transcutaneous (e.g., cosmetic appealing with no protruding abutment, lower rate of soft tissue complications) and percutaneous (e.g., direct bone conduction without attenuation of high-frequency energy that occurs when mechanical oscillations are delivered through the skin) implantable bone conduction implant. The BONEBRIDGE implant surgery required about one hour to complete, and the SAMBA sound processor may be activated within two to four weeks after surgery.

The MED-EL ADHEAR is unique, because it is not an implantable bone conduction device (Figure 26–38). The MED-EL ADHEAR contains an Adhesive Adapter, which is a soft pad with a sticky surface that is placed on the hairless area just behind the auricle. The Adhesive Adapter contains a plastic connector that is used to couple to the sound processor and to deliver mechanical oscillations to the mastoid bone. The Adhesive Adapter is designed to optimize delivery of mechanical oscillations to the head without placing uncomfortable pressure on the underlying

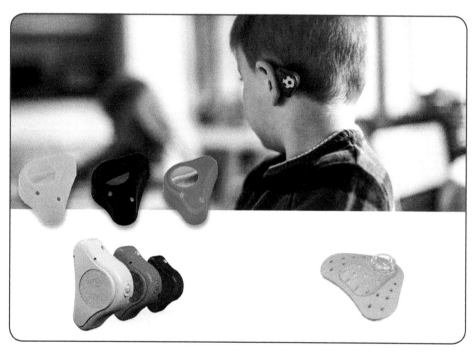

FIGURE 26–38. MED-EL ADHEAR bone conduction device. Image provided courtesy of MED-EL Corporation.

skin. Each adhesive pad may be used for three to seven days and is water resistant (e.g., may be used during showering, exercise).

The MED-EL ADHEAR Audio Processor is used with the Adhesive Adapter. It contains a snap coupler that is coupled to the connector of the Adhesive Adapter. The ADHEAR Audio Processor contains a dual-microphone system that may be used to provide both omnidirectional and adaptive directional beamforming. The ADHEAR Audio Processor also contains automatic noise reduction and feedback cancellation. Additionally, it contains a telecoil, a three-prong Euro-port connector for remote microphone receivers, and may be connected with personal audio devices via Bluetooth. A push button allows the user to change between up to four different programs.

Programming Modern Implantable Bone Conduction Devices

The audiologist must program the bone conduction sound processor to meet the unique needs of each recipient of an implantable bone conduction implant.

The following sections describe the steps involved in programming modern implantable bone conduction sound processors.

Programming the Cochlear Baha 5 Series

Cochlear Baha 5 bone conduction sound processors are programmed in the Cochlear Baha Fitting Suite software, which may be used in a stand-alone version or within the NOAH hearing aid programming software system. Baha 5 sound processors are programmed with use of the ReSound Airlink 2 wireless programming interface. Of note, the Baha 5 and Baha 5 Power processors may also be programmed with use of the ReSound Airlink programming interface. Once the Cochlear Baha Fitting Suite software is launched, the audiologist must select whether a Baha 5 series or a Baha 3 or 4 series processor is being programmed (Figure 26–39). This text will only discuss the steps involved in the programming of a Baha 5 series sound processor. The audiologist must click on the arrow in the upper right corner of the Baha 5 pane to launch the software used to program Baha 5 processors. Once the software is launched, the audiologist

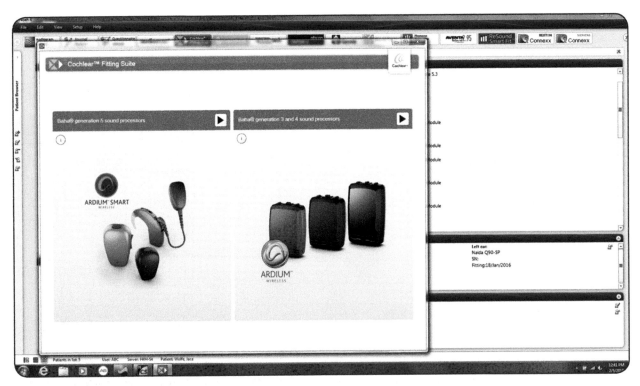

FIGURE 26–39. Cochlear Baha Fitting software. Image provided courtesy of Cochlear Americas, ©2018.

must identify which Baha 5 series sound processor is being programmed for the recipient (Figure 26–40). Then, the audiologist must select whether the sound processor programming session will be based on the settings already contained within the sound processor, on the settings the software recommends to best meet the recipient's needs based on audiometric profile, age, wearing configuration, and so forth, or on the factory default settings (Figure 26–41). For a new recipient, the audiologist should typically select the "Fitting Software" option, whereas the audiologist should select the "Sound Processor" option for existing recipients. Selecting the "Detect" option will trigger the Airlink 2 interface to communicate with the Baha 5 series sound processor, and the software will prompt the audiologist to connect with a Baha 5 series sound processor by opening and then closing the battery door of the sound processor to facilitate the wireless connection.

For new fittings, the next step following the connection to the sound processor is to indicate whether the recipient is an adult or a child and whether the recipient is a monaural or binaural Baha user (Figure 26–42). Next, the audiologist indicates whether the Baha 5 processor is being fitted for a recipient with a conductive/mixed hearing loss or single-sided sensorineural hearing loss (Figure 26–43). Then, the audiologist indicates whether the Baha 5 sound processor is being fitted with the transcutaneous Attract implant, the percutaneous Connect implant, the Soundband (or test band), or with the SoftArc. If the Baha sound processor is being used with the Softband or SoundArc, the audiologist must indicate whether the Baha 5 processor is being fitted for everyday use or for a demonstration in the clinic (Figure 26–44).

Additionally, the audiologist may enter the bone conduction thresholds into the "Audiogram" section of the "Prescribe" menu (Figure 26–45). Of note, the bone conduction thresholds will be imported from NOAH if the Cochlear Baha Fitting Suite is launched from the NOAH software. Inclusion of the bone conduction thresholds is necessary for the Cochlear Baha Fitting Suite software to calculate prescribed gain settings to meet the recipient's individual needs.

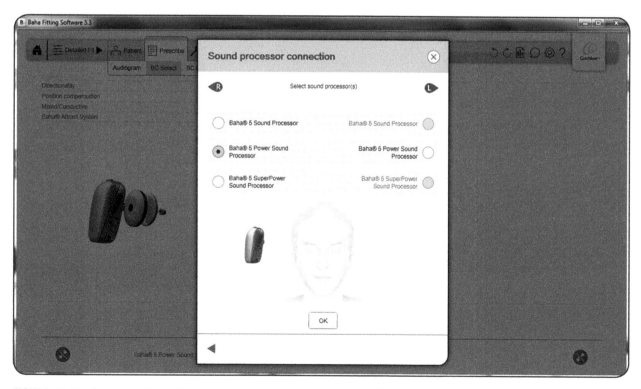

FIGURE 26–40. Selection of Baha 5 sound processor in the Cochlear Baha Fitting software. Image provided courtesy of Cochlear Americas, ©2018.

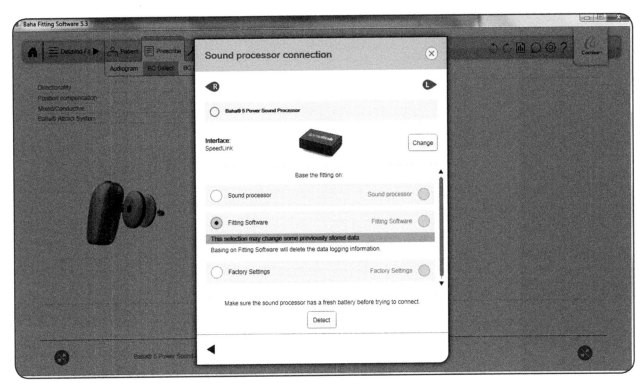

FIGURE 26–41. Determination of whether the sound processor settings will be based on a previous program session, a new fitting, or factory settings. Image provided courtesy of Cochlear Americas, ©2018.

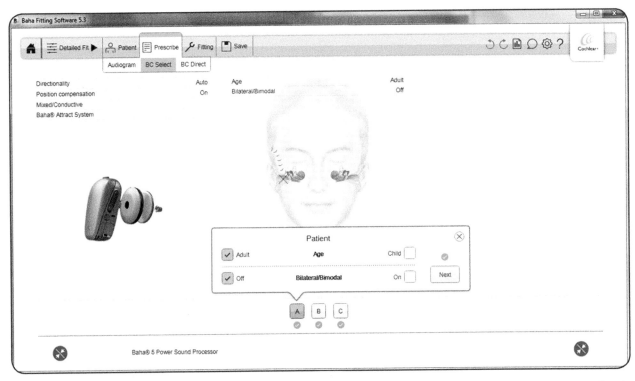

FIGURE 26–42. Entry of patient-specific information for Baha 5 programming. Image provided courtesy of Cochlear Americas, ©2018.

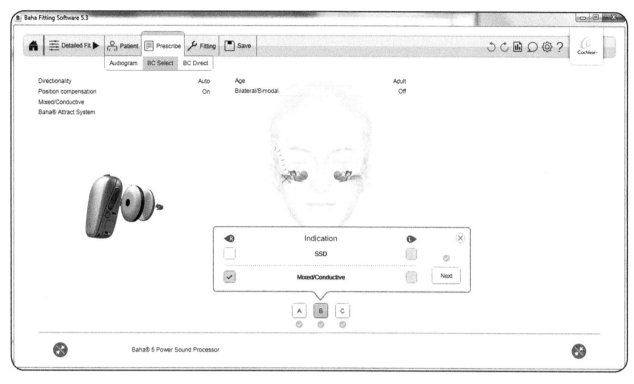

FIGURE 26–43. Entry of patient-specific information for Baha 5 programming. Image provided courtesy of Cochlear Americas, ©2018.

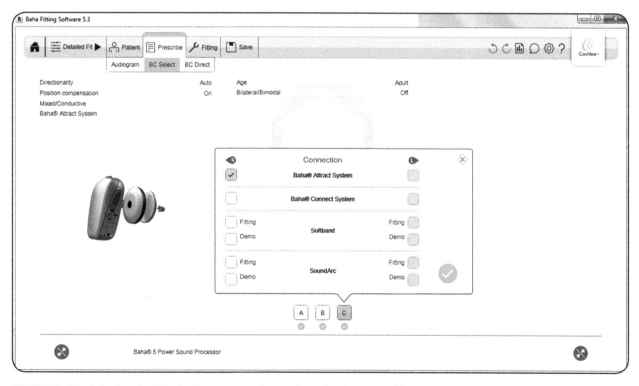

FIGURE 26–44. Selecting the Baha implant and wearing configuration. Image provided courtesy of Cochlear Americas, ©2018.

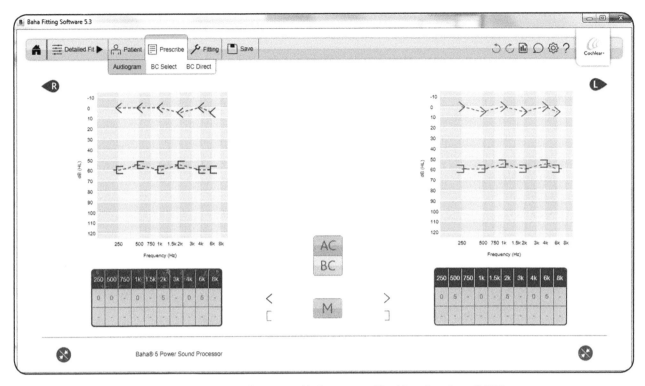

FIGURE 26–45. Entry of the recipient's audiogram. Image provided courtesy of Cochlear Americas, ©2018.

Ideally, the audiologist should also utilize the "BC Direct" feature to measure in situ bone conduction thresholds (Figure 26–46). In short, the BC Direct feature allows for the measurement of bone conduction thresholds with the stimuli delivered via the sound processor as it is worn in the wearing configuration in which the recipient will use it for daily use (e.g., Baha 5 attached to Connect abutment, on Attract magnet, or to the Softband or SoundArc). Measuring the bone conduction thresholds with the sound processor located at the recipient's customary position of use allows for a determination of the attenuation of sound as it is transmitted from the processor to the cochlea via bone conduction (e.g., skull transfer function, transcranial attenuation), and across the skin in the case of the Attract and Softband configurations. The BC Direct in situ bone conduction thresholds are used along with the recipient's audiometric thresholds, the connection type, and indication of use (conductive vs. single-sided sensorineural) to calculate prescribed gain based on the proprietary Cochlear Baha Prescription formula. Of note, cochlear hearing loss is characterized by abnormal loudness growth (i.e., loudness recruitment), and as a result, gain is

not prescribed in a linear (1:1) fashion per decibel of hearing loss. In contrast, the Cochlear Baha Prescription formula compensates for bone conduction transmission loss (e.g., skull transmission attenuation, transcranial attenuation, soft tissue attenuation) in a 1:1 manner. To be clear, the Cochlear Baha Prescription formula does account for sensorineural hearing loss by compensating for cochlear hearing loss with a gain prescription similar to what is employed by traditional hearing aid fitting prescriptions (e.g., DSL 5.0, NAL-NL2).

After the measurement tasks are completed in the "Prescribe" menu, the audiologist proceeds to the "Fitting" menu to make any necessary programming adjustments to fine-tune the Baha 5 sound processor to optimize recipient performance and benefit. Within the Fitting menu, the audiologist can access the "Fine Tuning" screen within the "Adjustments" platform to make frequency-specific changes to the gain for 40 and 60 dB SPL inputs and to the maximum power output (MPO) (Figure 26–47). Additionally, the audiologist may click on the program numbers from "1" to "4" to add a new program for the recipient to use in speech situations (e.g., "Noise," Music") (Figure 26–48).

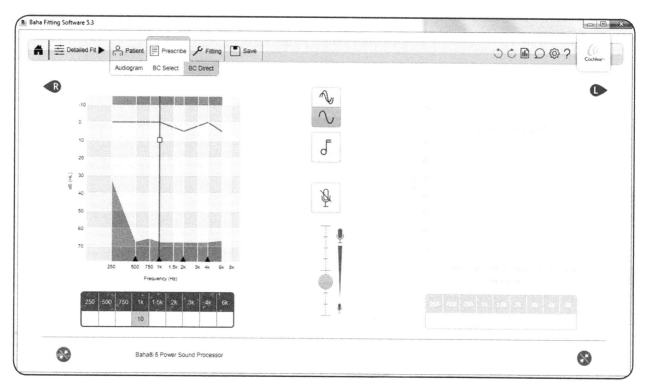

FIGURE 26–46. BC Direct in situ audiometric assessment. Image provided courtesy of Cochlear Americas, ©2018.

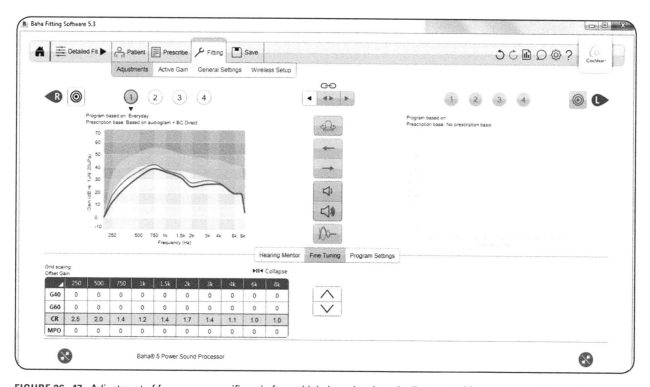

FIGURE 26–47. Adjustment of frequency-specific gain for multiple input levels and adjustment of frequency-specific maximum output force level. Image provided courtesy of Cochlear Americas, ©2018.

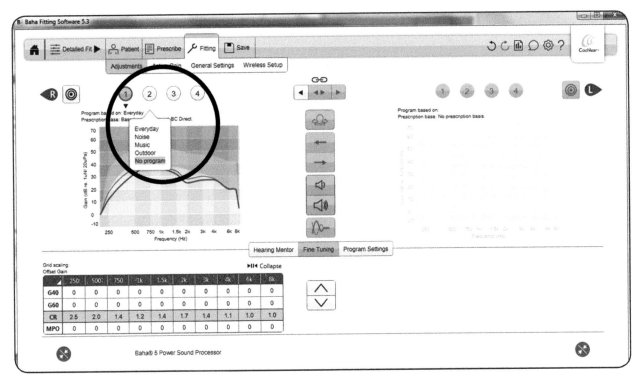

FIGURE 26–48. Creation of situation-specific programs. Image provided courtesy of Cochlear Americas, ©2018.

Also within the Adjustments menu, the audiologist may access the "Hearing Mentor" program to make broad adjustments to address subjective complaints that the recipient has regarding overall loudness, sound quality, his/her own voice, and performance in noise (Figure 26–49). Moreover, within the Adjustments menu, the audiologist can access the "Program Settings" tab to adjust the microphone mode, the operation of the noise reduction system, the magnitude of the noise reduction, and the aggressiveness of the feedback reduction feature (Figure 26–50).

Furthermore, within the Fitting menu, the audiologist may make adjustments (±3 dB) to the "Active Gain" feature to increase or decrease the output for each of the seven acoustic scenes within the SmartSound iQ Scene Classifier (Figure 26–51). These adjustments would be made to address an individual recipient's complaint about a specific listening situation that corresponds to one of the seven acoustic scenes (e.g., soft speech, loud noise). The "General Settings" screen (Figure 26–52) within the Fitting menu allows the audiologist to adjust a variety of different features, including:

- Control Sync: Allows for an adjustment that is made on one processor to simultaneously be

made to the other processor of binaural Baha 5 users

- Position Compensation: Allows the audiologist to enable or disable Position Compensation
- Mic relative Wireless Acc. (dB): Allows the audiologist to attenuate the sound processor microphone by 6 dB when a wireless accessory is being used
- Allows the audiologist to enable or disable the low battery alarm, the volume indicator tones, the volume control, and LED visual indicator
- Allows the audiologist to adjust the loudness and pitch of the indicator tones

Within the "Wireless Setup" screen of the Fitting menu, the audiologist may pair the recipient's wireless accessories to the Baha 5 series sound processor and determine the wireless program slot in which each wireless accessory may be accessed (Figure 26–53). Finally, after all necessary adjustments have been completed to optimize recipient performance, the audiologist should proceed to the "Save" menu to download the recipient's program(s) to the Baha 5 series sound processor(s) and to save the settings to the Cochlear Baha Fitting Suite software (Figure 26–54). Of note, data logging may be enabled and/or reset within the Save menu.

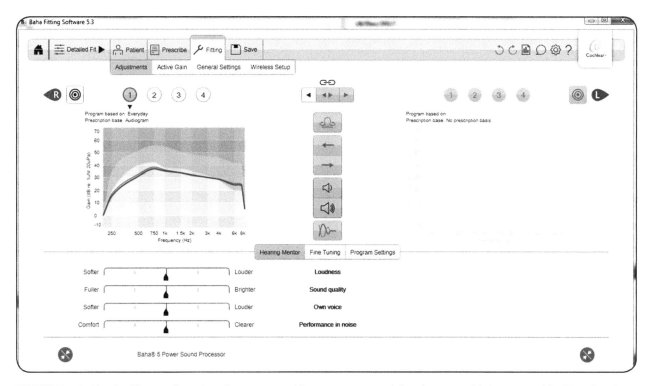

FIGURE 26–49. Hearing Mentor: allows for adjustments to address common complaints. Image provided courtesy of Cochlear Americas, ©2018.

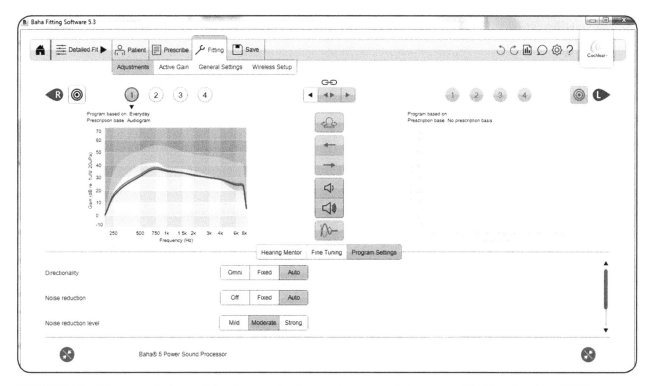

FIGURE 26–50. Adjustment of advanced signal processing features. Image provided courtesy of Cochlear Americas, ©2018.

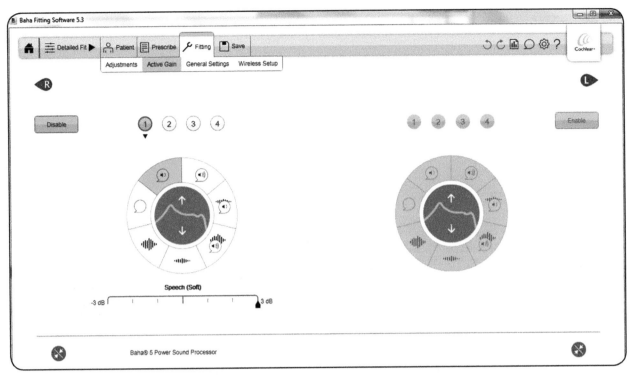

FIGURE 26–51. Active Gain: allows adjustment of gain within each of the SmartSound iQ seven acoustic scenes (e.g., soft speech in quiet, speech in noise, etc.). Image provided courtesy of Cochlear Americas, ©2018.

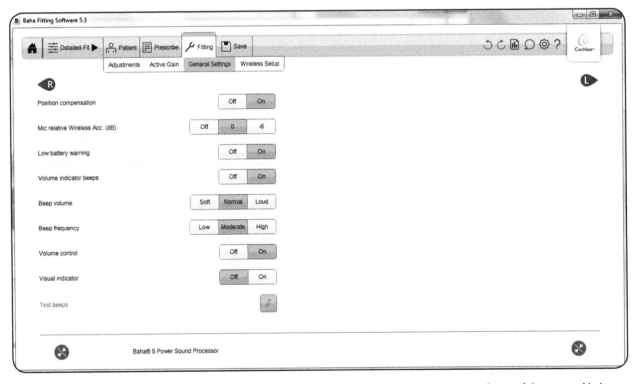

FIGURE 26–52. Adjustment of processor configuration settings (e.g., indicators, microphone compensation, etc.). Image provided courtesy of Cochlear Americas, ©2018.

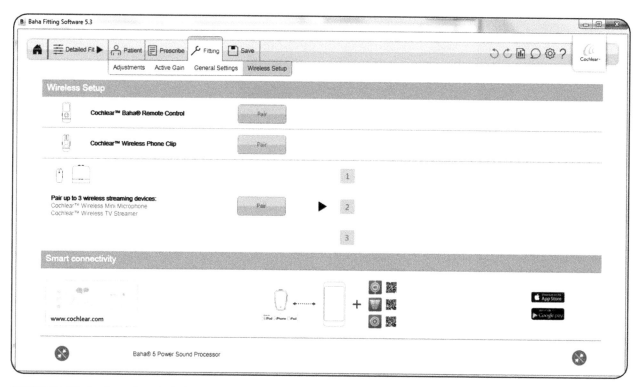

FIGURE 26–53. Configuration of wireless hearing assistive technologies. Image provided courtesy of Cochlear Americas, ©2018.

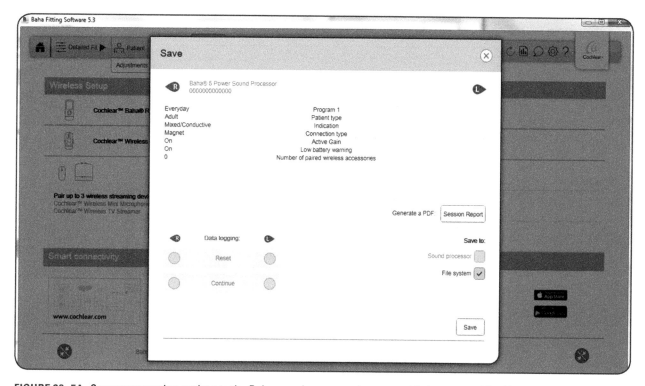

FIGURE 26–54. Save programming settings to the Baha sound processor. Image provided courtesy of Cochlear Americas, ©2018.

Programming the Oticon Ponto 3 Series

Oticon Medical bone conduction sound processors are programmed in the Oticon Medical fitting software, which may be used in a stand-alone version or within the NOAH hearing aid programming software system. Oticon Medical Ponto sound processors are programmed with use of the NOAHLink, NOAH HI-PRO, and EXPRESSlink programming interfaces. To program an Oticon Medical Ponto processor, the audiologist must insert a battery into the Ponto processor and connect the processor to the Oticon cable (Oticon #2 cable for NOAHLink and Oticon #3 cable for NOAH HI-PRO and the EXPRESSlink that is connected to the programming interface. Of note, this text will only discuss the steps involved in the programming of the Oticon 3 series sound processor (which is the latest Oticon sound processor), but the programming of earlier Oticon Ponto processors is similar to the steps described here.

Once the Oticon Medical fitting software is launched, the audiologist will begin the programming process in the "Selection" menu. First, the audiologist must select "Detect" in the Selection screen to establish a connection to the processor (Figure 26–55). If the Ponto is being fitted for a recipient with single-sided sensorineural deafness, then the audiologist should select the "Single-sided deafness" option in the lower corner of the "Selection screen." For recipients with single-sided deafness, less gain will be prescribed in the low-frequency range, and a relatively greater amount of gain will be prescribed in the high-frequency range. If the recipient will be using the Ponto on a soft band, headband, or test band, then the audiologist should select the "Soft band" option in the lower corner of the "Selection" screen. For recipients who use the Ponto on a soft band, headband, or test band, more gain will be provided (particularly in the high-frequency range) to overcome the attenuation that occurs as the mechanical oscillations are transmitted through the skin. Of note, if neither the single-sided deafness nor soft band options are selected, the software prescription will be based on an abutment fitting for a conductive/mixed hearing loss.

Also within the Selection menu, the audiologist may create additional user programs by accessing the "Program Manager" tab (Figure 26–56). As many as four user programs may be loaded onto the Ponto 3 series sound processors. The audiologist can create a "General" program that uses the processor micro-

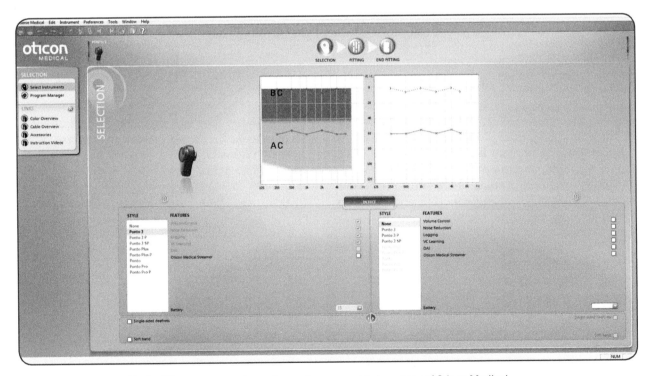

FIGURE 26–55. Oticon Medical Ponto programming software. Image provided courtesy of Oticon Medical.

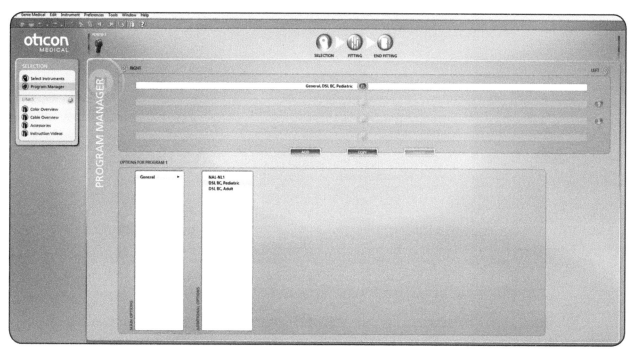

FIGURE 26–56. Selecting prescriptive fitting method used to determine the gain that will be prescribed for the Ponto user. Image provided courtesy of Oticon Medical.

phone to capture audio signals. Additionally, programs may be created for telecoil (T), direct auditory input (DAI), remote microphone (FM), and processor microphone plus remote microphone (FM+M) use. Of note, the telecoil, DAI, and remote microphone (FM) signals may also be activated from the Oticon Medical Streamer. Moreover, within the Program Manager screen, the gain prescribed by the Ponto software may be based on NAL-NL1, DSL Bone Conduction for Children, and DSL Bone Conduction for Adults.

Once the instrument is selected, the type of fitting is specified, and the programs have been determined, the audiologist must proceed to the "Fitting" menu to make any adjustments that are necessary to optimize an individual recipient's hearing performance (Figure 26–57). The first step that is typically completed in the Fitting menu is to conduct a feedback measurement in the "Feedback Manager" screen (Figure 26–58). The Feedback Manager measurement generates a signal encompassing the entire bandwidth of the processor to determine the recipient's maximum gain available prior to feedback. Based on the results of the measurement, the Feedback Manager limits the gain of the Ponto 3 sound processor with the objective of avoiding providing a gain level that

would generate acoustic feedback. The information obtained from the feedback measurement maximizes the capacity of the Dynamic Feedback Cancellation (DFC) system and is used to optimize the function of the volume control. Furthermore, the audiologist may adjust the DFC settings by selecting from one of three options:

- Off—adaptive feedback cancellation is disabled
- Medium—feedback cancellation with phase inversion is enabled but frequency shift feedback cancellation is disabled
- Maximum—feedback cancellation with phase inversion and frequency shift are both enabled

After the DFC is optimized, the audiologist should proceed to the "BC In-situ Audiometry" tab to measure the recipient's bone conduction thresholds with signals delivered to the Ponto 3 sound processor while it is worn on the recipient's head (Figure 26–59). The in-situ bone conduction thresholds are measured in a similar fashion to how bone conduction thresholds are measured during diagnostic assessment. The audiologist simply uses the keyboard's arrow keys or the mouse to change the

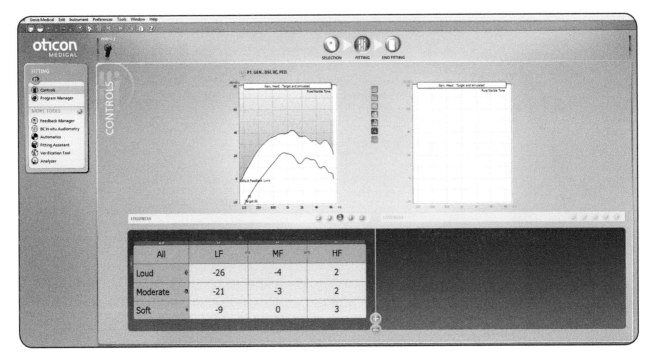

FIGURE 26–57. Oticon Ponto fitting menu. Image provided courtesy of Oticon Medical.

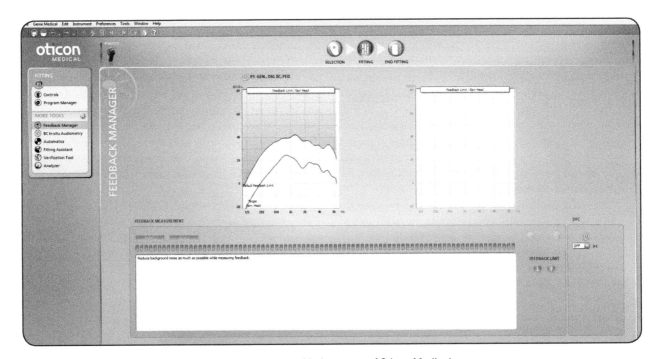

FIGURE 26–58. Oticon Ponto feedback manager. Image provided courtesy of Oticon Medical.

presentation level and frequency of the test signal. The signal may be presented by using the mouse to select the "Play Tone" radio button or by pressing the keyboard's space bar. The last signal that is presented at each frequency is the value that is saved in the BC in-situ measurement.

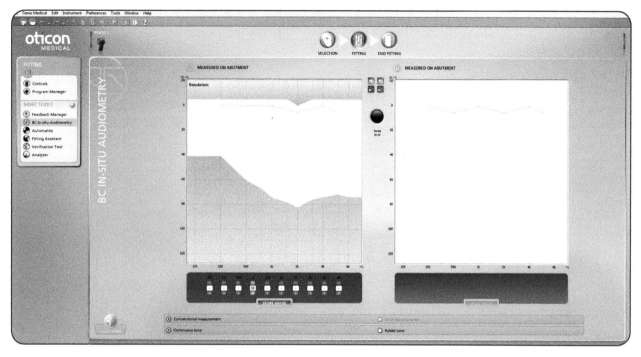

FIGURE 26–59. Oticon Ponto bone conduction in situ audiometry. Image provided courtesy of Oticon Medical.

The BC in-situ measurement should be completed in a quiet environment. The indicator bar next to the picture of the sound processor in the BC In-situ Audiometry screen will turn red when ambient noise levels are too high. The audiologist may use the "Talk Over" button to speak to the recipient during the measurement. Of note, if the recipient switches from using the Ponto 3 on a soft band to using it on an abutment, the BC in-situ measurement should be re-measured. The gain prescribed by the software will be recalculated after the BC in-situ measurement is completed.

Once the feedback and BC in-situ measurements are completed, the audiologist may proceed to the "Controls" section of the Fitting menu to make frequency-specific adjustments to the gain provided for soft, moderate, and loud inputs as well as to the maximum force output (MFO) (Figure 26–60). Of note, the MFO is always prescribed to the maximum setting, but some recipients may wish to have the MFO decreased if the output generated in response to high-level inputs is too loud. The Fitting screen also contains a "Loudness" adjustment control which adjusts the overall gain. The Loudness control is set to "0" by default but can be increased or decreased by two steps. Oticon Medical recommends a decrease of the Loudness control if the recipient indicates that incoming sound is too loud or that his/her own voice is too

"boomy" or loud. A decrease of the Loudness control primarily decreases low-frequency gain. Oticon recommends increasing the Loudness control if incoming sounds are too soft. An increase of the Loudness control primarily increases high-frequency gain.

Several types of fitting graphs are available within the Fitting screen. The "Head" and "Skull" graphs simulate the gain or output for the Ponto 3 when worn on an abutment or when measured on a skull simulator, respectively (Figure 26–61). The FLogram is similar to the SPLogram that audiologists use to view air conduction hearing aid output relative to a wearer's hearing thresholds in dB SPL. The FLogram shows the recipient's bone conduction thresholds and the sound processor output with force levels converted to dB SPL. As a result, the FLogram provides an indication of whether the Ponto 3 output signal is audible to the recipient. However, it is important to note that all of the aforementioned graphs provide a simulation of the output of the Ponto 3 and not a measurement of the actual output level.

The "Automatics" section of the Fitting menu allows the audiologist to make adjustments to the noise management technologies of the Oticon Ponto 3 processor (Figure 26–62). In the Automatics menu, the audiologist may select the microphone mode that will be used by the recipient. The Auto (tri-mode) option is

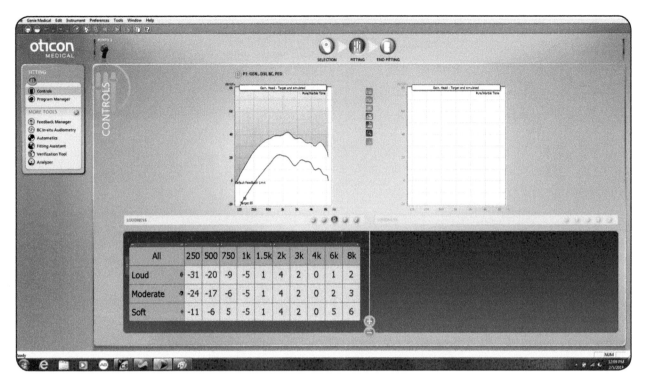

FIGURE 26–60. Oticon Ponto "Controls" section allows for frequency-specific adjustment of gain at multiple input levels. Image provided courtesy of Oticon Medical.

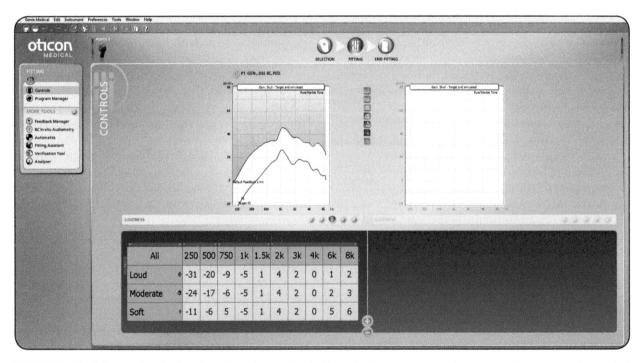

FIGURE 26–61. Fitting graphs simulate the gain and output for the Ponto 3 when worn on an abutment or when measured on a skull simulator. Image provided courtesy of Oticon Medical.

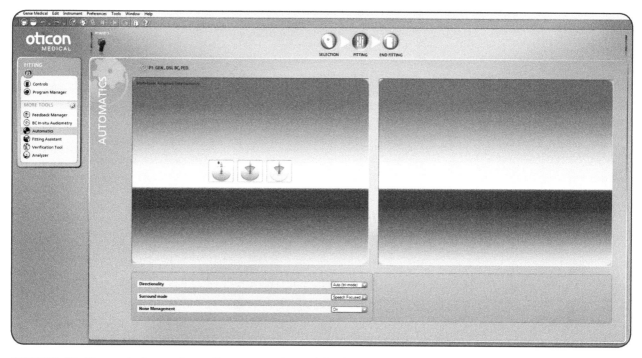

FIGURE 26–62. "Automatics" menu allows adjustments to advanced signal processing features. Image provided courtesy of Oticon Medical.

the default option and automatically selects the microphone mode that provides the most favorable SNR for the recipient. Additionally, the audiologist may choose whether the noise reduction technologies are enabled or disabled. Furthermore, for bilateral Ponto 3 users, the audiologist can enable/disable the binaural synchronization option that automatically synchronizes the directional mode and noise reduction technologies used by each sound processor.

The "Fitting Assistant" screen allows the audiologist to make quick adjustment to select common recipient complaints (Figure 26–63). The "Soft Sound Perception" adjustment allows the audiologist to increase or decrease high-frequency gain for low-level inputs. The "LF Compression Ratio" allows the audiologist to change the low-frequency compression ratio to adjust gain for moderate- to high-level low-frequency inputs. The "LF Roll-off" adjusts the low-frequency gain linearly for all input levels. The audiologist may hover the mouse over the setting of each slider bar to receive an indication of the specific adjustment that is being made (Figure 26–64).

The "Verification Tool" menu allows the audiologist to complete electroacoustic verification measurements without the advanced technologies of the Ponto 3 compromising the measurement results (Figure 26–65). Many of the active features may be dis-

abled to allow for electroacoustic measurements to be completed with nonspeech signals and a skull simulator. The Memory/Analyzer tab allows the audiologist to review the results of the data logging collected by the Ponto 3 sound processor (e.g., program usage, volume control, microphone mode) (Figure 26–66). Of note, a unique feature of the Oticon Ponto sound processor is the Learning volume control (VC). The Learning VC logs the recipient's volume control adjustments across nine different environments and then makes automatic adjustments to the gain settings as the recipient changes environments with the goal of providing an output level that is satisfactory to the recipient and does not lead to a need to manually adjust the VC. The Learning VC activity may be reviewed in the Memory/Analyzer screen.

Once the fitting is complete, the audiologist proceeds to the "End Fitting" menu to finalize the programming session (Figure 26–67). By selecting the "Buttons and Beeps" tab, the audiologist may enable/disable audible indicators associated with various functions (e.g., program change, low battery, etc.) as well as adjust the frequency and level of the audible indicators. The audiologist may also demonstrate the audible indicators to the recipient. Additionally, the audiologist may select the "ConnectLine" tab to manage the recipient's wireless streaming accessories.

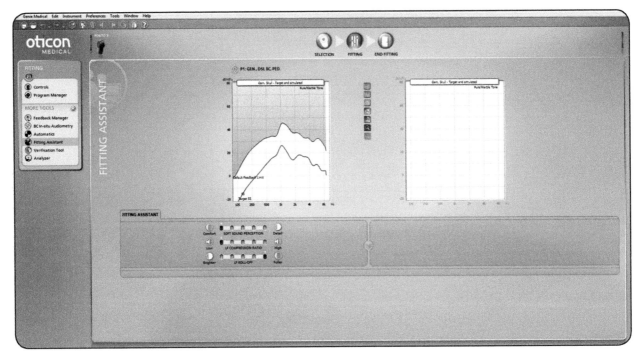

FIGURE 26–63. "Fitting Assistant" allows for adjustments to address common complaints of Ponto users. Image provided courtesy of Oticon Medical.

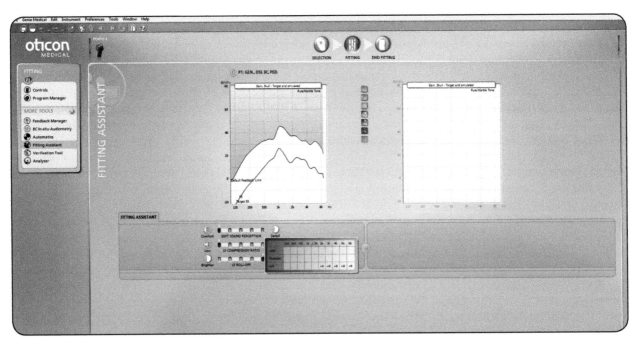

FIGURE 26–64. "Fitting Assistant" allows for adjustments to address common complaints of Ponto users. Hovering the mouse over the area of adjustment shows the magnitude of the adjustment that will be made. Image provided courtesy of Oticon Medical.

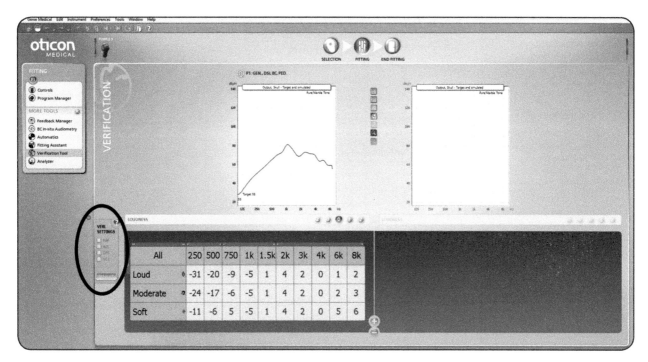

FIGURE 26–65. "Verification" section allows audiologist to disable active features for the purpose of completing electroacoustic analysis or other types of verification. Image provided courtesy of Oticon Medical.

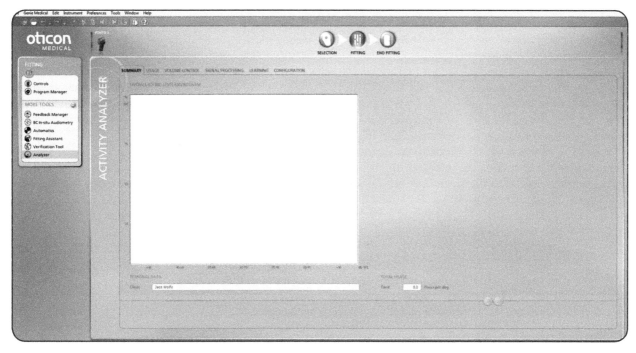

FIGURE 26–66. Data logging. Image provided courtesy of Oticon Medical.

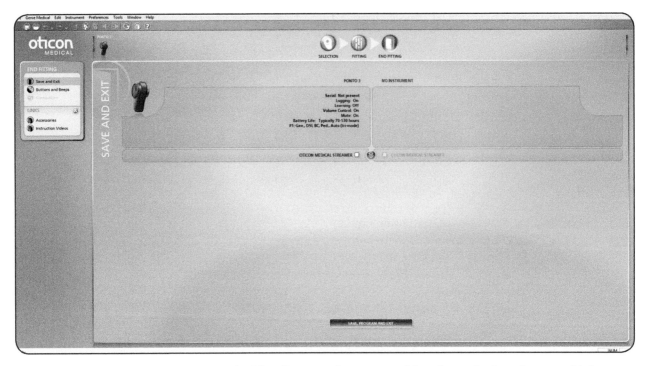

FIGURE 26–67. Save programming changes to the Oticon Ponto sound processor and the software database. Image provided courtesy of Oticon Medical.

The ConnectLine screen allows the audiologist to customize the operation of the Oticon Medical Streamer and to adjust the mixing settings of the sound processor microphone and wireless streaming device. Furthermore, the audiologist can access videos within the "Instructional Videos" tab to demonstrate to the recipient the proper function of the Oticon Ponto 3 sound processor and wireless accessories. Once the audiologist is finished with optimizing the sound processor and with instructing the recipient, the program settings may be saved to the sound processor within the "Save and Exit" screen. As shown in Figure 26–67, a summary of the programming session is provided in the Save and Exit screen.

Programming the Medtronic Alpha 2 MPO ePlus™

Medtronic Alpha 2 MPO ePlus™ bone conduction sound processors are programmed in the Sophono fitting software, which may be used in a stand-alone version or within the NOAH hearing aid programming software system. Medtronic Alpha 2 MPO ePlus sound processors are programmed with use of the NOAHLink or NOAH HI-PRO. To program a Medtronic Alpha 2 MPO ePlus processor, the audiologist must insert a battery into the processor and connect the processor to the proper programming cable (Siemens or Oticon #3 cable). Then, the audiologist must ensure that the volume control is in the "on" position. Of note, this text will only discuss the steps involved in the programming of the Medtronic Alpha 2 MPO ePlus sound processor (which is the latest Medtronic Sophono sound processor), but the programming of earlier Sophono processors is similar to the steps described here.

Once the Sophono fitting software is launched, the audiologist begins by entering recipient information into the "Patient Information" space. Also within the Patient Information Space, the audiologist must enter the recipient's pure-tone bone conduction thresholds. If the Sophono software is operated within the NOAH hearing aid fitting software, then the audiologist enters the patient information into NOAH and that information is imported into the Sophono software. After the patient information is entered into the fitting software, the audiologist must identify whether the fitting is a bilateral fitting and whether it is for a recipient with conductive/mixed hearing loss or single-sided deafness (Figure 26–68). The audiometric information is necessary to generate the prescriptive target gain.

Next, the audiologist must select "Device Detection" to establish a connection to the processor. The audiologist should select "Fitting" to initiate the fitting process. The initial gain settings will be based upon the bone conduction thresholds, the type of hearing loss (conductive or single-sided deafness), and whether the fitting is unilateral or bilateral.

Then, the audiologist may make several adjustments in the "Initial Fit" tab of the "Fitting" menu (Figure 26–69). The audiologist may adjust the overall gain to optimize loudness and access to speech and environmental sounds. Also, the "Feedback Canceller" feature may be used to reduce the likelihood of acoustic feedback. The active feedback canceller may be enabled/disabled, and the volume control may also be enabled/disabled. Additionally, the audiologist may adjust the microphone mode and may also create multiple programs for the recipient to use in different listening situations.

Within the "Bands" tab of the "Fitting" menu, the audiologist may make frequency-specific adjustments to the gain settings (Figure 26–70). Within the "Filters" tab, the audiologist may make adjustments

to each of the six notch filters of the Alpha 2 MPO ePlus sound processor in order to reduce acoustic feedback (Figure 26–71). The "Hz" slider allows the audiologist to adjust the center frequency of these notch filters. The "dB" slider allows the audiologist to adjust the magnitude of the attenuation provided by the filter, and the "Sharpness" slider allows the audiologist to adjust the range of the frequencies to be filtered within the notch filter. Of note, Medtronic recommends that the audiologist use a spectral analyzer to determine the frequency of the acoustic feedback. Spectral analyzers may be used on smartphones or tablets (e.g., iTunes "Feedback Detector," Google Play "Spectrum Analyzer"). Once the frequency of the acoustic feedback is identified, the audiologist can make adjustments in the corresponding notch filter to reduce the feedback.

Within the "Features" tab, the audiologist may adjust the levels of the indicator tones that the recipient hears when the program is switched and/or the battery life is low (Figure 26–72). Also, within the "Advanced Features" tab, the audiologist may adjust the kneepoint of the AGC, the aggressiveness of the noise reduction, and the operation of data logging (i.e., enabled/disabled) (Figure 26–73). The "Manage Memories" option allows the audiologist to select the number of programs available to the recipient and to make adjustments within each program (Figure 26–74).

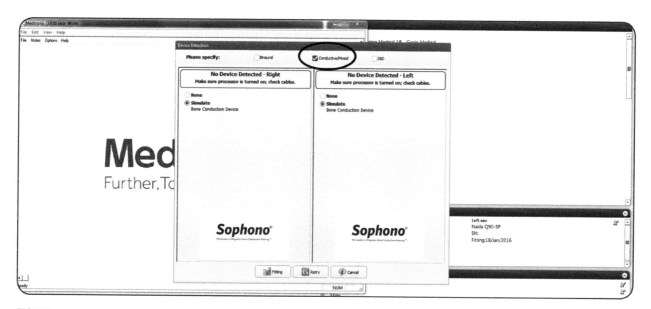

FIGURE 26–68. Medtronic Sophono fitting software. Image provided courtesy of Medtronic Sophono.

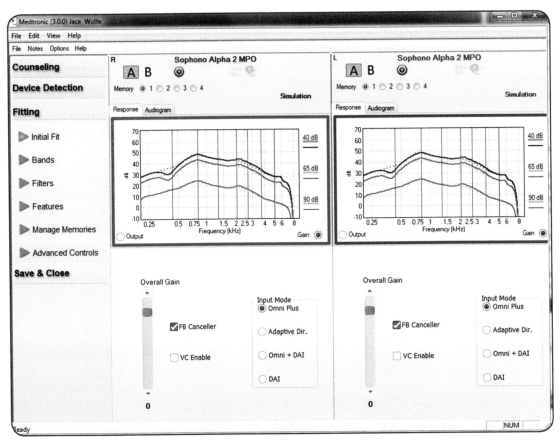

FIGURE 26–69. "Initial Fit" section allows adjustment of overall gain and microphone mode. The feedback canceller and volume control may also be enabled/disabled. Image provided courtesy of Medtronic Sophono.

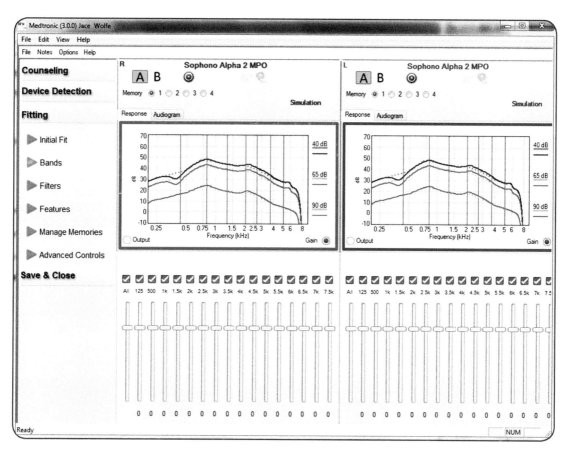

FIGURE 26–70. "Bands" section allows frequency-specific gain adjustments. Image provided courtesy of MedtronicSophono.

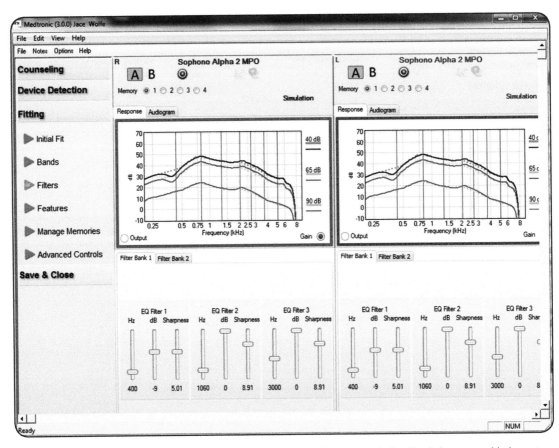

FIGURE 26–71. "Filters" allows for adjustment of notch filters to address acoustic feedback. Image provided courtesy of Medtronic Sophono.

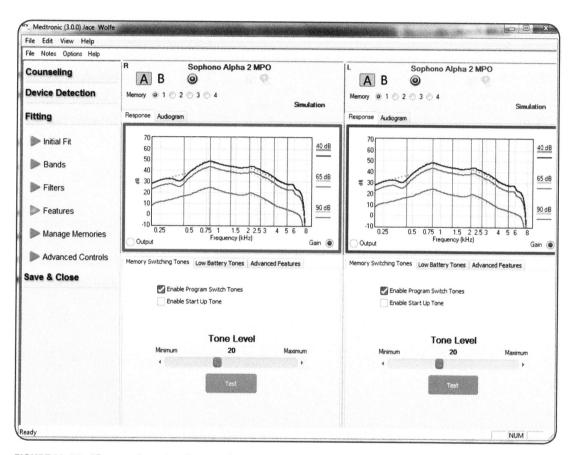

FIGURE 26–72. "Features" section allows audiologist to adjust features of audible indicators (e.g., low battery alarm, program switch, and so forth). Image provided courtesy of Medtronic Sophono.

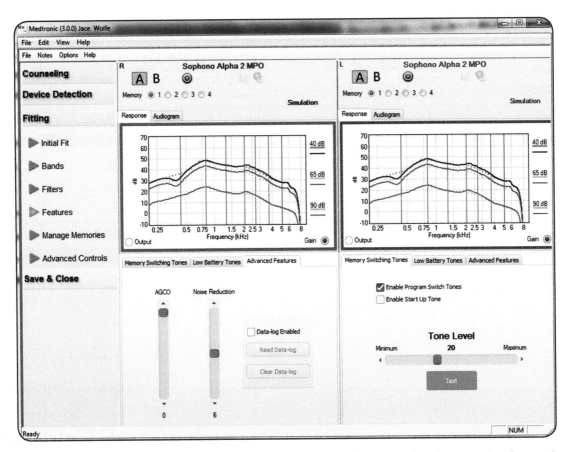

FIGURE 26–73. "Features" section allows audiologist to adjust advanced features such as the automatic gain control, noise reduction activation, data logging, and so forth. Image provided courtesy of Medtronic Sophono.

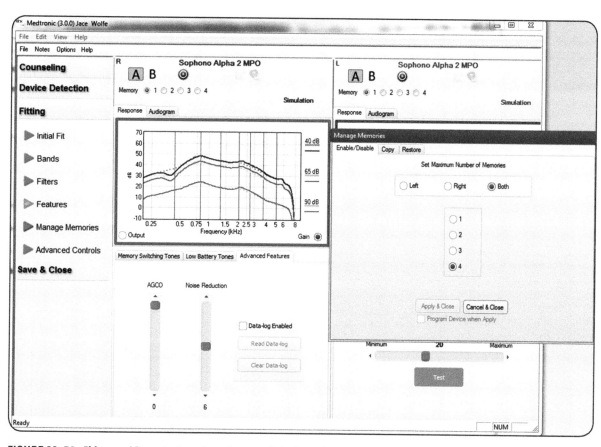

FIGURE 26–74. "Manage Memories" section allows audiologist to determine the number of programs the user will have in his/her sound processor. Image provided courtesy of Medtronic Sophono.

The "Advanced Controls" screen allows the audiologist to adjust a number of different advanced signal processing parameters, including the compression ratio, the low-level gain, the compression kneepoint ("Lth"), the expansion threshold (to reduce gain for very low-level sounds if the recipient complains that low-level ambient noise or microphone noise is bothersome), the expansion ratio, and the crossover frequencies that determine the bandwidth of the channels over which expansion and compression processing are implemented (Figure 26–75). The audiologist may use the "Counseling" tab to access video tutorials to educate the recipient regarding the care, use, and maintenance of his/her new sound processor (Figure 26–76). During the fitting session, all changes made to the recipient's program are saved to the sound processor. However, the audiologist uses the "Save and Close" tab to save programming changes to the database, finalize the programming session, and close out of the fitting software.

Key Concepts

- Implantable bone conduction implants can be very beneficial for individuals with chronic conductive and mixed hearing loss and single-sided deafness.
- Implantable bone conduction implants are available in percutaneous and transcutaneous configurations. There are advantages and limitations of both the percutaneous and transcutaneous implants. The audiologist and surgeon should counsel the bone conduction implant candidate so that the appropriate implant may be selected to meet his/her needs.
- Modern implantable bone conduction implant technology is quite sophisticated. Each manufacturer offers advanced technology with multiple wearing options. The audiologist is tasked with selecting the options that best meet the needs of each individual user.

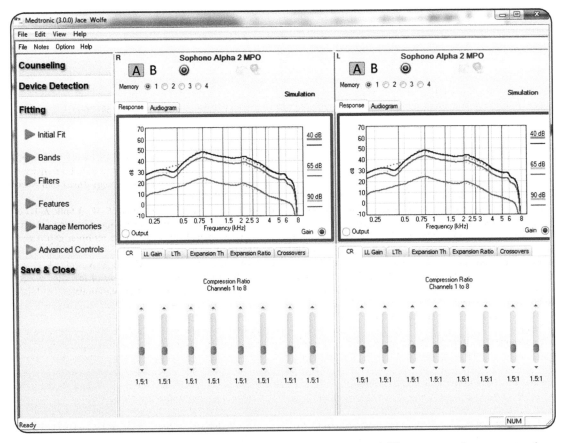

FIGURE 26–75. "Advanced Controls" section allows audiologist to adjust several different processing parameters (e.g., compression ratio, expansion threshold, etc.). Image provided courtesy of Medtronic Sophono.

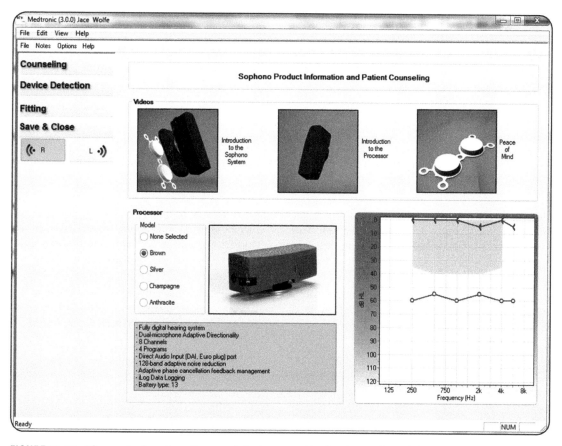

FIGURE 26–76. "Counseling" section allows audiologist to provide visual examples to inform the user of how to properly care for, maintain, and use his/her sound processor. Image provided courtesy of Medtronic Sophono.

References

Bosman, A. J., Hol, M. K., Snik, A. F., Mylanus, E. A., & Cremers, C. W. (2003). Bone-anchored hearing aids in unilateral inner ear deafness. *Acta Otolaryngology, 123*(2), 258–260.

Bosman, A. J., Snik, A. F., van der Pouw, C. T., Mylanus, E. A., & Cremers, C. W. (2001). Audiometric evaluation of bilaterally fitted bone-anchored hearing aids. *Audiology, 40*(3), 158–167.

Chen, S. Y., Mancuso, D., & Lalwani, A. K. (2017). Skin necrosis after implantation with the BAHA Attract: A case report and review of the literature. *Otology and Neurotology, 38*(3), 364–367.

Cochlear. (2014). *Cochlear Baha 4 Systems candidate selection guide 2014.*

Colquitt, J. L., Loveman, E., Baguley, D. M., Mitchell, T. E., Sheehan, P. Z., Harris, P., . . . Welch, K. (2011), Bone-anchored hearing aids for people with bilateral hearing impairment: A systematic review. *Clinical Otolaryngology, 36,* 419–441.

Cone-Wesson, B. (1995). Bone-conduction ABR tests. *American Journal of Audiology, 4*(3), 14–19.

Danhauer, J. L., Johnson, C. E., & Mixon, M. (2010). Does the evidence support use of the Baha implant system (Baha) in patients with congenital unilateral aural atresia? *Journal of the American Academy of Audiology, 21*(4), 274–286.

Davids, T., Gordon, K. A., Clutton, D., & Papsin, B. C. (2007). Bone-anchored hearing aids in infants and children younger than 5 years. *Archives of Otolaryngology–Head and Neck Surgery, 133*(1), 51–55.

De Wolf, M. J., Hendrix, S., Cremers, C. W., & Snik, A. F. (2011). Better performance with bone-anchored hearing aid than acoustic devices in patients with severe air-bone gap. *Laryngoscope, 121*(3), 613–616.

De Wolf, M. J., Hol, M. K., Mylanus, E. A., Snik, A. F., & Cremers, C. W. (2011). Benefit and quality of life after bone-anchored hearing aid fitting in children with unilateral or bilateral hearing impairment. *Archives of Otolaryngology–Head and Neck Surgery, 137*(2), 130–138.

Edwards, C. G., Durieux-Smith, A., & Picton, T. W. (1985). Neonatal auditory brainstem responses from ipsilateral and contralateral recording montages. *Ear and Hearing, 6*(4), 175–178.

Flynn, M. C. (2015). Smart and small–innovative technologies behind the Cochlear™ Baha® 5 Sound Processor. *Cochlear Bone Anchored Solutions AB,* 629761.

Foxe, J. J., & Stapells, D. R. (1993). Normal infant and adult auditory brainstem responses to bone-conducted tones. *Audiology, 32*(2), 95–109.

Godbehere, J., Carr, S. D., Moraleda, J., Edwards, P., & Ray, J. (2017). A comparison study of complications and initial follow-up costs of transcutaneous and percutaneous bone conduction devices. *Journal of Laryngology and Otology, 131*(8), 667–670.

Gravel, J. S., & Traquina, D. N. (1992). Experience with the audiologic assessment of infants and toddlers. *International Journal of Pediatric Otorhinolaryngology, 23*(1), 59–71.

Hakansson, B. E. (2003). The balanced electromagnetic separation transducer, a new bone conduction transducer. *Journal of the Acoustical Society of America, 113*(2), 818–825.

Hakansson, B., Tjellström, A., & Carlsson, P. (1990). Percutaneous vs transcutaneous transducers for hearing by direct bone conduction. *Otolaryngology–Head and Neck Surgery, 102*, 339–344.

Hall, J. W., & Swanepoel, D. W. (2010). *Objective assessment of hearing.* San Diego, CA: Plural.

Hatton, J. L., Janssen, R. M., & Stapells, D. R. (2012). Auditory brainstem responses to bone-conducted brief tones in young children with conductive or sensorineural hearing loss. *International Journal of Otolaryngology, 2012*, 284864.

Hol, M. K., Bosman, A. J., Snik, A. F., Mylanus, E. A., & Cremers, C. W. (2004). Bone-anchored hearing aid in unilateral inner ear deafness: A study of 20 patients. *Audiology and Neuro-Otology, 9*(5), 274–281.

Hol, M. K., Bosman, A. J., Snik, A. F., Mylanus, E. A., & Cremers, C. W. (2005). Bone-anchored hearing aids in unilateral inner ear deafness: An evaluation of audiometric and patient outcome measurements. *Otology and Neurotology, 26*(5), 999–1006.

Hol, M. K., Snik, A. F., Mylanus, E. A., & Cremers, C. W. (2005a). Does the bone-anchored hearing aid have a complementary effect on audiological and subjective outcomes in patients with unilateral conductive hearing loss? *Audiology and Neurotology, 10*(3), 159–168.

Hol, M. K., Snik, A. F., Mylanus, E. A., & Cremers, C. W. (2005b). Long-term results of bone-anchored hearing aid recipients who had previously used air-conduction hearing aids. *Archives of Otolaryngology–Head and Neck Surgery, 131*(4), 321–325.

Hol, M. K., Spath, M. A., Krabbe, P. F., van der Pouw, C. T., Snik, A. F., Cremers, C. W., & Mylanus, E. A. (2004). The bone-anchored hearing aid: Quality-of-life assessment. *Archives of Otolaryngology–Head and Neck Surgery, 130*(4), 394–399.

Iseri, M., Orhan, K. S., Tuncer, U., Kara, A., Durgut, M., Guldiken, Y., & Surmelioglu, O. (2015). Transcutaneous bone-anchored hearing aids versus percutaneous ones: Multicenter comparative clinical study. *Otology and Neurotology, 36*(5), 849–853.

Iseri, M., Orhan, K. S., Yariktas, M. H., Kara, A., Durgut, M., Ceylan, D. S., . . . Deger, K. (2015). Surgical and audiological evaluation of the Baha BA400. *Journal of Laryngology and Otology, 129*(1), 32–37.

Janssen, R. M., Hong, P., & Chadha, N. K. (2012). Bilateral bone-anchored hearing aids for bilateral permanent conductive hearing loss: A systematic review. *Otolaryngology–Head and Neck Surgery, 147*(3), 412–422.

Jerger, J. (1984). *Pediatric audiology: Current trends.* San Diego, CA: College-Hill Press.

Johansson, M. L., Stokroos, R. J., Banga, R., Hol, M. K., Mylanus, E. A., Savage Jones, H., . . . Hultcrantz, M. (2017). Short-term results from seventy-six patients receiving a bone-anchored hearing implant installed with a novel minimally invasive surgery technique. *Clinical Otolaryngology, 42*(5), 1043–1048.

Johansson, P., Jimbo, R., Kozai, Y., Sakurai, T., Kjellin, P., Currie, F., & Wennerberg, A. (2015). Nanosized hydroxyapatite coating on peek implants enhances early bone formation: A histo-

logical and three-dimensional investigation in rabbit bone. *Materials (Basel), 8*(7), 3815–3830.

Kilpadi, K. L., Chang, P. L., & Bellis, S. L. (2001). Hydroxylapatite binds more serum proteins, purified integrins, and osteoblast precursor cells than titanium or steel. *Journal of Biomedical Materials Research, 57*(2), 258–267.

Kohan, D. (2015, February). *Implantable auditory devices.* Presented at the Ultimate Colorado Midwinter Meeting, Vail, Colorado.

Krempaska, S., Koval, J., Schmid, C., Pfiffner, F., Kurz, A., & Kompis, M. (2014). Influence of directionality and maximal power output on speech understanding with bone-anchored hearing implants in single sided deafness. *European Archives of Oto-rhinolaryngology, 271*(6), 1395–1400.

Kunst, S. J., Hol, M. K., Mylanus, E. A., Leijendeckers, J. M., Snik, A. F., & Cremers, C. W. (2008). Subjective benefit after BAHA system application in patients with congenital unilateral conductive hearing impairment. *Otology and Neurotology, 29*(3), 353–358.

Kunst, S. J., Leijendeckers, J. M., Mylanus, E. A., Hol, M. K., Snik, A. F., & Cremers, C. W. (2008). Bone-anchored hearing aid system application for unilateral congenital conductive hearing impairment: Audiometric results. *Otology and Neurotology, 29*(1), 2–7.

Kurz A, Flynn M, Caversaccio M, Kompis M. (2014). Speech understanding with a new implant technology: A comparative study with a new nonskin penetrating Baha system. *BioMedical Research International, 2014*, 416205.

Lin, L. M., Bowditch, S., Anderson, M. J., May, B., Cox, K. M., & Niparko, J. K. (2006). Amplification in the rehabilitation of unilateral deafness: speech in noise and directional hearing effects with bone-anchored hearing and contralateral routing of signal amplification. *Otology and Neurotology, 27*(2), 172–182.

Madell, J. R., & Flexer, C. A. (2008). *Pediatric audiology: Diagnosis, technology, and management.* New York, NY: Thieme.

Mavrogenis, A. F., Dimitriou, R., Parvizi, J., & Babis, G. C. (2009). Biology of implant osseointegration. *Journal of Musculoskeletal and Neuronal Interactions, 9*(2), 61–71.

McDermott, H. J., Henshall, K. R., & McKay, C. M. (2002). Benefits of syllabic input compression for users of cochlear implants. *Journal of the American Academy of Audiology, 13*(1), 14–24.

Naunton, R. F. (1960). A masking dilemma in bilateral conductive deafness. *Archives of Otolaryngology, 72*, 753–757.

Nelissen, R. C., Stalfors, J., de Wolf, M. J., Flynn, M. C., Wigren, S., Eeg-Olofsson, M., Hol, M. K. (2014). Long-term stability, survival, and tolerability of a novel osseointegrated implant for bone conduction hearing: 3-year data from a multicenter, randomized, controlled, clinical investigation. *Otology and Neurotology, 35*(8), 1486–1491.

Nelissen, R. C., den Besten, C. A., Faber, H. T., Dun, C. A., Mylanus, E. A., & Hol, M. K. (2016). Loading of osseointegrated implants for bone conduction hearing at 3 weeks: 3-year stability, survival, and tolerability. *European Archives of Otorhinolaryngology, 273*(7), 1731–1737.

Nelissen, R. C., den Besten, C. A., Mylanus, E. A., & Hol, M. K. (2016). Stability, survival, and tolerability of a 4.5-mm-wide bone-anchored hearing implant: 6-month data from a randomized controlled clinical trial. *European Archives of Otorhinolaryngology, 273*(1), 105–111.

Nelissen, R. C., Agterberg, M. J., Hol, M. K., & Snik, A. F. (2016). Three-year experience with the Sophono in children with congenital conductive unilateral hearing loss: Tolerability, audiometry, and sound localization compared to a bone-anchored hearing aid. *European Archives of Otorhinolaryngology, 273*(10), 3149–3156.

OIHP. (2008). *Ontario Infant Hearing Program audiologic assessment protocol.* Retrieved from https://www.mountsinai.on.ca/care/infant-hearing-program/documents/IHPAudiologicAssessmentProtocol3.1FinalJan2008.pdf

Priwin, C., Jonsson, R., Hultcrantz, M., & Granstrom, G. (2007). BAHA in children and adolescents with unilateral or bilateral conductive hearing loss: A study of outcome. *International Journal of Pediatric Otorhinolaryngology, 71*(1), 135–145.

Priwin, C., Stenfelt, S., Granstrom, G., Tjellstrom, A., & Hakansson, B. (2004). Bilateral bone-anchored hearing aids (BAHAs): An audiometric evaluation. *Laryngoscope, 114*(1), 77–84.

Rompen, E., Raepsaet, N., Domken, O., Touati, B., & Van Dooren, E. (2007). Soft tissue stability at the facial aspect of gingivally converging abutments in the esthetic zone: A pilot clinical study. *Journal of Prosthetic Dentistry, 97*(6 Suppl.), S119–S125.

Saroul, N., Akkari, M., Pavier, Y., Gilain, L., & Mom, T. (2013). Long-term benefit and sound localization in patients with single-sided deafness rehabilitated with an osseointegrated bone-conduction device. *Otology and Neurotology, 34*(1), 111–114.

Small, S. A., Ishida, I. M., & Stapells, D. R. (2017). Infant cortical auditory evoked potentials to lateralized noise shifts produced by changes in interaural time difference. *Ear and Hearing, 38*(1), 94–102.

Snik, A. F., Mylanus, E. A., & Cremers, C. W. (2002). The bone-anchored hearing aid in patients with a unilateral air-bone gap. *Otology and Neurotology, 23*(1), 61–66.

Snik, A. F., Mylanus, E. A., Proops, D. W., Wolfaardt, J. F., Hodgetts, W. E., Somers, T., . . . Tjellstrom, A. (2005). Consensus statements on the BAHA system: Where do we stand at present? *Annals of Otology, Rhinology, and Laryngology Supplement, 195*, 2–12.

Stanford, C. M., & Keller, J. C. (1991). The concept of osseointegration and bone matrix expression. *Critical Review in Oral Biology in Medicine, 2*(1), 83–101.

Stapells, D. R., & Mosseri, M. (1991). Maturation of the contralaterally recorded auditory brainstem response. *Ear and Hearing, 12*(3), 167–173.

Stapells, D. R., & Ruben, R. J. (1989). Auditory brain stem responses to bone-conducted tones in infants. *Annals of Otology, Rhinology, and Laryngology , 98*(12 Pt. 1), 941–949.

Stevens, J., Sutton, G., Wood, S., Feirn, R., Lightfoot, G., Meredith, R., . . . Booth, R. (2013). *Screening programmes guidelines for the early audiological assessment and management of babies referred from the Newborn Hearing Screening Programme.* Retrieved from https://www.thebsa.org.uk/wp-content/uploads/2014/08/NHSP_NeonateAssess_2014.pdf

Sutton, G., Lightfoot, G., Stevens, J., Booth, R., Brennan, S., Feirn, R., & Meredith, R. (2013). *Newborn hearing screening and assessment guidance for auditory brainstem response testing in babies.* Retrieved from https://www.thebsa.org.uk/wp-content/uploads/2014/08/NHSP_ABRneonate_2014.pdf

Thompson, G., & Folsom, R. C. (1985). Reinforced and nonreinforced head-turn responses of infants as a function of stimulus bandwidth. *Ear and Hearing, 6*(3), 125–129.

Tjellstrom, A. (1990). Osseointegrated implants for replacement of absent or defective ears. *Clinics in Plastic Surgery, 17*(2), 355–366.

Tjellstrom, A., Hakansson, B., & Granstrom, G. (2001). Bone-anchored hearing aids: Current status in adults and children. *Otolaryngology Clinics of North America, 34*(2), 337–364.

Valeriote, H, & Small. S.A. (2015). *Comparison of air- and bone-conduction auditory brainstem and multiple 80-Hz auditory steady-state responses in infants with normal hearing and conductive hearing loss.* Abstracts of the XXIV Biennial Symposium of the International Evoked Response Audiometry Study Group IERASG

Van der Pouw, K. T., Snik, A. F., & Cremers, C. W. (1998b). Audiometric results of bilateral bone-anchored hearing aid application in patients with bilateral congenital aural atresia. *Laryngoscope, 108*(4 Pt. 1), 548–553.

Van der Pouw, C. T., Carlsson, P., Cremers, C. W., & Snik, A. F. (1998a). A new more powerful bone-anchored hearing aid: First results. *Scandinavian Audiology, 27*(3), 179–182.

Verstraeten, N., Zarowski, A. J., Somers, T., Riff, D., & Offeciers, E. F. (2009). Comparison of the audiologic results obtained with the bone-anchored hearing aid attached to the headband, the testband, and to the "snap" abutment. *Otology and Neurotology, 30*(1), 70–75.

Wazen, J. J., Spitzer, J. B., Ghossaini, S. N., Fayad, J. N., Niparko, J. K., Cox, K., & Soli, S. D. (2003). Transcranial contralateral cochlear stimulation in unilateral deafness. *Otolaryngology–Head and Neck Surgery, 129*(3), 248–254.

Westerkull, P., & Jinton, L. (2012). The new wide Ponto implant design-clinical and surgical aspects. *Oticon Medical White Paper.*

27

Medical Considerations for Osseointegrated Bone Conduction Implants

Mark Wood

Introduction and Overview

Over the past several decades, hearing technology has advanced to the point that more patients now have access to a wider variety of hearing technology, designed to meet their hearing needs. Although acoustically fit hearing aids have improved in quality and can fit a wider range of hearing losses, many patients cannot benefit adequately from this technology because of the severity of their loss or physical characteristics that impair acoustic hearing aid function. Bone anchored technologies have provided the opportunity to meet more patients' hearing needs, despite anatomic variations that might prohibit the use or diminish the hearing outcomes of acoustically fit hearing aids.

Bone anchored devices are indicated for patients with conductive, mixed, and sensorineural hearing loss. Specific indications for these devices are discussed in other sections of this book, and each device has manufacturers' recommended applications, specified by FDA guidelines. Patient age, history of ear disease, history of ear surgery, and hearing profile can also affect which devices may be best suited to meet a specific patient's hearing needs.

Bone anchored devices can be divided into two broad categories: osseointegrated implants and bone fixture implants. Osseointegrated implants have, as part of their mechanical base, an implant screw, which is surgically placed. This implant screw becomes osseointegrated to the temporal bone and is precisely placed behind the pinna. This means that after surgical placement, the bone of the implant site grows onto the implant screw forming a biologic attachment. These implant screws are made of titanium, which allows the development of this biologic association of metal and bone (Hakansson et al., 1985). The biologic integration of the implant allows physical loading of the implant through either a transcutaneous abutment or a magnetic attachment. The two commercially available devices in this category include the Baha implant (Cochlear Ltd.) and the Ponto implant (Oticon Medical). The Audiant implant (Xomed), developed in the 1980s, is no longer commercially produced.

Bone fixture implants are attached to the bone of the skull, but do not rely on osseointegration for the function of the device. The Sophono implant (Medtronic Corporation) is the only bone fixture implant currently approved by the FDA in the United States. The BONEBRIDGE (MED-EL Corporation), another bone fixture device, is available in Europe and will not be discussed in this chapter because it is not currently approved by the FDA in the United States.

Each of these devices relies on a fixed, subcutaneous implant and an attached, external processor. The implant is inert, whereas the external processor is electronically active. The electronic component interacts with the implanted portion in one of two ways. Either there is a direct physical connection with a transcutaneous abutment or there is a magnetic "connection" with aligned magnets across an intact skin barrier. The Cochlear Baha system can be provided in both a transcutaneous model, the Connect, and a magnetic model, the Attract. The Oticon Ponto implant is only available in a transcutaneous abutment model, whereas the Sophono is only available in a magnetic model.

Other implantable devices such as the Envoy Esteem implant and the MED-EL SOUNDBRIDGE (MED-EL Corporation) are not discussed in this chapter because the primary mode of hearing amplification that they provide does not rely on bone fixation or bone conduction through the skull. The MED-EL SOUND-BRIDGE device relies on an activator attached to the ossicular chain or specifically placed in the middle ear. The Envoy Esteem device is fixed in the mastoid cavity, to the lateral temporal bone, but its activator relies on an attachment to the ossicular chain. Our focus, in this chapter, will be on the devices that are surgically attached to the post-auricular temporal bone area, relying on the transmission of acoustic energy through this bone attachment via bone conduction.

Surgical Preparation

In the United States, most of the implant devices in this category are placed in an operating room, under general anesthesia. The surgery could be performed under local anesthesia with or without sedation for cooperative patients, but most patients undergo a brief general anesthesia for comfort and medical safety. All patients must be healthy enough for anesthesia, and so a medical screening is required by the surgeon, and occasionally in a preoperative setting, with the anesthesia team who will be sedating the patient. Surgical time for these procedures varies from 25 to 60 minutes depending on device being placed and the speed of the surgeon. These procedures are usually performed in an ambulatory or outpatient setting.

Careful preoperative protocols require patient acknowledgment of the planned surgery and surgeon marking of the surgical side, right or left, and last minute discussion with the patient and the family regarding postoperative care. Once the patient is positioned on the operating room table and under stable anesthesia, a standard surgical routine is followed for all devices. Skin markings are made for device placement and surgical incision placement,

since each device has an optimal placement position behind the pinna. The hair is shaved in a small, surrounding area of skin to keep hair out of the way, to allow good visualization for any incisions, and to be able to achieve good surgical antisepsis.

Skin thickness measurements are important for all of these devices, since this will affect device function. Abutment length is chosen based on the skin thickness for percutaneous models, and transcutaneous magnetic performance is affected by skin thickness. For magnetic devices, 6 mm of skin thickness is optimal for device retention and implant performance. For transcutaneous devices, skin thickness determines optimal abutment selection for proper skin health and maintenance after device placement. Both Baha and Ponto abutment lengths vary from 8 to 14 mm. Optimally, abutments protrude about 2 to 3 mm beyond the surface of the skin in the final healed condition. Skin thickness can easily be determined using a small needle, a clamp, and a measuring tool (Figure 27–1). For transcutaneous abutments, measurement of one site is adequate because the abutment protrudes in only one area. For magnetic devices, measurements must be made in several areas to ensure the whole area of skin covering the magnetic surface has the recommended skin thickness (Figure 27–2). Once skin thickness has been determined, local anesthesia with epinephrine is injected to achieve vasoconstriction to help control operative

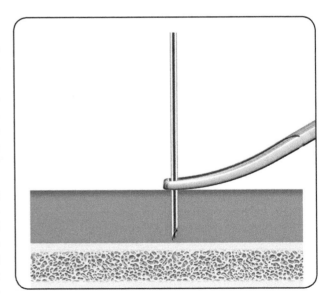

FIGURE 27–1. Measurement of soft tissue thickness. Image provided courtesy of Cochlear, Ltd.

bleeding, and for perioperative pain control. The surgical site is cleansed with a surgical solution and the area is partitioned with surgical drapes.

Osseointegrated implants require the use of proprietary torque controlled drills for placement of the implant screw. Once the skin has been incised and the periosteal surface exposed, the periosteum is incised and elevated (Figure 27–3). The edges of the periosteum are elevated and the bone surface is exposed. The drill is then used with burs to create a guide hole and then an implant hole specifically sized to allow placement of the implant screw. While using the drill, the wound is irrigated thoroughly to wash away bone fragments and to cool the bone, because

overheating of the bone can contribute to failure of osseointegration.

The drill is used at high speed to first drill a guide hole, perpendicular to the surface of the skin (Figure 27–4). Guide bur depth varies from 3 to 4 mm. Both Baha and Ponto have guide burs which allow 3 and 4 mm holes to be drilled, but both companies recommend 4 mm implant screws for maximal strength of the osseointegrated screw. If there is bone at the bottom of the hole using the 3-mm guide bur, the 4 mm bur is used to allow placement of a 4-mm implant screw. In children or adults with thin bone, emissary blood vessels or dura of the cranial vault can be encountered. If these soft tissues are identified

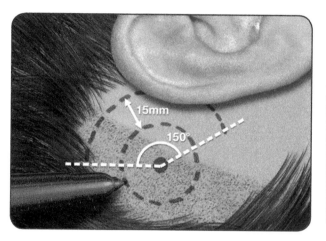

FIGURE 27–2. Marking the incision and implant site prior to surgery. Image provided courtesy of Cochlear, Ltd.

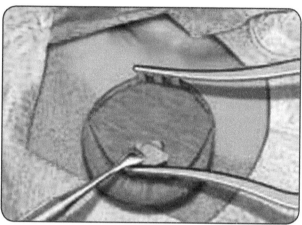

FIGURE 27–3. The periosteum is incised and elevated. Image provided courtesy of Cochlear, Ltd.

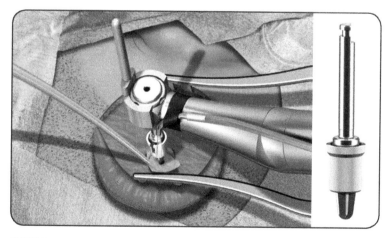

FIGURE 27–4. A drill is used at high speed to drill a guide hole. Image provided courtesy of Cochlear, Ltd.

at the bottom of a 3-mm hole, the implant site must be moved or a 3-mm implant may have to be placed.

Next, a widening bur is used to widen the hole for implant placement (Figure 27–5). For both the Baha and the Ponto implant, the bur produces a 4-mm deep hole and a precise width, along with an external lip at the surface of the bone, to allow the screw head to achieve a "countersink" at the surface of the bone (Figure 27–6). This allows the screw head to be flush with the surface of the bone once it is placed.

The screws used for both the Baha and the Ponto implants are self-taping; this means that the grooves of the screw cut the bone as it is placed, achieving a tight and very specific placement in the implant hole. The implant drill is set for a torque control, which allows a specific amount of force to be applied to the screw as it is being placed. The head turns at a slower rate and the drill stops automatically once the maximal preset force setting is achieved by the drill. This setting prevents overinsertion of the implant screw, which would destroy the self-taping cuts that are made in the bone. Over-insertion can lead to failure of osseo-integration and an unusable implant screw. Irrigation is also used during this part of the procedure to ensure the bone is cooled. The same drill can be used for both the Baha and the Ponto implant screw.

Most transcutaneous abutments come from the manufacturer attached to the implant screw (Figure 27–7). This allows a single stage procedure, placing the implant with the abutment in one surgical setting.

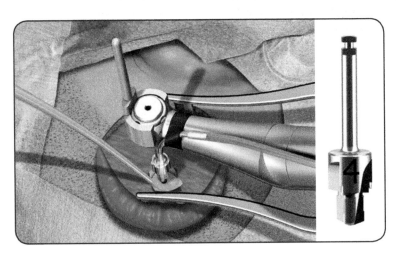

FIGURE 27–5. A widening bur is used to widen the hole for implant placement. Image provided courtesy of Cochlear, Ltd.

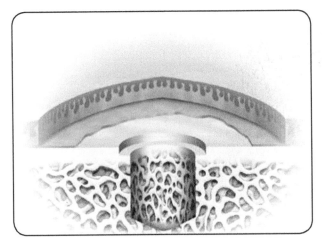

FIGURE 27–6. A "countersink" is created at the surface of the bone. Image provided courtesy of Cochlear, Ltd.

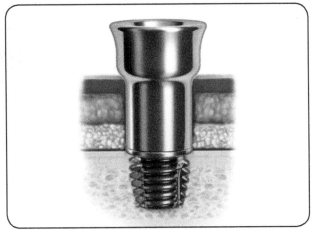

FIGURE 27–7. A percutaneous abutment attached to the implant fixture. Image provided courtesy of Oticon Medical.

Once the implant is placed, a skin hole is created to allow the abutment to protrude through the skin. The traditional method utilizes a generic 4-mm skin punch at the site of the implant, about 5 mm behind the incision (Figure 27–8). Once the skin is removed from the punch hole, the abutment is worked through the hole with gentle stretching of the skin. The skin incision is then closed with suture (Figure 27–9).

Magnetic devices require the same surgical preoperative preparations, but skin incisions vary according to device and will be discussed individually. Both the Baha Attract and the Sophono manufacturers provide skin thickness gauges in their surgical equipment to assist with skin thickness assessment. Needle skin thickness is determined preoperatively, and then after skin flap elevation, a skin thickness gauge can be used to ensure the proper skin thickness, after elevation of the flap (Figure 27–10).

After the device is placed and the wound is closed, surgical wounds require a bandage to collect drainage and to provide a light compression to the area in order to help control bleeding and swelling (Figure 27–11). These bandages are usually left in place for 24 to 72 hours. Each surgeon's routine will vary related to the length of necessary compression.

In the postoperative period, after the removal of the bandage, patients are instructed how to clean and care for the wound as it heals. Surgical follow-up usually occurs 5 to 10 days after implant placement and sutures are removed at this follow-up visit.

Device activation refers to the postoperative episode with the audiology team when the patient is fit with the external electronic components. Current FDA guidelines specify that activation can occur at one month for the Baha Attract implant and the Sophono implant. As their function does not rely on

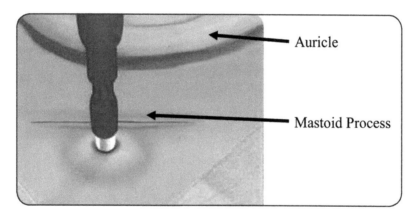

FIGURE 27–8. A skin punch is made at the site of the implant. Image provided courtesy of Oticon Medical.

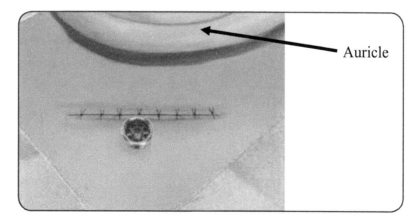

FIGURE 27–9. The skin incision is closed with suture. Image provided courtesy of Oticon Medical.

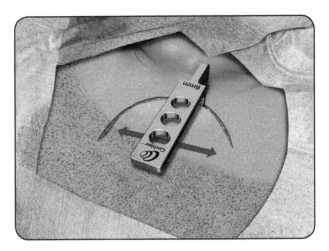

FIGURE 27–10. A skin thickness gauge is used to ensure the proper soft tissue thickness. Image provided courtesy of Cochlear, Ltd.

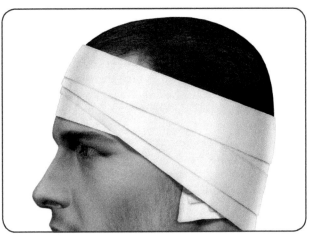

FIGURE 27–11. A compression bandage placed over the implant site. Image provided courtesy of Cochlear, Ltd.

osseointegration, they can be activated once the skin swelling has resolved and the wound appears stable. Current FDA guidelines specify that the Baha Connect and the Ponto implant devices may be activated at 90 days after surgery. This longer period of healing provides sufficient time for osseointegration of the implant screw, which will bear an external load because of their transcutaneous design. This allows optimal long-term health of the implant site soft tissues and bone.

Surgical Technique

Each device has published surgical technique that is regulated by FDA guidelines. The following descriptions follow each company's published surgical instructions that are regulated by the FDA.

Each device has a recommended, optimal location behind the pinna, determined by bone thickness needs, the location of attached external components, and the location of other personal accessories such as glasses or hats. Measurements are usually made from the posterior edge of the external auditory meatus and the relationship to the top of the pinna if it is present.

Skin thickness is easily measured after skin markings are made but prior to any infusion of local anesthetic or surgical manipulation. Using a small needle, the skin can be pierced until the needle strikes bone, and then a clamp is placed across the needle at the skin surface. When the needle is withdrawn, the thickness can be measured on a ruler

(see Figure 27–1). The order of device presentation is done alphabetically.

Cochlear Baha Attract

The Attract is placed 50 to 70 mm from the posterior edge of the external auditory canal meatus (Figure 27–12). The upper edge of the magnet is positioned at about the level of the top of the pinna and the processor template is used to ensure that the processor will not touch the pinna or glasses. The site for the implant screw is marked on the skin, and then the template is used to mark the outline of the magnet, centered on the implant screw (see Figure 27–2). The proposed skin incision is outlined approximately 15 mm from the edge of the magnet placement. After infiltration of local anesthetic with epinephrine and pre-surgical cleansing, the skin incision is made using about a 50 to 60 degree arc (Figure 27–13). The skin flap is elevated and then the periosteum is incised at the site of the implant, and elevated (see Figure 27–3). The implant site is developed using the guide bur and the widening bur, and then the screw is placed using the torque control Baha drill.

A bone bed indicator is then attached to the implant screw to ensure that the magnet can be placed with sufficient clearance for the magnet mounting (Figure 27–14). If necessary, bone can be removed from the area to allow proper magnet mounting on the implant screw. The implant magnet is then placed and positioned with the correct magnet orientation and then tightened using the torque control screw-

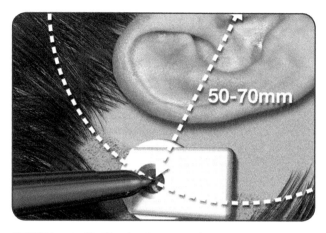

FIGURE 27–12. Marking the placement of the Baha Attract implant. Image provided courtesy of Cochlear, Ltd.

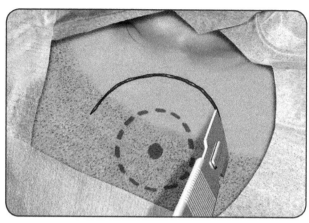

FIGURE 27–13. The skin incision for the Baha Attract is made using about a 50 to 60 degree arc. Image provided courtesy of Cochlear, Ltd.

driver (Figure 27–15). The skin thickness should then be checked to ensure a 6-mm thickness overlying the magnet (see Figure 27–10). Excess soft tissue can be removed from under the flap with scissors to ensure proper flap thickness. The wound is then closed in layers with suture and then a pressure dressing is placed (Cochlear, 2017).

Cochlear Baha Connect

The Connect is placed 50 to 55 mm behind the posterior edge of the canal meatus at about the level of the top of the pinna. The processor template is used to ensure that the processor will not touch the pinna or any glasses (Figure 27–16). The skin is marked for placement of the implant and then an incision line is

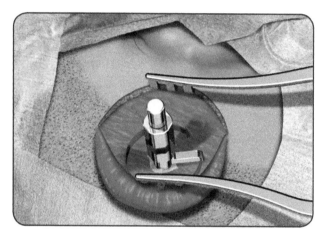

FIGURE 27–14. A bone bed indicator is used to ensure that the magnet can be placed with sufficient clearance for the magnet mounting. Image provided courtesy of Cochlear, Ltd.

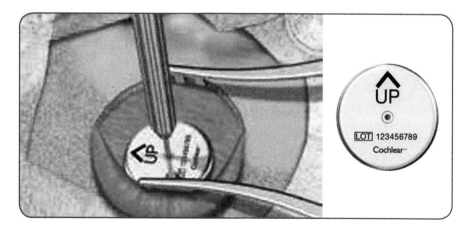

FIGURE 27–15. Tightening of the implant fixture using the torque control screwdriver. Image provided courtesy of Cochlear, Ltd.

marked 5-mm anterior to the implant site. After skin depth measurement, the skin is infiltrated with local anesthetic with epinephrine and surgically cleansed and draped. A 2-cm skin incision is made anterior to the implant site, and the flap elevated posteriorly to allow access to the implant site (Figure 27–17). The periosteum is incised and the implant site is prepared with the guide bur and widening bur.

For adults with healthy skin and bone, the implant screw and attached abutment can be placed together with one surgery (Figure 27–18). Once the implant

with attached abutment is placed, a skin punch is used to place a hole through the skin to allow the abutment to be exteriorized (Figure 27–19). The incision is closed and a healing cap with surgical dressing is placed on the abutment, and then a pressure dressing is placed (Figure 27–20).

For some patients it may be necessary to stage this procedure by placing the implant screw first and then allowing the wound to heal and the implant to osseointegrate. After placement of the implant screw, a cover screw is placed into the implant screw to

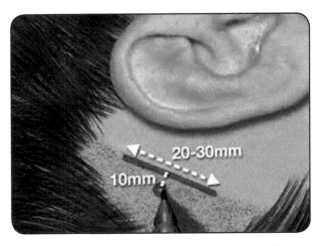

FIGURE 27–16. Marking the incision site for the Baha Connect implant. Image provided courtesy of Cochlear, Ltd.

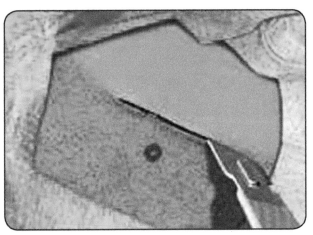

FIGURE 27–17. An incision is made for the Baha Connect implant. Image provided courtesy of Cochlear, Ltd.

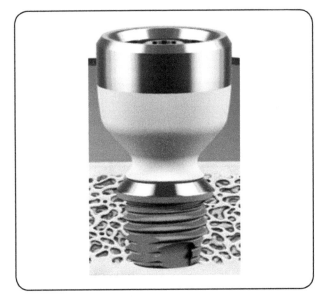

FIGURE 27–18. The Cochlear Baha Connect implant with abutment attached to fixture. Image provided courtesy of Cochlear, Ltd.

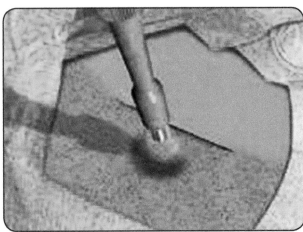

FIGURE 27–19. A skin punch is used to place a hole through the skin. Image provided courtesy of Cochlear, Ltd.

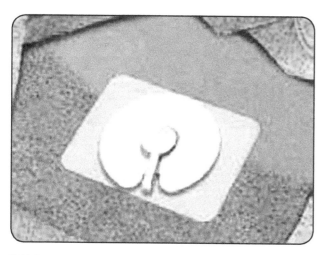

FIGURE 27–20. Surgical dressing is placed on the abutment. Image provided courtesy of Cochlear, Ltd.

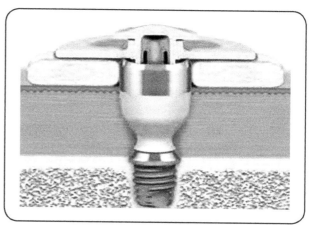

FIGURE 27–21. A cover screw is placed into the implant screw to protect from ingrowth of scar tissue. Image provided courtesy of Cochlear, Ltd.

protect from ingrowth of scar tissue (Figure 27–21). After waiting 90 days for osseointegration, the abutment can then be placed about a week prior to activation of the device, by removing the skin overlying the implant with a skin punch, removing the cover screw, and then attaching the appropriate abutment (Cochlear, 2015).

Oticon Medical Ponto

The Oticon Medical Ponto is placed 50 to 55 mm behind the posterior edge of the external auditory canal meatus just below the level of the upper edge of the pinna (Figure 27–22). The processor template is used to ensure that the processor will not touch the pinna or glasses.

The implant can be placed using two surgical techniques: the traditional method follows the same steps as the Baha Connect as illustrated above. The Minimally Invasive Ponto Surgery (MIPS) uses a special insertion kit, which alleviates the need for an open skin incision.

For the MIPS procedure, the implant site is marked, skin thickness measured, and local anesthetic with epinephrine is injected at the implant site in the same way, followed by surgical cleansing and draping of the site (Figure 27–23). A 5-mm biopsy punch is used to remove the skin and soft tissues down to the periosteum at the implant site and the periosteum is removed (Figures 27–24 and 27–25).

A guide cannula is placed and held at the implant site (Figure 27–26) and the sequence of drilling the

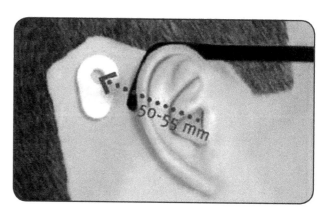

FIGURE 27–22. Marking the implant site for the Oticon Medical Ponto. Image provided courtesy of Oticon Medical.

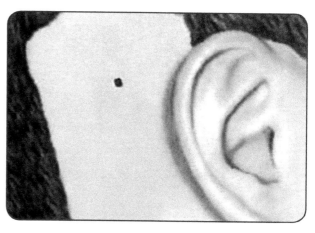

FIGURE 27–23. Marking the implant site for the Oticon Medical Ponto for the Minimally Invasive Ponto Surgery (MIPS). Image provided courtesy of Oticon Medical.

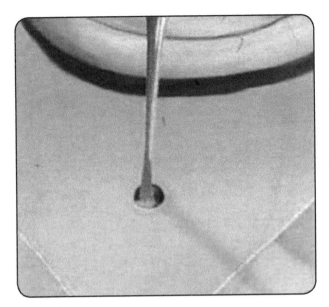

FIGURE 27–24. A 5-mm biopsy punch is used to remove the skin and soft tissues down to the periosteum. Image provided courtesy of Oticon Medical.

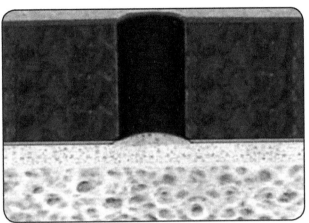

FIGURE 27–25. A visual example of the soft tissue after the completion of the skin punch. Image provided courtesy of Oticon Medical.

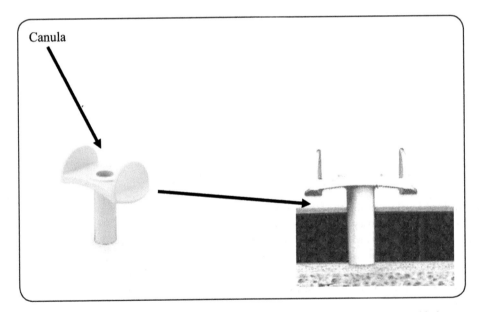

Canula

FIGURE 27–26. The cannula is placed in the hole created by the skin punch. Image provided courtesy of Oticon Medical.

guide hole and then the implant hole is done with MIPS burs (Figure 27–27). The guide and widening burs are designed to work through the cannula guide and are precisely measured to ensure proper bone drilling depth (Figure 27–28). Care must be taken to hold the cannula guide perpendicular to the surface of the scalp for correct placement and skin orientation. The implant with attached abutment is then placed using the torque control drill and insertion indicator (Figure 27–29). A hand counter torque wrench

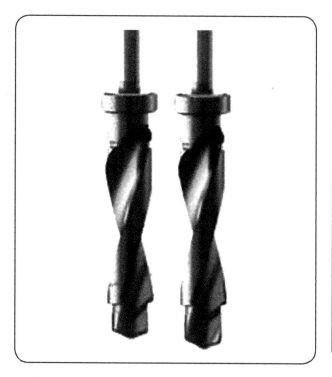

FIGURE 27–27. Oticon Ponto guide and widening burs. Image provided courtesy of Oticon Medical.

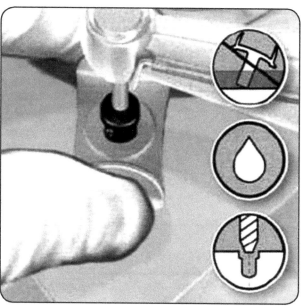

FIGURE 27–28. Drilling into the cannula to ensure proper drilling depth. Image provided courtesy of Oticon Medical.

is then used to ensure a tight fixture of the implant (Figure 27–30). The healing cap with gauze dressing around the abutment is then placed, followed by a sterile dressing (Figure 27–31) (Oticon, 2014, 2015).

Medtronic Sophono

The Sophono implant is placed 5.5 cm from the posterior edge of the external auditory canal meatus. The implant surgical template is used to mark the skin for device location and to plan the incision, and then the skin depth is measured (Figure 27–32). The area is infiltrated with local anesthetic with epinephrine and then the area is surgically cleansed and draped. A curving skin incision is made posterior to the implant site and the skin flap is elevated (Figure 27–33). The implant template is then placed on the periosteum and the area marked for the two recesses and then the sites are drilled for implant placement (Figure 27–34). The implant is then placed into the recesses and five screws are used to anchor the device to the bone (Figure 27–35). The wound is closed with suture and a dressing is placed (Sophono, 2015).

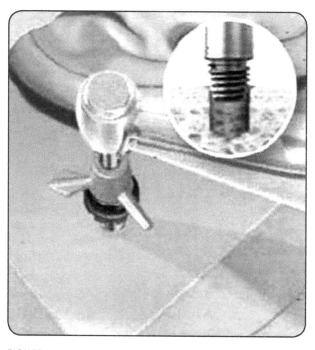

FIGURE 27–29. A torque control drill is used to implant fixture (with abutment attached) into the skull. Image provided courtesy of Oticon Medical.

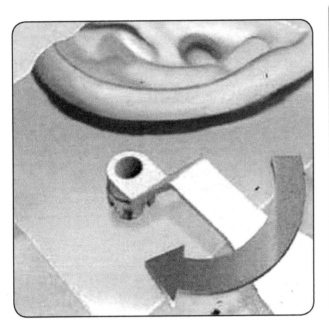

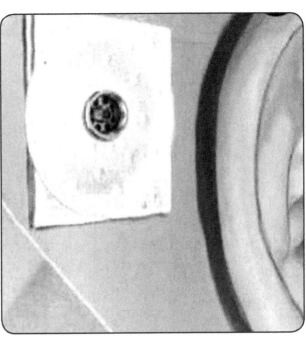

FIGURE 27–30. A hand counter torque wrench is used to ensure tight stabilization of the implant. Image provided courtesy of Oticon Medical.

FIGURE 27–31. A sterile dressing is placed at the implant site. Image provided courtesy of Oticon Medical.

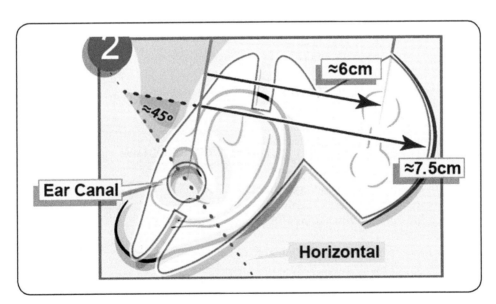

FIGURE 27–32. The implant surgical template is used to mark the skin for device location and to plan the incision for the Medtronic Sophono implant. Image provided courtesy of Medtronic Sophono.

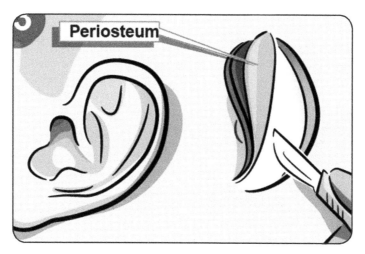

FIGURE 27–33. A curved skin incision is made posterior to the implant site, and the skin flap is elevated. Image provided courtesy of Medtronic Sophono.

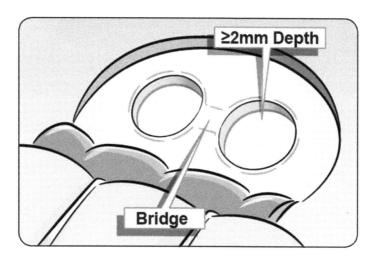

FIGURE 27–34. Two recesses are created in the skull to house the Medtronic Sophono implant. Image provided courtesy of Medtronic Sophono.

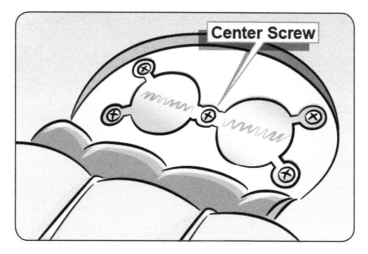

FIGURE 27–35. Screws are inserted into the skull to hold the Sophono implant in place. Image provided courtesy of Medtronic Sophono.

Key Concepts

- Implantable bone conduction implants are indicated for patients with conductive/mixed hearing loss and for individuals with single-sided sensorineural hearing deafness.
- The otologic surgeon should conduct a thorough medical and physical evaluation to ensure that the bone conduction implant candidate is suitable for a bone conduction implant and is likely to benefit from the device.
- The manufacturers of implantable bone conduction implants provide detailed protocols that guide the surgeon in executing a series of technical steps to ensure the successful implantation of the bone conduction implant.
- Regulatory bodies provide oversight of the indications of use for bone conduction implants. Otologic surgeons and audiologists should consider these indications for use along with the information obtained from the medical and audiologic evaluation of the individual to determine whether an implantable bone conduction implant is in the best interests of the individual.

References

Cochlear. (2015). *Surgery guide: Cochlear Baha Dermalock surgical procedure.* Centennial, CO: Cochlear Americas.

Cochlear. (2017). *Surgery guide: Cochlear Baha Attract System surgical procedure.* Centennial, CO: Cochlear Americas.

Hakansson, B., Tjellstrom, A., Rosenhall, U., & Carlsson, P. (1985). The bone-anchored hearing aid. Principal design and psychoacoustical evaluation. *Acta Oto-Laryngologica, 100,* 229–239.

Oticon. (2014). *Surgical manual including linear incision with tissue preservation.* Sweden: Oticon Medical AB.

Oticon. (2015). *Addendum to surgical manual including minimally invasive ponto surgery (MIPS).* Sweden: Oticon Medical AB.

Sophono. (2015). *Quick reference for Sophono implant procedure.* Sophono, Inc. by Medtronic.

28

Middle Ear Implantable Hearing Devices

Jace Wolfe

Introduction

Middle ear implantable hearing devices are quite unique and heterogeneous in their design and operation, but all middle ear implants share a defining characteristic, which is a surgically implanted component that is coupled to a structure in the middle ear and that mechanically oscillates to facilitate stimulation of the cochlea. Unlike conventional hearing aids, which convert an electrical signal from the hearing aid's digital signal processor back to an amplified acoustic signal, middle ear implantable hearing devices convert an electrical signal from the system's digital signal processor into mechanical oscillatory energy. In most cases, this amplified mechanical oscillating energy is delivered to one of the middle ear ossicles, but it may also be delivered to other structures within the middle ear such as the tympanic membrane or the round window membrane. Because of the assorted differences that exist in the composition and function of middle ear implants, a detailed description of middle ear implantable hearing systems is most effectively provided in a discussion of each individual system that has been developed over the past several decades. The objective of this chapter is to provide a basic overview of middle ear implantable hearing devices and to discuss the audiologic principles associated with middle ear implantable hearing technology.

Overview of Middle Ear Implantable Hearing Devices

In 2000, the Symphonix Vibrant Soundbridge was the first middle ear implantable hearing device to receive FDA approval for commercial use. The Symphonix Vibrant Soundbridge contained two components, (1) an external sound processor with a microphone that captured sound and sent it to a digital signal processor that then delivered the processed signal to an external coil which transmitted the signal via electromagnetic induction, and (2) the internal coil of the middle ear implant which processed the signal and delivered it to a vibrating mechanical component that was coupled to the ossicular chain. Figure 28–1 provides an example of technology that is similar to the components that made up the Symphonix Vibrant Soundbridge.

At that time, digital hearing aids were just being introduced for clinical use, and as a result, many patients received limited benefit from conventional air conduction hearing aids. For instance, active feedback cancellation technology was in its infancy, so even digital hearing aids were fairly limited in the amount of high-frequency gain that could be provided prior to acoustic feedback. Additionally, the bandwidth of air conduction hearing aids did not extend much beyond 4000 Hz, and frequency lowering technology was not available in the hearing

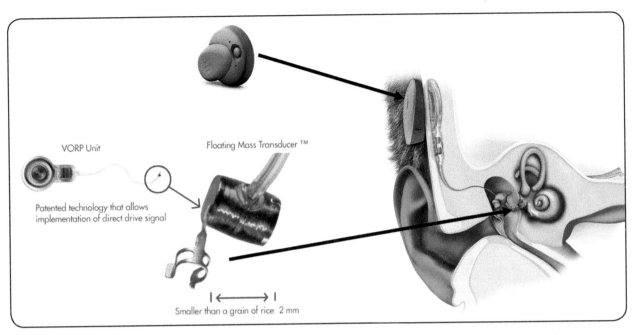

VORP Unit

Floating Mass Transducer ™

Patented technology that allows
implementation of direct drive signal

|←——→|
Smaller than a grain of rice: 2 mm

FIGURE 28–1. An example of the VIBRANT SOUNDBRIDGE middle ear implant with the transducer coupled to the ossicular chain. Image provided courtesy of MED-EL Corporation.

aids of major manufacturers. As a result, persons with moderate to severe high-frequency hearing loss often experienced inadequate audibility from the use of air conduction hearing aids. Furthermore, receiver-in-the-canal (RIC) and thin-tube miniaturized behind-the-ear (BTE) hearing aids had yet to be developed, so persons with low-frequency hearing sensitivity in the normal to mild hearing loss range often had complaints related to the occlusion effect when fitted with air conduction hearing aids.

In the 1990s and early 2000s, middle ear implantable hearing devices were seen as a solution to the aforementioned limitations that plagued analog and early-model digital hearing aids. Specifically, the theoretical advantages of middle ear implantable hearing devices include:

- Greater available gain prior to acoustic feedback; it should be noted that the threat of acoustic feedback is reduced but not eliminated with the use of middle ear implantable hearing devices. In short, the enhanced mechanical oscillation of the middle ear structures can generate acoustical or mechanical energy that may leak back to the microphone (or other sensor) of the implant, resulting in an oscillating feedback loop.
- Avoidance of the occlusion effect, although some middle ear implants do require the use of

a component in the external auditory meatus; it is important to note that middle ear implantable hearing devices that do not require use of a component in the external auditory meatus may be the only suitable option for a person with chronic external otitis or severe skin allergies that prohibit the use of a hearing aid in the ear. Also, some persons cannot tolerate the physical presence of a hearing aid, earmold, or RIC dome in their external auditory meatus. Additionally, middle ear implantable hearing devices that do not require use of a component in the external auditory meatus are not prone to problems from cerumen.

- Improved comfort, although again, some devices do require a component to be worn in or on the ear while many commercial devices require, at the least, a component to be worn on the head.
- Theoretically, many manufacturers of middle ear implantable hearing devices have claimed that middle ear implants can provide higher-fidelity sound with less distortion relative to air conduction hearing aids.
- Some persons may prefer the aesthetics of a middle ear device, particularly if all of the components are implanted under the skin.
- Fully implantable middle ear devices allow the recipient to hear with the implant 24 hours a

day, 7 days a week and may be used during daily activities such as showering, swimming, exercise, etc. and may also be worn comfortably during sleep without a great threat for acoustic feedback.

There are also some theoretical disadvantages of middle ear implantable hearing devices, including:

- The recipient must undergo an invasive surgery requiring one to two hours (but possibly more) for most devices. Most middle ear implantable hearing devices are implanted while the recipient is under general anesthesia, although exceptions do exist. As a result, the risks involved with any otologic surgery (e.g., facial nerve injury, infection, soft tissue complications, cochlear trauma secondary to manipulation of the middle ear) and anesthesia are present with surgery for middle ear implantable hearing devices. However, the complication rate associated with middle ear implant surgery is generally considered to be relatively low (Bittencourt et al., 2014). Moreover, with many middle ear implantable hearing devices, the recipient must wait up to 8 to 10 weeks for healing to occur before the middle ear implant is activated for daily use.
- The cost of middle ear implantable hearing devices is higher than conventional air conduction hearing aids, and surgical costs are usually fairly expensive. In the majority of cases, health insurance does not cover the costs associated with middle ear implantable hearing devices. Furthermore, an audiologist must program the middle ear implant to meet the recipient's needs, and the patient typically must pay out-of-pocket for the audiologist's services.
- Some middle ear implantable hearing devices require the surgeon to disarticulate the ossicular chain, which results in a maximum conductive hearing loss. As a result, when the device is not in use, the recipient is likely to hear worse than prior to the surgery.
- Because most middle ear implantable hearing devices contain a magnet that is coupled to the ossicular chain, recipients of most middle ear implants cannot typically undergo MRI assessment without removal of the implant. However, it should be noted that the MED-EL VIBRANT SOUNDBRIDGE is designed to allow the recipient to undergo a 1.5-tesla MRI without removal of the implant.

- Because middle ear implantable hearing devices do not produce an acoustic output in the ear canal, real-ear probe microphone measurements cannot be used to measure the output of a middle ear implant. As a result, there is no readily accepted method to verify the appropriateness of the program (i.e., gain/output settings) provided by the audiologist.

Estimates are not readily available for number of persons worldwide to have received middle ear implantable hearing devices. However, it is conservative to suggest that the number of middle ear implant recipients lags far behind the number of recipients of cochlear implants and osseointegrated bone conduction implants. A major reason for the disparity in the number of middle ear implant and cochlear implant recipients is the fact that the costs associated with the former is not typically covered by health insurance, whereas the costs associated with the latter are. Moreover, the theoretical technical advantages that were touted by the early developers of middle ear implants to provide superior performance over air conduction hearing aids in the 1990s and early 2000s no longer clearly exist today. Advances in digital hearing aid technology have resulted in higher levels of available gain before acoustic feedback, and as a result, most persons with moderately severe to severe high-frequency hearing loss can receive adequate audibility through the use of modern air conduction hearing aids. Additionally, research has indicated that many persons with severe to profound high-frequency hearing loss receive limited benefit from audibility provided by high-gain, high-frequency amplification (Convery & Keidser, 2011; Keidser et al., 2007). Consequently, any improvement in audibility provided by a middle ear implant (relative to an air conduction hearing aid) for a person with severe to profound high-frequency hearing loss may not improve the hearing performance of the recipient.

Also, the development of open-canal, miniaturized BTE hearing aids (e.g., RIC, thin-tube) in the mid-2000s successfully addressed the problems related to the occlusion effect for many persons with normal to near-normal low-frequency hearing. Furthermore, modern digital hearing aids are now equipped with receivers that can provide high gain and output levels with a wideband frequency response (i.e., >7000 Hz) and low levels of distortion. Modern digital hearing aids also feature advanced noise management technologies (e.g., adaptive directional beam-formers, automatic noise reduction, wind noise reduction) that have provided improved hearing performance and listening comfort in many challenging listening situations. Collectively, the advancement of digital hearing aid technology has addressed many of the limitations that existed almost 20 years ago and has allowed for satisfactory hearing performance for most persons with mild to severe sensorineural hearing loss. Similarly (and as mentioned earlier in this text), cochlear implant technology and hybrid cochlear implant technology have also improved considerably over the past two decades and the indications for use have expanded. As a result, many persons who have significant high-frequency hearing loss and are unable to achieve satisfactory performance with modern air conduction hearing aids have received considerable benefit from cochlear implantation.

Because of the improvements in modern air conduction hearing aids as well as the expansion of cochlear implant candidacy, most persons with sensorineural hearing loss have not elected to pursue middle ear implantable hearing devices. The potential benefits of middle ear implantable hearing devices relative to contemporary hearing aids or cochlear implants often do not outweigh the financial costs associated with middle ear implants along with the need to undergo an invasive surgery. The typical recipient of a middle ear implantable hearing device is one who strongly prefers a totally implantable (or partially implantable) hearing device for cosmetic or lifestyle reasons (e.g., 24/7 use during exercise, swimming, sleeping). Also, middle ear implantable devices may be medically necessary for persons who cannot tolerate the presence of a hearing aid in or on the external ear (e.g., external otitis, excessive cerumen production, etc.). Although rare, middle ear implants may be the ideal solution for the person who is unsatisfied with the performance obtained with air conduction hearing aids and does not have enough hearing loss to warrant cochlear implantation.

Assessment of Candidacy for Middle Ear Implantable Hearing Devices

As with cochlear implants and osseointegrated bone conduction implants, middle ear implantable hearing devices have manufacturer-specific indications for use that are approved by the U.S. FDA (or the respective regulatory bodies of countries other than the United States). In general, middle ear implantable hearing devices are considered for adults (18 years and older) who have sensorineural hearing loss. The ideal candidate is likely to have a moderate to moderately severe hearing loss with reasonably good open-set word recognition capacity. Persons with mild hearing loss are unlikely to be willing to incur the expensive cost and invasive surgery required to receive a middle ear implantable hearing device. Persons with severe to profound hearing loss (i.e., pure-tone thresholds of 75 to 80 dB HL and poorer) are likely to be better candidates for cochlear implants, because the severity of their hearing loss may limit the benefit they will obtain from a middle ear implant. Likewise, persons with fair to poor open-set speech recognition (e.g., word recognition scores <60% correct) measured in optimal conditions (i.e., in quiet at a presentation level that optimizes speech recognition—"PB Max") are not ideal candidates for middle ear implants because their limited speech recognition capacity (which is possibly due to cochlear dysfunction and/or auditory processing deficits) will restrict hearing performance with a middle ear implant. It is important to acknowledge that the health care providers of the implantable hearing device team (e.g., otologist, audiologist) may decide that a middle ear implant is medically appropriate for a person who does not meet the FDA-approved indications for use. In such a case, an off-label decision would be made to recommend a middle ear implantable hearing device for the patient.

Persons with chronic conductive hearing loss have historically been considered to be poor candidates for middle ear implants. In particular, chronic middle ear effusion is a contraindication for middle ear implantation, because the presence of the middle ear fluid would hamper the mechanical oscillation of the transducer placed in the middle ear space. Of note, however, middle ear implantable hearing devices may still be considered for some adults with conductive hearing loss provided the middle ear space is aerated and there is no threat of chronic middle ear effusion or cholesteatoma. For example, the oscillating transducer of some middle ear implants may be coupled to the round window rather than the middle ear ossicles (Figure 28–2) (Olszewski et al., 2017; Skarzynski et al., 2014), a method that effectively bypasses the middle ear and provides direct stimulation to the cochlea. Such an approach may be ideal for a candidate who has otosclerosis or some other ossicular chain pathology.

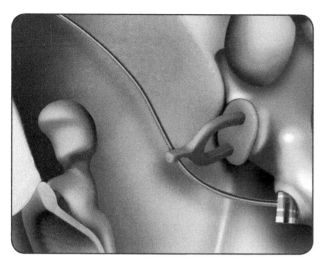

FIGURE 28–2. An example of the VIBRANT SOUNDBRIDGE middle ear implant with the transducer coupled to the round window. Image provided courtesy of MED-EL Corporation.

The assessment battery for evaluation of candidacy for middle ear implantable hearing devices should include air and bone conduction pure-tone audiometry at octave and interoctave frequencies from 250 to 8000 Hz. Middle ear measurements (e.g., tympanometry, acoustic reflex threshold assessment, wideband reflectance) should also be conducted to evaluate the conductive properties of the middle ear system. The candidate should have completed a trial with the most suitable conventional air conduction hearing aids available to meet his/her needs. Real ear probe microphone measurements should be completed to confirm that the output of the candidate's hearing aids has been optimized to meet his/ her needs (i.e., a close match (±5 dB is obtained between the output of the hearing aids and evidence-based prescriptive targets). Additionally, aided word recognition assessment should be completed at presentation levels consistent with speech levels encountered during daily listening situations (e.g., 60–65 dB SPL and 50 dB SPL). Of course, the otologic surgeon will also complete a thorough medical evaluation to ensure that the candidate meets otologic and medical criteria for consideration for a middle ear implantable hearing device. Moreover, the otologist will typically order a CT scan to evaluate the anatomy of the middle ear to ensure that the patient is a good candidate for a middle ear implant and to assist in planning for the surgery. Finally, some otologists may order an MRI to evaluate the central nervous system preoperatively,

because the presence of a middle ear implant complicates the completion and interpretation of an MRI conducted postoperatively.

General Types of Middle Ear Implantable Hearing Devices

Modern middle ear implantable hearing devices typically contain one of three different types of transducers: (1) piezoelectric, (2) electromagnetic, and (3) electromechanical.

Piezoelectric

Piezoelectric materials possess a unique property when they come in contact with electricity. Specifically, when a voltage is applied to a piezoelectric material, the crystal will oscillate. When the piezoelectric material is coupled to a middle ear structure, the movement of the piezoelectric material delivers mechanical energy to the middle ear. Likewise, when physically displaced (i.e., moved back and forth), some piezoelectric materials will generate an electrical voltage. These natural properties of piezoelectric materials make them attractive for use in implantable hearing devices. For instance, a piezoelectric material may be coupled to the tympanic membrane or ossicular chain, and when sound causes the middle ear to vibrate, the associated movement of the piezoelectric material generates an electrical current that may be delivered to the processor of the middle ear implant. As a result, the piezoelectric material takes the place of a microphone as the transducer that can capture sound and convert it to an electric signal. Alternatively, the processed electrical signal from the middle ear implant's processor may be delivered to a piezoelectric material that is coupled to the ossicular chain or round window. When the piezoelectric component receives the electrical signal, it will oscillate and the resultant mechanical energy will be delivered to the middle ear or cochlea. Of note, the intensity and frequency of an electrical signal generated by a piezoelectric material is essentially proportional to the intensity and frequency of the driving force. Also, the intensity and frequency of the oscillations of a piezoelectric component that is stimulated by an electrical current is essentially proportional to the intensity and frequency of the driving current.

Examples of piezoelectric materials include lead titanium zirconate (also known as PZT), barium titanate, quartz, and Rochelle salt. Lead titanium zirconate is a commonly used piezoelectric in middle ear implants (Beleites et al., 2014a, 2014b; Carlson, Pelosi, & Haynes, 2014; Dumon et al., 1995a, 1995b). An advantage of piezoelectric devices is that no power source is required to convert the mechano-acoustic signal into an electrical signal. Another advantage is the fact that piezoelectric crystals have a relatively robust stability and durability. The primary disadvantage of a piezoelectric transducer is that it has a relatively low output and narrow bandwidth relative to electromagnetic and electromechanical transducers. Consequently, a piezoelectric stimulator may not provide enough amplification for a recipient with a moderately severe to severe hearing loss.

Electromagnetic

Middle ear implants operating on the principle of **electromagnetic** induction contain a biocompatible magnet that is coupled to the ossicular chain (or some other middle ear structure) and is positioned in close proximity to a wired coil. An electrical current is delivered to the coil to create a fluctuating magnetic field around the coil. The fluctuating magnetic field alternatively attracts and repels the magnet, causing it to oscillate. The mechanical energy created by the oscillation of the magnet is delivered to the ossicular chain. The intensity and frequency of the movement of the magnet is essentially proportional to the intensity and frequency of the electrical current that is sent to the wired coil.

Electromagnetic transducers are commonly used in electronic applications and may be successfully used to transmit audio signals across the speech frequency bandwidth. A potential disadvantage of an electromagnetic transducer is the fact that the output is dependent upon the magnet being in close proximity to the stimulating coil (Beleites et al., 2014a, 2014b). Specifically, the output of the magnet decreases by the square of the distance between the coil and magnet. For example, if the distance between the coil and magnet is doubled, the output level produced by the oscillating magnet is only one-quarter of what it was with the original separation between the two components. As such, the surgeon must be certain to position the coil and magnets at the recommended distance from one another. Still, however, it is possible that head and mouth movements may temporarily alter the distance between the magnet and coil, resulting in a momentary change in the output of the magnet.

Electromechanical

Electromechanical transducers are a variant of electromagnet transducers and were designed to eliminate the limitation that occurred with the latter when a suboptimal distance existed between the coil and the magnet. Electromechanical transducers comprise a biocompatible magnet that is surrounded by a wire coil. In other words, the coil and the magnet are housed together in one package, a design which optimizes and stabilizes the spatial separation between the coil and magnet. The electromechanical transducer is physically coupled to the ossicular chain (or conceivably to the round window). An electrical current is delivered from the middle ear implant's processor to the coil, creating an electromagnetic field that alternatively attracts and repels the underlying magnet. The mechanical energy created by the oscillating magnet is delivered to the structure to which the transducer is coupled.

An advantage of an electromechanical transducer is the potential to generate a higher output level and wider frequency response. Furthermore, electromechanical transducers are not prone to variable output that may potentially plague an electromagnetic transducer when the distance between the magnet and coil is altered. A theoretical disadvantage of an electromechanical transducer is the fact that the use of multiple components housed within one package creates a device that is more complex and potentially more prone to mechanical failure. However, this potential limitation is fairly negligible because modern manufacturing practices reduce the likelihood of failure.

Modern Middle Ear Implantable Hearing Devices

A number of middle ear implantable hearing devices have been approved for commercial use. These devices are quite diverse in both their design and their application for use. Some are partially implantable and require use of an externally worn sound processor, whereas others are totally implantable. In the following section, a review will be provided of modern middle ear implantable devices that are FDA approved for commercial use for persons with hearing loss.

MED-EL VIBRANT SOUNDBRIDGE

The MED-EL VIBRANT SOUNDBRIDGE is a partially implantable middle ear implant system that contains two basic components: (1) an external sound processor known as the Amadè (Figure 28–3) and

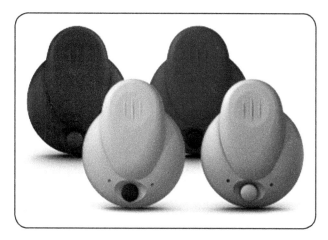

FIGURE 28–3. The Amadè sound processor. Image provided courtesy of MED-EL Corporation.

(2) the MED-EL VIBRANT SOUNDBRIDGE implant (Figure 28–4). The VIBRANT SOUNDBRIDGE **Vibrating Ossicular Prosthesis** (VORP 502x) implant has the same general appearance of a cochlear implant and comprises: (1) a receiving coil that surrounds a biocompatible magnet, (2) an internal processor and stimulator (i.e., the "demodulator"), (3) a lead (the Conductor Link) that delivers electrical current from the stimulator to the transducer, and (4) the Floating Mass Transducer (FMT).

Sound is captured by the microphones of the Amadè sound processor and analyzed by the Amadè's digital signal processor. The processed signal is converted to an electrical current that is delivered to the Amadè's transmitting coil, where it is delivered across the recipient's skin via electromagnetic induction (i.e., short range radio frequency [RF] transmission). The coil of the VORP 502x receives the RF signal and converts it to an electrical signal that is delivered to the VORP 502x implant's processor for analysis. Then, the VORP 502x delivers an electrical current down the Conductor Link lead to the FMT. The FMT is an electromechanical transducer that contains a wire coil that surrounds a magnet, which is housed in a titanium case. The electrical current travels from the Conducting Link through the FMT's coil, creating a magnetic field that attracts and repels the magnet within the FMT. In conventional use, the

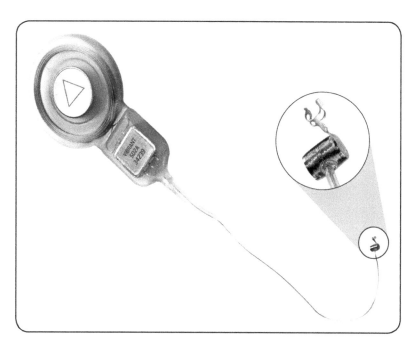

FIGURE 28–4. The VIBRANT SOUNDBRIDGE implant with the Vibrating Ossicular Prosthesis (VORP 502x). Image provided courtesy of MED-EL Corporation.

FMT is coupled to the long process of the incus (Figure 28–5A), and as a result, the amplified mechanical energy of the oscillating magnet is delivered to the ossicular chain, resulting in greater displacement of the ossicular chain and cochlea. The FMT may also be coupled to the body of the incus (Figure 28–5B), and for recipients with mixed/conductive hearing loss, it may be coupled to the round window (via a special round window coupler or with the placement of fascia) to deliver mechanical stimulation directly to the cochlea (see Figure 28–2).

Of note, at the time of this writing, MED-EL had developed the VORP 503 implant, which is approved for use in most European countries but not by the FDA for use in the United States. The VORP 503 contains several design improvements that may potentially provide benefit for the recipient:

- MED-EL suggests the VORP 503 is compatible with 1.5-T MRI because the poles of the magnets are designed to react neutrally to the magnetic field of the MRI and to avoid aligning with the magnetic field. As a result, the magnetic field of the MRI does not apply stress to the magnets of the SOUNDBRIDGE VORP 503 implant. The magnet technology contained within the VORP 503 is similar to the MRI-compatible magnet technology used in the MED-EL SYNCHRONY cochlear implant.
- The VORP 503 possesses a lower profile than its predecessor.

- The VORP 503 contains two "fixation holes" through which titanium screws may be inserted into the skull to facilitate stability of the implant's receiving coil and demodulator.
- The VORP 503 contains a shorter conductor link length with increased tensile strength to allow for easier handling by the surgeon.
- The VORP 503 provides an array of couplers to allow the surgeon to choose the coupling apparatus that will optimize connection to the desired location (e.g., short process of incus, long process of incus, stapes head, round window).

The FDA-approved indications for use for the MED-EL VIBRANT SOUNDBRIDGE VORP 502x are:

- Adults (18 years and older)
- Audiologic results consistent with sensorineural hearing loss
- Unaided pure-tone air conduction thresholds within the following ranges:
  ○ 500 Hz: 30–65 dB HL
  ○ 1000 Hz: 40–75 dB HL
  ○ 1500 Hz: 45–80 dB HL
  ○ 2000 Hz: 45–80 dB HL
  ○ 3000 Hz: 50–85 dB HL
  ○ 4000 Hz: 50–85 dB HL
- Word recognition equal to or better than 50% correct (recorded materials) in best aided condition (65 dB SPL presentation level) or when

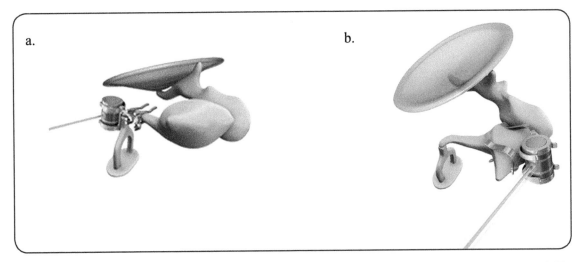

FIGURE 28–5. A. The VIBRANT SOUNDBRIDGE Floating Mass Transducer coupled to the long process of the incus. **B.** The Floating Mass Transducer coupled to the body of the incus. Images provided courtesy of MED-EL Corporation.

tested under earphones at most comfortable presentation level
- Normal middle ear anatomy
- Psychologically and motivationally suitable with realistic expectations of the benefits and limitations of the device

Contraindications for the MED-EL VIBRANT SOUND-BRIDGE include:

- Conductive hearing loss
- Retrocochlear or central auditory disorder
- Active middle ear infections
- Tympanic membrane perforations associated with recurrent middle ear infections
- A skin or scalp condition that may preclude attachment of the audio processor

Also of note, at the time of this writing, the SAMBA sound processor was available for MED-EL SOUNDBRIDGE recipients but was not yet approved by the FDA for use in the United States (Figure 28–6). The SAMBA features wireless connectivity that allows users to connect to personal electronic devices via Bluetooth or telecoil. For Bluetooth use, SAMBA users must have the Siemens miniTek wireless interface, which sends and receives audio information from Bluetooth devices and delivers audio information to the SAMBA via near-field magnetic induction. The SAMBA also possesses the "Intelligent Sound Adapter," which is an acoustic scene classifier that analyzes the user's environment and automatically selects the most appropriate settings (e.g., microphone mode, noise reduction) for the environment. Additionally, the "Intelligent Sound Adapter" keeps track of the user's manual adjustments (i.e., volume control changes) and automatically changes the processor settings based on the user's previous adjustments. The SAMBA also contains adaptive directional microphone technology and "Speech Tracking," which seeks to focus toward the direction from which speech is arriving.

Many otologic surgeons will elect to proceed with implantation of the VIBRANT SOUNDBRIDGE for persons who are likely to benefit from the device even though they may not meet the exact indications for use of the implant. For instance, the SOUND-BRIDGE is routinely considered for persons who have thresholds better than 30 dB HL at 500 Hz with moderately severe to severe high-frequency hearing loss. Additionally, and as previously discussed, the VIBRANT SOUNDBRIDGE is considered for persons with conductive hearing loss in Europe and other countries outside of the United States with placement of the FMT on the round window. Furthermore, otologic surgeons in Europe may consider the VIBRANT SOUNDBRIDGE implant for children over the age of 5 years (Lim et al., 2012; Minovi et al., 2014; Strenger & Stark, 2012).

The Amadè sound processor contains two omnidirectional microphones that may be used for directional beam-forming. The Amadè also possesses an 8-channel (with 16 bands for audiologists to adjust gain) wide dynamic range compressor. Additionally, the Amadè contains automatic noise reduction, speech enhancement processing, adaptive feedback cancellation, and wind noise reduction. The user may select from up to three programs that may be accessed via a push button that is located between the two microphone ports. The Amadè is powered by a zinc-air 675 disposable battery and has a removable magnet that is available in various strengths.

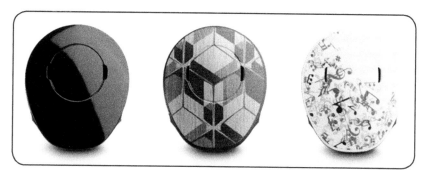

FIGURE 28–6. SAMBA sound processor for the VIBRANT SOUNDBRIDGE middle ear implant. Image provided courtesy of MED-EL Corporation.

The Amadè sound processor is programmed with use of the MED-EL SOUNDBRIDGE software, which may be used within the NOAH fitting system or in a stand-alone version. The NOAH HI-PRO and NOAHLink programming interfaces may be used to connect the sound processor to the programming computer. In order to program the device, the audiologist must insert a new power zinc-air 675 battery into the Amadè sound processor and connect a Siemens Connex 02 programming cable to the programming interface and processor. Then, the battery door of the Amadè sound processor must be positioned so that the door is right next to the programming cable without touching the cable. The battery door must be in the proper position in order for the sound processor to be in programming mode and detected by the programming computer. If the Amadè is not detected by the programming computer, then the audiologist should attempt to re-position the battery door and attempt to detect the sound processor again. Figures 28–7 through 28–11 provide screenshots from the programming software. When the sound processor is initially fitted for the recipient, the prescribed gain and output values may be based on one of three different evidence-based fitting methods (DSL-I/O, NAL-NL1, NAL-NL2) (Figure 28–8). After the initial fitting is applied, the audiologist may make general adjustments to the gain/output settings in the "Basic Tuning" menu (Figure 28–9). In the "Fine Tuning" menu, the audiologist may adjust overall and band-specific gain, overall maximum power output, compression characteristics, microphone mode, noise reduction properties, and so on (Figure 28–10). Additionally, the "**Vibrogram**" feature may be used to measure in situ thresholds, which are then used to prescribe individually specific gain/output values based on the output level from the device required to elicit an auditory response from the recipient (Figure 28–11).

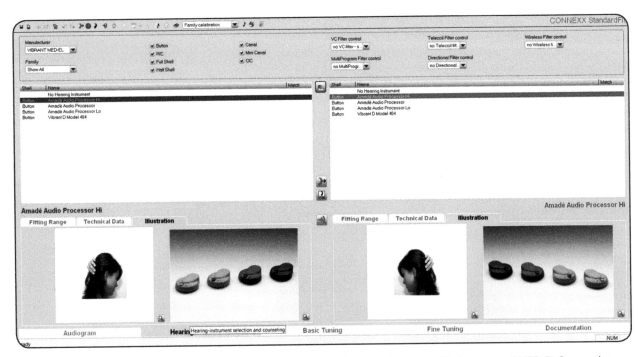

FIGURE 28–7. Fitting software for VIBRANT SOUNDBRIDGE middle ear implants. Image provided courtesy of MED-EL Corporation.

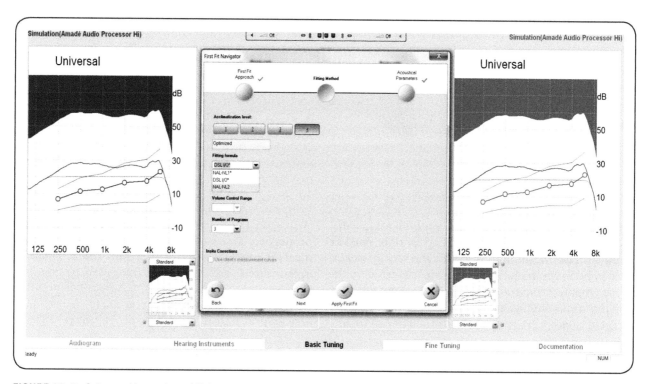

FIGURE 28–8. Select evidence-based fitting method used to prescribe gain for VIBRANT SOUNDBRIDGE implant recipients. Image provided courtesy of MED-EL Corporation.

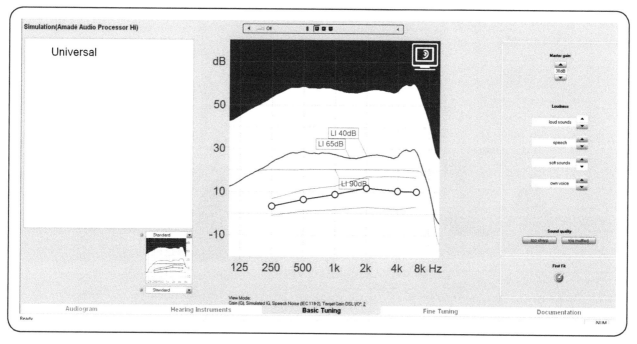

FIGURE 28–9. "Basic Tuning" section allows for programming adjustments to address reports that VIBRANT SOUNDBRIDGE recipients commonly make about sound quality and their listening experience. Image provided courtesy of MED-EL Corporation.

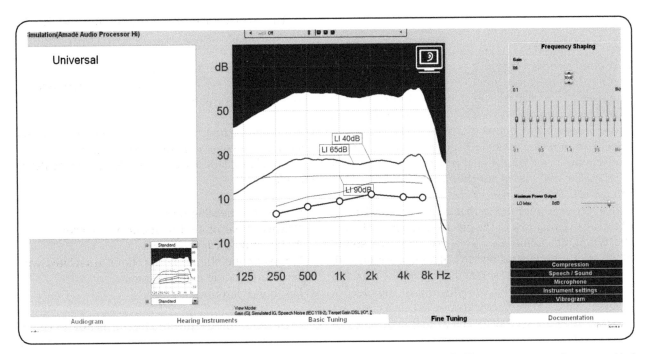

FIGURE 28–10. "Fine Tuning" section allows audiologist to make adjustments to a variety of different parameters. Image provided courtesy of MED-EL Corporation.

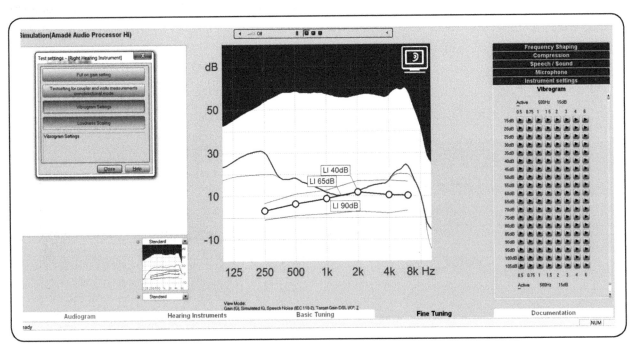

FIGURE 28–11. The Vibrogram allows the audiologist to make in situ measurements of hearing threshold with tonal signals delivered directly from the implant. Image provided courtesy of MED-EL Corporation.

MAXUM (Ototronix, LLC)

The Ototronix MAXUM middle ear implant contains two components (Figure 28–12): (1) an externally worn ear-level sound processor, and (2) a neodymium-iron-boron magnet that is housed in a titanium case. The externally worn sound processor is known as the Integrated Processor and Coil (IPC) and consists of an in-the-canal style hearing aid that contains a microphone, a digital signal processor, and an electromagnetic coil that is attached to the medial end of the device. The objective of the MAXUM fitting is to take a deep ear impression that allows the fabrication of the device that places the electromagnetic coil near the tympanic membrane. The IPC captures sound at the microphone, analyzes the incoming sound with the digital signal processor, and converts the signal to an electrical current that is delivered to the electromagnetic coil. As the electrical current travels through the coil, it is converted to electromagnetic lines of flux that emanate across the tympanic membrane and toward the MAXUM's magnet, which is coupled to the incudostapedial joint at the neck of the stapes. The fluctuating electromagnetic field from the IPC's coil alternatively repels and attracts the magnet, and this oscillating movement of the magnet delivers mechanical energy to the ossicular chain.

The FDA-approved indications for use for the Ototronix MAXUM are:

- Adults (18 years and older)
- Audiologic results consistent with moderate to severe sensorineural hearing loss

It is recommended that the individual have "experience with appropriately fit hearing aids."

Contraindications for the Ototronix MAXUM include:

- Conductive hearing loss
- Retrocochlear or central auditory disorder
- Active middle ear infections
- Tympanic membrane perforations associated with recurrent middle ear infections
- Disabling tinnitus

Of note, the candidate should ideally have air-bone gaps of no more than 10 dB. Also, the candidate's preoperative word recognition scores should be 60% correct or better (Pelosi, Carlson, & Glasscock III, 2014).

The Ototronix MAXUM is based on the SOUNDTEC Direct Drive Hearing System originally developed by Jack Hough and colleagues at the Hough Ear Institute

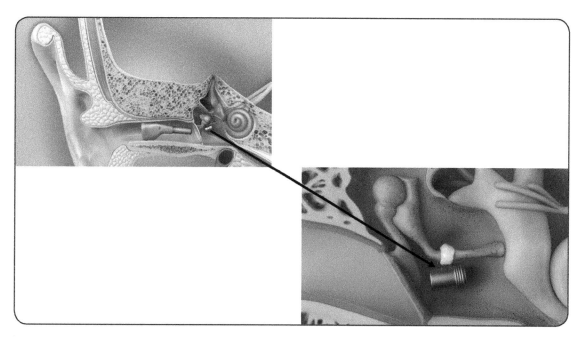

FIGURE 28–12. The Ototronix MAXUM middle ear implant. Image provided courtesy of Ototronix.

(Hough et al., 2001). A unique feature of the MAXUM implant is that it may be implanted under local anesthesia through the tympanic membrane (i.e., transcanal approach). Conceivably, the MAXUM device can be implanted in the surgeon's clinic without the need for general anesthesia and without a mastoidectomy approach. As a result, the MAXUM surgery is less invasive than the surgery required for other middle ear implantable devices. In order to ensure optimal efficiency of the electromagnetic signal from the coil to the magnet, the coil must be positioned close to the tympanic membrane, and the magnet must be positioned parallel to the coil.

The IPC device is generally fitted about 3 weeks after surgery (Pelosi, Carlson, & Glasscock III, 2014). Heat (e.g., hairdryer) may be used to bend/shape the coil of the IPC if needed to facilitate a parallel orientation with the implanted magnet to optimize stimulus delivery. The audiologist may program the MAXUM IPC using Ototronix's proprietary fitting software.

Envoy Esteem

The Envoy Esteem middle ear implant is the only totally implantable hearing device approved for commercial distribution by the United States FDA. The Envoy Esteem implant contains four components which are all contained within one implantable device (Figure 28–13): (1) the Esteem Sensor, (2) the Esteem Sound Processor, (3) the Esteem Driver, and (4) a non-rechargeable lithium-iodide battery. All of these components are implanted in the temporal bone. In other words, the Envoy Esteem does not contain an externally worn component. The Esteem Sound Processor and battery are implanted in a "bed" that the surgeon hollows out in the temporal bone just behind the auricle. The Esteem Sensor and Driver are placed in the middle ear space. The Esteem Sensor is coupled to the body of the incus and contains a piezoelectric transducer that converts the movement of the incus into an electrical signal which is delivered via a lead to the Esteem Sound Processor. The signal is analyzed by the Esteem Sound Processor and then delivered via a separate lead to the Esteem Driver, which also contains a piezoelectric transducer that converts the electrical signal into mechanical oscillations. The Esteem Driver is coupled to the head of the stapes, and the mechanical energy from the oscillating driver is delivered back to the ossicular chain. Because the signal is captured at a lateral location of the ossicular chain and then delivered back to a medial location

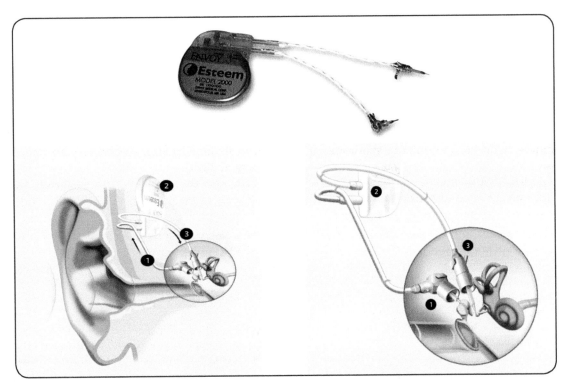

FIGURE 28–13. The Envoy Esteem totally implantable middle ear implant. Image provided courtesy of Envoy Medical.

of the ossicular chain, the surgeon must disarticulate the ossicles between the incus and stapes in order to avoid a feedback loop between the sensor and driver. As a result, the recipient will have a maximum conductive hearing loss after the procedure. Of note, the Esteem Sound Processor and nonrechargeable battery may be detached from the sensor and driver. The lithium-iodide battery is intended to last for 4.5 to 9 years, but it may last as little as 2.8 years for recipients who are continuously exposed to high-level sound. The surgeon can replace the battery and Esteem Sound Processor in an outpatient procedure under local anesthetic or general anesthesia, depending upon the preference of the surgeon and recipient.

The FDA-approved indications for use for the Envoy Esteem are:

- Adults (18 years and older)
- Stable bilateral sensorineural hearing loss
- Moderate to severe sensorineural hearing loss defined by pure-tone average
- Unaided speech discrimination test score greater than or equal to 40%
- Normally functioning eustachian tube
- Normal middle ear anatomy
- Adequate space for Esteem implant as determined via high resolution CT scan
- A minimum of 30 days of "experience with appropriately fit hearing aids"

Contraindications for the Envoy Esteem include:

- History of postadolescent chronic middle ear infections, inner ear disorders, or recurring vertigo requiring treatment, disorders such as mastoiditis, hydrops, or Meniere's syndrome or disease
- Known history of fluctuating air conduction and/or bone conduction hearing loss over the past one-year period of 15 dB in either direction at two or more frequencies from 500 to 4000 Hz.
- History of otitis externa or eczema of the external auditory meatus
- Cholesteatoma or destructive middle ear disease
- Retrocochlear or central auditory disorder
- Disabling tinnitus defined as tinnitus that requires treatment
- History of keloid formation
- Hypersensitivity to silicone rubber, polyurethane, stainless steel, titanium, and/or gold
- A pre-existing medical condition or undergoing a treatment that may affect healing process
- Pregnancy

The Envoy Esteem is not MRI compatible, so the device should not be considered for persons who must undergo serial MRI assessment. Also, monopolar cautery should be avoided after implantation. Financial cost is another consideration that prohibits many individuals from pursuing the Envoy Esteem implant. Health insurance does not typically cover the costs associated with middle ear implants, and the typical cost associated with implantation of an Envoy Esteem is about $35,000 to $40,000 per ear.

Envoy has developed three different instruments that may be used to evaluate and/or adjust the Esteem implant. The Esteem Intraoperative System Analyzer may be used to evaluate the function (e.g., ensure that transducers are operating, check for presence of feedback loop between sensor and driver) of the Esteem implant both intraoperatively and postoperatively. The Esteem Programmer may be used by the audiologist to program the Esteem implant to meet the recipient's needs. The Esteem Personal Programmer is a remote control that is used by the recipient to adjust the volume control, switch programs, and place the device in standby mode (i.e., turn the device on/off). Use of standby mode during situations in which the recipient does not need to hear with the implant will prolong battery life. The Esteem implant is typically activated about six to eight weeks after surgery (Marzo, Sappington, & Shohet, 2014). Typically, the Envoy Esteem recipient is seen multiple times by the audiologist over the first few months of device use for programming to optimize hearing performance, which usually reaches optimal levels four to six months after surgery (Marzo, Sappington, & Shohet, 2014).

Of note, the candidate should ideally have air-bone gaps of no more than 10 dB. Also, the candidate's preoperative word recognition scores should be 60% correct or better (Pelosi, Carlson, & Glasscock III, 2014).

Other Middle Ear Implantable Hearing Devices

Aside from the middle ear implants mentioned above, there are several other middle ear implants that have been developed but have not received approval by the FDA to be commercially distributed in the United States.

Otologics Carina (Cochlear Ltd.)

The Otologics Carina (Figure 28–14) was developed by Otologics, LLC, which encountered financial hardship and was acquired by Cochlear, Ltd. The Otologics Carina is a fully implantable middle ear implant that contains five components: (1) a receiver coil that surrounds a biocompatible magnet, (2) a microphone that is placed under the skin just above and behind the auricle in close proximity to the receiver coil, (3) a digital signal processor, (4) a rechargeable battery, and (5) an electromechanical transducer that is coupled to a lead and connected to the processor via the IS-1 connector.

The electromechanical transducer functions in a piston-like manner when stimulated and is coupled to a hole that the surgeon drills into the long process of the incus. The implanted microphone captures audio signals, converts them to an electrical signal, and delivers the electrical signal to the digital signal processor for analysis and determination of the stimulation needed for the recipient to hear the audio signal. Then, the processed electrical signal is delivered via a lead to the electromechanical transducer. The oscillating, piston-like movement of the transducer delivers mechanical energy to the ossicular chain.

The rechargeable battery is charged with use of an external charging coil that is placed on the head over the implant's receiver coil. The implant is designed to allow for one full day of use on a full battery charge. The recipient may hear with the Carina implant while the charging coil is being worn to charge the battery. The rechargeable battery is designed to last for up to eight years. When the battery expires or if the processor fails, the implant, battery, and receiving coil may be removed from the IS-1 Connector so that the electromechanical transducer may be left in place.

The Carina is intended for use in adults who have mild to severe sensorineural hearing loss and monosyllabic word recognition scores greater than 40% correct at 80 dB HL under earphones or a sensation level of 40 dB. The hearing loss should be stable and of postlingual onset. The recipient should have undergone at least a three-month trial with hearing aids fitted to evidence-based prescriptive targets (i.e., NAL-NL2, DSL 5.0 Adults, etc.). Although the Carina is not approved by the FDA for commercial distribution in the United States, Cochlear has received a CE-mark for use of the Carina in Europe.

The Carina implant may be programmed using the manufacturer's proprietary programming software and the NOAH-link programming interface.

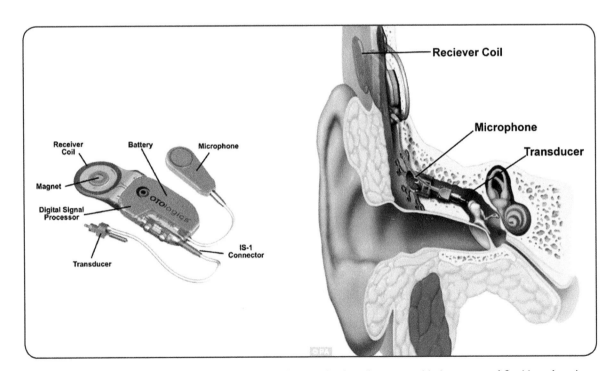

FIGURE 28–14. Otologics Carina totally implantable middle ear implant. Image provided courtesy of Cochlear Americas, ©2018.

An electromagnetic short-range radio frequency coil with a magnet in the center of the coil is connected to the NOAHlink and placed over the receiver coil of the implant. Radio frequency signals are delivered from the programming system to the implant to allow the audiologist to optimize the gain/output settings to meet the recipient's needs. The recipient is also provided with a remote control that may be held next to the implant to deliver radio frequency signals to the implant to adjust volume settings, switch programs, and place the device in standby mode.

The surgery for the fully implantable Carina typically takes two to three hours to complete. Implantation of the Carina requires a mastoid approach similar to what is used in cochlear implant surgery. The implant is activated approximately eight weeks after surgery. Of note, the skin over the microphone will likely thin over time, resulting in improved sensitivity of the microphone (Jenkins & Uhler, 2014). The Desired Sensation Level prescriptive method is used to assign gain/output values based on the recipient's audiometric thresholds. Ideally, the audiologist should complete an in situ audiogram with use of the Carina implant. Additionally, a feedback measurement may be completed to determine whether acoustic feedback is a potential threat and limit gain settings to avoid feedback. The Carina contains data logging that informs the audiologist of device use as well as the operation of the implant (e.g., battery current drain, impedance of the transducer) (Jenkins & Uhler, 2014). It should be noted that the Otologic Carina was approved for commercial use in Europe in 2006. Also, the Otologic Carina has been used for recipients who have conductive hearing loss by delivering stimulation from the transducer directly to the round window.

Codacs™ Direct Acoustic Cochlear Stimulation (DACS)

Codacs™ Direct Acoustic Cochlear Stimulation (DACS) was developed via a joint venture between Cochlear Ltd. and Phonak AG/Sonova. The DACS implant is a partially implantable device that was designed for persons with severe to profound mixed hearing loss caused by otosclerosis. The DACS system contains five components (Figure 28–15): (1) an external ear-level sound processor that contains a transmitting coil that surrounds a magnet, (2) an internal receiving coil that surrounds a magnet, (3) a digital signal processor/stimulator, (4) an electromechanical transducer (actuator), and (5) a middle ear ossicle prosthesis.

The audio signal is captured by the microphones of the sound processor, delivered to the digital signal processor for analysis, and then delivered to the

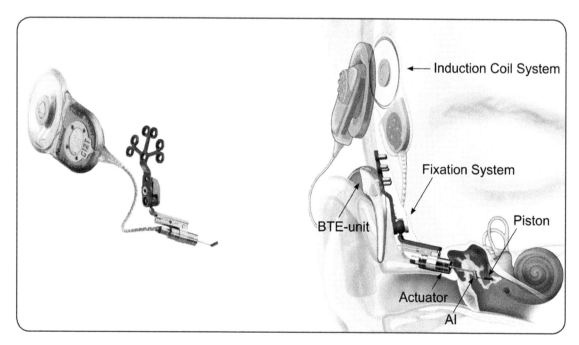

FIGURE 28–15. The Codacs™ Direct Acoustic Cochlear Stimulation (DACS) implant for severe to profound mixed hearing loss. Image provided courtesy of Cochlear Americas, ©2018.

external transmitting coil, where it is converted to an electromagnetic signal and transmitted to the internal receiving coil via short-range radio frequency transmission. The internal receiving coil receives the signal, converts it to an electrical signal, and delivers it to the implant's processor, where it is analyzed and converted to an electrical signal that drives the transducer (actuator). The driving oscillation of the transducer delivers mechanical energy to the middle ear prosthesis or directly to the round window (Grossohmichen et al., 2015). The DACS is a clever and potentially beneficial hearing technology solution for persons who have severe otosclerosis with residual cochlear function allowing for satisfactory speech recognition with sufficient stimulation. It is designed for adults who have severe to profound air conduction thresholds with bone conduction thresholds in the moderate to severe hearing loss range. However, it is not currently approved by the FDA for use in the United States. Cochlear does have approval for a CE-mark for the DACS for use in Europe.

Audiologic Management of Recipients of Middle Ear Implantable Hearing Devices

As previously noted, several weeks typically elapse between middle ear implant surgery and activation of the device. The audiologist should conduct otoscopy at each programming session and inspect the status of the implant site for signs of inflammation or distress. As previously discussed, the audiologist must use the manufacturer's proprietary fitting software and instruments to program middle ear implantable devices. Unfortunately, in contrast to the standard of care for the fitting of conventional air conduction hearing aids, a verification measure does not exist (such as real ear probe microphone measurements) to evaluate the output of the middle ear implant relative to an evidence-based prescriptive target (e.g., DSL 5.0, NAL-NL2). In the absence of the availability of a proven verification measure, audiologists should complete behavioral assessment to determine whether the recipient is receiving adequate benefit from and achieving satisfactory hearing performance with the middle ear implant. Sound-field detection thresholds for warbled tones should be measured, and the device should be programmed to optimize audibility for low-level sounds. Ideally, sound-field warbled tone thresholds should be in the 20 to 30 dB

HL range, but it is quite possible that thresholds will not be obtained at 30 dB HL or better for persons who have hearing thresholds in the moderately severe hearing loss range or poorer.

Ideally, the audiologist should also administer speech recognition assessment and assessment of functional hearing performance via standardized questionnaires. The author recommends evaluation of aided monosyllabic word recognition in the sound-field at presentation levels of 50 and 60 dBA. The audiologist should make programming adjustments to optimize aided speech recognition for low- and moderate-level speech inputs. Additionally, the author recommends evaluation of sentence recognition in noise. The recipient's ability to understand speech in noise will assist the audiologist in determining whether additional assistance may be required to aid the recipient in communicating effectively in noise (e.g., counseling regarding communication strategies to optimize performance in noise, use of program directional microphone, use of hearing assistive technology if available). Finally, the audiologist should administer standardized questionnaires (e.g., APHAB, COSI) to evaluate the recipient's hearing performance with the implant during everyday use.

A number of research studies have explored the outcomes obtained with a variety of different middle ear implants (Barbara, Manni, & Monnini, 2009; Chen et al., 2004; Fraysse et al., 2001; Hough et al., 2001; Jenkins et al., 2004; Kahue et al., 2014; Sterkers et al., 2003; Todt et al., 2002; Uziel et al., 2003; Verhaegen et al., 2008). An exhaustive review of this research is beyond the scope of this chapter and is unnecessary because the findings and conclusions of these studies of modern middle ear implants have been fairly uniform. In general, the use of middle ear implantable hearing devices allows for better hearing performance than the unaided condition. However, research has generally found that recipients obtain similar speech recognition in quiet and in noise and aided soundfield thresholds between middle ear implants and well-fitted modern air conduction hearing aids (Barbara, Manni, & Monnini, 2009; Chen et al., 2004; Fraysse et al., 2001; Hough et al., 2001; Jenkins et al., 2004; Kahue et al., 2014; Martin et al., 2009; Siegert, Mattheis, & Kasic, 2007; Sterkers et al., 2003; Todt et al., 2002; Uziel et al., 2003; Verhaegen et al., 2008). In many cases, middle ear implant recipients do report favorable subjective satisfaction with and benefit from the use of middle ear implants (Chen et al., 2004; Jenkins et al., 2008; Luetje et al., 2002).

Key Concepts

- Middle ear implants are generally intended for use by persons with moderate to moderately severe sensorineural hearing loss.
- Middle ear implants are intended to overcome many of the historical limitations of hearing aids, including limited gain before acoustic feedback and the occlusion effect.
- A variety of different middle ear implants have been developed. Some are partially implantable, whereas others are totally implantable. Research has generally failed to show significant improvement in hearing performance with middle ear implants relative to modern digital hearing aids. Most health insurance policies will not provide coverage for middle ear implants, so the recipient often has to pay "out-of-pocket" for a middle ear implant. Consequently, middle ear implants are not used as commonly as conventional hearing aids or cochlear implants.

References

Barbara, M., Manni, V., & Monini, S. (2009). Totally implantable middle ear device for rehabilitation of sensorineural hearing loss: Preliminary experience with the Esteem, Envoy. *Acta Otolaryngologica, 129*(4), 429–432.

Beleites, T., Bornitz, M., Neudert, M., & Zahnert, T. (2014a). [The Vibrant Soundbridge as an active implant in middle ear surgery]. *HNO, 62*(7), 509–519.

Beleites, T., Neudert, M., Bornitz, M., & Zahnert, T. (2014b). Sound transfer of active middle ear implants. *Otolaryngology Clinics of North America, 47*(6), 859–891.

Bittencourt, A. G., Burke, P. R., Jardim Ide, S., Brito, R., Tsuji, R. K., Fonseca, A. C., & Bento, R. F. (2014). Implantable and semi-implantable hearing aids: A review of history, indications, and surgery. *International Archives of Otorhinolaryngology, 18*(3), 303–310.

Carlson, M. L., Pelosi, S., & Haynes, D. S. (2014). Historical development of active middle ear implants. *Otolaryngology Clinics of North America, 47*(6), 893–914.

Chen, H., & Zeng, F. G. (2004). Frequency modulation detection in cochlear implant subjects. *Journal of the Acoustical Society of America, 116*(4 Pt 1), 2269–2277.

Chen, X., Han, D., Zhao, X., Kong, Y., Liu, S., Mo, L., & Wu, Y. (2004). [The psychophysical tests in different age of patients with cochlear implants]. *Lin Chuang Er Bi Yan Hou Ke Za Zhi, 18*(4), 215–218.

Convery, E., & Keidser, G. (2011). Transitioning hearing aid users with severe and profound loss to a new gain/frequency response: Benefit, perception, and acceptance. *Journal of the American Academy of Audiology, 22*(3), 168–180.

Dumon, T., Zennaro, O., Aran, J. M., & Bebear, J. P. (1995a). [Development of a piezo-electrical vibrator for middle ear implant. State of research]. *Review of Laryngology, Otology, Rhinology (Bord), 116*(4), 309–312.

Dumon, T., Zennaro, O., Aran, J. M., & Bebear, J. P. (1995b). Piezo-electric middle ear implant preserving the ossicular chain. *Otolaryngology Clinics of North America, 28*(1), 173–187.

Fraysse, B., Lavieille, J. P., Schmerber, S., Enee, V., Truy, E., Vincent, C., . . . Sterkers, O. (2001). A multicenter study of the Vibrant Soundbridge middle ear implant: Early clinical results and experience. *Otology and Neurotology, 22*(6), 952–961.

Grossohmichen, M., Salcher, R., Kreipe, H. H., Lenarz, T., & Maier, H. (2015). The Codacs direct acoustic cochlear implant actuator: Exploring alternative stimulation sites and their stimulation efficiency. *PLoS One, 10*(3), e0119601.

Hough, J. V., Dyer, R. K., Jr., Matthews, P., & Wood, M. W. (2001a). Early clinical results: SOUNDTEC implantable hearing device phase II study. *Laryngoscope, 111*(1), 1–8.

Hough, J. V., Dyer, R. K., Jr., Matthews, P., & Wood, M. W. (2001b). Semi-implantable electromagnetic middle ear hearing device for moderate to severe sensorineural hearing loss. *Otolaryngology Clinics of North America, 34*(2), 401–416.

JJenkins, H. A., Atkins, J. S., Horlbeck, D., Hoffer, M. E., Balough, B., Alexiades, G., & Garvis, W. (2008). Otologics fully implantable hearing system: Phase I trial 1-year results. *Otology and Neurotology, 29*(4), 534–541.

enkins, H. A., Niparko, J. K., Slattery, W. H., Neely, J. G., & Fredrickson, J. M. (2004). Otologics middle ear transducer ossicular stimulator: performance results with varying degrees of sensorineural hearing loss. *Acta Otolaryngologica, 124*(4), 391–394.

Jenkins, H. A., & Uhler, K. (2014). Otologics active middle ear implants. *Otolaryngology Clinics of North America, 47*(6), 967–978.

Kahue, C. N., Carlson, M. L., Daugherty, J. A., Haynes, D. S., & Glasscock, M. E., 3rd. (2014). Middle ear implants for rehabilitation of sensorineural hearing loss: A systematic review of FDA approved devices. *Otology and Neurotology, 35*(7), 1228–1237.

Keidser, G., Dillon, H., Dyrlund, O., Carter, L., & Hartley, D. (2007). Preferred low- and high-frequency compression ratios among hearing aid users with moderately severe to profound hearing loss. *Journal of the American Academy of Audiology, 18*(1), 17–33.

Lim, L. H., Del Prado, J., Xiang, L., Yusof, A. R., & Loo, J. H. (2012). Vibrant Soundbridge middle ear implantations: Experience at National University Hospital Singapore. *European Archives of Otorhinolaryngology, 269*(9), 2137–2143.

Luetje, C. M., Brackman, D., Balkany, T. J., Maw, J., Baker, R. S., Kelsall, D., . . . Arts, A. (2002). Phase III clinical trial results with the Vibrant Soundbridge implantable middle ear hearing device: A prospective controlled multicenter study. *Otolaryngology–Head and Neck Surgery, 126*(2), 97–107.

Martin, C., Deveze, A., Richard, C., Lefebvre, P. P., Decat, M., Ibanez, L. G., . . . Tringali, S. (2009). European results with totally implantable carina placed on the round window: 2-year follow-up. *Otology and Neurotology, 30*(8), 1196–1203.

Marzo, S. J., Sappington, J. M., & Shohet, J. A. (2014). The Envoy Esteem implantable hearing system. *Otolaryngology Clinics of North America, 47*(6), 941–952.

Minovi, A., & Dazert, S. (2014). [Diseases of the middle ear in childhood]. *Laryngorhinootologie, 93*(Suppl. 1), S1–S23.

Olszewski, L., Jedrzejczak, W. W., Piotrowska, A., & Skarzynski, H. (2017). Round window stimulation with the Vibrant Soundbridge: Comparison of direct and indirect coupling. *Laryngoscope, 127*(12), 2843–2849.

Pelosi, S., Carlson, M. L., & Glasscock, M. E., 3rd. (2014). Implantable hearing devices: The Ototronix MAXUM system. *Otolaryngology Clinics of North America, 47*(6), 953–965.

Siegert, R., Mattheis, S., & Kasic, J. (2007). Fully implantable hearing aids in patients with congenital auricular atresia. *Laryngoscope, 117*(2), 336–340.

Skarzynski, H., Olszewski, L., Skarzynski, P. H., Lorens, A., Piotrowska, A., Porowski, M., . . . Pilka, A. (2014). Direct round window stimulation with the Med-El Vibrant Soundbridge: 5 years of experience using a technique without interposed fascia. *European Archives of Otorhinolaryngology, 271*(3), 477–482.

Sterkers, O., Boucarra, D., Labassi, S., Bebear, J. P., Dubreuil, C., Frachet, B., . . . Vaneecloo, F. M. (2003). A middle ear implant, the Symphonix Vibrant Soundbridge: Retrospective study of the first 125 patients implanted in France. *Otology and Neurotology, 24*(3), 427–436.

Strenger, T., & Stark, T. (2012). [The application of implantable hearing aids using the Vibrant Soundbridge as an example]. *HNO, 60*(2), 169–176; quiz 176–168.

Todt, I., Seidl, R. O., Gross, M., & Ernst, A. (2002). Comparison of different Vibrant Soundbridge audioprocessors with conventional hearing AIDS. *Otology and Neurotology, 23*(5), 669–673.

Uziel, A., Mondain, M., Hagen, P., Dejean, F., & Doucet, G. (2003). Rehabilitation for high-frequency sensorineural hearing impairment in adults with the Symphonix vibrant soundbridge: A comparative study. *Otology and Neurotology, 24*(5), 775–783.

Verhaegen, V. J., Mylanus, E. A., Cremers, C. W., & Snik, A. F. (2008). Audiological application criteria for implantable hearing aid devices: A clinical experience at the Nijmegen ORL clinic. *Laryngoscope, 118*(9), 1645–1649.

Index